THE WASHINGTON MANUAL™ OF SURGERY

Sixth Edition

Department of Surgery
Washington University
School of Medicine
St. Louis, Missouri

Editors

Mary E. Klingensmith, MD

Abdulhameed Aziz, MD

Ankit Bharat, MD

Amy C. Fox, MD

Matthew R. Porembka, MD

Foreword by
Timothy J. Eberlein, MD
Bixby Professor and Chair of Surgery
Director, Siteman Cancer Center
Washington University
School of Medicine
St. Louis, Missouri

Wolters Kluwer | Lippincott Williams & Wilkins
Health

Philadelphia • Baltimore • New York • London
Buenos Aires • Hong Kong • Sydney • Tokyo

Acquisitions Editor: Brian Brown
Product Manager: Brendan Huffman
Production Manager: Bridgett Dougherty
Senior Manufacturing Manager: Benjamin Rivera
Marketing Manager: Lisa Lawrence
Design Coordinator: Doug Smock
Production Service: Aptara, Inc.

Library of Congress Cataloging-in-Publication Data
The Washington manual of surgery / [edited by] Mary E. Klingensmith. — 6th ed.
    p. ; cm.
    Manual of surgery
    Includes bibliographical references and index.
    ISBN 978-1-4511-1594-9 (alk. paper)
    I. Klingensmith, Mary E.   II. Washington University (Saint Louis, Mo.).
Dept. of Surgery.   III. Title: Manual of surgery.
    [DNLM: 1. Surgical Procedures, Operative–methods.   WO 500 W317 2008]
    LC classification not assigned
    617'.91—dc23

                                                                                    2011032666

Care has been taken to confirm the accuracy of the information presented and to describe generally accepted practices. However, the authors, editors, and publisher are not responsible for errors or omissions or for any consequences from application of the information in this book and make no warranty, expressed or implied, with respect to the currency, completeness, or accuracy of the contents of the publication. Application of the information in a particular situation remains the professional responsibility of the practitioner.

The authors, editors, and publisher have exerted every effort to ensure that drug selection and dosage set forth in this text are in accordance with current recommendations and practice at the time of publication. However, in view of ongoing research, changes in government regulations, and the constant flow of information relating to drug therapy and drug reactions, the reader is urged to check the package insert for each drug for any change in indications and dosage and for added warnings and precautions. This is particularly important when the recommended agent is a new or infrequently employed drug.

Some drugs and medical devices presented in the publication have Food and Drug Administration (FDA) clearance for limited use in restricted research settings. It is the responsibility of the health care providers to ascertain the FDA status of each drug or device planned for use in their clinical practice.

To purchase additional copies of this book, call our customer service department at (800) 638-3030 or fax orders to (301) 223-2320. International customers should call (301) 223-2300.

Visit Lippincott Williams & Wilkins on the Internet: at LWW.com. Lippincott Williams & Wilkins customer service representatives are available from 8:30 am to 6 pm, EST.

10 9 8 7 6 5 4 3 2

Contributors

Christopher Anderson, MD
Associate Professor of Surgery
University of Mississippi Medical Center
Jackson, Mississippi

Michael Avidan, MBBCh
Professor of Anesthesiology and
  Cardiothoracic Surgery
Washington University School of Medicine
St. Louis, Missouri

Abdulhameed Aziz, MD
Resident in Surgery
Washington University School of Medicine
St. Louis, Missouri

Ankit Bharat, MD
Fellow in Cardiothoracic Surgery
Washington University School of Medicine
St. Louis, Missouri

Alejandro Bribiesco, MD
Resident in Surgery
Washington University School of Medicine
St. Louis, Missouri

L. Michael Brunt, MD
Professor of Surgery
Washington University School of Medicine
St. Louis, Missouri

Brian Bucher, MD
Resident in Surgery
Washington University School of Medicine
St. Louis, Missouri

Arnold Bullock, MD
Professor of Surgery
Washington University School of Medicine
St. Louis, Missouri

William Chapman, MD
Professor of Surgery
Washington University School of Medicine
St. Louis, Missouri

Michael Chicoine, MD
Associate Professor of Neurological Surgery
Washington University School of Medicine
St. Louis, Missouri

Kendra Conzen, MD
Resident in Surgery
Washington University School of Medicine
St. Louis, Missouri

Travis Crabtree, MD
Assistant Professor of Surgery
Washington University School of Medicine
St. Louis, Missouri

Ralph Damiano, MD
John M. Shoenberg Professor of Surgery
Washington University School of Medicine
St. Louis, Missouri

Charl De Wet, MD
Associate Professor of Anesthesiology and
  Cardiothoracic Surgery
Washington University School of Medicine
St. Louis, Missouri

Patrick Dillon, MD
Associate Professor of Surgery
Washington University School of Medicine
St. Louis, Missouri

Bernard DuBray, MD
Resident in Surgery
Washington University School of Medicine
St. Louis, Missouri

J. Christopher Eagon, MD
Associate Professor of Surgery
Washington University School of Medicine
St. Louis, Missouri

Oluwadamilola Fayanju, MD, MPHS
Resident in Surgery
Washington University School of Medicine
St. Louis, Missouri

Elizabeth Fialkowski, MD
Fellow in Pediatric Surgery
Washington University School of Medicine
St. Louis, Missouri

James Fleshman, MD
Professor of Surgery
Washington University School of Medicine
St. Louis, Missouri

Amy Fox, MD
Fellow in Endocrine Surgery
University of Michigan
Ann Arbor, Michigan

Bradley Freeman, MD
Professor of Surgery
Washington University School of Medicine
St. Louis, Missouri

Noopur Gangopadhyay, MD
Resident in Plastic and Reconstructive
  Surgery
Washington University School of Medicine
St. Louis, Missouri

Michael Gardner, MD
Assistant Professor of Orthopedic Surgery
Washington University School of Medicine
St. Louis, Missouri

Patrick Geraghty, MD
Associate Professor of Surgery and Radiology
Washington University School of Medicine
St. Louis, Missouri

Bruce Hall, MD, PhD, MBA
Professor of Surgery
Washington University School of Medicine
St. Louis, Missouri

Nicholas Hamilton, MD
Resident in Surgery
Washington University School of Medicine
St. Louis, Missouri

Bruce Haughey, MBChB, MS
Kimbrough Professor of Otolaryngology
Washington University School of Medicine
St. Louis, Missouri

William Hawkins, MD
Associate Professor of Surgery
Washington University School of Medicine
St. Louis, Missouri

Laureen Hill, MD
Professor of Anesthesiology and
  Cardiothoracic Surgery
Emory School of Medicine
Atlanta, Georgia

David Hoganson, MD
Resident in Surgery
Washington University School of Medicine
St. Louis, Missouri

Ashley Holder, MD
Resident in Surgery
Washington University School of Medicine
St. Louis, Missouri

Richard Hotchkiss, MD
Professor of Anesthesiology, Medicine, Surgery,
  Molecular Biology and Pharmacology
Washington University School of Medicine
St. Louis, Missouri

Steven Hunt, MD
Assistant Professor of Surgery
Washington University School of Medicine
St. Louis, Missouri

Samay Jain, MD
Resident in Urologic Surgery
Washington University School of Medicine
St. Louis, Missouri

Fabian Johnston, MD
Fellow in Surgical Oncology
Johns Hopkins School of Medicine
Baltimore, Maryland

Enjae Jung, MD
Resident in Surgery
Washington University School of Medicine
St. Louis, Missouri

Jason Keune, MD, MBA
Resident in Surgery
Washington University School of Medicine
St. Louis, Missouri

Alicia Kieninger, MD
Attending Surgeon
Saint Joseph's Mercy Health System
Oakland, Michigan

John Kirby, MD
Associate Professor of Surgery
Washington University School of Medicine
St. Louis, Missouri
Assistant Professor of Surgery
Washington University School of Medicine
St. Louis, Missouri

Mary E. Klingensmith, MD
Mary Culver Distinguished Professor of Surgery
Washington University School of Medicine
St. Louis, Missouri

Lindsay Kuroki, MD
Resident in Obstetrics and Gynecology
Washington University School of Medicine
St. Louis, Missouri

Anson Lee, MD
Resident in Surgery
Washington University School of Medicine
St. Louis, Missouri

Jeremy Leidenfrost, MD
Resident in Surgery
Washington University School of Medicine
St. Louis, Missouri

Jennifer Leinecke, MD
Resident in Surgery
Washington University School of Medicine
St. Louis, Missouri

David Linehan, MD
Professor of Surgery
Washington University School of Medicine
St. Louis, Missouri

Jeffrey Lowell, MD
Professor of Surgery and Pediatrics
Washington University School of Medicine
St. Louis, Missouri

Malcolm MacConamara, MD
Resident in Surgery
Washington University School of Medicine
St. Louis, Missouri

Susan Mackinnon, MD
Shoenberg Professor of Plastic and Reconstructive Surgery
Washington University School of Medicine
St. Louis, Missouri

Julie Margenthaler, MD
Associate Professor of Surgery
Washington University School of Medicine
St. Louis, Missouri

Brent Matthews, MD
Professor of Surgery
Washington University School of Medicine
St. Louis, Missouri

Kathleen Mckeon, MD
Resident in Orthopedic Surgery
Washington University School of Medicine
St. Louis, Missouri

Lora Melman, MD
Resident in Surgery
Washington University School of Medicine
St. Louis, Missouri

Bryan Meyers, MD, MPH
Patrick and Joy Williamson Professor of Surgery
Washington University School of Medicine
St. Louis, Missouri

Jonathan Mitchem, MD
Resident in Surgery
Washington University School of Medicine
St. Louis, Missouri

Jeffrey Moley, MD
Professor of Surgery
Washington University School of Medicine
St. Louis, Missouri

Susan Pitt, MD
Resident in Surgery
Washington University School of Medicine
St. Louis, Missouri

Matthew Porembka, MD
Resident in Surgery
Washington University School of Medicine
St. Louis, Missouri

Babafemi Pratt, MD
Resident in Surgery
Washington University School of Medicine
St. Louis, Missouri

Matthew Reynolds, MD
Resident in Neurological Surgery
Washington University School of Medicine
St. Louis, Missouri

T. Elizabeth Robertson, MD
Attending Surgeon
Saint Anthony's Medical Center
St. Louis, Missouri

Kathryn Rowland, MD
Resident in Surgery
Washington University School of Medicine
St. Louis, Missouri

Brian Rubin, MD
Professor of Surgery
Washington University School of Medicine
St. Louis, Missouri

Luis Sanchez, MD
Gregorio A. Sicard Professor of Surgery
Washington University School of Medicine
St. Louis, Missouri

Douglas Schuerer, MD
Associate Professor of Surgery
Washington University School of Medicine
St. Louis, Missouri

Sunitha Sequira, MD
Resident in Otolaryngology
Washington University School of Medicine
St. Louis, Missouri

Gergorio Sicard, MD
Eugene M. Bricker Professor of Surgery
Washington University School of Medicine
St. Louis, Missouri

Robert Southard, MD
Assistant Professor of Surgery
Washington University School of Medicine
St. Louis, Missouri

Lauren Steward, MD
Resident in Surgery
Washington University School of Medicine
St. Louis, Missouri

Steven Strasberg, MD
Pruett Professor of Surgery
Washington University School of Medicine
St. Louis, Missouri

William Symons, MD
Resident in Surgery
Washington University School of Medicine
St. Louis, Missouri

Marcus Tan, MD
Fellow in Surgical Oncology
Memorial Sloan-Kettering Cancer Center
New York, New York

Premal Thaker, MD, MS
Assistant Professor of Obstetrics and
  Gynecology
Washington University School of Medicine
St. Louis, Missouri

Amber Traugott, MD
Resident in Surgery
Washington University School of Medicine
St. Louis, Missouri

Thomas Tung, MD
Associate Professor of Surgery
Washington University School of Medicine
St. Louis, Missouri
Assistant Professor of Surgery
Washington University School of Medicine
St. Louis, Missouri

Isaiah Turnbull, MS
Resident in Surgery
Washington University School of Medicine
St. Louis, Missouri

Derek Wakeman, MD
Resident in Surgery
Washington University School of Medicine
St. Louis, Missouri

Foreword

Welcome to the sixth edition of *The Washington Manual*^{TM} *of Surgery*. The most important focus of our Department of Surgery is medical education of students, residents, fellows, and practicing surgeons. This commitment is no more evident than in the current edition of *The Washington Manual*^{TM} *of Surgery*.

The educational focus of our Department of Surgery has a rich tradition. The first full-time Head of the Department of Surgery at Washington University was Dr. Evarts A. Graham (1919–1951). Dr. Graham was a superb educator. Not only was he an outstanding technical surgeon but his insightful comments at conferences and ward rounds were well-known and appreciated by a generation of surgeons who learned at his elbow. Dr. Graham was a founding member of the American Board of Surgery and made many seminal contributions to the management of surgical patients. His work in the development of oral cholecystography actually helped establish the Mallinckrodt Institute of Radiology at Washington University. Dr. Graham was among the first to identify the epidemiological link of cigarette smoking to lung cancer and was instrumental in raising public health consciousness about the deleterious effect on health from cigarette smoke.

Dr. Carl Moyer (1951–1965) succeeded Dr. Graham. Dr. Moyer is still regarded as a legendary educator at Washington University. He was particularly known for his bedside teaching techniques, as well as for linking pathophysiology to patient care outcomes. Dr. Walter Ballinger (1967–1978) came from the Johns Hopkins University and incorporated the Halsted traditions of resident education. Dr. Ballinger introduced the importance of laboratory investigation and began to foster development of the surgeon/scientist in our department. Dr. Samuel A. Wells (1978–1997) is credited with establishing one of the most accomplished academic Departments of Surgery in the United States. Not only did he recruit world-class faculty but he increased the focus on research and patient care. Dr. Wells also placed a great emphasis on educating the future academic leaders of surgery.

As in previous editions, this sixth edition of *The Washington Manual*^{TM} *of Surgery* combines authorship of residents ably assisted by faculty coauthors and our senior editor, Dr. Mary Klingensmith, who is vice-chair for education in our department. This combination of resident and faculty participation has helped focus the chapters on issues that will be particularly helpful to the trainee in surgery. This new edition of the manual provides a complete list of updated references that will serve medical students, residents, and practicing surgeons who wish to delve more deeply into a particular topic. This manual does not attempt to extensively cover pathophysiology or history, but it presents brief and logical approaches to the management of patients with comprehensive surgical problems. In each of the chapters, the authors have attempted to provide the most up-to-date and important diagnostic and management information for a given topic. We have attempted to standardize each of the chapters so that the reader will be able to most easily obtain information regardless of subject matter.

The sixth edition has undergone a reorganization of chapters with an emphasis on clarity and consistency. As with the past edition, evidence-based medicine has been incorporated into each of the chapters, with updated information and references to reflect current knowledge and practice. All of the sections have been updated and rewritten to reflect the most current standards of practice in each topic. These updates have been carefully edited and integrated so that the volume of pages remains approximately the same. Our goal is to keep this volume concise, portable, and user-friendly.

I am truly indebted to Dr. Klingensmith for her passion for education and her specific devotion to this project. In addition, I am proud of the residents in the Department of Surgery at Washington University who have done such an outstanding job with their faculty members in this sixth edition. I hope that you will find *The Washington Manual*^{TM} *of Surgery* a reference you commonly utilize in the care of your patient with surgical disease.

Timothy J. Eberlein, MD
St. Louis, Missouri

Preface

As with the previous five editions, this sixth edition of *The Washington Manual™ of Surgery* is designed to complement *The Washington Manual of Medical Therapeutics*. Written by resident and faculty members of the Department of Surgery, it presents a brief, rational approach to the management of patients with surgical problems. The text is directed to the reader at the level of the 2nd- or 3rd-year surgical resident, although surgical and nonsurgical attendings, medical students, physician assistants, nurse practitioners, and others who provide care for patients with surgical problems will find it of interest and assistance. The book provides a succinct discussion of surgical diseases, with algorithms for addressing problems based on the opinions of the physician authors. Although multiple approaches may be reasonable for some clinical situations, this manual attempts to present a single, effective approach for each. We have limited coverage of diagnosis and therapy; this is not an exhaustive surgical reference. Coverage of pathophysiology, the history of surgery, and extensive reference lists have been excluded from most areas.

This is the sixth edition of the manual; the first edition was published in 1997, followed by editions in 1999, 2002, 2005, and 2007. New to this volume is a chapter on "emergencies in surgical patients" as well as updated evidence-based medicine, with the latest information and treatment algorithms in each section. As with previous editions, this sixth edition includes updates on each topic as well as substantial new material.

This is a resident-prepared manual. Each chapter was updated and revised by a resident with assistance from a faculty coauthor. Editorial oversight for the manual was shared by four senior resident coeditors (Ankit Bharat, MD, Chapters 1, 3, 4, 7 to 9, 30, 31, and 38; Amy Fox, MD, Chapters 2, 21 to 25, 29, 32, 36, and 37; Abdulhameed Aziz, MD, Chapters 5, 6, 17 to 20, 26, 28, and 34; and Matthew Porembka, MD, Chapters 10 to 16, 27, 33, and 35). The tremendous effort of all involved—residents and faculty members and particularly the senior resident coeditors—is reflected in the quality and consistency of the chapters.

I am indebted to the former senior editor of this work, Gerard M. Doherty, MD, who developed and oversaw the first three editions, then handed over to me an exceptionally well-organized project. I am grateful for the continued tremendous support from Lippincott Williams & Wilkins, who have been supportive of the effort and have supplied dedicated assistance. Brian Brown has been tremendously helpful, and Brendan Huffman has been a terrific developmental editor, keeping me in line and on schedule.

Finally, I am grateful to have an outstanding mentor and friend in my department chair, Timothy J. Eberlein, MD. Dr. Eberlein has a very full professional life, overseeing both a productive department and a cancer center. Despite this, he continues to appreciate the individuals with whom he interacts. He is an inspiration for his friendship, leadership, and dedication.

M.E.K.

Contents

1 General and Perioperative Care of the Surgical Patient

Oluwadamilola M. Fayanju and Mary E. Klingensmith

I. PREOPERATIVE EVALUATION AND MANAGEMENT

A. **General Evaluation of the Surgical Patient.** The goals of preoperative evaluation are to (1) identify the patient's medical problems, (2) determine if further information is needed to characterize the patient's medical status, (3) establish if the patient's condition is medically optimized, and (4) confirm the appropriateness of the planned procedure.

   1. **History and physical examination.** A thorough history and physical are essential in evaluating surgical patients. Key elements of the history should include preexisting medical conditions known to increase operative risk, such as ischemic heart disease, congestive heart failure (CHF), renal insufficiency, prior cerebrovascular accident (CVA), and diabetes mellitus. Prior operations, operative complications, medication allergies, and the patient's use of tobacco, alcohol, and/or drugs should also be noted.

   2. **Routine diagnostic testing.** Minor surgical procedures and procedures on young, healthy patients often require minimal or no diagnostic testing. Table 1-1 lists routine preoperative diagnostic tests and reasons for their use. Inclusion or exclusion of these tests should be selected on a case-by-case basis with consideration of the probability that results will alter management.

   3. **Preoperative medications.** In general, patients should continue their medications in the immediate preoperative period. Exceptions to this rule include diabetic medications (see Section I.B.6), anticoagulants (see Section I.B.8.a), and antiplatelet agents. The use of some medications such as statins and angiotensin-converting enzyme (ACE) inhibitors should be individualized. It is important to query patients regarding their use of over-the-counter and herbal medications.

B. **Specific Considerations in Preoperative Management**

   1. **Cerebrovascular disease.** Perioperative stroke is an uncommon surgical complication, occurring in less than 1% of general patients and in 2% to 5% of cardiac surgical patients. The majority (>80%) of these events are postoperative, and they are most often caused by hypotension or cardiogenic emboli during atrial fibrillation. Acute surgical stress might cause focal signs from a previous stroke to recur, mimicking acute ischemia.

      a. **Risk factors** for perioperative stroke include previous CVA, age, hypertension, coronary artery disease (CAD), diabetes, and tobacco

TABLE 1-1	Routine Preoperative Testing
Test	**Comment**
Complete blood cell count	History of recent blood loss, sickle cell disease/thalassemia, bleeding disorder, thrombocytopenia, or liver disease/splenomegaly; all intermediate and major procedures (cases where EBL ≥500 mL is anticipated). Consider for patients with history of anemia, renal insufficiency, coronary artery disease, and recent chemotherapy.
Urinalysis	All implant cases.
Serum electrolytes, creatinine, and blood urea nitrogen	History of renal disease (can do point-of-care hemoglobin/hematocrit, K+, Na+ on day of surgery for patients on dialysis), diabetes mellitus, or hypertension; patients taking diuretics/digoxin/ACE inhibitors/ARBs. Creatinine should be obtained for all vascular surgery patients on day of surgery (unless prior result within 24 hours prior to operation).
Coagulation studies	History of bleeding disorder, liver disease, or excessive alcohol use; patients receiving anticoagulants (in particular, should check PT/INR on morning of surgery for patients instructed to discontinue warfarin); cardiothoracic, vascular, angiographic, and craniotomy procedures.
Biochemical and profiles (including liver enzymes)	History of liver disease/jaundice, biliary disease, bleeding disorder, or excessive alcohol use; cholecystectomy, cardiopulmonary bypass procedures. Consider in patients with pulmonary hypertension and right heart failure. Albumin is a strong predictor of perioperative morbidity and mortality and should be considered for major procedures.
Pregnancy testing	Menstruating women unable to assure (by history) that they are not pregnant or if >30 days have passed since last menstrual period; females <18 years of age.
Chest X-ray	Presence of acute cardiac or pulmonary symptoms. Patients undergoing cardiothoracic procedures should receive a CXR within 2 weeks of surgery; history of a chest CT within 2 weeks precludes the need for an additional CXR.

| TABLE 1-1 | Routine Preoperative Testing *(Continued)* |

Test	Comment
Electrocardiogram	Within 12 weeks of surgery (or less if condition warrants) for patients with known heart disease; within 6 months prior to surgery for all patients >50 years of age.
Type and cross/type and screen	None if very low risk of blood loss; type and screen if risk of substantial blood loss is low to moderate; type and cross if moderate to high risk of substantial blood loss (greater than 500 mL).

ACE, angiotensin-converting enzyme; ARB, angiotensin receptor blocker; CXR, chest X-ray; EBL, estimated blood loss.

Adapted from the "Minimum Requirements for Preoperative Diagnostic Testing" issued by the Center for Preoperative Assessment & Planning (CPAP) with permission from Dr. Laureen Hill, Vice Chairperson of the Department of Anesthesiology, Washington University in St. Louis.

use. Known or suspected cerebrovascular disease requires special consideration.

   (1) **The asymptomatic carotid bruit** is relatively common, occurring in approximately 14% of surgical patients older than 55 years. However, fewer than 50% of bruits reflect hemodynamically significant disease. No increase in risk of stroke has been demonstrated during noncardiac surgery in the presence of an asymptomatic bruit.

   (2) **Patients with recent transient ischemic attacks (TIAs)** are at increased risk for perioperative stroke and should have preoperative neurologic evaluation [e.g., computed tomography (CT) of the head, echocardiography, carotid Doppler]. Patients with symptomatic carotid artery stenosis should have an endarterectomy or carotid stenting before elective surgery.

   (3) **Elective surgery for patients with a recent CVA** should be delayed for a minimum of 2 weeks, ideally for 6 weeks.

  2. **Cardiovascular disease** is one of the leading causes of death after noncardiac surgery. Patients who experience a myocardial infarction (MI) after noncardiac surgery have a hospital mortality rate of 15% to 25% (*CMAJ*. 2005;173:627). A study of 4,315 patients older than 50 years between 1989 and 1994 undergoing nonemergent, noncardiac surgery with expected postoperative stays greater than 48 hours found that major perioperative cardiac events occur in 1.4% of the patients (*Circulation*. 1999;100:1043). Since more than 100 million adults worldwide undergo noncardiac surgery annually, approximately 500,000 to 900,000 patients each year experience perioperative cardiac death, a nonfatal MI, or nonfatal cardiac arrest postoperatively. Risk stratification by the operating surgeon, anesthesiologist, and consulting internist is important.

a. **Risk factors.** The following risk factors have been associated with perioperative cardiac morbidity:

(1) **The patient's age** (>70 years) has been identified as an independent multivariate risk factor for cardiac morbidity.

(2) **Unstable angina** is defined as chest pain that does not correlate with the level of physical activity and, therefore, occurs at rest or with minimal physical exertion. Elective operation in patients with unstable angina is contraindicated and should be postponed pending further evaluation.

(3) **Recent MI** is a well-defined risk factor for cardiac morbidity. The risk of reinfarction is significant if an operation is performed within 6 months of an MI (11% to 16% at 3 to 6 months). This risk is still increased substantially after 6 months, in contrast to patients without a history of MI (4% to 5% vs. 0.13%).

(4) **Untreated CHF** is a predictor of perioperative cardiac morbidity. Consequently, these patients should be optimized before any operative procedures are performed.

(5) **Diabetes mellitus,** especially in those requiring insulin, is thought to confer additional independent risk for an adverse cardiac outcome.

(6) **Valvular heart disease.** Aortic stenosis is a significant risk factor and may confer a 14-fold increase in relative risk independent of the manifestations of CHF. Patients with unexplained symptoms of dyspnea on exertion, shortness of breath, chest pain, syncope, or an uncharacterized systolic ejection murmur should undergo further diagnostic evaluation before elective operation. All patients with valvular heart disease, even hemodynamically insignificant disease (excluding patients with only mitral valve prolapse and no murmur), should receive prophylactic antibiotics before any operation that can introduce bacteria into the bloodstream or any dental procedure to reduce the risk of infectious endocarditis (Table 1-2).

(7) **Arrhythmias and conduction defects.** Both supraventricular and ventricular arrhythmias have been identified as independent risk factors for perioperative coronary events. The existence of a preoperative arrhythmia should prompt a search for underlying cardiac or pulmonary disease.

(8) **Peripheral vascular disease (PVD).** Because of the high coexistence of CAD with PVD, a lower threshold for obtaining diagnostic testing is warranted.

(9) **Type of procedure.** Patients who are undergoing thoracic surgery, vascular surgery, or upper abdominal surgery are at higher risk for adverse cardiac outcomes. Other procedures considered high risk include emergent major operations,

TABLE 1-2	Antibiotic Prophylaxis of Bacterial Endocarditis for Adult Patients	

Procedure	Situation	Regimen
Dental, oral, respiratory, esophageal	Standard	**Amoxicillin** 2 g PO 1 hr before procedure
	Unable to take PO	**Ampicillin** 2 g IM or IV 30 min before procedure
	Penicillin-allergic	**Clindamycin** 600 mg PO 1 hr before procedure; or **cephalexin**[a] or **cefadroxil**[a] 2 g PO 1 hr before procedure; or **clarithromycin** or **azithromycin** 500 mg PO 1 hr before procedure
	Penicillin-allergic and unable to take PO	**Clindamycin** 600 mg IV within 30 min before procedure or **cefazolin**[a] 1 g IV within 30 min before procedure
Gastrointestinal and genitourinary	High-risk patients	**Ampicillin** 2 g IM or IV, plus **gentamicin** 1.5 mg/kg (max 120 mg) within 30 min before procedure; 6 hr later, **ampicillin** 1 g IV/IM or **amoxicillin** 1 g PO
	High-risk, penicillin-allergic patients	**Vancomycin** 1 g IV plus **gentamicin** 1.5 mg/kg (max 120 mg) timed to finish within 30 min of starting procedure
	Moderate-risk patients	**Amoxicillin** 2 g PO 1 hr before procedure or **ampicillin** 2 g IM or IV 30 min before procedure
	Moderate-risk, penicillin allergic patients	**Vancomycin** 1 g IV timed to finish within 30 min of starting procedure

[a]Cephalosporins should not be used in patients with anaphylactic or urticarial reactions to penicillin.
IM, intravascular; IV, intravenous; PO, by mouth.

especially in the elderly, and prolonged procedures associated with large fluid shifts or significant blood loss.

(10) **Functional impairment.** Patients with a poor functional capacity have a significantly higher risk of experiencing a postoperative cardiac event. Poor function is an indication for more aggressive preoperative evaluation, whereas patients who exercise regularly generally have sufficient cardiac reserve to withstand stressful operations.

b. **Revised cardiac risk index.** See Table 1-3.

TABLE 1-3	Revised Cardiac Risk Index[a]
Risk factor	**Comment**
High-risk surgery	Intrathoracic, intraperitoneal, major vascular
Ischemic heart disease	History of myocardial infarction, positive exercise test, angina, nitrate therapy, electrocardiogram with abnormal Q waves
History of CHF	History of CHF, pulmonary edema, or paroxysmal nocturnal dyspnea, bilateral rales, S_3 gallop, chest X-ray showing pulmonary vascular redistribution
History of cerebrovascular disease	History of transient ischemic attack or stroke
Preoperative insulin therapy for diabetes	
Preoperative serum creatinine >2 mg/dL	

[a]Rates of major cardiac complication with 0, 1, 2, or 3 of these factors were 0.4%, 0.9%, 7.0%, and 11.0%, respectively.

CHF, congestive heart failure.

Adapted with permission from Lee TH, Marcantonio ER, Mangione CM, et al. Derivation and prospective validation of a simple index for prediction of cardiac risk of major noncardiac surgery. *Circulation* 1999;100:1043.

 c. **Preoperative testing.** Patients at intermediate risk for a perioperative myocardial event may require additional studies to determine if further therapy is needed to optimize their status.

  (1) **A preoperative electrocardiogram (ECG)** is warranted in intermediate- or high-risk patients with a history of recent chest pain scheduled for an intermediate- or high-risk procedure. In addition, our policy is to obtain an ECG on any patients with a cardiac history, concerning symptoms, or significant risk factors, especially diabetes and renal failure. A screening ECG is obtained on all patients over the age of 50 years.

  (2) **Noninvasive testing.** Patients who are identified to be at risk of a perioperative cardiovascular event by the revised cardiac risk index or who have other risk factors (e.g., PVD, unexplained chest pain, diabetes, and ECG abnormalities) should undergo further evaluation.

   (a) **Exercise stress testing** provides useful information for risk stratification. An inability to achieve even modest levels of exercise or the presence of exercise-induced ECG changes identifies patients at significant risk for an adverse outcome.

   (b) **Dipyridamole thallium imaging** has a very high negative predictive value of approximately 99% but a moderate positive predictive value ranging from 4% to 20%.

   (c) **Dobutamine stress echocardiography** is believed to provide similar adrenergic stimulus to perioperative stress. A meta-analysis of eight studies and 1,877 patients suggested a trend toward superior prognostic accuracy with dobutamine stress echocardiography compared to other tests, with a sensitivity of 85% and a specificity of 70% for predicting perioperative cardiac death or non-fatal MI in patients undergoing vascular surgery (*Heart.* 2003;89:1327).

(3) **Invasive testing.** Patients identified as high risk on noninvasive testing can be further evaluated with angiography. Patients with significant cardiac lesions should have definitive treatment [angioplasty or coronary artery bypass grafting (CABG)] prior to an elective surgical procedure.

d. **Preoperative management**

   (1) **Patients with pacemakers** should have their pacemakers turned to the uninhibited mode (e.g., DOO) before surgery. In addition, a bipolar cautery should be used when possible in these patients. If unipolar cautery is necessary, the grounding pad should be placed away from the heart.

   (2) **Patients with internal defibrillators** should have these devices turned off during surgery.

   (3) **Perioperative beta-blockade** should be considered as part of a thorough evaluation of each patient's clinical and surgical risk. Preoperative evaluation should involve identification of active cardiac conditions that would require intensive management and may result in delay or cancelation of nonemergent operations. Over the past 15 years, there has been conflicting and poorly supported evidence regarding the efficacy of beta-blockers in reducing perioperative cardiac events. However, recent studies, including the PeriOperative ISchemic Evaluation (POISE) trial, suggest that beta-blockers reduce perioperative ischemia and may reduce the risk of MI and cardiovascular death in high-risk patients (*Lancet.* 2008;371:1839–1847; see Table 1-3 for revised cardiac risk index). However, in the case of beta-blocker-naïve patients, routine administration of higher-dose long-acting metoprolol on the day of surgery and without dose titration should be avoided as its use is associated with an overall increase in mortality. Ideally, in appropriate patients, beta-blockers should be started days to weeks before elective surgery. Preoperatively, each patient's dose should be titrated to achieve adequate heart rate control so that there is a greater likelihood of the patient's benefiting from beta-blockade while

avoiding the risks of hypotension and bradycardia. Titrated rate control with beta-blockers should continue during and after the operation to maintain a heart rate between 60 and 80 beats per minute in the absence of hypotension, as this regimen has been demonstrated to be efficacious (*Circulation.* 2009;120:2123–2151).

(4) **Patients with recent angioplasty or stenting.** Over the past two decades, use of coronary angioplasty and stenting has increased dramatically. Several studies have shown a high incidence of cardiovascular complications when noncardiac surgery is performed shortly after coronary angioplasty or stenting. A study of 216 consecutive patients who underwent noncardiac surgery within 3 months of percutaneous coronary intervention demonstrated that significantly more adverse clinical events (acute MI, major bleeding, and death) occurred when noncardiac surgery was performed within 2 weeks of percutaneous coronary intervention (*Am J Cardiol.* 2006;97:1188). Current guidelines are to delay noncardiac surgery at least 6 weeks after coronary angioplasty or stenting.

3. **Pulmonary disease.** Preexisting lung disease confers a dramatically increased risk of perioperative pulmonary complications.

a. **Preoperative evaluation and screening**

(1) **Risk factors**

(a) **Chronic obstructive pulmonary disease (COPD)** is by far the most important risk factor, increasing rates of pulmonary complications three- to fourfold.

(b) **Smoking** is also a significant risk factor. Operative risk reduction has only been documented after 8 weeks of smoking cessation; however, there are physiologic benefits to stopping as little as 48 hours before surgery.

(c) **Advanced age,** that is, older than 60 years.

(d) **Obesity.** Body mass index (BMI) greater than 30 kg/m^2.

(e) **Type of surgery.** Pulmonary complications occur at a much higher rate for thoracic and upper abdominal procedures.

(f) **Acute respiratory infections.** Postoperative pulmonary complications occur at a much higher rate for patients with acute respiratory infections; therefore, elective operations should be postponed in these individuals.

(g) **Functional status.** In the patient with pulmonary disease or a history of smoking, a detailed evaluation of the patient's ability to climb stairs, walk, and perform daily duties is vital to stratify risk. Clinical judgment has been shown to be of equal or greater value relative to pulmonary function testing for most patients.

(2) **Physical examination** should be performed carefully, with attention paid to signs of lung disease (e.g., wheezing, prolonged expiratory–inspiratory ratio, clubbing, or use of accessory muscles of respiration).

    (3) Diagnostic evaluation

       (a) Chest X-ray (CXR) should be done for acute symptoms related to pulmonary disease.

       (b) An **arterial blood gas (ABG)** should be considered in patients with a history of lung disease or smoking to provide a baseline for comparison with postoperative studies.

       (c) Preoperative pulmonary function testing is controversial and probably unnecessary in stable patients with previously characterized pulmonary disease undergoing nonthoracic procedures.

  b. Preoperative prophylaxis and management

    (1) Pulmonary toilet. Increasing lung volume by the use of preoperative incentive spirometry is potentially effective in reducing pulmonary complications.

    (2) Antibiotics do not reduce pulmonary infectious complications in the absence of preoperative infection. Elective operations should be postponed in patients with respiratory infections. If emergent surgery is required, patients with acute pulmonary infections should receive intravenous (IV) antibiotic therapy.

    (3) Cessation of smoking. All patients should be encouraged to and assisted in smoking cessation before surgery.

    (4) Bronchodilators. In the patient with obstructive airway disease and evidence of a significant reactive component, bronchodilators may be required in the perioperative period. When possible, elective operation should be postponed in the patient who is actively wheezing.

4. Renal disease

  a. Preoperative evaluation of patients with existing renal insufficiency

    (1) Risk factors

       (a) Additional underlying medical disease. A substantial percentage of patients who require chronic hemodialysis for chronic renal insufficiency (CRI) have diabetes or hypertension. The incidence of CAD is also substantially higher in these patients. Much of the perioperative morbidity and mortality arises from these coexisting illnesses.

       (b) Metabolic and physiologic derangements of CRI. A variety of abnormalities in normal physiology that occur as a result of CRI can affect operative outcome adversely; these include alterations in electrolyte concentrations, acid–base balance, platelet function, the cardiovascular system, and the immune system. Specifically, the most common abnormalities in the perioperative period include hyperkalemia, intravascular volume overload, and infectious complications.

       (c) Type of operative procedure. Minor procedures under local or regional anesthesia are usually well tolerated in patients with CRI; however, major procedures are associated with increased morbidity and mortality.

(2) Evaluation

(a) History. It is important to ascertain the specific etiology of CRI because patients with hypertension or diabetes and CRI are at a substantially increased risk of perioperative morbidity and mortality. The timing of last dialysis, the amount of fluid removed, and the preoperative weight provide important information about the patient's expected volume status. In nonanuric patients, the amount of urine (s)he makes on a daily basis should also be documented.

(b) Physical examination should be performed carefully to assess the volume status. Elevated jugular venous pulsations or crackles on lung examination can indicate intravascular volume overload.

(c) Diagnostic testing

(i) Laboratory data. Serum sodium, potassium, calcium, phosphorus, magnesium, and bicarbonate levels should be measured, as well as blood urea nitrogen (BUN) and creatinine levels. A complete blood cell count (CBC) should be obtained to evaluate for significant anemia or a low platelet level. Normal platelet numbers can mask platelet dysfunction in patients with chronic uremia.

(ii) Supplemental tests such as noninvasive cardiac evaluation may be warranted in patients with CRI and other risk factors.

(3) Management

(a) Timing of dialysis. Dialysis should be performed within 24 hours of the planned operative procedure.

(b) Intravascular volume status. CAD is the most common cause of death in patients with CRI. Consequently, because of the high incidence of coexisting CAD, patients with CRI undergoing major operations may require invasive monitoring in the intraoperative and postoperative periods. Hypovolemia and volume overload are both poorly tolerated.

b. Patients at risk for perioperative renal dysfunction. The reported incidence of acute renal failure (ARF) after operations in patients without preexisting CRI ranges from 1.5% to 2.5% for cardiac surgical procedures to more than 10% for patients undergoing repair of supraceliac abdominal aortic aneurysms (AAAs).

(1) Risk factors for the development of ARF include elevated preoperative BUN or creatinine, CHF, advanced age, intraoperative hypotension, sepsis, aortic cross-clamping, and intravascular volume contraction. Additional risk factors include administration of nephrotoxic drugs, such as aminoglycosides, and the administration of radiocontrast agents.

(2) Prevention

(a) Intravascular volume expansion. Adequate hydration is the most important preventive measure for reducing the incidence of ARF because all mechanisms of renal failure are exacerbated by renal hypoperfusion caused by intravascular volume contraction.

(b) **Radiocontrast dye administration.** Patients undergoing radiocontrast dye studies have an increased incidence of postoperative renal failure. Fluid administration (1 to 2 L of isotonic saline) alone appears to confer protection against ARF. Additional measures for reducing the incidence of contrast dye-mediated ARF include the use of low-osmolality contrast agents, a bicarbonate drip, and oral *N*-acetylcysteine (600 mg orally two times a day on the day of and the day after contrast agent administration). A prospective, single-center, randomized trial conducted from 2002 to 2003 of 119 patients with stable serum creatinine levels of at least 1.1 mg/dL demonstrated that patients randomized to receive an infusion of sodium bicarbonate before and after IV contrast administration had a significantly lower rate of contrast-induced nephropathy than patients randomized to receive sodium chloride (13.5% vs. 1.7%) (*JAMA.* 2004;291:2376). A meta-analysis of 7 studies and 805 patients found that compared with preprocedural hydration alone, the administration of *N*-acetylcysteine and hydration significantly reduced the relative risk of contrast nephropathy by 56% in patients with CRI (*Lancet.* 2003;362:598). However, a follow-up meta-analysis of 13 randomized trials including 1,892 patients did not find conclusive evidence that *N*-acetylcysteine administration before coronary angiography in patients with impaired renal function reduced the incidence of contrast nephropathy (*Am J Heart.* 2006;151:140). *N*-acetylcysteine has minimal toxicity, and further studies are needed to define its exact role.

(c) **Other nephrotoxins**—including aminoglycoside antibiotics, nonsteroidal anti-inflammatory drugs (NSAIDs), and various anesthetic drugs—can predispose to renal failure and should be used judiciously in patients with other risk factors for the development of ARF.

5. **Infectious complications.** Infectious complications may arise in the surgical wound itself or in other organ systems. They may be initiated by changes in the physiologic state of the respiratory, genitourinary, or immune systems associated with surgery. It is impossible to overemphasize the importance of frequent hand washing or antiseptic foam use by all health care workers to prevent the spread of infection.

a. **Assessment of risk.** Risk factors for infectious complications after surgery can be grouped into procedure-specific and patient-specific risk factors.

(1) **Procedure-specific risk factors** include the type of operation, the degree of wound contamination (see Table 1-4), and the duration and urgency of the operation.

TABLE 1-4   Classification of Surgical Wounds

Wound Class	Definition	Examples of Typical Procedures	Wound Infection Rate (%)	Usual Organisms
Clean	Nontraumatic, elective surgery; no entry of GI, biliary, tracheobronchial, respiratory, or GU tracts	Wide local excision of breast mass	2	*Staphylococcus aureus*
Clean-contaminated	Respiratory, genitourinary, GI tract entered but minimal contamination	Gastrectomy, hysterectomy	<10	Related to the viscus entered
Contaminated	Open, fresh, traumatic wounds; uncontrolled spillage from an unprepared hollow viscus; minor break in sterile technique	Ruptured appendix; resection of unprepared bowel	20	Depends on underlying disease
Dirty	Open, traumatic, dirty wounds; traumatic perforated viscus; pus in the operative field	Intestinal fistula resection	28–70	Depends on underlying disease

GI, gastrointestinal.

(2) **Patient-specific risk factors** include age, diabetes, obesity, immunosuppression, malnutrition, preexisting infection, and other chronic illness.

b. **Prophylaxis**

(1) **Nonantimicrobial strategies** documented to decrease the risk of postoperative infection include strict sterile technique, maintaining normal body temperature, maintaining normal blood glucose levels, and hyperoxygenation.

(2) **Surgical wound infection.** Antibiotic prophylaxis has contributed to a reduction in superficial wound infection rates (see Table 1-5 for specific recommendations). To ensure the highest blood concentration of medication at the time the operation begins, antibiotic infusions should end immediately prior to, that is, within 0–60 minutes of, incision (Casabar E, Portell J. *The Tool Book: Drug Dosing and Treatment Guidelines, Barnes-Jewish Hospital.* 8th ed. St. Louis, MO: Department of Pharmacy, Barnes-Jewish Hospital; 2010). A prospective study of 2,847 patients undergoing elective clean or clean-contaminated surgical procedures in a community hospital demonstrated that prophylactic administration of antibiotics 2 hours before surgery significantly reduced the risk of postoperative wound infection to 1.4% compared to 3.3% and 3.8%, respectively, in patients who received antibiotics postoperatively and prior to 2 hours before surgery (*N Engl J Med.* 1992;326:281–286). Repeat doses should be administered according to the usual dosing protocol during prolonged procedures.

(3) **Preoperative skin antisepsis** also plays an important role in preventing postsurgical infection. A recent randomized-controlled trial demonstrated the superiority of prepping with chlorhexidine–alcohol scrub over prepping with povidone–iodine scrub and paint in decreasing rates of both superficial (4.2% vs. 8.6%) and deep (1% vs. 3%) incisional infections (*N Engl J Med.* 2010;362:18–26).

(4) **Respiratory infections.** Risk factors and measures for preventing pulmonary complications are discussed in Section I.B.3.

(5) **Genitourinary infections** may be caused by instrumentation of the urinary tract or placement of an indwelling urinary catheter. Preventive measures include sterile insertion of the catheter and removal of the catheter as soon as possible postoperatively. A prophylactic dose of antibiotics should be given after a difficult catheter insertion or if excessive manipulation of the urinary tract has occurred.

6. **Diabetes mellitus.** Diabetic patients experience significant stress during the perioperative period and are at an estimated 50% increased risk of morbidity and mortality versus nondiabetic patients. They experience more infectious complications and have impaired wound healing. Most importantly, vascular disease is common in diabetics, and silent CAD must always be considered. MI, often with an atypical presentation, is the leading cause of perioperative death among diabetic patients.

TABLE 1-5 Recommendations for Antibiotic Prophylaxis

Nature of Operation	Likely Pathogens	Recommended Antibiotics	Adult Dose Before Surgery[a]
Cardiac: prosthetic valve and other procedures	Staphylococci, corynebacteria, enteric Gram-negative bacilli	Vancomycin and Cefazolin Vancomycin and Aztreonam[a]	1 g IV or 15 mg/kg IV 1–2 g IV 1 g IV or 15 mg/kg IV 1 g IV
Thoracic	Staphylococci	Cefazolin Vancomycin[a]	1–2 g IV 1 g IV or 15 mg/kg IV
Vascular: peripheral bypass or aortic surgery with prosthetic graft	Staphylococci, streptococci, enteric Gram-negative bacilli, clostridia	Cefazolin Vancomycin and Aztreonam[a]	1–2 g IV 1 g IV or 15 mg/kg IV 1 g IV
Orthopedic: total joint replacement or internal fixation of fractures	Staphylococci	Cefazolin Vancomycin[a]	1–2 g IV 1 g IV or 15 mg/kg IV
Gastrointestinal			
Upper GI and hepatobiliary	Enteric Gram-negative bacilli, enterococci, clostridia	Cefazolin Cefotetan Cefoxitin Clindamycin and Gentamicin[a] Ciprofloxacin and Metronidazole[a]	1–2 g IV 1–2 g IV 1–2 g IV 900 mg IV 1.5 mg/kg IV 400 mg IV 500 mg IV
Colorectal	Enteric Gram-negative bacilli, anaerobes, enterococci	Cefoxitin Cefotetan Ciprofloxacin and Metronidazole[a]	1–2 g IV 1–2 g IV 400 mg IV 500 mg IV
Appendectomy (no perforation)	Enteric Gram-negative bacilli, anaerobes, enterococci	Cefoxitin Cefotetan Ciprofloxacin and Metronidazole[a]	1–2 g IV 1–2 g IV 400 mg IV 500 mg IV

TABLE 1-5	Recommendations for Antibiotic Prophylaxis *(Continued)*		
Nature of Operation	Likely Pathogens	Recommended Antibiotics	Adult Dose Before Surgery[a]
Obstetrics/ gynecology	Enteric Gram-negative bacilli, anaerobes, group B streptococci, enterococci	Cefotetan Cefoxitin Cefazolin Clindamycin and Gentamicin[a]	1–2 g IV 1–2 g IV 1–2 g IV 900 mg IV 1.5 mg/kg IV

[a]Indicated for patients with penicillin/cephalosporin allergy.

IV, intravenous.

Source: Casabar E, Portell J. *The Tool Book: Drug Dosing and Treatment Guidelines, Barnes-Jewish Hospital.* 8th ed. St. Louis, MO: Department of Pharmacy, Barnes-Jewish Hospital; 2010.

    a. Preoperative evaluation. All diabetic patients should have their blood glucose checked on call to the operating room and during general anesthesia to prevent unrecognized hyperglycemia or hypoglycemia.

      (1) Patients with **diet-controlled diabetes mellitus** can be maintained safely without food or glucose infusion before surgery.

      (2) Patients who are taking oral hypoglycemic agents should discontinue these medications the evening before scheduled surgery. Patients who take long-acting agents such as chlorpropamide or glyburide should discontinue these medications 2 to 3 days before surgery.

      (3) Patients who normally take insulin require insulin and glucose preoperatively to prevent ketosis and catabolism. Patients undergoing major surgery should receive one half of their morning insulin dose and 5% dextrose intravenously at 100 to 125 mL/hour. Subsequent insulin administration by either subcutaneous (SC) sliding-scale or insulin infusion is guided by frequent (every 4 to 6 hours) blood glucose determinations. SC insulin pumps should be inactivated the morning of surgery.

  7. Adrenal insufficiency and steroid dependence

    a. Exogenous steroids are used to treat a variety of diseases that are encountered in surgical patients. Perioperative management of these individuals requires knowledge of the dose amount and frequency for each type of steroid (long-acting vs. short-acting) as well as the length of preoperative treatment with exogenous steroids.

    b. Perioperative stress-dose steroids are indicated for patients undergoing major surgery who have received chronic steroid replacement or immunosuppressive steroid therapy within the preceding year.

c. **Dosage recommendations** for perioperative steroids reflect estimates of normal adrenal responses to major surgical stress. The normal adrenal gland produces 250 to 300 mg cortisol per day under maximal stress, peaking at 6 hours after stress commences and returning to baseline after 24 hours unless stress continues. A regimen of hydrocortisone sodium succinate (100 mg IV) on the evening before major surgery, at the beginning of surgery, and every 8 hours on the day of surgery approximates the normal adrenal stress response. Tapering is not necessary in uncomplicated cases. Patients who are undergoing minor surgery or diagnostic procedures usually do not require stress-dose steroids.

8. **Anticoagulation.** The most common indications for warfarin therapy are atrial fibrillation, venous thromboembolism (VTE), and mechanical heart valves. Mitigation of warfarin's anticoagulant effect occurs only after several days of cessation of the drug, and several days are required to reestablish the effect after warfarin is resumed. Recommendations for the management of anticoagulation in the perioperative period require weighing the risks of subtherapeutic anticoagulation (e.g., thromboembolic events) against the benefits (e.g., reduced incidence of perioperative bleeding).

   a. **Preoperative anticoagulation.** It is generally considered safe to perform surgery when the international normalized ratio (INR) value is below 1.5. Patients whose INRs are maintained between 2.0 and 3.0 normally require withholding of the medication for 4 days preoperatively. For patients whose INRs are maintained at a value greater than 3.0, withholding medication for a longer period of time is necessary. The INR should be measured the day before surgery, if possible, to confirm that the anticoagulation is reversed. Alternate prophylaxis should be considered for the preoperative period when the INR is less than 2.0.

   b. **Postoperative anticoagulation.** The anticoagulant effects of warfarin require several doses before therapeutic levels are reached. For this reason, in patients who can tolerate oral or nasogastric medications, warfarin therapy can be resumed on postoperative days 1 or 2. In patients with atrial fibrillation, mechanical heart valve, or VTE, those deemed to be at high risk for thromboembolism should be bridged with therapeutically dosed SC low molecular weight heparin (LMWH) or therapeutically dosed IV unfractionated heparin (UFH) until INR is therapeutic; moderate-risk patients can be bridged with therapeutically dosed SC LMWH, therapeutically dosed IV UFH, or prophylactically dosed SC LMWH. Low-risk patients do not need to be bridged to warfarin therapy (*Chest.* 2008;133(6, suppl):299S–339S; Table 1-6 in this chapter provides suggested risk stratification for likelihood of developing arterial or VTE). Despite these guidelines, however, the decision as to when and whether to anticoagulate postoperatively ultimately needs to be made after a collaborative risk–benefit analysis by a patient's surgeon and cardiologist or internist.

c. **Emergent procedures.** In urgent or emergent situations in which there is no time to reverse anticoagulation before surgery, plasma products must be administered. In addition, Factor VII can have immediate effects, whereas vitamin K will have observable effects within 8 hours.

II. POSTOPERATIVE CARE OF THE PATIENT. This section summarizes general considerations in all postoperative patients.

A. **Routine Postoperative Care**

1. **Intravenous fluids.** The intravascular volume of surgical patients is depleted by both insensible fluid losses and redistribution into the third space. As a general rule, patients should be maintained on IV fluids until they are tolerating oral intake. Extensive abdominal procedures require aggressive fluid resuscitation. Insensible fluid losses associated with an open abdomen can reach 500 to 1,000 mL/hour.

2. **Deep venous thrombosis prophylaxis.** Many postoperative patients are not immediately ambulatory. In these individuals, it is important to provide prophylactic therapy to reduce the risk of deep venous thrombosis (DVT) and pulmonary embolism (PE) (see Table 1-6). Prophylaxis should be started preoperatively in patients undergoing major procedures because venous stasis and relative hypercoagulability occur during the operation. The American College of Chest Physicians (ACCP) recommends the use of pharmacologic methods combined with the use of intermittent pneumatic compression devices in high-risk general surgery patients with multiple risk factors. Prophylaxis and management of patients with a history of DVT or PE are discussed in Chapter 20.

3. **Pulmonary toilet.** Pain and immobilization in the postoperative patient decrease the clearance of pulmonary secretions and the recruitment of alveoli. Patients with inadequate pulmonary toilet can develop fevers, hypoxemia, and pneumonia. Early mobilization, incentive spirometry, and cough and deep breathing exercises are indispensable to avoid these complications.

4. **Medications**

   a. **Antiemetics.** Postoperative nausea is common in patients after general anesthesia and in patients receiving narcotics.

   b. **Ulcer prophylaxis.** Patients with a history of peptic ulcer disease (PUD) should have some form of ulcer prophylaxis in the perioperative period with either acid-reducing agents or cytoprotective agents, such as sucralfate. Routine ulcer prophylaxis in patients without a history of PUD has only been of proven benefit in those with a coagulopathy or prolonged ventilator dependence.

   c. **Pain control.** Inadequate pain control can slow recovery or contribute to complications in postoperative patients. Individuals whose pain is poorly controlled are less likely to ambulate and take deep breaths and are more likely to be tachycardic.

TABLE 1-6	Levels of Thromboembolism Risk and Recommended Thromboprophylaxis in Hospital Patients		
Level of Risk		Approximate DVT Risk w/o Prophylaxis (%)	Suggested Thromboprophylaxis Options
Low	Minor surgery in mobile patients Medical patients who are fully mobile	<10	Early and "aggressive" ambulation
Moderate	Most general, open gynecologic or urologic surgery patients Medical patients who are on bed rest, "sick"	10–40	LMWH, unfractionated SC heparin BID or TID, fondaparinux
	Moderate VTE risk plus high bleeding risk		Mechanical thromboprophylaxis
High	THA, TKA, HFS Major trauma Spinal cord injury	40–80	LMWH, fondaparinux, warfarin (INR 2–3)
	High VTE risk plus high bleeding risk		Mechanical thromboprophylaxis

THA, total hip arthroplasty; TKA, total knee arthroplasty; HFS, hip fracture surgery; LMWH, low molecular weight heparin; VTE, venous thromboembolism; INR, international normalized ratio.
Adapted with permission from Geerts WH et al. *Prevention of Venous Thromboembolism: American College of Chest Physicians Evidence-Based Clinical Practice Guidelines.* 8th ed. Chest 2008;133:381S–453S.

    d. Antibiotics. Surgeon preferences often dictate the use of postoperative antibiotics in particular cases. Recommendations for specific procedures are given in Table 1-5. Antibiotic therapy for specific infectious etiologies is discussed in Section III.E.2.

  5. Laboratory tests. Postoperative laboratory tests should be individualized; however, the following considerations are important when planning laboratory evaluations:

    a. A **CBC** should be obtained in the immediate postoperative period and on subsequent postoperative days in any procedure in which significant blood loss occurred. If there is a concern for ongoing blood loss, serial hematocrits should be followed.

b. Serum electrolytes, BUN, and creatinine are important postoperatively in patients on nothing-by-mouth (NPO) status, with renal insufficiency, or who are receiving large volumes of IV fluids, total parenteral nutrition (TPN), or transfusions. In patients with large transfusion requirements, it is important to keep track of calcium and magnesium levels.

c. Coagulation studies are important in patients who have had insults to the liver or large transfusion requirements.

d. Daily **ECGs** and a series of three **troponin I** levels 8 hours apart are appropriate ways to monitor for myocardial ischemia in patients with significant cardiac risk factors.

e. CXRs, preferably in the PACU, are necessary after any procedure in which the thoracic cavity is entered or when central venous access is attempted. CXRs on subsequent postoperative days should be considered on an individual basis if significant pulmonary or cardiovascular disease is present.

III. COMPLICATIONS

A. Neurologic Complications

1. Perioperative stroke

a. Presentation. Patients usually describe a rapid onset of focal loss of neurologic function (unilateral weakness or clumsiness, sensory loss, speech disorder, diplopia, or vertigo). Massive strokes can present with altered mental status.

b. Examination. A thorough neurologic examination, in addition to vital signs, finger-stick glucose, and pulse oximetry, should be assessed.

c. Evaluation

(1) Laboratory evaluation should include a CBC, electrolytes, BUN, creatinine, and coagulation studies. An ECG should be done to rule out cardiac arrhythmia.

(2) A **CT scan of the head** should be obtained urgently to rule out a hemorrhagic stroke.

(3) Further studies including echocardiography, carotid and transcranial ultrasound, and magnetic resonance imaging (MRI) may be ordered in consultation with a neurologist.

2. Treatment

a. General supportive measures include supplemental oxygen and IV fluid.

b. Aspirin (325 mg orally) should be given immediately in ischemic stroke.

c. Thrombolysis has been proven effective in improving outcomes from ischemic strokes; however, it is usually contraindicated in postoperative patients and should only be initiated in close consultation with a neurologist.

3. Seizures. Evaluation and treatment of postoperative seizures involve the same principles as those encountered in other settings. Most seizures in surgical patients without a history of seizure can be attributed to metabolic derangements including electrolyte abnormalities (e.g., hyponatremia and hypocalcemia), hypoglycemia, sepsis, fever, and drugs (e.g., imipenem).

a. Determine from patient history whether a true seizure was witnessed; if so, note its type, characteristics (i.e., general vs. focal), and similarity to any previous seizures. New-onset seizures are worrisome and iatrogenic causes (e.g., medications) and CVA must be considered. A history of preoperative alcohol use may indicate withdrawal.

b. Complete physical and neurologic examination should focus on airway, oxygenation, and hemodynamics and then on any sequelae of seizure, including trauma, aspiration, or rhabdomyolysis. A focally abnormal neurologic examination, especially in the setting of a new-onset focal seizure, suggests a possible cerebrovascular event.

c. Laboratory and diagnostic studies. The immediate evaluation of a patient should consist of vital signs, a blood glucose determination, CBC, and serum chemistries, including calcium and magnesium. Serum levels of anticonvulsants should be measured in patients who normally take these medications. Patients with new-onset seizures who do not have identifiable metabolic or systemic causes warrant further evaluation with a head CT scan followed by a lumbar puncture.

d. Treatment of new-onset, single, nonrecurring seizures or recurrent generalized seizures with identifiable metabolic or systemic causes usually requires only correction of the underlying abnormality.

    (1) Recurrent generalized tonic–clonic seizures require anticonvulsant therapy. A regimen beginning with a 15- to 20-mg/kg load of phenytoin, given parenterally in three divided doses, and followed by maintenance dosing of 5 mg/kg/day in three divided doses controls most seizures. Therapeutic serum levels are 10 to 20 mg/mL.

    (2) Status epilepticus, defined as a seizure lasting more than 5 minutes or a series of multiple, continuous seizures without return to baseline mental status, is a medical emergency.

        (a) Monitor cardiopulmonary parameters and stabilize the patient's airway with a soft oral or nasal airway. Endotracheal intubation might be required to protect the airway. Phenobarbital and benzodiazepines in combination severely depress the respiratory drive. IV access should be established immediately.

        (b) Administer parenteral anticonvulsants promptly.

            (i) Lorazepam (2 to 4 mg IV at a rate of 2 mg/min) should be administered to patients with generalized convulsions lasting longer than 5 minutes. Either lorazepam or fosphenytoin may be given intramuscularly in emergent situations if IV access has not yet been established. Results are usually seen within 10 minutes. A second parenteral anticonvulsant should be started concurrently, and a neurology consult should be obtained immediately (Casabar E, Portell J. *The Tool Book: Drug*

Dosing and Treatment Guidelines, Barnes-Jewish Hospital. 8th ed. St. Louis, MO: Department of Pharmacy, Barnes-Jewish Hospital; 2010).

   (ii) **Fosphenytoin** (prescribed in phenytoin equivalents) administered parenterally is the first choice to supplement benzodiazepines in this setting.

   (iii) **Phenobarbital** is a second-line agent and should be used when fosphenytoin is contraindicated (e.g., heart block) or ineffective. A loading dose of 20 mg/kg IV can be given at 100 mg/minute. Maintenance doses of 1 to 5 mg/kg/day intravenously or orally are required to achieve therapeutic plasma levels. Institution of a phenobarbital coma should be considered if status epilepticus continues.

4. Delirium. Delirium is fairly common in patients (especially the elderly) who undergo the stress of an operation. An underlying cause usually can be identified, and in most cases it involves medications or infection. Other causes include hypoxemia, electrolyte abnormalities, cardiac arrhythmias, MI, and stroke. Alcohol withdrawal, discussed in Section III.A.4, is another common cause of postoperative delirium.

   a. Symptoms include impaired memory, altered perception, and paranoia. Altered sleep patterns result in drowsiness during the day and wakefulness and agitation at night (i.e., sundowning). Disorientation and combativeness are common.

   b. Management begins with eliminating the possibility of an underlying physiologic or metabolic derangement. Heart rate, blood pressure (BP), temperature, and oxygen saturation should be assessed, and a thorough physical exam should be performed with attention to the possibility of infection. CBC and electrolytes should be obtained. Other testing, including ECG, ABG, urinalysis (UA), and CXR, is dictated by clinical suspicion. Medications should be reviewed carefully, with consideration directed toward anticholinergic agents, opiate analgesics, and antihistamines. If no underlying organic cause is identified, alteration in sleep patterns or sensory deprivation can be invoked, and haloperidol (1 to 5 mg orally or intramuscularly) can be prescribed. Often, family reassurance or transfer to a room with natural light is curative. Physical restraints might be necessary to prevent self-harm.

5. Alcohol withdrawal carries a significant risk of morbidity and mortality and requires a high level of vigilance.

   a. Symptoms. Minor withdrawal can begin 6 to 8 hours after cessation of alcohol intake and is characterized by anxiety, tremulousness, anorexia, and nausea. Signs include tachycardia, hypertension, and hyperreflexia. These signs and symptoms generally resolve within 24 to 48 hours. **Delirium tremens** typically occurs 72 to 96 hours or longer after cessation of alcohol intake and is characterized by disorientation, hallucinations, and autonomic lability that includes tachycardia, hypertension, fever, and profuse diaphoresis.

b. Treatment

(1) Benzodiazepines—such as chlordiazepoxide, 25 to 100 mg orally every 6 hours; oxazepam, 5 to 15 mg orally every 6 hours; or diazepam, 5 to 20 mg orally or IV every 6 hours—can be used as prophylaxis in alcoholics who have a history of withdrawal or to alleviate symptoms of minor withdrawal. Patients with delirium tremens should be given diazepam, 5 to 10 mg IV every 10 to 15 minutes, to control symptoms. Oversedation must be avoided through close monitoring. The dose of benzodiazepines should be reduced in patients with liver impairment. Moderate alcohol intake with meals can be a simple way to prevent and treat alcohol withdrawal.

(2) Clonidine, 0.1 mg orally four times a day, or atenolol, 50 to 100 mg orally every day, can be used to treat tachycardia or hypertension resulting from autonomic hyperactivity. Close hemodynamic monitoring is required during therapy.

(3) General medical care. Fluid and electrolyte abnormalities should be corrected, and fever should be treated with acetaminophen or cooling blankets as needed. Thiamine, 100 mg intramuscularly for 3 days followed by 100 mg orally every day, should be given to all suspected alcoholic patients to prevent development of Wernicke encephalopathy. Many chronic alcoholics have hypomagnesemia; if present, magnesium sulfate should be administered to patients with normal renal function. Folate should be given 1 mg intramuscularly or orally every day.

(4) Restraints should be used only when necessary to protect the patient from self-harm.

(5) Alcohol withdrawal seizures occur 12 to 48 hours after cessation of alcohol and are most often generalized tonic–clonic. They are usually brief and self-limited, although status epilepticus occurs in approximately 3% of cases. Benzodiazepines are most helpful in preventing recurrent seizures.

B. Cardiovascular Complications

1. Myocardial ischemia and infarction

a. The **presentation** of myocardial ischemia in the postoperative patient is often subtle. Frequently, perioperative MI is silent or presents with dyspnea, hypotension, or atypical pain.

b. In postoperative patients who present with chest pain, the **differential diagnosis** includes myocardial ischemia or infarction, PE, pneumonia, pericarditis, aortic dissection, and pneumothorax.

c. Evaluation

(1) Physical examination should be performed carefully to assess BP, heart rate, and organ and tissue perfusion. The lungs should be auscultated for signs of pulmonary edema and diminished or absent breath sounds unilaterally (concerning for pneumothorax). Auscultation of the heart can reveal a new murmur suggestive of ischemic mitral regurgitation or a pericardial friction rub suggestive of pericarditis.

(2) Diagnostic testing

    (a) An **ECG** is warranted in virtually all cases of postoperative chest pain, with comparison to prior tracings. Sinus tachycardia is one of the most common rhythms associated with myocardial ischemia.

    (b) Laboratory data

        (i) Cardiac enzymes. An elevated troponin I level is diagnostic of MI. A series of three samplings of troponin I 6–9 hours apart has a sensitivity and specificity of greater than 90% for detecting myocardial injury (*N Engl J Med.* 2009;361:868–877).

        (ii) Routine serum chemistries and CBC.

        (iii) Oxygen saturation should be determined via pulse oximetry, and supplemental oxygen should be administered. Significant hypoxia can be seen with MI, CHF, pneumonia, and PE.

    (c) CXRs should be obtained to evaluate for pneumothorax, infiltrate, or evidence of pulmonary edema.

    (d) Further diagnostic evaluation (e.g., echocardiography, coronary catheterization, ventilation–perfusion (V/Q) scintigraphy, or CT scan) should be pursued as indicated by the diagnostic workup.

(3) Treatment

    (a) Telemetry should be used in all patients with suspected myocardial ischemia.

    (b) Oxygen therapy. Arterial oxygen saturation should be kept greater than 90% with supplemental oxygen. Endotracheal intubation and mechanical ventilation are indicated for patients with respiratory fatigue, hypoxia that is refractory to supplemental oxygen therapy, and/or progressive hypercapnia.

    (c) Pharmacologic therapy

        (i) Nitrates. In the absence of hypotension (systolic BP <90 mm Hg), initial management of patients with chest pain of presumed cardiac origin includes the use of sublingual nitroglycerin (0.4 mg), which can be repeated every 5 minutes until pain resolves. Additionally, topical nitrate therapy (0.5 to 2 inches every 6 hours) can be instituted. Ongoing myocardial ischemia or infarction should be treated with IV nitroglycerin, starting with an infusion rate of 5 μg/minute and increased at 5-μg/minute increments until the chest pain is relieved or significant hypotension develops.

        (ii) Beta-adrenergic receptor antagonists, that is, beta-blockers. In the absence of significant contraindications (e.g., heart failure, bradycardia, heart block, or significant COPD), patients should be treated with IV beta-adrenergic receptor antagonists (e.g., metoprolol,

15 mg IV, in 5-mg doses every 5 minutes, followed by a 50- to 100-mg oral dose every 12 hours).

(iii) **Morphine sulfate** (1 to 4 mg IV every hour) is also useful in the acute management of chest pain to decrease the sympathetic drive of an anxious patient.

(iv) **Antiplatelet therapy** in the form of a nonenteric-coated aspirin (325 mg) can also be given if the patient is at low risk of perioperative bleeding.

(d) **Other therapeutic measures.** Thrombolytic therapy, anticoagulation, or coronary catheterization should be considered on an individual basis in consultation with a cardiologist.

2. **Congestive heart failure**
   a. **Differential diagnosis** of shortness of breath or hypoxia in the perioperative period includes CHF, pneumonia, atelectasis, PE, reactive airway disease (asthma, COPD exacerbation), and pneumothorax. These pulmonary conditions are discussed in Section III.C.
   b. **Evaluation**
      (1) **History.** CHF can occur immediately postoperatively as a result of excessive intraoperative administration of fluids or 24 to 48 hours postoperatively related to mobilization of fluids that are sequestered in the extracellular space. Myocardial ischemia or infarction can also result in CHF. Net fluid balance and weight for the preceding days should be assessed.
      (2) **Physical examination** should be directed toward signs and symptoms of fluid overload and myocardial ischemia.
      (3) **Diagnostic testing**
         (a) **Laboratory data.** Troponin I, B-type natriuretic peptide (BNP), ABG, CBC, electrolytes, and renal function tests should be obtained.
         (b) **Pulse oximetry.**
         (c) **ECG.**
         (d) **CXR.**
         (e) An **echocardiogram** is frequently indicated in patients with new CHF to evaluate valves, assess the contractility and dimensions of each cardiac chamber, and rule out tamponade.
         (f) Invasive measurement of cardiac output with a **pulmonary artery catheter** may be of use in assessing volume status.
   c. **Management of congestive heart failure**
      (1) **Supplemental oxygen** should be administered. Mechanical ventilation is indicated in patients with refractory hypoxemia.
      (2) **Diuretics.** Treatment should be initiated with furosemide (20 to 40 mg IV push), with doses up to 200 mg every 6 hours as necessary to achieve adequate diuresis. Furosemide drips can be effective in promoting diuresis. Fluid intake should be limited, and serum potassium should be monitored closely.
      (3) **Morphine** (1 to 4 mg IV pushed every hour)

(4) **Arterial vasodilators.** To reduce afterload and help the failing heart in the acute setting, sodium nitroprusside or ACE inhibitors can be used to lower the systolic BP to 90 to 100 mm Hg.

(5) **Inotropic agents.** Digoxin increases myocardial contractility and can be used to treat patients with mild failure. Patients with florid failure may need invasive monitoring and titration of drips if they do not respond to these measures. If there is a low cardiac index (<2.5 L/minute/m^2) with elevated filling pressures, inotropic agents are indicated. Therapy can be initiated with dobutamine (3 to 20 μg/kg/minute) to increase the cardiac index to a value near 3 L/minute/m^2. Milrinone is also a useful agent for refractory CHF. (A loading dose of 50 μg/kg is administered over 10 minutes, followed by a continuous infusion of 0.375 to 0.750 μg/kg/minute titrated for clinical response.) If hypotension is accompanied by low systemic vascular resistance, vasopressors may be useful (Table 1-7).

TABLE 1-7	Doses of Commonly Used Vasopressors		
Vasopressor	**Preparation**	**Infusion**	**Comments**
Dobutamine	250 mg/250 mL NS or D5 W	Start at 3 μg/kg/min and titrate up to 20 μg/kg/min based on clinical response	Beta-agonist
Dopamine	800 mg in 500 mL NS or D5 W	Start at 3 μg/kg/min and titrate to systolic BP	Beta-adrenergic effects dominate at lower infusion rates
Epinephrine	5 mg/500 mL NS or D5 W	1–4 μg/min and titrate to effect	Alpha and beta
Norepinephrine	8 mg in 500 mL D5 W	Start at 2 μg/min and titrate to systolic BP	Strong alpha-adrenergic agonist
Phenylephrine (Neo-Synephrine)	10 mg in 250 mL D5 W or NS	Start at 10 μg/min and titrate to systolic BP	May be ineffective in severe distributive shock

BP, blood pressure; D5 W, 5% dextrose in water; NS, normal saline.

C. **Pulmonary Complications**
   1. The **differential diagnosis** of dyspnea includes atelectasis, lobar collapse, pneumonia, CHF, COPD, asthma exacerbation, pneumothorax, PE, and aspiration.

   2. **Evaluation**
      a. **History.** Additional factors that help to differentiate disease entities include the presence of a fever, chest pain, and the time since surgery.
      b. **Physical examination** with attention to jugular venous distention, breath sounds (wheezing, crackles), symmetry, and respiratory effort.
      c. **Diagnostic testing**
         (1) **Laboratory.** CBC, chemistry profile, and pulse oximetry or ABG.
         (2) **ECGs** should be obtained for any patient older than 30 years with significant dyspnea or tachypnea to exclude myocardial ischemia and in any patient who is dyspneic in the setting of tachycardia.
         (3) **CXRs** are mandatory in all dyspneic patients.
         (4) **V/Q scan, spiral CT scan of the chest,** or **pulmonary angiogram** may be helpful.

   3. **Management** of specific diagnoses
      a. **Atelectasis** commonly occurs in the first 36 hours after operation and typically presents with dyspnea and hypoxia. Therapy is aimed at reexpanding the collapsed alveoli. For most patients, deep breathing and coughing along with the use of incentive spirometry are adequate. Postoperative pain should be sufficiently controlled so that pulmonary mechanics are not significantly impaired. In patients with significant atelectasis or lobar collapse, chest physical therapy and nasotracheal suctioning might be required. In rare cases, bronchoscopy can aid in clearing mucus plugs that cannot be cleared using less invasive measures.
      b. **Pneumonia** is discussed in Section III.E.2.b.
      c. **Pulmonary embolism** is discussed in Section III.F.
      d. **Gastric aspiration** usually presents with acute dyspnea and fever. CXR might be normal initially but subsequently demonstrate a pattern of diffuse interstitial infiltrates. Therapy is supportive, and antibiotics are typically not given empirically.
      e. **Pneumothorax** is treated with tube thoracostomy. If tension pneumothorax is suspected, immediate needle decompression through the second intercostal space in the midclavicular line using a 14-gauge needle should precede controlled placement of a thoracostomy tube.
      f. **COPD and asthma exacerbations** present with dyspnea or tachypnea, wheezing, hypoxemia, and possibly hypercapnia. Acute therapy includes administration of supplemental oxygen and inhaled beta-adrenergic agonists (albuterol, 3.0 mL (2.5 mg) in 2 mL normal saline every 4 to 6 hours via nebulization). Beta-adrenergic agonists are indicated primarily for acute exacerbations

rather than for long-term use. Anticholinergics such as ipratropium bromide metered-dose inhaler (Atrovent, 2 puffs every 4 to 6 hours) can also be used in the perioperative period, especially if the patient has significant pulmonary secretions. Patients with severe asthma or COPD may benefit from parenteral steroid therapy (methylpred-nisolone, 50 to 250 mg intravenously every 4 to 6 hours) as well as inhaled steroids (beclomethasone metered-dose inhaler, 2 puffs four times a day), but steroids require 6 to 12 hours to take effect.

D. Renal Complications
1. Acute renal failure
  a. **Causes.** The etiologies of postoperative renal insufficiency can be classified as prerenal, intrinsic renal, and postrenal (Table 1-8).
    (1) **Prerenal azotemia** results from decreased renal perfusion that might be secondary to hypotension, intravascular volume contraction, or decreased effective renal perfusion.
    (2) **Intrinsic renal** causes of ARF include drug-induced acute tubular necrosis, pigment-induced renal injury, radiocontrast dye administration, acute interstitial nephritis, and prolonged ischemia from suprarenal aortic cross-clamping.
    (3) **Postrenal causes** of ARF can result from obstruction of the ureters or bladder. Operations that involve dissection near the ureters, such as colectomy, colostomy closure, or total abdominal hysterectomy, have a higher incidence of ureteral injuries. In addition to ureteral injuries or obstruction, obstruction of the bladder from an enlarged prostate, narcotic use for management of postoperative pain, or an obstructed urinary catheter can contribute to postrenal ARF.
  b. **General evaluation**
    (1) **History and physical examination**
    (2) **Laboratory evaluation**
      (a) **Urinalysis with microscopy and culture** (as indicated) can help to differentiate between etiologies of renal failure.
      (b) **Serum chemistries.**

TABLE 1-8	Laboratory Evaluation of Oliguria and Acute Renal Failure				
Category	FE_{Na}	U_{Osm}	RFI	U_{Cr}/P_{Cr}	U_{Na}
Prerenal	<1	>500	<1	>40	<20
Renal (acute tubular necrosis)	>1	<350	>1	<20	>40
Postrenal	>1	<50	>1	<20	>40

FE_{Na}, fractional excretion of sodium; RFI, renal failure index; U_{Cr}/P_{Cr}, urine–plasma creatinine ratio; U_{Na}, urine sodium; U_{Osm}, urine osmolality.

(c) **Urinary indices** help to classify ARF into prerenal, postrenal, or intrinsic renal categories (Table 1-8). Fractional excretion of sodium (FE_{Na}) can be calculated from

$$FE_{Na} = (U_{Na}/P_{Na})/(U_{Cr}/P_{cr}),$$

where U_{Na} is urine sodium, P_{Na} is plasma sodium, and U_{Cr}/P_{Cr} is urine–plasma creatinine ratio. The renal failure index (RFI) is $(U_{Na})(P_{Cr})/U_{Cr}$. These measurements must be obtained before diuretic administration.

(3) **Other diagnostic testing**

(a) **Renal ultrasonography** can be used to exclude obstructive uropathy, assess the chronicity of renal disease, and evaluate the renal vasculature with Doppler ultrasonography.

(b) **Radiologic studies** using IV contrast are contraindicated in patients with suspected ARF due to potential exacerbation of renal injury.

c. **Management of specific problems**

(1) **Oliguria** (<500 mL/day) in the postoperative period.

(a) **Evaluation.** The goal of this evaluation is to determine the patient's intravascular volume status and to differentiate the causes of oliguria. Cardiac echocardiography, central venous pressures, and pulmonary artery pressures can assist with the evaluation of volume status.

(b) **Management**

(i) **Prerenal.** In most surgical patients, oliguria is caused by hypovolemia. Initial management includes fluid challenges (e.g., normal saline boluses of 500 mL). Patients with adequate fluid resuscitation and CHF may benefit from invasive monitoring and optimization of cardiac function.

(ii) **Intrinsic renal.** Treat the underlying cause, if possible, and manage volume status.

(iii) **Postrenal.** Ureteral injuries or obstruction can be treated with percutaneous nephrostomy tubes and generally are managed in consultation with a urologist. Urinary retention and urethral obstruction can be managed by placement of a Foley catheter or, if necessary, a suprapubic catheter.

(2) **Elevated creatinine and ARF**

(a) **Evaluation.** The laboratory and diagnostic evaluation for patients with a rising creatinine is similar to the evaluation for patients with oliguria.

(b) **Management** includes careful attention to the intravascular volume status. The patient should be weighed daily, and intakes and outputs should be recorded carefully. Serum electrolytes should be monitored closely. The patient should be maintained in a euvolemic state. Hyperkalemia, metabolic acidosis, and hyperphosphatemia are common problems in patients with ARF and should be managed as discussed in Chapter 4. Medication doses should be adjusted appropriately and potassium removed from maintenance IV fluids.

  (i) **Dialysis.** Indications for dialysis include intravascular volume overload, hyperkalemia, severe metabolic acidosis, and complications of uremia (encephalopathy, pericarditis).

E. **Infectious Complications**
  1. **Management of infection and fever**
    a. **Evaluation of fever** should take into account the amount of time that has passed since the patient's most recent operation.
      (1) **Intraoperative fever** may be secondary to malignant hyperthermia, a transfusion reaction, or a preexisting infection.
        (a) **Diagnosis and management** of a transfusion reaction are discussed in Chapter 5.
        (b) **Malignant hyperthermia** is discussed in Chapter 3.
        (c) **Preexisting infections** should be treated with empiric IV antibiotics.
      (2) **High fever (>39°C) in the first 24 hours** is commonly the result of a streptococcal or clostridial wound infection, aspiration pneumonitis, or a preexisting infection.
        (a) **Streptococcal wound infections** present with severe local erythema and incisional pain. Penicillin G (2 million units IV every 6 hours) or ampicillin (1 to 2 g IV every 6 hours) is effective therapy. Patients with a **severe necrotizing clostridial infection** present with systemic toxemia, pain, and crepitus near the incision. Treatment includes emergent operative débridement and metronidazole (500 mg IV every 6 hours) or clindamycin (600 to 900 mg IV every 8 hours).
      (3) **Fever that occurs more than 72 hours after surgery** has a broad differential diagnosis, including pneumonia, urinary tract infection, thrombophlebitis, wound infection, intraabdominal abscess, and drug allergy.
    b. **Diagnostic evaluation.** The new onset of fever or leukocytosis without an obvious source of infection requires a thorough history and physical examination (including inspection of all wounds, tubes, and catheter sites) and selected laboratory tests.
    c. **Specific laboratory tests**
      (1) **CBC.**
      (2) **Urinalysis.**
      (3) **CXR.**
      (4) **Gram stain/culture.** Cultures of the blood, sputum, urine, and/or wound should be dictated by the clinical situation.
    d. **Antibiotics.** Empiric antibiotics can be initiated after collection of cultures, with therapy directed by clinical suspicion.
    e. **Imaging studies** such as ultrasound or CT should be chosen based on clinical context.

2. **Management of specific infectious etiologies**
   a. **Wound infection** is diagnosed by local erythema, swelling, pain, tenderness, and wound drainage. Fever and leukocytosis are usually present but may be absent in superficial wound infections. The primary treatment is to open the wound to allow drainage. The wound should be cultured. If the infection is contained in the superficial tissue layers, antibiotics are not required. In the case of a clean procedure that did not enter the bowel, the usual pathogens are staphylococcal and streptococcal species. If surrounding erythema is extensive, parenteral antibiotics should be initiated. Wound infections in the perineum or after bowel surgery are more likely to be caused by enteric pathogens and anaerobes. More aggressive infections with involvement of underlying fascia require emergent operative débridement and broad-spectrum IV antibiotics.
   b. **Respiratory infections.** Pneumonia is diagnosed by the presence of fever, leukocytosis, purulent sputum production, and an infiltrate on CXR. After Gram stain and culture of the sputum and blood is performed, empiric antibiotics can be started. Pneumonias that occur in postoperative patients should be treated as nosocomial infections. Patients requiring mechanical ventilation for longer than 48 hours are at risk for ventilator-associated pneumonia (VAP), which may require bronchoscopy for diagnosis.
   c. **Gastrointestinal infections** may present with fever, leukocytosis, and diarrhea. *Clostridium difficile* is a common cause of diarrhea in hospitalized patients, and there should be a low threshold for performing an assay for the *C. difficile* organism or toxin. Initial therapy includes fluid resuscitation and metronidazole (500 mg orally or IV every 6 to 8 hours) or vancomycin (250 to 500 mg orally every 6 hours).
   d. **Intraabdominal abscess or peritonitis** present with fever, leukocytosis, abdominal pain, and tenderness. If the patient has generalized peritonitis, emergency laparotomy is indicated. If the inflammation appears to be localized, a CT scan of the patient's abdomen and pelvis should be obtained. The primary management of an intraabdominal abscess is drainage. In many circumstances, this can be performed percutaneously with radiologic guidance. In other situations, operative débridement and drainage are required. Empiric antibiotic therapy should cover enteric pathogens and anaerobes.
   e. **Genitourinary infections.** After the urine is cultured, simple lower-tract infections can be managed with oral antibiotics. Ill patients or those with pyelonephritis require more aggressive therapy.
   f. **Prosthetic-device–related infections** may present with fever, leukocytosis, and systemic bacteremia. Infection of prosthetic valves may present with a new murmur. Management may require removal of the infected device and the use of long-term antibiotics.
   g. **Catheter-related infections** also are diagnosed by the presence of fever, leukocytosis, and systemic bacteremia. Local erythema and purulence may be present around central venous catheter insertion sites. Erythema, purulence, a tender thrombosed vein, or lymphangitis may

be present near an infected peripheral IV line. Management includes removal of the catheter and IV antibiotic coverage.

h. **Fascial or muscle infections** may result from gross contamination of a surgical wound or from a previously infected wound. Fasciitis and deep-muscle infections can present with hemorrhagic bullae over the infected area, rapidly progressive edema with foul-smelling "dishwater" pus, erythema, pain, and/or crepitus. Fever, tachycardia, and ultimately cardiovascular collapse occur in rapid succession. Therapy includes emergent operative débridement, management of shock, and broad-spectrum antibiotics (including anaerobic coverage). Necrotizing fasciitis is a surgical emergency; death may result within a few hours of the development of symptoms.

i. **Viral infections** complicating operations are uncommon in immunocompetent patients.

j. **Fungal infections** (primarily with *Candida* species) occur most commonly after long-term antibiotic administration. In these patients, evaluation of persistent fever without an identified bacterial source should include several sets of routine and fungal blood cultures, removal of all IV catheters, and examination of the retina for *Candida endophthalmitis*. Therapy includes amphotericin B, fluconazole, or micafungin.

F. **Deep Venous Thrombosis and Pulmonary Embolism**
   1. **Diagnosis and treatment of DVT**
      a. **Diagnosis**
         (1) **Symptoms** of DVT vary greatly, although classically they include pain and swelling of the affected extremity distal to the site of venous obstruction. Signs of DVT on physical examination may include edema, erythema, warmth, a palpable cord, or calf pain with dorsiflexion of the foot (Homan's sign). Physical examination alone is notoriously inaccurate in the diagnosis of DVT.
         (2) **Noninvasive studies** of the venous system, most notably B-mode ultrasonography plus color Doppler (duplex scanning), have revolutionized the diagnosis and management of suspected DVT. Reported sensitivity and specificity of this test for the detection of proximal DVT are greater than 90% with nearly 100% positive predictive value. This modality is less reliable in the detection of infrapopliteal thrombi, and a negative study in symptomatic patients should be followed by repeat examination in 48 to 72 hours to evaluate for propagation of clot proximally. Patients in whom a negative study contrasts with a strong clinical suspicion may require contrast venography, the gold standard for diagnosis of DVT.
      b. **Treatment.** See Chapter 20.
   2. **Diagnosis and treatment of PE**
      a. **Diagnosis**
         (1) **Symptoms** of PE are neither sensitive nor specific. Mental status changes, dyspnea, pleuritic chest pain, and cough can occur, and hemoptysis is encountered occasionally. Signs of PE most

commonly include tachypnea and tachycardia. Patients with massive PE may experience syncope or cardiovascular collapse. PE should be considered in any postoperative patient with unexplained dyspnea, hypoxia, tachycardia, or dysrhythmia.

(2) **Laboratory studies.** Initial evaluation of patients with suspected PE must include noninvasive assessment of arterial oxygen saturation, ECG, and CXR. Findings that are suggestive of PE include arterial oxygen desaturation, nonspecific ST-segment or T-wave changes on ECG, and atelectasis, parenchymal abnormalities, or pleural effusion on CXR. Such classic signs as $S_1Q_3T_3$ on ECG or a prominent central pulmonary artery with decreased pulmonary vascularity (Westermark's sign) on CXR are uncommon. ABG determination is a helpful adjunctive test; a decreased arterial oxygen tension (Pao_2) (<80 mm Hg), an elevated alveolar–arterial oxygen gradient, or a respiratory alkalosis may support clinical suspicion. Data that are obtained from these initial studies collectively may corroborate clinical suspicion but none of these alone is either sensitive or specific for PE. **D-Dimer** assays have a high negative predictive value; however, positive values, particularly in the setting of recent surgery, are less helpful because the postoperative period is one of many conditions that can cause an elevation of this test.

(3) **Imaging studies**

(a) **Spiral CT scan** is becoming the primary diagnostic modality for PE. The advantages of CT scans for PE include increased sensitivity, the ability to simultaneously evaluate other pulmonary and mediastinal abnormalities, greater after-hours availability, and the ability to obtain a CT venogram with the same dye load. This study subjects the patient to a contrast dye load and requires a large (18 g or higher) IV in the antecubital vein, but it is not invasive. There are still wide variations in technology and institutional expertise with this modality, with reported sensitivities ranging from 57% to 100% and specificity ranging from 78% to 100%.

(b) A **V/Q scan** that demonstrates one or more perfusion defects in the absence of matched ventilation defects is abnormal and may be interpreted as high, intermediate, or low probability for PE, depending on the type and degree of abnormality. V/Q scans alone are neither sensitive nor specific for PE, and their interpretation may be difficult in patients with preexisting lung disease, especially COPD. Nevertheless, high-probability scans are 90% predictive and suffice for diagnosis of PE. In the appropriate clinical setting, a high-probability V/Q scan should prompt treatment. Likewise, a normal scan virtually excludes PE (96%). Scans of intermediate probability require additional confirmatory tests.

(c) **Pulmonary angiography** is the reference standard for the diagnosis of PE, but it is an invasive test with some element of risk. This test is rapidly being supplanted by spiral CT for most circumstances. Its use should be reserved for (1) resolution of conflicting or inconclusive clinical and non-invasive data; (2) patients with high clinical suspicion for PE and extensive preexisting pulmonary disease in whom interpretation of V/Q scans is difficult without access to spiral CT; and (3) confirmation of clinical and noninvasive data in patients who are at high risk for anticoagulation or in unstable patients being considered for thrombolytic therapy, pulmonary embolectomy, or vena caval interruption.

(d) Treatment

(1) Supportive measures include administration of oxygen to correct hypoxemia and use of IV fluids to maintain BP. Hypotensive patients with high clinical suspicion of PE (i.e., high-risk patients, patients with acute right heart failure or right ventricular ischemia on ECG) require immediate transfer to an intensive care unit, where hemodynamic monitoring and vasoactive medications may be required.

(2) Anticoagulation with intravenous UFH or SC LMWH should be started immediately with a target activated partial thromboplastin time (PTT) of 50 to 80 seconds. Oral warfarin can be started concurrently while heparin is continued until a therapeutic PT is achieved. Anticoagulation should continue for 6 months unless risk factors persist or DVT recurs.

(3) Thrombolytic therapy is not indicated in the routine treatment of PE in surgical patients because the risk of hemorrhage in individuals with recent (<10 days) surgery outweighs the uncertain long-term benefits of this therapy. Surgical patients with shock secondary to angiographically proven massive PE that is refractory to anticoagulation should be considered for either transvenous embolectomy or open pulmonary embolectomy. These aggressive measures are rarely successful.

(4) Inferior vena caval filter placement is indicated when a contraindication to anticoagulation exists, a bleeding complication occurs while receiving anticoagulation, or a DVT or PE recurs during anticoagulation therapy.

G. Complications of Diabetes

1. Tight blood glucose control. A landmark prospective study of 1,548 patients who were admitted to a surgical intensive care unit on mechanical ventilation randomly assigned patients to tight control with intensive insulin therapy (blood glucose between 80 and 110 mg/dL) versus conventional control (blood glucose between 180 and 200 mg/dL and treatment only for levels >215 mg/dL). This study showed nearly a two-fold decrease in mortality in the tight-glucose-control group. Intensive insulin therapy also reduced overall in-hospital mortality, bloodstream infections, ARF, the median number of red blood cell transfusions, and critical illness polyneuropathy (*N Engl J Med.* 2001;345:1359).

2. **Diabetic ketoacidosis (DKA)** may occur in any diabetic patient who is sufficiently stressed by illness or surgery. DKA patients who require an operation should be provided every attempt at correction of metabolic abnormalities before surgery, although in cases such as gangrene, surgery may be essential for treatment of the underlying cause of DKA. DKA may occur without excessive elevation of the blood glucose. Management of this disorder should emphasize volume repletion, correction of acidosis and electrolyte abnormalities, and regulation of blood glucose with insulin infusion.

   a. **Laboratory tests** should include blood glucose, CBC, serum electrolytes, serum osmolarity, and ABG.

   b. **Restoration of intravascular volume** should be initiated with isotonic (0.9%) saline or lactated Ringer's solution without glucose. Patients without cardiac disease should receive 1 L or more of fluid per hour until objective evidence of normalization of intravascular volume is demonstrated by a urine output greater than 30 mL/hour and stabilization of hemodynamics. Invasive hemodynamic monitoring may be required to guide fluid replacement in some circumstances (i.e., CHF, MI, and renal failure). Maintenance fluids of 0.45% NaCl with potassium (20 to 40 mEq/L) can be instituted when intravascular volume has been restored. Dextrose should be added to fluids when the blood glucose is less than 400 mg/dL.

   c. **Correction of acidosis** with bicarbonate therapy is controversial but should be considered if the blood pH is less than 7.1 or shock is present. Two ampules (88 mEq $NaHCO_3$) of bicarbonate can be added to 0.45% NaCl and given during the initial resuscitation.

   d. **Potassium replacement** should be instituted immediately unless hyperkalemia with ECG changes exists. In nonoliguric patients, replacement should begin with 30 to 40 mEq/hour of KCl for serum potassium of less than 3; 20 to 30 mEq/hour of KCl for serum potassium of 3 to 4; and 10 to 20 mEq/hour of KCl for potassium of greater than 4 mEq/L.

   e. **Blood glucose** can be controlled with 10 units of insulin as an IV bolus followed by insulin infusion at 2 to 10 units per hour to a target range of 200 to 300 mg/dL. When the blood glucose falls below 400 mg/dL, 5% dextrose should be added to the IV fluids. Therapy is guided by hourly blood glucose determinations.

3. **Nonketotic hyperosmolar syndrome** is characterized by severe hyperglycemia and dehydration without ketoacidosis. This occurs most often in elderly noninsulin-dependent diabetes mellitus patients with renal impairment and may be precipitated by surgical illness or stress. Laboratory findings include blood glucose that exceeds 600 mg/dL and serum osmolarity of greater than 350 mOsm/L. Therapy is similar to that for DKA but with two notable exceptions: (1) Fluid requirements are often higher, and replacement should be with 0.45% saline; and (2) total insulin requirements are less.

H. Hypertension

1. **Definition.** Postoperative hypertension should be defined by the patient's preoperative BP. Patients with chronic hypertension have a shift in their cerebral autoregulatory system that may not allow for adequate cerebral perfusion at normotensive BPs. A reasonable goal of therapy for acute postoperative hypertension is within 10% of the patient's normal BP.

2. **Treatment.** Before using antihypertensive drugs in the treatment of postoperative hypertension, it is essential to diagnose and treat potentially correctable underlying causes, such as pain, hypoxemia, hypothermia, and acidosis. Acute hypertension can be managed with clonidine (0.1 mg orally every 6 hours), hydralazine (10 to 20 mg intravenously every 6 hours), labetalol (10 to 20 mg intravenously every 10 minutes, to a total dose of 300 mg), or a nitroprusside drip (0.25 to 8 µg/kg/minute intravenously). In situations in which the patient is unable to take oral medications and IV medications are not appropriate, nitroglycerin paste (0.5 to 2 inches every 6 hours) can be used.

IV. DOCUMENTATION.
Optimal patient care requires not only appropriate management but also effective communication and documentation. Documentation is essential for communication among members of the health care team, risk management, and reimbursement. All documentation should include a date, time, legible signature, and contact information (such as phone or pager number) in case clarification is necessary.

A. Hospital Orders

1. **Admission orders** should detail every aspect of a patient's care. **ADCVAANDIML** is a simple mnemonic to help in organizing admission, postoperative, and transfer orders:

   a. **Admit.** Include nursing division, surgical service, attending physician, and admission status (in-patient vs. 23-hour observation).

   b. **Diagnosis.** The principal diagnosis and, if relevant, care path. Include the operation or procedure performed.

   c. **Condition.** Distinguish among stable, guarded, and critical.

   d. **Vitals.** Include the frequency with which vital signs should be obtained and special instructions for additional monitoring such as pulse oximetry and neurologic and vascular checks.

   e. **Allergies.** Include specific reactions if known.

   f. **Activity.** Include necessary supervision and weight-bearing status, if applicable. If mobilizing the patient, include specific instructions for ambulation. Patients on bedrest should be considered for DVT prophylaxis.

   g. **Nursing orders.** These may include dressing care, drain care, urine output monitoring, antiembolic stockings, and sequential compression devices. Include specific parameters for physician notification for abnormal results (such as low urine output or low BP). Daily weights, intake and output, pulmonary toilet (such as incentive spirometry), and regimens for turning patients should be addressed here. So should **ventilator settings,** if applicable. Include mode, rate, tidal volume or pressure support, positive end-expiratory pressure (PEEP), and oxygen percentage (FiO_2).

h. Diet. Include diet type (e.g., regular, American Diabetes Association, and renal) and consistency (e.g., clear liquids, full liquids, and pureed) as well as supervision instructions, if applicable. Patients are NPO after midnight if a procedure requiring sedation is planned for the following day.

i. IV fluids. Include fluid type, rate, and time interval.

j. Medications. Include home medications if appropriate. Reference to patient-controlled anesthesia forms should be made here. Indications for new medications should be provided. Include the dose, route, and frequency of each medication ordered.

k. Laboratories. All necessary laboratory and radiographic investigations should be listed here, as well as ECGs, cardiac diagnostic laboratory testing, pulmonary function tests, and other special procedures.

2. **Review orders with nursing staff.** All orders should be reviewed with the nursing staff, particularly any unusual orders or orders that must be expedited.

3. **STAT (immediate) orders** should be designated as such on the order form and brought to the attention of the nursing staff. This is especially true for orders for new medicines because the pharmacy must be notified and the medicine brought to the floor.

4. **Discharge orders**

   a. Discharge should include location and condition. If a transfer to another institution is planned, copies of all medical records and a copy of current orders should be included.

   b. Activity limitations, if applicable, should be included. Workplace or school documentation may also be necessary.

   c. Medicines. Prescriptions for new medicines as well as detailed instructions are required.

   d. Follow-up. Follow-up plans with the appropriate physicians should be clearly indicated, with contact information for their offices.

   e. Special. Wound care, catheter care, physical therapy, home health care needs, or special studies should be described before discharge.

B. Hospital Notes

1. **History and physical examination.** The admission history and physical examination should be a complete record of the patient's history. Include past medical and surgical history, social history and family history, allergies, and home medications with doses and schedules. A complete review of systems should be documented. Outpatient records are often helpful and should be obtained if possible.

2. **Preoperative notes** summarize the results of pertinent laboratory tests and other investigations before one proceeds to the operating room (Table 1-9).

TABLE 1-9	Preoperative Note
Preoperative diagnosis	
Procedure planned	
Attending physician	
Laboratory investigations	
Electrocardiogram (if applicable)	
Chest X-ray and other radiology (if applicable)	
Informed consent	
NPO (nothing by mouth) past midnight	
Type and screen/cross (if applicable)	

3. **Operative notes.** A brief operative note should be placed in the written medical record immediately following the operation, including the operative findings and the patient's condition at the conclusion of the procedure (Table 1-10). The surgeon should also complete a dictated operative note immediately after the operation. This dictated note should include specific operative indications, antibiotic administration, preparation and drape position, sponge and instrument count, and copy distribution.

4. **Postoperative check.** Several hours after an operation, a patient should be examined, with vital signs and urine output reviewed. Documentation in the medical record in the form of a SOAP (subjective-objective-assessment-plan) note should be included.

5. **Discharge summary.** A detailed account of a patient's hospitalization should be dictated at the time of discharge (Table 1-11). If a dictation confirmation number is provided, it should be recorded in the written medical record as the final note of the hospitalization. A discharge summary must accompany any patient who is being transferred to another institution.

V. INFORMED CONSENT

A. **Obtaining Informed Consent.** Recognition of patient autonomy dictates that physicians provide adequate information so that patients can make informed decisions regarding their medical care. Patients should understand the disease process, the natural course of the disease, the risks and benefits of the procedure under consideration, and potential alternative therapies.

TABLE 1-10	Brief Operative Note
Preoperative diagnosis	
Postoperative diagnosis	
Procedure performed	
Attending surgeon	
Assistant/resident surgeons	
Type of anesthesia	
Operative findings and complications	
Specimens removed	
Packs, drains, and catheters	
Estimated blood loss	
Urine output	
Fluids administered	
Blood products administered	
Antibiotics administered	
Documentation that "time-out" to verify correct patient, procedure, and site was performed	
Patient disposition and condition	

The most common and serious risks of the procedure as well as aspects of the patient's condition that might affect the outcome of a planned procedure or might place the patient at increased risk should all be discussed. Recovery time, including amount and expected duration of postoperative pain, hospitalization, and future functional status, should also be reviewed. The use of invasive monitoring devices, including arterial and pulmonary artery catheters, should be explained. These discussions should use terms that are readily understood by the patient. This is also an important opportunity for a physician to learn about the patient's wishes for aggressive treatment and acceptance of limitations to functional status.

TABLE 1-11	Discharge Summary (Dictated)
Your name, date, and time of dictation	
Patient name	
Patient registration number	
Attending physician	
Date of admission	
Date of discharge	
Principal diagnosis	
Secondary diagnosis	
Brief history and physical examination	
Laboratory/radiographic findings	
Hospital course	
List of procedures performed with dates	
Discharge instructions	
Discharge condition	
Copy distribution	

B. **Documentation of Informed Consent.** An informed consent form is completed and signed by the patient before any elective operative procedure. In addition to the generic consent form, informed consent discussions should be documented in the progress notes section of the medical record. These notes should document the salient features of the informed consent discussion and specifically document that the potential complications and outcomes were explained to the patient. The patient's refusal to undergo a procedure that has been recommended by the physician should be documented clearly in the chart. In certain situations, such as a medical emergency, it is impossible to obtain informed consent. Inability to obtain consent should be documented carefully in the medical record. Local medical bylaws generally have provisions for these types of situations and should be consulted on a case-by-case basis.

VI. **ADVANCE DIRECTIVES.** These are legal documents that allow patients to provide specific instructions for health care treatment in the event that the patient is unable to make or communicate these decisions personally. Advance directives commonly include standard living wills and durable powers of attorney for health care. With the growing realization that medical technology can prolong life considerably and sometimes even indefinitely beyond the point of significant or meaningful recovery, the importance of these issues is clear. Patients should be offered the opportunity to execute an advance directive on admission to the hospital.

A. **Living Wills.** Provide specific instructions for the withdrawal of medical treatment in the event that a patient is unable to make treatment decisions and is terminally ill. Living wills do not include withdrawal or withholding of any procedure to provide nutrition or hydration.

B. **Durable Powers of Attorney for Health Care.** These directives allow a patient to legally designate a surrogate or proxy to make health care decisions if the patient is unable to do so. Because of the difficulty of predicting the complexities of aggressive medical management, powers of attorney are often more helpful than living wills in making difficult treatment decisions.

C. **Implementation.** Advance directives are personal documents and therefore differ from patient to patient. These documents should be reviewed carefully before implementation. Advance directives are also legal documents, and they should be displayed prominently in the medical record. To be legally binding, the documents must be executed properly. If there is any question of validity, the risk management or legal staff of the hospital should be consulted. The most effective advance directives include specific instructions for health care decisions. Important issues to be addressed include the following:

1. **Intravenous fluids**
2. **Enteral and parenteral nutrition**
3. **Medicines**
4. **Inotropic support**
5. **Renal dialysis**
6. **Mechanical ventilation**
7. **Cardiopulmonary resuscitation**

D. **Conflicts.** Although advance directives can be helpful in the management of critically ill patients, their implementation often is difficult. Advance directives, by their nature, cannot provide for every medical situation. For this reason, it is important to communicate with the patient and family before the execution of an advance directive and with the family in the event that a patient becomes incapacitated. If no advance directive is available, the physician and family must consider carefully when life-prolonging medical treatments are no longer beneficial to the patient. In such a case, the state's interest in preserving life might conflict with the desires of the family and physician. If the family and physician do not agree, the hospital ethics committee or risk management staff should be consulted.

2 Nutrition

Bernard J. DuBray Jr and J. Chris Eagon

The human body is an engine designed to burn fuel in order to perform work. The fuels we utilize are called nutrients, which come in three flavors: **carbohydrates, lipids,** and **protein.** Oxidation releases potential energy stored in the chemical bonds of nutrients, which is then harnessed in the form of ATP. Our bodies use ATP as energy currency in order to perform everything from ion transport and biomolecular synthesis to locomotion.

Dietary nutrition supplies the nutrients that drive cellular metabolism. The chemical processes that maintain cellular viability consist of catabolic (breakdown) and anabolic (synthesis) reactions. Catabolism produces energy, whereas anabolism requires energy. While both processes occur concomitantly, our collective metabolism can be driven in either direction to balance our energy needs. Feeding drives synthesis and storage, whereas starvation promotes the mobilization of energy. In preparation to "fight or flight," physiological stressors also mobilize energy stores. Populations stressed by surgery are at a unique metabolic disadvantage since they are often nutritionally restricted perioperatively. A through understanding of metabolism and its influences is necessary to assess for nutritional adequacy in surgical patients.

NUTRIENT METABOLISM

I. **CARBOHYDRATES. Glucose** is the functional unit of carbohydrate metabolism. It is the body's primary energy source, providing 30% to 40% of calories in a typical diet. The brain and red blood cells rely almost exclusively on a steady supply of glucose to function. Whereas each gram of enteral carbohydrate provides **4 kcal** of energy, parenteral formulations are hydrated and thus provide only **3.4 kcal/g.**

A. **Glucose stores.** During fed states, hyperglycemia leads to insulin secretion, which promotes glycogen synthesis. About **12 hours** worth of glycogen is available in the **liver and skeletal muscles,** which can provide a steady supply of glucose in between meals. In times of starvation and stress, depleted glycogen stores cause the release of glucagon, which promotes hepatic gluconeogenesis from amino acids. If dietary carbohydrates are not resumed, glucagon promotes ketone body formation from lipids, which the brain can utilize. A minimum intake of 400 calories of carbohydrate per day minimizes protein breakdown, which can be given in maintenance intravenous (IV) fluids during times of nil per os (NPO).

B. **Carbohydrate digestion** is initiated by the action of salivary amylase, and absorption is generally completed within the first 1 to 1.5 m of small intestine. Salivary and pancreatic amylases cleave starches into oligosaccharides. Surface oligosaccharidases then hydrolyze and transport these molecules across the gastrointestinal (GI) tract mucosa. Diseases that result in generalized mucosal flattening (e.g., celiac sprue, Whipple disease, and hypogammaglobulinemia) may cause diminished uptake of carbohydrates because of resultant deficiencies in oligosaccharidases.

II. **LIPIDS.** **Fatty acids** are the functional units of lipid metabolism. They comprise 25% to 45% of calories in the typical diet. During starvation, lipids provide the majority of energy in the form of ketone bodies converted by the liver from long-chain fatty acids. Each gram of lipid provides **9 kcal** of energy.

A. **Lipid Storage.** Bound to a glycerol backbone, free fatty acids join to form triacylglycerols during fed states. **Triglycerides** are stored in adipocytes and can be mobilized in times of stress or starvation. Lipids are important energy sources for the heart, liver, and skeletal muscle. Lipolysis is stimulated by steroids, catecholamines, and glucagon. Insulin promotes synthesis and storage.

Roles of lipids. Whereas carbohydrates are used exclusively for fuel, lipids have additional functional and structural roles. In addition to energy storage, lipids **comprise membranes in cells,** serve as **signaling factors,** and are contained in certain **vitamins.**

B. **Digestion and absorption of lipids** is complex and utilizes nearly the entire GI tract. Coordination between **biliary and pancreatic secretions** as well as a functional jejunum and ileum are necessary. Fat in the duodenum stimulates cholecystokinin and secretin release, which leads to gallbladder contraction and pancreatic enzyme release, respectively. **Pancreatic secretions** contain a combination of lipase, cholesterol esterase, and phospholipase A_2. In the alkaline environment of the duodenum, lipase hydrolyzes triglycerides to one monoglyceride and two fatty acids. Bile salts emulsify fat into micelles, which facilitates absorption across the intestinal mucosal barrier by creating a hydrophilic outer coating. Bile salts are then reabsorbed in the terminal ileum to maintain the bile salt pool **(i.e., the enterohepatic circulation).** The liver is able to compensate for moderate intestinal bile salt losses by increased synthesis from cholesterol. Major ileal resection may lead to depletion of the bile salt pool and subsequent fat malabsorption. Clinical lipid deficiency results in a generalized scaling rash, poor wound healing, hepatic steatosis, and bone changes. This condition is usually a consequence of long-term fat-free parenteral nutrition, in which high glucose levels stimulate relative hyperinsulinemia, thus inhibiting lipolysis and preventing peripheral essential fatty acid liberation. This can be avoided by providing at least 3% of caloric intake as parenteral lipid.

III. **PROTEIN.** **Amino acids** are the functional units of protein metabolism. Whereas the body has energy reserves for carbohydrates and lipids, there are no stores of protein. All of the body's protein serves a functional purpose. Proteins are important for the biosynthesis of enzymes, structural molecules, and immunoglobulins. When energy needs are unmet by nutrition, muscle breakdown yields amino acids for hepatic gluconeogenesis, which can lead to wasting and deconditioning in severe circumstances. Each gram of protein can be converted into **4 kcal** of energy.

Daily protein requirements in the average healthy adult without excessive losses are approximately 0.8 g/kg body weight. In the United States, the

Figure 2-1. Distribution and utilization of total body protein. (Adapted from Mulholland MW, Lillemoe KD, Doherty GM, et al. Whole body protein metabolism in a normal 70 kg man. In: Greenfield LJ, Mulholland MW. *Greenfield's Surgery: Scientific Principles and Practice.* 5th ed., Philadelphia: Wolters Kluwer Health/Lippincott Williams & Wilkins; 2010:56.)

typical daily intake averages twice this amount. Requirements for patients with acute illness increase to 1.2 g/kg/day and up to 2.5 g/kg/day in severely physiologically stressed patients in the intensive care unit (Fig. 2-1).

A. **Digestion of proteins** yields dipeptides and single amino acids, which are actively absorbed. Gastric pepsin initiates the process of digestion. Pancreatic proteases, activated on exposure to enterokinase found throughout the duodenal mucosa, are the principal effectors of protein degradation. Once digested, almost 50% of protein absorption occurs in the duodenum, and complete protein absorption is achieved by the midjejunum. Protein absorption can effectively occur at every level of the small intestine; therefore, clinically significant protein malabsorption is relatively infrequent, even after extensive intestinal resection. The 20 amino acids are divided into essential and nonessential groups, depending on whether they can be synthesized *de novo* in the body.

   1. **Major roles of amino acids** include the following:
      a. **Synthesis and recycling** of proteins.
      b. **Catabolic reactions,** resulting in energy generation and CO_2 production.
      c. **Incorporation of nitrogen** into nonessential amino acids and nucleotides.
      d. **Transport and storage** of small molecules and ions.

   B. **Metabolism of absorbed amino acids** occurs initially in the liver where portions of amino acids are extracted to form circulating proteins. Excess amino acids can have their carbon skeletons oxidized for energy. In addition to dietary metabolism, existing structural protein is continuously recycled. Daily protein turnover is 250 to 300 g, or approximately 3% of total body protein. The primary site of turnover is the GI tract, where shed enterocytes and secreted digestive enzymes are regularly lost. Obligate nitrogen losses also occur from an inability to reuse nitrogen with 100% efficiency. Nitrogen loss of 10 to 15 g/day occurs through urinary excretion.

STRESS METABOLISM

Alterations in metabolism due to physiologic stress share similar patterns with simple starvation. Regardless of the stimulus, our conserved response to stress is the same—catabolic shifts mobilize energy stores in order to prepare us to "fight or flight."

   A. **Simple Starvation.** After an overnight fast, liver glycogen is rapidly depleted as glucagon responds to falling serum glucose levels. Carbohydrate stores are exhausted after 24 hours. For the first few days during starvation, caloric needs are met by fat and protein degradation. Most of the protein is from breakdown of skeletal and visceral muscle, which is converted to glucose via hepatic gluconeogenesis. The brain preferentially uses this endogenously produced glucose, with the remainder consumed by red blood cells and leukocytes. Within approximately 10 days of starvation, the brain adapts and uses fat in the form of ketoacids as its fuel source. Produced by the liver from free fatty acids, the use of ketoacids has a protein-sparing effect.

   B. **Physiologic stress.** The interaction of metabolic and endocrine responses that result from major operation, trauma, or sepsis can be divided into three phases.

      1. **Catabolic phase.** After major injury, the metabolic demand is dramatically increased, as reflected in a significant rise in the urinary excretion of nitrogen (beyond that seen in simple starvation). Following a major surgical procedure, protein depletion inevitably occurs because patients are commonly prevented from eating in addition to having an elevated basal metabolic rate. The hormonal response of physiologic stress includes elevation in the serum levels of glucagon, glucocorticoids, and catecholamines and reduction in insulin.

      2. The **early anabolic phase** is also called the *corticoid withdrawal phase* as the body shifts from catabolism to anabolism. The timing of this event

is variable, depending on the severity of stress, and ranges from several days to several weeks. The period of anabolism can last from a few weeks to a few months, depending on many factors, including the ability of the patient to obtain and use nutrients and the extent to which protein stores have been depleted. This phase is marked by a positive nitrogen balance, and there is a rapid and progressive gain in weight and muscular strength. The total amount of nitrogen gained is equivalent to the amount lost in the catabolic phase; however, the rate of repletion is much slower than the rapid rate of protein depletion after the original insult.

3. The **late anabolic phase** is the final period of recovery and may last from several weeks to months. Adipose stores are replenished gradually and nitrogen balance equilibrates. Weight gain is much slower during this period than in the early anabolic phase due to the higher caloric content of fat—the primary energy stores deposited during the early anabolic phase—as compared to protein.

NUTRITIONAL ASSESSMENT

Nutrition plays a vital and often underappreciated role in the recovery of patients from surgery. It is estimated that between 30% and 50% of hospitalized patients are malnourished. While most healthy patients can tolerate 7 days of starvation, subjects to major trauma, surgery, sepsis, or other critical illness require nutritional intervention earlier. Poor nutrition has deleterious effects on wound healing and immune function, which increases postoperative morbidity and mortality. Identification of those at risk for malnutrition is made through ongoing clinical assessments by vigilant clinicians.

I. TYPES OF MALNUTRITION

A. **Overnutrition.** Obesity as defined by body mass index >30

B. **Undernutrition**

1. Caloric
   a. **Marasmus** is characterized by inadequate protein *and* caloric intake, typically caused by illness-induced anorexia. It is a chronic nutritional deficiency marked by losses in weight, body fat, and skeletal muscle mass. Visceral protein stores remain normal, as do most lab indices.

2. Noncaloric
   a. **Kwashiorkor** is characterized by catabolic protein loss, resulting in **hypoalbuminemia** and generalized **edema.** This form of malnutrition develops with prolonged starvation or severe stress. Even in a well-nourished patient, a severe stress (e.g., major burn or prolonged sepsis) may rapidly lead to depletion of visceral protein stores and impairment in immune function.
   b. **Vitamins and trace elements.** In addition to the principle sources of energy, our metabolic machinery also requires various other substances in order to function efficiently. Vitamins are involved with

TABLE 2-1	Vitamins	
Vitamin	**Function**	**Deficiency State**
Fat Soluble		
A (Retinol)	Rhodopsin synthesis	Xerophthalmia, keratomalacia
D (Cholecalciferol)	Intestinal calcium absorption, bone remodeling	Rickets (children), osteomalacia (adults)
E (α-Tocopherol)	Antioxidant	Hemolytic anemia, neurologic damage
K (Naphthoquinone)	τ-Carboxylation of glutamate in clotting factors	Coagulopathy (deficiency in factors II, VII, IX, and XI)
Water Soluble		
B$_1$ (Thioamide)	Decarboxylation and aldehyde transfer reactions	Beriberi, neuropathy, fatigue, heart failure
B$_2$ (Riboflavin)	Oxidation-reduction reactions	Dermatitis, glossitis
B$_5$ (Niacin)	Oxidation-reduction reactions	Pellagra (dermatitis, diarrhea, dementia, death)
B$_6$ (Pyridoxal phosphate)	Transamination and decarboxylation reactions	Neuropathy, glossitis, anemia
B$_7$ (Biotin)	Carboxylation reactions	Dermatitis, alopecia
B$_9$ (Folate)	DNA synthesis	Megaloblastic anemia, glossitis
B$_{12}$ (Cyanocobalamin)	DNA synthesis, myelination	Megaloblastic anemia, Neuropathy
C (Ascorbic acid)	Hydroxylation of hormones, hydroxylation of proline in collagen synthesis, antioxidant	Scurvy

Adapted from Atluri P, Karakousis GC, Porrett PM, Kaiser LR. Vitamins. In: *The Surgical Review: An Integrated Basic Science and Clinical Science Study Guide*. 2nd ed. Philadelphia: Lippincott Williams & Wilkins; 2006:252.

wound healing and healthy immune function while many trace elements are important as cofactors and enzymatic catalysts. **These substances cannot be synthesized *de novo*** and therefore must be part of dietary intake. Deficiencies can have a multitude of detrimental effects (Tables 2-1 and 2-2).

TABLE 2-2	Minerals	
Trace Element	**Function**	**Deficiency**
Chromium	Promotes normal glucose utilization in combination with insulin	Glucose intolerance, peripheral neuropathy
Copper	Component of enzymes	Hypochromic microcytic anemia, neutropenia, bone demineralization, diarrhea
Fluorine	Essential for normal structure of bones and teeth	Caries
Iodine	Thyroid hormone production	Endemic goiter, hypothyroidism, myxedema, cretinism
Iron	Hemoglobin synthesis	Hypochromic microcytic anemia, glossitis, stomatitis
Manganese	Component of enzymes, essential for normal bone structure	Dermatitis, weight loss, nausea, vomiting, coagulopathy
Molybdenum	Component of enzymes	Neurologic abnormalities, night blindness
Selenium	Component of enzymes, antioxidant	Cardiomyopathy
Zinc	Component of enzymes involved in metabolism of lipids, proteins, carbohydrates, nucleic acids	Alopecia, hypogonadism, olfactory and gustatory dysfunction, impaired wound healing, acrodermatitis enteropathica, growth arrest

Adapted from Atluri P, Karakousis GC, Porrett PM, Kaiser LR. Trace elements. In: *The Surgical Review: An Integrated Basic Science and Clinical Science Study Guide*. 2nd ed. Philadelphia: Lippincott Williams & Wilkins; 2006:253.

II. CLINICAL ASSESSMENT

A. **History.** Every good clinical assessment should begin with a thorough history from the patient. Specific inquiries pertinent to nutritional status include recent history of weight fluctuation with attention as to the timing and intent.

Recent weight loss (5% in the last month or 10% over 6 months) or a current body weight of 80% to 85% (or less) of ideal body weight suggests significant malnutrition. Anorexia, nausea, vomiting, dysphagia, odynophagia, gastroesophageal reflux, or a history of generalized muscle weakness should prompt further evaluation. A complete history of current medications is essential to alert caretakers to potential underlying deficiencies as well as drug–nutrient interactions.

B. **Physical examination** may identify muscle wasting (especially thenar and temporal muscles), loose or flabby skin (indicating loss of subcutaneous fat), and peripheral edema and/or ascites (as a result of hypoproteinemia). Subtler findings of nutritional deficiency include skin rash, pallor, glossitis, gingival lesions, hair changes, hepatomegaly, neuropathy, and dementia (*The A.S.P.E.N. nutrition support practice manual,* 1998).

Adjuncts to physical examination:

Anthropometric measurements such as triceps skinfold thickness and midarm muscle circumference reflect body-fat stores and skeletal muscle mass, respectively. These values are standardized for gender and height and should be reported as a percentage of the predicted value. Along with body mass index, these values allow the clinician to assess the patient's visceral and somatic protein mass and fat reserve.

Creatinine-height index can be used to determine the degree of malnutrition. A 24-hour urinary creatinine excretion is measured and compared to normal standards. The creatinine height index is calculated using the following equation:

$$\text{CHI} = \frac{\text{Actual 24-hour creatinine excretion}}{\text{Predicted creatinine excretion}}.$$

> Greater than 80% represents no to mild protein depletion, 60% to 80% represents moderate depletion, and less than 60% represents severe depletion.

C. **Laboratory tests** associated with nutrition are nonspecific indicators of the *degree of illness* rather than strict markers of nutrition. **Albumin, prealbumin, and transferrin** vary with the hepatic metabolic (decreased synthesis) and capillary leak (diluted serum levels) response to inflammation as well as the nutritional status (*J Am Diet Assoc.* 2004;104(8):1258–1264). Levels associated with illness are as follows:

1. **Serum albumin** of less than 3.5 g/dL (35 g/L) in a stable, hydrated patient; half-life is 14 to 20 days.

2. **Serum prealbumin** may be a more useful indicator of acute changes: 10 to 17 mg/dL corresponds to mild depletion, 5 to 10 mg/dL to moderate depletion, and less than 5 mg/dL to severe depletion; half-life is 2 to 3 days.

3. **Serum transferrin** of less than 200 mg/dL; half-life is 8 to 10 days.

III. ESTIMATION OF ENERGY NEEDS

A. **Basal energy expenditure** can be predicted by using the Harris-Benedict equation (in kilocalories per day):

> For **men** equals
> $66.4 + [13.7 \times \text{weight (kg)}] + [5 \times \text{height (cm)}] - [6.8 \times \text{age (years)}]$.
> For **women** equals
> $65.5 + [9.6 \times \text{weight (kg)}] + [1.7 \times \text{height (cm)}] - [4.7 \times \text{age (years)}]$.

These equations provide a reliable estimate of the energy requirements in approximately 80% of hospitalized patients. The actual caloric need is obtained by multiplying basal energy expenditure by specific stress factors (Table 2-3). Most stressed patients require 25 to 35 kcal/kg/day. In obese patients, these equations tend to overestimate caloric needs.

TABLE 2-3	Disease Stress Factors Used in Calculation of Total Energy Expenditure
Clinical Condition	**Stress Factor**
Starvation	0.80–1.00
Elective operation	1.00–1.10
Peritonitis or other infections	1.05–1.25
Adult respiratory distress syndrome or sepsis	1.30–1.35
Bone marrow transplant	1.20–1.30
Cardiopulmonary disease (noncomplicated)	0.80–1.00
Cardiopulmonary disease with dialysis or sepsis	1.20–1.30
Cardiopulmonary disease with major surgery	1.30–1.55
Acute renal failure	1.30
Liver failure	1.30–1.55
Liver transplant	1.20–1.50
Pancreatitis	1.30–1.80

Adapted from Shoppell JM, Hopkins B, Shronts EP. Nutrition screening and assessment. In: Gottschlich M, ed. *The Science and Practice of Nutrition Support: A Case Based Core Curriculum.* Dubuque, IA: Kendall/Hunt; 2001:107–140.

TABLE 2-4	Estimated Protein Requirements in Various Disease States

Clinical Condition	Protein Requirements (g/kg ideal body weight per day)
Healthy, nonstressed	0.80
Bone marrow transplant	1.40–1.50
Liver disease without encephalopathy	1.00–1.50
Liver disease with encephalopathy	0.50–0.75 (advance as tolerated)
Renal failure without dialysis	0.60–1.00
Renal failure with dialysis	1.00–1.30
Pregnancy	1.30–1.50

Simplified Estimates	
Mild metabolic stress (elective hospitalization)	1.00–1.10
Moderate metabolic stress (complicated postoperative care, infection)	1.20–1.40
Severe metabolic stress (major trauma, pancreatitis, sepsis)	1.50–2.50

Adapted from Nagel M. Nutrition screening: identifying patients at risk for malnutrition. *Nutr Clin Pract*. 1998;8:171–175.

B. **Estimates of protein requirements.** The appropriate calorie:nitrogen ratio is approximately 150:1 (calorie:protein ratio of 24:1), which increases to 300:1 to 400:1 in uremia. In the absence of severe renal or hepatic dysfunction, approximately **1.5 g protein per kilogram body weight** should be provided daily (Table 2-4).

Twenty-four-hour nitrogen balance is calculated by subtracting nitrogen loss from nitrogen intake. Nitrogen intake is the sum of nitrogen delivered from enteral and parenteral feedings. Nitrogen is lost through urine, fistula drainage, diarrhea, and so on. The usual approach is to measure the urine urea nitrogen concentration of a 24-hour urine collection and multiply by urine volume to estimate 24-hour urinary loss. Nitrogen loss equals 1.2 × [24-hour urine urea nitrogen (g per day)] + 2 g per day as a correction factor to account for nitrogen losses in stool and skin exfoliation.

NUTRITION ADMINISTRATION

Surgical patients present a unique set of challenges to clinicians who must determine **when, how, and what** to feed them. Safe administration of an oral diet requires that the patient should have an intact chewing/swallowing mechanism along with a functioning alimentary tract. The timing, route, and type of nutrition are important considerations in surgical patients.

A. **Initial timing of administration.** Open abdominal surgery produces a **paralytic ileus** of variable length that alters the digestion and absorption of nutrients. Resolution, marked by the passage of flatus, occurs in most patients within 72 hours of surgery and is symptomatic of functional GI continuity. Traditionally, postoperative patients were maintained on dextrose-containing IV fluids and kept NPO for up to 7 days until evidence of bowel function returned. Several strategies have recently emerged to shorten postoperative ileus.

Strategies to hasten GI recovery following abdominal surgery:

1. **Laparoscopic surgery** is less traumatic and has been associated with shorter periods of ileus versus open approaches.

2. **Epidural analgesia** with an infusion of local anesthetic minimizes narcotic dependence on pain control and thus its adverse effects on gut motility (*Cleve Clin J Med.* 2009;76(11):641–648). In addition, thoracic epidurals are efficient at blocking many of the sympathetic reflex arcs that inhibit gut motility. Clinicians should be aware of the side effects of epidurals, which include hypotension and urinary retention.

3. **Selective use of nasogastric tubes** has been shown to decrease rates of pneumonia, fever, and atelectasis while hastening resumption of oral feeding (*Ann Surg.* 1995;221(5):469–476).

4. **Early enteral feeding** has been evaluated in a meta-analysis of 13 RCTs consisting of 1,173 patients undergoing GI surgery (*J Gastrointest Surg.* 2009;13(3):569–575). There were no significant differences in morbidity between groups fed within 24 hours and those fed after traditional return of bowel function.

> It is important to note that an ileus must be distinguished from more ominous conditions, such as an obstruction. A prolonged ileus may be the result of intra-abdominal pathology.

B. **Route of administration.** Oral administration of nutrition is the preferred route since it is the most physiologic and the least invasive. In patients with a functioning GI tract, several requirements must still be met, however, before initiating an oral diet.

1. **Mental alertness and orientation.** Patients who have altered mentation are at increased risk for aspiration and should not begin an oral nutrition regimen.

2. **Intact chewing/swallowing mechanism.** Patients who have had a stroke or undergone pharyngeal surgery may have difficulty swallowing. They may be candidates for modified oral diets, such as mechanical soft, or pureed.

C. **Diet selection**

1. **Transitional diets** minimize digestive stimulation and colonic residue while providing more calories than IV fluids alone in patients recovering from postoperative ileus. Advancement to the next stage should be predicated on frequent assessment of the patient's bowel function in the absence of nausea, vomiting, or distention (*Manual of Clinical Nutrition Management,* 2009).

Clear liquids provide fluids mostly in the form of sugar and water. Patients with evidence of bowel function or who have undergone laparoscopic surgery can be given clear liquids and expect between 700 and 1,000 additional kcal per day. Examples include most juices, coffee, and tea.

Full liquids are a bit more substantive and include foods that are liquid at body temperature, such as gels and frozen liquids. In addition, full liquids contain dairy products and would not be appropriate in patients who are lactose intolerant. Transition to full liquids is good for patients who have undergone head and neck surgery and thus may have some difficulty swallowing postoperatively. At goal, full liquids provide approximately 1,200 kcal and 40 g of protein per day (*Manual of Clinical Nutrition Management,* 2009).

Regular diet represents an unrestricted regimen that includes various foods designed to meet all caloric, protein, and elemental needs.

2. **Surgery-specific diets**
   a. **Postgastrectomy diet.** Procedures that reduce the reservoir capacity of the stomach can produce a "dumping syndrome" postoperatively. When undigested, hyperosmolar, food reaches the small bowel, massive fluid shifts lead to diaphoresis, abdominal cramping, and diarrhea. The postgastrectomy diet encourages small, frequent meals that minimize fluid intake and simple carbohydrates. Caloric needs are met mostly by protein and lipids (*Manual of Clinical Nutrition Management,* 2009).

Procedures that can cause dumping syndrome

Standard Whipple procedure
Partial/total gastrectomy/antrectomy
Esophagectomy
Pyloromyotomy

---

   b. **Postgastric bypass.** Patients who undergo bariatric surgery have unique postoperative nutritional needs as well as long-term goals of sustained weight loss.

   Postbariatric surgery transitional diets emphasize small meals without added sugar to avoid stretching the pouch and dumping syndrome, respectively. Patients progress from clear liquid to the regular bariatric diet in approximately 6 weeks. During this time, patients are taught to eat 3 to 5 small meals per day **slowly** over a period of 45 minutes in order to stay fuller longer. This pattern is preferred to "grazing" (small, frequent meals), which leads to higher caloric intake.

   Long-term nutritional goals promote healthy food choices that maintain weight loss while minimizing dyspepsia. Foods such as chicken, fish, fruit, vegetables, and salad are well tolerated by bariatric patients, whereas steak, rice, bread, soda, and ice cream are associated with dyspepsia and should be avoided.

   c. **Low-residue diet** is essentially a low-fiber diet (<10g/day) and is intended to delay transit, reduce residue, and allow bowel rest in times of colonic inflammation and/or irritation. Patients who benefit from a low-residue diet include those going through an acute phase of **IBD, diverticulitis, or regional enteritis** (*Manual of Clinical Nutrition Management,* 2009).

NUTRITIONAL SUPPORT

The need for nutritional support should be assessed continually in patients both preoperatively and postoperatively. Most elective surgical patients have adequate fuel reserves to withstand common catabolic stresses and partial starvation for up to 7 days and do not benefit from perioperative nutritional support (*Nutrition.* 2000;16(9):723–728). For these patients, IV fluids with appropriate electrolytes and a minimum of 100 g glucose daily (to minimize protein catabolism) is adequate. However, even well-nourished patients can quickly become malnourished following a major operation or trauma (*Curr Probl Surg.* 1995;32(10):833–917). Without nutritional intervention, these patients may suffer complications related to impaired immune function and poor wound healing from depleted visceral protein stores. Patients with a significant degree of preoperative malnutrition have less reserve, tolerate catabolic stress and starvation poorly, and are at higher risk for postoperative complications.

ROUTES OF NUTRITIONAL SUPPORT

A. **Enteral.** In general, the enteral route is preferred to the parenteral route. Enteral feeding is simple, physiologic, and relatively inexpensive. Enteral feeding maintains the GI tract cytoarchitecture and mucosal integrity (via trophic effects), absorptive function, and normal microbial flora. This results in less bacterial translocation and endotoxin release from the intestinal lumen into the bloodstream (*Nutrition.* 2000;16(7–8):606–611). Choice of appropriate feeding site, administration technique, formula, and equipment may circumvent these problems.

> Enteral feedings are **indicated** for patients who have a functional GI tract but are unable to sustain an adequate oral diet.
> Enteral feedings may be **contraindicated** in patients with an intestinal obstruction, ileus, GI bleeding, severe diarrhea, vomiting, enterocolitis, or a high-output enterocutaneous fistula.

1. **Feeding tubes.** Nasogastric, nasojejunal (e.g., Dobhoff), gastrostomy, and jejunal tubes are available for the administration of enteral feeds. Percutaneous gastrostomy tubes can be placed endoscopically or under fluoroscopy.
2. **Enteral feeding products.** Various commercially available enteral formulas are available. Standard solutions provide 1 kcal/mL; calorically concentrated solutions (>1 kcal/mL) are available for patients who require volume restriction. The available dietary formulations for enteral feedings can be divided into polymeric (blenderized and nutritionally complete commercial formulas), chemically defined formulas (elemental diets), and modular formulas (Table 2-5).

TABLE 2-5 Enteral Formulas

Per 1,000 mL

Product	Description	kcal/mL	mOsm	Protein g (% kcal)	Carbohydrates g (% kcal)	Fat g (% kcal)	H_2O (mL)	Na (mEq)	K (mEq)	Ca (mg)	PO_4 (mg)	Vitamin K (mg)
Standard												
Ensure	Lactose-free, low residue	1.06	470	37.2 (14)	145 (54.5)	37.2 (31.5)	845	36.8	40	530	530	43
Osmolite	Isotonic, lactose-free, low residue	1.06	300	37.2 (14)	145 (54.6)	38.5 (31.4)	841	27.6	25.9	530	530	43
Jevity	Isotonic, lactose-free, high dietary fiber (14.4 g/L), high nitrogen content	1.06	310	44.4 (16.7)	151.7 (53.3)	36.8 (30)	833	40.4	40	909	756	61
Glucerna	Lactose-free, low carbohydrates, high fiber (14.4 g/L)	1	375	41.8 (16.7)	93.7 (33.3)	55.7 (50)	873	40.3	40	703	703	57
Low Volume												
Ensure Plus	Lactose-free, low residue	1.5	690	54.9 (14.7)	200 (53.3)	53.3 (32)	769	45.9	49.7	704	704	57
Magnacal	Lactose-free, low residue	2	590	70 (14)	250 (50)	80 (34)	690	43.5	32	1,000	1,000	300
Low Volume, High Nitrogen												
Ensure Plus HN	Lactose-free, low residue	1.5	650	62.6 (16.7)	199.9 (53.3)	50 (30)	769	51.5	46.5	1,056	1,056	85
Perative	Lactose-free, low residue	1.3	425	66.6 (20.5)	177 (54.5)	37.3 (25)	789	45.2	44.3	867	867	70

Very High Nitrogen

Replete with Fiber	Lactose-free, high fiber (14 g/L)	1	300	62.5 (25)	113 (45)	34 (30)	840	21.7	40	1,000	1,000	80
Sustacal	Lactose-free, low residue	1.01	650	61 (24)	140 (55)	23 (21)	840	40	54	1,010	930	240
Elemental												
Vivonex TEN	Elemental, low fat, low residue	1	630	38.2 (15.3)	205.6 (82.2)	2.77 (2.5)	845	20	20	500	500	22.3
Pudding (per 5-oz serving)												
Ensure Pudding	Contains lactose		250	6.8	34.0	9.7		10.4	8.5	200	200	12
Modulars (analysis per tablespoon)												
Polycose Liquid	Glucose polymer	30			7.5							
ProMod	Protein supplement	17	3		0.4	0.4		0				
Microlipid	Fat supplement	67.5				7.5			1	15.6	15.6	
MCT Oil	MCT supplement	115.5				14				15.6		

MCT, medium-chain triglycerides.

3. **Enteral feeding protocols.** It is recommended to start with a full-strength formula at a slow rate, which is steadily advanced. This reduces the risk of microbial contamination and achieves goal intake earlier. Conservative initiation and advancement are recommended for patients who are critically ill, those who have not been fed for some time, and those receiving a high-osmolarity or calorie-dense formula.

   a. **Bolus feedings** are reserved for patients with nasogastric or gastrostomy feeding tubes. Feedings are administered by gravity, begin at 50 to 100 mL every 4 hours, and are increased in 50-mL increments until goal intake is reached (usually 240 to 360 mL every 4 hours). Tracheobronchial aspiration is a potentially serious complication because feedings are prepyloric. To reduce the risk of aspiration, the patient's head and body should be elevated to 30 to 45 degrees during feeding and for 1 to 2 hours after each feeding. The gastric residual volume should be measured before administration of the feeding bolus. If this volume is greater than 50% of the previous bolus, the next feeding should be held. The feeding tube should be flushed with approximately 30 mL of water after each use. Free water volume can be adjusted as needed to treat hypo- or hypernatremia.

   b. **Continuous infusion** administered by a pump is generally required for nasojejunal, gastrojejunal, or jejunal tubes. Feedings are initiated at 20 mL/hour and increased in 10- to 20-mL/hour increments every 4 to 6 hours until the desired goal is reached. The feeding tube should be flushed with approximately 30 mL of water every 4 hours. Feedings should be held or advancement should be slowed if abdominal distension or pain develops. For some patients, the entire day's feeding can be infused over 8 to 12 hours at night to allow the patient mobility free from the infusion pump during the day.

4. **Conversion to oral feeding.** When supplementation is no longer needed, an oral diet is resumed gradually. In an effort to stimulate appetite, enteral feeding can be modified by the following measures:

   a. **Providing fewer feedings.**

   b. **Holding daytime feedings.**

   c. **Decreasing the volume of feedings.** When oral intake provides approximately 75% of the required calories, tube feedings can be stopped.

5. **Complications**

   a. **Metabolic derangements.** Abnormalities in serum electrolytes, calcium, magnesium, and phosphorus can be minimized through vigilant monitoring. **Hypernatremia** may lead to the development of mental lethargy or obtundation. This is treated with the slow administration of free water by giving either dextrose 5% in water (D_5W) intravenously or additional water in the tube feedings. **Hyperglycemia** may occur in patients receiving tube feeds and is particularly common in preexisting diabetics or in the setting of sepsis. A sliding scale insulin protocol along with long-acting agents should be used to treat hyperglycemia in tube-fed patients.

b. **Clogging** can usually be prevented by careful routine flushing of the feeding tube. Instillation of carbonated soda, cranberry juice, or pancreatic enzyme replacement is sometimes useful for unclogging feeding tubes. Note the use of a 1 mL syringe with stopcock and IV tubing will generate a greater pressure than 60 mL GU syringe ($P = F/A$).

c. **Tracheobronchial aspiration** of tube feeds may occur with patients who are fed into the stomach or proximal small intestine and can lead to major morbidity. Patients at particular risk are those with central nervous system abnormalities and those who are sedated. Precautions include frequent assessment of gastric residuals as well as head of bed elevation.

d. **High gastric residuals** as a result of outlet obstruction, dysmotility, intestinal ileus, or bowel obstruction may limit the usefulness of nasogastric or gastrostomy feeding tubes. Treatment of this problem should be directed at the underlying cause. Gastroparesis frequently occurs in diabetic or head-injured patients. Promotility agents such as metoclopramide or erythromycin may aid in gastric emptying. If gastric retention prevents the administration of sufficient calories and intestinal ileus or obstruction can be excluded, a nasojejunal or jejunostomy feeding tube may be necessary.

e. **Diarrhea** occurs in 10% to 20% of patients; however, other causes of diarrhea (e.g., *Clostridium difficile* colitis) should be considered. Diarrhea may result from an overly rapid increase in the volume of hyperosmolar tube feedings, medications (e.g., metoclopramide), a high-fat diet, or the presence of components not tolerated by the patient (e.g., lactose). If other causes of diarrhea can be excluded, the volume or concentration of tube feedings should be decreased. If no improvement occurs, a different formula should be used. Antidiarrheal agents such as loperamide should be reserved for patients with severe diarrhea who have had infectious etiologies excluded.

B. **Parenteral nutrition** is indicated for patients who require nutritional support but cannot meet their needs through oral intake and for whom enteral feeding is contraindicated or not tolerated.

1. **Peripheral parenteral nutrition (PPN)** is administered through a peripheral IV catheter. The osmolarity of PPN solutions generally is limited to 1,000 mOsm (approximately 12% dextrose solution) to avoid phlebitis. Consequently, unacceptably large volumes (>2,500 mL) are necessary to meet the typical patient's nutritional requirements. Temporary nutritional supplementation with PPN may be useful in selected patients but is not typically indicated.

2. **Total parenteral nutrition (TPN)** provides complete nutritional support (*Surgery.* 1968;64(1):134–142). The solution, volume of administration, and additives are individualized on the basis of an assessment of the nutritional requirements.

a. **Access.** TPN solutions must be administered through a central venous catheter. A dedicated single-lumen catheter or a multilumen catheter can be used. Catheters should be replaced for unexplained fever or bacteremia.

    b. TPN solutions are generally administered as a 3-in-1 admixture of protein, as amino acids (10%; 4 kcal/g); carbohydrate, as dextrose (70%; 3.4 kcal/g); and fat, as a lipid emulsion of soybean or safflower oil (20%; 9 kcal/g). Alternatively, the lipid emulsion can be administered as a separate IV "piggyback" infusion. Special solutions that contain low, intermediate, or high nitrogen concentrations as well as varying amounts of fat and carbohydrate are available for patients with diabetes, renal or pulmonary failure, or hepatic dysfunction.

    Additives. Other elements can be added to the basic TPN solutions.

    (1) Electrolytes (i.e., sodium, potassium, chloride, acetate, calcium, magnesium, phosphate) should be adjusted daily. The number of cations and anions must balance; this is achieved by altering the concentrations of chloride and acetate. The calcium:phosphate ratio must be monitored to prevent salt precipitation.

    (2) Medications such as albumin, H_2-receptor antagonists, heparin, iron, dextran, insulin, and metoclopramide can be administered in TPN solutions. Regular insulin should initially be administered subcutaneously on the basis of the blood glucose level. After a stable insulin requirement has been established, insulin can then be administered via TPN solution—generally at two thirds the daily subcutaneous insulin dose.

    (3) Vitamins and trace elements are added daily using a commercially prepared mixture (e.g., 10 mL MVI-12; 1 mL trace element-5: 1 mg copper, 12 μg chromium, 0.3 μg manganese, 60 μg selenium, and 5 mg zinc). Vitamin K is not included in most multivitamin mixtures and must be added separately (10 mg once a week).

C. Administration of TPN is most commonly a **continuous infusion.** A new 3-in-1 admixture bag of TPN is administered daily at a constant infusion rate over 24 hours. Additional maintenance IV fluids are unnecessary, and total infused volume should be kept constant while nutritional content is increased. Serum electrolytes should be obtained and TPN adjusted until the patient can be maintained on a stable regimen.

    1. Cyclic administration of TPN solutions may be useful for selected patients, including (1) those who will be discharged from the hospital and subsequently receive home TPN, (2) those with limited IV access who require administration of other medications, and (3) those who are metabolically stable and desire a period during the day when they can be free of an infusion pump. Cyclic TPN is administered for 8 to 16 hours, most commonly at night. This should not be done until metabolic stability has been demonstrated for patients on standard, continuous TPN infusions.

D. Discontinuation of TPN should take place when the patient can satisfy 75% of his or her caloric and protein needs with oral intake or enteral feeding. The calories provided by TPN can be decreased in proportion to calories from the patient's increasing enteral intake. To discontinue TPN, the infusion rate should be halved for 1 hour, halved again the next hour, and then discontinued. Tapering in this manner prevents rebound hypoglycemia from hyperinsulinemia. It is not necessary to taper the rate if the patient demonstrates glycemic stability when TPN is abruptly discontinued (i.e., cycled TPN) or receives less than 1,000 kcal/day.

E. **Complications associated with TPN**

1. **Catheter-related complications** can be minimized by strict aseptic technique and routine catheter care (*Surg Clin North Am.* 1985; 65(4):835–865).

2. **Metabolic complications** include electrolyte abnormalities and glucose homeostasis. Strict maintenance of serum glucose level below 110 mg/dL improves mortality and reduces infectious complications in surgical intensive care unit patients (*N Engl J Med.* 2001;345(19):1359–1367).

   Cholestasis is another common metabolic complication of long-term parenteral nutrition. This is due to the lack of enteral stimulation for gallbladder contraction. Cholestatic liver disease may ultimately lead to biliary cirrhosis, which is treated with transplantation.

DISEASE-SPECIFIC NUTRITION

A. The increase in metabolic demands following **thermal injury** correlates with the extent of ungrafted body surface area. Providing analgesia and thermoneutral environments lowers the accelerated metabolic rate and helps to decrease catabolic protein loss until the surface can be grafted (*Compr Ther.* 1991;17(3):47–53).

B. **Diabetes** often complicates nutritional management. Hyperglycemia with glycosuria causes osmotic diuresis and loss of electrolytes in urine, whereas hypoglycemia can result in shock, seizures, or vascular instability. The goal in patients with diabetes is to maintain the serum glucose within the normal range. Adjustments in insulin dosing should be made with the understanding that insulin requirements will decrease as the patient recovers from the initial stress.

C. Patients with marginal pulmonary reserve who are ventilator dependent may be particularly **difficult to wean** (*JAMA.* 1980;243(14):1444–1447). Excessive carbohydrate administration increases CO_2 production, which is compensated by increasing minute ventilation. In patients with marginal reserve, increasing minute ventilation may lead to fatigue and difficulty weaning.

The respiratory quotient (**RQ**) represents the balance between CO_2 production and O_2 consumption and is a general indicator of metabolism.

$$RQ = \frac{\dot{V}_{CO_2}}{\dot{V}_{O_2}}.$$

D. Patients with **renal failure** can have excessive protein loss through dialysis, which may result in a negative nitrogen balance. These patients should be nutritionally replenished according to their calculated needs. Patients who receive peritoneal dialysis absorb approximately 80% of the dextrose in the dialysate fluid (assuming a normal serum glucose level).

E. Nutritional complications of **hepatic failure** include wasting of lean body mass, fluid retention, vitamin and trace metal deficiencies, anemia, and encephalopathy. Branched-chain amino acids (BCAA) are metabolized by skeletal muscle and may be helpful in limiting the severity of encephalopathy (*J Nutr.* 2006;136(1 suppl):295S–298S). The largest randomized controlled trial evaluating BCAA-enriched therapy including 646 cirrhotic patients showed a significant decrease in complication rates (progression of liver failure, development of liver cancer, rupture of esophageal varices) in patients receiving oral supplementation with BCAA (*Clin Gastroenterol Hepatol.* 2005;3(7):705–713).

F. **Cancer-related cachexia** is a syndrome of lean muscle wasting, peripheral insulin resistance, and increased lipolysis. More than two thirds of patients with cancer experience significant weight loss (*JPEN J Parenter Enteral Nutr.* 2002;26(5 suppl):S63–S71). Antineoplastic therapies, such as chemotherapy, radiation, or operative extirpation, can worsen malnutrition. While adding TPN improves weight, nitrogen balance, and biochemical markers, there is little support for a survival benefit. Megestrol acetate (Megace) improves food intake, fat gain, and patient mood but does not affect outcome.

G. **Short-bowel syndrome** occurs in patients with less than 180 cm of functional small bowel. Dietary management includes consuming frequent small meals, avoiding hyperosmolar foods, restricting fat intake, and limiting consumption of foods high in oxalate (precipitates nephrolithiasis). In addition to glutamine, recombinant human growth hormone (r-HGH) assists these patients in weaning from parenteral nutrition (*J Clin Gastroenterol.* 2006;(40 suppl 2):S99–S106). Definitive therapy involves either isolated intestinal or multivisceral (cases complicated by concomitant TPN-induced liver dysfunction) transplantation.

Life Support and Anesthesia

3

Jason D. Keune and Charl J. De Wet

LIFE SUPPORT

Sudden cardiac arrest continues to be a leading cause of death. The **time** from cardiopulmonary arrest to the initiation of **basic life support (BLS)** and **advanced cardiac life support (ACLS)** is critical to outcome. The following guidelines were developed by the American Heart Association (AHA) to standardize treatment for adults (*Circulation.* 2010; 122, Supplement). These guidelines were revised in 2010, and differ from those previously published.

LIFE SUPPORT AND CARDIOPULMONARY ARREST ALGORITHMS

I. **BLS.** The first three steps in the BLS algorithm are **recognition and activation,** early **cardiopulmonary resuscitation** (CPR) and rapid **defibrillation,** when appropriate:

A. **Determine unresponsiveness** by tapping the victim on the shoulder and shouting at the victim.

B. The **emergency response system** should be activated, whether in the community or in an institution with an emergency response system. A manual defibrillator or an automated external defibrillator (AED) should be obtained, if possible. If **two providers** are present, then one should proceed to CPR, and the other should perform these tasks.

C. Time to initiation of **CPR** is associated with higher likelihood of survival (*Circ Cardiovasc Qual Outcomes.* 2010;3:63–81); therefore, high-quality chest compressions should be initiated as early as possible. Providers should push **hard** and fast (since the resulting stroke volume is limited, maintenance of cardiac output relies on compression rate) and allow **complete recoil** of the chest.

D. **Rapid defibrillation** should be performed. If a manual defibrillator is used, then a shockable rhythm must be identified before proceeding with this step. If an AED is used, the device will identify a shockable rhythm and deliver a shock, if appropriate.

E. **Rescue breaths** should not be performed until after high-quality chest compressions have been initiated.

F. The **pulse check** has been removed from the algorithm for lay rescuers. Health-care providers should take no more than 10 seconds to detect a pulse.

G. The **AHA BLS algorithm for Health-care providers** is given in Figure 3-1.

Figure 3-1. Adult basic life support algorithm, American Heart Association.

II. **ACLS.** Properly performed BLS is critical to the successful performance of ACLS, which is a team effort that depends on effective supervision by a team leader. The leader should ensure that the sequential actions of ACLS are expediently executed by the team.

A. **Sudden Cardiac Arrest**

1. **Airway**

a. The provider should open the airway with a **head tilt-chin** lift maneuver.

b. Airway adjuncts include **cricoid pressure, the oropharyngeal airway,** and **the nasopharyngeal airway.**

c. The risks of the use of an **advanced airway** should be considered along with its benefits. The interruption in chest compressions that may be needed for airway placement should be minimized. Effective use of advanced airways is dependent on provider knowledge and practice. Care should be taken to ensure that airway placement and placement verification does not compromise high-quality CPR.

d. Endotracheal intubation remains the procedure of choice for the unconscious and/or apneic patient. When intubation is not possible, several alternative airway ventilation methods, such as the **Laryngeal Mask Airway** or the **Esophageal-Tracheal Combitube,** may provide more effective ventilation than a bag-mask apparatus.

e. Continuous waveform capnography and **clinical assessment** are recommended as the most reliable way to verify proper placement of an advanced airway.

2. **Breathing**
   a. When a **lone provider** is ventilating the patient, mouth-to-mouth or mouth-to-mask techniques are the most efficient.
   b. Bag-mask ventilation is an acceptable method of providing oxygenation and ventilation during CPR when two providers are present.
   c. If the patient is being ventilated with a **mask,** then one provider should open the airway and provide a tight seal between the mask and face, and the other should squeeze the bag. Two one-second breaths should be given during a brief pause after every 30 chest compressions.
   d. If an advanced airway has been placed, the provider should give one breath every 6 to 8 seconds without a pause in chest compressions.

3. **Circulation**
   a. In low blood flow states, **oxygen delivery** to the heart and brain is more dependent on blood flow than arterial oxygen content; therefore, an emphasis should be placed on **chest compressions** during the initial phase of resuscitation.

4. **Defibrillation**
   a. The only rhythms shown to increase survival to hospital discharge when defibrillated are **ventricular fibrillation** (VF) and **pulseless ventricular tachycardia** (VT).
   b. If a **biphasic defibrillator** is used, the initial shock should be delivered at the manufacturer's recommended dose. The provider may deliver a maximal dose if unsure as to the manufacturer's recommended initial dose. Subsequent energy doses should be equal to or greater than earlier doses.
   c. If a **monophasic defibrillator** is used, a 360-J initial shock should be delivered, with that dose being used for all subsequent shocks.

5. **Pulseless electrical activity (PEA) and asystole**
   a. If a rhythm check reveals an **organized, nonshockable rhythm,** a pulse check should be performed.
   b. If a pulse is detected, post–cardiac arrest care should be initiated.
   c. If a pulse is absent, or the rhythm is asystole, CPR should be resumed.

    d. PEA is almost uniformly fatal unless an underlying cause can be identified and treated. Potentially reversible causes follow the acronym 6 H 5 T:

    e. Hypovolemia, especially resulting from hemorrhage, is the most common cause of PEA.

    f. Hypoxia.

    g. Hypothermia.

    h. Hydrogen ions (severe acidosis).

    i. Hyperkalemia or hypokalemia.

    j. Hypoglycemia.

    k. Tablets/toxins.

    l. Tension pneumothorax, evidenced by tracheal deviation and decreased ipsilateral breath sounds, should be treated by insertion of a large-bore angiocatheter (14-gauge) into the pleural space through the second intercostal space in the midclavicular line, followed by a thoracostomy tube.

    m. Tamponade (pericardial) is treated by pericardiocentesis.

    n. Thrombosis of coronary vessels (acute coronary syndromes).

    o. Thrombosis of pulmonary vessels (pulmonary embolism).

6. Vasopressor use

    a. Epinephrine (Adrenalin) has been shown, in retrospective analysis, to improve return of spontaneous circulation, when compared to no epinephrine for sustained VT and PEA/asystole. No difference in survival between treatment groups was seen (*Resuscitation.* 1995;29:195–201).

    b. Epinephrine should be given intravenous/intraosseous (IV/IO) at a dose of 1 mg every 3 to 5 minutes during cardiac arrest.

    c. If IV/IO access cannot be established, epinephrine can be given endotracheally at a dose of 2 to 2.5 mg.

    d. Amiodarone (Pacerone, Cordarone) can be given for VF or pulseless VT unresponsive to CPR, defibrillation and vasopressor. The initial dose is 300 mg IV/IO. A second dose of 150 mg IV/IO can be given.

    e. One dose of **vasopressin (Pitressin)** 40 units IV/IO may replace either the first or second dose of epinephrine.

7. The **AHA ACLS algorithm for adult cardiac arrest** is given in Figure 3-2.

B. Acute Symptomatic Arrhythmias. It is important to emphasize that electrocardiography (ECG) should be interpreted in the context of clinical assessment of the patient when evaluating acute symptomatic arrhythmias.

1. Bradycardia

    a. Bradycardia is defined as heart rate less than 60 beats per minute.

    b. The **symptoms** of unstable bradycardia include acutely altered mental status, angina, acute heart failure, hypotension, or shock that persists despite an adequate airway and breathing.

    c. If unstable bradycardia is present, the primary treatment is **atropine** (at an initial dose of 0.5 mg IV. The dose can be repeated every 3 to 5 minutes to a maximum of 3 mg.

Figure 3-2. Adult advanced cardiac life support algorithm for adult cardiac arrest, American Heart Association.

    d. If atropine is not effective, then either dopamine or epinephrine infusion or transcutaneous pacing (TP) should be initiated.

        (1) Dopamine (Intropin) should be given at a dose of 2 to 10 mcg/kg/minute.

        (2) Epinephrine should be given at a dose of 0.02 to 0.3 mcg/kg/minute.

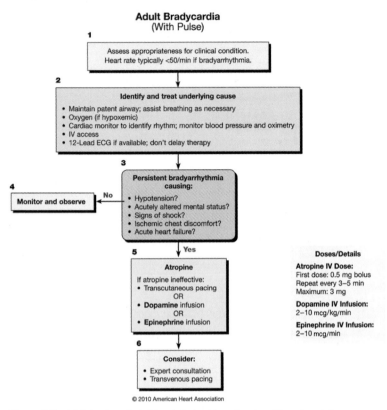

Figure 3-3. Adult bradycardia (with pulse) algorithm, American Heart Association.

      (3) TP is a temporizing measure that is painful in conscious patients. After initiation of TP, preparations for transvenous pacing should be made, and expert consultation should be sought.

   e. The **AHA ACLS bradycardia (with pulse) algorithm** is given in Figure 3-3.

 2. Tachycardia

   a. Tachycardia is defined as a heart rate greater than 100 beats per minute.

   b. The **symptoms** of unstable tachycardia include acutely altered mental status, angina, acute heart failure, hypotension or shock that persists despite an adequate airway and breathing.

   c. If unstable tachycardia is present, **synchronized cardioversion** should be performed, when indicated (see below).

      (1) If possible, IV access should be obtained and the patient should be sedated prior to proceeding. Cardioversion should not be delayed in the extremely unstable patient.

(2) Synchronized cardioversion is indicated for **unstable supraventricular tachycardia (SVT), unstable atrial fibrillation, unstable atrial flutter,** and **unstable monomorphic VT.**

(3) For cardioversion of **atrial fibrillation,** an initial biphasic energy dose of 120 to 200 J is recommended. The dose should be increased in a stepwise fashion if the initial shock fails.

(4) For cardioversion of **atrial flutter** or **SVT,** an initial biphasic energy dose of 50 to 100 J is recommended. The dose should be increased in a stepwise fashion if the initial shock fails.

(5) For cardioversion of **monomorphic VT,** an initial energy dose of 100 J is recommended. The dose can be increased in a stepwise fashion if the initial shock fails, but there is no evidence addressing this issue, and this recommendation is based on expert opinion alone.

(6) For **wide, irregular tachycardias,** unsynchronized defibrillation doses should be delivered.

d. **Sinus tachycardia** is usually caused by an underlying physiologic condition. Therapy should be directed at treatment of this underlying cause.

e. If the patient is **not hypotensive** and has a **narrow-complex SVT,** the following therapy should be attempted:

(1) A **vagal maneuver** (valsalva maneuver or carotid sinus massage) alone will terminate up to 25% of paroxysmal SVTs and should be performed first (not indicated if patient has significant carotid disease).

(2) If the vagal maneuver is unsuccessful, **adenosine** should be administered at a dose of **6 mg IV,** given by **rapid** IV push through a large vein, followed by a 20-mL flush.

(3) If the rhythm does not convert within 1 to 2 minutes, a dose of **12 mg IV** should be given using the same method.

(4) **Expert consultation** should be obtained.

f. If the patient is **stable,** an ECG should be obtained and the QRS complex evaluated to determine whether it is ≥0.12 seconds.

(1) If the QRS complex is ≥0.12 seconds (a **wide-complex tachycardia**), a determination should be made as to whether it is **regular** or **irregular**.

(2) If **regular,** the **wide-complex tachycardia** can be treated with **adenosine,** as above.

(3) If **irregular,** or **polymorphic,** adenosine should never be given, as it can precipitate degeneration to VF.

g. If the **regular, wide-complex tachycardia** is not terminated with adenosine, then antiarrhythmic infusion should be considered. A continuous ECG should be obtained as these drugs are given, to facilitate diagnosis.

(1) **Procainamide (Pronestyl, Procan, Procanbid)** can be administered at 20 to 50 mg/minute until either the rhythm is suppressed, hypotension ensues, QRS duration increases 50%, or the maximum dose is given (17 mg/kg). A maintenance dose is 1 to 4 mg/minute. Procainamide **should not be given** to patients   prolonged QT or congestive heart failure.

  (2) **Amiodarone** can be given at a dose of 150 mg IV over 10 minutes, with repeated dosing as needed to a maximum dose of 2.2 g IV per 24 hours. A maintenance infusion is 1 mg/minute over the first 6 hours.

  (3) **Sotalol (Betapace)** can be given at a dose of 1.5 mg/kg over 5 minutes. Sotalol **should not be given** to patients with a prolonged QT interval.

  (4) If one drug is not successful at termination of the rhythm, another drug should not be started without **expert consultation.**

 h. If the wide-complex tachycardia is **irregular,** it is likely **atrial fibrillation** with aberrancy, **atrial fibrillation** using an accessory pathway, or **polymorphic VT/torsades de pointes.**

3. Atrial fibrillation

 a. Management of **atrial fibrillation** should center around control of the ventricular rate or conversion of the arrhythmia to sinus rhythm. **Cardioversion** should be attempted if unstable.

 b. Since patients with atrial fibrillation are at higher risk for **cardioembolic events** if the arrhythmia should persist for longer than **48 hours,** cardioversion or pharmacologic conversion should not be attempted in these patients, unless the patient is grossly unstable. It should be kept in mind that patients with atrial fibrillation of a shorter duration are not precluded from having such events. An alternative strategy in stable patients with atrial fibrillation persisting longer than 48 hours is to anticoagulate with heparin and perform transesophageal echocardiography to ensure absence of a left atrial thrombus prior to cardioversion.

 c. **Rate control** can be established in several ways.

  (1) **IV β-blockers** or **nondihydropyridine calcium channel blockers (e.g., diltiazem)** can be given for atrial fibrillation with rapid ventricular response.

  (2) **Amiodarone** or **digoxin (Digitek, Lanoxin, Lanoxicaps)** can be used for rate control in patients with congestive heart failure; however, providers should be mindful of the potential for rhythm conversion with the use of amiodarone.

 d. The AHA guidelines recommend expert consultation for **rhythm control** of atrial fibrillation.

4. Polymorphic (irregular) VT/torsades de pointes

 a. **Unstable polymorphic VT** should be treated with immediate defibrillation.

 b. If a long QT interval is observed during sinus rhythm, then the **irregular, wide-complex tachycardia** is likely **torsades de pointes.**

  (1) **Medications** known to prolong the QT interval should be stopped.

  (2) **Electrolyte imbalances** should be corrected.

  (3) **IV magnesium** can be given for torsades de pointes.

  (4) **Isoproterenol (Isuprel)** or **ventricular pacing** can be effective in terminating the arrhythmia associated with drug-induced QT prolongation.

Figure 3-4. Adult tachycardia (with pulse) algorithm, American Heart Association.

(5) If the arrhythmia is due to **familial long-QT syndrome, IV magnesium, pacing, and/or β-blockers** can be used. Isoproterenol should be avoided in this situation.

c. If a long QT interval is not observed, then the **irregular, wide-complex tachycardia** may be VT due to myocardial ischemia.

(1) **IV amiodarone** and **β-blockers** can be given to reduce the frequency of recurrence of this arrhythmia; however, efforts should be made to address revascularization.

d. If **cardiac arrest** develops any time during the bradycardia or tachycardia algorithms, providers should implement the ACLS Cardiac Arrest Algorithm.

e. **The AHA ACLS adult tachycardia (with pulse) algorithm** is given in Figure 3-4.

C. Post–Cardiac Arrest Care

The initial goals of post–cardiac arrest care are as follows:

1. To **optimize** cardiopulmonary function and vital organ perfusion.

2. To **determine** the underlying cause of the arrest so as to prevent its recurrence.

3. To **transfer** the patient to a setting in which acute coronary interventions, neurologic care, goal-directed critical care, and hypothermia are available.

Figure 3-5. Adult post–cardiac arrest care algorithm, American Heart Association.

Subsequent goals include the following:

1. Control of **body temperature** to optimize neurologic recovery and overall survival
2. Treatment of **acute coronary syndromes**
3. Optimization of **mechanical ventilation**
4. Assessment of **prognosis**
5. **Provision** of rehabilitation services.

The **adult immediate post–cardiac arrest care algorithm** is given in Figure 3-5.

ANESTHESIA

Preparing the Patient

I. **PATIENT PREPARATION FOR OPERATION**

A. **Preoperative evaluation**

1. A **comprehensive preoperative evaluation** is critical to the safe administration of anesthetic care.

a. A **complete history,** including medication usage and prior anesthetic usage, should be obtained.

   b. An **examination of airway,** vascular access, and other pertinent anatomy tailored to the anticipated operation should be undertaken.
2. In **patients without preexisting disease,** preoperative screening and testing are determined primarily by age.
   a. **Hemoglobin or hematocrit** may be the only test required in some healthy patients younger than 40 years.
   b. A **serum pregnancy test** should be obtained for female patients of childbearing age.
   c. A **screening chest X-ray and ECG** are obtained for patients who are 50 years or older, unless an indication is found from the history or physical examination, or both.
3. **Additional testing** may be required when clinically indicated.
   a. **Serum electrolytes** must be evaluated in patients with diabetes or renal insufficiency and in patients who are taking diuretics.
   b. **Coagulation studies** (prothrombin time, partial thromboplastin time, bleeding time) must be evaluated in patients who are receiving anticoagulation therapy or have a personal or family history that is suggestive of abnormal bleeding.
   c. **Additional testing or consultation** may be required in patients with evidence of severe coexisting disease, especially those with cardiac, pulmonary, or renal compromise.
4. Unstable or uncontrolled medical conditions, upper respiratory infections, and solid food ingestion within 6 hours of surgery are **indications to cancel or postpone elective surgery.**
5. **American Society of Anesthesiologists (ASA) criteria** (see Table 3-1)

TABLE 3-1	American Society of Anesthesiologists (ASA) Criteria
ASA Grade	**Description**
I	There is no organic, physiologic, biochemical, or psychiatric disturbance; the pathologic process for which the operation is to be performed is localized and is not a systemic disturbance.
II	Mild-to-moderate systemic disturbance caused by either the condition to be treated or other pathophysiologic processes
III	Severe systemic disturbance or disease for whatever cause, even though it may not be possible to define the degree of disability
IV	Indicative of the patient with severe systemic disorder that is already life-threatening and not always correctable by the operative procedure
V	The moribund patient who has little chance of survival but is submitted to operation in desperation

An E is added after a grade to indicate emergency surgery (e.g., IVE).

B. **Nothing by mouth (NPO) status**

1. For all patients, it is customary to abstain from any oral intake except for medications with sips of water for 8 hours before elective surgery. However, for adult patients who are not considered to be at increased risk for aspiration of gastric contents, the following **aspiration prophylaxis regimens** can be used.

   a. **Solid food** is permitted until 6 hours before surgery.

   b. **Clear liquids** (which do not include milk or juices containing pulp) are permitted until 2 hours before surgery (*Anesthesiology.* 1999;90:896).

2. **Patients with slowed or incomplete gastric emptying** (e.g., those who are morbidly obese, diabetic, or on narcotic therapy) **may require longer fasting periods and additional pretreatment with metoclopramide, histamine H_2-receptor antagonists, and/or oral sodium citrate.** Rapid-sequence induction should be considered in these patients. Maintenance IV fluids should be considered in NPO inpatients.

C. **Medications**

1. Patients can receive **benzodiazepines or narcotics** to alleviate preoperative anxiety and pain.

2. **Cardiovascular or other pertinent medications** usually are administered on the morning of surgery with small sips of water. Inpatients who normally receive scheduled insulin doses should instead be placed on sliding-scale insulin, with blood sugars checked frequently every 2 to 6 hours while NPO, depending on difficulty of their diabetic control. Outpatients should be instructed to take one-half to one-third of their regular insulin dose the morning of surgery and to check blood sugars frequently. **It is essential to avoid hypoglycemia.**

3. In general, antiplatelet medications such as **aspirin** or **clopidogrel** should be held 5 days prior to surgery unless otherwise specified.

D. **Obstructive sleep apnea (OSA)**

1. **Over the last few years,** OSA has been recognized as a significant source of perioperative morbidity and mortality in the United States. The American Society of Anesthesiology guidelines for the perioperative management of OSA are shown in Tables 3-2 and 3-3 (*Anesthesiology.* 2006;104:1081).

TYPES OF ANESTHESIA

I. **LOCAL ANESTHETICS** are categorized into two groups. **Esters (one i)** include tetracaine, procaine, cocaine, and chloroprocaine. **Amides (two i's)** include lidocaine, bupivacaine, ropivacaine, and mepivacaine. Characteristics of commonly used local anesthetic agents are summarized in Table 3-4.

A. **Mechanism of action**

1. **Local anesthetics** work by diffusing through the nerve plasma membrane and causing blockade of sodium channels. The nerve cell is unable to depolarize, and axonal conduction is inhibited.

TABLE 3-2 Identification and Assessment of Obstructive Sleep Apnea[a]

A. Clinical signs and symptoms suggesting the possibility of OSA
1. Predisposing physical characteristics
   a. BMI 55 kg/m^2 (95th percentile for age and gender)
   b. Neck circumference 17 in. (men) or 16 in. (women)
   c. Craniofacial abnormalities affecting the airway
   d. Anatomic nasal obstruction
   e. Tonsils nearly touching or touching in the midline
2. History of apparent airway obstruction during sleep (two or more of the following are present; if patient lives alone or sleep is not observed by another person, then only one of the following needs to be present)
   a. Snoring (loud enough to be heard through closed door)
   b. Frequent snoring
   c. Observed pauses in breathing during sleep
   d. Awakens from sleep with choking sensation
   e. Frequent arousals from sleep
   f. Intermittent vocalization during sleep
   g. Parental report of restless sleep, difficulty breathing, or struggling respiratory efforts during sleep
3. Somnolence (one or more of the following is present)
   a. Frequent somnolence or fatigue despite adequate "sleep"
   b. Falls asleep easily in a nonstimulating environment (e.g., watching TV, reading, riding in or driving a car, despite adequate "sleep")
   c. Parent or teacher comments that child appears sleepy during the day, is easily distracted, is overly aggressive, or has difficulty concentrating
   d. Child often difficult to arouse at usual awakening time

   If a patient has signs or symptoms in two or more of the foregoing categories, there is a significant probability that he or she has OSA. The severity of OSA may be determined by sleep study (see following tabulation). If a sleep study is not available, such patients should be treated as though they have moderate sleep apnea unless one or more of the foregoing signs or symptoms is severely abnormal (e.g., markedly increased BMI or neck circumference, respiratory pauses that are frightening to the observer, patient regularly falls asleep within minutes after being left unstimulated). In these cases, patients should be treated as though they have severe sleep apnea.
B. If a sleep study has been done, the results should be used to determine the perioperative anesthetic management of a patient. However, because sleep laboratories differ in their criteria for detecting episodes of apnea and hypopnea, the Task Force believes that the sleep laboratory's assessment (none, mild, moderate, or severe) should take precedence over the actual AHI (the number of episodes of sleep-disordered breathing per hour). If the overall severity is not indicated, it may be determined by using the following table.

(continued)

TABLE 3-2	Identification and Assessment of Obstructive Sleep Apnea[a] *(continued)*	
Severity of OSA	Adult AHI	Pediatric AHI
None	0–5	0
Mild OSA	6–20	1–5
Moderate OSA	21–40	6–10
Severe OSA	>40	>10

[a]Items in brackets refer to pediatric patients.

AHI, apnea-hypopnea index; BMI, body mass index; OSA, obstructive sleep apnea; TV, television.

With permission from Gross JB, Bachenberg KL, Benumof JL, et al. Practice guidelines for the perioperative management of patients with obstructive sleep apnea. *Anesthesiology.* 2006;104:1081–1093.

    2. **Local tissue acidosis** (e.g., from infection) slows the onset and decreases the intensity of analgesia by causing local anesthetic molecules to become positively charged and less able to diffuse into the neuron.

  B. **Toxicity (dose dependent, except for allergic reactions)**

    1. **Central nervous system (CNS) toxicity**

      a. **Signs and symptoms** include mental status changes, dizziness, perioral numbness, a metallic taste, tinnitus, visual disturbances, and seizures. Seizures resulting from inadvertent intravascular injection usually last only minutes. Continuous infusion of local anesthetics may result in high plasma levels and prolonged seizures.

      b. **Treatment** involves airway support and ventilation with 100% oxygen, which should always be available. Prolonged seizures may require administration of benzodiazepines [midazolam (Versed), 1 to 5 mg intravenously; diazepam (Valium), 5 to 15 mg intravenously; or lorazepam (Ativan), 1 to 4 mg intravenously]. Intubation may be required to ensure adequate ventilation.

    2. **Cardiovascular toxicity**

      a. **Signs and symptoms** range from decreased cardiac output to hypotension and cardiovascular collapse. Most local anesthetics cause CNS toxicity before cardiovascular toxicity. Bupivacaine (Marcaine) is an exception, and its intravascular injection can result in severe cardiac compromise.

      b. **Treatment** includes fluid resuscitation, administration of vasopressors, and CPR, if necessary.

    3. **Hypersensitivity reactions,** although rare, have been described with **ester**-based local anesthetics and are attributed to the metabolite *p*-aminobenzoic acid. True amide-based local anesthetic anaphylactic reactions are questionable.

TABLE 3-3	Obstructive Sleep Apnea Scoring System	
		Points
A. Severity of sleep apnea based on sleep study (or clinical indicators if sleep study not available). Point score – $(0–3)^{a,b}$ Severity of OSA (Table 3-3)		
	None	0
	Mild	1
	Moderate	2
	Severe	3
B. Invasiveness of surgery and anesthesia. Point score – $(0–3)$ Type of surgery and anesthesia		
	Superficial surgery under local or peripheral nerve block anesthesia without sedation	0
	Superficial surgery with moderate sedation or general anesthesia	1
	Peripheral surgery with spinal or epidural anesthesia (with no more than moderate sedation)	1
	Peripheral surgery with general anesthesia	2
	Airway surgery with moderate sedation	2
	Major surgery, general anesthesia	3
	Airway surgery, general anesthesia	3
C. Requirement for postoperative opioids. Point score – $(0–3)$ Opioid requirement		
	None	0
	Low-dose oral opioids	1
	High-dose oral opioids, parenteral, or neuraxial opioids	3
D. Estimation of perioperative risk. Overall score = score for A plus the greater of the score for either B or C. Point score – $(0–6)^c$		

Note: A scoring system similar to this table can be used to estimate whether a patient is at increased perioperative risk of complications from obstructive sleep apnea (OSA). This example, which has not been clinically validated, is meant only as a guide, and clinical judgment should be used to assess the risk of an individual patient.

[a]One point may be subtracted if a patient has been on continuous positive airway pressure (CPAP) or noninvasive positive-pressure ventilation (NIPPV) before surgery and will be using his or her appliance consistently during the postoperative period.

[b]One point should be added if a patient with mild or moderate OSA also has a resting arterial carbon dioxide tension (Pa_{CO_2}) >60 mm Hg.

[c]Patients with score of 4 may be at increased perioperative risk from OSA; patients with a score of 5 or 6 may be at significantly increased perioperative risk from OSA.

With permission from *Anesthesiology.* 2006;104:1081–1093.

    a. Signs and symptoms can range from urticaria to bronchospasm, hypotension, and anaphylactic shock.

    b. Treatment is similar to that for hypersensitivity reactions from other etiologies. Urticaria responds to diphenhydramine, 25 to 50 mg intravenously. Bronchospasm is treated with inhaled bronchodilators

TABLE 3-4	Local Anesthetics for Infiltration			
	Maximum Dose (mg/kg)		**Length of Action (hr)**	
Agent	**Plain**	**With Epinephrine**[a]	**Plain**	**With Epinephrine**[a]
Procaine	—	8	0.25–1	0.5–1.5
Lidocaine	5	7	0.5–1	2–6
Mepivacaine	5	7	0.75–1.5	2–6
Bupivacaine	2.5	3	2–4	3–7
Tetracaine	1.5		24	

[a]1:200,000.

(e.g., albuterol) and oxygen. Hypotension is treated with fluid resuscitation and vasopressors [e.g., phenylephrine hydrochloride (Neo-Synephrine)] or small incremental doses of epinephrine as required. Anaphylactic cardiovascular collapse should be treated with epinephrine, 0.5 to 1 mg, administered as an IV bolus.

C. **Epinephrine** (1:200,000, 5 µg/mL) is mixed with local anesthetic solutions to prolong the duration of neural blockade and reduce systemic drug absorption. Its use is **contraindicated** in areas where arterial spasm would lead to tissue necrosis (e.g., nose, ears, fingers, toes, and penis).

II. REGIONAL ANESTHESIA

A. **In the operating room**

1. **General considerations**

a. The **importance of preoperative communication between anesthesiologist and surgeon** cannot be overemphasized. The extent and duration of the procedure must be appreciated by the anesthesiologist so that the appropriate area and duration of anesthesia can be achieved. If the possibility of a prolonged or involved operative procedure is likely, a combined anesthetic technique (local/regional and general anesthesia), or general anesthetic only, may be more appropriate. Certain surgical positions are poorly tolerated by awake patients (e.g., steep Trendelenburg may cause respiratory compromise); in these instances, a general anesthetic is appropriate.

b. **Supplements to regional anesthesia.** No regional anesthetic technique is foolproof, and local infiltration by the surgeon may be required if there is an incomplete block. IV sedation using short-acting benzodiazepines, narcotics, barbiturates, or propofol can also be helpful. General anesthesia may be required when a regional technique provides inadequate analgesia.

c. **NPO status.** Because any regional anesthetic may progress to a general anesthetic, NPO requirements for regional and general anesthetics are identical.

d. **Monitoring requirements** are no different from those for general anesthesia. Heart rhythm, blood pressure (BP), and arterial oxygen saturation should be monitored regularly during regional or general anesthesia. Other monitoring may be indicated, depending on coexisting disease states.

2. **Types of regional anesthesia**

   a. **Spinal anesthesia** involves the injection of small volumes (low doses) of local anesthetic solution into the subarachnoid space at the level of the lumbar spine.

   (1) **Anatomy and placement** (Fig. 3-6)

   (a) With the use of sterile technique and after local anesthetic infiltration of the skin and subcutaneous tissues, a small (22- to 27-gauge) **spinal needle is passed between two adjacent lumbar spinous processes.** The needle is passed through the following structures: supraspinous ligament, interspinous ligament, ligamentum flavum, dura mater, and arachnoid mater. Cerebrospinal fluid (CSF) is aspirated, and the appropriate local anesthetic solution is injected.

   (2) **Level of analgesia**

   (a) **Multiple variables** affect the spread of analgesia. The **baricity** of the agent (solution density compared to that of CSF) and the position of the patient immediately after

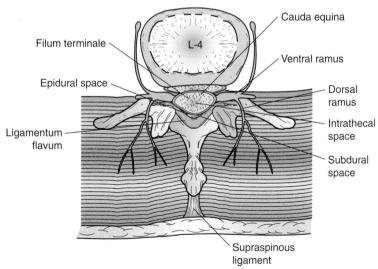

Figure 3-6. Anatomy for spinal and epidural anesthesia.

injection are major determinants of level. The **total dose injected** (increased dose results in higher spread) and the **total volume injected** (increased volume results in higher spread) are also important determinants of anesthetic level.

(b) **Older patients** tend to have greater spread of anesthesia by a few dermatomes, but clinical significance is variable.

(3) **Onset and duration of analgesia**

(a) The **specific characteristics of the local anesthetic** used and the **total dose injected** are the primary determinants of onset and duration of action. Epinephrine added to the solution increases the duration of analgesia.

(b) **The variability in length of analgesia** is significant, ranging from as little as 30 minutes [lidocaine (Xylocaine)] to up to 6 hours [tetracaine with epinephrine (Pontocaine, Dicaine)].

(4) **Complications**

(a) **Hypotension** may occur as a result of sympatholytic-induced vasodilation (decreased venous return to the heart followed by bradycardia). It may be more severe in hypovolemic patients or in those with preexisting cardiac dysfunction. Treatment includes volume resuscitation with crystalloid, vasopressors (epinephrine, 5 to 10 μg intravenously or phenylephrine hydrochloride, 50 to 100 μg intravenously), and positive inotropic and chronotropic drugs. It is advisable to administer 500 to 1,000 mL of crystalloid prior to spinal block to avoid hypotension due to spinal anesthesia. In refractory cases elevating the legs or placing the patient in Trendelenburg position may prevent cardiac arrest from decreased venous return to the heart. Under no circumstances should a hypotensive patient be placed in reverse Trendelenburg as this may lead to cardiac arrest.

(b) **High spinal blockade.** Inadvertently high levels of spinal blockade may result in hypotension (blocking dermatomes T1–4: preganglionic cardioaccelerator nerves), dyspnea (loss of chest proprioception or intercostal muscle function), or apnea (decreased medullary perfusion secondary to hypotension). Treatment consists of ventilatory support and/or intubation, fluid bolus, and chrono- and inotropic support of the heart. Once a high spinal block has occurred reversed, Trendelenburg position will be of no immediate benefit and is probably contraindicated since decreased venous return may lead to cardiac arrest.

(c) **Headache** after spinal anesthesia or diagnostic lumbar puncture is encountered with higher frequency in young or female patients. This is usually the result of leakage of CSF from the puncture site. A postural component is always present (i.e., symptoms worsened by sitting up or standing). The recent use of smaller-gauge spinal needles has reduced the frequency of this complication. Treatment includes oral or IV fluids, oral analgesics, and caffeinated beverages. Severe refractory headache may require placement of an epidural blood patch to prevent ongoing leakage of CSF.

(d) **CNS infection** after spinal anesthesia, although extremely rare, may result in meningitis, epidural abscess, or arachnoiditis.

(e) **Permanent nerve injury** is exceedingly rare and is seen with the same frequency as in general anesthesia.

(f) **Urinary retention with bladder distention** occurs in patients with spinal anesthesia whose bladders are not drained by urethral catheters, which should remain in place until after the spinal anesthesia has been stopped and full sensation has returned.

(5) **Contraindications**

(a) **Absolute contraindications** to spinal anesthesia are localized infection at the planned puncture site, increased intracranial pressure, generalized sepsis, coagulopathy, and lack of consent.

(b) **Relative contraindications** include hypovolemia, preexisting CNS disease, chronic low back pain, platelet dysfunction, and preload-dependent valvular lesions such as aortic and mitral stenosis.

b. **Epidural anesthesia**

(1) **Anatomy and placement (Fig. 3-6)**

(a) Inserting an epidural needle is similar to placing a spinal needle except that the **epidural needle is not advanced through the dura.** No CSF is obtained. The tip of the epidural needle lies in the epidural space between the ligamentum flavum posteriorly and the dura mater anteriorly. Local anesthetic solution can then be injected.

(b) Either the **needle is removed** (single-shot method) or, more commonly, **a flexible catheter is passed through the needle** into the space and the needle is withdrawn over the catheter (continuous catheter technique). Local anesthetics or opioids can be infused as needed.

(2) **Level of analgesia**

(a) Once injected into the epidural space, the local anesthetic solution diffuses through the dura and into the spinal nerve roots, usually resulting in a **bilateral dermatomal distribution of analgesia.**

(b) The spread of nerve root blockade is primarily determined by the **volume** of injection and, to a lesser degree, by patient **position and age** and **area of placement.**

(3) **Onset and duration of analgesia**

(a) **Epidural anesthesia develops more slowly than does spinal anesthesia** because the local anesthetic solution must diffuse farther. The rate of onset of sympathetic blockade and hypotension also is slowed, enabling more precise titration of hemodynamic therapy compared with spinal anesthesia.

(b) The **dosing interval** depends on the agent used.

(4) **Complications** are similar to those encountered with spinal anesthesia.

(a) **Spinal headache** may result from inadvertent perforation of the dura.

(b) **Epidural hematoma** is rare and usually occurs with coexisting coagulopathy. Emergent laminectomy may be required to decompress the spinal cord and avoid permanent neurologic injury.

(c) If a patient with an epidural catheter in place becomes **hypotensive,** stopping the infusion of anesthetic will often correct the BP. Alternatively a vasoconstrictor or chronotropic drug may be used to ameliorate the sympathetic blockade.

c. **Combined spinal and epidural anesthesia**
   (1) **Anatomy and placement**
      (a) A **small-gauge spinal needle** is placed through an epidural needle once the epidural space has been located. The dura is punctured only by the spinal needle, and placement is verified by CSF withdrawal. Subarachnoid local anesthetics or preservative-free opioids can then be administered via the spinal needle.
      (b) The **spinal needle** is withdrawn after the initial dosing, and an epidural catheter is threaded into the epidural space through the existing epidural needle.
   (2) **Onset and duration.** This procedure combines the quick onset of spinal analgesia with the continuous dosing advantages of epidural analgesia.
   (3) **Complications** are similar to those seen in spinal and epidural anesthesia.

d. **Comparison of spinal or epidural anesthesia with general anesthesia.** Although the incidence of thromboembolic complications and total blood loss is reduced in certain surgical procedures with spinal or epidural anesthesia, there is no evidence that long-term mortality is reduced compared with general anesthesia (*Br J Anaesth.* 1986;58:284; *Cochrane Database Syst Rev.* 2000;(4):CD000521).

e. **Brachial plexus blockade.** Injection of local anesthetic solution into the sheath surrounding the brachial plexus results in varying degrees of upper extremity blockade. This technique is indicated for any procedure involving the patient's shoulders, arms, or hands. Electrical nerve stimulation with/without ultrasound-guidance is now frequently used to aid in placement of these blocks. The approach taken depends on the distribution of blockade desired.

   (1) **Axillary block.** The needle is placed into the brachial plexus sheath from the axilla. Blockade above the patient's elbow is unreliable.

(2) Supraclavicular blockade. The needle is directed caudally from behind the posterior border of the inner one-third of the clavicle. This technique reliably blocks the entire upper extremity, sparing the patient's shoulder. There is a risk of pneumothorax.

(3) Interscalene blockade involves the cervical as well as brachial plexus and reliably blocks the patient's shoulder. There is a high incidence of phrenic nerve block, which increases the risk of pulmonary complications in patients with chronic obstructive pulmonary disease. This also serves as a contraindication to bilateral blockade.

f. Cervical plexus blockade blocks the anterior divisions of C1 to C4 and is the anesthetic method of choice for carotid endarterectomy at many institutions. Inadvertent blockade of neighboring structures does occur.

(1) Phrenic nerve blockade may result in transient diaphragmatic paralysis. Simultaneous bilateral cervical plexus blockade is therefore contraindicated.

(2) Ipsilateral cervical sympathetic plexus blockade may result in Horner syndrome, producing transient ptosis, miosis, and facial anhidrosis.

B. Outside the operating room

1. Intercostal nerve block is indicated after thoracotomy or before chest tube placement.

a. Anatomy and placement (Fig. 3-7)

(1) The **posterior axillary line is identified,** and with the use of sterile technique, a 23-gauge needle is placed perpendicular to the patient's skin until contact is made with his or her rib. The needle is then walked caudad off the patient's rib and advanced several millimeters. After negative aspiration, 5 mL of bupivacaine 0.25% to 0.50% with epinephrine (1:200,000) is injected.

(2) Usually, **five interspaces** (including two above and two below the interspace of interest) are injected.

b. Complications include pneumothorax and intravascular injection causing myocardial suppression and serious life-threatening arrhythmias. Bradycardia, asystole or heart block may result from inadvertent intravascular injection or rapid absorption of bupivacaine. Treatment should focus on hemodynamic support and with 20% intralipid. Injection into the nerve sheath with retrograde spread back to the spinal cord can produce a high spinal or epidural block.

2. Digital block is indicated for minor procedures of the fingers.

a. Anatomy and placement

(1) From the **dorsal surface of the hand,** a 23-gauge needle is placed on either side of the metatarsal head and inserted until the increased resistance of the palmar connective tissue is felt. An injection of 1 to 2 mL of lidocaine 1% to 2% is made as the needle is withdrawn.

Figure 3-7. Anatomy and placement for intercostal nerve block. **(A)** The provider's hand closest to the patient's head (cephalic) first locates the target interspace and then **(B)** retracts the skin over the rib above. **(C)** The hand closest to the patient's feet (caudad) places the needle and attached syringe containing local anesthetic through the skin onto the rib at approximately a 30-degree angle, with the needle bevel directed cephalad. **(D)** The cephalic hand then grasps the needle while maintaining contact with the patient and allows the tension of the retracted skin to walk the needle off the inferior edge of the rib and advance 2 to 3 mm.

(2) **Supplemental injection** of 0.5 to 1 mL of lidocaine 1% to 2% in the interdigital web on either side may be required.
b. Epinephrine is contraindicated.

C. **Local infiltration**

1. **In the operating room,** the area of incision can be infiltrated before incision or at the conclusion of the operation. Evidence suggests that there is no difference in postoperative discomfort or analgesic use between pre- and postoperative infiltration with local anesthetic (*Arch Surg.* 1997;132(7):766–799). Bupivacaine is frequently used.
2. **Outside the operating room,** local anesthetic infiltration may also be useful during wound débridement, central venous catheter placement, or repair of minor lacerations. The agent of choice is lidocaine 1% to

2% due to its quick onset and low toxicity. The area of interest should be injected liberally. Frequent aspiration helps to avoid intravascular injection. Injection should be repeated as necessary.

3. Local anesthetics containing **epinephrine** are **contraindicated** in areas where arterial spasm would lead to tissue necrosis (e.g., nose, ears, fingers, toes, and penis).

III. **GENERAL ANESTHESIA.** A balanced general anesthetic can provide hypnosis (unconsciousness), analgesia, amnesia, and skeletal muscle relaxation.

A. All patients who are undergoing general anesthesia require an appropriate **preoperative evaluation** and optimization of any coexisting medical problems (see "Preparing the Patient," Sections I.A.1 and I.A.2).

B. **Monitoring.** Basic monitoring requirements for general anesthesia are similar to those for regional anesthesia.

C. **Induction of general anesthesia.** IV agents are most widely used owing to rapid onset and ease of administration.

1. Thiopental (Pentothal), a barbiturate (3 to 5 mg/kg intravenously), has a rapid onset and redistribution. However, there is often an associated decrease in cardiac output, BP, and cerebral blood flow. It should be used with caution in patients with hypotension or active coronary ischemia.

2. Propofol (Diprivan), a phenol derivative (1 to 3 mg/kg intravenously), is used for both induction and maintenance of anesthesia. Onset of action is immediate. It has hemodynamic properties that are similar to those of thiopental but is associated with a low incidence of postoperative nausea and vomiting. The pharmacokinetics is not changed by chronic hepatic or renal failure. A water-soluble *prodrug* form, *fospropofol*, has recently been approved by the FDA. Fospropofol is rapidly broken down by the enzyme *alkaline phosphatase* to form propofol. This new formulation may not produce the pain at injection site that often occurs with the traditional form of the drug.

3. Etomidate (Amidate), an imidazole derivative (0.3 mg/kg intravenously), has an onset of 30 to 60 seconds and has only mild direct hemodynamic depressant effects. Adrenal insufficiency may result from a single administration.

4. Ketamine (Ketalar), a phencyclidine derivative (1 to 4 mg/kg intravenously), increases cardiac output and BP in patients who are not catecholamine depleted and provides dissociative anesthesia. It is also an excellent analgesic but raises intracranial pressure and is not used in patients with head trauma. The use of ketamine is limited owing to **emergence delirium** and nightmares and is often reserved for use in the pediatric population and has the advantage that it can be given **intramuscularly.**

D. **Airway management.** Ventilation during general anesthesia may be spontaneous, assisted, or controlled.

1. Mask ventilation with spontaneous respiratory effort can be used during limited (usually peripheral) procedures that do not require neuromuscular relaxation. Because the airway is unprotected, this technique is contraindicated in patients at risk for aspiration.

2. **Endotracheal intubation** secures the airway, allows control of ventilation, and protects against aspiration. Although frequently performed orally with the laryngoscope, intubation can also be accomplished nasally and, in anatomically challenging patients, can be performed with the aid of a fiberoptic bronchoscope via oral or nasal routes. Newer video laryngoscopes may be helpful aids in difficult intubations.

3. The **Laryngeal Mask Airway (LMA)** is an alternative airway device used for anesthesia and airway support consisting of an inflatable silicone mask and rubber connecting tube. It is inserted blindly into the pharynx, forming a low-pressure seal around the laryngeal inlet and permitting gentle positive pressure ventilation. It is an appropriate airway choice when mask ventilation can be used but endotracheal intubation is not necessary. The use of LMA is contraindicated in non-fasted patients, morbidly obese patients, and patients with obstructive or abnormal lesions of the oropharynx.

E. **Neuromuscular blockade** facilitates tracheal intubation and is required for many surgical procedures. It provides the surgeon with improved working conditions and optimizes ventilatory support. Its use may increase the risk for intraoperative awareness and postoperative neuromuscular weakness. It should only be used when clinically indicated and normal neuromuscular function should be ascertained prior to extubation or stopping the anesthetic. Agents that produce neuromuscular blockade act on postsynaptic receptors in the neuromuscular junction to antagonize the effects of acetylcholine competitively. Agents are categorized as either depolarizing or nondepolarizing (Table 3-5).

1. **Succinylcholine (Anectine, Quelicin)** is a rapidly acting (60 seconds), rapidly metabolized [by plasma cholinesterase (a.k.a. pseudocholinesterase or butyrylcholinesterase)] depolarizing agent that allows return of neuromuscular function in 5 to 10 minutes. In certain patients, the normally mild hyperkalemic response that is almost immediate will be greatly exaggerated leading to cardiac arrest. Its use is therefore usually contraindicated in patients with severe burns, trauma, or paralysis or patients with other neuromuscular disorders or prolonged bedrest. In addition, it can cause increases in intraocular, intracranial, and gastric pressures. It is also contraindicated in those with a personal or family history of **malignant hyperthermia** – a rare but deadly complication (see Section H.1.). In patients with inherited pseudocholinesterase deficiency administration will result in prolonged neuromuscular blockade (up to 8 hours).

2. **Nondepolarizing muscle relaxants** can be divided into short-, intermediate-, and long-acting agents. Associated hemodynamic effects and elimination pathways vary.

   a. **These agents are sometimes used in an intensive care setting** when paralysis is necessary for adequate ventilation of an intubated patient. Such patients must have adequate sedation and analgesia before and during paralysis. Duration of therapy should be as short as clinically feasible and dosage response should be monitored by train-of-four stimulus every 4 hours, with the goal being **at least**

TABLE 3-5 Agents Producing Neuromuscular Blockade

Agent	Initial Dose (mg/kg)	Duration (min)	Elimination	Associated Effects
Depolarizing				
Succinylcholine	1–1.5	3–5	Plasma cholinesterase	Fasciculations, increase or decrease in heart rate, transient hyperkalemia, known malignant hyperthermia trigger agent
Nondepolarizing				
Mivacurium	0.15	8–10	Plasma cholinesterase	Flushing, decrease in BP
Atracurium	0.2–0.4	20–35	Ester hydrolysis	Histamine release
Cisatracurium	0.1–0.2	20–35	Ester hydrolysis	—
Vecuronium	0.1–0.2	25–40	Primarily hepatic	—
Rocuronium	0.6–1.2	30	Primarily hepatic	—
d-Tubocurare	0.5–0.6	75–100	Primarily renal	Histamine release, decrease in BP
Pancuronium	0.04–0.1	45–90	Primarily renal	Increase in heart rate, mean arterial BP, and cardiac output
Doxacurium	0.05–0.08	90–180	Primarily renal	Decrease in BP

BP, blood pressure.

one out of four twitches. Corticosteroids, aminoglycosides, and long-term use of neuromuscular blockers potentiate the risk of a prolonged critical level of neuromyopathy.

   b. Reversal of neuromuscular blockade for patients who are receiving nondepolarizing muscle relaxants usually is performed before extubation to ensure full return of respiratory muscle function and protective airway reflexes. The diaphragm is less sensitive to muscle relaxants than are the muscles of the head and neck. A spontaneously ventilating patient **may be unable to protect the airway.** The definitive test for assessing the degree of remaining paralysis is to have the patient raise the head from the bed for 5 seconds or more. **Acetylcholinesterase inhibitors** (neostigmine, 0.06 to 0.07 mg/kg, and edrophonium, 0.1 mg/kg) act to increase the availability of acetylcholine at the neuromuscular junction, thereby reducing the binding frequency to the nicotinic receptors of the nondepolarizing muscle relaxant (competitive antagonism). Accumulation of acetylcholine also binds to muscarinic receptors. Muscarinic cholinergic side effects (bradycardia, bronchospasm, gastrointestinal hypermotility, excessive sweating and secretions, etc.) of these reversal drugs should always be prevented by combining these reversal agents with a muscarinic anticholinergic agent such as atropine or glycopyrrolate.

F. Maintenance of anesthesia

   1. The **goal of anesthesia** is to provide unconsciousness, amnesia, analgesia, and, usually, muscle relaxation. Balanced anesthesia involves the combined use of inhalational agents, narcotics, and muscle relaxants to attain this goal.

   2. Inhalational agents

   a. All inhalational agents provide varying degrees of unconsciousness, amnesia, and muscle relaxation.

   b. Isoflurane (Forane) has a relatively low rate of metabolism. It causes less cardiovascular depression than previously used agents. Newer agents are now commonly used. Sevoflurane (non-irritating – great for inhalational induction) and desflurane (more irritating to the airway, but less fat soluble and therefore faster clearance) are now much more commonly used.

   c. Halothane (Fluothane) use has decreased significantly. It has a rapid onset of action. Its use is excellent for asthmatics because of its bronchial smooth muscle-relaxing properties. However, it does sensitize the myocardium to catecholamines, increasing the rate of ventricular arrhythmias. Halothane should also be used with caution in patients with brain lesions because it is a potent vasodilator and can increase cerebral perfusion and intracranial pressure. It is rarely used in adult patients but is still used as an induction agent for pediatric patients because of the decreased irritating effects of halothane on the airway. Sevoflurane is now more commonly used in children for the same reason.

   d. Nitrous oxide by itself cannot provide surgical anesthesia. When combined with other inhalational agents, it reduces the required dose and subsequent side effects of the other agents. Nitrous oxide is extremely soluble and readily diffuses into any closed gas space, increasing its pressure. As a result, this agent should not be administered to patients with intestinal obstruction or suspected pneumothorax.

3. **IV agents**
   a. **Narcotics** can be administered continuously or intermittently. These agents provide superior analgesia but unreliable amnesia. Commonly used narcotics include fentanyl, sufentanil, alfentanil, remifentanil, morphine, and meperidine.
   b. **Hypnotics, benzodiazepines, and propofol.** Propofol infusion provides excellent hypnosis (unconsciousness) but insignificant analgesia and unreliable amnesia. It causes significant pain on injection and even small bolus doses may induce apnea in susceptible patients. The rapid dissipation of its effects and the low incidence of postoperative nausea have contributed to its widespread use in outpatient surgery. The maintenance dose is 0.1 to 0.2 mg/kg/minute. Lower-dose infusions can be used in the ICU setting. Prolonged infusions may cause hypertriglyceridemia.
   c. **Ketamine** by itself can provide total anesthesia. The associated emergence of delirium and nightmares limits its use. It provides excellent analgesia and is frequently used for burn patients requiring frequent dressing changes.

G. **Recovery from general anesthesia.** The goal at the conclusion of surgery is to provide a smooth, rapid return to consciousness, with stable hemodynamics and pulmonary function, protective airway reflexes, and continued analgesia.

1. **Preparation for emergence from anesthesia** usually begins before surgical closure, and communication between the surgeon and anesthesiologist facilitates prompt emergence of the patient at the procedure's termination.

2. Patients recover from the effects of sedation or general or regional anesthesia in the **postanesthesia care unit.** Once they are oriented, comfortable, hemodynamically stable, ventilating adequately, and without signs of anesthetic or surgical complications, they are discharged to the appropriate ward or to home.

H. **Complications of general anesthesia**

1. **Malignant hyperthermia** is a hypermetabolic disorder of skeletal muscle that is characterized by intracellular hypercalcemia and rapid adenosine triphosphate consumption. This condition is initiated by exposure to one or more anesthetic-triggering agents, including desflurane, enflurane, halothane, isoflurane, sevoflurane, and succinylcholine. Its incidence is approximately 1 in 50,000 in adults and 1 in 15,000 in children. The Malignant Hyperthermia Association of the United States (MHAUS) may be called at anytime with questions: **1–800-MH-HYPER.**
   a. **Signs and symptoms may occur in the operating room or more than 24 hours postoperatively** and include tachycardia, tachypnea,

hypertension, hypercapnia, hyperthermia, acidosis (metabolic with/without respiratory component), and skeletal muscle rigidity.

b. **Treatment** involves immediate administration of dantrolene (Dantrium, Dantamacrin) (1 mg/kg intravenously up to a cumulative dose of 10 mg/kg). This attenuates the rise in intracellular calcium. Repeat doses are given as needed if symptoms persist. Each vial commonly contains 20 mg of dantrolene and 3 g of mannitol and must be mixed with 50 mL of sterile water. Acidosis and hyperkalemia should be monitored and treated appropriately. Intensive care monitoring for 48 to 72 hours is indicated after an acute episode of malignant hyperthermia to evaluate for recurrence, acute tubular necrosis, pulmonary edema, and disseminated intravascular coagulation.

2. Laryngospasm

a. **During emergence from anesthesia,** noxious stimulation of the vocal cords can occur at light phases of anesthesia. In addition, blood or other oral secretions can irritate the larynx. As a result, the vocal cords may be brought into forceful apposition, and the flow of gas through the larynx may then be restricted or prevented completely. This alone may cause airway compromise or may lead to **negative-pressure pulmonary edema.**

b. **Treatment** involves the use of positive-pressure ventilation by mask to break the spasm. Such therapy usually is sufficient. Succinylcholine may be required in refractory cases to allow successful ventilation.

3. Nausea and vomiting

a. **Cortical** (pain, hypotension, hypoxia), **visceral** (gastric distention, visceral traction), **vestibular,** and **chemoreceptor trigger zone** (narcotics) afferent stimuli all can play a role in postoperative nausea and vomiting. The overall incidence is approximately 30%. It is more common in 11- to 14-year-old preadolescents, women, and obese patients. Narcotics, etomidate, inhalational gasses, and reversal agents such as neostigmine have also been implicated.

b. **Treatment** includes avoiding gastric distention during ventilation as well as administering agents such as prochlorperazine (Compazine), an antidopaminergic agent, 10 mg intravenously or orally every 4 to 6 hours as needed. Other useful agents include ondansetron (Zofran), 4 mg intravenously (dosing can be repeated every 6 to 8 hours if symptoms persist), or droperidol (Droleptan, Dridol) (0,625 mg IV). Droperidol is highly effective but may lead to sedation and the FDA has issued a black box warning because of possibility of prolonging the QT-interval and therefore the patient's ECG has to be monitored.

4. Urinary retention

a. Although very common with spinal anesthesia [see Section II.A.2.a(4)(f)], **urinary retention occurs in only 1% to 3% of cases involving general anesthesia.** It most commonly occurs after pelvic operations and in conjunction with benign prostatic hypertrophy.

    b. Treatment ranges from conservative (early ambulation, having patient sit or stand while attempting to micturate) to aggressive (bladder catheterization).

5. Hypothermia

    a. General anesthesia induction causes **peripheral vasodilation,** which leads to internal redistribution of heat, resulting in an increase in peripheral temperature at the expense of the core temperature. The core temperature then decreases in a linear manner until a plateau is reached. Such hypothermia is more pronounced in the elderly. Hypothermia may lead to cardiac arrhythmias and coagulopathy.

    b. Treatment should be preventative: the most effective being warming the operating room overnight or prior to the patient's arrival in the OR and minimizing unnecessary length and extent of exposure of the patient prior to draping. Other measures include passive warming during an operation by insulation of all exposed surfaces. In addition, active warming with forced-air convective warmers is effective, but care should be taken in using warmers with patients with vascular insufficiency (warmers should not be used on ischemic extremities).

6. Nerve injury

    a. Nerve palsies can occur secondary to improper positioning of the patient on the operating table or insufficient padding of dependent regions. Such palsies can be long lasting and debilitating.

    b. Prophylactic padding of sensitive regions and attention to **proper positioning** remain the most effective preventative therapies.

7. Postanesthesia shaking/shivering

    a. Meperidine (Demerol) and other narcotics (less effective) may relieve the clonic–tonic postanesthesia shivering, which occurs in up to two thirds of patients emerging from anesthesia. The clonic component from residual inhalational anesthetic is also triggered by hypothermia and accentuates the shivering. It has significant metabolic effects including acidosis and myocardial ischemia and may also be painful to the patient.

INTUBATION AND SEDATION

I. EMERGENT INTUBATION BY RAPID-SEQUENCE INDUCTION

    A. Patients in respiratory distress outside the operating room may require intubation to ensure adequate oxygenation and ventilatory support. Whenever possible, an anesthesiologist should be alerted and present at the time of intubation to assist if necessary; however, intubation should not be unduly delayed while waiting for an anesthesiologist to arrive.

    B. Airway support with 100% oxygen mask ventilation should be initiated before intubation. In the emergent setting or with the hemodynamically unstable patient, rapid-sequence induction of anesthesia with etomidate followed by succinylcholine may be preferred. Succinylcholine should be avoided in patients with severe burns, intracranial bleeds, and eye trauma. Intubation can then be performed via laryngoscopy using an endotracheal tube of appropriate size—in general, a size 8 tube for men and a size 7 tube for women. After inflation of the cuff, bilateral and equal breath sounds should be auscultated, end-tidal CO_2 and pulse oximetry measured, and a portable chest X-ray ordered to ensure proper placement. The patient should be continued on 100% oxygen until transfer to an intensive care setting.

II. SEDATION FOR PROCEDURES

A. Monitored anesthesia care

1. In monitored anesthesia care or local standby cases, **an anesthesiologist is present** to monitor and sedate the patient during the procedure. The surgeon is responsible for analgesia, which is accomplished with local infiltration or peripheral nerve blockade. Sedating or hypnotic medications (e.g., propofol) provide sedation only, and when given in conjunction with inadequate analgesia, they may result in a disinhibited, uncooperative patient.

2. **Monitoring is identical to that required for general or regional anesthesia.** Supplemental oxygen is provided by facemask or nasal cannula.

3. **NPO criteria** are identical to those for general or regional anesthesia.

4. **Considerable variation exists** regarding the response of patients to sedating medications, and protective airway reflexes may be diminished with even small doses.

B. Local procedures in the operating room

1. *Local* implies that **an anesthesiologist is not required** to monitor the patient or provide sedation. It still is advisable for the physician performing the procedure to monitor the ECG, arterial oxygen saturation, and BP even if sedation is not given.

2. **Painful stimuli** can increase vagal tone, resulting in bradycardia, hypotension, and hypoventilation.

C. Sedation outside the operating room

1. **Indications** are to relieve patient anxiety and avoid potentially detrimental hemodynamic sequelae during invasive procedures or diagnostic tests.

2. **Oxygen** should be supplied by nasal cannula or facemask when sedation is given. When benzodiazepines and narcotics are combined, even healthy patients breathing room air may become hypoxic.

3. **Monitoring** should include pulse oximetry, continuous ECG, and BP.

4. The end result should be a calm, easily arousable, cooperative patient. Oversedation may result in hypoventilation, airway obstruction, or disinhibition. Doses of commonly used sedatives are summarized in Table 3-6.

TABLE 3-6	Medications for Short-Term Sedation and Analgesia During Procedures		
Agent	**Route**	**Dose (as needed)**	**Comments**
Midazolam (Versed)	IV	0.5–1 mg q15 min	Benzodiazepines provide sedation only
Meperidine (Demerol)	IV	25–50 mg q10–15 min	Narcotics provide analgesia with unpredictable sedative effects
Fentanyl	IV	25–50 µg q5–10 min	Narcotics provide analgesia with unpredictable sedative effects
Propofol (Diprivan)	IV	10–20 mg over 3–5 min q10 min	May cause hypotension, especially with boluses

IV, intravenous; q, every.

5. **Side effects** that result from benzodiazepine administration include oversedation, respiratory depression, and depressed airway reflexes. Flumazenil (Romazicon), a benzodiazepine antagonist, can be used to reverse such effects. A dose of 0.2 mg intravenously should be administered and repeated every 60 seconds as required to a total dose of 1 mg. It can produce seizures and cardiac arrhythmias. Sedation can recur after 30 to 60 minutes, requiring repeated dosing.

POSTOPERATIVE MEDICATION AND COMPLICATIONS

I. **POSTOPERATIVE ANALGESIA** is provided to minimize patient discomfort and anxiety, attenuate the physiologic stress response to pain, enable optimal pulmonary toilet, and enable early ambulation. Analgesics can be administered by the oral, IV, or epidural route.

A. **IV route.** Many patients are unable to tolerate oral medications in the immediate postoperative period. For these patients, narcotics can be administered intravenously by several mechanisms.
   1. **As needed (PRN)**
      a. **Narcotics**
         (1) The **intermittent administration of IV or intramuscular narcotics by nursing staff** has the disadvantage that the narcotics may be given too infrequently, too late, and in insufficient amounts to provide adequate pain control. This may be the only choice in patients who are functionally unable to operate a patient-controlled analgesia (PCA) device.

(2) Morphine (Duramorph), 2 to 4 mg intravenously every 30 to 60 minutes, or **meperidine,** 50 to 100 mg intravenously every 30 to 60 minutes, should provide adequate analgesia for most patients. Orders should be written to withhold further injections for a respiratory rate of less than 12 breaths/minute or in cases of oversedation.

b. Nonsteroidal anti-inflammatory drugs (NSAIDs)

(1) Ketorolac (Toradol) is an NSAID that is available in oral and in injectable forms and is an effective adjunct to opioid therapy. The usual adult dose is 30 mg intramuscularly, followed by 15 to 30 mg every 6 hours for no longer than 48 hours.

(2) Ketorolac shares the potential side effects of other NSAIDs and should be used cautiously in the elderly and in patients with a history of peptic ulcer disease, renal insufficiency, steroid use, or volume depletion.

2. PCA

a. With PCA, the patient has the ability to self-deliver analgesics within **preset safety parameters.** It is imperative to stress to family and friends that only the patient should administer the analgesic.

b. Patients initially receive **morphine** (100 mg in 100 mL, with each dose delivering 1 mg), **hydromorphone (Dilaudid)** (50 mg in 100 mL, with each dose delivering 0.25 mg), or **meperidine** (1,000 mg in 100 mL, with each dose delivering 20 mg), with a maximum of one dose every 10 minutes. If this treatment provides inadequate pain control, the concentration of the drug can be increased and/or the lockout time period can be reduced.

3. Continuous "basal" narcotic infusions are rarely used in the surgical population. Respiratory arrest can occur with the "buildup" of narcotic levels.

B. Epidural infusions are useful for treating postoperative pain caused by thoracotomy, extensive abdominal incisions, or orthopedic lower-extremity procedures. Narcotics, local anesthetics, or a mixture of the two can be infused continuously through catheters placed in the patient's lumbar or thoracic epidural space.

C. Oral agents. There are multiple oral agents and combination analgesics.

D. Side effects and complications

1. Oversedation and respiratory depression

a. Arousable, spontaneously breathing patients should be given supplemental oxygen and be monitored closely for signs of respiratory depression until mental status improves. Medications for pain or sedation should be decreased accordingly.

b. Unarousable but spontaneously breathing patients should be treated with oxygen and naloxone (Narcan). One vial of naloxone (0.4 mg) should be diluted in a 10-mL syringe, and 1 mL (0.04 mg) should be administered every 30 to 60 seconds until the patient is arousable. Too much naloxone may result in severe pain and/or severe hypertension with possible pulmonary edema. Adequate ventilation should be confirmed by arterial blood gas measurement. Current opioid administration should be stopped and the regimen decreased. In addition to continuous-pulse oximetry, the patient should be monitored closely for potential recurrence of sedation as the effects of naloxone dissipate.

2. **Apnea**
   a. **Treatment** involves immediate supportive mask ventilation and possible intubation if no improvement in clinical status.
   b. **Naloxone,** 0.2 to 0.4 mg intravenously, should be considered. The same precautions need to be taken into account as mentioned above.

3. **Hypotension and bradycardia**
   a. **Local anesthetics administered via lumbar epidurals** decrease sympathetic tone to the abdominal viscera and lower extremities and greatly increase venous capacitance. Thoracic epidurals can additionally block the cardioaccelerator fibers, resulting in bradycardia.
   b. The **treatment** of choice for any of these situations (excluding bradycardia) is cessation of epidural infusion followed by volume resuscitation. Epinephrine can be used to raise BP acutely; 10 mg is diluted in 100 mL and given intravenously 1 mL at a time. If needed, this mixture can be infused intravenously starting at 15 mL/hour (25 μg/minute). Bradycardia can be treated with atropine, 0.4 to 1 mg intravenously, or glycopyrrolate (Robinul) given intravenously in 0.2-mg increments every 3 to 5 minutes as needed.

4. **Nausea and vomiting**
   a. **Naloxone** in small doses (0.04 to 0.1 mg intravenously as needed).
   b. **Prochlorperazine** (Compazine) 10 mg intravenously or orally every 4 to 6 hours.
   c. **Promethazine** (Phenergan) is a phenothiazine derivative that competitively blocks histamine H_1 receptors. Accidental intra-arterial injection can result in gangrene and there is therefore significant concerns regarding its use.
   d. **Ondansetron** (Zofran) 4 mg intravenously every 6 to 8 hours.
   e. **Metoclopramide** (Reglan) 10 mg intravenously every 6 to 8 hours. It should never be used as a first-line agent because of risk of extrapyramidal side effects.

5. **Pruritus**
   a. **Naloxone,** 0.04 to 0.1 mg intravenously, is effective.
   b. **Diphenhydramine (Benadryl),** 25 to 50 mg intravenously as needed, may provide symptomatic relief.

6. **Monoamine oxidase inhibitors** (e.g., isocarboxazid, phenelzine, and even hydralazine) may **interact adversely with** Phenylpiperidine derivative *Opioids* such as *Meperidine/(Pethidine), Tramadol, Methadone, Fentanyl.* This interaction may result in severe hemodynamic swings, respiratory depression, seizures, diaphoresis, hyperthermia, and coma. Meperidine has been most frequently implicated and should be avoided.

4 Fluid, Electrolyte, and Acid–Base Disorders

Ashley M. Holder and Richard S. Hotchkiss

DIAGNOSIS AND TREATMENT OF FLUID, ELECTROLYTE, AND ACID–BASE DISORDERS

I. **DEFINITION OF BODY FLUID COMPARTMENTS.** Water constitutes 50% to 70% of lean body weight. Total body water content is slightly higher in men, is most concentrated in skeletal muscle, and declines steadily with age. Total body water is divided into an intracellular fluid compartment and an extracellular fluid compartment, which consists of an intravascular compartment and an interstitial compartment, as illustrated in Figure 4-1. The extracellular and intracellular compartments have distinct electrolyte compositions. The principal extracellular cation is Na^+, and the principal extracellular anions are Cl^- and HCO_3^-. In contrast, the principal intracellular cations are K^+ and Mg^{2+}, and the principal intracellular anions are phosphates and negatively charged proteins.

II. **OSMOLALITY AND TONICITY.** *Osmolality* refers to the number of osmoles of solute particles per kilogram of water. Total osmolality is comprised of both effective and ineffective components. Effective osmoles cannot freely permeate cell membranes and are restricted to either the intracellular or extracellular fluid compartments. The asymmetric accumulation of effective osmoles in either extracellular fluid (e.g., Na^+, glucose, mannitol, and glycine) or intracellular fluid (e.g., K^+, amino acids, and organic acids) causes transcompartmental movement of water. Because the cell membrane is freely permeable to water, the osmolalities of the extracellular and intracellular compartments are equal. The effective osmolality of a solution is equivalent to its tonicity. Ineffective osmoles, in contrast, freely cross cell membranes and therefore are unable to affect the movement of water between compartments. Such ineffective solutes (e.g., urea, ethanol, and methanol) contribute to total osmolality but not to tonicity. *Tonicity*, not osmolality, is the physiologic parameter that the body attempts to regulate.

III. **COMMON ELECTROLYTE DISORDERS**

   A. **Sodium**

   1. **Physiology.** The normal individual consumes 3 to 5 g of NaCl (130 to 217 mmol Na^+) daily. Sodium balance is maintained primarily by the kidneys. Normal Na^+ concentration is 135 to 145 mmol/L (310 to 333 mg/dL). Potential sources of significant Na^+ loss include sweat,

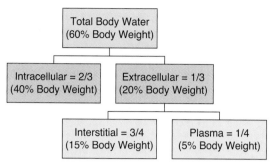

Figure 4-1. Body fluid compartments.

urine, and gastrointestinal secretions (Table 4-1). The Na^+ concentration largely determines the plasma osmolality (P_{osm}), which can be approximated by the following equation:

$$P_{osm}\left(\frac{mOsm}{L}\right) = 2 \times serum\left[Na^+\left(\frac{mmol}{L}\right) + K^+\left(\frac{mmol}{L}\right)\right]$$
$$+ \frac{glucose\left(\frac{mg}{dL}\right)}{18} + \frac{BUN\left(\frac{mg}{dL}\right)}{2}.8,$$

where BUN is blood urea nitrogen. Normal P_{osm} is 290 to 310 mOsm/L. In general, hypotonicity and hypertonicity coincide with hyponatremia and hypernatremia, respectively. However, Na^+ concentration and total body water are controlled by independent mechanisms. As a consequence, hyponatremia or hypernatremia may occur in conjunction with hypovolemia, hypervolemia, or euvolemia.

2. **Hyponatremia**
   a. **Causes and diagnosis.** The diagnostic approach to hyponatremia is illustrated in Figure 4-2. Hyponatremia may occur in conjunction with hypertonicity, isotonicity, or hypotonicity. Consequently, it is necessary to measure the serum osmolality to evaluate patients with hyponatremia.
      (1) **Isotonic hyponatremia.** Hyperlipidemic and hyperproteinemic states result in an isotonic expansion of the circulating plasma volume and cause a decrease in serum Na^+ concentration, although total body Na^+ remains unchanged. The reduction in serum sodium (mmol/L) can be estimated by multiplying the measured plasma lipid concentration (mg/dL) by 0.002 or the increase in serum protein concentration above 8 g/dL by 0.25. Isotonic, sodium-free solutions of glucose, mannitol, and glycine are restricted initially to the extracellular fluid and may similarly result in transient hyponatremia [see Section III.A.2.c (5)].
      (2) **Hypertonic hyponatremia.** Hyperglycemia may result in a transient fluid shift from the intracellular to the extracellular compartment, thereby diluting serum Na^+ concentration.

TABLE 4-1	Composition of Gastrointestinal Secretions				
Source	Volume (mL/24 hr)[a]	Na$^+$ (mmol/L)[b]	K$^+$ (mmol/L)[b]	Cl$^-$ (mmol/L)[b]	HCO$_3$ (mmol/L)[b]
Salivary	1,500 (500–2,000)	10 (2–10)	26 (20–30)	10 (8–18)	30
Stomach	1,500 (100–4,000)	60 (9–116)	10 (0–32)	130 (8–154)	0
Duodenum	(100–2,000)	140	5	80	0
Ileum	3,000	140 (80–150)	5 (2–8)	104 (43–137)	30
Colon	(100–9,000)	60	30	40	0
Pancreas	(100–800)	140 (113–185)	5 (3–7)	75 (54–95)	115
Bile	(50–800)	145 (131–164)	5 (312)	100 (89–180)	35

[a]Average volume (range).
[b]Average concentration (range).
Reprinted with permission from Faber MD, Schmidt RJ, Bear RA, et al. Management of fluid, electrolyte, and acid-base disorders in surgical patients. In: Narins RG, ed. *Clinical Disorders of Fluid and Electrolyte Metabolism*. New York: McGraw-Hill; 1994:1424.

Figure 4-2. Diagnostic approach to hyponatremia. CHF, congestive heart failure; ECF, extracellular fluid; GI, gastrointestinal; SIADH, syndrome of inappropriate antidiuretic hormone secretion; TURP, transurethral resection of the prostate. (Adapted from Narins RG, Jones ER, Stom MC, et al. Diagnostic strategies in disorders of fluid, electrolyte, and acid-base homeostasis. *Am J Med.* 1982;72:496–520.)

The expected decrease in serum Na^+ is approximately 1.3 to 1.6 mmol/L (2.99 to 3.68 mg/dL) for each 100-mg/dL increase in blood glucose above 200 mg/dL. Rapid infusion of hypertonic solutions of glucose, mannitol, or glycine may have a similar effect on Na^+ concentration [see Section III.A.2.c (5)].

(3) **Hypotonic hyponatremia** is classified on the basis of extracellular fluid volume. Hypotonic hyponatremia generally develops as a consequence of the administration and retention of hypotonic fluids [e.g., dextrose 5% in water (D5 W) and 0.45% NaCl] and rarely from the loss of salt-containing fluids alone.

(a) **Hypovolemic hypotonic hyponatremia** in the surgical patient most commonly results from replacement of sodium-rich fluid losses (e.g., from the GI tract, skin, or lungs) with an insufficient volume of hypotonic fluid (e.g., D5 W and 0.45% NaCl).

(b) **Hypervolemic hypotonic hyponatremia.** The edematous states of congestive heart failure, liver disease, and nephrosis occur in conjunction with inadequate circulating blood volume. This serves as a stimulus for the renal retention of sodium and of water. Disproportionate accumulation of water results in hyponatremia.

(c) **Isovolemic hypotonic hyponatremia**

   (i) **Water intoxication** typically occurs in the patient who consumes large quantities of water and has mildly impaired renal function (primary polydipsia). Alternatively, it may be the result of the administration of large quantities of hypotonic fluid in the patient with generalized renal failure.

   (ii) **K^+ loss,** either from GI fluid loss or secondary to diuretics, may result in isovolemic hyponatremia due to cellular exchange of these cations.

   (iii) **Reset osmostat.** Normally, the serum "osmostat" is set at 285 mOsm/L. In some individuals, the osmostat is "reset" downward, thus maintaining a lower serum osmolality. Several chronic diseases (e.g., tuberculosis and cirrhosis) predispose to this condition. These patients respond normally to water loads with suppression of antidiuretic hormone (ADH) secretion and excretion of free water.

   (iv) **SIADH** (syndrome of inappropriate ADH) is characterized by low plasma osmolality (<280 mOsm/L), hyponatremia (<135 mmol/L), low urine output with concentrated urine (>100 mOsm/kg), elevated urine sodium (>20 mEq/L), and clinical euvolemia. The major causes of SIADH include pulmonary disorders (e.g., atelectasis, empyema, pneumothorax, and respiratory failure), central nervous system disorders (e.g., trauma, meningitis, tumors, and subarachnoid hemorrhage), drugs (e.g., cyclophosphamide, cisplatin, and nonsteroidal anti-inflammatory drugs), and ectopic ADH production (e.g., small-cell lung carcinoma).

(4) **Transurethral resection syndrome** refers to hyponatremia in conjunction with cardiovascular and neurologic manifestations, which infrequently follow transurethral resection of the prostate. This syndrome results from intraoperative absorption of significant amounts of irrigation fluid (e.g., glycine, sorbitol, or mannitol). Isotonic, hypotonic, or hypertonic hyponatremia may occur. Management of these patients may be complicated.

b. **Clinical manifestations.** Symptoms associated with hyponatremia are predominantly neurologic and result from hypoosmolality. A decrease in P_{osm} causes intracellular water influx, increased intracellular volume, and cerebral edema. Symptoms include lethargy, confusion, nausea, vomiting, seizures, and coma. The likelihood that symptoms will occur is related to the degree of hyponatremia and to the rapidity with which it develops. Chronic hyponatremia is often asymptomatic until the serum Na^+ concentration falls below 110 to 120 mEq/L (253 to 276 mg/dL). An acute drop in the serum Na^+ concentration to 120 to 130 mEq/L (276 to 299 mg/dL), conversely, may produce symptoms.

c. **Treatment**

(1) **Isotonic and hypertonic hyponatremia** correct with resolution of the underlying disorder.

(2) **Hypovolemic hyponatremia** can be managed with administration of 0.9% NaCl to correct volume deficits and replace ongoing losses.

(3) **Water intoxication** responds to fluid restriction (1,000 mL/day).

(4) For **SIADH,** water restriction (1,000 mL/day) should be attempted initially. The addition of a loop diuretic (furosemide) or an osmotic diuretic (mannitol) may be necessary in refractory cases.

(5) **Hypervolemic hyponatremia** may respond to water restriction (1,000 mL/day) to return Na^+ to greater than 130 mmol/L (299 mg/dL). In cases of severe congestive heart failure, optimizing cardiac performance may assist in Na^+ correction. If the edematous hyponatremic patient becomes symptomatic, plasma Na^+ can be increased to a safe level by the use of a loop diuretic (furosemide, 20 to 200 mg intravenously every 6 hours) while replacing urinary Na^+ losses with 3% NaCl. A reasonable approach is to replace approximately 25% of the hourly urine output with 3% NaCl. Hypertonic saline should not be administered to these patients without concomitant diuretic therapy. Administration of synthetic brain natriuretic peptide (BNP) is also useful therapeutically in the setting of acute heart failure because it inhibits Na^+ reabsorption at the cortical collecting duct and inhibits the action of vasopressin on water permeability at the inner medullary collecting duct.

(6) In the presence of symptoms or extreme hyponatremia [Na^+ <110 mmol/L (253 mg/dL)], hypertonic saline (3% NaCl) is indicated. Serum Na^+ should be corrected to approximately 120 mmol/L (276 mg/dL). The quantity of 3% NaCl that is required to increase serum Na^+ to 120 mmol/L (276 mg/dL) can be estimated by calculating the Na^+ deficit:

$$Na^+ \text{ deficit (mmol)} = 0.60 \times \text{lean body wt (kg)}$$
$$\times \left[120 - \text{measured } Na^+ \left(\frac{mmol}{L} \right) \right]$$

(Each liter of 3% NaCl provides 513 mmol Na^+). The use of a loop diuretic (furosemide, 20 to 200 mg intravenously every 6 hours) may increase the effectiveness of 3% NaCl administration. Central pontine demyelination can occur in the setting of correction of hyponatremia. The risk factors for demyelination are controversial but appear to be related to the chronicity of hyponatremia (>48 hours) and the rate of correction. The serum Na^+ should be increased by no more than 12 mmol/L (27.6 mg/dL) in 24 hours of treatment [i.e., Na^+ <0.5 mmol (1.15 mg/dL)/hour]. For acute hyponatremia (<48 hours), the serum Na^+ may be corrected more rapidly [i.e., Na^+ = 1 to 2 mmol (2.3 to 4.6 mg/dL)/hour]. The patient's volume status should be carefully monitored over this time, and the serum Na^+ should be measured frequently (every 1 to 2 hours). Once the serum Na^+ concentration reaches 120 mmol/L (276 mg/dL) and symptoms have resolved, administration of hypertonic saline can be discontinued.

3. **Hypernatremia**
    a. **Diagnosis.** Hypernatremia is uniformly hypertonic and typically the result of water loss in excess of solute. Patients are categorized on the basis of their extracellular fluid volume status. The diagnostic approach to hypernatremia is illustrated in Figure 4-3.

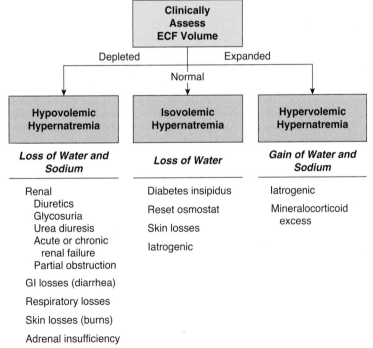

Figure 4-3. Diagnostic approach to hypernatremia. ECF, extracellular fluid; GI, gastrointestinal. (Adapted from Narins RG, Jones ER, Stom MC, et al. Diagnostic strategies in disorders of fluid, electrolyte, and acid-base homeostasis. *Am J Med.* 1982;72:496–520.)

(1) **Hypovolemic hypernatremia.** Any net loss of hypotonic body fluid results in extracellular volume depletion and hypernatremia. Common causes in the surgical patient include diuresis as well as GI, respiratory, and cutaneous (e.g., burns) fluid losses. Chronic renal failure and partial urinary tract obstruction also may cause hypovolemic hypernatremia.

(2) **Hypervolemic hypernatremia** in the surgical patient is most commonly iatrogenic and results from the parenteral administration of hypertonic solutions (e.g., $NaHCO_3$, saline, medications, and nutrition).

(3) **Isovolemic hypernatremia**

   (a) **Hypotonic losses.** Constant evaporative losses from the skin and respiratory tract, in addition to ongoing urinary free water losses, require the administration of approximately 750 mL of electrolyte-free water (e.g., D5 W) daily to parenterally maintained afebrile patients. Inappropriate replacement of these hypotonic losses with isotonic fluids is the most common cause of isovolemic hypernatremia in the hospitalized surgical patient.

   (b) **Diabetes insipidus** is characterized by polyuria and polydipsia in association with hypotonic urine (urine osmolality <200 mOsm/kg or a specific gravity of <1.005) and a high plasma osmolality (>287 mOsm/kg). *Central diabetes insipidus* (CDI) describes a defect in the hypothalamic secretion of ADH and is commonly seen after head trauma or hypophysectomy. CDI may also occur as a result of intracranial tumors, infections, vascular disorders (aneurysms), hypoxia, or medications (e.g., clonidine and phencyclidine). *Nephrogenic diabetes insipidus* (NDI) describes renal insensitivity to normally secreted ADH. NDI may be familial or drug induced (e.g., lithium, demeclocycline, methoxyflurane, and glyburide) or may occur as a result of hypokalemia, hypercalcemia, or intrinsic renal disease. If CDI and NDI are not distinguishable clinically, they can be differentiated by dehydration testing.

   (c) **Therapeutic.** Hypertonic saline may be administered for deliberate hypernatremia to control elevated intracranial pressure (ICP) and cerebral edema after head injury. Apart from osmotic properties, hypertonic saline also has hemodynamic, vasoregulatory, and immunomodulatory effects. Two prospective, randomized studies demonstrated the efficacy of using hypertonic saline to reduce ICP. A study of adult patients with brain injury in an intensive care unit (ICU) comparing a 7.5% saline/6% dextran solution (HSD) and a 20% mannitol solution showed that HSD lowered ICP more effectively and for a longer duration than did mannitol (*Crit Care Med.* 2005;33:196). Another study in children with severe head injury comparing hypertonic saline (Na^+ 268 mmol/L) with lactated

Ringer's solution (Na^+ 131 mmol/L) demonstrated that an increase in serum sodium concentration was correlated with a reduction in ICP and an elevation in cerebral perfusion pressure. The children receiving hypertonic saline had fewer complications and a shorter ICU stay than the children receiving lactated Ringer's solution (*Crit Care Med.* 1998;26:1265).

b. Clinical manifestations. Symptoms of hypernatremia that are related to the hyperosmolar state are primarily neurologic. These initially include lethargy, weakness, and irritability and may progress to fasciculations, seizures, coma, and irreversible neurologic damage.

c. Treatment

(1) Water deficit associated with hypernatremia can be estimated using the following equation where TBW = Total body weight:

$$\text{Water deficit (L)} = 0.60 \times \text{TBW(kg)} \times [(\text{serum } Na^\uparrow + (\text{mmol/L}))/140 - 1]$$

Rapid correction of hypernatremia can result in cerebral edema and permanent neurologic damage. Consequently, only one half of the water deficit should be corrected over the first 24 hours, with the remainder being corrected over the following 2 to 3 days. Serial Na^+ measurements are necessary to ensure that the rate of correction is adequate but not excessive. Oral fluid intake is acceptable for replacing water deficits. If oral intake is not possible, D5 W or D5 0.45% NaCl can be substituted. In addition to the actual water deficit, insensible losses and urinary output must be replaced.

(2) Diabetes insipidus

(a) Central diabetes insipidus can be treated with desmopressin acetate administered intranasally [0.1 to 0.4 mL (10 to 40 μg) daily] or subcutaneously or intravenously [0.5 to 1 mL (2 to 4 μg) daily].

(b) Nephrogenic diabetes insipidus treatment requires removal of any potentially offending drug and correction of electrolyte abnormalities. If these measures are ineffective, dietary sodium restriction in conjunction with a thiazide diuretic may be useful (hydrochlorothiazide, 50 to 100 mg/day orally).

B. Potassium

1. Physiology. K^+ is the major intracellular cation, with only 2% of total body K^+ located in the extracellular space. The normal serum concentration is 3.3 to 4.9 mmol/L (12.9 to 19.1 mg/dL). Approximately 50 to 100 mmol (195 to 390 mg/dL) K^+ is ingested and absorbed daily. Ninety percent of K^+ is renally excreted, with the remainder eliminated in stools.

2. Hypokalemia

a. Causes. K^+ depletion from inadequate intake alone is rare. Common causes of K^+ depletion in the surgical patient include GI losses (e.g., diarrhea, persistent vomiting, and nasogastric suctioning), renal losses (e.g., diuretics, fluid mobilization, and amphotericin B), and cutaneous losses (e.g., burns). Other causes of hypokalemia include acute intracellular K^+ uptake (associated with insulin excess, metabolic alkalosis, myocardial infarction, delirium tremens, hypothermia, and theophylline toxicity). Hypokalemia may also occur in the malnourished patient after initiation of total parenteral nutrition (refeeding syndrome), caused by the incorporation of K^+ into rapidly dividing cells.

b. **Clinical manifestations.** Mild hypokalemia [K^+ >3 mmol/L (11.7 mg/dL)] is generally asymptomatic. Symptoms occur with severe K^+ deficiency [K^+ <3 mmol/L (11.7 mg/dL)] and are primarily cardiovascular. Early electrocardiogram (ECG) manifestations include ectopy, T-wave depression, and prominent U waves. Severe depletion increases susceptibility to re-entrant arrhythmias.

c. **Treatment.** In mild hypokalemia, oral replacement is suitable. Typical daily therapy for the treatment of mild hypokalemia in the patient with intact renal function is 40 to 100 mmol (156 to 390 mg) KCl orally in single or divided doses. Parenteral therapy is indicated in the presence of severe depletion, significant symptoms, or oral intolerance. K^+ concentrations (administered as chloride, acetate, or phosphate) in peripherally administered intravenous fluids should not exceed 40 mmol/L (156 mg/dL), and the rate of administration should not exceed 20 mmol (78 mg)/hour. However, higher K^+ concentrations [60 to 80 mmol/L (234 to 312 mg/dL)] administered more rapidly (with cardiac monitoring) are indicated in cases of severe hypokalemia, for cardiac arrhythmias, and in the management of diabetic ketoacidosis. Administration of high K^+ concentrations via subclavian, jugular, or right atrial catheters should be avoided because local K^+ concentrations may be cardiotoxic. Hypomagnesemia frequently accompanies hypokalemia and generally must be corrected to replenish K^+ effectively.

3. **Hyperkalemia**

a. **Causes and diagnosis.** Hyperkalemia may occur with normal or elevated stores of total body K^+. Pseudohyperkalemia is a laboratory abnormality that reflects K^+ release from leukocytes and platelets during coagulation. Spurious elevation in K^+ may result from hemolysis or phlebotomy from a strangulated arm. Abnormal redistribution of K^+ from the intracellular to the extracellular compartment may occur as a result of insulin deficiency, β-adrenergic receptor blockade, acute acidemia, rhabdomyolysis, cell lysis (after chemotherapy), digitalis intoxication, reperfusion of ischemic limbs, and succinylcholine administration.

b. **Clinical manifestations.** Mild hyperkalemia [K^+ = 5 to 6 mmol/L (19.5 to 23.4 mg/dL)] is generally asymptomatic. Signs of significant hyperkalemia [K^+ >6.5 mmol/L (25.4 mg/dL)] are, most notably, ECG abnormalities: symmetric peaking of T waves, reduced P-wave voltage, and widening of the QRS complex. If untreated, severe hyperkalemia ultimately may cause a sinusoidal ECG pattern.

c. **Treatment**

(1) **Mild hyperkalemia** [K^+ = 5 to 6 mmol/L (19.5 to 23.4 mg/dL)] can be treated conservatively by the reduction in daily K^+ intake and, if needed, the addition of a loop diuretic (e.g., furosemide) to promote renal elimination. Any medication that is capable of impairing K^+ homeostasis (e.g., nonselective β-adrenergic antagonists, angiotensin-converting enzyme inhibitors, K^+-sparing diuretics, and nonsteroidal anti-inflammatory drugs) should be discontinued, if possible.

(2) **Severe hyperkalemia** [K^+ >6.5 mmol/L (25.4 mg/dL)]

(a) **Temporizing measures** produce shifts of potassium from the extracellular to the intracellular space.

(i) **$NaHCO_3$** [1 mmol/kg or 1 to 2 ampules (50 mL each) of 8.4% $NaHCO_3$] can be infused intravenously over a 3- to 5-minute period. This dose can be repeated after 10 to 15 minutes if ECG abnormalities persist.

(ii) **Dextrose** (0.5 g/kg body weight) infused with insulin (0.3 unit of regular insulin/g of dextrose) transiently lowers serum K^+ (the usual dose is 25 g dextrose, with 6 to 10 units of regular insulin given simultaneously as an intravenous bolus).

(iii) **Inhaled β-agonists** [e.g., albuterol sulfate, 2 to 4 mL of 0.5% solution (10 to 20 mg) delivered via nebulizer] have been shown to lower plasma K^+, with a duration of action of up to 2 hours. Although only modest increases in heart rate and blood pressure have been reported when the nebulized form of this drug is used, caution is warranted in patients with known or suspected cardiovascular disease.

(iv) **Calcium gluconate 10%** (5 to 10 mL intravenously over 2 minutes) should be administered to patients with profound ECG changes who are not receiving digitalis preparations. Calcium functions to stabilize the myocardium.

(b) **Therapeutic measures** to definitively decrease total body potassium by increasing potassium excretion:

(i) **Sodium polystyrene sulfonate** (Kayexalate), a Na^+-K^+ exchange resin, can be administered orally (20 to 50 g of the resin in 100 to 200 mL of 20% sorbitol every 4 hours) or rectally (as a retention enema, 50 g of the resin in 50 mL of 70% sorbitol added to 100 to 200 mL of water every 1 to 2 hours initially, followed by administration every 6 hours) to promote K^+ elimination. A decrease in serum K^+ level typically occurs 2 to 4 hours after administration.

(ii) **Hydration** with 0.9% NaCl in combination with a **loop diuretic** (e.g., furosemide, 20 to 100 mg intravenously) should be administered to patients with adequate renal function to promote renal K^+ excretion.

(iii) **Dialysis** is definitive therapy in severe, refractory, or life-threatening hyperkalemia.

C. Calcium

1. **Physiology.** Serum calcium (8.9 to 10.3 mg/dL or 2.23 to 2.57 mmol/L) exists in three forms: ionized (45%), protein bound (40%), and in a complex with freely diffusible compounds (15%). Only free ionized Ca^{2+} (4.6 to 5.1 mg/dL or 1.15 to 1.27 mmol/L) is physiologically active. Daily calcium intake ranges from 500 to 1,000 mg, with absorption varying considerably. Normal calcium metabolism is under the influence of parathyroid hormone (PTH) and vitamin D. PTH promotes calcium resorption from bone and reclamation of calcium from the glomerular filtrate. Vitamin D increases calcium absorption from the intestinal tract.

2. **Hypocalcemia**

   a. **Causes and diagnosis** Hypocalcemia most commonly occurs as a consequence of calcium sequestration or vitamin D deficiency. Calcium sequestration may occur in the setting of acute pancreatitis, rhabdomyolysis, or rapid administration of blood (citrate acting as a calcium chelator). Transient hypocalcemia may occur after total thyroidectomy, secondary to vascular compromise of the parathyroid glands, and after parathyroidectomy. In the latter case, serum Ca^{2+} reaches its lowest level within 48 to 72 hours after operation, returning to normal in 2 to 3 days. Hypocalcemia may occur in conjunction with Mg^{2+} depletion, which simultaneously impairs PTH secretion and function. Acute alkalemia (e.g., from rapid administration of parenteral bicarbonate or hyperventilation) may produce clinical hypocalcemia with a normal serum calcium concentration due to an abrupt decrease in the ionized fraction. Because 40% of serum calcium is bound to albumin, hypoalbuminemia may decrease total serum calcium significantly—a fall in serum albumin of 1 g/dL decreases serum calcium by approximately 0.8 mg/dL (0.2 mmol/L). Ionized Ca^{2+} is unaffected by albumin. As a consequence, the diagnosis of hypocalcemia should be based on ionized, not total serum, calcium.

   b. **Clinical manifestations.** Tetany is the major clinical finding and may be demonstrated by Chvostek's sign (facial muscle spasm elicited by tapping over the branches of the facial nerve). The patient may also complain of perioral numbness and tingling. In addition, hypocalcemia can be associated with QT-interval prolongation and ventricular arrhythmias.

   c. **Treatment**

      (1) **Parenteral therapy.** Asymptomatic patients, even those with moderate hypocalcemia (calcium 6 to 7 mg/dL or 1.5 to 1.75 mmol/L), do not require parenteral therapy. Symptoms such as overt tetany, laryngeal spasm, or seizures are indications for parenteral calcium. Approximately 200 mg of elemental calcium is needed to abort an attack of tetany. Initial therapy consists in the administration of a calcium bolus (10 to 20 mL

of 10% calcium gluconate over 10 minutes) followed by a maintenance infusion of 1 to 2 mg/kg elemental calcium/hour. Calcium chloride contains three times more elemental calcium than calcium gluconate; one 10-mL ampule of 10% calcium chloride contains 272 mg (13.6 mEq) elemental calcium, whereas one 10-mL ampule of 10% calcium gluconate contains only 90 mg (4.6 mEq) elemental calcium. The serum calcium level typically normalizes in 6 to 12 hours with this regimen, at which time the maintenance rate can be decreased to 0.3 to 0.5 mg/kg/hour. In addition to monitoring calcium levels frequently during therapy, one should check Mg^{2+}, phosphorus, and K^+ levels and replete as necessary. Calcium should be administered cautiously to patients who are receiving digitalis preparations because digitalis toxicity may be potentiated. Once the serum calcium level is normal, oral therapy can be initiated.

   (2) **Oral therapy.** Calcium salts are available for oral administration (calcium carbonate, calcium gluconate). Each 1,250-mg tablet of calcium carbonate provides 500 mg of elemental calcium (25.4 mEq), and a 1,000-mg tablet of calcium gluconate has 90 mg (4.6 mEq) of elemental calcium. In chronic hypocalcemia, with serum calcium levels of 7.6 mg/dL (1.9 mmol/L) or higher, the daily administration of 1,000 to 2,000 mg of elemental calcium alone may suffice. When hypocalcemia is more severe, calcium salts should be supplemented with a vitamin D preparation. Daily therapy can be initiated with 50,000 IU of calciferol, 0.4 mg of dihydrotachysterol, or 0.25 to 0.50 μg of 1,25-dihydroxyvitamin D_3 orally. Subsequent therapy should be adjusted as necessary.

3. Hypercalcemia

   a. Causes and diagnosis. Causes of hypercalcemia include malignancy, hyperparathyroidism, hyperthyroidism, vitamin D intoxication, immobilization, long-term total parenteral nutrition, thiazide diuretics, and granulomatous disease. The finding of an elevated PTH level in the face of hypercalcemia supports the diagnosis of hyperparathyroidism. If the PTH level is normal or low, further evaluation is necessary to identify one of the previously cited diagnoses.

   b. Clinical manifestations. Mild hypercalcemia (calcium <12 mg/dL or <3 mmol/L) is generally asymptomatic. The hypercalcemia of hyperparathyroidism is associated infrequently with classic parathyroid bone disease and nephrolithiasis. Manifestations of severe hypercalcemia include altered mental status, diffuse weakness, dehydration, adynamic ileus, nausea, vomiting, and severe constipation. The cardiac effects of hypercalcemia include QT-interval shortening and arrhythmias.

   c. Treatment of hypercalcemia depends on the severity of the symptoms. Mild hypercalcemia (calcium <12 mg/dL or <3 mmol/L) can be managed conservatively by restricting calcium intake and treating the underlying disorder. Volume depletion should be corrected if present, and vitamin D, calcium supplements, and thiazide diuretics should be discontinued. The treatment of more severe hypercalcemia may require the following measures:

(1) **NaCl 0.9% and loop diuretics** may rapidly correct hypercalcemia. In the patient with normal cardiovascular and renal function, 0.9% NaCl (250 to 500 mL/hour) with furosemide (20 mg intravenously every 4 to 6 hours) can be administered initially. The rate of 0.9% NaCl infusion and the dose of furosemide should subsequently be adjusted to maintain a urine output of 200 to 300 mL/hour. Serum Mg^{2+}, phosphorus, and K^+ levels should be monitored and repleted as necessary. The inclusion of KCl (20 mmol) and $MgSO_4$ (8 to 16 mEq or 1 to 2 g) in each liter of fluid may prevent hypokalemia and hypomagnesemia. This treatment may promote the loss of as much as 2 g of calcium over 24 hours.

(2) **Salmon calcitonin,** in conjunction with adequate hydration, is useful for the treatment of hypercalcemia associated with malignancy and with primary hyperparathyroidism. Salmon calcitonin can be administered either subcutaneously or intramuscularly. Skin testing by subcutaneous injection of 1 IU is recommended before progressing to the initial dose of 4 IU/kg intravenously or subcutaneously every 12 hours. A hypocalcemic effect may be seen as early as 6 to 10 hours after administration. The dose may be doubled if unsuccessful after 48 hours of treatment. The maximum recommended dose is 8 IU/kg every 6 hours.

(3) **Pamidronate disodium,** in conjunction with adequate hydration, is useful for the treatment of hypercalcemia associated with malignancy. For moderate hypercalcemia (calcium 12 to 13.5 mg/dL or 3 to 3.38 mmol/L), 60 mg of pamidronate diluted in 1 L of 0.45% NaCl, 0.9% NaCl, or D5 W should be infused over 24 hours. For severe hypercalcemia, the dose of pamidronate is 90 mg. If hypercalcemia recurs, a repeat dose of pamidronate can be given after 7 days. The safety of pamidronate for use in patients with significant renal impairment is not established.

(4) **Plicamycin** (25 μg/kg, diluted in 1 L of 0.9% NaCl or D5 W, infused over 4 to 6 hours each day for 3 to 4 days) is useful for treatment of hypercalcemia associated with malignancy. The onset of action is between 1 and 2 days, with a duration of action of up to 1 week.

D. Phosphorus

1. **Physiology.** Extracellular fluid contains less than 1% of total body stores of phosphorus at a concentration of 2.5 to 4.5 mg/dL (0.81 to 1.45 mmol/L). Phosphorus balance is regulated by a number of hormones that also control calcium metabolism. As a consequence, derangements in concentrations of phosphorus and calcium frequently

coexist. The average adult consumes 800 to 1,000 mg of phosphorus daily, which is predominantly renally excreted.

2. Hypophosphatemia

a. Causes

(1) Decreased intestinal phosphate absorption results from vitamin D deficiency, malabsorption, and the use of phosphate binders (e.g., aluminum-, magnesium-, calcium-, or iron-containing compounds).

(2) Renal phosphate loss may occur with acidosis, alkalosis, diuretic therapy (particularly acetazolamide), during recovery from acute tubular necrosis, and during hyperglycemia as a result of osmotic diuresis.

(3) Phosphorus redistribution from the extracellular to the intracellular compartment occurs principally with respiratory alkalosis and administration of nutrients such as glucose (particularly in the malnourished patient). This transient decrease in serum phosphorus is of no clinical significance unless there is a significant total body deficit. Significant hypophosphatemia may also occur in malnourished patients after the initiation of total parenteral nutrition (refeeding syndrome) as a result of the incorporation of phosphorus into rapidly dividing cells.

(4) Hypophosphatemia may develop in **burn patients** as a result of excessive phosphaturia during fluid mobilization and incorporation of phosphorus into new tissues during wound healing.

b. Clinical manifestations. Moderate hypophosphatemia (phosphorus 1 to 2.5 mg/dL or 0.32 to 0.81 mmol/L) is usually asymptomatic. Severe hypophosphatemia (phosphorus <1 mg/dL or 0.32 mmol/L) may result in respiratory muscle dysfunction, diffuse weakness, and flaccid paralysis.

c. Treatment. A study of patients at Barnes-Jewish Hospital's surgical ICU (Saint Louis, MO) demonstrated that the use of an aggressive phosphorus repletion protocol based on a patient's admission weight (kg) and most recent phosphorus level (mg/dL) leads to more successful treatment of hypophosphatemia than physician-directed therapy (see Table 4-2). Adequate repletion of phosphorus is especially important in critically ill patients, who are more likely to experience adverse physiologic consequences from hypophosphatemia, including the inability to be weaned from the ventilator, organ dysfunction, and death. Phosphorus replacement should begin with intravenous therapy, especially for moderate (1 to 1.7 mg/dL) or severe (<1 mg/dL) hypophosphatemia (*J Am Coll Surg.* 2004;198:198). Risks of intravenous therapy include hyperphosphatemia, hypocalcemia, hypotension, hyperkalemia (with potassium phosphate), hypomagnesemia, hyperosmolality, metastatic calcification, and renal failure. Five to 7 days of intravenous repletion may be required before intracellular stores are replenished. Once the serum phosphorus level exceeds 2 mg/dL (0.65 mmol/L), oral therapy can be initiated with a sodium-potassium phosphate salt [e.g., Neutra-Phos, 250 to 500 mg (8 to 16 mmol phosphorus)

TABLE 4-2	Phosphorus Repletion Protocol		
Phosphorus Level	Weight 40–60 kg	Weight 61–80 kg	Weight 81–120 kg
1 mg/dL	30 mmol Phos IV	40 mmol Phos IV	50 mmol Phos IV
1–1.7 mg/dL	20 mmol Phos IV	30 mmol Phos IV	40 mmol Phos IV
1.8–2.2 mg/dL	10 mmol Phos IV	15 mmol Phos IV	20 mmol Phos IV

If the patient's potassium is <4, use potassium phosphorus.
If the patient's potassium is >4, use sodium phosphorus.
IV, intravenous; Phos, phosphorus.
Adapted with permission from Taylor BE, Huey WY, Buchman TG, et al. Effectiveness of a protocol based on patient weight and serum phosphorus levels in repleting hypophosphatemia in a surgical ICU. *J Am Coll Surg* 2004;198:198–204.

orally four times a day; each 250-mg tablet of Neutra-Phos contains 7 mmol each of K^+ and Na^+].

3. **Hyperphosphatemia**

   a. **Causes** include impaired renal excretion and transcellular shifts of phosphorus from the intracellular to the extracellular compartment (e.g., tissue trauma, tumor lysis, insulin deficiency, or acidosis). Hyperphosphatemia is also a common feature of postoperative hypoparathyroidism.

   b. **Clinical manifestations,** in the short term, include hypocalcemia and tetany. In contrast, soft tissue calcification and secondary hyperparathyroidism occur with chronicity.

   c. **Treatment** of hyperphosphatemia, in general, should eliminate the phosphorus source, remove phosphorus from the circulation, and correct any coexisting hypocalcemia. Dietary phosphorus should be restricted. Urinary phosphorus excretion can be increased by hydration (0.9% NaCl at 250 to 500 mL/hour) and diuresis (acetazolamide, 500 mg every 6 hours orally or intravenously). Phosphate binders (aluminum hydroxide, 30 to 120 mL orally every 6 hours) minimize intestinal phosphate absorption and can induce a negative balance of greater than 250 mg of phosphorus daily, even in the absence of dietary phosphorus. Hyperphosphatemia secondary to conditions that cause phosphorus redistribution (e.g., diabetic ketoacidosis) resolves with treatment of the underlying condition and requires no specific therapy. Dialysis can be used to correct hyperphosphatemia in extreme conditions.

E. **Magnesium**

   1. **Physiology.** Mg^{2+} (1.3 to 2.2 mEq/L or 0.65 to 1.10 mmol/L) is predominantly an intracellular cation. Renal excretion and retention play the major physiologic role in regulating body stores. Mg^{2+} is not under direct hormonal regulation.

2. **Hypomagnesemia**

   a. **Causes.** Hypomagnesemia on the basis of dietary insufficiency is rare. Common etiologies include excessive GI or renal Mg^{2+} loss. GI loss may result from diarrhea, malabsorption, vomiting, or biliary fistulas. Urinary loss occurs with marked diuresis, primary hyperaldosteronism, renal tubular dysfunction (e.g., renal tubular acidosis), chronic alcoholism, or as a drug side effect (e.g., loop diuretics, cyclosporine, amphotericin B, aminoglycosides, and cisplatin). Hypomagnesemia may also result from shifts of Mg^{2+} from the extracellular to the intracellular space, particularly in conjunction with acute myocardial infarction, alcohol withdrawal, or after receiving glucose-containing solutions. After parathyroidectomy for hyperparathyroidism, the redeposition of calcium and Mg^{2+} in bone may cause dramatic hypocalcemia and hypomagnesemia. Hypomagnesemia is usually accompanied by hypokalemia and hypophosphatemia and is frequently encountered in the trauma patient.

   b. **Clinical manifestations.** Symptoms of hypomagnesemia are predominantly neuromuscular and cardiovascular. With severe depletion, altered mental status, tremors, hyperreflexia, and tetany may be present. The cardiovascular effects of hypomagnesemia are similar to those of hypokalemia and include T-wave and QRS-complex broadening as well as prolongation of the PR and QT intervals. Ventricular arrhythmias most commonly occur in patients who receive digitalis preparations. We recommend maintaining a patient's magnesium at the upper limit of normal (2 to 2.5 mEq/L to prevent QT prolongation and arrhythmias.

   c. **Treatment**

      (1) **Parenteral therapy** is preferred for the treatment of severe hypomagnesemia (Mg^{2+} <1 mEq/L or 0.5 mmol/L) or in symptomatic patients. In cases of life-threatening arrhythmias, 1 to 2 g (8 to 16 mEq) of $MgSO_4$ can be administered over 5 minutes, followed by a continuous infusion of 1 to 2 g/hour for the next several hours. The infusion subsequently can be reduced to 0.5 to 1 g/hour for maintenance. The normal range of Mg^{2+} (1.3 to 2.2 mEq/L or 0.65 to 1.10 mmol/L) is probably below its physiologic optimum. Thus, except in cases of renal failure, vigorous correction of either severe or symptomatic hypomagnesemia is warranted. In less urgent situations, $MgSO_4$ infusion may begin at 1 to 2 g/hour for 3 to 6 hours, with the rate subsequently adjusted to 0.5 to 1 g/hour for maintenance. Mild hypomagnesemia (1.1 to 1.4 mEq/L or 0.5 to 0.7 mmol/L) in an asymptomatic patient can be treated initially with the parenteral administration of 50 to 100 mEq (6 to 12 g) of $MgSO_4$ daily until body stores are replenished. Treatment should be continued for 3 to 5 days, at which time the patient can be switched to an oral maintenance dose. Intravenous $MgSO_4$ remains the initial therapy of choice for torsades de pointes (polymorphologic ventricular

tachycardia). Furthermore, it is used to achieve hypermagnesemia that is therapeutic for eclampsia and pre-eclampsia.

    (2) Oral therapy. Magnesium oxide is the preferred oral agent. Each 400-mg tablet provides 241 mg (20 mEq) of Mg^{2+}. Other formulations include magnesium gluconate [each 500-mg tablet provides 27 mg (2.3 mEq) of Mg^{2+}] and magnesium chloride [each 535-mg tablet provides 64 mg (5.5 mEq) of Mg^{2+}]. Depending on the level of depletion, oral therapy should provide 20 to 80 mEq of Mg^{2+}/day in divided doses.

    (3) Prevention of hypomagnesemia in the hospitalized patient who is receiving prolonged parenteral nutritional therapy can be accomplished by providing 0.35 to 0.45 mEq/kg of Mg^{2+}/day [i.e., by adding 8 to 16 mEq (1 to 2 g) of $MgSO_4$ to each liter of intravenous fluids].

3. Serum Mg^{2+} levels should be monitored during therapy. The dose of Mg^{2+} should be reduced in patients with renal insufficiency.

4. Hypermagnesemia

    a. Causes. Hypermagnesemia occurs infrequently, is usually iatrogenic, and is seen most commonly in the setting of renal failure.

    b. Clinical manifestations. Mild hypermagnesemia (Mg^{2+} 5 to 6 mEq/L or 2.5 to 3 mmol/L) is generally asymptomatic. Severe hypermagnesemia (Mg^{2+} >8 mEq/L or 4 mmol/L) is associated with depression of deep tendon reflexes, paralysis of voluntary muscles, hypotension, sinus bradycardia, and prolongation of PR, QRS, and QT intervals.

    c. Treatment. Cessation of exogenous Mg^{2+} is necessary. Calcium gluconate 10% (10 to 20 mL over 5 to 10 minutes intravenously) is indicated in the presence of life-threatening symptoms (e.g., hyporeflexia, respiratory depression, or cardiac conduction disturbances) to antagonize the effects of Mg^{2+}. A 0.9% NaCl (250 to 500 mL/hour) infusion with loop diuretic (furosemide, 20 mg intravenously every 4 to 6 hours) in the patient with intact renal function promotes renal elimination. Dialysis is the definitive therapy in the presence of intractable symptomatic hypermagnesemia.

IV. PARENTERAL FLUID THERAPY. The composition of commonly used parenteral fluids is presented in Table 4-3.

    A. Crystalloids, in general, are solutions that contain sodium as the major osmotically active particle. Crystalloids are relatively inexpensive and are useful for volume expansion, maintenance infusion, and correction of electrolyte disturbances.

    1. Isotonic crystalloids (e.g., lactated Ringer's solution and 0.9% NaCl) distribute uniformly throughout the extracellular fluid compartment so that after 1 hour, only 25% of the total volume infused remains in the intravascular space. Lactated Ringer's solution is designed to mimic extracellular fluid and is considered a balanced salt solution. This solution provides a HCO_3^- precursor and is useful for replacing GI losses

TABLE 4-3	Composition of Common Parenteral Fluids[a]								
Solution	Volume[b]	Na^+	K^+	Ca^{2+}	Mg^{2+}	Cl^-	HCO_3 (as lactate)	Dextrose (g/L)	mOsm/L
Extracellular fluid	—	142	4	5	3	103	27	—	280–310
Lactated Ringer's	—	130	4	3	—	109	28	—	273
0.9% NaCl	—	154	—	—	—	154	—	—	308
0.45% NaCl	—	77	—	—	—	77	—	—	154
D5 W	—	—	—	—	—	—	—	50	252
D5/0.45% NaCl	—	77	—	—	—	77	—	50	406
D5LR	—	130	4	3	—	109	28	50	525
3% NaCl	—	513	—	—	—	513	—	—	1,026
7.5% NaCl	—	1,283	—	—	—	1,283	—	—	2,567

6% hetastarch	500	154	—	—	—	154	—	—	310
10% dextran-40	500	0/154[c]	—	—	—	0/154[c]	—	—	300
6% dextran-70	500	0/154[c]	—	—	—	0/154[c]	—	—	300
5% albumin	250,500	130–160	<2.5	—	—	130–160	—	—	330
25% albumin	20,50,100	130–160	<2.5	—	—	130–160	—	—	330
Plasma protein fraction	250,500	145		—	—	145	—	—	300

[a]Electrolyte concentrations in mmol/L.
[b]Available volumes (mL) of colloid solutions.
[c]Dextran solutions available in 5% dextrose (0 Na+, 0 Cl) or 0.9% NaCl (154 mmol Na+, 154 mmol Cl).
D5LR, 5% dextrose in lactated Ringer's solution; D5/0.45% NaCl, 5% dextrose per 0.45% NaCl; D5 W, 5% dextrose in water.

and extracellular fluid volume deficits. In general, lactated Ringer's solution and 0.9% NaCl can be used interchangeably. However, 0.9% NaCl is preferred in the presence of hyperkalemia, hypercalcemia, hyponatremia, hypochloremia, or metabolic alkalosis.

2. **Hypertonic saline solutions** alone and in combination with colloids, such as dextran, have generated interest as a resuscitation fluid for patients with shock or burns. These fluids are appealing because, relative to isotonic crystalloids, smaller quantities are required initially for resuscitation. A randomized, double-blinded study of a 250-mL dose of hypertonic saline (7.5% NaCl, 6% dextran-70) compared to placebo (0.9% NaCl) given to patients in hemorrhagic shock after sustaining blunt trauma showed that the patients receiving the hypertonic saline bolus had significant blunting of neutrophil activation and alteration of the pattern of monocyte activation and cytokine secretion with a only a transient increase in serum sodium that normalized within 24 hours. This immunomodulatory effect of hypertonic saline plus dextran may help to prevent widespread tissue damage and multiorgan dysfunction seen after traumatic injury (*Ann Surg.* 2006;243:47). However, another recent randomized controlled trial of patients with blunt trauma in hypovolemic shock that compared resuscitation with either lactated Ringer solution or 7.5% hypertonic saline and 6% dextran 70 demonstrated no significant difference in ARDS-free survival (*Arch Surg.* 2008;143(2):139). The possible side effects of hypertonic solutions include hypernatremia, hyperosmolality, hyperchloremia, hypokalemia, and central pontine demyelination with rapid infusion and should be administered with caution until more research becomes available.

B. **Hypotonic solutions** (D5 W, 0.45% NaCl) distribute throughout the total body water compartment, expanding the intravascular compartment by as little as 10% of the volume infused. For this reason, hypotonic solutions should not be used for volume expansion. They are used to replace free water deficits.

C. **Colloid solutions** contain high-molecular-weight substances that remain in the intravascular space. Early use of colloids in the resuscitation regimen may result in more prompt restoration of tissue perfusion and may lessen the total volume of fluid required for resuscitation. However, there are no situations in which colloids have unequivocally been shown to be superior to crystalloids for volume expansion. In fact, the SAFE (Saline versus Albumin Fluid Evaluation) study, which randomized 6,997 patients in the ICU to receive either 4% albumin or normal saline for fluid resuscitation, found no significant difference in outcomes, including mortality and organ failure, between the two groups (*N Engl J Med.* 2004;350:2247). Because colloid solutions are substantially more expensive than crystalloids, their routine use in hypovolemic shock is controversial. In addition, a post hoc study of ICU patients with traumatic brain injury revealed that patients who underwent fluid resuscitation with albumin compared to saline had significantly higher mortality rates (*N Engl J Med.* 2007;357:874). The use of colloids is indicated when crystalloids fail to sustain plasma volume because of low colloid osmotic pressure (e.g., increased protein loss from the vascular space, as in burns and peritonitis).

1. **Albumin preparations** ultimately distribute throughout the extracellular space, although the initial location of distribution is the vascular compartment. Preparations of 25% albumin (100 mL) and 5% albumin (500 mL) expand the intravascular volume by an equivalent amount (450 to 500 mL). Albumin 25% is indicated in the edematous patient to mobilize interstitial fluid into the intravascular space. The cost per liter of albumin is more than that of other colloid solutions and 30 times the cost of the intravascular volume-equivalent amount of crystalloid solutions; thus, albumin preparations should be used judiciously. They are not indicated in the patient with adequate colloid oncotic pressure (serum albumin >2.5 mg/dL, total protein >5 mg/dL), for augmenting serum albumin in chronic illness (cirrhosis or nephrotic syndrome), or as a nutritional source.

2. **Dextran** is a synthetic glucose polymer that undergoes predominantly renal elimination. In addition to its indications for volume expansion, dextran also is used for thromboembolism prophylaxis and promotion of peripheral perfusion. Dextran solutions expand the intravascular volume by an amount equal to the volume infused. Side effects include renal failure, osmotic diuresis, coagulopathy, and laboratory abnormalities (i.e., elevations in blood glucose and protein and interference with blood cross-matching). Preparations of 40- and 70-kD dextran are available (dextran-40 and dextran-70, respectively).

3. **Hydroxyethyl starch (hetastarch)** is a synthetic molecule resembling glycogen that is available as a 6% solution in 0.9% NaCl. Hetastarch, like 5% albumin, increases the intravascular volume by an amount equal to or greater than the volume infused. Hetastarch is less expensive than albumin and has a more favorable side effect profile than dextran formulations, making it an appealing colloid preparation. Hextend is a colloid that contains 6% hetastarch, balanced electrolytes, a lactate buffer, and physiologic levels of glucose. Relative to hetastarch in saline, Hextend seems to have a more beneficial coagulation profile, less antigenicity, and antioxidant properties.

   a. **Indications** include use as a plasma volume-expanding agent in shock from hemorrhage, trauma, sepsis, and burns. Urine output typically increases acutely secondary to osmotic diuresis and must not be misinterpreted as a sign of adequate peripheral perfusion in this setting.

   b. **Elimination** is hepatic and renal. Patients with renal impairment are particularly subject to initial volume overload and tissue accumulation of hetastarch with repeated administration. In these patients, initial volume resuscitation accomplished with hetastarch should be maintained with another plasma volume expander, such as albumin or crystalloid.

   c. **Laboratory abnormalities** include elevations in serum amylase to approximately twice normal without alteration in pancreatic function.

d. **Dosing** of hetastarch 6% solution is 30 to 60 g (500 to 1,000 mL), with the total daily dose not exceeding 1.2 g/kg (20 mL/kg) or 90 g (1,500 mL). In hemorrhagic shock, hetastarch solution can be administered at a rate of 1.2 g/kg/hour (20 mL/kg/hour). Slower rates of administration generally are used in patients with burns or septic shock. In individuals with severe renal impairment (creatinine clearance <10 mL/minute), the usual dose of hetastarch can be administered initially, but subsequent doses should be reduced by 50% to 75%.

D. **Principles of fluid management.** A normal individual consumes an average of 2,000 to 2,500 mL of water daily. Daily water losses include approximately 1,000 to 1,500 mL in urine and 250 mL in stool. The minimum amount of urinary output that is required to excrete the catabolic end products of metabolism is approximately 800 mL. An additional 750 mL of insensible water loss occurs daily via the skin and respiratory tract. Insensible losses increase with hypermetabolism, fever, and hyperventilation.

1. **Maintenance.** Maintenance fluids should be administered at a rate that is sufficient to maintain a urine output of 0.5 to 1 mL/kg/hour. Maintenance fluid requirements can be approximated on the basis of body weight as follows: 100 mL/kg/day for the first 10 kg, 50 mL/kg/day for the second 10 kg, and 20 mL/kg/day for each subsequent 10 kg. Maintenance fluids in general should contain Na^+ (1 to 2 mmol/kg/day) and K^+ [0.5 to 1 mmol/kg/day (e.g., D5/0.45% NaCl + 20 to 30 mmol K^+/L)].

2. **Preoperative management.** Pre-existing volume and electrolyte abnormalities should be corrected before operation whenever possible. Consideration of duration and route of loss provides important information regarding the extent of fluid and electrolyte abnormalities.

3. **Intraoperative fluid management** requires replacement of preoperative deficit as well as ongoing losses (Table 4-4). Intraoperative losses include maintenance fluids for the duration of the case, hemorrhage, and "third-space losses." The maintenance fluid requirement is calculated as detailed previously (see Section IV.D.1). Acute blood loss can be replaced with a volume of crystalloid that is three to four times the blood loss or with an equal volume of colloid or blood. Intraoperative insensible and third-space fluid losses depend on the size of the incision and the extent of tissue trauma and dissection and can be replaced with an appropriate volume of lactated Ringer's solution. Small incisions with minor tissue trauma (e.g., inguinal hernia repair) result in third-space losses of approximately 1 to 3 mL/kg/hour. Medium-sized incisions with moderate tissue trauma (e.g., uncomplicated sigmoidectomy) result in third-space losses of approximately 3 to 7 mL/kg/hour. Larger incisions and operations with extensive tissue trauma and dissection (e.g., pancreaticoduodenectomy) can result in third-space losses of approximately 9 to 11 mL/kg/hour or greater.

4. **Postoperative fluid management** requires careful evaluation of the patient. Sequestration of extracellular fluid into the sites of injury or operative trauma can continue for 12 or more hours after operation. Urine output should be monitored closely and intravascular volume repleted to maintain a urine output of 0.5 to 1 mL/kg/hour. GI losses that exceed 250 mL/day from nasogastric or gastrostomy tube suction

TABLE 4-4	Estimation of Intraoperative Fluid Loss and Guide for Replacement
Preoperative deficit	
Maintenance IVF × hr NPO, plus preexisting deficit related to disease state	
Maintenance fluids	
Maintenance IVF × duration of case	
Third-space and insensible losses	
1–3 mL/kg/hr for minor procedure (small incision)	
3–7 mL/kg/hr for moderate procedure (medium incision)	
9–11 mL/kg/hr for extensive procedure (large incision)	
Blood loss	
1 mL blood or colloid per 1 mL blood loss, or 3 mL crystalloid per 1 mL blood loss	

IVF, intravenous fluids; NPO, nothing by mouth.

should be replaced with an equal volume of crystalloid. Mobilization of perioperative third-space fluid losses typically begins 2 to 3 days after operation. Anticipation of postoperative fluid shifts should prompt careful evaluation of the patient's volume status and, if needed, consideration of diuresis before the development of symptomatic hypervolemia.

V. ACID–BASE DISORDERS

A. **Diagnostic approach**

1. **General concepts**

   a. **Acid–base homeostasis** represents equilibrium among the concentration of H^+, partial pressure of CO_2 (PCO_2), and HCO_3^-. Clinically, H^+ concentration is expressed as pH.

   b. **Normal pH** is 7.35 to 7.45. **Acidemia** refers to pH of less than 7.35, and **alkalemia** refers to pH of greater than 7.45.

   c. **Acidosis and alkalosis** describe processes that cause the accumulation of acid or alkali, respectively. The terms *acidosis* and *acidemia* and the terms *alkalosis* and *alkalemia* are often used interchangeably, but such usage is inaccurate. A patient, for example, may be acidemic while alkalosis is occurring.

   d. **Laboratory studies** that are necessary for the initial evaluation of acid–base disturbances include arterial pH, arterial PCO_2 ($PaCO_2$) (normal is 35 to 45 mm Hg), and serum electrolytes [HCO_3^-

TABLE 4-5	Expected Compensation for Simple Acid–Base Disorders		
Primary Disorder	Initial Change	Compensatory Response	Expected Compensation
Metabolic acidosis	HCO_3^- decrease	P_{CO_2} decrease	P_{CO_2} decrease $= 1.2 \times \Delta HCO_3^-$
Metabolic alkalosis	HCO_3^- increase	P_{CO_2} increase	P_{CO_2} increase $= 0.7 \times \Delta HCO_3^-$
Respiratory acidosis	P_{CO_2} increase	HCO_3^- increase	Acute: HCO_3^- increase $= 0.1 \times \Delta P_{CO_2}$ Chronic: HCO_3^- increase $= 0.35 \times \Delta P_{CO_2}$
Respiratory alkalosis	P_{CO_2} decrease	HCO_3^- decrease	Acute: HCO_3^- decrease $= 0.2 \times \Delta P_{CO_2}$ Chronic: HCO_3^- decrease $= 0.5 \times \Delta P_{CO_2}$

(normal is 22 to 31 mmol/L)]. Although base-excess or base-deficit calculations can be made, this information does not add substantially to the evaluation.

2. **Compensatory response to primary disorders.** Disorders that initially alter Pa_{CO_2} are termed *respiratory acidosis* or *alkalosis*. Alternatively, disorders that initially affect plasma HCO_3^- concentration are termed *metabolic acidosis* or *alkalosis*. Primary metabolic disorders stimulate respiratory responses that act to return the ratio of P_{CO_2} to HCO_3^- (and therefore the pH) toward normal. Similarly, primary respiratory disturbances elicit countervailing metabolic responses that also act to normalize pH. As a general rule, these compensatory responses do not normalize pH because to do so would remove the stimulus for compensation. By convention, these compensating changes are termed *secondary, respiratory,* or *metabolic* compensation for the primary disturbance. The amount of compensation to be expected from either a primary respiratory or metabolic disorder is presented in Table 4-5. Significant deviations from these expected values suggest the presence of a mixed acid–base disturbance.

B. **Primary metabolic disorders**

1. **Metabolic acidosis** results from the accumulation of nonvolatile acids, reduction in renal acid excretion, or loss of alkali. The most common causes of metabolic acidosis are listed in Table 4-6. Metabolic acidosis

TABLE 4-6	Causes of Metabolic Acidosis
Increased anion gap	Renal tubular dysfunction
Increased acid production	Renal tubular acidosis
Ketoacidosis	Hypoaldosteronism
Diabetic	Potassium-sparing diuretics
Alcoholic	Loss of alkali
Starvation	Diarrhea
Lactic acidosis	Ureterosigmoidostomy
Toxic ingestion (salicylates, ethylene glycol, methanol)	Carbonic anhydrase inhibitors
Renal failure	Administration of HCl (ammonium chloride, cationic amino acids)
Normal anion gap (hyperchloremic)	

has few specific signs. The appropriate diagnosis depends on the clinical setting and laboratory tests.

a. **The anion gap** (AG; normal = 12 ± 2 mmol/L) represents the anions, other than Cl^- and HCO_3^-, which are necessary to counterbalance Na^+ electrically (all values are in mmol/L):

$$AG = Na^+ - [Cl^- + HCO_3^-]$$

It is useful diagnostically to classify metabolic acidosis into increased or normal AG metabolic acidosis.

(1) **Increased AG metabolic acidosis** (Table 4-6).

(2) **Normal AG (hyperchloremic) metabolic acidosis** (Table 4-6).

b. **Treatment of metabolic acidosis** must be directed primarily at the underlying cause of the acid–base disturbance. Bicarbonate therapy should be considered in patients with moderate-to-severe metabolic acidosis only after the primary cause has been addressed. The HCO_3^- deficit (mmol/L) can be estimated using the following equation:

$$HCO_3^- \text{ deficit} \left(\frac{mmol}{L} \right) = \text{body weight (kg)} \times 0.4$$

$$\times \left[\text{desired } HCO_3^- \left(\frac{mmol}{L} \right) - \text{measured } HCO_3^- \left(\frac{mmol}{L} \right) \right]$$

This equation serves to provide only a rough estimate of the deficit because the volume of HCO_3^- distribution and the rate of ongoing H^+ production are variable.

- (1) **Rate of HCO_3^- replacement.** In nonurgent situations, the estimated HCO_3^- deficit can be repaired by administering a continuous intravenous infusion over 4 to 8 hours [a 50-mL ampule of 8.4% $NaHCO_3$ solution (provides 50 mmol HCO_3^-) can be added to 1 L of D5 W or 0.45% of NaCl]. In urgent situations, the entire deficit can be repaired by administering a bolus over several minutes. The goal of HCO_3^- therapy should be to raise the arterial blood pH to 7.20 or the HCO_3^- concentration to 10 mmol/L. One should not attempt to normalize pH with bicarbonate administration because the risks of bicarbonate therapy (e.g., hypernatremia, hypercapnia, cerebrospinal fluid acidosis, or overshoot alkalosis) are likely to be increased. Serial arterial blood gases and serum electrolytes should be obtained to assess the response to HCO_3^- therapy.
- (2) **Lactic acidosis.** Correction of the underlying disorder is the primary therapy for lactic acidosis. Reversal of circulatory failure, hypoxemia, or sepsis reduces the rate of lactate production and enhances its removal. Because the use of $NaHCO_3$ in lactic acidosis is controversial, no definite recommendations can be made.

2. **Metabolic alkalosis (Table 4-7)**
   a. **Causes**
   - (1) **Chloride-responsive metabolic alkalosis** in the surgical patient is typically associated with extracellular fluid volume deficits. The most common causes of metabolic alkalosis in the surgical patient include inadequate fluid resuscitation or diuretic therapy (e.g., contraction alkalosis), acid loss through GI secretions (e.g. nasogastric suctioning and vomiting), and the exogenous administration of HCO_3^- or HCO_3^- precursors (e.g. citrate in blood). Posthypercapnic metabolic alkalosis occurs after the rapid correction of chronic respiratory acidosis. Under normal circumstances, the excess in bicarbonate that is generated by any of these processes is excreted rapidly in the urine. Consequently, maintenance of metabolic alkalosis requires impairment of renal HCO_3^- excretion, most commonly due to volume and chloride depletion. Because replenishment of Cl^- corrects the metabolic alkalosis in these conditions, each is classified as Cl^--responsive metabolic alkalosis.
   - (2) **Chloride-unresponsive metabolic alkalosis** is encountered less frequently in surgical patients and usually results from mineralocorticoid excess. Hyperaldosteronism, marked hypokalemia, renal failure, renal tubular Cl^- wasting (Bartter syndrome), and chronic edematous states are associated with chloride-unresponsive metabolic alkalosis.
   b. **Diagnosis.** Although the cause of metabolic alkalosis is usually apparent in the surgical patient, measurement of the urinary

TABLE 4-7	Causes of Metabolic Alkalosis
Associated with extracellular fluid volume (chloride) depletion	
Vomiting or gastric drainage	
Diuretic therapy	
Posthypercapnic alkalosis	
Associated with mineralocorticoid excess	
Cushing syndrome	
Primary aldosteronism	
Bartter syndrome	
Severe K^+ depletion	
Excessive alkali intake	

chloride concentration may be useful for differentiating these disorders. A urine Cl^- concentration of less than 15 mmol/L suggests inadequate fluid resuscitation, ongoing GI loss from emesis or nasogastric suctioning, diuretic administration, or post-hypercapnia as the cause of the metabolic alkalosis. A urine Cl^- concentration of greater than 20 mmol/L suggests mineralocorticoid excess, alkali loading, concurrent diuretic administration, or the presence of severe hypokalemia.

   c. **Treatment principles** in metabolic alkalosis include identifying and removing underlying causes, discontinuing exogenous alkali, and repairing Cl^-, K^+, and volume deficits. Because metabolic alkalosis generally is well tolerated, rapid correction of this disorder usually is not necessary.

   (1) **Initial therapy** should include the correction of volume deficits (with 0.9% NaCl) and hypokalemia. Patients with vomiting or nasogastric suctioning also may benefit from H_2-receptor antagonists or other acid–suppressing medications.

   (2) **Edematous patients.** Chloride administration does not enhance HCO_3^- excretion because it does not correct the reduced effective arterial blood volume. Acetazolamide (5 mg/kg/day intravenously or orally) facilitates fluid mobilization while decreasing renal HCO_3^- reabsorption. However, tachyphylaxis may develop after 2 to 3 days.

(3) **Severe alkalemia** (HCO_3^- >40 mmol/L), especially in the presence of symptoms, may require more aggressive correction. The infusion of acidic solutions is occasionally indicated in the patient with severe refractory metabolic alkalosis and chloride loss, typically due to massive nasogastric drainage or complete prepyloric obstruction. Ammonium chloride (NH_4Cl) is hepatically converted to urea and HCl. The amount of NH_4Cl that is required can be estimated using the following equation:

$$NH_4Cl \text{ (mmol)} = 0.2 \times \text{weight (kg)} \times [103 - \text{serum } Cl^- \text{ (mmol)}].$$

NH_4Cl is prepared by adding 100 or 200 mmol (20 to 40 mL of the 26.75% NH_4Cl concentrate) to 500 to 1,000 mL of 0.9% NaCl. This solution should be administered at a rate that does not exceed 5 mL/minute. Approximately one half of the calculated volume of NH_4Cl should be administered, at which time the acid–base status and Cl^- concentration should be repeated to determine the necessity for further therapy. NH_4Cl is contraindicated in hepatic failure.

(4) **HCl** [0.1 N (normal), administered intravenously] corrects metabolic alkalosis more rapidly. The amount of H^+ to administer can be estimated using the following equation:

$$H^+ \text{ (mmol)} = 0.5 \times \text{weight (kg)} \times [103 - \text{serum } Cl^- \text{ (mmol/L)}].$$

To prepare 0.1 N HCl, mix 100 mmol of HCl in 1 L of sterile water. The calculated amount of 0.1 N HCl must be administered via a central venous catheter over 24 hours. The HCO_3^- concentration can be safely reduced by 8 to 12 mmol/L over 12 to 24 hours.

(5) **Dialysis** can be considered in the volume-overloaded patient with renal failure and intractable metabolic alkalosis.

C. **Primary respiratory disorders**

1. **Respiratory acidosis** occurs when alveolar ventilation is insufficient to excrete metabolically produced CO_2. Common causes in the surgical patient include respiratory center depression (e.g., drugs and organic disease), neuromuscular disorders, and cardiopulmonary arrest. Chronic respiratory acidosis may occur in pulmonary diseases, such as chronic emphysema and bronchitis. Chronic hypercapnia may also result from primary alveolar hypoventilation or alveolar hypoventilation related to extreme obesity (e.g., Pickwickian syndrome) or from thoracic skeletal abnormalities. The diagnosis of acute respiratory acidosis usually is evident from the clinical situation, especially if respiration is obviously depressed. Appropriate therapy is correction of the underlying disorder. In cases of acute respiratory acidosis, there is no indication for $NaHCO_3$ administration.

2. **Respiratory alkalosis** is the result of acute or chronic hyperventilation. The causes of respiratory alkalosis include acute hypoxia (e.g.,

TABLE 4-8	Common Causes of Mixed Acid–Base Disorders

Metabolic acidosis and respiratory acidosis

Cardiopulmonary arrest

Severe pulmonary edema

Salicylate and sedative overdose

Pulmonary disease with superimposed renal failure or sepsis

Metabolic acidosis and respiratory alkalosis

Salicylate overdose

Sepsis

Combined hepatic and renal insufficiency

Metabolic alkalosis and respiratory acidosis

Chronic pulmonary disease, with superimposed:
    Diuretic therapy
    Steroid therapy

Vomiting

Reduction in hypercapnia by mechanical ventilation

Metabolic alkalosis and respiratory alkalosis

Pregnancy with vomiting

Chronic liver disease treated with diuretic therapy

Cardiopulmonary arrest treated with bicarbonate therapy and mechanical ventilation

Metabolic acidosis and alkalosis

Vomiting superimposed on
    Renal failure
    Diabetic ketoacidosis
    Alcoholic ketoacidosis

pneumonia, pneumothorax, pulmonary edema, and bronchospasm), chronic hypoxia (e.g., cyanotic heart disease and anemia), and respiratory center stimulation (e.g., anxiety, fever, Gram-negative sepsis, salicylate intoxication, central nervous system disease, cirrhosis, and pregnancy). Excessive ventilation may also cause respiratory alkalosis in the mechanically ventilated patient. Depending on its severity and acuteness, hyperventilation may or may not be clinically apparent. Clinical findings are nonspecific. As in respiratory acidosis, the only effective treatment is correction of the underlying disorder.

D. **Mixed acid–base disorders.** When two or three primary acid–base disturbances occur simultaneously, a patient is said to have a mixed acid–base disorder. As summarized in Table 4-5, the respiratory or metabolic compensation for a simple primary disorder follows a predictable pattern. Significant deviation from these patterns suggests the presence of a mixed disorder. Table 4-8 lists some common causes of mixed acid–base disturbances. The diagnosis of mixed acid–base disorders depends principally on evaluation of the clinical setting and on interpretation of acid–base patterns. However, even normal acid–base patterns may conceal mixed disorders.

5 Hemostasis and Transfusion Therapy

Alejandro Bribriesco and Michael Avidan

There are two main goals of hemostasis: (1) **prevent bleeding from defects in vessel walls via the temporary formation of localized, stable clot** and (2) **repair of the injured vessel wall.**

I. **MECHANISMS OF HEMOSTASIS.** Hemostasis is centered on the creation and destruction of a fibrin-cross-linked platelet plug (thrombus). Thrombus formation is **limited to the area of vessel injury** and **is temporary** in nature. This involves a complex interplay of thrombotic, anticoagulant, and fibrinolytic processes that occur simultaneously. Injury, disease, medications, and scores of other factors can tip the homeostatic balance resulting in life-threatening hemorrhagic or thrombotic complications.

A. **Thrombus formation** occurs in response to endothelial damage that exposes collagen (subendothelial matrix) and tissue factor (TF) (smooth muscle) to circulating blood (*N Engl J Med.* 2008;359:938). Two critical and interdependent events occur simultaneously to create a stable, fibrin-cross-linked thrombus: (1) platelet plug formation and (2) blood coagulation.

1. **Platelet plug formation:** Exposed subendothelial collagen interacts with glycoprotein (GP) Ia/IIA and VI on platelets leading to tethering at an injured site. Platelet adhesion is reinforced by Von Willebrand factor (vWF) interaction with GP Ib/V/IX. Engaged GP receptors further activate platelets leading to release of vasoactive agents and expression of important adhesions molecules, such as GP IIb/IIIa involved in fibrin cross-linking of platelets.

2. **Blood coagulation** refers to the **generation of fibrin via thrombin** as the end-product of activation of serine proteases known as coagulation "factors." These include both enzymatic proteins and cofactors (e.g., factors V and VIII). As with platelet plug formation, blood coagulation is initiated by endothelial disruption with uncovering of TF, a membrane protein expressed on multiple cell types including vascular cells such as fibroblasts and medial smooth-muscle cells. Importantly, TF is the **sole initiator of thrombin generation** and therefore fibrin formation.

3. **Cell-based model of coagulation (*Thromb Haemost.* 2001;85:958):** Traditionally, the coagulation network was divided into intrinsic and extrinsic pathways (Fig. 5-1). Although useful for *in vitro* studies, this dichotomy does not reflect the *in vivo* environment. Recently a

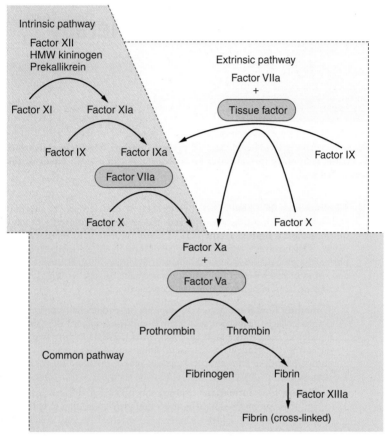

Figure 5-1. Blood coagulation cascade. Plasma zymogens are sequentially converted to active proteases (*arrows*). Nonenzymatic protein cofactors (*ovals*) are required at several stages of the cascade. Factors IX and X and prothrombin are activated on phospholipid surfaces. Thrombin cleaves fibrinogen, yielding fibrin monomers that polyme rize to form a clot. HMW, high molecular weight.

cell-based model of coagulation has developed that focuses on three critical steps (initiation, activation, propagation) with cellular TF as key.

    a. Initiation: Cells bearing TF are exposed to circulating factor VIIa creating a complex (extrinsic pathway) that activates both factor Xa and factor XIa (intrinsic pathway). This Xa–Va complex (prothrombinase complex) initiates thrombin activation as "the common pathway."

    b. Amplification: As noted above, vessel injury localizes and activates platelets at a site of vascular injury. In the amplification stage, thrombin fully activates platelet that allows accumulation of activated factors V, VIII, and XI on the platelet's phospholipid surface membrane.

   c. **Propagation:** Finally, the congregated factors assemble into the "Tenase" complex (VIIIa, IXa) and the prothrombinase complex that leads to large-scale production of thrombin **(thrombin burst).** Large amounts of thrombin are then available to (1) activate factors V, VIII, IX for further coagulation propagation (2) convert fibrinogen to fibrin, and (3) activate platelets via Par4 receptor, and (4) activate factor XIII that ultimately cross-links fibrin into a "mesh" that is required for stable platelet–platelet adhesion (thrombus). **Fibrinogen (factor I)** is important for thrombus strength and can compensate for low platelet levels.

B. **Endogenous anticoagulants** are important to restrict coagulation to the specific area of vascular injury and prevent pathologic thrombosis.

   1. **The endothelium** serves as a physical barrier sequestering subendothelial factors (TF, collagen) from platelets and circulating coagulation factors. Endothelial cells actively release antiplatelet factors [nitric oxide, prostacyclin (PGI_2)] as well as express surface enzymes that degrade ADP, a platelet-activating factor. Intact endothelial cells are also coated with thrombomodulin (see below) and heparin-like glycosaminoglycans that facilitate antithrombin (AT) activation.

   2. **AT (previously known as antithrombin III)** inhibits coagulation by binding several clotting factors (e.g., thrombin and factor Xa) and producing complexes that are cleared from the circulation. Heparin markedly accelerates AT-induced factor inhibition, increasing factor clearance, and leading to anticoagulation.

   3. **The thrombomodulin–protein C–protein S system:** Thrombomodulin, an endothelial membrane protein, binds with thrombin creating "anticoagulant thrombin" that accelerates the activation of protein C, a vitamin K-dependent proenzyme. Activated protein C inactivates factors Va and VIIIa in the presence of protein S.

   4. **Other anticoagulant factors** include TF pathway inhibitor (TFPI) that inactivates the TF/VIIa/Xa complex.

C. **Fibrinolysis** involves the dissolution and remodeling of thrombus (clot busting). Plasminogen is a plasma zymogen that is incorporated into a forming thrombus. Tissue plasminogen activator (tPA) converts plasminogen to its active form plasmin, breaks down clot, and allows for subsequent wound healing. Other plasminogen activators include urokinase and streptokinase. As with thrombus formation, fibrinolysis involves a complex interplay of positive and negative regulatory mechanisms. Negative feedback includes (1) α-2 antiplasmin in blood, (2) plasminogen activator inhibitor (PAI-1) from platelets and endothelial cells and (3) thrombin-activated fibrinolytic inhibitor (TAFI).

II. **EVALUATION OF HEMOSTASIS.** A detailed history and physical examination constitute the most important screening tools for hemostasis disorders in

TABLE 5-1 Preoperative Evaluation of Hemostasis, Bleeding Disorder, and Anemia

	History	Physical Exam	Drugs	Labs

Platelets	• Easy bruising
	• Frequent nosebleeds
	• Prolonged bleeding after:
	  • Minor injury
	  • Dental procedures
	  • Surgery
	  • Childbirth
		• Mucosal bleeding
		• Petechiae
		• Purpura
			• ASA
			• Clopidogrel
			• NSAIDs
				CBC with differential

Coagulation	• After unrecognized injury, **delayed** development of:
	  • Hematomas
	  • Hemarthrosis
	• Nutritional status (i.e., vitamin K)
	• Family history of males with bleeding disorder (i.e., hemophilia)
	• Atrial fibrillation, DVT/PE, or other conditions requiring anticoagulant therapy
		• Joint fullness, bruising
		• Hematomas
		• Broad/large scar formation
			• Warfarin
			• Heparin, LMWH
			• Herbs, supplements
				PT/INR
				PTT

Global	• Need for previous transfusions • Melena, hematochezia • Hematemesis • Hemoptysis • Family history of bleeding disorders	• Skin, conjunctival pallor • Tachycardia • Hypotension • Flow murmur		CBC Reticulocyte count Iron studies

Abbreviations: ASA, Aspirin; CBC, complete blood count; DVT, deep vein thrombosis; LMWH, low molecular weight heparin; NSAID, nonsteroidal anti-inflammatory drug; PE, pulmonary embolism; PT/INR, prothrombin time/international normalized ratio; PTT, partial thromboplastin time.

surgical patients (Table 5-1). A family history of bleeding or bleeding disorders should be elicited. Laboratory studies can further characterize or identify clinical suspicion. Although surgical patients can have hereditary disorders of hemostasis, acquired defects and medications affecting hemostasis are most common in this patient population. In cases of hereditary hemostasis disorders, it is often helpful to work with the patient's hematologist in perioperative management. Below, evaluation is divided into evaluation of platelets, coagulation, and global hemostasis.

A. **Evaluation of platelets**
 1. **Laboratory evaluation**
    a. **Platelet count** (140,000 to 400,000/μL). Abnormalities in platelet number should be confirmed with a peripheral smear. Both thrombocytopenia and significant thrombocytosis require further investigation. It should be noted that the average life span of a normal platelet is **7 days.**
    b. **Platelet function.** No single test is adequate for screening platelet dysfunction due to limited sensitivity; therefore, the risk or severity of surgical bleeding cannot be reliably assessed. **Bleeding time** (2.5 to 9 minutes) measures the duration of bleeding to stop after a standardized superficial cut. Qualitative platelet disorders, von Willebrand disease (vWD), vasculitides, and connective tissue disorders prolong bleeding time.

 2. **Platelet disorders**
    a. **Thrombocytopenia** is defined as a platelet count of less than 140,000/μL. If platelet function is normal, thrombocytopenia is infrequently the cause of bleeding unless counts are below 50,000/μL. Severe spontaneous bleeding occurs with platelet counts under 10,000/μL. Intramuscular injections, rectal examinations, suppositories, or enemas should be limited in patients with severe thrombocytopenia (<10,000/μL). Occult liver disease must be considered for thrombocytopenia of unknown etiology.
    b. **Drug-induced thrombocytopenia.** Many drugs can affect platelet production or cause increased platelet destruction thereby causing or exacerbating bleeding. Common drugs include antibiotics (trimethoprim–sulfamethoxazole, penicillins, rifampin), thiazide diuretics, and chemotherapeutic agents. Increased destruction of platelets is most commonly the result of an immune mechanism in which platelets are destroyed by complement activation by drug–antibody complexes. **All nonessential drugs should be discontinued until the cause of the thrombocytopenia is identified.** Drug-induced thrombocytopenia typically resolves within 7 to 10 days after cessation and clearance of the offending agent. Prednisone (1 mg/kg/day orally) may facilitate recovery of platelet counts.
    c. **Heparin-induced thrombocytopenia (HIT)** is a unique form of drug-induced thrombocytopenia in which two different forms have been recognized.

(1) **HIT type I** is a nonimmune, heparin-associated thrombocytopenia that typically begins within 4 days of initiation of heparin therapy. Platelet counts range between 100,000 and 140,000/μL. The incidence ranges from 5% to 30%. This form of HIT may not require cessation of heparin.

(2) **HIT type II** is a severe immune-mediated syndrome caused by heparin-dependent antiplatelet antibodies (anti-PF4-heparin complex) occurring 5 to 10 days after initial exposure to heparin but within hours after re-exposure. Platelet counts are often less than 100,000/μL or drop by more than 30% from baseline. In a minority of cases, thrombotic events ensue, including extensive arterial and venous thrombosis (*N Engl J Med.* 2006;355:809). If HIT is suspected, **all heparin products should be stopped immediately** until the diagnosis is refuted. Sources of heparin include flushes and heparin-coated catheters.

(a) **Lab tests:** HIT is a clinical diagnosis with laboratory findings. The enzyme-linked immunosorbent assay (ELISA, HIT panel) and serotonin release assay (SRA) may suggest the diagnosis if the associated clinical features are present. The ELISA is a sensitive test that is useful for screening but has low specificity. The SRA is the gold standard due to its high sensitivity and specificity and often used as a confirmatory test. However, SRA is expensive and not widely available.

(b) **Treatment:** Because thrombotic complications can continue even after the cessation of heparin, anticoagulation with nonheparin anticoagulants such a direct thrombin inhibitor (lepirudin or argatroban; see Section III.D.3) is recommended if there are no contraindications to anticoagulation. Platelet transfusion will exacerbate the process and is contraindicated. **If HIT is present, warfarin administration can potentiate a hypercoagulable state and has been associated with the development of venous limb gangrene.** Therefore, warfarin therapy should not be initiated until (1) platelet count >150K and (2) adequate alternative anticoagulant control have been achieved.

(3) **Dilutional thrombocytopenia** can occur with rapid blood product replacement for massive hemorrhage. No formula predicts accurate platelet requirements in this setting (see section on "Massive Transfusion" for further discussion).

(4) **Other causes of thrombocytopenia** include disseminated intravascular coagulation (DIC), sepsis, immune thrombocytopenic purpura (ITP), thrombotic thrombocytopenic purpura (TTP), hemolytic uremic syndrome (HUS), dialysis, and hematopoietic disorders.

3. **Thrombocytosis** is defined as a platelet count greater than 600,000/μL. Essential thrombocytosis is caused by myeloproliferative disease. Secondary thrombocytosis occurs with splenectomy, iron deficiency,

malignancy, or chronic inflammatory disease. Aspirin therapy (81 mg/day orally) is useful in prevention of thrombotic events in patients with myeloproliferative disorders and in decreasing fetal loss in pregnant women. Secondary thrombocytosis is generally not associated with an increased thrombotic risk and usually requires no specific therapy.

4. **Qualitative platelet dysfunction**

   a. **Acquired defects of platelets** are caused by uremia, liver disease, or cardiopulmonary bypass. Desmopressin acetate (DDAVP, $0.3 \mu g/kg$ intravenously 1 hour before operation) may limit bleeding from platelet dysfunction, particularly in uremic patients. Conjugated estrogens (0.6 mg/kg/day intravenously for 5 days) also can improve hemostatic function.

   b. **Hereditary defects** of platelet dysfunction (e.g., vWD, Bernard–Soulier syndrome, Glanzmann thrombasthenia, and storage pool defects) are less common and usually warrant consultation with a hematologist.

5. **Antiplatelet medications**

   a. **Aspirin** irreversibly acetylates cyclooxygenase, inhibiting platelet synthesis of thromboxane A2 and causing decreased platelet function. It is often used in the prevention and treatment of acute transient ischemic attacks, stroke, myocardial infarction, and coronary and vascular graft occlusion. Aspirin should be discontinued about 1 week before elective nonvascular operations to allow new, functional platelets to form.

   b. **Clopidogrel (Plavix)** is a thienopyridine that irreversibly inhibits platelet function by binding to the adenosine diphosphate (ADP) receptor that promotes aggregation and secretion. It is used to decrease thrombotic events in percutaneous coronary and vascular stenting and patients with unstable angina. Although the half-life of clopidogrel is 8 hours, the bleeding time remains prolonged over 3 to 7 days, demonstrating that complete recovery of platelet function takes 5 days. Therefore, patients should discontinue clopidogrel therapy 7 days prior to elective operations to decrease the risk of bleeding complications. Specifically, clopidogrel has become more prevalent with the increased use of coronary artery stents that require a full year of antiplatelet treatment for drug-eluting stents and at least 4 weeks with bare metal stents (*Chest*. 2008;133:776S). Discontinuation of clopidogrel within this time period carries a significant risk of stent thrombosis with resultant myocardial infarction. Continuation of aspirin, consultation with a cardiologist and consideration of preoperative "bridge" with GP IIb/IIIa inhibitors (see below) should be considered.

   c. **GP IIb/IIIa inhibitors include** abciximab (ReoPro), tirofiban (Aggrastat), and eptifibatide (Integrilin) and function by blocking platelet adhesion to fibrin. These agents are used in preventing coronary artery thrombosis after coronary angioplasty or in unstable angina. Although they have relatively short half-lives (0.5 to 2.5 hours), the bleeding time may remain elevated for longer periods. It is recommended that surgery be delayed 12 hours after discontinuing abciximab and 4 hours after discontinuing tirofiban or eptifibatide. Zero-balance ultrafiltration may be beneficial in patients who need immediate surgical interventions (*Perfusion.* 2002;17:33).

d. **Other medications: Dextran** is used to reduce perioperative thrombotic events such as bypass graft occlusion because of its ability to decrease platelet aggregation and adhesion. **Nonsteroidal anti-inflammatory drugs (NSAIDS)** such as ketorolac (Toradol) inhibit cyclooxygenase, reversibly inhibiting platelet aggregation. **Hetastarch** can cause a transient decrease in platelet counts and should be used judiciously for perioperative colloid blood volume expansion

6. **Platelet transfusions**

a. **Indications.** Platelet transfusions are used to control bleeding that is caused by thrombocytopenia or platelet dysfunction and to prevent spontaneous bleeding in situations of severe thrombocytopenia (<10,000/μL). In cases of bleeding or for minor surgical procedures, the transfusion threshold is often increased to a platelet count of less than 50,000/μL. For severe ongoing hemorrhage, before major operations and trauma, platelet counts greater than 100,000/μL should be the goal (*Ann Surg.* 2010;251:604). Preparations, volumes, and expected response are summarized in Table 5-2.

b. **Complications associated with platelet transfusions**

(1) **Alloimmunization** occurs in 50% to 75% of patients receiving repeated platelet transfusions and presents as a failure of the platelet count to increase significantly after a transfusion. In patients who need long-term platelet therapy, human leukocyte antigen-matched single-donor platelets slow the onset of alloimmunization.

(2) **Post-transfusion purpura** is a rare complication of platelet transfusions seen in previously transfused individuals and multiparous women. It is usually caused by antibodies that develop in response to a specific platelet antigen Pl[A1] from the donor platelets. This condition presents with severe thrombocytopenia, purpura, and bleeding occurring 7 to 10 days after platelet transfusion. Although fatal bleeding can occur, the disease is typically self-limiting. Plasmapheresis or an infusion of intravenous immunoglobulin may be helpful.

B. **Evaluation of coagulation**

1. **Laboratory evaluation**

a. **Prothrombin time (PT)** (11 to 14 seconds) is the clotting time measured after the addition of thromboplastin, phospholipids, and calcium to citrated plasma. This test assesses the extrinsic and common pathways and is most sensitive to factor VII deficiency. Test reagents vary in their responsiveness to warfarin-induced anticoagulation; therefore, the **international normalized ratio (INR)** is used to standardize PT reporting between laboratories.

TABLE 5-2	Blood Products			
Blood Product	Volume (mL)	Additional Factors	Expected Response	Common Use
PRBC 1 unit	200–250	Fibrinogen: 10–75 mg Clotting factors: none	Increase: 1 mg/dl Hgb 3% HCT	ABLA MTP Surgical blood loss
Platelets SDP (apheresis) RDP[b]	300–500 50 per unit	Fibrinogen: 2–4 mg/mL (360–900 mg) Clotting factors: equivalent of 200–250 mL of plasma (hemostatic level) "6 pack" of pooled RDP similar to SDP	Increase: 30–60 K/mm^3 Increase: 7–10 K/mm^3 per unit	Plt count <10K MTP Bleeding with known qualitative plt defect
FFP[a] 1 unit	180–300	Fibrinogen: 400 mg Clotting factors: 1 mL contains 1 active unit of each factor	Decrease: PT/INR PTT	Coagulopathy Warfarin overdose DIC
Cryo 10 pack		Fibrinogen: 1200–1500 Clotting factors: VIII, vWF, XII	Decrease: PT/INR PTT Increase: fibrinogen level	vWD DIC Hemophilia A

[a]Note: Duration of FFP effect is approximately 6 hours. INR of FFP is 1.6 to 1.7.
[b]4–10 RDP units are pooled prior to transfusion.
Abbreviations: ABLA, acute blood loss anemia; Cryo, cryoprecipitate; FFP, fresh-frozen plasma; Hbg, hemoglobin; HCT, hematocrit; MTP, massive transfusion protocl; PRBC, packed red blood cells; plt, platelet; RDP, random donor platelets; SDP, single donor platelets.

b. **Partial thromboplastin time (PTT)** (26 to 36 seconds) is the clotting time for plasma that is pre-incubated in particulate material (causing contact activation) followed by the addition of phospholipid and calcium. Inhibitors or deficiencies of factors in the intrinsic or common pathways cause prolongation of the PTT. A prolonged PTT should be evaluated by a 50:50 mixture with normal plasma. Factor deficiencies are corrected by the addition of normal plasma, whereas PTT prolongation due to inhibitors remains abnormal.

c. **Activated clotting time (ACT)** assesses the clotting time of whole blood. A blood sample is added to a diatomate-containing tube, leading to activation of the intrinsic pathway. The ACT is used to follow coagulation in patients requiring high doses of heparin (i.e., vascular procedures, percutaneous coronary interventions, or cardiopulmonary bypass). Automated systems are available for intraoperative use, allowing accurate and rapid determinations of the state of anticoagulation. Normal ACT is less than 130 seconds, with therapeutic target values ranging from 400 to 480 seconds for cardiac bypass procedures and 250 to 350 seconds for noncardiac vascular procedures.

d. **Thrombin time (TT)** (11 to 18 seconds) is the clotting time for plasma after the addition of thrombin. Patients with a fibrinogen level of less than 100 mg/dL or with abnormal fibrinogen will have a prolonged TT. The presence of fibrin degradation products (FDPs) or heparin can also elevate the TT. Prolongation of the TT by heparin can be confirmed by the addition of protamine sulfate to the assay, resulting in normalization of the test.

e. **Factor assays.** Individual assays for specific coagulation factors can be useful in certain situations. Factor Xa activity may be used to assess the effect of low molecular weight heparin (LMWH). Factor VIII and IX levels are assessed in hemophiliacs prior to an operative procedure to guide transfusion of appropriate blood products. A fibrinogen level (150 to 360 mg/dL) can be measured directly by functional or immunologic quantitative assays. This level can be underestimated by the TT. FDP elevations (>8 μg/mL) occur in many disease states with increased fibrinogen turnover, including DIC, thromboembolic events, and during administration of fibrinolytic therapy. D-dimer levels reflect fibrinolysis and are useful in outpatient evaluations for pulmonary embolism (PE). The utility in surgical patients is less clear due to its nonspecific elevation in response to inflammation.

2. **Disorders of coagulation**

a. **Acquired factor deficiencies**

(1) **Vitamin K deficiency** leads to the production of inactive, noncarboxylated forms of **factors II (prothrombin), VII, IX, X, and proteins C and S.** The diagnosis should be considered in a patient with a prolonged PTT that corrects with a 50:50 mixture of normal plasma. Vitamin K deficiency can occur in patients without oral intake within 1 week, with biliary

obstruction, with malabsorption, and in those receiving antibiotics or warfarin.

(2) **Liver dysfunction** leads to complex alterations in coagulation through decreased synthesis of most clotting and anticlotting factors with the notable exceptions of factor VIII and vWF (from endothelium). Coagulopathy is worsened by uremic platelet dysfunction as well as thrombocytopenia from portal hypertension-associated hypersplenism. Spontaneous bleeding is infrequent, but coagulation defects should be corrected prior to invasive procedures. Fresh-frozen plasma (FFP) administration often improves the coagulopathy transiently. Any patient with liver disease should be thoroughly evaluated preoperatively including assessment of liver function (Childs-Pugh class; MELD score).

(3) **Sepsis** overstimulates the coagulation cascade reflected by decreased levels of anticoagulant factors such as protein C, protein S, and AT. This imbalance in hemostasis causes microvascular thrombi to form. These thrombi further amplify injury resulting in distal tissue ischemia and hypoxia. Therapy with activated protein C (drotrecogin alfa, Xigris) has been reported to decrease mortality in patients with severe sepsis as defined by an Acute Physiology and Chronic Health Evaluation (APACHE) II score greater than or equal to 25. However, higher rates of bleeding have been noted in patients receiving activated protein C compared to placebo (*N Engl J Med.* 2001;344:699). However, controversy exists regarding the use of activated protein C given the results of subsequent studies that question its efficacy and highlight the risks of bleeding (*N Engl J Med.* 2005;355:1332).

b. **Hemophilia** is an inherited factor deficiency of either factor VIII (hemophilia A) or factor IX (hemophilia B, Christmas disease). The diagnosis is suggested by patient history (Table 5-1) and an elevated PTT, normal PT, and normal bleeding time. Factor activity assays confirm the diagnosis and is an indicator of disease severity. Minor bleeding can often be controlled locally without the need for factor replacement therapy. DDAVP stimulates the release of vWF into the circulation, which increases factor VIII levels two- to six-fold. This may control minor bleeding in patients with mild disease. Major bleeding (e.g., during a surgical procedure) requires factor VIII replacement. Recombinant factor VIIa is FDA approved for the treatment of patients who have developed inhibitors to factor VIII or IX (see Section II.B.5.c). Cryoprecipitate contains factor VIII, vWF, and fibrinogen (Table 5-1) and can be used to treat patients with hemophilia A for control of bleeding. Purified factor IX is the treatment of choice for hemophilia B.

c. **vWD** is the **most common** inherited bleeding disorder with a prevalence as high as 1% of the general population. vWD is subcategorized (type 1 to 3) by the type of abnormality present in vWF.

DDAVP is effective to increase plasma vWF in type 1 disease but is ineffective for types 2 and 3. These disorders require replacement via blood products with high amounts of vWF and factor VIII, such as cryoprecipitate (Table 5-2).

   d. **Other inherited factor deficiencies** account for fewer than 10% of severe factor deficiencies. Deficiencies of factor XII, HMWK, or prekallikrein do not cause bleeding and require no treatment.

   e. **Inherited hypercoagulable disorders** place patients at risk for thrombosis (venous and/or arterial) and include deficiencies in body anticoagulants (AT, protein C, and protein S deficiencies), hyperhomocystinemia, and prothrombin gene mutations.

      (1) **Activated protein C resistance (factor V Leiden)** is the most common hereditary coagulation disorder accounting for 40% to 50% of inherited hypercoagulable disorders. Factor V Leiden is caused by a genetic mutation in factor V that renders it resistant to breakdown by activated protein C leading to venous thrombosis. Routine preoperative screening in asymptomatic patients is unnecessary. Therapy for venous thrombosis consists of anticoagulation with heparin followed by warfarin therapy. The role of long-term warfarin anticoagulation for patients with a single thrombotic event is undefined.

      (2) **AT deficiency** is an autosomal-dominant disorder (prevalence 1:500) that presents with recurrent venous and occasionally arterial thromboembolism, usually in the second decade of life. Assays for AT levels are typically decreased in the setting of acute thrombosis and also if the patient is receiving heparin. Patients with acute thromboembolism or previous history of thrombosis are typically anticoagulated. AT-deficient patients should have the AT level restored to more than 80% of normal activity with AT concentrate prior to operation or childbirth.

      (3) **Protein C deficiency and protein S deficiency** are risk factors for venous thrombosis. In a state of protein C or S deficiency, factors Va and VIIIa are not adequately inactivated, thereby allowing unchecked coagulation. Besides the inherited type, protein C deficiency is encountered in patients with liver failure and in those who are receiving warfarin therapy. Symptomatic patients are treated with heparin [or low-molecular-weight heparin (LMWH)] anticoagulation followed by warfarin therapy. In individuals with diminished protein C activity, effective heparin anticoagulation must be confirmed before warfarin initiation because warfarin transiently lowers protein C levels further and potentially worsens the hypercoagulable state manifested as warfarin-induced skin necrosis (see below). Patients with protein C or S deficiency but with no history of thrombosis typically do not require prophylactic anticoagulation.

   f. **Acquired hypercoagulable disorders**
      (1) **Antiphospholipid antibodies** are immunoglobulins that are targeted against antigens composed in part of platelet and

endothelial cell phospholipids. Antiphospholipid antibody disorders may be detected by **lupus anticoagulant, anticardiolipin, or other antiphospholipid antibodies.** Patients with these antibodies are at risk for arterial and venous thrombosis, recurrent miscarriages, and thrombocytopenia.

- **g. Other acquired hypercoagulable states** include malignancies, pregnancy or the use of estrogen therapy, intravascular hemolysis (e.g., hemolytic anemia or after cardiopulmonary bypass), and the localized propensity for thrombosis in arteries that have recently undergone endarterectomy, angioplasty, or placement of prosthetic vascular grafts.

3. Anticoagulation medications

- **a. Principles and indications.** Anticoagulation is used to prevent and treat thrombosis and thromboembolic events. Before therapy is instituted, careful consideration must be given to the risk of thromboembolism and to anticoagulation-induced bleeding complications. Specific indications for anticoagulation therapy are discussed in detail in other chapters. Table 5-3 summarizes selected anticoagulant medications. Relative contraindications to anticoagulation therapy include recent surgical intervention, severe trauma, intracranial bleeding, and patients at risk of falling.

- **b. Heparin**
  - **(1) Unfractionated heparin**
    - **(a) Administration.** Heparin is administered parenterally, either subcutaneously or intravenously. PTT should be measured before initiation of heparin, 6 hours after the initial bolus, and 6 hours after each change in dosing. Platelet counts should be measured daily until a maintenance dose of heparin is achieved and periodically thereafter to monitor for development of HIT.
    - **(b) Complications** that occur with heparin therapy include bleeding and HIT. If bleeding occurs, heparin should be discontinued, and immediate assessment of the PT, PTT, and complete blood count (CBC) should be undertaken. Gastrointestinal (GI) bleeding that occurs while a patient is therapeutically anticoagulated suggests an occult source and warrants further evaluation. HIT is an uncommon but potentially devastating complication of heparin therapy and must be recognized early (see Section II.A.2.c).
    - **(c) Heparin clearance** is rapid, occurring with a half-life of about 90 minutes. Reversal can be achieved more quickly with intravenous protamine sulfate. Each milligram of protamine sulfate reverses about 100 units of heparin. The PTT or ACT can be used to assess the adequacy of the reversal. Protamine should be used with caution because it can induce anaphylactoid reactions and other complications.
  - **(2) LMWH** preparations include enoxaparin, dalteparin, and tinzaparin. The anticoagulant effect of LMWH is **predominantly**

TABLE 5-3 Anticoagulant Medications

Drug	Mechanism	Metabolism	Dose for DVT Prophylaxis	Dose for Therapeutic Anticoagulation	Therapeutic Target	Reversal Agent
Heparin	Potentiates antithrombin: IIa, Xa, IXa, XIa, XIIa inhibition	Hepatic, RES and 50% renal excretion	5000 U SC twice to thrice daily	Bolus = 80 u/kg Infusion = 18 u/kg/hr; adjust to target PTT	APTT = 60–80 s	Protamine: start with 25–50 mg
LMWH (e.g., Enoxaparin)	Potentiates antithrombin: Xa inhibition	Mainly renal excretion	40 mg SC once daily	1 mg/kg SC twice daily	Chromogenic anti-Xa assay: 0.6–1 anti-Xa U/mL	None
Fondaparinux	Potentiates antithrombin: Xa inhibition	Renal	2.5 mg SC once daily	5 or 7.5 or 10 mg SC once daily	Chromogenic anti-Xa assay	None
Rivaroxiban	Direct Xa inhibition	Likely liver	10 mg PO once daily		Chromogenic anti-Xa assay	None
Warfarin	Prevents carboxylation of X, IX, VII, II, protein C and S	Hepatic, marked genetic variability		2–10 mg PO daily; adjust to target INR.	INR = 2–4	Vitamin K: 1–10 mg PO or plasma; start with 2–4 units

Agent	Mechanism	Metabolism/Excretion	Dose	Monitoring	Reversal agent
Lepirudin	Direct thrombin inhibition	Renal	Bolus = 0.4 mg/kg; Infusion = 0.15 mg/kg/hr; adjust to target PTT	APTT = 60–80 (1.5–2.5 times control)	None
Bivalirudin	Direct thrombin inhibition	Proteolytic cleavage and renal (20%)	Bolus = 1 mg/kg; Infusion = 0.2 mg/kg/hr; adjust to target PTT	APTT = 60–80 s	None
Desirudin	Direct thrombin inhibition	Renal	10–15 mg SC twice daily	Prolongs the APTT	None
Argatroban	Direct thrombin inhibition	Hepatic	Infusion = 2 mcg/kg/min; adjust to target PTT	APTT = 60–80 s; may prolong INR	None
Dabigatran etexilate	Direct thrombin inhibition	Renal (unchanged) and some conjugation with glucuronic acid	150 mg PO twice daily; 150 mg PO once daily		None

due to **factor Xa inhibition** via potentiation of AT, and LMWH results in less thrombin inhibition than unfractionated heparin. The advantages of LMWH include a more predictable anticoagulant effect, less platelet interaction, and a longer half-life. Dosing is based on weight, and laboratory monitoring is not typically needed. LMWH may be used for longer-term therapy in patients with a contraindication to oral anticoagulant treatment (e.g., pregnant patients who cannot take warfarin). Because LMWH has a longer half-life and no effective antidote, it must be used with caution in surgical patients and in those in whom a bleeding risk has been substantiated.

c. **Direct thrombin inhibitors** are a class of compounds that bind to free and fibrin-bound thrombin. These agents inhibit thrombin activation of clotting factors, fibrin formation, and platelet aggregation.

(1) **Hirudin,** an anticoagulant originally derived from leeches, has been formulated as lepirudin and bivalirudin. **Lepirudin,** recombinant hirudin, binds irreversibly to thrombin, providing effective anticoagulation. The drug is approved in patients with HIT but may be considered in other severe clotting disorders. **Bivalirudin** is a truncated form of recombinant hirudin that targets only the active site of thrombin. Bivalirudin is FDA approved for HIT as well as for use during percutaneous coronary angioplasty and stenting.

(2) **Argatroban** is a synthetic thrombin inhibitor that is also approved for treatment of HIT.

d. **Warfarin** is an oral vitamin K antagonist that causes anticoagulation by inhibiting vitamin K-mediated carboxylation of factors II, VII, IX, and X as well as proteins C and S. The vitamin K-dependent factors decay with varying half-lives, so the full warfarin anticoagulant effect is not apparent for 5 to 7 days. When immediate anticoagulation is necessary, heparin or another agent must be used initially.

(1) **Administration.** Warfarin usually is initiated with a loading dose of 5 to 10 mg/day for 2 days, followed by dose adjustment based on daily INR results. The smaller dose is more likely to produce an INR of 2 to 3 with less excess anticoagulation and decreases the risk of a hypercoagulable state caused by precipitous drops in protein C levels during initiation of warfarin therapy (*Arch Int Med.* 1999;159:46). Elderly patients, those with hepatic insufficiency, and those who are receiving parenteral nutrition or broad-spectrum antibiotics, should be given lower initial doses of warfarin. A daily dose of warfarin needed to achieve therapeutic anticoagulation usually ranges from 2 to 15 mg/day. An INR of 2 to 3 is therapeutic for most indications, but patients with prosthetic heart valves should be maintained with an INR of 2.5 to 3.5. Once a stable INR is obtained on a stable warfarin dose, it can be monitored biweekly or monthly.

(2) **Complications.** The bleeding risk in patients who are treated with warfarin is estimated to be approximately 10% per year. The risk of bleeding correlates directly with the INR. Warfarin-induced

skin necrosis, caused by dermal venous thrombosis, occurs rarely when warfarin therapy is initiated in patients who are not already anticoagulated and is often associated with hypercoagulability caused by protein C deficiency. Warfarin can produce significant birth defects and fetal death and should not be used during pregnancy. Changes in medications and diet may affect warfarin or vitamin K levels and require more vigilant INR monitoring and dose adjustment.

(3) **Reversal of warfarin-induced anticoagulation** requires up to 1 week after discontinuation of therapy. Vitamin K administration can be used to reverse warfarin anticoagulation within 1 to 2 days, but the effect can last for up to 1 week longer. The appropriate vitamin K dose depends on the INR and the urgency with which correction must be accomplished. For patients with bleeding or extremely high INR levels (>10), 10 mg of vitamin K should be administered intravenously. Serial INR levels should be followed every 6 hours. In addition, FFP can be administered to patients with ongoing hemorrhage. Recombinant human factor VIIa (see below) has also been used (100 μg/kg) off label in cases of life-threatening bleeding.

e. **Indirect factor Xa inhibitors (Fondaparinux)** are small, synthetic, heparin-like molecules that enhance AT-mediated inhibition of factor Xa. Fondaparinux has been shown to be as effective in preventing DVT after hip and knee replacement. Monitoring of coagulation parameters is usually not necessary.

4. Fibrinolytic therapy

a. Thrombolytic therapy is most often used for iliofemoral deep venous thrombosis (DVT), superior vena caval thrombosis, PE resulting in a hemodynamically unstable patient, acute thrombosis of peripheral, mesenteric, and coronary arteries, acute vascular graft occlusion, thrombosis of hemodialysis access grafts, and occlusion of venous catheters. Contraindications to fibrinolytic therapy are listed in Table 5-4. tPA (alteplase) or a recombinant analog (reteplase), as well as urokinase (Abbokinase), are used for lysis of catheter, venous, and peripheral arterial thrombi.

5. Transfusion products for coagulopathy (Table 5-2)

a. **FFP** contains all the coagulation factors. However, factors V and VIII may not be stable through the thawing process and are not reliably recovered from FFP. Therefore, it can be used to correct coagulopathies that are due to deficiencies of any other coagulation factor and is particularly useful when multiple factor deficiencies exist (e.g., liver disease or massive transfusion). FFP effects are immediate and typically **last about 6 hours.** Factor VIII and IX deficiencies are best treated using specific factor concentrates.

b. **Cryoprecipitate** is the cold-insoluble precipitate of fresh plasma and is rich in factor VIII and vWF as well as fibrinogen, fibronectin, and factor XIII. Cryoprecipitate may be used as second-line therapy in vWD or hemophilia but is most often used to correct fibrinogen deficiency in DIC or during massive transfusion.

TABLE 5-4	Contraindications to Fibrinolytic Therapy

Absolute Contraindications

Intolerable ischemia (for arterial thrombosis)

Active bleeding (not including menses)

Recent (<2 mo) stroke or neurosurgical procedure

Intracranial pathology such as neoplasm

Relative Contraindications

Recent (<10 d) major surgery, major trauma, parturition, or organ biopsy

Active peptic ulcer or recent gastrointestinal bleeding (within 2 wk)

Uncontrolled hypertension (blood pressure >180/110 mm Hg)

Recent cardiopulmonary resuscitation

Presence or high likelihood of left heart thrombus

Bacterial endocarditis

Coagulopathy or current use of warfarin

Pregnancy

Hemorrhagic diabetic retinopathy

c. **Recombinant human factor VIIa (rhFVIIa, NovoSeven)** is FDA approved for the treatment of hemophilia with inhibitors of factors VIII or XI. The recommended dose for this indication is 90 to 120 µg/kg, which can be repeated every 2 hours for 24 hours. However, the off-label use of rhFVIIa has exponentially grown as "rescue therapy" for patients with severe or dangerous bleeding that is not responsive to routine transfusion therapy. Although rhFVIIa used in blunt trauma was shown to reduce the overall blood transfusion requirement and reduce the incidence of multisystem organ failure and acute respiratory distress syndrome (*Crit Care.* 2006;10:R178; *J Trauma.* 2006;60:242), the safety of the drug is still in question. rhVIIa at pharmacologic doses may lead to unexpected thromboembolic events (stroke, MI, PE, DVT) due to its supraphysiologic activity and so NovoSeven should be used with caution (*J Am Coll Surg.* 2009;209:659). And point of fact, a recent meta-analysis of off-label rhVIIa use demonstrated an increased risk of arterial thrombosis **(including coronary artery thrombosis)** with a dose-dependent effect observed with doses >80 µg/kg (*N Engl J Med.* 2010;363:1791).

C. **Evaluation of global hemostasis**

1. **Laboratory tests:** Traditional *in vitro* tests such as PT/INR, PTT, and ACT are useful in the diagnosis and management of bleeding diathesis; however, abnormal values obtained in a test tube are not always indicative or representative of underlying hemostatic perturbation. Thromboelastrograph (TEG) evaluates hemostasis as a dynamic process where functional attributes such as kinetics of clot formation, growth, strength, and stability, are measured, thereby providing pertinent *in vivo* characterization of clot. This modality functions well in point of care situations such as during liver transplantation given the need for close monitoring and rapid evaluation of hemostasis and is currently being advocated as a tool for guiding and monitoring trauma resuscitation (*Ann Surg.* 2010;251:604) and cardiac surgery (*Anesth Analg.* 1999;88:312).

2. **Global disorders of hemostasis**

a. **DIC** has many inciting causes, including sepsis and extensive trauma or burns. The pathogenesis involves inappropriate generation of thrombin within the vasculature, leading to platelet activation, formation of fibrin thrombi, and increased fibrinolytic activity. DIC often presents with complications from microvascular thrombi that involve the vascular beds of the kidney, brain, lung, and skin. In some patients, the consumption of coagulation factors, particularly fibrinogen, and the activation of the fibrinolytic pathway can lead to bleeding. Laboratory findings in DIC include thrombocytopenia, hypofibrinogenemia, increased FDPs, and prolonged TT and PTT. Therapy begins with treatment of the underlying cause. Management of hemodynamics and oxygenation is critical. Correction of coagulopathy with platelet transfusions, FFP, and cryoprecipitate should be undertaken for bleeding complications but should not be given empirically given the potential risk of worsening inappropriate coagulation due to DIC.

III. ANEMIA

A. **Evaluation.** Anemia is defined as a hemoglobin level of less than 12 g/dL in women and less than 14 g/dL in men. A history and physical examination may determine the cause and acuity of anemia. Initial laboratory evaluation is usually a CBC, but a peripheral blood smear, reticulocyte count, and mean cell volume (MCV) may further help to identify the cause of the anemia. The blood smear is used to identify abnormalities in red blood cells (RBCs), white blood cells (WBCs), and platelets. The reticulocyte count assesses the bone marrow response to anemia. A normal or low reticulocyte count in the presence of anemia suggests an inadequate bone marrow response. The MCV differentiates different types of anemia.

B. **Anemias associated with RBC loss or increased RBC destruction**

1. **Bleeding** is the most frequently encountered cause of RBC loss. Most postoperative patients have an obvious etiology for blood loss; however,

sources of occult bleeding include the GI tract, uterus, urinary tract, and retroperitoneum. The hematocrit is not a reliable method to determine acute blood loss because the patient loses plasma in addition to RBCs.

2. **Sepsis.** Anemia is common is sepsis and is partially due to a decreased expression of the erythropoietin gene, but treatment with recombinant human erythropoietin has failed to demonstrate an increase in survival. Transfusions for a hematocrit level lower than 30% earlier in the stages of sepsis is associated with a decreased risk of mortality (*N Engl J Med.* 2001;345:1368).

C. **Hemolytic anemias**

1. **Acquired hemolytic anemias** are caused by autoimmune disorders, medications, or trauma. The direct Coombs test usually identifies autoimmune hemolytic anemia. Idiosyncratic drug-induced hemolytic anemia is rare but cefotetan-induced hemolysis is noteworthy because of its frequency and severity in surgical patients. Traumatic hemolytic anemias are often induced by malfunctioning prosthetic heart valves or vascular grafts.

2. **Hereditary hemolytic anemias** include the hemoglobinopathy of sickle cell disease, which is caused by abnormal hemoglobin that polymerizes under decreased oxygen tension. Dehydration and hypoxia must be avoided to prevent sickling, which is critical in patients who undergo general anesthesia. Other hereditary hemolytic anemias include RBC membrane abnormalities (e.g., hereditary spherocytosis) and RBC enzymopathies (e.g., glucose 6-phosphate dehydrogenase deficiency).

D. **Anemias associated with decreased RBC production**

1. **Iron-deficiency anemia** is most commonly caused by menstrual bleeding or occult GI blood loss. Sources of GI blood loss include gastritis, peptic ulcer disease, angiodysplasia, hemorrhoids, and colon adenocarcinoma. In men and postmenopausal women with iron-deficiency anemia, a complete GI evaluation for a potential source of blood loss is strongly recommended. Iron requirements for women increase during pregnancy owing to the transfer of iron to the fetus. Patients with a gastrectomy, achlorhydria, chronic diarrhea, or intestinal malabsorption may have diminished intestinal absorption of iron. The diagnosis is suggested by a hypochromic microcytic (MCV <80) anemia, low serum iron levels (<60 μg/dL), increased total iron-binding capacity (>360 μg/dL), and low serum ferritin levels (<14 ng/L). A trial of iron therapy typically establishes the diagnosis. Oral iron replacement (ferrous sulfate 325 mg orally three times a day) is usually sufficient treatment. Iron dextran also can be administered intramuscularly (100 mg/day) or as a single-dose intravenous preparation (1 to 2 g over 3 to 6 hours) in patients with malabsorption, poor compliance, or intolerance of oral preparations. IV administration of iron dextran must be closely monitored given the risk of severe anaphylactic reactions.

2. **Megaloblastic anemias (anemia with MCV >100)** are associated with a deficiency of cobalamin (vitamin B_{12}) or folic acid. Cobalamin, derived in the diet from meat and dairy products, is dependent on

intrinsic factor (IF) for absorption. IF is produced by gastric parietal cells, and the IF-cobalamin complex is absorbed in the terminal ileum. **Pernicious anemia** in which anti-IF antibodies occur places patients at risk. In addition, patients with gastrectomy, ileal resection or ileitis, intestinal parasites, or bacterial overgrowth can develop vitamin B_{12} deficiency. However, because only a small portion of the body's stores is used each day, vitamin B_{12} deficiency takes several years to manifest. In addition to anemia, vitamin B_{12} deficiency often causes a neuropathy (extremity paresthesias), weakness, ataxia, and poor coordination. In contrast to vitamin B_{12} deficiency, folic acid deficiency can develop within weeks from decreased intake (e.g., alcohol abuse), malabsorption, or increased use (e.g., pregnancy or hemolysis). Clinical suspicion, CBC and serum vitamin B_{12}, or folate levels establish the diagnosis. Therapy for vitamin B_{12} deficiency involves replacement with cyanocobalamin (1 mg/day intramuscularly for 7 days, then weekly for 2 months, then monthly). Folic acid is replenished (1 mg/day orally) until the deficiency is corrected. An incomplete response to therapy might indicate a coexisting iron deficiency, which occurs in one-third of patients with megaloblastic anemia.

3. **Other anemias** associated with decreased RBC production include anemia due to renal insufficiency, chronic disease, chemotherapy, and the thalassemias. Aplastic anemia is an acquired defect of bone marrow stem cells and is associated with pancytopenia. The majority of cases are idiopathic or autoimmune, but approximately 20% are drug related (e.g., gold, benzene, chemotherapeutics, anticonvulsants, sulfonamides, and chloramphenicol). Some are associated with an antecedent viral infection. A bone marrow biopsy helps to establish the diagnosis.

IV. **TRANSFUSION THERAPY.** The risks and benefits of transfusion therapy must be considered carefully in each situation. Informed consent should be obtained before blood products are administered. The indications for transfusion should be noted in the medical record. Before elective procedures that are likely to require blood transfusion, the options of autologous or directed blood donation should be discussed with the patient in time to allow for the collection process.

A. **Indications.** RBC transfusions are used to treat anemia and improve the oxygen-carrying capacity of the blood. A hemoglobin level of 7 to 8 g/dL is adequate for tissue oxygenation in most normovolemic patients. However, therapy must be individualized based on the clinical situation rather than a hemoglobin level. The patient's age, cardiovascular and pulmonary status, volume status, the type of transfusion (i.e., homologous vs. autologous), and the expectation of further blood loss should guide transfusion decisions. Of note, algorithm-guided approaches to transfusion that utilize laboratory and POC values (i.e., TEG) have been shown to be safe and decrease the number blood products transfused in cardiac surgery (*Br J Anesth.* 2004;92:178) and are being evaluated for trauma (*Ann Surg.* 2010;251: 604).

B. **Transfusions in critically ill patients.** Critically ill patients may be at increased risk for the immunosuppressive complications of transfusions and may benefit from a more restrictive transfusion protocol. This was demonstrated in the TRICC (Transfusion Requirements in Critical Care) trial, a randomized, controlled trial that showed significantly lower mortality rates with a restrictive transfusion strategy (transfusion for hemoglobin between 7 and 9 g/dl) (*N Engl J Med.* 1999;340:409). Patients with active cardiac ischemia or infarction may benefit from a higher hemoglobin level to improve oxygen delivery.

C. **Preparation.** Before administration, both donor blood and recipient blood are tested to decrease transfusion reactions. Blood typing tests the recipient's RBCs for antigens (A, B, and Rh) and screens the recipient's serum for the presence of antibodies to a panel of known RBC antigens. Each unit to be transfused is then cross-matched against the recipient's serum to check for preformed antibodies against antigens on the donor's RBCs. In an emergency situation, type O/Rh-negative blood that has been prescreened for reactive antibodies may be administered prior to blood typing and cross-matching. After blood typing, type-specific blood can be given. Certain populations of patients require specially prepared blood products. For example, patients who need chronic transfusion therapy and organ transplant should be administered leukocyte-depleted blood. Immunocompromised patients and those receiving blood from first-degree relatives should be given irradiated blood to prevent graft versus host disease (GVHD).

D. **Administration (Table 5-2).** Proper identification of the blood and patient is necessary to prevent transfusion errors. Packed RBCs should be administered through a standard filter (170 to 260 μm) and an 18-gauge or larger intravenous catheter. The rate of transfusion is determined by the clinical situation; typically, however, each unit of blood must be administered within 4 hours to prevent infection. Patients are monitored for adverse reactions during the first 5 to 10 minutes of the transfusion and frequently thereafter.

E. **Alternatives to homologous transfusion** exist and may provide advantages in safety and cost when used in elective procedures with a high likelihood of significant blood loss.

1. **Autologous predonation** is the preferred alternative for elective transfusions. Up to 20% of patients still require allogeneic transfusion, however, and transfusion reactions may still result from clerical errors in storage. Despite its intrinsic advantages, predonation is not cost-effective when the risk of transfusion is moderate or low.

2. **Isovolemic hemodilution** is a technique in which whole fresh blood is removed and crystalloid is simultaneously infused in the immediate preoperative period. The blood is stored at room temperature and reinfused after acute blood loss has ceased. Moderate hemodilution (hematocrit 32% to 33%) is as effective as autologous predonation in reducing the need for allogeneic transfusion and is much less costly.

3. **Intraoperative autotransfusion (Cell Saver)** in which blood from the operative field is returned to the patient can decrease allogeneic transfusion requirements. Equipment to separate and wash recovered

RBCs is required. Contraindications include neoplasm and enteric or purulent contamination.

4. Erythropoietin may be effective in decreasing allogeneic transfusion requirements when given preoperatively. Appropriate dose can be calculated based on anticipated transfusion requirements and is administered weekly over 2 to 4 weeks. Adjunctive use with autologous predonation has not consistently been shown to be effective. Chronic anemia, particularly anemia due to renal disease, is usually treated with erythropoietin (50 to 100 U/kg subcutaneously three times a week) rather than with transfusions. Erythropoietin should be used with caution in critically ill patients as it is associated with an increased risk of thrombotic events (*N Engl J Med.* 2007;357:965).

F. **Complications of transfusions**

1. **Infections.** Current methods of blood screening have greatly reduced the transmission rate of viral disease. Hepatitis B transmission is in the range of 1 in 205,000 units transfused. The risk of HIV or hepatitis C transmission is in the range of 1 in 2 million units transfused. Cytomegalovirus (CMV) transmission is a risk in CMV-negative immunocompromised patients and can be lowered by using either leukocyte-depleted or CMV-negative blood products. Bacteria and endotoxins can be infused with blood products, particularly in platelets that are stored at room temperature. Parasitic infections also can be transmitted, although rarely, with blood products.

2. **Transfusion reactions**

   a. **Allergic reactions** are the most common type of transfusion reactions and occur when the patient reacts to donated plasma proteins in the blood. Symptoms include itching or hives and can often be treated with antihistamines such as diphenhydramine (25 to 50 mg orally or intravenously). Prophylactic administration of diphenhydramine (Benadryl) and prednisone prior to a transfusion may be considered in patients with a previous history of allergic reaction. Rarely, severe reactions may involve bronchospasm or laryngospasm, which should prompt discontinuation of the infusion. Steroids and subcutaneous epinephrine may also be required.

   b. **Febrile nonhemolytic reactions** involve the development of a high fever during or within 24 hours of a transfusion. This reaction is mediated by the body's response to WBCs in donated blood. General malaise, chills, nausea, or headaches may accompany the fever. Because fever can be the first manifestation of a more serious transfusion reaction, the situation must be promptly evaluated. Patients with a previous history of a febrile reaction should receive leukoreduced blood products.

   c. **Acute immune hemolytic reactions** are the most serious transfusion reactions, in which patient antibodies react to transfused RBC antigens causing intravascular hemolysis. This typically occurs with ABO or Rh incompatibility. Symptoms include nausea, chills, anxiety, flushing, and chest or back pain. Anesthetized or comatose patients may show signs of excessive incisional bleeding or oozing from mucous membranes. The reaction may progress to shock or renal failure with hemoglobinuria. If a transfusion reaction is suspected, the infusion should be stopped immediately. Identities of the donor unit and recipient should be rechecked because clerical error is the most common cause. A repeat cross-match should be performed in addition to a CBC, coagulation studies, and serum bilirubin. Treatment includes maintenance of intravascular volume, hemodynamic support as needed, and preservation of renal function. Urine output should be maintained at greater than 100 mL/hour using volume resuscitation and possibly diuretics if resuscitation is attained. Alkalinization of the urine to a pH of greater than 7.5 by adding sodium bicarbonate to the intravenous fluids (two to three ampules of 7.5% sodium bicarbonate in 1,000 mL of D5W) helps to prevent precipitation of hemoglobin in the renal tubules.

d. **Delayed hemolytic reactions** result from an anamnestic antibody response to antigens other than the ABO antigens to which the recipient has been previously exposed. Transfused blood cells may take days or weeks to hemolyze after transfusion. Typically there are few signs or symptoms other than a falling RBC count or elevated bilirubin. Specific treatment is rarely necessary, but severe cases should be treated like acute hemolytic reactions, with volume support and maintenance of urine output.

e. **Transfusion-related acute lung injury (TRALI)** may be one of the most common causes of morbidity and mortality associated with transfusion. TRALI typically occurs within 1 to 2 hours of transfusion but can occur any time up to 6 hours later. Patients complain of shortness of breath and may have a fever. Support can vary from supplemental oxygen to intubation and ventilation. Although most cases resolve on their own, severe cases can be fatal.

f. **GVHD** can occur after transfusion of immunocompetent T cells into immunocompromised recipients or human leukocyte antigen-identical family members. GVHD presents with a rash, elevated liver function tests and pancytopenia. It has an associated mortality of greater than 80%. Irradiation of donor blood from first-degree relatives of immunocompetent patients and all blood for immunocompromised patients prevents this complication.

3. **Volume overload after blood transfusion** can occur in patients with poor cardiac or renal function. Careful monitoring of the volume status and judicious use of diuretic therapy can reduce the risk of this complication.

4. **Massive transfusion,** usually defined as the transfusion of blood products that are greater in volume than a patient's normal blood volume in less than 24 hours, creates several risks not encountered with a lesser volume or rate of transfusion. **Coagulopathy** might arise as a result of platelet or coagulation factor depletion. This has led to the use of transfusion ratios in the trauma setting that involve the transfusion of platelets and FFP in concert with packed red blood cells (PRBCs). No definitive ratio has been established but ratios of 1:1 or 1:2 FFP:PRBC

are common. Blood products should be guided by the clinical situation and lab values (including TEG if available) rather than empirically based. **Hypothermia** can result from massive volume resuscitation with chilled blood products but can be prevented by using blood warmers. Hypothermia can lead to cardiac dysrhythmias and coagulopathy. **Citrate toxicity** can develop after massive transfusion in patients with hepatic dysfunction. Hypocalcemia can be treated with intravenous administration of 10% calcium gluconate. **Electrolyte abnormalities,** including acidosis and hyperkalemia, occur rarely after massive transfusions, especially in patients with preexisting hyperkalemia.

V. **LOCAL HEMOSTATIC AGENTS.** Local hemostatic agents can aid in the intraoperative control of bleeding from needle punctures, vascular suture lines, or areas of extensive tissue dissection. Anastomotic bleeding usually is best controlled with local pressure or a simple suture. Local hemostatic agents promote hemostasis by providing a matrix for thrombus formation.

A. **Gelatin sponge** (e.g., Gelfoam) can absorb many times its weight of whole blood by capillary action and provides a platform for coagulation. Gelfoam itself is not intrinsically hemostatic. It resorbs in 4 to 6 weeks without a significant inflammatory reaction.

B. **Oxidized cellulose** (e.g., Surgicel) is a knitted fabric of cellulose that allows clotting by absorbing blood and swelling into a scaffold. Its slow resorption can create a foreign body reaction.

C. **Collagen sponge** (e.g., Helistat) is produced from bovine tendon collagen and promotes platelet adhesion. It is slowly resorbed and creates a foreign body reaction similar to that of cellulose.

D. **Microfibrillar collagen** (e.g., Avitene and Hemotene) can be sprayed onto wounds and anastomoses for hemostasis, particularly in areas that are difficult to reach. It stimulates platelet adhesion and promotes thrombus formation. Because microfibrillar collagen can pass through autotransfusion device filters, it should be avoided during procedures that utilize the cell saver.

E. **Topical thrombin** can be applied to the various hemostatic agents or to dressings and placed onto bleeding sites to achieve a fibrin-rich hemostatic plug. Topical thrombin, usually of bovine origin, is supplied as a lyophilized powder and can be applied directly to dressings or dissolved in saline and sprayed onto the wound. Repeated use of bovine thrombin may result in formation of inhibitors to thrombin or factor V, which is not usually associated with a clinical bleeding disorder, although there may be dramatic alterations in the coagulation testing. Topical thrombin can be used effectively in anticoagulated patients.

F. **Gelatin matrices** (e.g., FloSeal) are often used in combination with topical thrombin intraoperatively. Typically, bovine thrombin (5,000 units) is sprayed onto the matrix, which is then applied to the site of bleeding.

G. **Fibrin sealants** (e.g., Tiseel and Evicel) are prepared by combining human thrombin and human fibrinogen. These components are separated prior to administration and are mixed during application to tissue via a dual-syringe system. An insoluble, cross-linked fibrin mesh is created with provides a matrix for thrombus formation.

Wound Healing and Care

Isaiah R. Turnbull, Thomas H. Tung, and John P. Kirby

Wound healing is the normal response to injury. Wound healing is divided into acute wound healing and chronic wound healing. *Acute wound healing* is the normal orderly process that occurs after an uncomplicated injury and requires minimal practitioner intervention. Chronic wound healing *does not* follow an orderly progression of healing and often necessitates a variety of interventions to facilitate closure.

ACUTE WOUND HEALING

I. **PHYSIOLOGY OF THE ACUTE WOUND.** Disruption of tissue integrity, whether surgical or traumatic, initiates a sequence of events directed at restoring the injured tissue to a normal state. Normal wound healing occurs in an orderly fashion and is a balance of repair and regeneration of tissue. Normal wound healing is affected by tissue type, the nature and extent of injury, and comorbid conditions. Wound healing is grouped into early, intermediate, and late stages.

A. **Early wound healing**

1. **Establishment of hemostasis.** Injury causes disruption of blood vessels with resulting hemorrhage. Severed blood vessels with smooth muscle in the vessel wall immediately constrict to minimize hemorrhage. Within minutes, the coagulation cascade is initiated and produces the end-product fibrin. The fibrin matrix binds and activates platelets, facilitating hemostasis. It also serves as the initial scaffold for wound healing. In later phases of wound healing, the fibrin matrix facilitates cell attachment and migration and serves as a reservoir for cytokines.

2. **Inflammatory phase** (days 1 to 4). The inflammatory phase is recognized at the skin level by the cardinal signs of *rubor* (redness), *calor* (heat), *tumor* (swelling), and *dolor* (pain). Injury immediately activates three plasma-based systems: the coagulation cascade, the complement cascade, and the kinin cascade. Proinflammatory factors attract leukocytes and facilitate their migration out of the intravascular space and into the wound. **Polymorphonuclear leukocytes (PMNs)** are the dominant inflammatory cells in the wound for the first 24 to 48 hours. They phagocytize bacteria, foreign material, and damaged tissue. They also release cytokines such as TNF-alpha and interleukin-1 that further stimulate the inflammatory response. The inflammatory phase progresses with the infiltration of circulating **monocytes** into the wound. Monocytes migrate into the extravascular space through capillaries and differentiate into **macrophages.** Macrophages are activated by the locally produced cytokines and are essential for normal healing

because of their important role in the coordination of the healing process. They phagocytize bacteria and damaged tissue, secrete enzymes for the degradation of tissue and extracellular matrix, and release cytokines for inflammatory cell recruitment and fibroblast proliferation. The inflammatory phase lasts a well-defined period of time in primarily closed wounds (approximately 4 days), but it continues indefinitely to the end-point of complete epithelialization in wounds that close by secondary or tertiary intention. Foreign material or bacteria can change a normal healing wound into one with chronic inflammation.

B. **Intermediate wound-healing** events involve mesenchymal cell migration and proliferation, angiogenesis, and epithelialization.

1. **Fibroblast migration** occurs 2 to 4 days after wounding. Chemotactic cytokines influence fibroblasts to migrate into the wound from undamaged tissue. Movement of cells occurs on the extracellular matrix, consisting of fibrin, fibronectin, and vitronectin.

2. While the wound is infiltrated by mesenchymal cells, **angiogenesis** takes place to restore the vasculature that has been disrupted by the wound.

3. **Epithelialization** restores the barrier between the wound and the external environment. Epithelialization of wounds occurs via the migration of epithelial cells from the edges of the wound and from remaining epidermal skin appendages. Migration of epithelial cells occurs at the rate of 1 mm/day in clean, open wounds. Primarily closed wounds have a contiguous epithelial layer at 24 to 48 hours.

C. **Late wound healing** involves the deposition of collagen and other matrix proteins and wound contraction. The primary function of the fibroblast at this stage becomes protein synthesis. Fibroblasts produce several proteins that are components of the extracellular matrix, including collagen, fibronectin, and proteoglycans. Glucocorticoids compromise wound healing by inhibiting protein production by fibroblasts.

1. **Collagen** is the main protein secreted by fibroblasts. It provides strength and structure and facilitates cell motility in the wound. Collagen is synthesized at an accelerated rate for 2 to 4 weeks, greatly contributing to the tensile strength of the wound. Oxygen, vitamin C, α-ketoglutarate, and iron are important cofactors for the cross-linkage of collagen fibers. If these are not present, wound healing may be poor.

2. **Wound contraction** is a decrease in the size of the wound without an increase in the number of tissue elements that are present. It involves movement of the wound edge toward the center of the wound through the action of myofibroblasts. It is differentiated from contracture, which is the pathologic and movement-limiting result of prolonged wound contraction across a joint primarily from scar formation. Wound contraction begins 4 to 5 days after wounding and continues for 12 to 15 days or longer if the wound remains open.

3. The final wound-healing event is **scar formation and remodeling.** It begins at approximately 21 days after wounding. At the outset of scar remodeling, collagen synthesis is downregulated, and the cellularity

of the wound decreases. During scar remodeling, collagen is broken down and replaced by new collagen that is denser and organized along the lines of stress. By 6 months, the wound reaches 80% of the bursting strength of unwounded tissue. It is important to note that a well-healed wound never achieves the strength of unwounded tissue. This process reaches a plateau at 12 to 18 months, but it may last indefinitely.

CHRONIC WOUND HEALING

I. **PHYSIOLOGY OF THE CHRONIC WOUND.** A chronic wound is a wound that fails to heal in a reasonable amount of time, given the wound's etiology, location, and tissue type. Prolonged or incomplete healing is caused by disruption of the normal process of acute wound healing. Most chronic wounds are slowed or arrested in the inflammatory or proliferative phases of healing and have increased levels of matrix metalloproteinases, which bind up or degrade the various cytokines and growth factors at the wound surface. Most often, there are definable causes of the failure of these wounds to heal. Treatment of these causes, along with maximal medical management of underlying medical problems, restores more normal healing processes. Treating a patient with a chronic wound involves identifying the type of wound, investigating the cause(s) of delayed healing, and improving the intrinsic (within the wound itself) and extrinsic (systemic) factors that lead to poor wound healing.

A. **Intrinsic or local factors** are abnormalities within the wound that prevent normal wound healing. These factors include (1) foreign body, (2) necrotic tissue, (3) repetitive trauma, (4) hypoxia/ischemia, (5) venous insufficiency, (6) infection, (7) growth factor deficit, (8) excessive matrix protein degradation, and (9) radiation. Factors that can be controlled by the surgeon include the blood supply to the wound; the temperature of the wound environment; the presence or absence of infection, hematoma, or seroma; the amount of local tissue trauma; and the technique used to close the wound.

B. **Extrinsic or systemic factors** also contribute to abnormal wound healing. Optimization of these factors is critical to healing a chronic wound: (1) diabetes mellitus, (2) steroids and antineoplastic drugs, (3) smoking, (4) collagen vascular disease, (5) repetitive trauma, and (6) chronic disease states in the kidney and liver.

II. **EVALUATION AND MANAGEMENT OF THE CHRONIC WOUND**

A. **Diagnosis.** Evaluation and management of a chronic wound must begin with a thorough history and physical examination.

1. **History.** One must establish whether the wound is new, recurrent, or chronic, how long it has been present, how it started, how quickly it developed, and whether it is improving or worsening. The patient must be questioned about existing comorbidities, with a focus on potential causes for immunosuppression (HIV,

steroids, chemotherapy), undiagnosed diabetes mellitus, peripheral vascular disease, coronary artery disease, rheumatologic disorders, and radiation exposure. Smoking and alcohol use should also be documented.

2. **Physical examination** should include the measured size and depth of the wound, and the tissues that are involved. The wound and the surrounding tissue should be evaluated for any signs of infection. The full extent of the wound should be defined including probing any undermined tissue flaps or drainage tracts with a sterile instrument. The surrounding tissue should also be evaluated for skin changes including maceration, hyperpigmentation, capillary refill, and pallor. For extremity wounds, a complete vascular assessment often requiring Doppler ultrasound of the arterial pulsations is a key component of the exam.

3. **Laboratory assessments** of serum electrolyte, hepatic transaminase, and bilirubin levels may aid with the diagnosis of diabetes and renal or hepatic dysfunction. A complete blood cell count may indicate infection with elevated white cell count or white cell abnormalities. Radiography can be performed to determine underlying bony pathology.

B. **Management** of the chronic wound must focus on optimization of host and local factors.

1. **Adequate nutrition** is necessary for appropriate wound healing. Sufficient calories, protein, vitamins, minerals, and water are necessary to aid in the healing. Patients who have severe malnutrition or whose gastrointestinal tract cannot be used should be placed on parenteral nutritional support.

2. **Underlying factors** that affect wound healing, such as chemotherapy, steroids, alcohol consumption, cigarette smoking, and blood glucose levels, must be modified as necessary to aid in the wound-healing process.

3. **Effective local wound care** is essential for the resolution of a chronic wound. Eradication of infection, aggressive debridement, and drainage of abscesses from the wound are important steps in local control.

4. **Antibiotics.** Systemic antibiotics should be administered to treat wounds that are actively infected with purulent discharge and or cellulitis. Topical antibiotics may be useful in slowly healing chronic wounds that are not actively infected but which have a quantitative bacterial count $>10^5$ CFU/mm^3 or which display secondary signs of infection such as friable granulation tissue, nonpurulent exudates, or abnormal foul odor (*Clin Infect Dis.* 2009;49:1541).

5. **Proper dressings** are an essential aspect of local care by helping to provide the appropriate environment for healing.
   a. Frequent damp-to-dry dressings are used when infection and drainage predominate. With the development of healthy granulation tissue, dressings should provide adequate protection and moisture to facilitate healing. Wounds with exudate should have this controlled by the dressing to protect the periwound from maceration.

     b. Negative pressure dressings (NPD) provide subatmospheric pressure a local wound though a porous foam sponge sealed over the wound with a semipermeable adhesive barrier. Vacuum is applied by an external pump. NPD are particularly useful for wounds with soft tissue deficits and can also be used to facilitate closure of open sternal or abdominal wounds. NPD should not be placed directly over exposed bowel, blood vessels, or cortical bone. NPD are also contraindicated when there is active infection or necrotic tissue in the wound. They can be placed safely over exposed fascia or fascia substitutes such as biologic or nonbiologic hernia repair mesh.

6. Edema control is often necessary for wounds of the lower extremity due to venous insufficiency. Elevation and wrapping in an elastic bandage reduce edema and venous hypertension. Unna boot, Jobst compression garments, and pneumatic compression devices can also be used.

7. Surgical therapy may be necessary to aid in the healing of a chronic wound. Besides surgical débridement or skin grafting on a healthy bed of granulation tissue, revascularization procedures may be necessary to provide adequate blood flow to distal circulation that supplies a non-healing/or chronic wound.

III. SPECIAL CATEGORIES OF CHRONIC WOUNDS. Chronic wounds are a heterogeneous group. Chronic wounds associated with vascular disease, diabetes, pressure necrosis, and radiation therapy are frequently encountered, cause great disability within the population, and place a great burden on the healthcare system.

    A. Diabetic foot ulcers

       1. Differential diagnosis. The first step to treating any lower-extremity ulcer is to identify the cause of the wound. The three most common causes of lower-extremity ulcers are diabetes mellitus, venous stasis, and arterial insufficiency. Diabetic ulcers most frequently result from undetected/untreated trauma to the neuropathic foot. They are typically associated with very thick callus and most often occur on the patient's heels or on the plantar surface of the metatarsal heads. Venous stasis ulcers most often occur on the medial aspect of the patient's lower leg or ankle (gaiter distribution) and are associated with the chronic edema and hyperpigmentation seen with venous insufficiency. Arterial insufficiency ulcers tend to occur distally on the tips of the patient's toes, but they can also occur at or near the lateral malleolus. The surrounding skin is thin, shiny, and hairless; these individuals typically relate symptoms of claudication or rest pain. Peripheral pulses are diminished or absent. Unfortunately, lower extremity ulcers frequently result from a combination of these common etiologies, which must be considered when devising a treatment plan.

       2. Pathogenesis of diabetic foot ulcers.

         a. Peripheral neuropathy is believed to be the most significant contributor to the development of lower-extremity ulcers in diabetic patients through impaired detection of injury from poorly fitting shoes or trauma. Diabetic motor neuropathy is also associated with abnormal weightbearing. The motor neuropathy results in abnormalities such as hammertoes or hallux valgus, which shift weightbearing more proximally than normal on the metatarsal heads. Additionally, the dorsum of the toes at the posterior inter-phalangeal joints is often traumatized by ill-fitting shoes in patients with hammertoes.

b. Autonomic neuropathy leads to failure of sweating and inadequate lubrication of the skin. Dry skin leads to mechanical breakdown that initiates ulcer formation. Autonomic neuropathy also contributes to failure of autoregulation in the microcirculation; therefore, arterial blood will shunt past capillaries into the venous blood flow. This reduces the nutritive blood flow to the skin and predisposes to ulcer formation.

c. Ischemia contributes to the development and progression of lower-extremity ulcers. Patients with diabetic foot ulcers should also be evaluated for proximal arterial insufficiency that may be amenable to intervention, improving the chances of healing of the ulcer.

3. Evaluation and treatment

a. Examination. The quality of the peripheral circulation, the extent of the wound, and the degree of sensory loss as assessed with a 10-gauge monofilament skin tester should be recorded. Web spaces should be examined for evidence of mycotic infection, which may lead to fissuring of the skin and subsequent infection. Mal perforans ulcers occur on the plantar surface of the metatarsals and extend to the metatarsal head, leaving exposed cartilage. Evaluation of diabetic foot ulcers should include plain x-rays of the foot to evaluate for osteomyelitis.

b. Treatment. With appropriate treatment, 24% of diabetic found wounds will heal by 12 weeks, and 31% by 20 weeks (*Diabetes Care.* 1999;22:692). Critical to treatment of any diabetic foot wound is complete offloading of the ulcer with an appropriate diabetic shoe or other orthotic device.

(1) Clean wounds are treated with minimal debridement and damp gauze or hydrogel-based dressing changes. Hydrogel dressings may be more effective than damp gauze (*Cochrane Cochrane Database Syst Rev.* 2010;20:CD003556). Exudative wounds may benefit from alginate, hydrocolloid, or NPD that minimize contact of the wound base with wound exudate, which is hypothesized to inhibit wound healing. Close follow-up is essential.

(2) Infected wounds are diagnosed based on clinical signs of infection. Plain x-rays may show osteomyelitis or gas in the soft tissues. The progression of infection in diabetic patients can occur rapidly. Patients with a suspected infected diabetic foot ulcer should be admitted for inpatient wound care and broad-spectrum antibiotic therapy. Infected wounds require a thorough exploration with drainage of all abscess cavities and debridement of infected, necrotic, or devitalized tissues. The clean wound can then be managed with local wound care as described above.

(3) **Antibiotic therapy.** For infected wounds, initial antibiotic therapy should be broad spectrum directed at both Gram-positive and Gram-negative organisms. In the acute phase parenteral treatment is indicated. Wound cultures should be obtained prior to initiation of antibiosis. Duration of antibiosis depends on severity of infection. For mild infections limited to the soft tissue 1 to 2 weeks of therapy is sufficient; moderate or severe infections require 2 to 4 weeks of total antibiotic therapy. For osteomyelitis involving viable bone, 4 to 6 weeks of IV therapy may be indicated. Consultation with an infectious disease specialist is helpful in guiding therapy (*Plast Reconstr Surg.* 2006;117:212S).

(4) **Prevention** remains one of the most important elements in the management of the diabetic foot. Meticulous attention to hygiene and daily inspection for signs of tissue trauma prevent the progression of injury. Podiatric appliances or custom-made shoes are helpful in relieving pressure on weightbearing areas and should be prescribed for any patient who has had neuropathic ulceration.

B. **Leg ulcers**

1. **Arterial insufficiency ulcers** tend to occur distally on the tips of the patient's toes or near the lateral malleolus. The surrounding skin is thin, shiny, and hairless. Patients frequently complain of claudication or rest pain. Peripheral pulses are diminished or absent. When **arterial ulcers** are suspected, obtain vascular evaluation including a peripheral and central pulse exam and segmental limb pressures with calculation of ankle-brachial indices and toe-pressures. Neglected chronic arterial insufficiency can result in dry gangrene and mummification of the toes. Critical to treatment of these wounds is restoration of arterial inflow (see Chapter 19). After optimization of arterial inflow, devitalized tissue can be resected to facilitate healing. Arterial insufficiency wounds and dry gangrene must be carefully assessed for signs of infection. If infection is suspected, obtain wound cultures, débride infected tissue, and institute appropriate antibiosis.

2. **Venous stasis ulcers** are among the most common types of leg ulcers and typically occur on the medial leg in the supramedial malleolar location. A patient with a venous stasis ulcer typically has a history of ulceration and associated leg swelling or of deep venous thrombosis. See Chapter 20 for complete description of venous stasis ulcers and their treatment.

C. **Skin tears** are often seen in the elderly with skin that is markedly thinned and in the chronic steroid-using patient. The hypermobile skin, with its poor subcutaneous connections, is prone to rip under shearing forces, and patients often present with a flap of skin that is torn away from its wound bed. One should follow the principles outlined previously, with this exception: The skin flap should be trimmed of obvious necrotic portions, and the remaining flap should be secured in place over the wound bed only to the extent that it can be without tension. It is rare that such a wound should be sutured closed because the flap will most likely necrose under the tension of the swelling that occurs over the following 2 to 4 days. Topical management of the area that is intentionally left open is often easily achieved with a hydrogel dressing.

D. Pressure ulcers

1. **Pathophysiology.** Prolonged pressure applied to soft tissue over bony prominences, usually caused by paralysis or the immobility associated with severe illness, predictably leads to ischemic ulceration and tissue breakdown. Muscle tissue seems to be the most susceptible. The prevalence of pressure ulcers is 10% of all hospitalized patients, 28% of nursing home patients, and 39% of spinal cord injury patients (*JAMA.* 2006;296:974). Pressure ulcers increase mortality rates more than twofold, and are the cause of death in 8% of paraplegics (*Am J Surg.* 2004;188:9S). The particular area of breakdown depends on the patient's position of immobility, with ulcers most frequently developing in recumbent patients over the occiput, sacrum, greater trochanter, and heels. In immobile patients who sit for prolonged periods on improper surfaces without pressure relief, ulcers often develop under the ischial tuberosities. **Pressure ulcers are described by stages (Table 6-1).** Such wounds do not necessarily proceed through each one of these stages during formation but can present at the advanced stages. Likewise, as these wounds heal, they do not go backward through the stages despite their present depth (e.g., a nearly healed stage IV ulcer does not become a stage II ulcer but rather a healing stage IV ulcer, signifying that the tissues of the healing wound are abnormal). When

TABLE 6-1	National Pressure Ulcer Advisory Panel Classification Scheme

Stage	Description
I	Nonblanchable erythema of intact skin; wounds generally reversible at this stage with intervention
II	Partial-thickness skin loss involving epidermis or dermis; may present as an abrasion, blister, or shallow crater
III	Full-thickness skin loss involving damage or necrosis of subcutaneous tissue but not extending through underlying structures or fascia
IV	Full-thickness skin loss with damage to underlying support structures (i.e., fascia, tendon, or joint capsule)

a full-thickness injury to the skin has occurred, one cannot adequately stage the wound until the eschar is incised and the actual depth is determined. The examiner must also look for underlying bony breakdown, osteomyelitis, or an overall physiologic decline as the root cause of a "pressure" ulcer whose actual etiology may be multifactorial in nature, and any successful healing regimen must be equally multifactorial. The clinician must also consider whether such regimens are realistic and discuss assessments and care plans openly with the patient and family regarding realistic expectations and treatment goals.

2. **Prevention**
   a. Skin care. Skin should be kept well moisturized but protected from excessive contact with extraneous fluids. Take care during transfers to avoid friction and shear stress.
   b. Frequent repositioning. High-risk patients should be repositioned at a minimum every 2 hours, either while seated or in bed.
   c. Appropriate support surfaces. Adequate support surfaces redistribute pressure from the bony prominences that cause pressure ulcers. The appropriate surface is determined by the patient risk stratification using the Norton Scale (*Decubitus.* 1989;2:24.) and Braden Scale (*Nurs Clin North Am.* 1987;22:417). Static support surfaces: foam, air, gel, and water-overlay support surfaces are appropriate for low-risk patients. Dynamic support surfaces: these are support modalities that are powered and actively redistribute pressure. These include alternating and low air-loss mattresses. These surfaces are appropriate for high-risk patients.

3. **Treatment**
   a. Debridement. Eschar and necrotic tissue should be débrided. Sharp debridement of small wounds can be done at the bedside. Larger wounds require operative debridement. Once the bulk of eschar and devitalized tissue is removed, debridement can be continued with damp-to-dry gauze dressings or with enzymatic debridement with topical agents such as collagenase.
   b. Wound cleansing. The base of uninfected ulcers should be cleaned with saline irrigation or a commercially available wound cleanser at each dressing change. Antiseptic solutions such as hydrogen peroxide, povidone–iodine, or Dakin's solution should not be routinely used as they are toxic to tissues and impede healing. For actively infected wounds, a short course (3 to 5 days) of damp to dry dressing changes with ¼ strength Dakins' solution may facilitate local bacterial control. However, topical antiseptic solutions cannot take the place of appropriate debridement and systemic antibiotic therapy.
   c. Dressing. Dressings should be selected to ensure the wound base remains moist while keeping the surrounding skin dry. Damp-to-dry gauze and hydrocolloid dressings are appropriate. NPD are also useful for pressure ulcers and may facilitate closure as compared to traditional dressings (*Br J Nurs.* 2004;13:135). See section on negative pressure dressing for indications/contraindications to NPD.

    d. Infection and bacterial colonization. All open ulcers are colonized with bacteria. Surface colonization is best controlled with topical wound cleansing. Superficial colonization does not require antibiotic therapy. Evidence of active infection (purulence, surrounding cellulitis or foul odor) should prompt reexploration of the wound with debridement of any necrotic or infected tissue. Bacterial infection with greater than 10^5 organisms per gram of tissue can impair wound healing. Quantitative tissue cultures should be obtained from wounds that fail to heal. The underlying bone should be evaluated for osteomyelitis with appropriate imaging.

    e. Nutrition. Successful treatment of pressure ulcers requires adequate nutrition. Patients should be provided with 30 to 35 kcal/kg body weight and 1.25 to 1.5 g protein/kg body weight (*National Pressure Ulcer Advisory Panel Quick Reference Guide;* 2009). These estimates should be adjusted for factors such as recent weight changes, BMI, and renal failure or other comorbid conditions. Patient with non-healing pressure ulcers will benefit from a formal nutrition assessment by a dietician.

4. Surgical treatment. Most pressure ulcers heal spontaneously when pressure is relieved. *This remains the most important factor in their healing.* The healing process may require up to 6 months. Unless the patient was only temporarily immobilized, recurrences are common. Surgical management may include simple closure, split-thickness skin grafting, or musculocutaneous flap, but these measures should be reserved for well-motivated patients in whom a real reduction in risk factors for recurrence is possible. Urinary and fecal diversion reduce soiling and maceration of perineal and sacral wounds, which facilitates healing of these wounds.

E. Ionizing radiation. Although ionizing radiation is a useful mode of cancer therapy, it produces detrimental local effects on tissue in the field of radiation and impairs normal wound healing. Radiation injures target and surrounding cells by damaging DNA, decreasing proliferative capacity of cells, and decreasing perfusion through damage to the small blood vessels. The **timing of radiation therapy** as it relates to operative therapy has been an important aspect of oncologic care. The primary factors that determine the effects of preoperative radiation therapy on wound healing are the timing and the dose. These vary from tissue to tissue. Postoperative radiation therapy has no effect on healing if it is administered 1 week after wounding. The intentional (surgical) wounding of a previously irradiated area needs careful planning and consideration. Many of the cells in such an area have been permanently damaged; therefore, their proliferative capacity is decreased. In addition, the wound has decreased vascularity, which creates a relative state of hypoxemia. Furthermore, the dermis of such a wound is more susceptible to bacterial invasion. The combined factors place a previously irradiated area at extreme risk for abnormal wound healing if it is subjected to surgical intervention. It has long been realized for the foregoing reasons that **radiation-damaged skin and wounds heal poorly.** Local measures that must be undertaken with wounds affected by radiation follow the same principles of good wound care. These measures include infection control through aggressive débridement and systemic antibiotics, topical antibiotics to promote epithelialization, moist dressings, and lubrication of dry skin. Optimal nutritional status must also be emphasized.

PROPHYLACTIC SURGICAL WOUND CARE

I. **PREOPERATIVE PREPARATION.** Even though antibiotic prophylaxis and sterile surgical technique have gained widespread acceptance, surgical site infections (SSIs) remain a persistent problem occurring in 2 to 5% of operations and affecting 750,000 people annually in the United States (*Surg Infect.* 2006;7:S1). Clean surgical operations typically result in SSIs from Gram-positive aerobes representing pathogens in common skin flora (*Curr Infect Dis Rep.* 2004;6:426). Clean-contaminated, contaminated, or dirty operations usually result in polymicrobial infections with enteric Gram-negative and anaerobic bacteria along with skin flora pathogens. Antibiotic resistance is an increasing problem. The rate of *Staphylococcus aureus* resistance to methicillin, oxacillin, or nafcillin (MRSA) now approaches 60%, and the rate of *Klebsiella pneumoniae* resistance to cephalosporins is 50% (*Expert Rev Anti Infect Ther.* 2006;4:223).

A. **Patient factors.** Whereas some characteristics, such as age, cannot be altered, other patient factors can be optimized.

   1. **Cigarette smoking** is a known risk factor for SSI (*J Am Coll Surg.* 2007;204:178) and a prospective, randomized trial demonstrated an 83% reduction in wound infections in the smoking cessation group compared to controls (*Lancet.* 2002;359:114). The Centers for Disease Control and Prevention (CDC) recommends smoking cessation at least 30 days prior to elective surgery.

   2. The impact of **nutrition** on wound healing depends on the wound type. Wounds closed by primary intention often heal even in emaciated patients as long as there are no wound infections (*Annu Rev Nutr.* 2003;23:263). In contrast, wounds that heal by secondary intention are heavily dependent on the patient's nutritional status. Malnourished patients have increased rates of infection and delayed wound healing, and there is ample evidence that tailored preoperative nutritional repletion reduces these complications (*Plast Reconstr Surg.* 2006;117:42S).

B. **Operative factors**

   1. **Chlorhexidine showers** the night before surgery reduce bacterial counts; however, no studies have demonstrated decreased SSI rates with preoperative showering (*Cochrane Database of Systematic Reviews* 2007: CD004985). Previous recommendations regarding showers as well as updates on other interventions as detailed in the following can be found on the CDC Web site.

   2. **Shaving** is associated with an increased risk of SSIs. Meta-analysis of the available studies on hair removal demonstrate that **clipping** performed immediately before surgery was associated with significantly fewer infections as compared to shaving (*J Perioper Pract.* 2007;17:118).

3. **Prophylactic antibiotics** are indicated for some clean cases and most clean-contaminated cases. Antibiotics should be administered prior to the incision, with many regulatory groups recommending administration within 60 minutes (*Expert Rev Anti Infect Ther.* 2006;4:223). Most guidelines recommend postoperative discontinuation of prophylactic antibiotics within 24 hours (*Surg Clin North Am.* 2005;85:1115). Recently, large prospective, randomized trials have demonstrated no evidence to support the use of antibiotic prophylaxis in hernia surgery (*Ann Surg.* 2004;240:955; *J Am Coll Surg.* 2005;200:393).

II. PERIOPERATIVE

A. **Surgeon hand antisepsis** has traditionally been performed with a 5- to 10-minute scrub. Current guidelines include use of either (1) a traditional scrub with antimicrobial soap for 2 to 6 minutes or (2) use of alcohol-based surgical hand scrub following the manufacturer's recommendation for use. No difference in SSI is seen between these two techniques (*JAMA.* 2002;288:722).

B. **Surgical site antisepsis** starts with cleansing and removing visible debris, followed by a prep of the intended incision site to the periphery in concentric circles using a sterile instrument. Current practices include using 7.5% povidone–betadine foaming solution, 10% povidone–betadine paint, alcohol solutions, chlorhexidine/alcohol preparations, and alcohol-containing iodophor solutions. Chlorhexidine-based solutions may be superior to iodine-based solutions for clean-contaminated surgical cases (*N Engl J Med.* 2010;362:18).

C. **Active warming** to prevent intraoperative hypothermia has been demonstrated to reduce surgical infections in prospective, randomized trials (*N Engl J Med.* 1996;334:1209; *Lancet.* 2001;358:876). Current recommendations are (1) temperature monitoring for all cases (2) forced-air warmers for procedures expected to last greater than 30 minutes, and (3) warmed IV fluids for procedures expected to last greater than 1 hour (*JACS.* 2009;209:492).

D. **Tight glycemic control** is recommended in the perioperative period, although the mechanisms explaining the detrimental effect of hyperglycemia remain largely unknown. In 2001, Van den Berghe reported a randomized, prospective study of 1,548 surgical patients in which stringent glycemic control between 80 and 110 mg/dL resulted in 34% decreased mortality versus maintenance of 180 to 200 mg/dL (*N Engl J Med.* 2001;345:1359). In addition, continuous intravenous insulin infusion has been shown significantly to reduce the incidence of sternal wound infections when compared to sliding-scale insulin (*Ann Thoracic Surg.* 1999;67:352). The American Diabetes Association and the American Association of Clinical Endocrinologists recommend glycemic targets between 80 and 110 mg/dL for critically ill patients in the intensive care unit. For patients with noncritical illness, a prandial glucose of less than 110 mg/dL and a random glucose level of less than 180 mg/dL were recommended in the perioperative period (*Endocr Pract.* 2004;10(suppl 2):4).

E. **Other controllable factors** include the length of operation, gentle tissue handling, and supplemental oxygen to diminish SSIs.

WOUND CLOSURE AND CARE

I. TIMING OF WOUND HEALING

A. **Primary intention** occurs when the wound is closed by direct approximation of the wound margins or by placement of a graft or flap. Direct approximation of the edges of a wound provides the optimal treatment on the condition that the wound is clean, the closure can be done without undue tension, and the closure can occur in a timely fashion. Wounds that are less than 6 hours old are considered in the "golden period" and are less likely to develop into chronic wounds. At times, rearrangement of tissues is required to achieve tension-free closure. Directly approximated wounds typically heal as outlined earlier, provided that there is adequate perfusion of the tissues and no infection. Primary intention also describes the healing of wounds created in the operating room that are closed at the end of the operative period. Epithelialization of surgical incisions occurs within 24 hours of closure. CDC guidelines dictate that a sterile dressing should be left in place during this susceptible period to prevent bacterial contamination.

B. **Secondary intention,** or spontaneous healing, occurs when a wound is left open and is allowed to close by epithelialization and contraction. Contraction is a myofibroblast-mediated process that aids in wound closure by decreasing the circumference of the wound (myofibroblasts are modified fibroblasts that have smooth muscle cell-like contractile properties). This method is commonly used in the management of wounds that are treated beyond the initial 6-hour "golden period" or of contaminated infected wounds with a bacterial count of greater than 10^5/g of tissue. These wounds are characterized by prolonged inflammatory and proliferative phases of healing that continue until the wound has either completely epithelialized or been closed by other means.

C. **Tertiary intention, or delayed primary closure,** is a useful option for managing wounds that are too heavily contaminated for primary closure but appear clean and well vascularized after 4 to 5 days of open observation so that the cutaneous edges can be approximated at that time. During this period, the normally low arterial partial pressure of oxygen (PaO_2) at the wound surface rises and the inflammatory process in the wound bed leads to a minimized bacterial concentration, thus allowing a safer closure than could be achieved with primary closure and a more rapid closure than could be achieved with secondary wound healing.

II. WOUND CLOSURE MATERIALS AND TECHNIQUES

A. **Skin adhesives.** Topical adhesives (e.g., Dermabond and Indermil) can be used to maintain skin edge alignment in wounds that are clean, can be closed without tension, and are in areas not subject to motion or pressure. When applied to an incision that has been closed by subcuticular sutures, it can provide a waterproof and antimicrobial barrier that prevents ingress of bacteria (*Infect Control Hosp Epidemiol.* 2004;25:664). Infection rates with Dermabond are similar to those with traditional closure methods (*Neurosurgery.* 2005;56(suppl 1):147), with the advantages that there are no staples or sutures to remove and that patients may shower immediately.

B. **Steri-Strips.** Skin tapes are the least invasive way to close a superficial skin wound; however, because they provide no eversion of wound edges, the cosmetic result may be suboptimal. In addition, skin tapes tend to loosen if moistened by serum or blood and therefore are seldom appropriate for all but the most superficial skin wounds in areas of minimal or no tension. Their most frequent use is in support of a skin closure after suture or staple removal.

C. **Suture**

1. **Needles.** Curved needles are designed for use with needle holders, whereas straight (Keith) needles can be used with or without a holder. Two types are in common use: circular (tapered, noncutting) and triangular (cutting). Cutting needles are preferable for closure of tough tissue, such as skin, and noncutting needles are preferable for placing sutures in delicate tissues, such as blood vessels or intestine.

2. **Suture material.** Several characteristics differentiate the various suture materials. They include the following:

   a. **Absorbable versus nonabsorbable.** Among the absorbable materials, wide variability is found with regard to tensile strength, rate of absorption, and tissue reaction.

   b. **Monofilament versus braided.** Braided suture has better handling characteristics than monofilament suture, but the interstices between the braided strands that compose the suture are easily colonized by bacteria and thus pose an infection risk.

   c. **Natural versus synthetic.** Characteristics of commonly used suture materials are summarized in Tables 6-2 and 6-3.

3. **Staples** allow for quick closure. In areas of lower cosmetic sensitivity, such as the thick skin of the back or anterior abdominal wall, staples may produce cosmetic results approximating those of sutures. They are particularly useful for closure of scalp wounds.

D. **Skin suture technique**

1. **Basic surgical principles apply** closure without tension, elimination of dead space, aseptic technique, and (when closing skin) eversion of the skin margins. A dog-ear occurs when unequal bites are taken on opposing sides of a wound or incision, causing the tissue to bunch up as the end of the wound is approached. This can be prevented by carefully aligning the wound at the time of deep tissue closure (elimination of dead space) with interrupted absorbable sutures and by taking equal bites of tissue on both sides of the wound.

2. **Suture removal.** Suture scars occur when stitches are left in place too long, allowing epithelialization of the suture tracts. This complication can be minimized by timely suture removal. Facial sutures should be removed at days 3 to 5; elsewhere, days 7 to 10 are appropriate. These guidelines should be modified for the individual patient. Application of skin tapes after suture removal provides further support.

TABLE 6-2 Characteristics of Absorbable Suture Materials

Suture (Trade Name)	Manufacturing Process	Effective Strength (d)	Complete Absorption (d)	Absorption Profile Tissue Reactivity	Handling	Application
Surgical gut	Collagen from sheep intestine submucosa	4–10	70	High	Poor	Used for quick-healing mucosa
Chromic gut	Catgut treated with chromic acid	10–14	90	Moderate	Poor	Used for quick-healing mucosa
Polyglycolic acid (Dexon)	Synthetic monofilament or braided	14–21	60–120	Minimal	Good	Subcutaneous sutures, mucosa, ligation of vessels
Polylactic acid (Vicryl)	Synthetic braided, lubricated with polyglactin 370; undyed or purple	20–30	60–90	Minimal	Excellent	Subcuticular and subcutaneous sutures
Polydioxane (PDS)	Monofilament polyester	40–60	180	Minimal	Good	Used for extended support
Polyglyconate (Maxon)	Synthetic monofilament	40–60	180–210	Minimal	Excellent	More supple than polydioxane

TABLE 6-3 Characteristics of Nonabsorbable Suture Materials

Suture (Trade Name)	Manufacturing Process	Tissue Reactivity	Handling	Application
Silk	Braided; derived from cocoon of silkworm larva	High	Excellent	Vessel ligation; high capillarity; should be avoided in areas prone to infection
Cotton	Braided	High	Excellent	Same as silk
Polyester	Braided terephthalate (Dacron), polyethylene (Mersilene), coated with Teflon (Tevdek), silicone (Ti-Cron), polybutilate (Ethibond)	Minimal	Good if uncoated; excellent if coated	Commonly used for fascia; uncoated sutures have excellent knot security; coated sutures require five throws for knot security
Nylon	Synthetic polyamide monofilament or braided (Nurolon, Surgilon)	Minimal	Good	Used for skin, fascia; requires five throws for knot security
Polypropylene (Prolene, Surgilene)	Plastic monofilament	Minimal	Good	High elasticity; commonly used for skin closure and vascular anastomoses; requires five throws
Polybutester (Novafil)	Plastic monofilament copolymer	Minimal	Good	Very high elasticity; used when tissue swelling is present
Steel	Alloy monofilament	None	Poor	Retention sutures, bone

III. **OPEN WOUND CARE OPTIONS (SEE TABLE 6-4).** This brief review is not meant to be comprehensive or an endorsement of any product or product category. It remains an area of intense research, clinical, and commercial interest in which availability and indications of both established and new products can be expected to change during the publication cycle of this manual. The clinician would do well to weigh each patient's response to treatment, the indications and risks of any particular product, and need for further treatment.

A. **Topical ointments.** Petroleum-based ointments that contain one or several antibiotics prevent adherence of dressings to the wound and, by maintaining moisture of the wound environment, accelerate epithelialization and healing of primarily approximated wounds.

B. **Impregnated gauze.** Gauze that is impregnated with petrolatum is used for the treatment of superficial, partial-thickness wounds to maintain moisture, prevent excessive loss of fluid, and, in the case of Xeroform, provide mild deodorizing. It can also be used as the first layer of the initial dressing on a primarily closed wound. The use of this type of gauze is contraindicated when infection of the wound is suspected and inhibition of wound drainage would lead to adverse consequences.

C. **Gauze packing.** The practice of packing an open wound with gauze prevents dead space, facilitates drainage, and provides varying degrees of débridement. The maximum amount of débridement is seen when the gauze is packed into the wound dry and removed after absorption and evaporation have taken place, leaving a dry wound with adherent gauze, which on removal extracts superficial layers of the wound bed (dry-to-dry dressing). This dressing is seldom indicated. Wounds that are in need of great amounts of débridement usually benefit most from sharp débridement in the operating room or at the bedside; dry-to-dry dressings are painful and violate the principle of maintaining a moist environment for the wounds. Moist-to-dry dressings provide a much gentler débridement, are less painful, and can include sterile normal saline or various additives. Dakin solution [in full (0.5% sodium hypochlorite), half, or quarter strength] can be used to pack infected open wounds for a brief period when antimicrobial action is desirable. Because of toxic effects upon keratinocytes, the use of Dakin solution is not indicated except in infected wounds for a short period (*Adv Skin Wound Care.* 2005;18:373). Improvement in the foul odor that often emanates from drained abscesses and other infected open wounds is an added benefit of using this additive.

D. **Hydrogels.** These water- or glycerin-based gels (e.g., IntraSite) can be used in shallow or deep, open wounds. The gel promotes healing by gently rehydrating necrotic tissue, facilitating its debridement, and absorbing exudate produced by the wounds, as well as maintaining a moist wound environment. A nonadherent, nonabsorbent secondary dressing is applied over the gel; dressings should be changed every 8 hours to 3 days, depending on the condition of the wound.

E. **Hydrocolloids.** These occlusive, adhesive wafers provide a moist and protective environment for shallow wounds with light exudate. They can remain in place for 3 to 5 days and can be used under compression dressings to treat venous stasis ulcers.

TABLE 6-4 Wound and Skin Care Products

Product/Trade Name	Advantages	Limitations	Applications
Gauze			
Kerlix (roll gauze)	Débride mechanically	May disrupt viable tissue during change	Moderately/heavily exudating wounds
	Manages exudates by capillarity	May cause bleeding on removal	Partial- and full-thickness chronic wounds (stages II, III, IV)
	Permeable to gases		
Gauze sponges	Fills dead space	May cause pain on removal	Acute wounds
	Conformable	Particulate matter may be left in wound	Secondary dressing
	Adaptable	Permeable to fluids and bacteria	
		Limited thermal insulation	
		May dehydrate wound bed (if allowed to dry)	
		Damp to dry dressings contraindicated—wound ostomy Continence nurses (WOCN) Society Standards of Care, 1992	
Transparent Adhesive Dressings			
Tegaderm (3M)	Manages exudates by moisture vapor	Manage light exudates only	IV entry sites

(continued)

TABLE 6-4 Wound and Skin Care Products *(Continued)*			
Product/Trade Name	Advantages	Limitations	Applications
Opsite (Smith & Nephew)	Impermeable to fluids and bacteria	May disrupt fragile skin	Minor burns or lacerations
	Permeable to gases	Application may be difficult	Reduces surface friction in high-risk areas (stage I)
	Visualization of wound		Lightly exudating partial-thickness chronic wounds (stage II)
	Conformable		Over eschar to promote autolytic débridement
	Low profile		Cover dressing
Hydrocolloids			
Restore Hydrocolloid (Hollister)	Forms moist gel in wound bed	Manages moderate exudates	Reduces surface friction in high-risk areas
DuoDerm (ConvaTec)	Impermeable to fluids and bacteria	Impermeable to gases	
Comfeel Ulcer Care Dressing (Coloplast)	Manages exudates by particle swelling	May traumatize fragile skin	Partial- and full-thickness wounds
Tegasorb (3M)		Do not use over eschar or puncture wounds	Moderately exudating wounds
	Thermal insulation good	Use with extreme caution on diabetic ulcers	Venous stasis ulcers in conjunction with Unna boot
	Conformable	Contraindicated in third-degree burns	

Wound Fillers

AcryDerm strands	Wound filler	Not recommended in dry wounds or wounds with sinus tracts or tunnels	
Absorbent Wound Dressing (AcryMed)	Absorbs exudate Forms moist wound bed		May be used in combination with other wound dressing to increase absorption or fill shallow areas

Hydrogels

Amorphous	Forms moist wound bed	May dehydrate	Partial- and full-thickness chronic wound (stages II, III)
Restore Hydrogel (Hollister)	Conformable	Minimal absorption	
IntraSite Gel (Smith & Nephew)	Manages exudates by swelling	Requires secondary dressing	Partial- and full-thickness burns Diabetic ulcers Lightly exudating wounds

Enzymatic Débriding Agents

Collagenase (Santyl, Smith & Nephew)	Liquefies necrotic tissue Contributes toward formation of granulation tissue and epithelialization of wounds	Conditions with pH higher or lower than 6–8 decrease enzyme activity	Débridement of chronic dermal ulcers and severely burned areas

(continued)

TABLE 6-4	Wound and Skin Care Products *(Continued)*		
Product/Trade Name	**Advantages**	**Limitations**	**Applications**
Accuzyme (Healthpoint)	Does not attack healthy tissue or newly formed granulation tissue		
Absorbent dressings			
Bard Absorption Dressing (Bard Medical)	Manages exudates by osmotic action	Permeable to fluids and bacteria	Heavily exudating wounds
	Cleans debris	May increase pH beyond physiologic levels	Full-thickness chronic wounds (stages III, IV)
	Reduces odor	May sting on application	Malodorous wounds
	Maintains moist wound bed	Requires secondary dressing	
	Permeable to gases		
	Molds to wound contour		
	Fills dead space		
	Extends life of secondary dressing		
	Daily dressing change		
	Inexpensive		
Alginate			
Restore CalciCare (Hollister)	Forms moist gel in wound bed	Permeable to fluids and bacteria	Moderately/heavily exudating wounds

Sorbsan (Dow Hickman Pharmaceuticals)	Manages exudates by capillarity Permeable to gases	May produce burning sensation on application	Partial- and full-thickness wounds (stages III, IV)
Kaltostat (ConvaTec)	Molds to wound contour Fills dead space Irrigates easily from wound bed Reduces wound pain Fibers left in wound are absorbed May be used on clinically infected wounds Nonirritating	Requires irrigation before removal if allowed to dry out	Partial-thickness burns Skin donor sites
Solutions			
Normal saline (0.9%)	Noncytotoxic solution for wound care	Wound dehydrates if allowed to dry out If dressing saturated, may macerate periwound skin	Partial- and full-thickness wounds Dressing changes two to three times daily
Hydrogen peroxide	Chemical débridement of necrotic tissue when used as an irrigating solution	Cytotoxic to fibroblasts Has been documented to result in air embolus if instilled into wound cavities under pressure	Wound irrigation—use only half-strength and always rinse wound with normal saline

(continued)

TABLE 6-4 Wound and Skin Care Products *(Continued)*

Product/Trade Name	Advantages	Limitations	Applications
Povidone–iodine (Betadine)	FDA has not approved for use in wounds	Cytotoxic to fibroblasts until diluted to 1:1,000 May cause acidosis in burn patients Lasting systemic effects include cardiovascular toxicity, renal toxicity, hepatotoxicity, and neuropathy Impairs wound's ability to fight infection and increases potential for wound infection	None for wound care
Antibacterial Cream			
Silver sulfadiazine (Silvadene)	Broad-spectrum antibacterial (*S. aureus, E. coli, P. aeruginosa, P. mirabilis,* β-hemolytic streptococci)	Never approved by FDA for wound management Should not be used in presence of hepatic or renal impairment	Apply 1/8 in to clean, débrided wound daily or twice daily

Platelet-Derived Growth Factor

Becaplermin (Regranex, Ortho-McNeil Pharmaceuticals)

May promote wound healing in otherwise recalcitrant neuropathic ulcer

Very few side effects

Dressing protocol may be confusing

Wound must have adequate blood supply

Wound must be free of infection

No osteomyelitis

Wound must be free of necrotic tissue

Complex dosing

Calculate dose by multiplying length by width of wound in cm and divide by 4

Wound is irrigated with NS

Apply precise amount of drug to wound, cover with NS dressing

Leave in place for 12 hr

Then irrigate wound with NS

Pack wound with NS dressing

Leave in place for 12 hr

FDA, Food and Drug Administration; *E. coli*, *Escherichia coli*; NS, normal saline; *P. aeruginosa*, *Pseudomonas aeruginosa*; *P. mirabilis*, *Proteus mirabilis*; *S. aureus*, *Staphylococcus aureus*; IV, intravenous.

Adapted with permission from Rolstad BS, Ovington LG, Harris A. Wound care product formulary. In: Bryand RA, ed. *Acute and Chronic Wounds: Nursing Management*, 2nd ed. St. Louis: Mosby; 2000.

F. **Alginates.** Complex carbohydrate dressings composed of glucuronic and mannuronic acid, derived from brown seaweed, are formed into ropes or pads that are highly absorbent (e.g., Kaltostat). Alginates are absorbable and are useful for the treatment of deep wounds with heavy exudate because they form a gel as they absorb wound drainage.

G. **Adhesive films.** These plastic membranes (e.g., Tegaderm) are self-adhering and waterproof, yet are permeable to oxygen and water vapor. They are appropriate for partial-thickness wounds, such as split-thickness skin graft donor sites or superficial abrasions. They can also be used as secondary dressings on wounds that are being treated with hydrocolloids or alginates.

H. **Collagen-containing products.** A number of collagen-containing products are available in powder, sheet, or fluid form. They are available as pure collagen, typically types 1 and 3, or combined with other materials such as calcium alginate (Fibracol). Some wounds respond better to collagen than to other dressing materials.

I. **Hydrofibers** represent a newer dressing category of strands; they are some of the most absorptive materials available for packing in a heavily draining wound.

J. **Growth factors.** Human recombinant platelet-derived growth factor (PDGF) is the only U.S. Food and Drug Administration-approved clinically available growth factor. Topically applied to a granulating wound, it promotes granulation tissue formation, angiogenesis, and epithelialization. A saline-moistened gauze dressing is applied daily at midday to help keep the wound bed moist. Although initial approval was for the treatment of diabetic plantar foot ulcers, the drug is often used on other wound types. Epidermal growth factor (EGF) is in clinical trials for the treatment of venous stasis ulcers.

K. **Skin substitutes.** There are many different types of biologically active materials and skin substitutes and a comprehensive review of their properties and use is beyond the scope of this chapter. The indication and usage of these products is guided by their biologic and material properties. Skin substitutes can be used to facilitate healing of chronic open wounds, to provide temporary or permanent wound coverage, and to bridge skin, soft tissue or fascial defects. The usage of individual products is guided by the manufacturer's recommendations and the nature of the wound.

1. **Xenograft products** (Permacol, EZ derm, Matriderm, Oasis) are derived from animal tissues and consist of a collagen and/or proteoglycan matrix designed to promote influx of fibroblasts.

2. **Allogeneic products** are acellular tissue substitutes derived from cadaveric sources (AlloDerm, Strattice, Graftjacket, GammaGraft) that can be used to provide wound coverage. Each of these products is differently processed and material properties guide usages including wound coverage and hernia repair.

3. **Bioengineered living tissues** are composites of a structural mesh and cultured keratinocytes. Cells can be derived from neonatal sources (Dermagraft, TransCyte, Apligraf, OrCel) or autologous skin (Epicel, Laserskin, Epidex, Hyalograft). These advanced products bring living, biologically active cells into the wound bed.

L. **Negative-pressure wound therapy.** Negative pressure created by vacuum-assisted closure devices (Wound VAC or Blue Sky or institutionally created dressings) appears to stimulate capillary ingrowth and the formation of granulation tissue in open wounds while keeping a relatively clean wound environment. VAC therapy is effective in the management of wounds as diverse as diabetic foot wounds, sacral ulcers, mediastinal dehiscence, perineum wounds, and wounds including prosthetic mesh (*Plast Reconstr Surg.* 2006;117:127S). Recently, VAC therapy has been reported to be successful in managing enterocutaneous fistulae (*J Wound Care.* 2003;12:343) and over areas with exposed bone (*Wounds.* 2005;17:137) or tendon (*J Burn Care Rehabil.* 2002;23:167). VAC therapy is contraindicated when there are exposed major blood vessels, untreated osteomyelitis, or cancer within the wound, and it is relatively contraindicated in anticoagulated patients.

M. **Hyperbaric oxygen.** Local hypoxia in wound tissue may contribute to delayed healing. Randomized clinical trials have demonstrated that hyperbaric oxygen treatment (HBOT) is successful in healing diabetic foot ulcers (*Diabetes Care.* 1987;19:81), preventing diabetic amputations (*Diabetes Care.* 1996;19:1338), and healing chronic ulcerations (*Plast Reconstr Surg.* 1996;93:829). Standard treatment protocols are based on appropriate debridement and wound care in conjunction with 90 minutes/day at 2 atmospheres of oxygen. The criteria for appropriate treatment are available on the Undersea and Hyperbaric Medical Society Web site, http://www.UHMS.org, and should be consulted for consideration to initiate treatment.

N. **Metallic silver-impregnated dressings.** The broad antimicrobial properties of silver have long been recognized. Silver-impregnated dressings are used extensively for burns, chronic leg ulcers, diabetic, and traumatic injuries. A variety of silver-based dressings are available with specific indications determined by the manufacturer.

IV. CARE OF WOUNDS IN THE EMERGENCY ROOM

A. **History and physical examination.** A careful history and physical examination of the whole patient should be performed, with attention to the time and mechanism of injury, initial treatments given, and prior or associated injuries. Medical, surgical, and immunization history and all known medication allergies should be documented. It is critically important that all injuries be identified, with appropriate prioritization of administered treatment plans. Careful neurologic and vascular examination should be performed distal to the site of injury and before administration of any anesthetics that could limit a later assessment.

B. **Anesthesia.** Lidocaine (Xylocaine) in concentrations from 0.5% to 2% is generally chosen for its rapidity of action (1 to 2 minutes). If longer duration is desired, bupivacaine (Marcaine) can be used; however, it may require up to 10 minutes to full onset. A 1:1 mixture of 1% lidocaine and 0.25% bupivacaine provides a rapid and reasonably long-acting local anesthetic to improve hemostasis and prolong the effect of the anesthetic. Mixtures containing epinephrine should not be used to treat wounds on distal extremities (nose, earlobes, fingers, toes, or penis) because the profound vasoconstriction may lead to ischemic tissue loss. Whenever local anesthetics are used, care should be taken to avoid intravascular injection by aspirating before infiltration. The maximum safe amount of anesthetic that can be administered to the patient should be calculated before starting treatment.

C. **Wound cleansing.** After adequate anesthesia is administered, the wound and surrounding skin should be cleansed in a gentle fashion. This is best accomplished with a standard wound-cleansing solution (e.g., Saf-Clens and Shur-Clens). It should be remembered that many standard scrub solutions are extremely toxic to all living cells; thus, they should never be used to wash the wound itself. A good rule to follow is that one should never place a solution in a wound that one would not place in one's eye. Wounds are best irrigated with saline or lactated Ringer's solution with pressures of 8 to 15 psi. An 18- or 19-gauge intravenous catheter or needle on a 35- to 60-mL syringe provides 8-psi irrigating pressure, which is adequate to irrigate most wounds. Battery-powered irrigation systems, available for portable use, deliver pressures of up to 15 psi and are easier to use when irrigating a wound with several liters of fluid. Abrasions should be scrubbed carefully with a gloved hand during cleansing to remove foreign material that might lead to traumatic skin tattooing.

D. **Wound hemostasis and exploration.** Direct pressure, elevation, and even the use of a blood pressure cuff as a tourniquet are effective means of limiting blood loss in the emergency setting. Electrocautery, suture ligation, or hemostat clamping of a bleeding site is best done by a practitioner who is familiar with the anatomy of the area because major nerves often lie adjacent to major arteries and any imprecision can lead to an iatrogenic injury worse than the initial trauma. Wounds should be explored carefully for foreign bodies and to determine the extent of injury. Multiplane x-ray views of the soft tissues of the wounded area can prove to be useful in locating radiopaque objects. If the wound contains difficult-to-locate or numerous foreign bodies, it can best be explored in the operating room.

E. **Débridement.** Traumatic breaks of the skin are often irregular, and the force of impact leaves a zone of surrounding skin and underlying tissue injury that is often best treated by judicious sharp débridement. All foreign material and devitalized tissue must be removed before wound closure is attempted. The goal of débridement is to obtain a clean wound with a bleeding skin margin that overlies healthy, viable tissue.

F. **Wound closure.** The decision to close a wound depends largely on the amount of contamination present and the amount of time that the wound has been open. Wounds that are older than 6 to 8 hours, puncture wounds, human bites, and wounds with gross infection should not be closed, with the possible exception of facial wounds, for in these the superior vascular supply can often overcome otherwise major contamination. At a microscopic level, wounds with greater than 10^5 bacteria/g of tissue are considered too heavily contaminated to close safely. Dog and cat bites should be allowed to heal by secondary intention, or they may be closed primarily over wicks only after thorough irrigation and débridement, with administration of appropriate antibiotics.

G. **Additional considerations for wounds in the emergency room**

   1. **Tetanus prophylaxis.** Tetanus is a potentially fatal disorder that is characterized by uncontrolled spasms of the voluntary muscles. It is caused by the neurotoxin of the anaerobic bacterium *Clostridium tetani.* A tetanus-prone wound has one or more of the following characteristics: (1) more than 6 hours old; (2) deeper than 1 cm; (3) contaminated by soil, feces, or rust; (4) stellate configuration (burst-type injury with marked soft-tissue injury); (5) caused by missile, crush, burn, or frostbite; (6) contains devitalized or denervated tissue; and (7) caused by an animal or human bite. Recommendations for tetanus prophylaxis are summarized in Table 6-5.

   2. **Antibiotics.** Antibiotic use does not allow closure of a wound that would otherwise be left open to heal secondarily, and it is not a substitute for good wound cleansing and débridement. Antibiotics should be chosen based on the indication (prophylactic or therapeutic), the location and age of the wound, and the mechanism of injury. In addition, one should consider the likely pathogen(s) that are most involved under the circumstances. Prophylactic antibiotics are indicated for immunocompromised patients and those with prosthetic heart valves or other permanently implanted prostheses. Prophylactic antibiotics should also be used when intestinal or genitourinary tract contamination is present, when an infection is likely to develop, or when an infection has potentially disastrous consequences (*Surg Clin North Am.*

TABLE 6-5	Summary of Immunization Practices Advisory Committee Recommendations for Tetanus Prophylaxis in Routine Wound Management			
Tetanus Immunization	Clean Minor Wounds		Tetanus-Prone Wounds	
	Td[a]	TIG[b]	Td	TIG
Unknown or less than three doses	Yes	No	Yes	Yes
Three doses or more	No (yes if >10 yr since last dose)	No	No (yes if >5 yr since last dose)	No

[a]Adsorbed tetanus and diphtheria toxoids, 0.5 mL intramuscularly. For children <7 yr, diphtheria-polio-tetanus is recommended.
[b]TIG (human), 250 units intramuscularly, given concurrently with the toxoid at separate sites. Heterologous antitoxin (equine) should not be given unless TIG is not available within 24 hr and only if the possibility of tetanus outweighs the danger of adverse reaction.
Td, tetanus-diphtheria toxoid (adult type); TIG, tetanus immune globulin.
Reprinted with permission from Centers for Disease Control and Prevention. Tetanus United States, 1987 and 1988. *MMWR.* 1990;39(3):37.

1997;77:3). For wounds that are likely to become infected, obtaining good wound cultures at the time of injury helps to better target the specific organism(s) that failed to respond to initial broad-spectrum antibiotic treatment.

3. **Furuncles and carbuncles.** Furuncles are small boils or abscesses caused by an infection of the hair follicle that extends into the subcutaneous tissue deep. Carbuncles are cutaneous infections of multiple hair follicles, characterized by the destruction of fibrous tissue septa. The usual causative organism is *S. aureus,* and the incidence and prevalence of skin abscesses has risen in parallel with the emergence of community-acquired MRSA (*Clin Infect Dis.* 2005;41:1373). Furuncles manifest as firm, tender, erythematous nodules. Predisposing factors include diabetes, corticosteroid use, impaired neutrophil function, or increased friction or perspiration as occurs in athletes or obese individuals. Whereas initial treatment can include oral antibiotics and warm compresses to promote drainage, if the furuncle exhibits fluctuance, an incision-and-drainage procedure is required. (1). Under local anesthesia and after site prep with chlorhexidine or an iodine-containing solution, the initial incision is made with a no. 11 scalpel with the blade oriented perpendicular to the skin and inserted into the area of maximum fluctuance. (2). A cruciform or elliptical incision will help to prevent premature epidermal closure with recurrent cavity formation. A hemostat or blunt finger dissection is used to probe and break up any loculations within the abscess cavity. (3). The cavity should be irrigated and packed with iodoform or plain gauze stripping, which will require regular packing change. The use of antibiotics after abscess drainage remains controversial and depends on appropriate clinical judgment. If antibiotics are administered and community-acquired MRSA is a possible cause of the infection, trimethoprim/sulfamethoxazole (TMP/SMX), doxycycline, clindamycin, or a third- or fourth-generation fluoroquinolone should be considered, and a 7-day course is generally sufficient (*Prim Care.* 2006;33:697). Oral, perirectal, or genital abscesses should be considered multibacterial, and agents such as amoxicillin–clavulanate or third- or fourth-generation fluoroquinolones should be used to cover Gram-positive, Gram-negative, and anaerobic organisms. Patients who are immunocompromised or diabetic may require intravenous antibiotic therapy. If oral or intravenous antibiotics are administered, a wound culture should be obtained from the abscess cavity prior to irrigation to determine whether the appropriate antibiotic has been selected. For all skin infections and drained abscesses, follow-up is extremely important.

H. **Bites.** The treatment of a bite wound beyond the basic treatment of copious irrigation and debridement is most dependent on the source of the bite.

1. **Human bites** typically occur during interpersonal conflict. Because the wound often seems relatively trivial, such as a small puncture wound or a laceration in a patient who is very upset or intoxicated, the patient may delay seeking treatment, which increases the likelihood

of the wound to become infected. A particularly troublesome bite is a small skin injury that is seen over the metacarpophalangeal joint of a patient who punched someone else in the mouth and sustained a tooth cut of the skin overlying the fisted knuckle. Such injuries often require operative joint irrigation and parenteral antibiotics. Unintentional bites of the lip or tongue sustained in a fall or during a seizure may also occasionally come to the attention of a surgeon. The oral flora of humans includes *Staphylococcus* and *Streptococcus* species, anaerobic bacteria, *Eikenella corrodens,* and anaerobic Gram-negative rods; antibiotic coverage should be directed initially toward these organisms.

2. **Mammalian animal bites.** Because infection is the most common complication of domestic animal bites, these bites should be considered contaminated and their immediate closure deferred. Infections that are caused by dog bites are usually polymicrobial, and pathogens include viridans streptococci, *Pasteurella multocida,* and *Bacteroides, Fusobacterium,* and *Capnocytophaga* species. Because these wounds are often larger open lacerations, only about 5% of dog bites become infected. The oral flora of the domestic cat is believed to be less complex, with *P. multocida* found in up to 60% of wounds caused by cat bites. Because these are smaller puncture wounds, up to 80% of these will become infected. Local laws require the confinement of animals to ensure that they do not manifest rabies. Rabies, a routinely fatal disease of the central nervous system, is caused by the rabies virus, which is a member of the rhabdovirus group and contains a single strand of RNA. Thanks in large part to an intensive immunization program, the incidence of rabies in the United States has been reduced greatly, to approximately five cases per year. Today, the major risk comes from wild animal bites. The recommendations for rabies prophylaxis and treatment are summarized in Table 6-6.

3. **Snake bites.** Ten percent of the snakes in the United States are venomous. Determining whether a venomous snake caused the bite is critical in the early management of bite injuries. Pit vipers usually leave two puncture wounds, whereas nonvenomous snakes generally leave a characteristic U-shaped bite wound. Poisonous snake venom contains many polypeptides that are damaging to human tissues, including phospholipase A, hyaluronidase, adenosine triphosphatase, 5-nucleotidase, and nicotinic acid dehydrogenase. The degree of envenomation and the time from injury determine the clinical manifestations. Immediate signs of envenomation include regional edema, erythema, and intense pain at the site of the bite. Systemic manifestations can ensue rapidly, especially with greater envenomation. The hematocrit and platelet count may fall, with concomitant elevation of the prothrombin time, partial thromboplastin time, and bleeding times. Without treatment, severe envenomation may lead to pulmonary edema, peripheral vascular collapse, direct cardiotoxicity, and acute renal failure. Coral snake venom is less toxic locally but can lead to profound neurologic sequelae. Early symptoms include nausea, euphoria, salivation, paresthesias, ptosis, and muscle weakness leading to respiratory arrest.

TABLE 6-6	Rabies Postexposure Prophylaxis Treatment Guide	
Species	**Condition of Animal**	**Treatment**[a]
Domestic cat or dog	Healthy and available for at least 10 d of observation	None; however, treatment should be initiated at the first sign of rabies[b]
	Suspected rabid[b]	Immediate
	Unknown	Contact public health department
Wild skunk, bat, fox, coyote, raccoon, or other carnivore	Regard as rabid; animal should be killed and tested as soon as possible	Immediate; however, discontinue if immunofluorescence test is negative

[a](1) Human rabies immune globulin, 20 IU/kg [if feasible, infiltrate half of dose around the wound(s), the rest intramuscularly in gluteal area] and (2) human diploid cell vaccine (HDCV), 1 mL intramuscularly in deltoid area (never in gluteal area) on days 0, 3, 7, 14, and 28. If the patient has previously been immunized, give booster HDCV only on days 0 and 3.
[b]Any animal suspected of being rabid should be killed and its brain studied with a rabies-specific fluorescent antibody.
Adapted with permission from Immunization Practices Advisory Committee. Rabies Prevention United States, 1991. *MMWR.* 1991;40(RR-3):1.

Treatment is most successful if administered promptly. Extremity wounds should be immobilized and a tourniquet applied proximal to the bite site to minimize the spread of the venom. Although small amounts of venom can be removed by suction through small incisions over the bite wound, a wider surgical excision of the bite removes even more, provided that it can be done in a timely fashion. Antivenom may help to neutralize the venom and should be administered intravenously as soon as possible after more severe bites or when systemic symptoms are noted. Current treatment includes CroFab, a Fab-segment–based product that lacks antigenic Fc antibody fragments. The antibody is produced by injecting sheep with one of four pit viper species indigenous to the United States: western diamondback rattlesnake, eastern diamondback rattlesnake, Mojave rattlesnake, and cottonmouth. The venoms of different species vary in composition and potency, but they are similar enough that CroFab can neutralize venom from many species, including those not included in the production process (*Am J Trop Med Hyg.* 1995;53:507). Indications for CroFab antivenom use are pit viper envenomation with worsening edema or any systemic symptom including coagulopathy. Relative contraindications include known hypersensitivity to CroFab, papain, or papaya (*Curr Opin Pediatr.* 2005;17:234). Shock is treated with circulatory support. Broad-spectrum antibiotics and tetanus prophylaxis are also indicated.

4. **Spider bites**
   a. The **black widow spider** *(Latrodectus mactans)* is found throughout the United States and prefers to inhabit dry, dark crevices. The female is distinguished by her shiny black body and a red hourglass mark on the abdomen. The actual bite may cause little pain, and victims often do not recall the event. The bite presents as a pale area surrounded by a red ring. The venom, a neurotoxin, causes muscular rigidity. Chest pain from muscular contraction follows upper-extremity bites, whereas lower-extremity bites may cause rigidity of the abdominal wall. Patients who present with abdominal wall rigidity, which might typically suggest an acute abdominal emergency, lack associated abdominal tenderness. Intense muscular spasms and pain are usually self-limiting and require no specific treatment. Severe cases may progress to respiratory arrest, which, along with shock, accounts for the observed mortality of approximately 5%. Therapy consists of respiratory and circulatory support, broad-spectrum antibiotics, narcotic analgesia, and muscle relaxants. Antivenin *(L. mactans)* is indicated for the very young or old and for patients with severe illness.
   b. The **brown recluse spider** *(Loxosceles reclusa)* is found throughout the central and southern United States, most often inhabiting dark, moist environments. It is 10 to 15 mm long, with a light tan to brown color, a flat body, and a violin-shaped band over the head and chest area of the back. Brown recluse venom is very locally toxic, containing hyaluronidase, and other elements that lead to coagulation necrosis of the area around the wound. Systemically, hemolysis with hemoglobinuria, hemolytic anemia, and renal failure may develop. Pain at the time of the bite is an inconsistent symptom; however, several hours after the bite, a characteristic lesion is seen, with a central zone of pale induration surrounded by an erythematous border. By this time, pain is severe. After approximately 1 week, a black eschar develops, which soon sloughs, leaving an ulcer that may continue to enlarge, with extensive necrosis of the underlying fat and subcutaneous tissues. Systemic illness most often occurs in children, with fever, malaise, nausea, and vomiting. Therapy is supportive, and mortality is rare. Many of these wounds will heal spontaneously. If necessary, excision of the wound should be deferred until the ulcer is well demarcated; broad-spectrum antibiotics are recommended.

Critical Care

Kendra D. Conzen and Laureen L. Hill

Patients are admitted to intensive care units (ICUs) because of either the presence or the risk of organ dysfunction. This chapter focuses on routine monitoring of the critically ill patient, the three most common reasons for surgical ICU admissions (respiratory, circulatory, and renal failure), and sepsis. It also addresses adjunctive topics, including sedation and analgesia, prophylaxis against stress-induced upper gastrointestinal (GI) hemorrhage, and the role of transfusion and glucose control in the care of the critically ill.

I. MONITORING OF THE CRITICALLY ILL PATIENT

A. **Temperature monitoring.** Critically ill patients are at increased risk for temperature alterations as a result of debilitation and predisposition to infection. All critically ill patients should have their core temperatures measured at least every 4 hours. While a rectal thermometer is the most accurate method of obtaining the core temperature, oral and bladder probes can reduce patient discomfort. Transcutaneous measurements are less reliable.

B. **Electrocardiographic (ECG) monitoring.** Continuous ECG monitoring with computerized dysrhythmia detection systems is standard in most ICUs. Continuous monitoring allows for rapid detection of dysrhythmias and assessment of heart rate and rhythm.

C. **Arterial pressure monitoring**

1. Indirect arterial pressure measurement with a sphygmomanometer should be performed at least hourly or more often during titration of vasoactive drips.

2. **Direct arterial pressure measurement** with intra-arterial catheters offers continuous measurement of arterial pressures and waveforms as well as easy, painless access for arterial blood gas (ABG) measurement. Arterial cannulation is warranted in patients with hemodynamic instability and in those who require frequent blood gas analysis. The most common site of insertion is the radial artery, which is chosen because of its accessibility and generally good collateral blood flow. If this is unavailable, alternatives include femoral and, less commonly, dorsalis pedis or axillary artery catheterization. These should be avoided in infants because occlusion may cause extremity ischemia and subsequent deformity. The extremity distal to the catheter should be assessed prior to insertion and frequently after insertion. The catheter should be removed immediately if there is evidence of distal ischemia. Rare infectious complications include local cellulitis and bacteremia, which may result from catheter colonization or contamination of the fluid-filled monitoring system.

D. **Central venous pressure (CVP) monitoring.** Central venous catheters provide access to measure CVP, CvO_2 and to administer vasoactive drugs and total parenteral nutrition. For techniques of catheter insertion, refer to Chapter 37.

E. **Pulmonary artery (PA) catheterization.** PA (also called *Swan-Ganz*) catheters are used to determine cardiac filling pressures, cardiac output (CO), PA pressures, systemic vascular resistance (SVR), and mixed venous oxygen saturation (SvO_2). They can be used in unstable patients with rapid changes in hemodynamic status to assess responses to treatment with fluid and cardioactive agents. It is important to note that the use of PA catheters has not been demonstrated to change mortality in prospective, randomized trials, in part due to error in interpretation and variation in management decisions.

1. **Continuous ECG and blood pressure monitoring and peripheral intravenous access** are required. An ECG must be checked prior to PA catheter placement to rule out left-bundle-branch block because PA catheter placement can induce transient right-bundle-branch block. If a patient with left-bundle-branch block needs a PA catheter, a transcutaneous pacemaker should be placed prior to PA catheter placement.

2. **Complications** associated with central venous access are described in Chapter 37. PA catheter **balloon rupture** exposes the patient to the risk of air and balloon fragment emboli. Balloon rupture should be suspected when air inflated into the balloon does not return; the diagnosis is confirmed if blood can be aspirated from the balloon port. If either of these occurs, the catheter should be removed immediately. **PA perforation** presents with hemoptysis, typically after balloon inflation. Management of this serious complication includes placement of the patient with his or her involved side in the dependent position and emergent thoracic surgical consultation. Atrial and ventricular **dysrhythmias** occur commonly during insertion of PA catheters and usually are self-limited.

3. **Esophageal Dopplers** (CardioQ, Deltex Medical) have been introduced as a less invasive alternative to PA catheters for goal-directed fluid therapy. Esophageal Dopplers measure descending aortic flow velocity over time, therefore SV is calculated by area under the velocity curve and a nomogram-based aortic diameter. Changes in SV with fluid can be used to titrate fluid administration. There has been no demonstration of improvement in outcomes associated with their use. Their potential risk is lower than with PA catheters; however, esophageal perforation can occur.

F. **Respiratory monitoring**

1. **Pulse oximetry** should be used in all critically ill patients. It provides quantitative, continuous assessment of arterial oxygen saturation (SaO_2). Probe malposition, motion, hypothermia, vasoconstriction, and hypotension may result in poor signal detection and unreliable measurements. Nail polish, dark skin, and elevated serum lipids falsely lower the SaO_2 measurement, whereas elevated carboxyhemoglobin

falsely raises the measurements. Methemoglobin results in a reading of 85%, regardless of oxygen saturation level.

2. **Capnography** provides quantitative, continuous assessment of expired CO_2 concentrations, and the gradient between arterial CO_2 partial pressure (Pa_{CO_2}) and end-tidal CO_2 ($ETCO_2$) measurements can be used to follow trends and the difference reflects the proportion of dead space ventilation. A rise in $ETCO_2$ can indicate a decrease in alveolar ventilation or an increase in CO_2 production, as seen with overfeeding, sepsis, fever, exercise, or acute increases in CO. A fall in $ETCO_2$ may indicate an increase in alveolar ventilation (when associated with a decrease in Pa_{CO_2}) or an increase in dead space (without a decreased Pa_{CO_2}), as seen with massive pulmonary embolism (PE) or air embolism, endotracheal tube (ET) or mainstem bronchus obstruction, ventilator circuit leak, or a sudden drop in CO.

II. **SEDATION AND ANALGESIA.** Altered mentation, which can span the spectrum from delirium to coma, is a common manifestation of acute illness. Delirium has independently been associated with increased ICU and in-hospital mortality (*Crit Care.* 2010;14:R210). Pain and emotional distress should be treated. Sedation allows critically ill patients to tolerate invasive supportive interventions such as intubation and mechanical ventilation. Titration of sedation is simplified by the use of an objective scoring system, such as the modified Ramsay scale (Table 7-1).

A. **Control of agitation.** The most frequently used agents are **benzodiazepines,** which are potent inducers of sedation, anxiolysis, and amnesia. The action of benzodiazepines appears to be mediated through γ-aminobutyric acid receptors, an inhibitory neurotransmitter. Effective doses of benzodiazepines may be higher in tolerant patients (e.g., those who have taken similar agents previously or who consume alcohol or smoke cigarettes regularly). Patients older than 50 years or those with preexisting

TABLE 7-1	Modified Ramsay Sedation Scale
Score	**Characteristics**
1	Anxious and agitated or restless, or both
2	Cooperative, oriented, and tranquil
3	Responds to commands only
4	Asleep, but responds to physical or auditory stimuli
5	Asleep, but responds sluggishly to physical or auditory stimuli
6	No response

cardiopulmonary, hepatic, or renal dysfunction are particularly susceptible to benzodiazepines and their metabolites. Initial doses should be reduced in these patients. Benzodiazepines have also been associated with higher rates of delirium (*Crit Care.* 2010;14:R38).

1. **Midazolam** has a short half-life (20 to 60 minutes) and a rapid onset (1 to 3 minutes) and offset of action. Although midazolam has a short half-life, when it is given as a continuous infusion for a prolonged period of time, metabolites accumulate, and patients may take a number of days to fully awaken.

2. **Lorazepam** has a longer half-life (10 to 20 hours) and a slower onset (10 to 20 minutes) of action. Unlike midazolam, lorazepam does not have active metabolites. However, similar to midazolam, the drug accumulates with prolonged use, and patients may remain sedated for a number of days after the agent is stopped. Lorazepam also precipitates in tubing over time due to the carrier vehicle used. Midazolam and lorazepam are acceptable alternatives for long-term sedation in the critically ill patient.

3. **Propofol** is a nonbenzodiazepine sedative-hypnotic that has an extremely short onset and offset of action and is usually delivered as a continuous infusion. It does not accumulate to the same degree as benzodiazepines and thus results in a shorter length of sedation after discontinuation. A major side effect of propofol is hypotension, especially in hypovolemic patients. Although it is more expensive than benzodiazepines, propofol is preferred for short-term sedation (<2 days) because of its rapid elimination. Prolonged use can cause hypertriglyceridemia and risk of pancreatitis or propofol infusion syndrome, evidenced by a metabolic acidosis.

4. **Dexmedetomidine** is a relatively selective α_2-adrenoreceptor agonist that may be helpful for short-term sedation of mechanically ventilated patients. Patients treated with this agent are more easily arousable than those sedated with either propofol or benzodiazepine infusions, experience less delirium, and have shorter ICU length of stay (*Intensive Care Med.* 2010;36:926; *Crit Care.* 2010;14:R38). Additionally, dexmedetomidine has analgesic and opiate-sparing properties. The main side effect is hypotension. Bradycardia has been observed in studies with loading doses and high maintenance doses. Dexmedetomidine is approved for use for a maximum of 24 hours, but has been safely administered for up to 5 days in clinical trials (*JAMA.* 2007;298:2644).

B. **Control of delirium**

1. **Antipsychotics: Haloperidol** is an antipsychotic medicine that can be used to treat delirium emergently. Major toxicities include hypotension, cardiac arrhythmias, prolongation of the QT interval, and extrapyramidal symptoms. Therefore, daily, scheduled dosing of atypical antipsychotics (e.g., olanzapine and quetiapine) may be preferable. ECGs should be checked daily in patients on long-term haloperidol.

C. Control of pain. Pain management is an important concern in the surgical ICU.

1. **Morphine** is administered as needed and for patient-controlled dosing because of its low cost and familiarity. Accumulation of active metabolites can occur in patients with renal impairment and its use should be avoided in those patients.

2. **Fentanyl** is the most commonly used opiate for continuous drips. It has a half-life of 30 to 60 minutes due to its rapid redistribution. Unlike morphine, fentanyl does not cause histamine release and is therefore less likely to cause hypotension.

3. **Hydromorphone** is a viable option for patients who are allergic to morphine or fentanyl. Hydromorphone has no active metabolites and can therefore be administered to patients with renal impairment.

4. **Meperidine** is used least frequently because of its side effects. Patients with renal or hepatic dysfunction are at risk for accumulation of normeperidine, a metabolite, which can cause neurotoxic side effects including seizures.

5. **Methadone** is a narcotic with a long half-life (8 to 59 hours) that can be used for pain management and to facilitate withdrawal from other narcotics. Substantial variability between individuals with regard to its pharmacokinetic properties mandates close monitoring of patients during initiation of treatment and conversion from other opioids.

6. **Thoracic or lumbar epidural catheters** are usually well tolerated, decrease the need for intravenous narcotics, and can substantially improve compliance with respiratory therapy. Significant risks include hypotension and intrathecal or intravascular catheter migration. Anticoagulation or active use of antiplatelet agents is relative contraindications due to risk for epidural hematoma and subsequent neurologic injury.

D. Regardless of which agents are used for sedation and analgesia, the presence of a **sedation protocol** decreases both length of stay in the ICU and the length of time a patient requires mechanical ventilation compared with physician-directed sedation.

E. For patients who require **long-term sedation and analgesia,** daily interruption of sedation to wakefulness produces decreased time on mechanical ventilation and shorter ICU stays, according to a prospective, randomized, controlled study (*N Engl J Med.* 2000;342:1477). However, this study did not include surgical patients, who have higher analgesia requirements than typical medical ICU patients. Therefore, the applicability of a "daily wakeup" to surgical ICU patients is less clear.

III. RESPIRATORY FAILURE

A. Etiology. Respiratory failure results from inadequate exchange of oxygen and/or carbon dioxide. Hypoxemia may be caused by ventilation/perfusion (V/Q) mismatch, hypoventilation, or impaired systemic delivery/extraction.

The extremes of V/Q mismatch are dead space ventilation (V/Q = ∞) and complete intrapulmonary shunt (V/Q = 0). Dead space ventilation refers to airflow within lung that does not equilibrate with blood gas content; this occurs in chronic obstructive pulmonary disease and PE. In contrast, intrapulmonary shunt results from perfusion of lung tissue that is poorly ventilated, such as in the setting of severe pulmonary edema, acute respiratory distress syndrome (ARDS), or pneumonia. Hypoventilatory hypoxemia may be caused by a failure of the mechanical ventilatory apparatus (e.g., neuromuscular disease, inspiratory muscle fatigue, and airway obstruction), which results in hypercapnia and hypoxemia. Although the etiology (possibly multifactorial) is important for longer-term treatment and prognosis, the early treatment of respiratory failure is similar regardless of the immediate cause.

B. **Diagnosis.** Signs or symptoms of respiratory impairment (e.g., tachypnea, dyspnea, or mental status changes) should prompt analysis of pulse oximetry and ABGs. Pulse oximetry monitoring results of less than 90% correspond to a partial arterial oxygen pressure (Pa_{O_2}) of less than 60 mm Hg, which seriously compromises tissue oxygenation. An acute rise in Pa_{CO_2} to greater than 50 mm Hg along with a pH of less than 7.35 (respiratory acidosis) implies a significant imbalance between carbon dioxide production and elimination (alveolar ventilation). **It is important to note that adequate oxygenation does not guarantee adequate ventilation.** A complete physical exam and portable chest x-ray are essential for figuring out the etiology of respiratory failure.

C. **Treatment**

1. **Oxygen therapy.** The objective of supplemental oxygen administration is to increase the relative concentration of oxygen in the alveoli. This is accomplished most commonly by delivering oxygen through a nasal cannula, simple face mask, or face mask with a reservoir (Table 7-2). The inspired oxygen concentration varies depending on the percentage of entrained air: The more air that is entrained (with an ambient oxygen concentration of 0.21), the lower the fraction of inspired oxygen (F_{IO_2}). When the required F_{IO_2} is high (~0.60), a high–air-flow system with oxygen enrichment via a jet-mixing or Venturi apparatus is used, and the oxygen is delivered by a tight-fitting mask with a reservoir. Whenever possible, inspired oxygen should be humidified to prevent drying of the airways and respiratory secretions.

2. **Airway management.** Securing and maintaining a patent airway is the first priority in an unstable patient. The most common source of airway obstruction in a patient with an altered sensorium is the tongue. This is corrected easily by the chin-lift or jaw-thrust maneuver or by placing an oropharyngeal or nasopharyngeal airway. In a conscious patient, an oropharyngeal airway can cause retching and is usually poorly tolerated. If uncertainty exists about whether the airway is patent or protected from aspiration, ET intubation is indicated. In most cases, intubation is not urgent. **Unless the physician is skilled in the placement of an artificial airway, the appropriate maneuver is to give supplemental oxygen and to assist with bag-mask ventilation if necessary until someone with airway expertise arrives.**

TABLE 7-2	Oxygen Delivery Systems	
Type	**F$_{IO_2}$ Capability**	**Comments**
Nasal cannula	24%–48%	At flow rates of 1–8 L/min; true F$_{IO_2}$ uncertain and highly dependent on minute ventilation; simple, comfortable, and can be worn during eating or coughing
Simple face mask	35%–55%	At flow rates of 6–10 L/min
High-humidity mask	Variable from 28% to nearly 100%	Flow rates should be 2–3 times minute ventilation; levels >60% may require additional oxygen bleed-in; excellent humidification
Reservoir mask		
Nonrebreathing	90%–95%	At flow rates of 12–15 L/min; incorporates directional valves that reduce room air entrainment and rebreathing of expired air
Partial rebreathing	50%–80%	At flow rates of 8–10 L/min
Ventimask	Available at 24%, 28%, 31%, 35%, 40%, and 50%	Provides controlled F$_{IO_2}$; useful in chronic obstructive pulmonary disease patients to prevent depression of respiratory drive; poorly humidified gas at maximum F$_{IO_2}$

F$_{IO_2}$, fraction of inspired oxygen.

a. **Oral and nasal ET intubation.** The oral route is usually the most expeditious. The nasal route can be used only when the patient is breathing spontaneously; significant skill is needed to direct the tip of the ET tube blindly past the vocal cords and into the trachea. Additionally, nasotracheal intubation poses a significant bleeding risk that can make subsequent airway management difficult. Once the tube is in the trachea, the adequacy of bilateral ventilation must be established using auscultation and a carbon dioxide indicator. A chest x-ray is used to document correct ET tube position.

b. **Noninvasive ventilation.** Biphasic positive airway pressure (BiPAP) is a form of ventilation that is delivered by means of a tight-fitting mask (no ET tube), which allows independent control of positive inspiratory and expiratory pressures. It is most useful as a bridge to aid respiratory efforts in patients with mild-to-moderate respiratory insufficiency of short duration (e.g., asthma or COPD exacerbations or pulmonary edema) and frequently can prevent the need for intubation in patients with rapidly reversible respiratory failure. BiPAP may result in gastric distension, thereby increasing the risk of aspiration, particularly in the patient with altered sensorium.

c. **Tracheostomy** should be considered in the presence of severe maxillofacial injury to ensure an adequate airway or if prolonged intubation is anticipated. Timing of tracheostomy has been found to be significantly correlated with length of mechanical ventilation, as well as duration of ICU and hospital stay (*Crit Care Med.* 2005;33:2513). Tracheostomy provides a more secure airway, improves patient comfort and oral hygiene, increases patient mobility, and enhances secretion removal. **If a tracheostomy falls out before an adequate tract has formed, the patient should be reintubated orotracheally rather than subjected to a blind attempt to replace the tracheostomy.**

d. **Cricothyroidotomy** is useful in emergency situations when attempts to ventilate by bag-valve-mask and ET tube are unsuccessful. The technique is described in Chapter 37. Percutaneous cricothyroidotomy may also be performed if a kit is available and someone with expertise is present.

e. **Complications.** Immediate complications include passage of the ET tube into either the esophagus or the tissue surrounding the trachea. Either can lead to death if not promptly recognized. Of these, esophageal intubation is substantially more common. When an ET tube is placed in tissue surrounding the trachea (most common when attempting to replace a tracheostomy that has fallen out), it can lead to hemorrhage, pneumothorax, pneumomediastinum, subcutaneous emphysema, and injury to the recurrent laryngeal nerve. Delayed complications of ET intubation include hemorrhage, which results from erosion of the tube into a vessel (usually the brachiocephalic artery). Immediate orotracheal intubation, removal of the tracheostomy tube, insertion of the surgeon's finger into the tracheostomy site, and anterior compression of the brachiocephalic artery against the clavicle can be used treat the hemorrhage. ET tube cuff pressures should be monitored frequently and kept below capillary filling pressures (i.e., <25 mm Hg) to prevent tracheal ischemia, which, if untreated, can lead to tracheomalacia or tracheal stenosis.

3. **Mechanical ventilation** is indicated for the treatment of respiratory failure. The goal of treatment is to improve alveolar ventilation and oxygenation and to reduce the work of breathing, while other therapies are instituted to treat underlying disease processes.

a. **Modes of mechanical ventilation** can be divided into volume-control and pressure-control modes. The key to understanding the differences between these modes lies in the relationship between pressure and volume and the variable that is controlled. The goal of volume-control modes is to deliver a set tidal volume to the patient to ensure adequate alveolar ventilation; airway pressure varies depending on compliance (compliance equals the change in volume divided by the change in pressure ($C = \Delta V/\Delta P$). In contrast, the goal of pressure-limited modes is to deliver a set airway pressure; tidal volume varies depending on compliance.

(1) **Volume-control modes**

(a) **Assist-control (A/C) ventilation** delivers a preset tidal volume at a set rate. As the machine senses each inspiratory effort by the patient, it delivers the set tidal volume. If the patient's respiratory rate is below the machine's set rate, ventilator-initiated breaths are delivered to make up the difference between the set rate and the patient's. A/C ventilation minimizes the work of breathing because the ventilator assists all breaths (hence, the term *full support*); however, for this reason, this mode is uncomfortable in the awake or minimally sedated patient if the patient's breaths are dyssynchronous with those delivered by the ventilator. Respiratory alkalosis from hyperventilation may develop in agitated patients.

(b) **Intermittent mandatory ventilation (IMV),** like A/C ventilation, delivers a preset tidal volume at a set rate. IMV will assist spontaneous respiratory efforts through the use of pressure support in which a spontaneously initiated breath triggers fresh gas flow until the level of set pressure support is achieved.

(2) **Pressure-control modes**

(a) **Pressure-support ventilation** delivers a preset inspiratory pressure but at no set rate. Constant inspiratory pressure continues until the inspiratory flow of gas falls below a predetermined level and the exhalation valve opens. Thus, tidal volumes are generated only when the patient is breathing spontaneously. This allows the patient to maintain control of inspiratory and expiratory time and thus tidal volume; as a result, this mode is the most comfortable for spontaneously breathing patients. The disadvantages of pressure-support ventilation are that (1) all ventilation depends on patient effort and (2) sudden increases in airway resistance decrease tidal volumes. Small amounts (5 to 8 cm H_2O) of pressure-support ventilation are used routinely to overcome the resistance to airflow caused by the ET tube and the inspiratory demand valves of the ventilator.

(b) **Pressure-control ventilation** delivers a preset inspiratory pressure (as opposed to tidal volume) at a set rate. This mode is used in patients with poor (low) lung compliance who develop high inspiratory pressures when they are ventilated with the more traditional modes described previously. Thus, the advantage of this mode is that it allows the physician to set the airway pressure and thereby minimize barotrauma. The disadvantage is that the tidal volume varies depending on compliance. The sudden development of an increase in airway resistance (coughing, thick secretions, a kink in the ET tube, a Valsalva maneuver), for example, increases airway pressures and decreases tidal volumes to dangerously low levels.

For patients in whom conventional mechanical ventilation is failing to achieve adequate oxygenation, open lung ventilation may be considered. Open lung ventilation attempts to minimize shearing forces due to alveolar collapse by stenting alveoli open at end expiration. Criteria for using an alternative mode of ventilation include F_{IO_2} greater than 70%, SpO_2 less than or equal to 88%, PEEP greater than 15, and plateau pressures greater than 30.

(3) **Airway pressure release ventilation (BiLevel)** is a style of ventilator support that allows a patient to breathe spontaneously at two levels of positive end-expiratory pressure (PEEP). The time at the lower PEEP level may be limited so that all breaths are taken at the upper PEEP level and the pressure is then released just long enough to allow the lung volume to decrease (airway pressure release). Alternatively, spontaneous breathing may occur at both levels. There is evidence to suggest that this improves patient comfort and synchrony with the ventilator.

(4) **High-frequency oscillatory ventilation** (HFOV) uses substantially faster rates (180 to 300/minute) and smaller tidal volumes than conventional modes. The result is a relative decrease in diaphragmatic excursion, lung movement, and airway pressures. The physical mechanisms responsible for gas movement are complex and incompletely understood. Although HFOV has not been demonstrated to improve survival, it is associated with a trend toward decreased mortality in ARDS in a recent prospective, randomized trial (52% vs. 37%, $p = 0.102$) and represents a viable "rescue" therapy for those failing with conventional ventilation (*Am J Respir Crit Care Med.* 2002;166:801). HFOV may be considered when F_{IO_2} requirements exceed 70% and mean airway pressure is approaching 20 cm H_2O or higher or when there is a PEEP of greater than 15 cm H_2O in ARDS. Patients do not always need to be paralyzed to undergo HFOV, but they do need to be deeply sedated (Ramsay 5 to 6). Adjustable variables include oscillatory frequency (Hz), F_{IO_2}, amplitude or power (tidal volume), and inspiratory time.

b. **Ventilator management**

(1) **Choice of ventilator mode.** Patient needs should be matched with the appropriate ventilator mode by considering each mode's advantages and disadvantages.

(2) F_{IO_2} should be adjusted to ensure adequate arterial oxygenation, which is a blood hemoglobin saturation of 92%. The lowest possible F_{IO_2} (ideally ≤0.40) should be used to achieve these levels of arterial saturation to prevent pulmonary oxygen toxicity.

(3) **Tidal volume.** There is no consensus on the optimal tidal volume for the postoperative patient who requires short-term mechanical ventilatory support. However, in ARDS, low tidal volumes are associated with improved survival. A multicenter, prospective, randomized trial demonstrated improved survival in patients who were ventilated with low tidal volumes (6 mL/kg ideal body weight) compared with high tidal volumes (12 mL/kg) (*N Engl J Med.* 2000;342:1301). As a result of this important study, the tidal volume should be adjusted to as low as 4 mL/kg ideal body weight as needed to maintain plateau pressures at less than 30 cm H_2O to minimize barotrauma but greater than 20 cm H_2O to minimize atelectasis.

(4) **Ventilatory rate.** Once the tidal volume has been determined, the rate is chosen (typically 8 to 16 breaths per minute) to provide adequate minute ventilation (the product of rate and tidal volume). The rate is adjusted to optimize arterial pH and $Paco_2$; an $ETCO_2$ monitor is useful in this regard.

(5) **Inspiratory–expiratory (I:E) ratio.** The normal I:E ratio is 1:2 to 1:3. Longer expiratory times allow patients with obstructive lung disease and decreased expiratory airflow to exhale fully and prevent stacking of breaths. In contrast, longer inspiratory times, which decrease peak airway pressures, are useful in patients with low pulmonary compliance. Inverse-ratio ventilation takes advantage of breath stacking, using I:E ratios from 1:1 to 4:1. Used only in patients with severe consolidating lung disease, inverse ratio ventilation is believed to improve gas exchange by progressive alveolar recruitment (mean airway pressures are higher, keeping a larger number of alveoli open for a greater percentage of the respiratory cycle). Inverse-ratio ventilation is used most commonly with pressure-control ventilation.

(6) **PEEP is intended to** increase functional residual capacity, increase lung compliance, and improve ventilation–perfusion matching by opening terminal airways and recruiting partially collapsed alveoli. PEEP of 5 cm H_2O is considered physiologic; higher levels are used when hypoxemia is moderate to severe. PEEP increases intrathoracic pressure and may decrease CO, reduces venous return to the heart, increases airway pressure, and alters pulmonary vascular resistance. PEEP levels of greater than 15 cm H_2O significantly increase the risk of barotrauma and spontaneous pneumothorax. Excess PEEP can also reduce lung compliance, decrease right ventricular (RV) filling, and increase RV afterload. PEEP applied to the spontaneously ventilating patient without inspiratory ventilatory support is called **continuous positive airway pressure (CPAP).**

(7) Sedation and neuromuscular paralysis. Sedation is often necessary in mechanically ventilated patients to control anxiety, allow the patient to rest, and synchronize breathing. However, a recent clinical trial demonstrated that patients who receive no sedation have more ventilator-free days and shorter ICU lengths of stay (*Lancet.* 2010;375:475). The need for paralysis is rare, except in patients with severe respiratory failure and decreased pulmonary compliance. If paralytics are necessary, they should be discontinued as soon as possible because long-term use is associated with paresis, which may last for weeks to months. Level of paralysis should routinely be assessed (e.g., with train-of-four neuromuscular testing).

(8) Prone positioning is one of several techniques that may have benefit as "rescue" strategies in patients with severe acute lung injury or ARDS. Patients are placed in a prone position for a scheduled period of time on a daily basis; theoretical benefits include recruitment of dorsal lung units, improved mechanics, decreased ventilation–perfusion mismatch, and increased secretion drainage (*JAMA.* 2005;294:2889). Although this therapy has been shown to benefit oxygenation, it has not been demonstrated to improve survival.

c. Complications

(1) ET tube dislodgment and patient self-extubation can produce a medical emergency characterized by life-threatening hypoxia and hypercarbia in those who are profoundly ill. For this reason, restraint of the patient's upper extremities is frequently required. If a patient does self-extubate, he or she should be closely observed because a surprising number of patients will be able to remain successfully extubated. If the patient shows any signs of respiratory distress, however, he or she should be immediately reintubated or placed on noninvasive ventilation, depending on the clinical scenario.

(2) ET tube cuff leaks should be suspected when there is an unexplained decrease in the returned expired volume associated with a fall in airway pressure. A cuff leak may indicate that the ET tube is at or partially above the vocal cords, and the tube may be advanced using a bronchoscope. A severe cuff leak should prompt change of the ET tube because there is increased risk of aspiration and decreased efficiency of ventilation.

(3) Respiratory distress may occur suddenly during mechanical ventilation due either to an acute change in the patient's status or to ventilator malfunction. The first priority is to disconnect the ventilator and switch to bag ventilation using 100% oxygen to ensure adequate ventilation and oxygenation. Increased airway pressures may indicate obstruction of the tube with secretions or a kink in the tube, bronchospasm, pneumothorax, inadequate patient sedation or migration of the ET tube into a mainstem bronchus. Check the ET tube for patency and suction; if there is a partial obstruction, use large-volume saline lavage to clear the tube. If the obstruction is complete, remove the ET tube and reintubate the patient. Listen closely for any change in breath sounds consistent with a pneumothorax, new lung consolidation, or pleural fluid collection. A less common but important cause of respiratory distress is PE. **Check the ventilator's function** and, if it is normal, return the patient to the ventilator, making any needed changes in ventilator settings to ensure adequate ventilation and oxygenation. The results of an ABG and a chest x-ray are frequently helpful.

(4) **Barotrauma** from very high peak airway pressures (≥ 50 cm H_2O) can lead to subcutaneous emphysema, pneumomediastinum, and pneumothorax. Whereas subcutaneous emphysema and pneumomediastinum usually are benign, a pneumothorax that develops while a patient is on positive-pressure ventilation is at high risk for tension pneumothorax and is usually treated emergently with tube thoracostomy.

(5) **Volutrauma is alveolar injury secondary to severe distention.**

(6) **Atelectrauma is alveolar damage caused by repetitive alveolar opening and closing in the setting of low surfactant or inadequate PEEP. In adults, this is most commonly associated with noncompliant alveoli in ARDS.**

(7) **Oxygen toxicity** refers to levels of intra-alveolar oxygen high enough to cause lung damage. The precise mechanism is not known, but it probably involves oxidation of cell membranes and generation of toxic oxygen radicals. An F_{IO_2} of 0.40 or less is considered safe even for long periods. Although experimental data demonstrate that microscopic damage to alveoli occurs after only a few hours of an F_{IO_2} of 1 in animals, convincing studies in human patients are impossible to perform due to ethical consideration. It appears prudent, however, to keep the F_{IO_2} at less than 0.60 whenever possible, often using higher levels of PEEP (8 to 12 cm H_2O) to help reduce the F_{IO_2}.

d. **Weaning off mechanical ventilation.** Although there are exceptions (e.g., immediate extubation of a healthy patient with normal lungs after general anesthesia), discontinuing mechanical ventilation may require weaning. In general, hemodynamic instability or high work of breathing (e.g., minute ventilation >15 L/minute) is contraindications to weaning. Reduction in the F_{IO_2} to 0.40 or less and of PEEP to 5 cm H_2O or less is accomplished first. The patient who has needed prolonged ventilatory support may require from several days to weeks to wean because of marginal respiratory muscle strength and the time required for the injured lungs to recover. The optimal strategy for weaning patients continues to be a topic of debate. The results of clinical trials indicate that the method of weaning from ventilator support is most likely of little consequence for patients who have been on mechanical ventilatory support for 2 weeks or less because the primary determinant of weaning success is simply resolution of the pathology that induced respiratory failure. At Washington University, patients are maintained on volume-control ventilation with daily CPAP trials to assess their suitability for extubation. The presence of a weaning protocol decreases patient time on the ventilator compared with physician-directed weaning.

IV. CIRCULATORY FAILURE: SHOCK

A. Shock is defined by global tissue hypoxia; it occurs when either the supply of or the ability to use oxygen is insufficient to meet metabolic demands. Shock can be recognized by evidence of end-organ dysfunction. If left uncorrected, shock leads to the death of cells, tissues, organs, and, ultimately, the patient. Understanding the **pathophysiology of shock** depends on an appreciation of the relationship of blood pressure [specifically, mean arterial pressure (MAP)] to CO and SVR: MAP is directly proportional to CO and SVR. Because CO is equal to stroke volume times heart rate, and stroke volume is proportional to preload, afterload, and myocardial contractility, MAP is usually proportional to heart rate, preload, afterload, and contractility. Compensatory changes in response to systemic hypotension include the release of catecholamines, aldosterone, renin, and cortisol, which act in concert to increase heart rate, preload, afterload, and contractility.

B. **Classification and recognition of shock** (Table 7-3). The morbidity and mortality of circulatory shock are related not only to the underlying cause

TABLE 7-3	Clinical Parameters in Shock					
Shock Classification	Skin	Jugular Venous Distension	Cardiac Output	Pulmonary Capillary Wedge Pressure	Systemic Vascular Resistance	Mixed Venous Oxygen Content
Hypovolemic	Cool, pale	↓	↓	↓	↑	↓
Cardiogenic	Cool, pale	↑	↓	↑	↑	↓
Septic						
Early	Warm, pink	↑↓	↑	↓	↓	↑
Late	Cool, pale	↓	↓	↓	↑	↑↓
Neurogenic	Warm, pink	↓	↓	↓	↓	↓

but also to the depth and duration of circulatory compromise. Early recognition and prompt intervention are therefore critical.

1. **Hypovolemic shock** results from loss of circulating blood volume (usually at least 20%) caused by acute hemorrhage, fluid depletion, or dehydration; these three are frequently distinguishable from one another by history. These patients typically are peripherally vasoconstricted, tachycardic, and have low jugular venous pressure.

2. **Distributive shock** is characterized by a hyperdynamic state consisting of tachycardia, vasodilation (with decreased cardiac filling pressures), decreased SVR, and increased CO; however, some patients present with hypodynamic septic shock and have decreased CO and hypoperfusion. Patients with hyperdynamic distributive shock feel warm. The most common causes of distributive shock include sepsis, the systemic inflammatory response syndrome (SIRS), neurogenic shock, adrenal insufficiency, and liver failure. **Neurogenic shock** results from interruption of the spinal cord at or above the thoracolumbar sympathetic nerve roots, which produces loss of sympathetic tone to the vascular system, causing vasodilation. The cardiovascular response is the same; patients are typically peripherally vasodilated (warm extremities) and tachycardic. Jugular venous pressure is usually low.

3. **Obstructive shock** results from etiologies that prevent adequate CO but are not intrinsically cardiac in origin. This type of shock may be caused by pulmonary embolus, tension pneumothorax, or cardiac tamponade. Jugular venous pressure is often elevated in these patients.

4. **Cardiogenic shock** results from inadequate CO due to intrinsic cardiac failure (e.g., acute myocardial infarction, valvular stenosis, regurgitation or rupture, ischemia, arrhythmia, cardiomyopathy, or acute ventricular septal defect). These patients typically are peripherally vasoconstricted and tachycardic. Their jugular venous pressure typically is elevated.

5. **Interventions common to all types of shock.** The goal of therapy is to ensure adequate delivery of oxygen to the peripheral tissues. Because oxygen delivery is proportional to the arithmetic product of Sao_2, hemoglobin concentration, and CO, each of these parameters should be optimized.

   a. **Sao_2.** It is necessary to administer supplemental oxygen, secure or provide an adequate airway, and check for adequate bilateral ventilation. A pulse oximetry (Sao_2) level that exceeds 92% should allow adequate delivery of oxygen at the periphery; however, levels should be maximized in the acute setting.

   b. **Hemoglobin concentration.** The hemoglobin concentration must be adequate to deliver oxygen to the tissues. One study indicated that for most critically ill patients, a transfusion trigger of 7 g/dL is appropriate, with the goal of keeping the hemoglobin concentration at 7 to 9 g/dL, except in patients with an ongoing myocardial infarction or severe ischemic cardiomyopathy (*N Engl J Med.* 1999;340:409). An important caveat is early goal-directed therapy in septic patients with SvO_2 less than 70 and hemoglobin less than 10 (*N Engl J Med.* 2001;345:1368).

c. **Cardiac output (CO).** The ECG tracing provides direct information about heart rate and several indirect clues about stroke volume. The atrial contraction provides approximately 15% to 25% of ordinary preload in normal patients and potentially up to 50% in patients with significant diastolic dysfunction, so the atrioventricular dyssynchrony observed in atrial fibrillation or third-degree atrioventricular block causes impairment of CO. This is clinically relevant for patients who have decreased ventricular compliance or decreased ejection fraction at baseline. Tachyarrhythmias decrease diastolic ventricular and coronary artery filling times. When it is severe (e.g., heart rate ~140 beats per minute), tachycardia predictably impairs preload, stroke volume, and CO. When treating tachycardia *per se,* it is imperative to distinguish between tachycardia as a compensatory response (e.g., sinus tachycardia secondary to hypovolemia) and tachycardia as a cause of shock (e.g., ventricular tachycardia). With the exception of the patient in pulmonary edema, *all* patients in circulatory shock should initially receive 10 to 20 mL/kg of a balanced salt solution, such as lactated Ringer's solution. The pace of volume infusion should reflect the depth of circulatory shock. To achieve rapid infusion rates, short, large-bore intravenous catheters (e.g., 14 or 16 gauge) in an peripheral vein are best. If this is not possible, an 8.5-French sheath inserted into a central vein is highly effective. **A multilumen central line is NOT an effective access for rapid volume resuscitation since resistance to flow is proportional to catheter length and inversely proportional to catheter lumen diameter raised to the 5th power.** The stopcocks should be removed from the venous lines to reduce flow resistance and deliver *warmed* fluids. Hypothermia is aggravated by rapid infusion of room temperature (i.e., 23 degrees centigrade) crystalloid and refrigerated blood, impairing the ability to unload oxygen from hemoglobin in the periphery and compromising all enzymatic processes, especially coagulation.

d. To assess the adequacy of resuscitation, peripheral pulses and urine output should be evaluated. Palpable pedal pulses or urine output that exceeds 1 mL/kg/ hour usually indicates a cardiac index of greater than 2 L/m^2/minute. These two simple techniques can be used to estimate cardiac performance in many patients. Patients who do not improve with initial resuscitative measures may require invasive hemodynamic monitoring. All patients in shock should be monitored with an indwelling bladder catheter. Metabolic acidosis, identified by an ABG determination and serum electrolytes, can reflect the depth of circulatory compromise and the adequacy of resuscitation; however, this is may not be true in patients with preexisting renal failure and baseline metabolic acidosis. Infusion of sodium bicarbonate should be reserved for patients with a pH of less than 7.15 because the sodium bicarbonate may actually worsen intracellular pH as the bicarbonate is converted to CO_2 at the tissue level, particularly if CO_2 elimination (i.e., effective ventilation) is impaired.

TABLE 7-4	Physiologic Changes in Hypovolemic Shock			
Blood loss (%)	<15	15–30	30–40	>40
Blood loss (mL)[a]	<750	750–1,500	1,500–2,000	>2,000
Heart rate (bpm)	NI	>100	>120	>140
Blood pressure	NI	SBP NI DBP ↑	SBP ↓ DBP ↓	SBP ↓↓ DBP ↓↓
Respiratory rate	NI	↑	↑↑	↑↑↑
Urine output	NI	↓	Oliguria	Anuria
Mental state	Minimal anxiety	Mild anxiety	Confusion	Lethargy

[a]Based on a 70-kg male patient.
bpm, beats per minute; DBP, diastolic blood pressure; NI, normal; SBP, systolic blood pressure.

6. **Specific therapy**
   a. **Hypovolemic shock.** Therapy focuses on control of ongoing volume loss and restoration of intravascular volume. External hemorrhage should be controlled by direct pressure. Internal hemorrhage may require further diagnostic tests and/or surgical intervention. The degree of volume deficit (Table 7-4) determines the type and volume of resuscitative fluid. Patients with blood losses of up to 20% of their circulating blood volume can be resuscitated using crystalloid solutions alone, typically lactated Ringer's solution. However, because salt solutions equilibrate with the interstitial space, volume replacement with these solutions alone requires three times the estimated volume deficit. Patients in whom diaphoresis, ashen facies, and hypotension develop have lost 30% or more of their blood volume and require urgent transfusion of blood. Individuals with severe dehydration often have profound metabolic and electrolyte abnormalities. Fluid administration should be modified once laboratory analysis of serum electrolytes is completed. With adequate volume resuscitation, vasoconstrictors and vasoactive agents can usually be avoided or discontinued.
   b. **Distributive shock**
      (1) **Septic shock (see Section V.C).**
      (2) **Critical illness-related corticosteroid insufficiency (CIRCI) can result from adrenal insufficiency or glucocorticoid resistance.** The diagnosis and treatment of adrenal insufficiency in septic shock are evolving and controversial. Per ACCM 2008

guidelines, adrenal insufficiency is best diagnosed by delta cortisol level < 9 ug/dL after a cosyntropin (synthetic ACTH, 250 ug) stimulation test or random total cortisol <10 ug/dL. There is a consensus that patients with primary adrenal insufficiency or those with septic shock refractory to fluid resuscitation and vasopressors should be treated with moderate dose hydrocortisone (50 mg IV every 6 hours) (*Crit Care Med.* 2008;36:1937). In many cases of CIRCI, dysfunction of the hypothalamic–pituitary axis is reversible and resolves with improvement in the underlying condition. Corticosteroids increase the risk of infection (*NEJM.* 2008;358:111).

(3) SIRS may result from noninfectious causes of inflammation (e.g., necrotizing pancreatitis, burns, and cardiopulmonary bypass). Treatment is supportive, with volume resuscitation, mechanical ventilation, and the administration of vasopressors as needed until the inflammatory process resolves.

c. Obstructive shock. Tension pneumo- or hemothoraces and pericardial tamponade require mechanical intervention. Tension pneumothorax is treated by needle decompression followed by tube thoracostomy. Hemothorax requires tube thoracostomy. Pericardial tamponade is treated by needle decompression, often with catheter placement for drainage. The treatment of PE varies based on the degree of hemodynamic compromise and must be individualized. Alternatives include systemic anticoagulation, thrombolysis, and surgical clot removal. Inferior vena cava (IVC) filters are used in patients who have a contraindication to systemic anticoagulation.

d. Cardiogenic shock. It is critical to distinguish shock caused by intrinsic myocardial dysfunction from extrinsic processes that interfere with venous return to the heart. Diagnosis may require echocardiography and cardiac catheterization. Management is directed toward maintaining adequate myocardial perfusion and CO with volume expansion and vasopressors, inotropes, or chronotropes (Table 7-5). Initial treatment is often guided by CVP measurements or, in severe cases, PA catheter data, while the precipitating cause of compromise is identified and treated. CVP is primarily useful for assessment of RV function and is not a reliable marker of volume status (*Chest.* 2008;134:172). Mechanical support with intra-aortic balloon counterpulsation may be necessary before and during recovery from definitive surgical treatment (see Chapter 30).

e. Neurogenic shock. As with septic shock, the initial intervention in neurogenic shock is volume infusion. A peripheral vasoconstrictor, such as phenylephrine or norepinephrine, is administered centrally to increase vascular tone if hypotension is refractory to volume infusion alone. Dopamine is useful in patients with neurogenic shock and bradycardia. Because patients with spinal shock tend to equilibrate body temperature with their environment, fluids and ambient room temperature must be kept warm.

TABLE 7-5 Vasoactive Drugs and Their Specific Actions

Class and Drug	Blood Pressure	Systemic Vascular Resistance	Cardiac Output	Heart Rate	Inotrope Low Dose	Inotrope High Dose	Renal Blood Flow	Coronary Blood Flow	Mvo₂
Alpha Only									
Phenylephrine	↑↑	↑↑↑↑	→	→	±	±	↓↓↓	± ↑↑	↑
Alpha and Beta									
Norepinephrine	↑↑↑	↑↑↑↑	↑↑↑	↑	↑	↑	↓↓↓	↑↑	↑↑
Epinephrine	↑↑↑	↑↑↑↑	↑↑↑↑	± ↑↑↑	↑↑	↑↑↑	→ ±	↑↑	↑↑↑
Dopamine	↑↑	↑↑	↑↑↑	↑↑	±	↑↑	↑↑↑	↑↑	↑↑
Beta Only									
Dobutamine	±	↓↓↓	↑↑↑↑	↑↑	↑↑↑	↑↑↑	±	↑↑↑	↑↑↑
Beta-Blocker									
Metoprolol	→	→	↓↓	↓↓↓	↓↓	↓↓↓	±	↓↓	↓↓
Other									
Nitroglycerine	± ↓	↓↓	↑↑	± ↓	±	±	± ↑↑	→	↓↓
Hydralazine	↓↓	↓↓↓	↑↑	↑↑	±	±	± ↑↑	→	↓↓
Nitroprusside	↓↓↓	↓↓↓	↑↑↑	± ↑	±	±	↑↑	±	↓↓

Mvo₂, mixed venous oxygen saturation.

V. SEPSIS

A. **Definition.** Sepsis is defined as SIRS resulting from infection. There is a consensus clinical definition of SIRS: body temperature greater than 38°C or less than 36°C, heart rate greater than 90 beats/minute, respiratory rate greater than 20/minute or Pa_{CO_2} less than 32, and white blood cell (WBC) count greater than 12 or less than 4 or greater than 10% bands. Severe sepsis is multiple-organ dysfunction or hypoperfusion resulting from infection.

B. Diagnosis

1. **Appropriate cultures** should be obtained as part of the initial evaluation. Two or more blood cultures are recommended, one of which should be drawn percutaneously.

2. **Additional radiologic imaging and diagnostic procedures** should be performed as warranted.

C. Treatment

1. **Addressing the infection**
   a. **Antibiotic therapy**
      (1) **Broad-spectrum intravenous antibiotics** should be initiated within the first hour after obtaining appropriate cultures. Failure to do so results in significantly increased mortality from severe sepsis (*Chest.* 2000;118:146). The use of antifungal therapies and agents directed at highly resistant Gram-negative rods, methicillin-resistant *Staphylococcus aureus,* vancomycin-resistant enterococcus, and resistant pneumococcus should be guided by the clinical situation and local patterns of susceptibility.
         (a) The following increase a patient's risk for infection with resistant organisms:
            (i) Prior treatment with antibiotics during the hospitalization.
            (ii) Prolonged hospitalization.
            (iii) Presence of invasive devices.
      (2) For pneumonias, the initial broad-spectrum antibiotic coverage should be narrowed to focus on the causative organism(s) identified on culture. For intra-abdominal infections, therapies remain broadly directed at the range of intra-abdominal organisms.
   b. **Source control: drainage, debridement, or removal of the infectious source** as appropriate, through surgical or other means.

2. **Circulatory support**
   a. **Early goal-directed therapy** involves adjustments of cardiac preload, afterload, and contractility to balance oxygen delivery with oxygen demand before the patient even arrives in the ICU. A recent study demonstrated a hospital mortality of 30.5% for patients presenting in the emergency department with sepsis when treated with early goal-directed therapy compared with 46.5% for patients treated with standard therapy (*N Engl J Med.* 2001;345:1368).

b. **In the first 6 hours,** the goals of resuscitation are as follows (*Crit Care Med.* 2008;36:296):
  (1) CVP 8 to 12 mm Hg.
  (2) MAP at least 65 mm Hg.
  (3) Urine output at least 0.5 mg/kg/hour.
  (4) Mixed SvO_2 at least 70%.

c. **Vasoactive medications.** To maintain CO, heart rate usually is increased. Septic patients who fail to achieve rapid hemodynamic stability with fluids and small doses of vasoconstrictors often undergo insertion of a PA catheter to optimize cardiac performance. Because PA catheters have not been demonstrated to improve outcome in either high-risk surgical patients or ARDS patients, placing this form of invasive monitoring should not be automatic but should be decided on an individual basis. If a PA catheter is placed, higher filling pressures are typically needed (pulmonary capillary wedge pressure of 14 to 18 mm Hg) to optimize performance in the dilated, septic heart.

  (1) Dopamine and norepinephrine are both commonly used; however, phenylephrine is not beneficial in the setting of sepsis. A recent randomized controlled trial did not show a mortality difference between use of dopamine and norepinephrine, but dopamine was associated with a significantly higher rate of dysrhythmias (*NEJM.* 2010;362:779; *Shock.* 2010;33:375).

  (2) Circulatory concentrations of endogenous **vasopressin** increase initially, then decrease (*Crit Care Med.* 2003;31:1752), and they are lower in septic shock than in cardiogenic shock. Low-dose vasopressin increases MAP, SVR, and urine output in septic patients who are hyporesponsive to catecholamines. This may spare patients from high-dose catecholamine requirements, although its impact on survival is unclear.

3. **Adjunctive treatments**
  a. **Activated protein C** has been demonstrated to reduce mortality in a large-scale prospective, randomized trial (*N Engl J Med.* 2001;344:699–709). Although this drug clearly improves survival in patients with severe sepsis and has a very short half-life, it is associated with an increase in serious bleeding and must be used with caution in patients in the immediate postoperative setting. Activated protein C can be started 12 hours after an operative procedure and should be held for approximately 1 hour before and after minor interventions such as central venous catheter placement. Of note, activated protein C is approved for use in patients with Acute Physiology and Chronic Health Evaluation (APACHE) II scores of greater than 25 and has not been documented to help patients with less severe forms of sepsis.

VI. **UPPER GASTROINTESTINAL HEMORRHAGE PROPHYLAXIS.** Patients in the ICU are at increased risk for stress-induced mucosal ulceration and resultant GI hemorrhage. Risk factors include head injury (Cushing ulcers); burns

(Curling ulcers); requirement for mechanical ventilation; previous history of peptic ulcer disease; use of nonsteroidal anti-inflammatory drugs or steroids; and the presence of shock, renal failure, portal hypertension, or coagulopathy. Strong data exist to support the use of drugs to maintain mucosal integrity in these patients at increased risk. In an evidence-based review of discordant meta-analyses, H_2-receptor antagonists (cimetidine, ranitidine, famotidine) were found to reduce significantly the incidence of clinically important GI bleeding in critically ill patients. Proton-pump inhibitors are useful in patients who bleed despite being on appropriate H_2-receptor antagonists.

VII. RENAL DYSFUNCTION

A. **Etiology and diagnosis.** Renal dysfunction commonly presents as progressive oliguria in the setting of increased renal function indices [blood urea nitrogen (BUN) and serum creatinine]. This can progress to renal failure and anuria (urine output <100 mL/day), which require renal replacement therapy (~5% of all ICU admissions). Renal insufficiency can also present as polyuria when decreased renal tubular function (fluid resorption) is not coupled with decreased glomerular filtration ("high-output" renal failure). Traditionally, the etiology of renal dysfunction has been divided into prerenal, intrarenal, and postrenal causes. A careful history and a review of the medical record are critical to making the correct diagnosis.

1. **Prerenal.** The glomerular and tubular function of the kidneys is normal, but clearance is limited as a result of decreased renal blood flow. This is the most common cause of renal insufficiency in the surgical ICU, and it is usually the result of inadequate volume resuscitation. The rise in the BUN typically is greater than that of the serum creatinine (BUN/creatinine ratio >20). The concentrating ability of the kidneys is normal, and thus the urine osmolality (>500 mOsm) and the fractional excretion of sodium (FE_{Na} <1) are normal.

   a. **Abdominal compartment syndrome** results from massive tissue (bowel) edema within the abdominal compartment or retroperitoneal hemorrhage, frequently although not exclusively as a complication of severe trauma and massive resuscitation. Increased intra-abdominal pressure decreases renal perfusion and retards renal venous and urinary outflow, inducing renal injury by a combination of pre-, intra-, and postrenal insults. Assessment of urinary bladder pressure via a Foley catheter serves as an indirect but accurate measure of intra-abdominal pressure (*J Trauma.* 1998;45:597). An acute increase in pressure greater than 25 cm H_2O demands intervention and typically surgical exploration (convert mm Hg to cm H_2O by multiplying mm Hg by 1.3).

2. **Intrarenal.** Tubular injury is most often caused by ischemia (i.e., prolonged prerenal state) or toxins. Nephrotoxins commonly encountered by ICU patients include aminoglycosides, intravenous radiocontrast agents, amphotericin, and chemotherapeutic drugs. Patients with pre-existing renal disease or diabetes are particularly susceptible. Intravenous

hydration before and during the administration of nephrotoxins should be used to decrease the incidence of renal insufficiency in patients at risk. The concentrating ability of the tubules is compromised, so the urine osmolality is low (<350 mOsm) and the FE_{Na} is greater than 1. Urinalysis and microscopic analysis of the urinary sediment may yield additional information about tubular pathology (e.g., presence of casts may indicate acute tubular necrosis).

    a. **N-Acetylcysteine,** an antioxidant, has been shown to prevent nephrotoxicity induced by intravenous dye in patients with preexisting renal dysfunction (*N Engl J Med.* 2000;343:180; *Am J Kidney Dis.* 2004;43:1).

    b. A prospective, single-center, randomized trial demonstrated that hydration with sodium bicarbonate is more effective than hydration with sodium chloride for prophylaxis of contrast-induced renal failure. The protocol was an infusion of 3 mL/kg/hour of 154 mEq/L of sodium bicarbonate in dextrose and water for the hour prior to contrast exposure, then 1 mL/kg/hour during the exposure and for 6 hours after (*JAMA.* 2004;291:2328).

  3. Postrenal. Bilateral obstruction of urinary flow can be caused by direct intraoperative injury or manipulation, prostatic hypertrophy, coagulated blood, or extrinsic compression (e.g., tumors). Urinary catheter malfunction must always be ruled out, typically by flushing the catheter with sterile saline. Ultrasound examination of the urinary system is used to rule out hydronephrosis.

B. Treatment

  1. Supportive measures. Initial therapy should be directed at minimizing ongoing renal injury by optimizing renal perfusion and discontinuing potentially nephrotoxic agents. Optimization of renal perfusion is usually accomplished by judicious volume resuscitation. If fluid resuscitation does not improve low urine output (<0.5 mL/kg/hour), measurement of pulmonary capillary wedge pressure or evaluation of cardiac function/filling with echocardiography can be used to guide fluid resuscitation and optimization of CO. Low-dose dopamine does not change progression to renal failure nor does it change mortality. **There is no role for "renal dose" dopamine in the ICU** (*Lancet.* 2000;356:2139). The doses or medications to be eliminated by the kidney should be adjusted for the degree of renal insufficiency. Refer to Chapter 4 for the treatment of the electrolyte (hyperkalemia) and acid–base disorders (metabolic acidosis) that accompany renal failure.

  2. Renal replacement therapy. Indications include complications of renal dysfunction that fail medical management, including hypervolemia, severe acidemia, refractory hyperkalemia, and uremia. Decisions about when and how to initiate renal replacement therapy are the subject of controversy and ongoing clinical trials.

    a. **Intermittent.** Because peritoneal dialysis is usually impractical in the surgical ICU, intermittent or continuous hemodialysis is the method of choice. Some hemodynamic impairment will ensue as a result of rapid, large shifts of fluid from the intravascular compartment through the dialysis filter. In healthy patients, this is usually well tolerated. However, hemodynamic deterioration (hypotension or dysrhythmias) can be induced in unstable patients due to decreased myocardial preload.

b. Continuous venovenous hemodialysis (CVVHD) (*N Engl J Med.* 1997;336:1303) is used in patients with preexisting hemodynamic instability, usually in the setting of shock. CVVHD decreases the rate of fluid shifts and thus has less risk of hemodynamic compromise relative to HD. The disadvantage of this type of dialysis is that CVVHD requires constant systemic anticoagulation to prevent clotting of blood in the filter and continuous sophisticated nursing surveillance.

VIII. ANEMIA. It is not uncommon for patients in the ICU to receive multiple units of packed red blood cells during their critical illness. The prospective Transfusion Requirements in Critical Care (TRICC) trial reported that **transfusing all patients to a hemoglobin of 10 mg/dL either has no effect or may actually decrease survival in the critically ill** (*N Engl J Med.* 1999;340:409). Multiple meta-analyses and systematic reviews have found an increased association of transfusions with infection, transfusion-related acute lung injury (TRALI), hospital and ICU length of stay, and mortality. A restrictive transfusion strategy (transfusion for hemoglobin <7 mg/dL) is recommended in critically ill patients; except in those with acute coronary syndrome, severe hypoxemia, or active hemorrhage. A recent randomized controlled trial demonstrated that administration of recombinant erythropoietin did not reduce the rate of transfusion or reduce mortality in critically ill patients, but increased the risk of thrombotic events (*NEJM.* 2007;357:965).

IX. BLOOD GLUCOSE CONTROL. A recent study of 1,548 surgical patients randomly assigned to tight glucose control with intensive insulin therapy (blood glucose between 80 and 110 mg/dL) versus conventional control (blood glucose between 180 and 200 mg/dL and treatment only above 215 mg/dL) showed nearly a twofold decrease in mortality in the tight-glucose-control group. Intensive insulin therapy also reduced overall in-hospital mortality, bloodstream infections, acute renal failure, the median number of red cell transfusions, and critical illness polyneuropathy (*N Engl J Med.* 2001;345:1359). However, a follow-up study in medical patients did not demonstrate a benefit (*N Engl J Med.* 2006;354:449). Hypoglycemia remains a major risk of tight glucose control and has been associated with increased mortality. A goal blood sugar of less than 140 mg/dL seems safe and beneficial; further study will be required to determine the response of different patient populations to varying intensities of insulin therapy.

X. COMMONLY USED DRUGS. Table 7-6 lists commonly used ICU drugs and their doses.

TABLE 7-6	Drugs Commonly Used in the Intensive Care Unit			
Drug	Dilution (Concentration)	Loading Dose	Initial Maintenance Dose	Comments
Diltiazem	125 mg/125 mL 0.9% NaCl or D5W (1 mg/mL)	0.25 mg/kg (followed by 0.35 mg/kg if needed)	5–10 mg/hr (max 15 mg/hr)	May cause hypotension
Dobutamine	250 mg/100 mL 0.9% NaCl (2,500 µg/mL)		2 µg/kg/min (max 20 µg/kg/min)	Selective inotropic (beta) effect; may cause tachycardia and arrhythmias
Dopamine	400 mg/250 mL 0.9% NaCl or D5W (1,600 µg/mL)		Dopa, 1–3 µg/kg/min; alpha, 3–10 µg/kg/min; beta, 10–20 µg/kg/min	Clinical response is dose and patient dependent; may cause arrhythmias and tachycardia
Epinephrine	5 mg/500 mL 0.9% NaCl or D5W, or 4 mg/100 mL 0.9% NaCl or D5W		0.01–0.05 µg/kg/min	Mixed alpha and beta effects; use central line; may cause tachycardia and hypotension
Esmolol	2.5 g/250 mL 0.9% NaCl or D5W (10 mg/mL)	500 µg/kg/min for 1 min (optional)	50 µg/kg/min (max 300 µg/kg/min)	Selective beta1-blocker; T1/2 9 min; not eliminated by hepatic or renal routes; may cause hypotension
Heparin	25,000 units/250 mL 0.45% NaCl (100 units/mL)	60 units/kg	14 units/kg/hr	Obtain PTT every 4–6 hr until PTT is 1.5–2 times control; may cause thrombocytopenia

Drug	Preparation	Loading	Infusion	Comments
Lidocaine	2 g/500 mL D5W (4 mg/mL)	1 mg/kg (can repeat two times if needed)	1–4 mg/min	Dose should be decreased in patients with hepatic failure, acute MI, CHF, or shock
Nitroglycerin	50 mg/250 mL D5W (200 μg/mL)		5–20 μg/min	Use cautiously in right-sided MI
Nitroprusside	50 mg/250 mL D5W (200 μg/mL)		0.25–0.50 μg/kg/min (max 10 μg/kg/min)	Signs of toxicity include metabolic acidosis, tremors, seizures, and coma; thiocyanate may accumulate in renal failure
Norepinephrine	8 mg/500 mL D5W (16 μg/mL)		0.2–1.3 μg/kg/min	Potent alpha effects; mainly beta1 effects at lower doses; use central line
Phenylephrine	10 mg/250 mL 0.9% NaCl or D5W (40 μg/mL)		10–100 μg/min	Pure alpha effects; use central line; may cause reflex bradycardia and decreased cardiac output
Vasopressin	20 units/100 mL NS (0.2 units/mL)		0.04 units/min	Do not titrate; higher doses may cause myocardial ischemia.

CHF, congestive heart failure; D5W, 5% dextrose in water; max, maximum; MI, myocardial infarction; PTT, partial thromboplastin time; T1/2, terminal half-life.

8 Esophagus

David M. Hoganson and Traves D. Crabtree

STRUCTURAL AND FUNCTIONAL DISORDERS OF THE ESOPHAGUS

I. **HIATAL HERNIA.** The distal esophagus normally is held in position by the *phrenoesophageal membrane,* a fusion of the endothoracic and abdominal transversalis fascia at the diaphragmatic hiatus. A hiatal hernia is present when a lax or defective phrenoesophageal membrane allows protrusion of the stomach up through the esophageal hiatus of the diaphragm.

A. **Epidemiology.** Hiatal hernia is the most common abnormality reported in upper gastrointestinal (GI) radiographic studies. An estimated 10% of the adult population in the United States has a hiatal hernia. The condition occurs most commonly in women in their fifth and sixth decades. Most hiatal hernias are asymptomatic; however, an estimated 5% of patients with a hiatal hernia have symptoms related to persistent gastroesophageal reflux (GER) disease.

B. The **type of hiatal hernia** is defined by the location of the gastroesophageal (GE) junction and the relationship of the stomach to the distal esophagus.

1. In **type I** or **sliding** hiatal hernia, the phrenoesophageal membrane is intact but lax, thereby allowing the distal esophagus and gastric cardia to herniate through the esophageal hiatus and placing the GE junction above the diaphragm. This is the most common type and is usually asymptomatic.

2. A **type II** or **paraesophageal** hiatal hernia occurs when a focal defect is present in the phrenoesophageal membrane, usually anterior and lateral to the esophagus, which allows a protrusion of peritoneum to herniate upward alongside the esophagus. The GE junction remains anchored within the abdomen, whereas the greater curvature of the stomach rolls up into the chest alongside the distal esophagus. Eventually, most of the stomach can herniate. Because the stomach is anchored at the pylorus and cardia, however, the body of the stomach undergoes a 180-degree organoaxial rotation, resulting in an upside-down intrathoracic stomach when it is herniated.

3. **Type III** represents a **combination** of types I and II. This type is more common than a pure type II and is characterized by herniation of both the greater curvature of the stomach and the GE junction into the chest.

4. A **type IV** hiatal hernia occurs when abdominal organs other than or in addition to the stomach herniate through the hiatus. Typically, these hernias are large and contain colon or spleen in addition to the stomach within the chest.

C. **Symptoms and complications** in patients with **sliding (type I)** hiatal hernias are related to GE reflux (GER; see Section II). **Paraesophageal and combined (types II, III, and IV) hernias** frequently produce post-prandial pain or bloating, early satiety, breathlessness with meals, and mild dysphagia related to compression of the distal esophagus by the adjacent herniated stomach. The herniated gastric pouch is susceptible to volvulus, obstruction, and infarction and can develop ischemic longitudinal ulcers (termed *Cameron ulcers*) with frank or occult bleeding.

D. **Diagnosis and evaluation**

1. **Chest x-ray.** The finding of an air-fluid level in the posterior medi-astinum on the lateral X-ray suggests the presence of a hiatal hernia. Differential diagnosis includes mediastinal cyst, abscess, or a dilated obstructed esophagus (as is seen in end-stage achalasia).

2. A **barium swallow** confirms the diagnosis and defines any coexisting esophageal abnormalities, including strictures or ulcers. It is the ini-tial diagnostic study of choice. The positions of the GE junction and proximal stomach define the type of hiatal hernia.

3. **Esophagogastroduodenoscopy (EGD)** is indicated in patients with symptoms of reflux or dysphagia to determine the degree of esophagitis and whether a stricture, Barrett esophagus, or a coexisting abnormality is present. EGD also establishes the location of the GE junction in rela-tion to the hiatus. A sliding hiatal hernia is present when greater than 2 cm of gastric mucosa is present between the diaphragmatic hiatus and the mucosal squamocolumnar junction.

4. **Esophageal manometry** to evaluate esophageal motility is essential in patients who are being considered for operative repair to rule out an esophageal motility disorder.

5. **CT scan** can be very useful for patients with large type III or type IV hernias to define the anatomy and guide preoperative planning.

E. **Management**

1. **Asymptomatic sliding hernias** require no treatment.

2. Patients with **sliding hernias** and **GER** with mild **esophagitis** should undergo an initial trial of medical management, consisting of H_2-blocking agents or proton pump inhibitors.

3. Patients who **fail** to obtain symptomatic relief with **medical therapy** or who have severe esophagitis should undergo esophageal testing to determine their suitability for an **antireflux procedure** (see Section II) **and hiatal hernia repair.** Additional indications for surgical evaluation are young patients who would require lifelong proton pump inhibitors, patients with ongoing regurgitation, patients with respiratory symp-toms (cough, aspiration pneumonia) and Barrett esophagus.

4. Patients who do not experience reflux but have symptoms related to their hernia (chest pain, intermittent dysphagia, or esophageal obstruc-tion) should undergo hiatal hernia repair.

5. All patients who are found to have a **type II, III, or IV hiatal her-nia** and who are operative candidates should be **considered for**

repair. The management of asymptomatic paraesophageal hernias is a controversial issue. Some surgeons believe that all paraesophageal hernias should be corrected electively, irrespective of symptoms, to prevent the development of complications. However, recent data suggest that observation of the asymptomatic patient, especially for those older than 65 years, may be the safest course (*Ann Surg.* 2002;236:492). Operative repair, which can be performed using either an abdominal or thoracic approach, consists in reduction of the hernia, resection of the sac, and closure of the hiatal defect. In type III hiatal hernias, the esophagus frequently is shortened, and thus a thoracic approach may be preferred.

6. **Paraesophageal hiatal hernias** are associated with a 60% incidence of GER. Furthermore, the operative dissection may lead to postoperative GER in previously asymptomatic patients. Therefore, an antireflux procedure should be performed at the time of hiatal hernia repair. A recent prospective, randomized trial showed that the addition of a biologic mesh to reinforce the crural repair resulted in a decreased recurrence at 6 months (*Ann Surg.* 2006;244:481). Biologic meshes are decellularized human or porcine tissues (subintestinal mucosa or dermis) that are used as hernia repair mesh. Use of Prolene or PTFE prosthetic mesh can lead to erosion into the esophagus (*Surg Endosc.* 2009;23:1219). Thus, if mesh is utilized, biologic mesh is favored in the current era.

II. GASTROESOPHAGEAL REFLUX

A. **Prevalence.** GER is a normal event after a meal and during belching. Symptoms of heartburn and excessive regurgitation are relatively common in the United States, occurring in approximately 7% of the population on a daily basis and in 33% at least once a month. Often, these individuals have x-ray evidence of a hiatal hernia with a portion of the stomach above the diaphragm. Reflux and hiatal hernia are not always related, and each can occur independently.

B. **Pathophysiology** in GER relates to abnormal exposure of the distal esophagus to refluxed stomach contents. In 60% of patients, a mechanically defective lower esophageal sphincter (LES) is responsible for the GER. The sphincter function of the LES depends on the integrated mechanical effect of the sphincter's intramural pressure and the length of esophagus exposed to intra-abdominal positive pressure. Other etiologies of GER are inefficient esophageal clearance of refluxed material, fixed gastric outlet obstruction, functional delayed gastric emptying, increased gastric acid secretion, and inappropriate relaxation of the LES.

C. The classic **symptom** of GER is posturally aggravated substernal or epigastric burning pain that is readily relieved by antacids. Additional common symptoms include regurgitation or effortless emesis, dysphagia, and excessive flatulence. Atypical symptoms may mimic laryngeal, respiratory, cardiac, biliary, pancreatic, gastric, or duodenal disease.

D. Diagnosis and evaluation

1. **Contrast radiography (upper GI)** demonstrates spontaneous reflux in only approximately 40% of patients with GER. However, it documents the presence or absence of hiatal hernia; can demonstrate some complications of reflux, such as esophageal stricture and ulcers; and is an appropriate initial study. The study should include a full view of the esophagus as well as a complete evaluation of the stomach, pylorus, and duodenum.

2. **EGD** is indicated in patients with symptoms of GER to evaluate for esophagitis and the presence of Barrett changes. **Esophagitis** is a pathologic diagnosis, but an experienced endoscopist can readily distinguish the more advanced stages. Four general grades of esophagitis occur.
   a. **Grade I:** normal or reddened mucosa
   b. **Grade II:** superficial mucosal erosions and some ulcerations
   c. **Grade III:** extensive ulceration with multiple, circumferential erosions with luminal narrowing; possible edematous islands of squamous mucosa present, producing the so-called cobblestone esophagitis
   d. **Grade IV:** fibrotic peptic stricture, shortened esophagus, columnar-lined esophagus.

3. **Esophageal manometric testing** is appropriate in the patient with reflux symptoms once surgery is being considered. Manometry defines the location and function of the LES and helps to exclude achalasia, scleroderma, and diffuse esophageal spasm from the differential diagnosis. Characteristics of a manometrically abnormal LES are (1) a pressure of less than 6 mm Hg, (2) an overall length of less than 2 cm, and (3) an abdominal length of less than 1 cm. These values are abnormal, and a patient with one or more of these abnormal values has a 90% probability of having reflux. Manometry also assesses the adequacy of esophageal contractility and peristaltic wave progression as a guide to the best antireflux procedure for the patient.

4. **Esophageal pH testing** over a 24-hour period is regarded as the gold standard in the diagnosis of GER. It is now used mainly when the data from the remainder of the evaluation are equivocal and diagnosis of reflux is in doubt. Twenty-four-hour pH testing can be performed on an outpatient or ambulatory basis: The patient has an event button to record symptoms and keep a diary of body position, timing of meals, and other activities. This allows correlation of symptoms with simultaneous esophageal pH alterations. A **DeMeester score** is derived based on the frequency of reflux episodes and the time required for the esophagus to clear the acid. The occurrences of low pH episodes are compared with patient recorded symptoms to determine symptomatic correlation of the acid reflux (*J Am Coll Surg.* 2010;210:345). Refluxing volume can also be recorded even if it is normal pH to measure symptom correlation with volume reflux.

5. A **gastric emptying study** can be useful in evaluating patients with reflux and symptoms of gastroparesis. It may be especially pertinent in patients considered for redo surgery when there is suspicion of vagus

nerve injury. Patients with gastroparesis may benefit from a pyloric drainage procedure (i.e., pyloroplasty or pyloromyotomy) in addition to an antireflux procedure.

E. Complications. Approximately 20% of patients with GER have complications, including esophagitis, stricture, or Barrett esophagus. Other, less common complications include acute or chronic bleeding and aspiration.

F. Treatment

1. **Medical treatment** aims to reduce the duration and amount of esophageal exposure to gastric contents and to minimize the effects on the esophageal mucosa.

   a. Patients are instructed to remain upright after meals, avoid postural maneuvers (bending, straining) that aggravate reflux, and sleep with the head of the bed elevated 6 to 8 inches. Patients are also encouraged to not lie down to sleep within an hour of eating.

   b. **Dietary alterations** are aimed at maximizing LES pressure, minimizing intragastric pressure, and decreasing stomach acidity. Patients are instructed to avoid fatty foods, alcohol, caffeine, chocolate, peppermint, and smoking and to eat smaller, more frequent meals. Obese patients are instructed to lose weight, avoid tight-fitting garments, and begin a regular exercise program. In addition, anticholinergics, calcium channel blockers, nitrates, beta-blockers, theophylline, alpha-blockers, and nonsteroidal anti-inflammatory medications may exacerbate reflux and should be replaced with other preparations or reduced in dose if possible.

   c. **Pharmacologic therapy** is indicated in patients who do not improve with postural or dietary measures. The goal is to lower gastric acidity or enhance esophageal and gastric clearing while increasing the LES resting pressure.

      (1) **Antacids** neutralize stomach acidity and thus raise intragastric pH.

      (2) **H_2-receptor antagonists** lower gastric acidity by decreasing the amount of acid that the stomach produces.

      (3) **Proton-pump inhibitors** act by selective noncompetitive inhibition of the H^+/K^+ pump on the parietal cell and are the standard therapy for erosive and non-erosive esophagitis (*J Clin Gastroenterol.* 2007;41:131).

      (4) **Prokinetic agents,** such as metoclopramide (dopaminergic antagonist), can decrease GER by increasing the LES tone and accelerating esophageal and gastric clearance.

   d. **Transoral endoscopic suturing** to plicate the GE junction and endoscopic application of **radiofrequency energy** (Stretta procedure) to the lower esophagus are two novel endoluminal therapies that can be performed on an ambulatory basis and generally with the patient under light sedation. These therapies, approved by the Food and Drug Administration, have been evaluated in several small, non–placebo-controlled trials with limited posttreatment evaluation. Studies have demonstrated improved quality of life over baseline but no difference compared to laparoscopic fundoplication. Freedom from acid suppression medication is lower than with laparoscopic fundoplication surgery. These options remain experimental and controversial.

2. **Surgical treatment** should be considered in patients who have symptomatic reflux, have manometric evidence of a defective LES, and fail to achieve relief with maximal medical management. Alternatively, surgical therapy should be considered in symptomatic patients who have achieved relief with medical therapy but to whom the prospect of a lifetime of medicine is undesirable (i.e., because of cost, side effects, inconvenience, or compliance). Surgical treatment consists of either a transabdominal or a transthoracic antireflux operation to reconstruct a competent LES and a crural repair to maintain the reconstruction in the abdomen.

   a. A **laparoscopic, transabdominal approach** is preferred in most patients, although the transthoracic approach may be beneficial in some patients with a shortened esophagus. A shortened esophagus should be suspected when a stricture is present and in patients who have had a failed antireflux procedure. The transabdominal approach is recommended for patients with a coexisting abdominal disorder, a prior thoracotomy, or severe respiratory disorder.

      (1) **Nissen fundoplication** is the most commonly performed procedure for GER. It consists of a 360-degree fundic wrap via open or laparoscopic technique. Long-term results in several series of open procedures are excellent, with 10-year freedom from recurrence of greater than 90%. Short-term results of the laparoscopic approach are as good as the open-repair results for relief of GER symptoms, with concomitant shorter hospital stay, better respiratory function, and decreased pain postoperatively (*Br J Surg.* 2004;91:975). The complete fundoplication in this repair is very effective at preventing reflux but is associated with a slightly higher incidence of inability to vomit, gas bloating of the stomach, and dysphagia. During surgery, care must be taken to ensure that the wrap is short, loose, and placed appropriately around the distal esophagus to minimize the incidence of these complications.

      (2) The **Hill posterior gastropexy** aims to anchor the GE junction posteriorly to the median arcuate ligament and creates a partial or 180-degree imbrication of the stomach around the right side of the intra-abdominal esophagus. In the original description, Hill recommended using intraesophageal manometry during placement of the sutures to achieve a pressure of 50 mm Hg in the distal esophagus.

      (3) The **Toupet fundoplication** is a partial 270-degree posterior wrap, with the wrapped segment sutured to the crural margins and to the anterolateral esophageal wall. For patients in whom esophageal peristalsis is documented to be markedly abnormal or absent preoperatively, a partial wrap has often been used to lessen the potential for postoperative dysphagia.

b. A **transthoracic approach** is a reasonable alternative in patients with esophageal shortening or stricture, coexistent motor disorder, obesity, coexistent pulmonary lesion, or prior antireflux repair.

(1) Nissen fundoplication can be done via a transthoracic approach, with results similar to those obtained with a transabdominal approach.

(2) The **Belsey Mark IV repair** consists of a 240-degree fundic wrap around 4 cm of distal esophagus. In cases of esophageal neuromotor dysfunction, it produces less dysphagia than may accompany a 360-degree (Nissen) wrap. Furthermore, the ability to belch is preserved, thereby avoiding the gas-bloat syndrome that may occur after a complete wrap. The Belsey wrap can be completed with an open thoracotomy or thoracoscopically (*Surg Endosc.* 2003;17:1212).

(3) Collis gastroplasty is a technique used to lengthen a shortened esophagus. To minimize tension on the antireflux repair, a gastric tube is formed from the upper lesser curvature of the stomach in continuity with the distal esophagus. The antireflux repair then is constructed around the gastroplasty tube. A gastroplasty should be considered preoperatively in patients with esophageal shortening, such as those with gross ulcerative esophagitis or stricture, failed prior antireflux procedure, or total intrathoracic stomach (*Surg Clin N Am.* 2005;85:433). However, in many of these patients, the esophagus can be adequately mobilized to allow more than 3 cm of intra-abdominal esophagus and thereby avoid the need to lengthen the esophagus. Development of an angled endoscopic stapler has made laparoscopic Collis gastroplasty technically feasible.

III. FUNCTIONAL ESOPHAGEAL DISORDERS comprise a diverse group of disorders involving esophageal skeletal or smooth muscle.

A. Motor disorders of esophageal skeletal muscle result in defective swallowing and aspiration. Potential causes can be classified into five major subgroups: neurogenic, myogenic, structural, iatrogenic, and mechanical. Most causes of oropharyngeal dysphagia are not correctable surgically. However, when manometric studies demonstrate that pharyngeal contractions, although weak, are still reasonably well coordinated, cricopharyngeal myotomy can provide relief.

B. Motor disorders of esophageal smooth muscle and LES can be subdivided into primary dysmotilities and disorders that involve the esophagus secondarily and produce dysmotility.

1. Primary dysmotility

a. Achalasia is rare (1/100,000 population) but is the most common primary esophageal motility disorder. It typically presents between the ages of 35 and 45 years. Chagas disease, caused by *Trypanosoma cruzi* and seen primarily in South America, can mimic achalasia and produce similar esophageal pathology. Achalasia is a disease of unknown etiology, characterized by loss of effective esophageal body peristalsis and failure of the LES to relax with swallowing, resulting in esophageal dilatation. LES pressure is often (but not invariably) elevated. The characteristic pathology is alteration in the ganglia of Auerbach plexus.

(1) **Symptoms** include progressive dysphagia, noted by essentially all patients; regurgitation immediately after meals (>70%); odynophagia (30%); and aspiration, with resultant bronchitis and pneumonia (10%). Some patients experience chest pain due to esophageal spasms.

(2) The **diagnosis** is suggested by a chest x-ray, which often shows a fluid-filled, dilated esophagus, and absence of a gastric air bubble. A **barium esophagogram** demonstrates tapering ("bird's beak") of the distal esophagus and a dilated proximal esophagus. The bird's-beak deformity is not specific for achalasia and can be seen in any process that narrows the distal esophagus (e.g., benign strictures or carcinoma). **Esophageal manometry** is the definitive diagnostic test for achalasia. Characteristic manometric findings include the absence of peristalsis, mirror-image contractions, and limited or absent relaxation of the LES with swallowing. Endoscopy should be performed to rule out benign strictures or malignancy, so-called pseudoachalasia.

(3) **Medical treatment** is aimed at decreasing the LES tone and includes nitrates, calcium channel blockers, and endoscopic injection of botulinum toxin (blocks acetylcholine release from nerve terminals) in the area of the LES but this is only beneficial in about 10% of patients.

(4) **Surgical treatment with a modified Heller esophagomyotomy** has been shown to produce excellent results in 90% to 98% of patients, using open or laparoscopic techniques (*J Thorac Cardiovasc Surg.* 2010;140:962). Many esophageal surgeons favor extending the myotomy onto the stomach to avoid a common cause of failure, an incomplete myotomy due to inadequate mobilization of the esophagogastric junction. A concomitant antireflux procedure with the esophagomyotomy helps avoid late stricture due to GER disease caused by the incompetent LES combined with the inability of the aperistaltic esophagus to evacuate refluxed material. **Laparoscopic esophagomyotomy** combined with a posterior 270-degree Toupet fundoplication or anterior 180-degree Dor fundoplication to limit postoperative reflux is currently the primary surgical approach (*J Clin Gastroenterol.* 2008;42:603–609).

b. *Vigorous achalasia* is a term used to describe a variant of achalasia in which patients present with the clinical and manometric features of classic achalasia and diffuse esophageal spasm. These patients have spastic pain and severe dysphagia, likely because of residual disordered peristalsis ineffective in overcoming the nonrelaxed LES. Treatment is the same as for classic achalasia, except that consideration should be given to performing a longer esophagomyotomy (to the aortic arch). With relief of the obstruction caused by the nonrelaxing LES, the pain usually disappears.

   c. Diffuse esophageal spasm is characterized by loss of the normal peristaltic coordination of the esophageal smooth muscle. This results in simultaneous contraction of segments of the esophageal body.

   (1) The primary **symptom** is severe spastic pain, which can occur spontaneously and at night. In addition, dysphagia, regurgitation, and weight loss are common.

   (2) The **diagnosis** is confirmed with esophageal manometry, which usually demonstrates spontaneous activity, repetitive waves, and prolonged, high-amplitude contractions. Characteristic broad, multipeaked contractions with or without propagation are seen, and normal peristaltic contractions also may be present. Intravenous injection with the parasympathomimetic bethanechol (Urecholine) can provoke pain and abnormal contractions.

   (3) **Treatment** with calcium channel blockers and nitrates can reduce the amplitude of the esophageal contractions but usually is not beneficial. Surgical treatment consists of a long esophagomyotomy, extending from the stomach to the aortic arch, and often a concomitant antireflux procedure.

   d. Nutcracker esophagus refers to a condition characterized manometrically by prolonged, high-amplitude peristaltic waves associated with chest pain that may mimic cardiac symptoms. Treatment with calcium channel blockers and long-acting nitrates has been helpful. Esophagomyotomy is of uncertain benefit.

   e. Hypertensive LES is characterized by an elevated basal pressure of the LES. In contrast to achalasia, the LES relaxes normally and the peristalsis of the esophagus is normal. However, in up to half of these patients, there is a degree of hypertensive contraction of the esophagus. Reduced compliance of the LES may result in dysphagia symptoms. Medical management consists of calcium channel blockers and nitrates although a myotomy may be indicated for refractory symptoms.

2. Secondary dysmotility represents the esophageal response to inflammatory injury or systemic disorders, such as scleroderma, multiple sclerosis, or diabetic neuropathy. Inflammation can produce fibrosis, which can lead to loss of peristalsis and esophageal contractility. The most common cause of secondary dysfunction is the reflux of gastric contents into the esophagus.

   a. Progressive systemic sclerosis, or scleroderma, produces esophageal manifestations in 60% to 80% of patients, and often the esophagus is the earliest site of GI involvement. It is characterized by atrophy of the smooth muscle of the distal esophagus, deposition of collagen in connective tissue, and subintimal arteriolar fibrosis. Normal contractions are present in the striated muscle of the proximal esophagus.

   b. In a subset of patients with severe long-standing GER disease, erosive esophagitis and stricture formation occur as a result of the combination of an incompetent LES and poor esophageal emptying secondary to low-amplitude, disordered peristaltic contractions. Intensive medical treatment of the reflux is essential before operation. Most surgeons prefer a Collis gastroplasty and a Belsey antireflux procedure for these patients because of the presence of esophageal shortening and impaired peristalsis.

IV. **ESOPHAGEAL STRICTURES** are either benign or malignant, and the distinction is critical. **Benign strictures** are either congenital or acquired.

A. **Congenital webs** are the only true congenital esophageal strictures. They represent a failure of appropriate canalization of the esophagus during development and can occur at any level. An imperforate web must be distinguished from a tracheoesophageal fistula, although a perforate web may not produce symptoms until feedings become solid.

B. Acquired strictures

1. **Esophageal rings** or **webs** occur at all levels in relation to the etiology of the webbing process. An example is **Schatzki ring,** which occurs in the lower esophagus at the junction of the squamous and columnar epithelium. A hiatal hernia is always present, and the etiology is presumed to be GER. Esophagitis is rarely present. Treatment generally consists of medical management of reflux with periodic dilation for symptoms of dysphagia.

2. **Strictures** of the esophagus can result from any esophageal injury, including chronic reflux, previous perforation, infection, or inflammation.

C. **Symptoms** associated with a stricture consist of progressive dysphagia to solid food and usually begin when the esophageal lumen narrows beyond 12 mm.

D. **Evaluation and treatment** of a stricture begins with the categorical **exclusion of malignancy.** The diagnosis usually is based on a barium swallow. Esophagoscopy is essential to assess the location, length, size, and distensibility of the stricture and to obtain appropriate biopsies or brushings. Because a peptic stricture secondary to reflux always occurs at the squamocolumnar junction, biopsy of the esophageal mucosa below a high stricture should demonstrate columnar mucosa. If squamous mucosa is found, the presumptive diagnosis of a malignant obstruction should be made, although strictures due to Crohn's disease, previous lye ingestion, or monilial esophagitis are among alternative diagnoses. Most strictures are amenable to **dilation,** and this relieves the symptoms. Attention is then directed at correcting the underlying etiology. **Resection** can be required for recurrent or persistent strictures or if malignancy cannot be ruled out.

V. **ESOPHAGEAL DIVERTICULA** are acquired conditions of the esophagus found primarily in adults. They are divided into traction and pulsion diverticula based on the pathophysiology that induced their formation.

A. A **pharyngoesophageal (or Zenker) diverticulum** is a pulsion diverticulum. It is the most common type of symptomatic diverticulum. **Symptoms** include progressive cervical dysphagia, cough on assuming a recumbent position, and spontaneous regurgitation of undigested food, leading to episodes of choking and aspiration. A hypertensive upper esophageal sphincter (UES) or uncoordinated pharyngeal contraction and opening of the UES results in increased pharyngeal intraluminal pressure. Herniation of the mucosa and submucosa results in this false diverticulum (not all layers of pharyngeal tissue present in diverticulum). **Diagnosis** with a barium swallow should prompt surgical correction with cricopharyngeal myotomy and diverticulectomy or suspension. **Endoscopic approaches** (i.e., stapling to produce a myotomy) have been reported with low recurrence rates (*Mayo Clin Proc.* 2010;85:719), although transcervical myotomy and diverticulectomy remain the treatment of choice.

B. A **traction or midesophageal or parabronchial diverticulum** occurs in conjunction with mediastinal granulomatous disease often due to histoplasmosis or tuberculosis. Symptoms are rare, but when they are present, they mandate operative excision of the diverticulum and adjacent inflammatory mass. On rare occasions, these diverticula present with chronic cough from an esophagobronchial fistula.

C. An **epiphrenic or pulsion diverticulum** can be located at almost every level but typically occurs in the **distal 10 cm** of the thoracic esophagus. Many patients are asymptomatic at the time of diagnosis, and in those who are symptomatic, it is difficult to determine whether the complaints stem from the diverticulum or from the underlying esophageal disorder.

   1. The **diagnosis** is made with a **contrast esophagogram;** however, endoscopic examination and esophageal function studies are essential in defining the underlying pathophysiology. In advanced disease, the diagnosis can be confused with achalasia owing to the dependency of the diverticulum and the lateral displacement and narrowing of the GE junction.

   2. **Operative treatment** is recommended for patients with progressive or incapacitating symptoms associated with abnormal esophageal peristalsis. Surgery consists of diverticulectomy or diverticulopexy, along with an extramucosal esophagomyotomy. The myotomy extends from the neck of the diverticulum down to the stomach. When the diverticulum is associated with a hiatal hernia and reflux, a concomitant nonobstructive antireflux procedure (Belsey Mark IV) is recommended. Any associated mechanical obstruction also must be corrected.

TRAUMATIC INJURY TO THE ESOPHAGUS

I. ESOPHAGEAL PERFORATION

A. Overall, perforation is associated with a 20% mortality rate. The **etiologies** may be broadly divided into intra- and extraluminal categories.

   1. **Intraluminal causes**

      a. **Instrumentation injuries** represent 75% of esophageal perforations and may occur during endoscopy, dilation, sclerosis of esophageal varices, transesophageal echocardiography, and tube passage. The most common sites are the anatomic sites of narrowing of the esophagus (e.g., at the cricopharyngeus and GE junction).

    b. Foreign bodies can cause acute perforation, or more commonly follow an indolent course with late abscess formation in the mediastinum or development of empyema.

    c. Ingested caustic substances, such as alkali chemicals, can produce coagulation necrosis of the esophagus.

    d. Cancer of the esophagus may lead to perforation.

    e. Barotrauma induced by external compression (e.g., Heimlich maneuver), forceful vomiting (Boerhaave syndrome), seizures, childbirth, or lifting can produce esophageal perforation. Almost all of these injuries occur in the distal esophagus on the left side.

  2. Extraluminal causes

    a. Penetrating injuries to the esophagus can occur from stab wounds or, more commonly, gunshot wounds.

    b. Blunt trauma may produce an esophageal perforation related to a rapid increase in intraluminal pressure or compression of the esophagus between the sternum and the spine.

    c. Operative injury to the esophagus during an unrelated procedure occurs infrequently but has been reported in association with thyroid resection, anterior cervical spine operations, proximal gastric vagotomy, pneumonectomy, and laparoscopic fundoplication procedures.

B. Esophageal perforations initially manifest with **dysphagia, pain,** and **fever** and progress to **leukocytosis, tachycardia, respiratory distress,** and **shock** if the perforation is left untreated. Cervical perforations may present with neck stiffness and subcutaneous emphysema, and an intrathoracic perforation should be suspected in patients with chest pain, subcutaneous emphysema, dyspnea, and a pleural effusion (right pleural effusion in proximal perforations, left effusion in distal perforations). Patients with intra-abdominal perforations usually present with **peritonitis.**

C. The **diagnosis** of esophageal perforation is suggested by pneumomediastinum, pleural effusion, pneumothorax, atelectasis, and soft-tissue emphysema on **chest x-ray** or mediastinal air and fluid on **computed tomography (CT) scan.** Rapid evaluation with water-soluble or dilute **barium contrast esophagography** is mandatory, although contrast studies carry a 10% false-negative rate for esophageal perforations. Because esophagoscopy is used primarily as an adjunctive study and can miss sizable perforations, any discoloration or submucosal hematoma should be considered highly suspicious for perforation after trauma to the posterior mediastinum. Whenever an esophageal perforation is suspected, diagnosis and treatment must be prompt because morbidity and mortality increase in direct proportion to the delay.

D. Principles of management include (1) adequate **drainage** of the leak, (2) intravenous **antibiotics,** (3) aggressive fluid **resuscitation,** (4) adequate **nutrition,** (5) **relief** of any distal obstruction, (6) **diversion** of enteric contents past the leak, and (7) **restoration** of GI integrity. Initially, patients are kept on nothing-by-mouth status, a nasogastric tube is placed carefully in the esophagus or stomach, and they receive intravenous hydration and broad-spectrum antibiotics.

E. **Definitive management** generally requires operative repair, although a carefully selected group of nontoxic patients with a locally contained perforation may be observed. Patients with an intramural perforation after endoscopic procedures or dilation have a characteristic radiographic finding of a thin collection of contrast material parallel to the esophageal lumen without spillage into the mediastinum. Management with a nasogastric tube and antibiotics almost always is successful in these patients.

1. **Cervical and upper thoracic perforations** usually are treated by cervical drainage alone or in combination with esophageal repair.

2. **Thoracic perforations** should be closed primarily and buttressed with healthy tissue, and the mediastinum should be drained widely. Even when perforations are more than 24 hours old, primary mucosal closure usually is possible. When primary closure is not possible, options include wide drainage alone or in conjunction with resection, or with exclusion and diversion in cases of severe traumatic injury to the esophagus.

3. **Abdominal esophageal perforations** typically result in peritonitis and require an upper abdominal midline incision to correct.

4. **Perforations associated with intrinsic esophageal disease** (e.g., carcinoma, hiatal hernia, or achalasia) require addressing the perforation as described previously and surgically correcting the associated esophageal disease concomitantly.

II. **CAUSTIC INGESTION.** Liquid alkali solutions (e.g., **Drano** and **Liquid-Plumr**) are responsible for most of the serious caustic esophageal and gastric injuries, producing coagulation necrosis in both organs. Acid ingestion is more likely to cause isolated gastric injury.

A. **Initial management** is directed at hemodynamic stabilization and evaluation of the airway and extent of injury.

1. **Airway compromise** can occur from burns of the epiglottis or larynx and may require tracheostomy.

2. **Fluid** resuscitation and broad-spectrum **antibiotics** should be instituted.

3. **Vomiting should not be induced,** but patients should be placed on nothing-by-mouth status and given an oral suction device.

4. Steroids are of no proven benefit.

B. **Evaluation** with water-soluble **contrast esophagography** and gentle **esophagoscopy** should be done early to assess the severity and extent of injury and to rule out esophageal perforation or gastric necrosis.

C. **Management**

1. Without perforation, management is supportive, with acute symptoms generally resolving over several days.

2. **Perforation, unrelenting pain,** or **persistent acidosis** mandate surgical intervention. A transabdominal approach is recommended to allow evaluation of the patient's stomach and distal esophagus. If it is necrotic, the involved portion of the patient's stomach and esophagus must be resected, and a cervical esophagostomy must be performed.

A feeding jejunostomy is placed for nutrition, and reconstruction is performed 90 or more days later.

3. **Late problems** include the development of **strictures** and an increased risk of **esophageal carcinoma** (1,000 times that of the general population).

ESOPHAGEAL TUMORS

I. **BENIGN ESOPHAGEAL NEOPLASMS** are rare, although probably many remain undetected. The most common lesions are mesenchymal tumors such as GI stromal tumors and leiomyomas, followed by polyps. Less common lesions include hemangioma and granular cell myoblastoma.

A. **Clinical features** depend primarily on the location of the tumor within the esophagus. **Intraluminal** tumors, such as polyps, cause esophageal obstruction, and patients present with dysphagia, vomiting, and aspiration. **Intramural** tumors, such as leiomyomas, usually are asymptomatic, but if they are large enough, they can produce dysphagia or chest pain.

B. **Diagnosis** usually involves a combination of barium swallow, esophagoscopy, and perhaps CT scanning or magnetic resonance (MR) scan studies.

C. **Treatment** of all symptomatic or enlarging tumors is **surgical removal.** Intraluminal tumors can be removed successfully via endoscopy, but if they are large and vascular, they should be resected via thoracotomy and esophagostomy. Intramural tumors usually can be enucleated from the esophageal muscular wall without entering the mucosa. This is done via a video-assisted thoracoscopic or open thoracotomy approach. Laparoscopic resection may be appropriate for distal lesions.

II. **BARRETT ESOPHAGUS** is defined as a metaplastic transformation of esophageal mucosa resulting from chronic GER. Histologically, the metaplastic epithelium must demonstrate **intestinal-type metaplasia** characterized by the presence of goblet cells. The columnar epithelium of Barrett esophagus may replace the normal squamous epithelium circumferentially, or it may be asymmetric and irregular.

A. **Prevalence.** Barrett esophagus is diagnosed in approximately 2% of all patients undergoing esophagoscopy and in 10% to 15% of patients with esophagitis. Autopsy studies suggest that the actual prevalence is much higher because many patients are asymptomatic and remain undiagnosed. Most patients diagnosed with Barrett esophagus are middle-aged white men.

B. The **symptoms** of Barrett esophagus arise from long-standing gastric reflux. Approximately 50% of patients with endoscopically proven Barrett have associated heartburn, 75% have dysphagia, and 25% have bleeding (*Ann Surg.* 1983;198:554).

C. **Diagnosis.** Barrett esophagus may be suggested on x-ray by the presence of a hiatal hernia (associated with 80% of cases of Barrett esophagus) with esophagitis and an esophageal stricture. Confirmation of the diagnosis requires endoscopy and careful correlation between the endoscopic and histologic appearances.

D. Complications

1. **Esophageal ulceration and stricture** are more likely to occur in patients with Barrett esophagus than in those with GER alone. This probably reflects the more severe nature of the GER in patients with Barrett esophagus.

   a. **Barrett ulcers** are distinctly different from the common erosions seen in esophagitis in that they penetrate the metaplastic columnar epithelium in a manner similar to that seen in gastric ulcers. They occur in up to 50% of patients with Barrett esophagus and, like gastric ulcers, can cause pain, bleed, obstruct, penetrate, and perforate.

   b. **A benign stricture** occurs in 30% to 50% of patients with Barrett esophagus. The stricture is located at the squamocolumnar junction, which may be found proximal to the GE junction. Strictures secondary to Barrett esophagus are located in the middle or upper esophagus, unlike the routine peptic strictures that usually occur in the distal esophagus.

2. **Dysplasia.** The metaplastic columnar epithelium of Barrett esophagus is prone to development of dysplasia that can be detected only by biopsy. Dysplasia is categorized as low or high grade, with high grade being pathologically indistinguishable from carcinoma *in situ.*

3. **Malignant degeneration** from benign to dysplastic to malignant epithelium has been demonstrated in Barrett esophagus. Low-grade dysplasia is present in 5% to 10% of patients with Barrett esophagus and can progress to high-grade dysplasia and malignancy.

4. **Adenocarcinomas** that arise within the esophagus above the normal GE junction are characteristic of malignant degeneration in Barrett esophagus. The risk of development of adenocarcinoma in Barrett esophagus is 50 to 100 times that of the general population. In several long-term series, the incidence of malignant degeneration in Barrett esophagus was estimated at between 1 in 50 and 1 in 400 patient-years of follow-up.

E. Treatment

1. Uncomplicated Barrett esophagus in **asymptomatic** patients requires no specific therapy, but endoscopic surveillance and biopsy should be performed at least annually. Neither medical nor surgical treatment of reflux has been demonstrated to reverse the columnar metaplasia of Barrett esophagus. However, elimination of reflux with an **antireflux procedure** may halt progression of the disease, heal ulceration, and prevent stricture formation.

2. Uncomplicated Barrett esophagus in **symptomatic** patients should be treated using the same principles that apply to patients with GER without Barrett esophagus. In addition, symptomatic patients should have annual surveillance endoscopy with biopsy. After laparoscopic antireflux surgery, patients with Barrett esophagus have symptomatic relief and reduction in medication use equivalent to non-Barrett patients. Absence of progression to high-grade dysplasia or adenocarcinoma suggests that laparoscopic surgery is an effective approach for the management of patients with Barrett esophagus (*Am J Surg.* 2003;186:6).

3. **Barrett ulcers** usually heal with medical therapy. Frequently, 8 weeks of treatment with an H_2-receptor antagonist or proton-pump inhibitor are necessary to achieve complete healing. Recurrence of ulcers is common after discontinuation of therapy. Ulcers that fail to heal despite 4 months of medical therapy are an indication for rebiopsy and antireflux surgery.

4. **Strictures** associated with Barrett esophagus are managed successfully with periodic esophageal dilation combined with medical management. Recurrent or persistent strictures warrant an antireflux operation combined with intraoperative stricture dilation. After surgery, several dilations can be required to maintain patency during the healing phase. Rarely, undilatable strictures require resection.

5. **Dysplasia** on biopsy of Barrett esophagus indicates that the patient is at risk for the development of adenocarcinoma.
   a. **Low-grade dysplasia** requires frequent (every 3 to 6 months) surveillance esophagoscopy and biopsy. Medical therapy for GER is recommended in these patients, even when asymptomatic.
   b. **High-grade dysplasia** is pathologically indistinguishable from carcinoma *in situ* and is an indication for esophagectomy. Patients who undergo esophagectomy for high-grade dysplasia have up to a 73% incidence of having a focus of invasive carcinoma present in the resected esophagus. Cure rates of nearly 100% can be expected in patients whose cancer is limited to the mucosa and who undergo esophagectomy. However, because of the morbidity and mortality associated with esophagectomy, other methods of treatment are emerging, such as radiofrequency ablation. A recent randomized, multicenter trial demonstrated the success of radiofrequency ablation of low-grade dysplasia and high-grade dysplasia Barrett's at rates of 90.5% and 81.0% compared to medical management control group dysplasia ablation rates of 22.7% and 19.0%, respectively (*N Engl J Med.* 2009;360:2277).

6. **Adenocarcinoma** in patients with Barrett esophagus is an indication for esophagogastrectomy. Early detection offers the best opportunity to improve survival after resection, which overall is 20% at 5 years.

III. ESOPHAGEAL CARCINOMA

A. **Epidemiology.** Carcinoma of the esophagus represents 1% of all cancers in the United States and causes 1.8% of cancer deaths. The two principal histologies are adenocarcinoma and squamous cell carcinoma.

1. **Risk factors** for squamous cell esophageal cancer include African American race, alcohol and cigarette use, tylosis, achalasia, caustic esophageal injury, Plummer–Vinson syndrome, nutritional deficiencies, and ingestion of nitrosamines and fungal toxins. Geographic location also represents a risk factor, likely as a result of local dietary customs, with a high incidence noted in certain areas of China, Western Kenya, South Africa, Iran, France, and Japan.

2. **Risk factors** for adenocarcinoma of the esophagus include white race, GER, Barrett esophagus, obesity, and cigarette smoking.

B. Pathology

1. **Squamous cell carcinoma** was previously the most common type of esophageal carcinoma. It tends to be multicentric and most frequently involves the middle third of the esophagus.

2. **Adenocarcinoma** now constitutes the majority of malignant esophageal tumors and is the carcinoma with the greatest rate of increase in the United States. It is less likely to be multicentric, but it typically exhibits extensive proximal and distal submucosal invasion. Adenocarcinoma most commonly involves the distal esophagus.

3. **Less common malignant esophageal tumors** include small-cell carcinoma, melanoma, leiomyosarcoma, lymphoma, and esophageal involvement by metastatic cancer.

C. Most patients with early-stage disease are asymptomatic or may have symptoms of reflux. Patients with esophageal cancer may complain of **dysphagia, odynophagia, and weight loss.** Symptoms that are suggestive of unresectability include hoarseness, abdominal pain, persistent back or bone pain, hiccups, and respiratory symptoms (cough or aspiration pneumonia suggesting possible esophagorespiratory fistula). Approximately 50% of presenting patients have unresectable lesions or distant metastasis, which is largely responsible for the generally poor prognosis.

D. The **diagnosis** is suggested by a barium swallow and confirmed with esophagoscopy and biopsy or brush cytology.

E. **Staging.** A system for staging esophageal cancer allows assignment of patients to groups with similar prognosis, helps to determine if local or systemic therapy is needed, and allows comparison of response to different types of therapy. In recently updated staging (*Cancer.* 2010;116:3763), esophageal adenocarcinoma and squamous cell carcinoma are staged differently with squamous cell carcinoma having additional variable of anatomical location. (Table 8-1). Evaluation for lymph node and distant-organ metastatic disease is performed by combined positron emission tomographic and CT scanning. Endoscopic ultrasonography is more accurate than radiographic studies for determining the depth of wall invasion and the involvement of peritumoral lymph nodes. Upper esophageal and midesophageal lesions require bronchoscopy to evaluate the airway for involvement by tumor.

F. Treatment

1. **Surgical resection** remains a mainstay of curative treatment of patients with localized disease. It offers the best opportunity for cure and provides substantial palliation when cure is not possible. The overall 5-year survival rate is 19% to 32%, with higher rates for patients with lower stages of disease (*Ann Thorac Surg.* 2006;82:1073–1077).

a. **Options for resection** include a standard transthoracic esophagectomy, a transhiatal esophagectomy, or an *en bloc* esophagectomy. Total esophagectomy with a cervical esophagogastric anastomosis and subtotal resection with a high intrathoracic anastomosis have become the most common resections and produce the best long-term functional results as well as the best chance for cure.

TABLE 8-1	TNM (Tumor, Node, Metastasis) Staging System for Esophageal Cancer

Definition of TNM

T: Primary Tumor

Tis	Carcinoma *in situ*/high-grade dysplasia
T1	Tumor invades the submucosa
T2	Tumor invades the muscularis propria
T3	Tumor invades adventitia
T4	Tumor invades adjacent structures
T4a Pleura, pericardium, diaphragm, or adjacent peritoneum	
T4b Other adjacent structures, e.g., aorta, cerebral body, trachea	

N: Regional Lymph Nodes

N0	No regional node metastasis
N1	1–2 regional lymph nodes
N2	3–6 regional lymph nodes
	N3 >6 regional lymph nodes

M: Distant Metastasis

M0	No distant metastasis
M1	Distant metastasis

G: Histologic Grade

GX: Grade cannot be assessed—
stage grouping as G1
G1: Well differentiated
G2: Moderately differentiated
G3: Poorly differentiated
G4: Undifferentiated—stage grouping
as G3 squamous

Adenocarcinoma Stage Grouping

Stage	T	N	M	G
0	Tis	0	0	1
IA	1	0	0	1–2
IB	1	0	0	3
	2	0	0	1–2
IIA	2	0	0	3
IIB	3	0	0	Any
	1–2	1	0	Any
IIIA	1–2	2	0	Any
	3	1	0	Any
	4a	0	0	Any
IIIB	3	2	0	Any
IIIC	4a	1–s2	0	Any
	4b	Any	0	Any
	Any	3	0	Any
IV	Any	Any	M1	Any

(continued)

TABLE 8-1	TNM (Tumor, Node, Metastasis) Staging System for Esophageal Cancer *(Continued)*

Squamous Cell Carcinoma Stage Grouping

Stage	T	N	M	G	Location
0	Tis	0	0	1	Any
IA	1	0	0	1	Any
IB	1	0	0	2–3	Any
IIA	2–3	0	0	1	Lower
IIB	2–3	0	0	1	Upper, middle
IIIA	2–3	0	0	2–3	Lower
IIIB	2–3	0	0	2–3	Upper, middle
IIIC	1–2	1	0	Any	Any
IV	1–2	2	0	Any	Any
	3	1	0	Any	Any
	4a	0	0	Any	Any
	3	2	0	Any	Any
	4a	1–2	0	Any	Any
	4b	Any	0	Any	Any
	Any	3	0	Any	Any
	Any	Any	1	Any	Any

Adapted from Rice TW, Rusch V, Ishwaran H, et al. Cancer of the esophagus and esophagogastric junction. *Cancer.* 2010;116:3763.

Esophagogastrectomy with anastomosis to the distal half of the esophagus is seldom used because troublesome postoperative reflux is common.

b. **Options for esophageal replacement** include the stomach, colon, and jejunum.

2. **Neoadjuvant therapy** with preoperative chemotherapy or chemoradiotherapy has been evaluated in a number of trials. Although it may enhance local control and resectability, the survival benefit is still debated. A recent prospective, randomized study demonstrated a survival advantage of trimodal neoadjuvant chemotherapy (cisplatin and fluorouracil) and radiation (50.4 Gy) followed by surgery versus surgery alone. Although the study only had 30 patients in the trimodal arm and 36 patients in the surgery alone arm, there was a 5-year survival advantage of 39% for trimodal therapy versus 16% for surgery alone (*J Clin Oncol.* 2008;26:1086).

3. **Radiotherapy** is used worldwide for attempted cure and palliation of patients with squamous cell esophageal cancer deemed unsuitable for resection. The 5-year survival rate is 5% to 10%. Palliation of dysphagia is successful temporarily in 80% of patients but rarely provides relief for longer than several months. Combination therapy involving radiation and concurrent administration of 5-fluorouracil with mitomycin C or cisplatin has been suggested to improve results and has replaced radiation alone in most protocols.

4. The goal of **palliative treatment** is the relief of obstruction and dysphagia.

    a. Radiotherapy and chemotherapy work best in patients with squamous cell carcinoma, particularly when it is located above the carina. Adenocarcinoma is less responsive to radiation, and the acute morbidity (nausea and vomiting) of external-beam irradiation of the epigastric area is substantial.

    b. Esophageal bypass procedures have been largely abandoned due to excessive complication rates.

    c. Intraluminal prostheses have been developed to intubate the esophagus and stent the obstruction. Self-expanding wire-mesh stents, often with a soft silicone (Silastic) coating, have been used with greater ease of insertion and satisfactory results. None of these prostheses allows normal swallowing, and in most cases no more than a pureed diet can be tolerated. Potential complications include perforation, erosion or migration of the stent, and obstruction of the tube by food or proximal tumor growth.

    d. Endoscopic laser techniques can restore an esophageal lumen successfully 90% of the time, with only a 4% to 5% perforation rate.

IV. COMPLICATIONS OF ESOPHAGEAL SURGERY. Esophageal surgery is fraught with potential complications, and consistently good results require meticulous attention to operative technique.

    A. Postthoracotomy complications can include atelectasis and respiratory insufficiency, pneumonia, wound infections, and persistent postoperative pain. Post-esophagectomy atrial fibrillation is particularly common at 17% (*J Thorac Cardiovasc Surg.* 2004;127:629).

    B. Complications related to an esophageal anastomosis consist primarily of leaks and strictures.

        1. Management of an **anastomotic leak** is based on the size of the leak, the location of the anastomosis, and the clinical status of the patient.

            a. A **cervical** anastomotic leak usually can be managed by opening the incision to allow drainage. Occasionally, the leak tracks below the thoracic inlet into the mediastinum, necessitating wider debridement and drainage. If a major leak occurs, esophagoscopy should be performed to rule out a significant ischemic injury to the stomach. If present, the anastomosis should be taken down and a cervical esophagostomy should be performed. The necrotic portion of the stomach should be resected, and the remaining stomach should be returned to the abdomen, with placement of a gastrostomy and feeding jejunostomy.

            b. Intrathoracic anastomotic leaks are associated with a high mortality rate. Small, well-drained leaks can be treated conservatively, but large or poorly drained leaks require operative exploration.

        2. Strictures usually are the result of a healed anastomotic leak, relative ischemia of the anastomosis, or recurrent cancer. Most can be dilated successfully.

C. **Complications of antireflux repairs** generally result from **preoperative** failure to recognize a confounding abnormality, such as poor gastric emptying or weak esophageal peristalsis, or **operative** miscalculations that result in too tight a fundoplication or excessive tension on the repair. Most of these complications require operative revision.

1. **Postoperative dysphagia** can result from a fundoplication that is too long or tight, a misplaced or slipped fundoplication that is positioned around the stomach rather than the distal esophagus, or a complete fundoplication in the setting of poor esophageal contractile function. It also can result from operative distortion of the GE junction, excessive narrowing of the diaphragmatic hiatus, or disruption of the crural closure and herniation of an intact repair into the chest.

2. **Persistent or recurrent reflux** after surgery suggests an inadequate or misplaced fundoplication, disruption of the fundoplication, or herniation of the repair into the chest.

3. **Breakdown of an antireflux repair** usually is recognized by a gradual recurrence of symptoms and can be confirmed by a contrast esophagram. Most commonly, disruption of a repair is due to inadequate mobilization of the cardia and excessive tension on the repair.

4. **Gas bloating** or gastric dilation secondary to swallowed air can occur if the fundoplication is too tight or if there is unrecognized gastric outlet obstruction or delayed gastric emptying.

9 Stomach

Fabian M. Johnston, J. Esteban Varela, and
William G. Hawkins

ANATOMY AND PHYSIOLOGY

The principal role of the stomach is to store and prepare ingested food for digestion
and absorption through a variety of motor and secretory functions. The stomach can
be divided into five regions based on external landmarks: the **cardia,** the region just
distal to the gastroesophageal (GE) junction; the **fundus,** the portion of the stomach
above and to the left of the GE junction; the **body,** or **corpus,** the largest portion of
the stomach; the **antrum,** the distal 25% to 30% of the stomach, located between
the incisura angularis and the pylorus; and the **pylorus,** a thickened ring of smooth
muscle forming the distal boundary of the stomach. The arterial blood supply to the
lesser curvature of the stomach is from the **left gastric** artery, a branch of the celiac
axis, and the **right gastric** artery, a branch of the common hepatic artery. The greater
curvature is supplied by the **short gastric** and **left gastroepiploic** arteries, branches of
the splenic artery, and the **right gastroepiploic** artery, a branch of the gastroduodenal
artery. Venous drainage of the stomach parallels arterial supply, with the left gastric
(coronary) and right gastric veins draining into the portal vein, the left gastroepiploic
vein draining into the splenic vein, and the right gastroepiploic draining into the
superior mesenteric vein. The principal innervation to the stomach is derived from
the right and left vagal trunks.

DISORDERS OF THE STOMACH

I. **PEPTIC ULCER DISEASE (PUD)** represents a spectrum of disease characterized
by ulceration of the stomach or proximal duodenum due to an imbalance
between acid secretion and mucosal defense mechanisms.

A. **Epidemiology.** In the United States, there are approximately 500,000
new cases of PUD each year, with an annual incidence of 1% to 2%
and lifetime prevalence between 8% and 14%. Although there has been
a steady decline in the incidence of PUD since the 1960s, ulcer-related
mortality remains approximately 10,000 cases annually.

B. **Location.** The location of peptic ulcers can differ but generally duodenal
ulcers are located at the antral–pylorus junction. Gastric ulcers usually fall
within one of five categories (Modified Johnson Classification).

1. Type 1. Lesser curvature 60% to 70%, associated with low mucosal
protection.

2. Type 2. Lesser curvature and duodenal 15%, associated with high acid
secretion.

3. Type 3. Prepyloric 20%, associated with high acid secretion.

4. Type 4. Proximal stomach/cardia, associated with low mucosal protection.

5. Type 5. Anywhere in stomach, medication induced.

C. **Pathogenesis.** Four etiologic factors are responsible for the vast majority of PUD.

1. ***Helicobacter pylori (H. pylori)* infection** is associated with 90% to 95% of duodenal ulcers and 70% to 90% of gastric ulcers. Infection produces chronic antral gastritis, increased acid and gastrin secretion, and decreased mucosal resistance to acid.

2. **Nonsteroidal anti-inflammatory drug (NSAID)** use confers an eightfold increase in risk of duodenal ulcers and a 40-fold increase in risk of gastric ulcers due to suppression of prostaglandin production. Dose-dependent relationship, ulcers do not recur when NSAID discontinued.

3. **Cigarette smoking** (*J Clin Gastro.* 1997;25:1)

4. **Acid hypersecretion** occurs in the majority of patients with duodenal ulcers.

D. **Presentation** in uncomplicated ulcer disease is usually burning, gnawing intermittent epigastric pain that is relieved by food or antacid ingestion for duodenal ulcers but exacerbated by intake for gastric ulcers. Pain may be accompanied by nausea, vomiting, and mild weight loss. **Differential diagnosis** is broad and includes GE reflux disease, biliary colic and related biliary tract disease, inflammatory and neoplastic pancreatic disease, and gastric neoplasms. In later stages, ulcers may present with bleeding, perforation, and obstruction.

E. **Diagnosis** can be made by barium contrast radiography or upper gastrointestinal (GI) endoscopy. **Esophagogastroduodenoscopy (EGD)** is more sensitive and specific than contrast examination for PUD. In addition, EGD offers therapeutic options (ligation of bleeding vessels) and diagnostic options (biopsy for malignancy, antral biopsy for *H. pylori*). Once the diagnosis of PUD is confirmed, further testing should be carried out to determine its etiology.

1. ***H. pylori* infection** can be detected noninvasively by radiolabeled **urea breath test** or **serologic antibody testing.** Antral tissue obtained during endoscopy can be subjected to direct **histologic examination** or rapid urease testing using the **cod liver oil (CLO) test.**

2. **Fasting serum gastrin levels** should be obtained in patients who have no history of NSAID use and are *H. pylori*-negative or who have recurrent ulcers despite adequate treatment, multiple ulcers, ulcers in unusual locations (i.e., second/third portions of the duodenum and small bowel), or complicated PUD (hemorrhage, perforation, obstruction). Such atypical presentations suggest the possibility of **Zollinger–Ellison syndrome,** a rare entity causing PUD in 0.1% to 1% of patients.

3. **Endoscopic biopsy of gastric** ulcers is mandatory to exclude malignancy if symptoms or signs (weight loss, anemia, obstructions), or appearance of ulcer (associated mass, folds around ulcer) are present. Multiple biopsies are necessary to exclude malignancy.

F. **Treatment** of PUD has changed dramatically with the development of antisecretory drugs [histamine$_2$-receptor blockers and proton-pump inhibitors (PPIs)], and *H. pylori*-eradication regimens greatly diminishing the role of elective surgery for PUD. Equally important is lifestyle modification.

1. **Medical therapy**
    a. ***H. pylori* eradication** is the cornerstone of medical therapy for PUD. Regimens typically consist of an acid-reducing medication (PPI, H2 blocker, bismuth salicylates) combined with two antibiotics administered for 10 to 14 days (triple therapy). These regimens are 85% to 90% effective in eradicating *H. pylori*. Antisecretory therapy is then continued until ulcer healing is complete.
    b. **NSAID-associated PUD** is treated by discontinuing the offending medication and initiating antisecretory therapy. If the NSAID must be continued, PPIs are most effective for facilitating ulcer healing.
    c. **Smoking cessation** greatly facilitates ulcer healing, but compliance rates are low.
    d. **Follow-up endoscopy** to ensure healing is essential for gastric ulcers because up to 3% harbor malignancy.
2. **Surgical therapy** for uncomplicated PUD is exceedingly rare. Indications for elective operation for PUD include bleeding (acute/chronic), perforation, obstruction, failure of medical therapy (intractability), and inability to exclude malignancy.
    a. **Duodenal ulcers** are treated by one of three acid-reducing operations: (1) truncal vagotomy with pyloroplasty, (2) truncal vagotomy with antrectomy and Billroth I (gastroduodenostomy) or Billroth II (gastrojejunostomy) reconstruction, or (3) highly selective vagotomy (HSV). Truncal vagotomy with antrectomy yields maximal acid suppression with lowest ulcer recurrence rates (1% to 2%) but carries the highest postoperative morbidity (15% to 30%) and mortality (1% to 2%) rates. HSV has the lowest postoperative morbidity (3% to 8%) and mortality rates but is technically demanding to perform and has higher recurrence rates (5% to 15%).
    b. **Gastric ulcers** are typically treated with either wedge excision or antrectomy with inclusion of the ulcer, depending on ulcer location. Concurrent acid-reducing operation is reserved for acid hypersecreting patients (type II and III) or patients who are known to have refractory ulcer disease despite maximal medical management; this is rare today.

II. **COMPLICATED PEPTIC ULCER DISEASE** refers to PUD complicated by hemorrhage, perforation, or obstruction. These complications represent the most common indications for surgery in PUD. Although there has been a sharp decline in elective surgery for PUD, the rates of emergency surgery for complicated PUD have been stable over time.

   A. **Hemorrhage** is the leading cause of death due to PUD, with associated 5% to 10% mortality. Evaluation and management begin with aggressive resuscitation and correction of any coagulopathy, followed by EGD. Although spontaneous cessation of bleeding occurs in 70% of patients, endoscopic therapy using thermal coagulation with or without epine-phrine is warranted in individuals who present with hemodynamic insta-bility, need for continuing transfusion, hematemesis or red stool, older than 60 years, and serious medical comorbidities, because these patients have a higher risk of recurrent bleeding. Endoscopic findings are impor-tant to note and can stratify the risk of rebleeding when noted. Risk of rebleeding increases with fresh or old clot, visible bleeding, visible vessel, or active bleeding in ascending order. **Indications for surgery** include repeated episodes of bleeding, continued hemodynamic instability, ongoing transfusion requirement of more than 4 to 6 units of packed red blood cells over 24 hours, and more than one unsuccessful endoscopic intervention.

1. **Bleeding duodenal ulcers** are usually located on the posterior duo-denal wall within 2 cm of the pylorus and typically erode into the gastroduodenal artery. Bleeding is controlled by duodenotomy and three-point ligation of the bleeding vessels. In hemodynamically sta-ble patients, consideration should be made for a concomitant acid-reducing procedure for those who have failed or are noncompliant with medical therapy. Postoperative *H. pylori* eradication is important to reduce the risk of recurrent bleeding.

2. **Bleeding gastric ulcers** present a diverse challenge because the patient's condition, comorbidities, and previous ulcer and medication history all play a role in surgical decision making. In unstable patients, biopsy followed by oversewing or wedge excision of the ulcer is gen-erally preferred. Stable patients are candidates for an acid reduction surgery such as antrectomy and vagotomy.

B. **Perforated peptic ulcer** typically presents with sudden onset of severe abdominal pain but may be less dramatic, particularly in hospitalized, eld-erly, and immunocompromised patients. The resulting peritonitis is often generalized but can be localized when the perforation is walled off by adja-cent viscera and structures. Examination reveals fever, tachycardia, and abdominal wall rigidity, and laboratory evaluation typically demonstrates leukocytosis. Abdominal X-ray reveals free subdiaphragmatic gas in 80% to 85% of cases. Aggressive fluid resuscitation and broad-spectrum antibi-otics followed by prompt operative repair are indicated in the vast majority of patients with perforated PUD. **Nonoperative treatment of perforated duodenal ulcer** can be considered in poor operative candidates in whom the perforation has been present for more than 24 hours, the pain is well localized, and there is no evidence of ongoing extravasation on upper GI water-soluble contrast studies (*Dig Surg.* 2010;27:161).

1. **Perforated duodenal ulcers** are best managed by simple omental patching and peritoneal debridement, followed by *H. pylori* eradica-tion. An acid-reducing procedure (preferably truncal vagotomy and pyloroplasty) should be added in stable patients who are known to be *H. pylori*-negative or have failed medical therapy.

2. **Perforated gastric ulcers** are best treated by simple wedge resection to eliminate the perforation and exclude malignancy. If wedge resection

of the ulcer cannot be performed due to its juxtapyloric location, multiple biopsies of the ulcer are taken and omental patching is performed.

C. **Gastric outlet obstruction** can occur as a chronic process due to fibrosis and scarring of the pylorus from chronic ulcer disease or as a consequence of acute inflammation superimposed on previous scarring of the gastric outlet. In general, gastric outlet obstruction secondary to PUD has become exceedingly rare with modern medical antisecretory therapy. Patients present with recurrent vomiting of poorly digested food, dehydration, and hypochloremic hypokalemic metabolic alkalosis. Management consists in correction of volume and electrolyte abnormalities, nasogastric suction, and intravenous antisecretory agents. EGD is necessary for evaluating the nature of the obstruction and for ruling out malignant etiology, and **endoscopic hydrostatic balloon dilation** can be performed at the same time. This is feasible in up to 85% of patients, but fewer than 40% have sustained improvement at 3 months (*Gastrointest Endosc.* 1996;43:98). **Indications for surgical therapy** include persistent obstruction after 7 days of nonoperative management and recurrent obstruction. Antrectomy to include the ulcer and truncal vagotomy is the ideal operation for most patients. In exceptional instances, truncal vagotomy with gastrojejunostomy may be preferred in those patients whose pyloroduodenal inflammation precludes safe management with Billroth I or II reconstructions.

III. **GASTRIC ADENOCARCINOMA** is the second most common cancer worldwide and the 10th most common malignancy in the United States. Its incidence has decreased dramatically over the last 60 years, perhaps secondary to improvements in refrigeration and diet. In addition, the anatomic pattern of gastric cancer is changing, with proximal or cardia cancers comprising a greater proportion of gastric cancers. Approximately one-third of gastric cancers are metastatic at presentation. The overall 5-year survival rate is 15%.

A. The **etiology** of gastric cancer is complex and multifactorial, involving a combination of genetic, environmental, and infectious risk factors. **Risk factors** for gastric cancer include male gender; family history; low socioeconomic status; polyposis syndromes; diets high in nitrates or salts, or pickled foods; adenomatous gastric polyps; previous gastric resection; Ménétrier disease; smoking; *H. pylori* infection; and chronic gastritis. Aspirin, fresh fruits and vegetables, selenium, and vitamin C may be protective against the development of gastric cancer.

B. **Classification.** Ninety-five percent of gastric cancers are adenocarcinomas arising from mucus-producing cells in the gastric mucosa. The **Lauren classification** system is most widely used and divides gastric cancers into two subtypes:

1. **Intestinal-type cancers** (30%) are glandular and arise from the gastric mucosa. Occurring more commonly in elderly men and in the distal stomach, they are associated with *H. pylori* and other environmental exposures that lead to chronic gastritis, intestinal metaplasia, and dysplasia. Hematogenous spread metastatic spread to distant organs is seen.

2. **Diffuse-type cancers** (70%) arise from the lamina propria and are associated with an invasive growth pattern with rapid submucosal spread. They occur more commonly in younger patients, females, and in the proximal stomach. Transmural and lymphatic spread with early metastases are more common, and diffuse-type cancers have worse overall prognosis.

C. **Presentation** of gastric cancer generally involves nonspecific signs and symptoms such as epigastric abdominal pain, unexplained weight loss, nausea, vomiting, anorexia, early satiety, and fatigue. Dysphagia is associated with proximal gastric cancers, whereas gastric outlet obstruction is more typical of distal cancers. Perforation and upper GI bleeding are the presenting manifestations in a minority of patients (1% to 4%) and generally portend advanced disease with poor prognosis. Classic physical findings in gastric cancer represent metastatic and incurable disease and include the following:

1. Enlarged supraclavicular nodes (Virchow's node).
2. Infiltration of the umbilicus (Sister Mary Joseph's node).
3. Fullness in the pelvic cul-de-sac (Blumer's shelf).
4. Enlarged ovaries on pelvic examination (Krukenberg's tumor).
5. Hepatosplenomegaly with ascites and jaundice.
6. Cachexia.

D. **Diagnosis** can be made by double-contrast upper GI barium contrast studies or by **EGD.** Endoscopy is generally the diagnostic method of choice because it permits direct visualization and multiple biopsies (≥7) of suspicious lesions. **Screening examination** by endoscopy or contrast studies is not cost-effective for the general US population, given the low incidence, but may be warranted in high-risk individuals, such as patients more than 20 years post-partial gastrectomy, patients with pernicious anemia or atrophic gastritis, immigrants from endemic areas (Russia, Asia), and patients with familial or hereditary gastric cancer. Mass screening in Japan, a country with a high incidence of gastric cancer, resulted in an increase in the detection of gastric cancer confined to mucosa and led to improvements in 5-year survival rates.

E. **Staging** is important in determining prognosis and appropriate treatment. The American Joint Committee on Cancer and International Union against Cancer (AJCC/UICC) jointly developed a staging system that is most widely used worldwide (Table 9-1). Once the diagnosis of gastric cancer is established, **computed tomography (CT) and endoscopic ultrasonography (EUS)** are the primary modalities employed for staging.

1. **CT scan of the abdomen and pelvis** is the best noninvasive modality for detecting metastatic disease in the form of malignant ascites or hematogenous spread to distant organs, most commonly the liver. Overall accuracy for tumor staging is 60% to 80% depending on the protocol used, but accuracy for determining nodal involvement is more limited and variable.

TABLE 9-1	TNM (Tumor, Node, Metastasis) Staging of Gastric Cancer

T: Primary Tumor

T0	No evidence of primary tumor
Tis	Carcinoma *in situ*
T1	Invasion of lamina propria or submucosa
T2	Invasion of muscularis propria or subserosa
T3	Penetration of serosa
T4	Invasion of adjacent structures

N: Regional Lymph Nodes

N0	No regional node metastasis
N1	Involved perigastric nodes within 3 cm of tumor
N2	Involved perigastric nodes >3 cm from tumor edge or involvement of left gastric, splenic, celiac, or hepatic nodes

M: Distant Metastasis

M0	No distant metastases
M1	Distant metastases present

Stage Grouping

Stage 0	Tis	N0	M0
Stage IA	T1	N0	M0
Stage IB	T1	N1	M0
	T2	N0	M0
Stage II	T1	N2	M0
	T2	N1	M0
	T3	N0	M0
Stage IIIA	T2	N2	M0
	T3	N1	M0
	T4	N0	M0
Stage IIIB	T3	N2	M0
	T4	N1	M0
Stage IV	T4	N2	M0
	Any T	Any N	Any M1

Adapted with permission from Fleming ID, Cooper JS, Henson DE, et al., eds. *AJCC Cancer Staging Manual,* 5th ed. Philadelphia: Lippincott Williams & Wilkins; 1998.

2. **EUS** adds to the preoperative evaluation of gastric cancer in several ways. It is superior to CT in delineating the depth of tumor invasion in the gastric wall and adjacent structures and identifying perigastric lymphadenopathy. EUS is the most accurate method available for T staging of gastric cancer, and accuracy for N staging approaches 70%. Addition of fine needle aspiration (FNA) of suspicious nodes increases accuracy even further and brings specificity to near 100%.

3. **Positron emission tomography (PET)/CT** combines the spatial resolution of CT with the contrast resolution of PET. It is most useful for its specificity in detecting nodal and distant metastatic disease not apparent on CT scan alone. Preliminary studies suggest that the use of PET/CT in staging patients with gastric cancer leads to upstaging in 6% and downstaging in 9% of patients.

4. **Laparoscopy** significantly enhances the accuracy of staging in patients with gastric cancer. Routine use of laparoscopy has been shown to detect small-volume peritoneal and liver metastases in 20% to 30% of patients believed to have locoregional disease, thereby avoiding unnecessary laparotomy in these patients (*J Gastro Liv Dis.* 2009;18:189; *J Minim Access Surg.* 2010;6:111). Although laparoscopic ultrasound enhances the accuracy of staging in other GI cancers, its role in gastric cancer awaits further study. Laparoscopy is not indicated in patients with T1 and T2 lesions, given the low incidence of metastases with these tumors (*J Am Coll Surg.* 2003;196:965).

F. **Treatment. Surgery** is the mainstay of curative therapy in the absence of disseminated disease.

1. **Extent of surgical resection** generally involves a wide resection to achieve negative margins with *en bloc* resection of lymph nodes and any structures involved by local invasion. In general, gross margins of 6 cm, confirmed to be negative intraoperatively with frozen section, are usually required to ensure microscopically negative margins on final histologic analysis.

    a. **Proximal tumors** of the stomach comprise up to half of all gastric cancers and can be resected by total gastrectomy or proximal subtotal gastrectomy. Total gastrectomy with Roux-en-Y esophagojejunostomy is generally the preferred option to avoid postoperative morbidity of reflux esophagitis and impaired gastric emptying associated with proximal subtotal gastrectomy. Tumors of the GE junction may require esophagogastrectomy with cervical or thoracic anastomosis.

    b. **Midbody tumors** comprise 15% to 30% of tumors and generally require total gastrectomy to achieve adequate margins.

    c. **Distal tumors** may be resected by distal subtotal gastrectomy or total gastrectomy with no difference in overall survival (*Ann Surg.* 1989;209:162; *Ann Surg.* 1994;220:176). However, nutritional status and quality of life are superior following subtotal gastrectomy, making it the preferred option when adequate margins can be obtained while maintaining an adequate gastric remnant (*Ann Surg.* 1997;226:613; *Ann Surg.* 2005;241:232).

  d. **Early gastric cancers,** defined as tumors confined to the mucosa, have limited propensity for lymph node metastasis and may be treated by limited gastric resections or **endoscopic mucosal resection.** Experience outside of Japan with early gastric cancers is limited.

  e. **Laparoscopic gastric resections** have been reported for the treatment of gastric cancer, with advantages of reduced pain, shorter hospitalization, and improved quality of life. Long-term outcome with respect to cancer recurrence awaits further study in a randomized, controlled fashion (*Ann R Coll Surg Engl.* 2010;92).

2. **Extent of lymphadenectomy** has long been a controversial issue in the surgical management of gastric cancer. Early retrospective Japanese studies showed improved survival with radical lymph node dissections. A standard (D1) lymphadenectomy entails removal of perigastric nodes, whereas an extended (D2) resection includes removal of nodes along the left gastric, hepatic, splenic, and celiac arteries. Although the results of major trials attempting to answer this question have yielded confounding results, it is generally agreed on that, at high-volume centers, D2 lymphadenectomies that preserve the distal pancreas and spleen can be performed without increased morbidity, and improves staging accuracy. D2 resection may yield a survival advantage in selected patients with stage II and III gastric cancers but available data are not convincing (*Am J Surg.* 2009;197:246; *Lancet Oncol.* 2010;11:439).

3. **Adjuvant therapy** for gastric cancer is important because the majority of patients with locoregional disease (all patients except those with T1–2N0M0 disease) are at high risk for local or systemic recurrence following curative surgery.

  a. **Adjuvant combined modality therapy.** Although adjuvant chemotherapy or radiation therapy alone has not shown much benefit in studies, recent trials have been able to demonstrate significant improvement in overall and disease-free survival rates in patients with resected gastric cancer treated postoperatively with 5-fluorouracil (5-FU)/leucovorin chemotherapy coupled with radiation therapy (*N Engl J Med.* 2001;345:725; *J Clin Oncol.* 2010;28:2430).

  b. **Neoadjuvant chemotherapy** for gastric cancer has the potential for improving patient tolerance, resectability rates (downstaging), and overall patient survival. A recently reported European trial demonstrated significant improvement in 5-year survival rates in patients with gastric cancer who were treated with six cycles of chemotherapy (three preoperatively and three postoperatively) compared to surgery alone (*N Engl J Med.* 2006;355:11). Chemotherapy regimen in this trial consisted of epirubicin, cisplatin, and 5-FU. Furthermore, preoperative chemotherapy improved curative resection rates.

4. **Palliative therapy** of gastric cancer is important due to overall low cure rates. Generally, patients with peritoneal disease, hepatic or nodal metastases, or other poor prognostic factors benefit most from endoscopic

palliation. Laparoscopic or open palliative surgical resection can be considered in patients with better prognosis and good performance status to prevent bleeding, obstruction, and perforation in patients with metastatic or otherwise unresectable cancer. Palliative surgical resections appear to provide superior relief of symptoms compared to surgical bypass. Palliative chemoradiation therapy also prolongs survival in patients and improves symptoms and quality of life when it can be administered safely.

IV. **PRIMARY GASTRIC LYMPHOMA (PGL)** accounts for fewer than 5% of gastric neoplasms. However, PGL comprises two thirds of all primary GI lymphomas because the stomach is the most commonly involved organ in extranodal lymphoma. PGLs are usually B-cell, non-Hodgkin lymphomas. Most PGLs occur in the distal stomach.

A. Patients typically present in their sixth decade with symptoms similar to those of gastric adenocarcinoma (epigastric pain, weight loss, anorexia, nausea, vomiting, and occult GI bleeding). Diagnosis is typically made using endoscopy, and staging to detect systemic disease is performed using CT of chest/abdomen/pelvis, bone marrow biopsy, and biopsy of enlarged peripheral lymph nodes.

B. Therapy of PGL has been advanced by the recognition that low-grade PGLs have features resembling mucosa-associated lymphoid tissue (MALT) and that the majority of low-grade MALT lymphomas are associated with *H. pylori* infection. Thus, **first-line therapy for low-grade MALT lymphomas is use of antibiotics directed at *H. pylori* eradication,** which leads to complete remission rates of 70% to 100%. Chemoradiation therapy is used as salvage therapy for failure of antibiotics. High-grade or non-MALT lymphomas are generally treated with chemoradiation therapy alone, with surgical resection reserved for those who fail chemoradiation or in emergency cases of hemorrhage or perforation.

V. **BENIGN GASTRIC TUMORS** account for fewer than 2% of all gastric tumors. They are usually located in the antrum or corpus. Presentation can be similar to that of peptic ulcer or adenocarcinoma, and diagnosis is made by EGD or contrast radiography.

A. **Gastric polyps** are classified by histologic findings. Endoscopic removal is appropriate if the polyp can be completely excised.

1. **Hyperplastic polyps** are regenerative rather than neoplastic and constitute 75% of gastric polyps. Risk of malignant transformation is minimal.

2. **Adenomatous polyps** are the second most common gastric polyp and are neoplastic in origin. The incidence of carcinoma within the polyp is proportional to its size, with polyps of greater than 2 cm having a 24% incidence of malignancy. Patients with familial adenomatous polyposis have a 50% incidence of gastroduodenal polyps and require endoscopic surveillance. Surgical resection with a 2- to 3-cm margin of

gastric wall can often be performed laparoscopically and is required if endoscopic excision is not possible.

VI. **GASTROINTESTINAL STROMAL TUMORS (GISTs)** comprise only 3% of all gastric malignancies and arise from mesenchymal components of the gastric wall. The median age at diagnosis is 60 years, with a slight male predominance. GISTs frequently display prominent extraluminal growth and can attain large sizes before becoming symptomatic.

   A. Presentation can be varied and includes asymptomatic masses found incidentally on physical exam or radiographic studies, vague abdominal pain and discomfort secondary to mass effect, and GI hemorrhage as a result of necrosis of overlying mucosa. Diagnosis is made by endoscopy and FNA biopsy. GISTs are graded according to tumor size and histologic frequency of mitoses. Staging is accomplished by CT of abdomen/pelvis and chest X-ray.

   B. **Treatment** is open or laparoscopic surgical resection with 2-cm margins of grossly normal gastric wall to ensure negative histologic margins. *En bloc* resection of any structures involved by local invasion should be attempted, although lymphadenectomy is not indicated because lymph node metastases are rare. Metastasis occurs by hematogenous route, and hepatic involvement is common, as is local recurrence after resection. GISTs are not radiosensitive or responsive to traditional chemotherapy. However, most GISTs express the **c-kit** receptor, a tyrosine kinase that acts as a growth factor receptor. **Imatinib mesylate (Gleevec™)** is a small-molecule inhibitor of the c-kit receptor that has become first-line therapy for metastatic or recurrent GIST. Approximately 60% of patients experience a partial response, and when maximal response is achieved, surgical therapy should be considered for patients in whom all gross disease can be removed.

VII. **GASTRIC CARCINOIDS** are rare neuroendocrine tumors accounting for less than 1% of all gastric neoplasms. Carcinoid tumors arise from enterochromaffin-like cells and can be secondary to hypergastrinemia associated with pernicious anemia or chronic atrophic gastritis. Tumors tend to be small, multiple, and asymptomatic, although larger solitary tumors may cause ulceration of overlying mucosa and symptoms similar to PUD. EGD with biopsy generally provides diagnosis. Treatment of large (>2 cm), solitary tumors is gastrectomy because these have the highest invasive potential. Treatment of smaller, multifocal tumors is less clear, with options ranging from observation, gastrectomy to include the tumors, and antrectomy without inclusion of tumors to reduce gastrin levels and induce tumor regression.

VIII. **POSTGASTRECTOMY SYNDROMES** are caused by changes in gastric emptying as a consequence of gastric operations. They may occur in up to 20% of patients who undergo gastric surgery, depending on the extent of resection, disruption of the vagus nerves, status of the pylorus, type of reconstruction, and presence of mechanical or functional obstruction. Clearly defining the syndrome that is present in a given patient is critical to developing a rational treatment plan (*World J Surg.* 2003;27:725). Most are treated nonoperatively and resolve with time.

A. **Nutritional disturbances** occur in 30% of patients after gastric surgery, either as a result of functional changes or postgastrectomy syndromes. Prolonged **iron, folate, vitamin B_{12}, calcium, and vitamin D deficiencies** can result in anemia, neuropathy, dementia, and osteomalacia. These can be prevented with supplementation.

B. **Dumping syndrome** is thought to result from the rapid emptying of a high-osmolar carbohydrate load into the small intestine. Gastric resection leads to the loss of reservoir capacity and the loss of pylorus function. Dumping syndrome is most common after Billroth II reconstruction.

  1. **Early dumping** occurs within 30 minutes of eating and is characterized by nausea, epigastric distress, explosive diarrhea, and vasomotor symptoms (i.e., dizziness, palpitations, flushing, and diaphoresis). It is presumably caused by rapid fluid shifts in response to the hyperosmolar intestinal load from the stomach to the small intestine. The resultant food bolus causes a rapid shift of extracellular fluid into the bowel lumen.

  2. **Late dumping** symptoms are primarily vasomotor and occur 1 to 4 hours after eating. The hormonal response to high simple carbohydrate loads results in hyperinsulinemia and reactive hypoglycemia. Symptoms are relieved by carbohydrate ingestion.

  3. **Treatment** is primarily nonsurgical and results in improvement in nearly all patients over time. Meals should be smaller in volume but increased in frequency, liquids should be ingested 30 minutes after eating solids, and simple carbohydrates should be avoided. Use of the long-acting somatostatin analog octreotide results in significant improvement and persistent relief in 80% of patients when behavioral modifications fail (*Nat Rev Gastro Hepatol.* 2009;6:583). If reoperation is necessary, conversion to Roux-en-Y gastrojejunostomy or an isoperistaltic/antiperistaltic jejunal loop is usually successful.

C. **Alkaline reflux gastritis** is most commonly associated with Billroth II gastrojejunostomy and requires operative treatment more often than other postgastrectomy syndromes. It is characterized by the triad of constant (not postprandial) epigastric pain, nausea, and bilious emesis. Vomiting does not relieve the pain and is not associated with meals. Endoscopy reveals inflamed, beefy red, friable gastric mucosa, and can rule out recurrent ulcer as a cause of symptoms. Bile reflux into the stomach is occasionally seen. Enterogastric reflux can be confirmed by hydroxy iminodiacetic acid (HIDA) scan. Mechanical obstruction is absent, distinguishing alkaline reflux gastritis from loop syndromes. **Nonoperative therapy** consists of frequent meals, antacids, and cholestyramine to bind bile salts but is usually ineffective. **Surgery** to divert bile flow from the gastric mucosa is the only proven treatment. The creation of a long-limb (45-cm) Roux-en-Y gastrojejunostomy effectively eliminates alkaline reflux and is the preferred option for most patients (*Gastroenterol Clin North Am.* 1994;23:281).

D. **Roux stasis syndrome** may occur in up to 30% of patients after Roux-en-Y gastroenterostomy. It is characterized by chronic abdominal pain, nausea, and vomiting that is aggravated with eating. It results from functional obstruction due to disruption of the normal propagation of pacesetter potentials in the Roux limb from the proximal duodenum, as well as altered motility in the gastric remnant. Near-total gastrectomy to remove the atonic stomach can improve gastric emptying and is occasionally useful in patients with refractory Roux stasis. Use of an "uncut" Roux-en-Y reconstruction (*Am J Surg.* 2001;182:52) may preserve normal pacemaker propagation and prevent the development of the syndrome.

E. **Loop syndromes** result from mechanical obstruction of either the **afferent** or **efferent** limbs of the Billroth II gastrojejunostomy. The location and etiology of the obstruction are investigated by plain abdominal X-rays, CT scan, upper GI contrast studies, and endoscopy. Relief of the obstruction may require adhesiolysis, revision of the anastomosis, occasionally bowel resection, or conversion of Billroth II to Roux-en-Y gastrojejunostomy.

1. **Afferent loop syndrome** can be caused acutely by bowel kink, volvulus, or internal herniation, resulting in severe abdominal pain and nonbilious emesis within the first few weeks after surgery. Lack of bilious staining of nasogastric drainage in the immediate postoperative period suggests this complication. Examination may reveal a fluid-filled abdominal mass, and laboratory findings may include elevated bilirubin or amylase. **Duodenal stump blowout** results from progressive afferent limb dilation, leading to peritonitis, abscess, or fistula formation. In the urgent setting, jejunojejunostomy can effectively decompress the afferent limb. A more **chronic form** of afferent loop syndrome results from partial mechanical obstruction of the afferent limb. Patients present with postprandial right upper quadrant pain relieved by bilious emesis that is not mixed with recently ingested food. Stasis can lead to bacterial overgrowth and subsequent bile salt deconjugation in the obstructed loop, causing **blind loop syndrome** (steatorrhea and vitamin B_{12}, folate, and iron deficiency) by interfering with fat and vitamin B_{12} absorption.

2. **Efferent loop syndrome** results from intermittent obstruction of the efferent limb of the gastrojejunostomy. Patients complain of abdominal pain and bilious emesis months to years after surgery, similar to the situation with regard to a proximal small bowel obstruction.

F. **Postvagotomy diarrhea** has an incidence of 20% after truncal vagotomy and is thought to result from alterations in gastric emptying and vagal denervation of the small bowel and biliary tree. The diarrhea is typically watery and episodic. Treatment includes antidiarrheal medications (loperamide, diphenoxylate with atropine, cholestyramine) and decreasing excessive intake of fluids or foods that contain lactose. Symptoms usually improve with time, and surgery is rarely indicated.

IX. **SEVERE OBESITY** is a condition characterized by the pathologic accumulation of excess body fat. It is defined as a body mass index [BMI = weight (kg)/ height (m^2)] equal to or greater than 40, which generally correlates with an actual body weight 100 lb greater than ideal body weight.

A. Epidemiology. Obesity is a disease process that has reached epidemic proportions worldwide, with the highest prevalence in the United States, where 5% of the adult population is morbidly obese (*JAMA.* 2010;303:235). Obesity is also becoming increasingly prevalent in the pediatric population (*JAMA.* 2010;303:242).

B. The **etiology** of morbid obesity is poorly understood and thought to result from an imbalance in biologic, psychosocial, and environmental factors governing caloric intake and caloric expenditure. Risk factors for the development of morbid obesity include **genetic predisposition,** diet, and culture.

C. Most patients with morbid obesity present with one or more of a number of weight-related comorbidities. Patients with **central** obesity (android or "apple" fat distribution) are at higher risk for development of obesity-related complications than those with **peripheral** obesity (gynecoid or "pear" fat distribution). This is due to increased visceral fat distribution, producing increased intra-abdominal pressure and increasing fat metabolism (with subsequent hyperglycemia, hyperinsulinemia, and peripheral insulin resistance). Table 9-2 lists some of the medical complications associated with morbid obesity. In addition to the aforementioned comorbidities, obesity also increases mortality. One study showed an increase in mortality among morbidly obese individuals (*NEJM.* 2006;355:8).

D. **Treatment** of morbid obesity is of paramount importance because of the many medical sequelae associated with obesity, nearly all are reversible on resolution of the obese state.

1. **Lifestyle changes** in diet, exercise habits, and behavior modification are first-line therapy for all obese patients. In combination, such changes can achieve 8% to 10% weight loss over a 6-month period, but losses are sustained at 1 year in only 60% of patients. However, certain comorbidities, such as diabetes, benefit from as little as 3% weight loss, and lifestyle changes alone may be sufficient in patients with BMI less than 27.

2. **Pharmacotherapy** is second-tier therapy used in patients with BMI greater than 27 and in combination with lifestyle changes. Currently, sibutramine, an appetite suppressant, and orlistat, a lipase inhibitor that reduces lipid absorption, are the only approved drugs for weight loss treatment. Weight loss with these agents is 6% to 10% at 1 year, but relapse rates after discontinuation of the drugs are high.

3. **Bariatric surgery** is the most effective approach for achieving durable weight loss in the morbidly obese. Multiple studies have confirmed the superiority of surgery to nonsurgical approaches in achieving and maintaining weight reduction in the morbidly obese (*N Engl J Med.* 2004;351:2683; *Surg Obes Relat Disord.* 2010;6:347). A National Institutes of Health Consensus Development Conference on morbid

TABLE 9-2	Complications of Morbid Obesity

Cardiac Hypertension Coronary artery disease Heart failure Arrhythmias	**Vascular** Deep venous thrombosis Venous stasis ulceration
Pulmonary Obesity hypoventilation syndrome Obstructive sleep apnea Respiratory insufficiency of obesity (pickwickian syndrome) Pulmonary embolism	**Infectious** Fungal infections Necrotizing soft tissue infections
Metabolic Type II diabetes Hyperlipidemia Hypercholesterolemia Nonalcoholic steatohepatitis	**Genitourinary** Nephrotic syndrome Stress urinary incontinence
	Gynecologic Polycystic ovary syndrome
Musculoskeletal Degenerative joint disease Lumbar disc disease Osteoarthritis	**Neurologic/psychiatric** Pseudotumor cerebri Depression Stroke Low self-esteem
Gastrointestinal Cholelithiasis Gastroesophageal reflux disease Hernias	**Oncologic** Cancers of uterus, breast, colon/ rectum, and prostate

obesity established guidelines for the evaluation and treatment of
morbidly obese patients with bariatric surgical procedures (*Ann Surg.*
2010;250:399).

a. **Indications.** Patients who have failed intensive efforts at weight
   control using medical means are candidates for bariatric surgery
   if they have a BMI index greater than 40 or greater than 35 with
   weight-related comorbidities.

b. **Preoperative evaluation.** A bariatric multidisciplinary team
   including primary care physicians, dietitians, physical therapists,
   anesthesiologists, nurses, and psychiatrists or psychologists evaluates a patient's weight history, dietary habits, motivation, social history, and comorbid medical conditions prior to surgery.

c. **Benefits** of surgery are related to reversal of the disease processes
   associated with severe obesity. Hypertension completely resolves
   in 62% of patients and resolves or improves in 79%. Diabetes is completely resolved in 77% of patients and resolves or
   improves in 86%. Obstructive sleep apnea resolves or improves
   in 85% of patients and hyperlipidemia improves in 70% (*Lancet.*

2009;10:653; *NEJM.* 2007;357:741). The quality of life is markedly better. Most importantly, recent studies demonstrate reduced mortality rates in morbidly obese patients undergoing bariatric surgery compared to matched controls (*NEJM.* 2004;351:2683; *Ann Surg.* 2010;250:399).

E. **Bariatric surgical procedures** can generally be divided into two types: **restrictive procedures,** which limit the amount of food that can be ingested, and **malabsorptive procedures,** which limit the absorption of nutrients and calories from ingested food by bypassing predetermined lengths of small intestine. The four standard operations used to produce weight loss in the morbidly obese include adjustable gastric banding (AGB) and vertical banded gastroplasty (restrictive procedures), biliopancreatic diversion (BPD) with and without duodenal switch (DS) (malabsorptive procedures), and Roux-en-Y gastric bypass (RYGBP) (combination). Sleeve gastrectomy, the first component of a DS operation, increasingly is being performed alone as a restrictive procedure.

1. **Adjustable gastric banding** (**AGB**) involves open or laparoscopic placement of a silicone band with an inflatable balloon around the proximal stomach at the angle of His. The band is connected to a reservoir that is implanted over the rectus sheath. The patient undergoes serial adjustments to inflate the band and create a small proximal gastric pouch. Excess weight loss is approximately 50%. Perioperative mortality is exceedingly low (0.05%), and overall complication rate is near 11%. Most complications are related to band slippage, which presents with obstructive symptoms or problems with the port (kinking or leaking of access tubing). Band erosion can occur but is far less frequent than the aforementioned complications. Advantages include safety, adjustability, and reversibility, whereas disadvantages include need for frequent postoperative visits (*JAMA.* 2010;303:316/519).

2. **Roux-en-Y gastric bypass (RYGBP)** is the most popular bariatric surgical procedure performed in the United States. A 30-mL proximal gastric pouch is created by either transection or occlusion using a stapling device. A 1-cm-diameter anastomosis is then performed between the pouch and a Roux limb of small bowel. This results in a small reservoir, a small passage for pouch emptying, and bypass of the distal stomach, duodenum, and proximal jejunum. The length of the Roux limb directly correlates with the degree of postoperative weight loss, with a 75-cm limb used for standard gastric bypasses and a 150-cm limb used for the superobese. Gastric bypass results in weight loss superior to that achieved with restrictive procedures, with mean excess weight loss of 70%. Perioperative mortality is 1%, and despite aggressive prophylaxis, **pulmonary embolism** (PE) remains the most common cause of death after bariatric surgery. Anastomotic leak at the gastrojejunostomy is another serious early complication, occurring in approximately 2% of cases. Unexplained **tachycardia** is often the only presenting sign of either complication in the perioperative period and warrants prompt investigation. Other early complications include wound infection (4% to 10%), gastric remnant dilation, and Roux limb obstruction. Late

complications include incisional hernia (15% to 25%), stomal stenosis (2% to 14%), marginal ulcer (2% to 10%), bowel obstruction (2%), and internal hernia (1%). Early or late **bowel obstruction** after RYGBP can be a life-threatening complication and generally requires prompt reoperation because of its association with internal hernia and potential for bowel strangulation. **CT scan with oral contrast** is the best diagnostic test to evaluate for leak or obstruction after RYGBP. Nutritional complications include folate, vitamin B_{12}, iron, and calcium deficiency. Dumping syndrome occurs in many patients and may reinforce dietary behavior modification to avoid sweets and high-calorie foods. Laparoscopic RYGBP is a technically challenging but safe procedure when performed by surgeons with advanced laparoscopic skills. Laparoscopic RYGBP produces equal excess weight loss and has similar mortality and leak rates as the open procedure. Its main advantages are reduced postoperative pain, reduced length of stay, and significantly reduced wound-related complications, such as wound infections, dehiscence, and incisional hernias (*NEJM.* 2009;361:445).

3. **Biliopancreatic diversion (BPD)** and **biliopancreatic diversion with duodenal switch (BPD-DS)** are two additional procedures for morbidly obese patients. BPD requires antrectomy with formation of a 200-cm alimentary channel and a 50- to 75-cm common channel. BPD-DS includes a sleeve gastrectomy, preservation of the pylorus, a 150-cm alimentary channel, and a 75- to 100-cm common channel. These procedures are done at select centers for the superobese and those who have failed to maintain weight loss following gastric bypass or restrictive procedures. Long-term outcomes indicate excess weight loss of 75% at 1 year, but nutritional deficiencies are more common than for RYGBP. Postoperative complications include anemia (30%), protein-calorie malnutrition (20%), dumping syndrome, and marginal ulceration (10%). These procedures are technically demanding and the applicability of these procedures to the obese population remains to be determined.

4. **Sleeve gastrectomy,** the first component of a DS operation, can be used alone as a purely restrictive procedure for the treatment of morbid obesity. It does not produce malabsorption and is technically easier to perform than BPD-DS or RYGBP. Preliminary reports have demonstrated 70% to 80% excess body weight loss at 1 year, but long-term outcomes and durability of this procedure remain unknown. It may be indicated as an initial procedure in the superobese population to induce enough weight loss to make BPD-DS or RYGBP technically more feasible (*Surg Obes Relat Disord.* 2010;6:1; *Ann Surg.* 2010;252:319).

10 Small Intestine

Susan C. Pitt and Steven R. Hunt

I. EMBRYOLOGY

A. Origin. The small intestine (SI) develops during the fourth week of fetal development. The duodenum arises from the foregut, while the jejunum and ileum derive from the midgut. The endoderm forms the absorptive epithelium and secretory glands. The remainder of the intestinal wall, including the muscularis and serosa, are created from the splanchnic mesoderm.

B. Rotation. During the fifth week of fetal development, the intestine herniates through the umbilicus and rotates 90 degrees around the axis of the vitelline duct and superior mesenteric artery (SMA). By the 10th week, the intestine returns to the abdominal cavity rotating an additional 180 degrees. This revolution positions the ligament of Treitz in the left upper quadrant and the cecum in the right upper quadrant. Cecal descent into the right lower quadrant later occurs at four months.

C. Lumen formation. Between the fourth and seventh weeks, the SI is lined by cuboidal cells. Rapid proliferation occasionally occludes the lumen, particularly in the duodenum, but patency is regained by the 10th week via apoptosis.

II. ANATOMY

A. Gross anatomy. The SI extends approximately 3 m from the pylorus to the ileocecal valve. The duodenum is only about 20 cm. The first portion or bulb is intraperitoneal, while the remaining second, third, and fourth portions are retroperitoneal. Biliary and pancreatic secretions enter the second portion of the duodenum at the ampulla of Vater. The jejunum and ileum are significantly longer and span approximately 100 and 150 cm, respectively. These segments of SI can be differentiated by examining the mesenteric blood supply. Jejunal arcades are larger, fewer in number, and have longer vessels between the arcades. The jejunum also has many circumferential mucosal folds called plicae circularis.

B. Vascular supply. The duodenum is supplied by the pancreaticoduodenal arteries that are branches of the gastroduodenal artery and SMA. The jejunum and ileum are supplied by the SMA. The superior mesenteric vein (SMV) runs parallel to the SMA, provides the venous drainage of the small bowel, and joins the splenic vein to form the portal vein.

C. Lymphatic drainage. The submucosal Peyer patches feed small lymphatics extending to the mesenteric lymph nodes. From there, drainage parallels the course of the named blood vessels and eventually accumulates at the subdiaphragmatic cisterna chyli before entering the thoracic duct.

D. **Innervation.** The vagus nerve supplies all abdominal parasympathetic fibers and plays an important role in regulating intestinal secretions and motility. These fibers cross mesenteric ganglia, particularly the celiac ganglion, and innervate the myenteric ganglion cells within the walls of the SI. Three sets of sympathetic nerves innervate the gut forming a plexus around the SMA. Sympathetic nerves modulate the intestinal blood supply, secretion, and motility as well as carry all pain signals from the intestine.

E. **Anatomy of the intestinal wall** is uniform from the duodenum to the ileocecal valve, consisting of four distinct tissue layers.

1. The **mucosa** is composed of the epithelium, lamina propria, and muscularis mucosae.

   a. The **epithelium** has both villi and crypts. The *villi* are protrusions of the epithelial layer into the lumen that act to dramatically increase absorptive capacity, while the *crypts* contain pluripotent cells that give rise to absorptive enterocytes (over 95% of the epithelial layer). *Paneth cells* secrete lysozyme, tumor necrosis factor (TNF), and cryptdin that provide nonspecific immunity. *Goblet cells* secrete mucus. More than 10 different subpopulations of *enteroendocrine cells* exist that secrete a variety of hormones. Of note, the entire intestinal lining is replaced every 3 to 5 days.

   b. The **lamina propria** is a layer of loose connective tissue that contains Peyer patches – collections of lymphocytes that span the lamina propria and submucosa and provide mucosal immunity.

   c. The **muscularis mucosa** is a layer of muscle separating the mucosa from the submucosa.

2. The **submucosa** is the strongest layer of the intestinal wall. Blood vessels and nerves run within this layer, including Meissner ganglion cells.

3. The **muscularis propria** consists of a thicker, inner circular layer and an outer longitudinal layer of smooth muscle cells. The Auerbach (myenteric) ganglion cells are located between these smooth muscle layers.

4. The **serosa** is a single layer of flat mesothelial cells composing the outermost layer of the small bowel. Serosa lines the extraluminal surface of the anterior duodenum and the entire jejunum and ileum.

F. **Enterocyte histology.** The absorptive capacity of enterocytes is due to the presence of microvilli and a glycocalyx coating outside the cell membrane. Digestive enzymes, such as disaccharidases, and Na-nutrient cotransporters are located in the apical membrane. Laterally, tight junctions prevent crossing of intraluminal contents across the epithelial layer. Intermediate junctions and desmosomes also help to maintain the barrier function of the intestinal epithelium. Na-K ATPases and passive nutrient transporters are found in the basal membrane.

III. **PHYSIOLOGY** of the SI involves a complex balance between absorption and secretion. The gut is also the largest endocrine organ in the human body.

A. **Absorption** is the principal function of the gastrointestinal (GI) tract.

1. **Water.** Under normal circumstances, approximately 7 to 10 L of fluid enter the SI each day, but only 1 L reaches the colon. Of this fluid, 2 L are derived from oral intake, 1 L from saliva, 2 L from gastric secretion, 2 L from pancreatic secretion, 1 L from bile, and 1 L from small-intestinal secretion. Alterations in small bowel permeability, tonicity of enteric substances, or rate of transit can result in diarrhea and large volume losses.

2. The majority of **electrolyte** absorption occurs in the SI. The most important electrolytes absorbed are sodium, chloride, and calcium. Sodium absorption occurs through passive diffusion, countertransport with hydrogen, and cotransport with chloride, glucose, and amino acids. Chloride is absorbed in exchange for bicarbonate, which accounts for the alkalinity of the luminal contents. Calcium is actively absorbed in the proximal SI by a process that is stimulated by vitamin D. Emesis, diarrhea, obstruction, and small-bowel ostomy effluent can result in impaired small-bowel electrolyte absorption.

3. **Bile salts** and **vitamin B_{12}-intrinsic factor** complexes are absorbed in the terminal ileum. Resection that leaves less than 100 cm of the ileum can result in bile acid deficiencies that limit absorption of the fat-soluble vitamins A, D, E, and K. Vitamin B_{12} deficiency can result in chronic megaloblastic anemia (pernicious anemia).

4. **Nutrients.** The absorption of carbohydrates, proteins, and fat is discussed in Chapter 2 and in the next section.

B. **Digestion.** Macronutrient digestion by salivary, gastric, biliary, and pancreatic secretions is covered in Chapter 2. This section discusses digestion at the level of the enterocyte.

1. **Brush border enzymes,** peptidases and disaccharidases, break down peptides and disaccharides into simple amino acids and monosaccharides.

2. **Active transport** via Na-K ATPases in the basolateral membrane of enterocytes keeps the intracellular Na concentration very low. This sodium gradient enables Na-nutrient cotransporters to move amino acids and monosaccharides into enterocytes.

3. **Passive transport.** After digestion by pancreatic lipases, triglycerides and fatty acids form micelles with bile salts. These micelles diffuse across the apical membrane and are reconstituted into chylomicrons, which subsequently enter submucosal lymphatics.

C. **Motility**

1. **Types of contractions.** *Circular muscle* contractions can temporarily segment the intestine for improved mixing of contents or they can propel food toward the colon if they progress caudad. When the *longitudinal muscle* contracts, sleeve contractions shorten the intestinal length helping to propel food forward.

2. **Neurohumoral effects.** Vagal cholinergic input and hormones such as motilin and cholecystokinin (CCK) stimulate contractions. Conversely, sympathetic neurons inhibit peristalsis.

3. During the **fasting state,** the migrating motor complex (MMC) performs the housekeeping function of clearing the lumen of debris. After a period of rest, random contractions of moderate strength are followed by several very strong contractions.

4. During the **fed state,** contractions occur more frequently and last longer, and multiple areas of the small bowel may contract at the same time. From each site of contraction, peristalsis proceeds caudally for a varying distance.

D. **Immunity.** Tight junctions between the enterocyte apical membranes provide a *barrier function* and prevent pathogens from crossing the epithelium. Mucosal plasma cells secrete immunoglobulin A (*IgA*), which binds intraluminal pathogens and targets them for destruction.

1. M cells are located in the epithelial layer over the Peyer patches. These cells facilitate direct antigen presentation to macrophages and lymphocytes thereby aiding acquired immunity to luminal pathogens.

2. T cells can be located within vacuoles of M cells and seem to have an immunosuppressive effect that may explain nonreactivity to ingested food.

E. **Endocrine** function is regulated by neural, hormonal (both autocrine and paracrine), and anatomic mechanisms.

1. **CCK** is produced by duodenal and jejunal I cells in response to intraluminal amino acids and fats. CCK causes gallbladder contraction, pancreatic enzyme secretion, and relaxation of the sphincter of Oddi.

2. **Enteroglucagon** from ileal and colonic L cells is released in response to intraluminal fat and bile acids and delays gastric emptying. Secretion can dramatically increase with inflammatory processes, such as Crohn's disease and celiac sprue.

3. **Gastric inhibitory peptide (GIP)** is secreted by duodenal and jejunal K cells in response to active transport of monosaccharides, long-chain fatty acids, and amino acids. GIP inhibits gastric acid and pepsinogen secretion and gastric emptying, but stimulates insulin release.

4. **Gastrin** is secreted in response to vagal stimulation and intraluminal peptides by duodenal G cells. Gastrin stimulates acid secretion by the gastric fundus and body and increases gastric mucosal blood flow.

5. **Motilin** is produced by duodenal and jejunal M cells in response to duodenal acid, vagal stimulation, and gastrin-releasing peptide. Motilin is involved in the MMC during the fasting state. Erythromycin is useful as a promotility agent due to its action as a motilin agonist.

6. **Secretin** is released by duodenal and jejunal S cells in response to acid, bile salts, and fatty acids in the duodenum. Secretin increases bicarbonate and water secretion from pancreatic ducts, and also inhibits gastric acid secretion and gastric motility.

7. **Somatostatin** broadly inhibits gut exocrine and endocrine function. Intestinal D cells and enteric neurons secrete somatostatin in response to intraluminal fat, protein, and acid.

8. **Vasoactive intestinal peptide (VIP)** is secreted throughout the SI in response to vagal stimulation. VIP increases mesenteric blood flow, intestinal motility, and pancreatic and intestinal secretions.

IV. SMALL-BOWEL OBSTRUCTION (SBO)

A. **Mechanical obstruction** of the SI can be partial, allowing some distal passage of gas or fluid, or complete, with total occlusion of the lumen. In a strangulated obstruction, the involved bowel has vascular compromise, which can ultimately lead to infarction and perforation of the intestinal wall. No clinical or laboratory values reliably differentiate simple from strangulated obstructions, although constant, as opposed to crampy, abdominal pain, fever, leukocytosis, and acidosis should raise the index of suspicion considerably. On the other hand, **ileus** implies failure of peristalsis without mechanical obstruction. Recent abdominal operations, electrolyte disturbances, trauma, peritonitis, systemic infections, bowel ischemia, and certain medications (i.e., narcotics) can all result in an ileus.

B. **Etiology**

1. **Adhesions** are the *most common* cause of SBO in US adults and mostly result from previous abdominal operations or inflammatory processes, although isolated congenital adhesions or bands can occur as well. Intra-abdominal adhesions occur in more than 90% of patients following major abdominal surgery and account for about 60% to 70% of SBOs (*Ann R Coll Surg Engl.* 1990;72:60–63; *Eur J Surg.* 1997;163(suppl 577):5–9).

2. **Incarcerated hernias** are the second most common cause of SBOs in industrialized nations and the most common cause of SBO worldwide. In children and patients without prior abdominal surgery, hernias are the most common cause of SBO in developed nations.

3. **Intussusception** occurs when one portion of bowel (the intussusceptum) telescopes into another (the intussuscipiens). Tumors, polyps, enlarged mesenteric lymph nodes, or a Meckel's diverticulum may serve as lead points of the telescoped segment. As opposed to intussusception in children, an adult with intussusception should prompt workup for bowel pathology. Asymptomatic, transient intussusception is occasionally seen incidentally on an abdominal CT scan performed for other reasons.

4. **Volvulus,** or the rotation of a segment of bowel around its vascular pedicle, is often caused by adhesions or congenital anomalies such as intestinal malrotation and more commonly occurs in the colon.

5. **Strictures** secondary to ischemia, inflammation (Crohn's disease), radiation therapy, or prior surgery may also cause obstruction.

6. **Gallstone ileus** occurs as a complication of cholecystitis. Fistulization between the biliary tree and the small bowel (cholecystoduodenal or choledochoduodenal fistula) allows one or more gallstones to travel distally and become lodged, typically at the ileocecal valve.

7. **External compression** from tumors, abscesses, hematomas, or other masses can cause functional SBO.

8. **Foreign bodies** typically pass without incident. Items presenting with obstruction may require operation if they cannot be retrieved endoscopically. Pathology due to swallowing foreign bodies is more common in institutionalized patients.

C. **Diagnosis** of SBO incorporates the full range of history, physical exam, and radiographic findings.

1. **Signs and symptoms.** Proximal SBOs present with early bilious **vomiting,** while distal obstructions present later, and emesis can be thicker and more feculent. Early in the disease course, **nausea** may be observed in the absence of vomiting. **Abdominal distention** typically increases the more distal the obstruction. **Abdominal pain** is poorly localized and often characterized as crampy and intermittent (i.e., colicky). **Obstipation,** complete absence of flatus and bowel movement, is observed once the distal bowel (beyond a complete obstruction) is evacuated. With a persistent obstruction, **hypovolemia** progresses due to impaired absorption, increased secretion ("third spacing"), and fluid losses from emesis. **Bloody bowel movements** suggest ischemia of the intestine or an alternative diagnosis.

2. **Physical examination.** Abnormal **vital signs** are generally indicative of hypovolemia (e.g., tachycardia and hypotension). **Abdominal exam** may reveal distension, prior surgical scars, and hernias. Palpation should make note of any masses. Peritoneal signs mandate prompt surgical evaluation and treatment due to the risk of bowel strangulation. Digital rectal examination may reveal the presence of an obstructing rectal tumor or impacted stool.

3. **Laboratory evaluation.** In the early stages of a SBO, laboratory values may be normal. As the process progresses, lab values commonly reflect dehydration demonstrating a contraction alkalosis (metabolic) with hypochloremia and hypokalemia. An elevated white blood cell (WBC) count, serum lactate level, and glucose, or an acidosis with a bicarbonate less than 20 may suggest strangulation (*Am Surg.* 2004;70:40; *Am J Surg.* 1994;167(6):575–578; *J Gastrointest Surg.* 2009;13(1):93–99).

4. **Radiologic evaluation**
   a. Characteristic findings of SBO on **abdominal plain films** are dilated loops of SI, air-fluid levels, and paucity of colorectal gas. These findings may be absent in early, proximal, and/or closed-loop obstructions. Gas within the bowel wall (pneumatosis intestinalis) or portal vein is suggestive of a strangulated obstruction and ischemia. Free intra-abdominal air indicates perforation of a hollow viscus. The findings of air in the biliary tree and a radiopaque gallstone in the right lower quadrant are pathognomonic of gallstone ileus. Paralytic ileus appears as gaseous distention uniformly distributed throughout the stomach, SI, and colon.
   b. **Contrast studies** (small-bowel follow-through [SBFT] or enteroclysis) can localize the site of obstruction and suggest an etiology. Barium

can be used if subtle mucosal lesions are suspected (i.e., lead point in a patient with recurring intussusceptions), but should be avoided in acute obstructions due to the risk of barium impaction. Water-soluble contrast agents are indicated as the initial contrast in most instances.

c. **Computed tomography (CT)** is an excellent imaging modality for diagnosing SBO. CT scans have the ability to localize and characterize the obstruction as well as provide information regarding the cause of the obstruction and the presence of other intra-abdominal pathology. Evidence suggests that CT scanning can improve the preoperative diagnosis of strangulation, with negative and positive predictive values greater than 90% (*J Gastrointest Surg.* 2005;9:690). In a recent study reviewing multiple preoperative clinical, laboratory, and radiologic findings at presentation, the most significant independent predictor of bowel strangulation in patients with SBO was the CT finding of reduced wall enhancement (sensitivity 56%, specificity 94%, likelihood ratio 9.3) (*J Gastrointest Surg.* 2009;13(1):93–99).

5. **Differential diagnosis**
   a. **Mesenteric vascular ischemia** can produce colicky abdominal pain, especially after meals. Acute occlusion often presents with marked leukocytosis and severe abdominal pain out of proportion to physical findings. Angiography confirms the diagnosis.
   b. **Colonic obstruction** can easily be confused with a distal SBO, especially if the ileocecal valve is incompetent. A water-soluble contrast enema can aid in diagnosis. The initial management and evaluation of large- and small-bowel obstructions are the same.
   c. **Paralytic ileus** is a common diagnosis in surgical patients. A thorough history, physical exam, and radiologic workup should differentiate ileus from obstruction. Narcotic and psychiatric medications, recent abdominal operations, and electrolyte abnormalities are common causes of ileus.
   d. As in paralytic ileus, radiography of primary **hypomotility** disorders reveals gas throughout the entire GI tract with particular distention of the small bowel. Treatment of these chronic diseases consists of prokinetic drugs and dietary manipulation.

D. **Treatment** of SBO is evolving and includes prevention at initial laparotomy.
   1. **Prevention.** The highest risk of adhesive SBO occurs after ileal pouch-anal anastomosis, open colectomy, and open gynecologic surgeries (class I evidence). Intraoperative preventative principles, including meticulous hemostasis; avoiding tissue ischemia, excessive dissection and damage; and reducing residual foreign bodies, may be of benefit (class III evidence). Excluding acute appendicitis, laparoscopy results in fewer adhesions than open techniques (class I evidence). Available bioabsorbable antiadhesion barriers, such as hyaluronic acid/carboxymethyl-cellulose (Seprafilm®, Genzyme, Cambridge, MA), and icodextrin 4% solution (Adept®, Baxter Healthcare S.A.), have

been shown to reduce adhesions (class I evidence) (*Am J Surg.* [published online ahead of print September 1, 2010]). While randomized studies demonstrate that these barriers are beneficial in reducing the severity and number of adhesions after surgery, whether or not they reduce the incidence and severity of later SBOs is unclear. A multicenter trial of 1,701 patients comparing Seprafilm® to no treatment found no difference in the overall rate of SBO (12% for both). However, at a mean follow-up of 3.5 years, a very modest reduction in the risk of SBO *requiring operation* was observed (1.8% vs. 3.4%; $P <0.05$) (*Dis Colon Rectum.* 2006;49(1):1–11).

2. **Nonstrangulated** obstructions can be treated nonoperatively if the patient is clinically stable. The cornerstone of treating any SBO is adequate fluid resuscitation to achieve a urine output of at least 0.5 mL/kg/hour. This resuscitation must meet maintenance fluid and electrolyte needs for a nothing-by-mouth (NPO) patient as well as replace prior and ongoing losses from nasogastric (NG) decompression. During any trial of nonoperative management, the patient must be observed closely and undergo serial abdominal examinations every 4 to 6 hours, preferably by the same person. If the patient deteriorates at any time (develops shock or peritonitis) or fails to improve within a few days, laparotomy is indicated. In patients with an SBO secondary to an incarcerated hernia, attempts to reduce the hernia can be made with mild sedation and manual pressure. If reduction is successful, the patient should be monitored carefully for evidence of bowel infarction or perforation. Severe initial tenderness or skin changes at the hernia site (erythema or ecchymosis) should increase the suspicion for strangulation. Inability to reduce the hernia requires urgent operation. Other situations that may warrant a trial of nonoperative therapy for a SBO include the early postoperative state, multiple prior SBOs, multiple previous abdominal operations with extensive adhesions or "frozen hostile abdomen," abdominal irradiation, Crohn's disease, and carcinomatosis.

3. **Strangulated** obstructions and the presence of peritonitis require prompt operative intervention. Mortality associated with gangrenous bowel approaches 30% if operation is delayed beyond 36 hours, but is closer to 10% when surgical interventions is prompt (*Am Surg.* 1988;54(9):565–569). Once again, fluid/electrolyte resuscitation with Foley catheter placement and NG tube decompression are crucial in the preoperative preparation of the patient.

4. **Fluid replacement** should begin with an isotonic solution. Serum electrolyte values, hourly urine output, and central venous pressure can be monitored to assess adequacy of resuscitation. Antibiotics should be given only as prophylaxis prior to surgery.

5. **Operative intervention** is generally performed via midline incision, though a standard groin incision can be used in the case of an incarcerated inguinal or femoral hernia. During the exploration and identification of the origin of obstruction, adhesiolysis is usually required and resection of gangrenous bowel may be necessary. The viability of

adjacent or compromised bowel must be determined, and a second-look operation within 24 to 48 hours should be planned if any doubt exists. If an obstructing lesion cannot be resected, an enteroenteric or enterocolonic anastomosis can bypass the area of obstruction. Placement of a gastrostomy tube for postoperative decompression should be considered in select cases, such as carcinomatosis or unresectable obstructing cancer.

E. **Prognosis.** The postoperative mortality from a nonstrangulating obstruction is very low. Obstructions associated with strangulated bowel carry a mortality of less than 10% if operation is performed shortly after presentation. Patients admitted to surgical services have been shown to have shorter hospital stays, earlier operative intervention, and reduced direct health-care costs when compared to patients admitted to a medical service (*Am Surg.* 2010;76(7):687–691). The same study also found that coronary artery disease and acute renal failure were associated with higher mortality.

V. **MECKEL'S DIVERTICULUM** is the most common congenital anomaly of the GI tract and occurs from failure of the vitelline or omphalomesenteric duct to obliterate by the sixth week of fetal development. A Meckel's lesion is a true diverticulum that contains all layers of the bowel wall and is located on the antimesenteric border of the ileum. Half of these lesions contain heterotopic mucosa, usually gastric (62%) or pancreatic (16%). The "*Rule of two's*" indicates that a 2% incidence; a 2:1 male:female ratio; patients usually present before 2 years of age; the location is about 2 feet from the ileocecal valve; and the base is typically 2 inches in width and often contains 2 types of mucosa.

A. **Presentation.** The vast majority of Meckel's diverticula are *asymptomatic.*

1. **Bleeding** is the most common presenting sign and tends to be episodic and painless. The source is typically from a peptic ulcer of the adjacent normal ileum caused by acid secretion from gastric mucosa within the diverticulum.

2. **Intestinal obstruction** from intussusception or an incarcerated hernia (Littré's hernia) is the second most common presentation. Obstruction can also occur due to volvulus of the small bowel around a fibrous band that connects the diverticulum to the anterior abdominal wall.

3. **Meckel's diverticulitis** occurs in 20% of symptomatic patients and is often mistaken for acute appendicitis. Intraluminal obstruction of the diverticulum leads to inflammation, edema, ischemia, necrosis, and perforation in a manner similar to appendicitis.

4. **Differential diagnosis** may include appendicitis, colonic diverticulitis, or Crohn's disease.

B. **Diagnosis.** In adults, the clinical diagnosis of a Meckel's diverticulum is extremely difficult except in the presence of bleeding. Preoperative diagnosis is made in under 10% of symptomatic patients (*J Am Coll Surg.* 2001;192:658–662).

1. **Radionuclide scans.** A *Meckel's scan* is based on the uptake of 99 m Tc-pertechnetate by ectopic gastric mucosa. In children, this test is the most accurate (90%) for diagnosing a Meckel's diverticulum, but is less accurate (46%) in adults because of the reduced prevalence of ectopic gastric mucosa within the diverticulum (*AJR.* 1996;166:567–573). The sensitivity and specificity of scintigraphy can be improved by pentagastrin and glucagon, or cimetidine. In the presence of bleeding, a tagged red blood cell scan can also be useful.

2. **Contrast studies.** SBFT and enteroclysis are diagnostic in up to 75% patients, but can be unreliable and variable between institutions.

3. **CT** and **sonography** are typically of little value because distinguishing between a diverticulum and intestinal loops can be very difficult.

C. Treatment

1. **Resection** is indicated in symptomatic patients. For patients who present with obstruction, simple diverticulectomy can be performed. Segmental small-bowel resections should be performed for acute diverticulitis, a wide-based diverticulum, volvulus with necrotic bowel, or bleeding.

2. **Incidental diverticulectomy** during surgery for other abdominal pathology is **not indicated.** Lifelong morbidity associated with the presence of a Meckel's diverticulum is extremely low.

VI. **SMALL-INTESTINAL BLEEDING** from small-bowel lesions is the most common cause of "obscure GI bleeding," which is defined as hemorrhage of unknown origin that persists or recurs after negative initial or primary endoscopic evaluation (colonoscopy and upper endoscopy). Obscure GI bleeding differs from "occult GI bleeding" in that occult bleeding refers to the initial presentation of a patient with a positive fecal occult blood test (FOBT) and/ or iron deficiency anemia (IDA), without visible fecal blood (*Gastroenterol.* 2000;118:201–221). Upper and lower GI bleedings are discussed in Chapters 9 and 12, respectively.

A. Diagnosis

1. **Enteroscopy**

a. **Push enteroscopy** employs a 400-cm enteroscope to visualize well into the jejunum, but efficacy is highly dependent on the skill of the endoscopist. The ability to perform biopsy or therapeutic maneuvers is an advantage. Intraoperative use of the scope via a small enterotomy distal to the ligament of Treitz can sometimes further localize a bleeding source.

b. **Extended small-bowel enteroscopy** depends on peristalsis to move the scope distally; thus, the procedure may require up to 8 hours for completion. Furthermore, therapeutic and biopsy capabilities are absent. When successful, as much as 70% of the SI can be visualized and may be more sensitive than conventional enteroclysis.

c. **Capsule endoscopy** is a disposable "camera pill" that images the entire GI tract as it passes from mouth to anus. While data demonstrate that capsule endoscopy is superior to push enteroscopy and barium small-bowel imaging for diagnosing obscure GI bleeding (*Am J Gastroenterol.* 2005;100(11):2407–2418), its diagnostic yield is around 50% (*J Gastrointest Liver Dis.* 2010;19(2):141–145). Nevertheless, capsule endoscopy is the third test of choice for obscure GI bleeding after traditional upper and lower endoscopy.

  d. Double-balloon enteroscopy (DBE) uses two inflatable balloons on the tip of an endoscope to relatively quickly negotiate the small bowel. The technique can be used antegrade or retrograde and allows therapeutic intervention. Although indications and clinical applications are evolving, DBE offers the promise that the SI may be fully accessible to endoscopic diagnosis and treatment in the same manner as the rest of the GI tract. In addition, endoscopic retrograde cholangiopancreatography (ERCP) can be performed in areas previously inaccessible due to surgery (i.e., post Roux-en-Y gastric bypass). DBE has a comparable diagnostic yield for obscure GI bleeding when compared to capsule endoscopy, though the latter is favored as the initial diagnostic test because of its noninvasive quality, tolerance, and ability to view the entire SI. Because of its therapeutic capabilities, DBE may be indicated in patients with a positive finding on capsule endoscopy or in patients with a normal capsule study and continued active bleeding (*Clin Gastroenterol Hepatol.* 2008;6(6):671–676).

2. Imaging

  a. A **tagged red blood cell** nuclear medicine scan is highly sensitive for the detection of GI bleeding, detecting rates of hemorrhage of 0.1 to 0.5 mL/minute. However, in the setting of SI bleeding, this test is of limited utility because of the lack of anatomic detail.

  b. Angiography has a better ability to localize small-bowel bleeding, although it is less sensitive than a nuclear medicine study (detects bleeding at 1 to 1.5 mL/min). The angiographer can also potentially therapeutically embolize the bleeding mesenteric vessel or leave a catheter in place to assist in intraoperative localization of the lesion. In addition, methylene blue can be selectively injected to stain the target segment of intestine immediately prior to or during surgery to aid in intraoperative localization.

B. Effective **surgical therapy** hinges on successful preoperative *localization* of the bleeding lesion. Unlike the remainder of the GI tract, the small bowel cannot be resected *en bloc* for intractable bleeding with a goal of long-term survival. Preoperative localization of the lesion for segmental resection is strongly advised because of the difficultly in identifying a source intraoperatively. The angiographic techniques described previously are invaluable in this regard. *Intraoperative enteroscopy* can be used to identify mucosal abnormalities in the majority of patients in whom upper endoscopy, colonoscopy, and push enteroscopy have failed to recognize as source of bleeding. However, the therapeutic efficacy in preventing recurrent hemorrhage has been reported to be less than 50% (*Am J Surg.* 1992;163(1):94–99).

VII. ENTERIC FISTULAS are a constant therapeutic challenge. A fistula is defined as a communication or tract between two epithelialized surfaces (e.g., bowel, skin, and bladder). Fistulas are categorized according to anatomy, output, and etiology.

A. **Anatomic considerations**

1. **External versus internal.** *External* fistulas are the most common and connect an internal organ system with the skin or atmosphere, for example, an enterocutaneous (ECF) or enteroatmospheric (EAF) fistula. *Internal* fistulas connect two hollow structures of the same or different organ systems. Examples include colovesicular and enteroenteric fistulas.

2. **Proximal versus distal.** *Proximal* fistulas are located in the stomach, duodenum, or jejunum and are usually associated with high outputs of 3 or more liters per day. Profound dehydration, malnutrition, and electrolyte disturbances are common with these fistulas. *Distal* fistulas arise in the ileum or colon and are associated with fewer complications than proximal fistulas, and they more often close with nonoperative treatment.

3. Anatomic, etiologic, and physiologic classifications are also used. Anatomical descriptions include the names of the organs involved such that a fistula between the small bowel and the colon is referred to as an enterocolonic fistula. These connections can be described based on the underlying etiology of the fistula as well (i.e., Crohn's, radiation-induced, postoperative, or cancer-based fistulae). Physiologic categorization of fistulas is centered on the *output* and is divided into *high* (>500 mL/day), *moderate* (200 to 500 mL/day), and *low* (<200 mL/day) output fistulas.

B. **Pathophysiology.** Fistula-associated complications may be life-threatening and require rapid intervention to avoid morbidity and mortality. The overall mortality for all enteric fistulas is 5% to 20%.

1. Loss of GI contents can lead to *hypovolemia* as well as *acid–base and electrolyte abnormalities.* High-output fistulas may release large volumes of fluid that cannot be adequately replaced by enteral means, leading to dehydration and intravascular volume depletion. Loss of large fluid volumes and associated electrolytes also results in metabolic derangements that correlate directly with the quantity of fistula output.

2. Malnutrition is caused by caloric intake insufficient to meet increased metabolic demands associated with fistula formation. In addition, substantial portions of the GI tract may be functionally excluded. The ensuing malabsorption leads to vitamin and mineral deficiency, as well as alterations in carbohydrate, fat, and protein metabolism.

C. **Etiology**

1. **Abdominal operations** are the leading cause of fistula formation. The risk is greatest for operations performed for inflammatory bowel disease, ischemia, malignancy, or extensive intestinal adhesions. Dissection may result in unrecognized enterotomies, devascularization, and

serosal disruption. Anastomotic disruption, leaks, and perianastomotic abscesses are also hazardous. Malnutrition and immunosuppression significantly increase the risk of fistula formation as well.

2. **Crohn's disease** of the small bowel is another common cause of ECFs or enteroenteric fistulas.

3. **Diverticular disease** results in fistula formation when localized abscesses drain into adjacent organs. Common examples include colovesical and colovaginal fistulas. Internal fistulas should be suspected in patients with diverticular disease who exhibit persistent or recurrent urinary tract infections or sepsis.

4. **Malignant** fistulas form when tumor perforates or invades adjacent structures. Healing does not occur if cancer is present, and resection is the only means of cure.

5. **Radiation enteritis** predisposes to fistula formation after operation, regardless of the temporal proximity of exposure.

6. **Trauma** (penetrating or blunt) to the abdomen or pelvis may also give rise to SB fistulas. Missed enteric injuries or those repaired in a contaminated field may be prone to leak and subsequent fistula formation. Unrecognized viscus rupture from blunt trauma that forms an abscess and drains into adjacent structures may have a similar result, seen most commonly with duodenum, colon, or pancreas injuries that infect the retroperitoneum.

7. **Other causes** of SB fistulas include a foreign body, vascular compromise, and various infectious diseases (amebiasis, tuberculosis, or actinomyces).

D. Diagnosis

1. **Imaging.** Anatomic definition via contrast radiography aids in determining prognosis and assists with the planning of operative repair. Fistulography is the best test that can be performed in mature fistula tracts (usually after 10 days) and typically provides good visualization of all tracts and sites of enteral communication (*Radiology.* 2002;224(1):9–23). Oral contrast studies, such as an upper GI with SBFT, can demonstrate contrast extravasation through the fistula, but are less sensitive than a fistulogram. SBFTs are valuable for assessing internal fistulas and sometimes distal obstructions. A contrast enema is the study of choice for rectal or colonic fistulas. In general, CT scanning is of limited value in assessing fistula anatomy, but should be used if an abscess or underlying malignancy is suspected.

2. **Endoscopy** can be useful to assess the bowel for underlying pathology, such as peptic ulceration, inflammatory bowel disease, or cancer. Fistula orifices themselves are, however, often difficult to identify by endoscopy.

E. Nonoperative treatment

1. **Spontaneous closure.** Approximately 40% of ECFs will close spontaneously typically after 4 to 6 weeks of sepsis-free, adequate nutritional support. A fistula with decreasing output and a healing wound should

be given additional time to close. Factors associated with increased rates of closure include low-output, long tract greater than 2 cm, small orifice less than 1 cm², a well-nourished state, and absence of abscess, sepsis, or active IBD. The difficult decision of how long to wait for spontaneous closure depends on individual circumstances and the complexity of the underlying illness. In a closed abdomen, waiting at least 3 to 6 months from the time of last laparotomy is advised before reoperating. For patients with enteroatmospheric fistulas, 6 to 12 months or longer may be needed before the underlying obliterative peritonitis subsides. Improved home intravenous (IV) therapy, parenteral nutrition, wound care, and somatostatin analogs have allowed longer periods of waiting for fistula closure to be possible. This time allows adhesions to attenuate and the patient to recover nutritional status and general health. If spontaneous healing does not appear likely, operative therapy is indicated after an appropriate waiting period.

2. **Fluid resuscitation and electrolyte correction.** The initial phase of ECF management focuses on hypovolemia correction followed by accurate measurement of ongoing fluid losses and prompt replacement. IV fluid administration is typically necessary because adequate enteral replacement of the increased fluid losses from the fistula is difficult. Electrolyte and acid–base status also must be followed closely. The composition of replacement fluids should be tailored to the type and the quantity of GI loses in order to meet the specific replacement demands (see Chapter 4, Table 4-1). In difficult cases, a basic metabolic profile can be measured on a sample of fistula output to direct fluid replacement.

3. **Sepsis control** is a mainstay of initial ECF treatment as sepsis remains the primary determinant of mortality from a fistula. Sepsis accompanies a large percentage of fistulas and is caused by undrained enteric leaks or abscesses. Furthermore, healing is impeded in the presence of sepsis.

   a. **Intra-abdominal abscess** presence should be excluded by a CT scan with PO and IV contrast in every patient presenting with a GI fistula. If found, percutaneous drainage should be performed.

   b. **IV antibiotics** directed against bowel flora are indicated when infection is present and used only when necessary. Reoperation for *source control* may be required to manage continuous bacterial seeding from the GI tract.

   c. **Infected wounds** are adequately opened and packed to allow complete drainage, debridement, and healing by secondary intention. Frequent dressing changes may be required.

4. **Nutritional support.** No level I evidence exists to support a nutritional route, although enteral feeding is widely preferred. Early, aggressive parenteral nutritional therapy has been shown to dramatically decreased mortality from fistulas (*Am J Surg.* 1964;108:157).

   a. **Complete bowel rest.** Initial NPO status reduces fistula drainage and simplifies the evaluation and stabilization of the patient. NG suction is beneficial only in the presence of distal obstruction.

b. **Enteral feeding** is preferred as long as fistula output does not increase. Patients with low-output colonic or distal SI fistulas are often safely fed with standard enteral formulas. However, if the available bowel is short, elemental feeding may maximize absorption. In proximal fistula patients, feeding distal to the fistula is typically very effective (e.g., feeding jejunostomy tube in a gastric fistula). Direct feeding an intestinal fistula or fistuloclysis via a radiologically placed feeding catheter is another option.

c. **Parenteral nutrition** can provide adequate nourishment when enteral feeding is not possible. Indications include intolerance to enteral nutrition, jejunal and ileal high-output fistulas, and proximal fistulas where distal enteral access is not possible. Complications of parenteral nutrition include biliary stasis, hepatic dysfunction, trace element (zinc, copper, chromium) and essential fatty acid deficiencies, and venous catheter-related difficulties.

5. **Control of fistula drainage.** Fistula effluent is corrosive to the skin and must be controlled. For low-output fistulas, dressings can sometimes be used to simply absorb the effluent, but may impede healing and cause skin breakdown if prolonged contact occurs. Therefore, intubation of matured fistula tracts may be beneficial. For high-output fistulas, a suction or sump drainage system is preferable. Use of *somatostatin analogs* has revealed mixed results and has not been shown to increase the rate of fistula closure. Reports have demonstrated a reduction in fistula output (*Gut.* 2002;49(suppl IV):iv11–iv20; *Arch Surg.* 1992;127:97–99) and a decreased time to fistula closure (*Akt Chir.* 1994;29:96–99), but these results have not been uniformly replicated. Common practice also employs H_2-receptor antagonists or proton-pump inhibitors to reduce gastric and duodenal fistula output and provide stress ulceration prophylaxis though their efficacy in fistula management is unproven.

6. **Skin protection.** Irritation and excoriation of the skin surrounding an ECF can be very painful, complicate wound management, and promote secondary infection. The skin surrounding a fistula should be examined and cleansed frequently as well as protected with a barrier device or powder. A vacuum-assisted wound closure device may help to control skin irritation and speed fistula closure (*World J Surg.* 2008;32:430–435). Early involvement of an enterostomal therapy nurse is critical in the management of fistula patients.

F. **Operative treatment** is indicated when a fistula fails to heal with nonoperative management, or when sepsis cannot be controlled. Common conditions under which fistulas fail to close can be remembered with the aid of the mnemonic FRIEND: Foreign body, Radiation, Inflammation or Infection, Epithelialization, Neoplasm, or Distal obstruction. The goals of surgery are to eradicate the fistula tract and to restore the epithelial continuity of the associated organ systems.

1. **Gastric fistulas** can arise from anastomotic breakdown or ulcer perforation. Most low-output gastric fistulas close spontaneously, such as occurs after removal of a gastrostomy tube. In cases where

surgery is needed, primary repair or serosal patch placement is usually successful.

2. **Duodenal fistulas** typically close spontaneously with nonoperative management. When operative intervention is required, primary closure of small duodenal wall disruptions may be performed, but a duodenal stricture may result with primary closure of large defects. Defects that are in close proximity to the ampulla may also prevent primary closure. In these cases, duodenal wall integrity may be restored by a serosal patch using another segment of bowel. Alternatively, a Roux-en-Y duodenoenterostomy may be performed to divert duodenal output into the bowel.

3. **Small-bowel fistulas** typically require bowel resection and primary reanastomosis. In rare severe cases, a temporary diverting enterostomy may be necessary. For enteroenteric or other internal fistulas, openings that are in close proximity to the involved region can be resected *en bloc.*

4. **Large-bowel fistulas** are associated with high spontaneous closure rates. Fluid and electrolyte abnormalities are rare because outputs tend to be low. However, sepsis rates may be greater. If operative closure is required, a mechanical bowel preparation may be desired. Primary closure is rarely appropriate and resection with primary reanastomosis is preferred, but the choice depends on associated conditions, the nutritional status of the patient, and the location and complexity of the lesion. A proximal, diverting loop ileostomy should be considered if the anastomosis is suboptimal.

5. **Enteral feeding tubes** placed at the time of definitive repair may facilitate postoperative management.

VIII. **SHORT-BOWEL SYNDROME (SBS)** is a malabsorptive state and symptom complex that follows massive small-bowel resection. In adults, the normal length of the SI varies from 300 to 600 cm and correlates directly with body surface area. The length of combined jejunum and ileum that increases the risk for developing SBS in adults is less than 200 cm of functional bowel or less than 30% of the initial SI length with the presence of the terminal ileum. SBS may be seen with greater lengths of SI if an underlying disease, such as Crohn's or radiation enteritis, is present. Several factors determine the severity of SBS, including the extent of resection, the portion of the GI tract removed, the type of disease necessitating the resection, the presence of coexistent disease in the remaining bowel, and the adaptability of the remaining bowel. If an end enterostomy is performed, resection resulting in less than 100 cm of intact SI generally leads to SBS. If greater than one-third of the colon is in place, SBS may not develop until less than 75 cm or 1 mg/kg of SI remains. Children tend to develop SBS when only 30% or less of normal SI length for age is left, and infants may survive resection of up to 85% of their bowel because of enhanced adaptation and growth. Because the ileum has specialized absorptive function, complete resection is not well tolerated. On the contrary, the entire jejunum can usually be resected without serious adverse nutritional sequela.

A. **Etiology.** In children, the most common etiologies for SBS include necrotizing enterocolitis, congenital intestinal atresia, midgut volvulus, and gastroschisis. The leading causes of massive intestinal resection in adults and elderly patients are mesenteric ischemia, trauma, inflammatory bowel disease, strangulated hernia, SI or mesenteric neoplasms, volvulus, and portal vein thrombosis.

B. **Pathophysiology.** SBS is characterized by diarrhea, dehydration, electrolyte disturbances, steatorrhea, malnutrition, and weight loss.

1. **Adaptation.** The SI undergoes several adaptive changes in response to massive SI resection in an attempt to counteract the development of SBS. Structural adaptations, including greater bowel caliber, increased villus height, deeper crypts, and enhanced enterocyte proliferation and apoptosis, act to increase the absorptive surface area and nutrient transport of the bowel. Slower transit and increased nutrient absorption occurs through functional adaptations such as temporary hypergastrinemia, increased gastric acid secretion, slower gastric emptying (especially if colon present), substantially increased colonic absorption of water and electrolytes, and colonocyte degradation of carbohydrates into short-chain fatty acids (SCFA), which increases caloric uptake up to 50%. With resection of the jejunum, the distal SI has the greatest adaptive potential and can assume nearly all of the absorptive properties of the proximal gut.

2. **Fluid and electrolyte response.** Of the 7 to 10 L of fluid presented daily to the SI, only 1 to 2 L are delivered into the colon. Significant quantities of electrolytes are absorbed in this process. With SBS, this physiology is altered. Fortunately, the right colon can absorb a significant amount of the increased fluid it encounters with SBS.

3. **Malabsorption and malnutrition**

   a. **Gastric hypersecretion,** seen early in the postoperative period, can persist for prolonged periods. Increased acid load may injure distal bowel mucosa, leading to hypermotility and impaired absorption. The severity of hypersecretion correlates directly with the extent of bowel resection, and is generally more pronounced after jejunal than after ileal resection. Loss of an intestinal inhibitory hormone has been implicated.

   b. **Cholelithiasis.** Altered bilirubin metabolism after ileal resection increases the risk of gallstone formation secondary to a decreased bile salt pool causing a shift in the cholesterol saturation index. Terminal ileum resection, steatorrhea, and osmotic diarrhea lead to decreased uptake of bile salts. Chronic total parenteral nutrition (TPN) and resultant cholestasis also increase risk of cholelithiasis.

   c. **Hyperoxaluria and nephrolithiasis.** Hyperoxaluria results from excessive fatty acids in the colonic lumen binding intraluminal calcium. Unbound oxalate, which is normally made insoluble by luminal calcium binding and excreted in the feces, is then readily absorbed. The result is hyperoxaluria and calcium oxalate nephrolithiasis.

    d. Diarrhea and steatorrhea. Rapid intestinal transit, hyperosmolar contents in the distal SI, disruption of the enterohepatic bile acid circulation, and bacterial overgrowth all promote steatorrhea and diarrhea. Fat absorption is severely impaired by ileal resection. Delivery of bile acids into the colon also produces a reactive, often severe watery diarrhea. Unabsorbed fats in the colon further inhibit absorption of water and electrolytes and stimulate secretion.

    e. Bacterial overgrowth. Loss of the ileocecal valve permits reflux of colonic bacteria into the SI leading to bacterial overgrowth that impairs digestion and absorption of nutrients as the bacteria compete for nutrients with the enterocytes. Intestinal dysmotility further promotes bacterial colonization. Bacterial overgrowth and changes in the indigenous microbial population result in pH alteration and deconjugation of bile salts, with resultant malabsorption, fluid loss, and decreased vitamin B_{12} absorption. Infectious diarrhea (bacterial or viral) is a main cause of morbidity.

C. Acute phase treatment. The primary goal in the acute phase (initial 4 weeks) is to stabilize the metabolic, respiratory, and cardiovascular parameters related to the fluid shifts and sepsis that frequently accompany massive small-bowel resection. TPN, strict intake and output records, and close monitoring of serum electrolytes are critical in the early management of patients with SBS.

    1. Prolonged ileus may result from deranged motility patterns and changes in intraluminal milieu. Parenteral nutrition should be provided until GI function resumes. If the ileus is unusually persistent, underlying mechanical obstruction or sepsis should be suspected and investigated.

    2. Gastric hypersecretion requires H_2-receptor antagonists or proton-pump inhibitors to reduce the hypersecretory response and protect against peptic ulceration. Antacids take effect immediately and should be administered routinely in patients with SBS.

    3. Nutritional support should be instituted early to maintain a positive nitrogen balance and to promote wound healing and adaptation of the remaining bowel. Enteral nutrition has a positive trophic effect on the bowel mucosa, stimulates the remaining intestine, and should be started as soon as possible, even if caloric goals are not met. Feeding tubes placed at laparotomy are often key. Initial feeds should be gradual, continuous low volume, low fat, and isosmotic. Isotonic salt-glucose solutions are useful.

D. Maintenance phase treatment. Maintenance therapy in SBS focuses on long-term nutritional goals, support of adaptation that takes place over the first 1 to 2 years, and addressing various clinical issues that arise.

    1. Nutritional support with supplemental vitamins, trace elements and minerals (zinc, selenium, and iron), and essential fatty acids (linoleic acid) should be given parenterally until adequate enteral absorption is achieved. Absorption of the fat-soluble vitamins A, D, E, and K is especially prone to compromise. Vitamin B_{12} and calcium uptake are also affected by altered fat absorption and should be supplemented. Potassium and magnesium losses should be closely monitored as well. Growth hormone and glutamine have been used with some success to treat inadequate adaptation and TPN dependence (*Ann Surg.* 2005;242:655–661). Nightly administration of chronic TPN can allow normal daily activity.

2. **Diarrhea** is often multifactorial in SBS, and dietary modifications can improve symptoms. H_2-receptor blockers reduce gastric acid production and secretory volume. Chelating resins like cholestyramine reduce intraluminal bile salts and resultant diarrhea but affect the systemic bile salt pool. Antisecretory medications, such as loperamide or somatostatin analogs, may be beneficial, although octreotide can inhibit the adaptation. Low-dose narcotics (diphenoxylate hydrochloride and atropine (Lomotil), codeine, or tincture of opium) are efficacious but addictive. Bacterial overgrowth should be evaluated by stool culture and antimicrobials, such as metronidazole or tetracycline, administered as needed.

3. **Late complications** are common and include nephrolithiasis, cholelithiasis, nutritional deficiencies (e.g., anemia, bone disease, and coagulopathy), liver dysfunction, TPN-related difficulties, and central venous catheter-related issues like thrombosis or sepsis. Anastomotic leaks, fistulas, strictures, and late bowel obstructions can also occur well beyond the early postoperative period and commonly require reoperation.

E. **Surgical therapy.** Various surgical procedures have been described for the management of SBS, but have not been widely adopted. The most commonly used intestinal lengthening procedures for patients with SBS are Serial Transverse Enteroplasty (STEP) and the Bianchi procedure that similarly have been shown to decrease TPN dependence, increase oral caloric intake, and reverse liver disease (*Ann Surg.* 2007;246(4):593–604). STEP is performed with a reusable GIA stapler that is applied to the bowel in sequence from opposite directions through small mesenteric windows creating a zig-zag like channel that lengthens the bowel. The Bianchi isolates the dual blood supply of the SI by separating the mesenteric borders, longitudinally divides the intestine, and creates an isoperistaltic end-to-end, handsewn anastomosis. Isolated small-bowel transplants or multivisceral transplantations (including the liver for patients with severe cholestatic cirrhosis from chronic TPN) are additional options for SBS. Prevention of complications and minimizing the extent of initial bowel resection that lead to SBS is extremely important.

IX. **CROHN'S DISEASE** is an idiopathic, chronic, granulomatous inflammatory disease that can affect any part of the GI tract from the mouth to the anus. This incurable, slowly progressive disease is characterized by episodes of exacerbation and remission. The incidence is 4/100,000, with a bimodal age distribution at 15 to 29 and 55 to 70 years old.

A. **Etiology.** The cause of Crohn's disease is unknown, but is believed to involve interplay between genetic and environmental factors. The genetic component is strong; Crohn's disease is 25 times more common among patients with a family history and has a concordance rate of 60% in monozygotic twins. Environmental aspects, such as smoking, also increase the risk of developing Crohn's disease. Pathogenesis likely relates to a defective mucosal barrier and/or dysregulated intestinal immunity that leads to a chronic inflammatory reaction within the intestinal wall.

B. **Bowel involvement.** The *terminal ileum* is the most common site of disease and is involved in 75% of cases. Three "patterns" of disease have been described.

   1. **Ileocolic** disease affects the terminal ileum (and in some cases the cecum) and is the most common form, affecting 40% of patients.

   2. **Small-bowel-only** disease (30% of patients) is confined to the more-proximal SI.

   3. **Colonic** disease (30% of patients) affects only the large intestine. Perianal involvement commonly coexists with more proximal forms, especially when the colon is affected. Anorectal disease confinement is rare (5%).

C. **Histology.** Grossly, diseased bowel is thickened, displays creeping fat and corkscrew vessels, and has a shortened fibrotic mesentery containing enlarged lymph nodes. Mucosal changes include pinpoint hemorrhages, aphthous ulcers, deep linear fissures, and *cobblestoning*. These findings commonly occur segmentally along the intestine rather than being contiguous causing *skip lesions*. Crohn's disease is characterized by full-thickness, *transmural inflammation* of the bowel wall that begins adjacent to the crypts and leads to the development of crypt abscesses, aphthous ulcers, and linear fissures. The transmural involvement can produce sinus tracts and fistulas between adjacent segments of bowel. *Granulomas* are also found in the bowel wall in 40% to 60% of patients and are detected in mesenteric lymph nodes in 25% of patients.

D. **Clinical presentation.** Crohn's disease has a highly variable presentation. Patient history is important in narrowing the differential diagnosis. Physical examination is performed with special attention to the abdominal and anorectal areas. No physical signs are pathognomonic for Crohn's disease, although the appearance of the perianal area may be highly suggestive. Laboratory evaluation is nonspecific.

   1. **Diarrhea** occurs in almost all patients and usually is not bloody unless the colon is involved. Patients with ileal disease may be bile salt deficient, resulting in steatorrhea. Mucosal inflammation with decreased absorption and increased secretion also results in diarrhea.

   2. **Abdominal pain** typically is intermittent, crampy, worse after meals, relieved by defecation, and poorly localized. A mass caused by thickened bowel, a phlegmon, or an abscess may be palpable.

   3. **Weight loss** occurs as a result of decreased oral intake, malabsorption, protein-losing enteropathy, and steatorrhea. Children with Crohn's disease develop vitamin and mineral deficiencies and growth retardation.

   4. **Constitutional symptoms** such as malaise and fever are common.

5. **Anorectal** disease is a common finding and may precede intestinal symptoms by several years. Such lesions include recurrent nonhealing anal fissures, large ulcers, complex anal fistulas, perianal abscesses, large, fleshy skin tags, and bluish skin discoloration. Perianal Crohn's disease is characterized by a multiplicity of lesions, lateral fissures, deep ulcers of the perianal skin and anal canal, and anal stricture.

6. **Extraintestinal manifestations** are numerous. The eyes may develop conjunctivitis, iritis, and uveitis. The skin may develop pyoderma gangrenosum, erythema nodosum multiforme, and aphthous stomatitis. Musculoskeletal manifestations include arthritis, ankylosing spondylitis, and hypertrophic osteoarthropathy. Finally, sclerosing cholangitis can lead to cirrhosis and liver failure.

E. **Imaging.** Radiological studies are indicated to help establish the diagnosis of Crohn's disease or to identify a complication that may require surgical intervention.

1. **Contrast radiography,** such as SBFT, enteroclysis (SBE), and water-soluble contrast enema, is valuable in the diagnosis of Crohn's disease and may reveal strictures or segments of ulcerated mucosa. SBE is considered the optimal investigation to exclude small-bowel disease in these patients, with a sensitivity of 93% and a specificity of 92% (*Eur Radiol.* 2000;10:1894–1898). However, in day-to-day practice, SBFT is simpler and may be preferred for its superiority in detecting mucosal disease, fistulas, or gastroduodenal involvement, but is operator dependent and not as good for strictures.

2. **Endoscopy** is most useful in diagnosis and for obtaining biopsy material in patients with terminal ileal and colonic disease. For patients with suspected Crohn's disease, ileocolonoscopy and biopsies from the terminal ileum as well as each colonic segment to look for microscopic evidence of disease are first-line procedures to establish the diagnosis. Similar to patients with ulcerative colitis, those with long-standing (>10 years) Crohn's colitis are at increased risk for adenocarcinoma, and surveillance colonoscopy for cancer is important. These patients also have an increased incidence of SI cancer.

3. **CT** with enteroclysis or enterography has improved significantly, leading to reports that it is complementary or even superior to barium studies for the detection of involved segments. CT is able to identify abscesses, focal inflammation, perforation, and wall thickening. Abscesses can be drained percutaneously under CT guidance.

4. **Magnetic resonance imaging (MRI)** is also useful for assessing the location, extent, and disease activity, particularly in specialized centers where MR has also undergone technical developments that may make it the method of choice complementary to ileocolonoscopy and biopsy. An added advantage of MRI is the ability to detect extramural complications including abscesses, fistulas, sacroiliitis, gallstones, and renal calculi. Magnetic resonance enteroclysis (**MRE**) has a reported sensitivity and specificity of 95% and 93%, respectively, for the primary diagnosis of Crohn's disease, but is more invasive than SBE (*Gut.* 2006;55:i1–i15).

F. **Complications.** Intestinal obstruction, stricture, fistula, perforation, intra-abdominal abscess, GI bleeding, and perirectal abscess and fistula can occur. Toxic colitis is a surgical emergency that can occur in these patients.

G. **Differential diagnosis.** Other inflammatory bowel diseases as well as common infectious abdominal conditions can mimic Crohn's disease.

1. **Ulcerative colitis.** Patients with Crohn's disease generally have less severe diarrhea, usually without gross blood. Perianal lesions, non-confluent skip lesions, transmural involvement, large mucosal ulcers and fissures, small-bowel involvement, *rectal sparing,* and the presence of granulomas all help to differentiate Crohn's disease from ulcerative colitis. Some patients who cannot be confidently diagnosed with either condition are labeled as having indeterminate colitis.

2. **Appendicitis.** Acute right-lower-quadrant abdominal pain due to Crohn's ileitis can mimic acute appendicitis.

3. **Infectious ileitis** presents with pain and bloody diarrhea. The diagnosis is made by stool culture.

4. **Other** diseases that present similarly to Crohn's disease include intestinal lymphoma, intestinal tuberculosis, ischemic enteritis, diverticulitis, severe gastroenteritis, pseudomembranous colitis, and irritable bowel syndrome.

H. **Treatment**

1. **Adequate nutrition** is essential both during and between disease flares, and enteral feeds should be continued whenever possible. A low-residue, high-protein, milk-free diet generally provides adequate nutrition. Vitamin and mineral supplementation may be necessary. Patients with severe or unresponsive disease should be given TPN and placed on total bowel rest.

2. **Medical management** is particularly important because Crohn's disease has no cure. Therefore, treatment seeks to palliate symptoms, correct nutritional disturbances, and reduce inflammation. Disease location, severity, and complications dictate therapeutic recommendations. Mild-to-moderate disease can be treated with oral aminosalicylates (sulfasalazine 3 to 6 g/day, or mesalamine 1 g four times/day). For ileal, colonic, or perianal disease, metronidazole, 500 mg three times/day, can be added. In patients with severe disease, steroid therapy should be initiated after active infection or abscess has been excluded. Prednisone, with initial daily doses of 40 to 60 mg orally, is a common outpatient treatment of acute flares; inpatients may receive hydrocortisone, 50 to 100 mg intravenously every 6 hours. Response to therapy should be evident within 7 days. Data show that infusions of infliximab (Remicade), a monoclonal antibody against (TNF), is effective for Crohn's flares and fistulas (*N Engl J Med.* 2004;350:876). Before receiving infliximab, no active source of infection should be present and purified protein derivative (PPD)-negative. Infliximab is particularly useful in poor surgical candidates who have failed medical management. After recovery from an acute flare, the medical regimen should be simplified

to prevent long-term complications. Steroids should be tapered as soon as possible to prevent side effects such as osteopenia, avascular necrosis, psychosis, and weight gain. The addition of immunomodulators, such as 6-mercaptopurine, may allow patients with refractory disease to taper off of prednisone.

3. **Surgical therapy** is indicated when medical therapy has failed to address acute complications of the disease, such as high-output fistulas, perforation, intra-abdominal abscess, severe colitis, bleeding, or obstruction from fibrotic strictures. Abdominal abscesses can usually be drained percutaneously with or without elective bowel resection later. Most Crohn's patients require operative treatment during their lifetime.

   a. At the time of operation, the most important principle is to correct the complication while *preserving bowel length* to prevent SBS. Resection to histologically negative margins does not significantly reduce the likelihood of disease recurrence; therefore, grossly normal margins of 2 cm are accepted. In the absence of free perforation, large abscesses, massively dilated bowel, severe malnutrition, or high-dose immunosuppression, primary anastomosis is safe. Stapling should be avoided in thick-walled bowel and a handsewn anastomosis is indicated. Recent series suggest that laparoscopic ileocolic resections are safe alternatives to open procedures, especially at the time of first operation (*Dis Colon Rectum.* 2003;46:1129). Issues that require special consideration beyond the scope of this chapter are duodenal disease, multiple skip lesions, and chronic fibrotic strictures in the setting of SBS.

   b. *Appendectomy.* Patients who are being explored for presumed acute appendicitis and are found to have Crohn's ileitis should have the appendix removed if the cecum is not inflamed. Conventional teaching has been that the terminal ileum should not be removed. This is controversial, however, given the low morbidity of ileocecal resection and the uncertainty of response to subsequent medical therapy.

   c. *Surgical complications* include anastomotic leaks, ECF fistulas, and sepsis related to intra-abdominal abscesses and wound infections.

I. **Prognosis.** Crohn's disease is a chronic, pan-intestinal disease that currently has no cure and requires chronic, lifelong treatment, with operation reserved for severe complications. Recently, however, specific "susceptibility genes" (e.g., *NOD2/CARD15*) have been identified in patients with Crohn's disease. Further study of the pathways involved may shed light on pathogenesis and lead to more effective medical treatments.

X. **NEOPLASMS** of the small bowel are uncommon and account for less than 2% of all GI cancers. Tumors of the SI present insidiously with vague, nonspecific symptoms, and, when benign, are often discovered incidentally. SI tumors can also be a lead point in an intussusception. The majority of malignant tumors eventually become symptomatic with weight loss, abdominal pain, obstruction, perforation, or hemorrhage.

A. **Benign tumors.** Benign small-bowel masses are more common than malignant.

1. **Leiomyoma** is the most common benign neoplasm of the SI and arises from mesenchymal cells. These tumors grow submucosally and project into the lumen of the small bowel. On a contrast studies, they appear as a smooth, eccentric filling defects with intact, normal-appearing mucosa. Histopathologic exam is needed to distinguish benign from malignant stromal tumors. Treatment consists of a segmental bowel resection.

2. **Adenomas** can occur sporadically as solitary lesions, or in association with familial adenomatous polyposis syndrome (Gardner variant). When symptomatic, these lesions can cause fluctuating pain secondary to intermittent obstruction, intussusception, or bleeding. Three types of SI adenomas exist: simple tubular, Brunner's gland, and villous adenomas. The duodenum is the most common site for all three types of adenomas. Tubular and Brunner's gland adenomas have a low malignant potential and can be treated with complete endoscopic polypectomy. Villous adenomas have significant malignant potential. If complete endoscopic resection is not possible, transduodenal excision with adequate margins is appropriate. Villous adenomas of the jejunum or ileum should be removed with a small-bowel resection.

3. **Hamartomas** arise in patients with Peutz–Jeghers syndrome, an autosomal-dominant, inherited syndrome of mucocutaneous melanotic pigmentation characterized by multiple GI polyps. Operative intervention is indicated only for symptoms. At surgery, all polyps larger than 1 cm should be resected. Because of an increased risk for *de novo* adenocarcinoma (arising separately from the hamartomas), patients need endoscopic screening.

4. **Other benign tumors** include **lipomas** that occur most often in the ileum and have no malignant potential. On CT, lipomas show fatty attenuation. **Hemangiomas** may be associated with Osler–Weber–Rendu disease and present with bleeding. Diagnosis can be made with enteroscopy, capsule endoscopy, or angiography. **Neurofibromas and fibromas** are less common tumors that can cause intussusception. **Endometriosis** can cause SI implants that appear as puckered, bluish-red, serosal-based nodules that can cause GI bleeding or obstruction.

B. **Malignant tumors**

1. **Adenocarcinoma** is the most common malignant small intestinal tumor. Forty percent occur in the duodenum, and their frequency decreases distally through the small bowel. Risk factors for the development of adenocarcinoma include villous adenomas, polyposis syndromes, Crohn's disease, and hereditary nonpolyposis colorectal cancer (HNPCC). Patients often remain asymptomatic for long periods of time and have distant metastases at diagnosis. The presenting symptoms depend on the location of the primary tumor. Periampullary tumors can present with painless jaundice, duodenal obstruction, or bleeding. More-distal tumors tend to present with abdominal pain and

weight loss from progressive obstruction. Contrast studies, CT, and endoscopy with or without ERCP can be used for diagnosis. *Treatment* consists of segmental small-bowel resection with excision of the adjacent lymph node-bearing mesentery. Any adherent structures should be resected *en bloc* if possible. Tumors of the terminal ileum should be resected along with the right colon. For carcinomas of the duodenum, a pancreaticoduodenectomy is usually required. In resections of duodenal adenocarcinomas, the 5-year survival rate is 56% for node-positive and 83% for node-negative disease, respectively (*Ann Surg Oncol.* 2004;11:380). Distal lesions tend to present at a later stage. Patients with metastatic disease at the time of diagnosis rarely survive past 6 months. 5-Fluorouracil–based chemotherapy regimens have been tried, but data on their efficacy are lacking.

2. **Gastrointestinal stromal tumors** (GISTs) arise from mesodermal-derived components of the SI and are equally distributed along the length of the intestine. These tumors grow extraluminally and cause symptoms late in their course. Because of their vascular nature, when these tumors outgrow their blood supply and necrose, they may hemorrhage into either the peritoneum or the lumen of the bowel. Mutations of **c-kit** (CD117; a tyrosine kinase responsible for neoplastic growth) allow diagnosis by immunohistochemistry. Curative *treatment* of GI stromal tumors is wide *en bloc* resection with tumor-free margins. Extensive lymph node resection is unnecessary because these tumors have a low potential for lymphatic spread. Traditional chemotherapy and radiation therapy are not effective in the treatment of metastatic GISTs. However, *imatinib mesylate (Gleevec)* is important in treatment and inhibits the overactive tyrosine receptor c-kit found on all GIST cells. Inhibition of this receptor has been shown to cause radiographic and histologic regression of metastatic lesions (*N Engl J Med.* 2001;344:1052). In the adjuvant setting following primary GIST resection, imatinib therapy improves recurrence-free survival (*Lancet.* 2009;373(9669):1097–1104. Sunitinib malate (Sutent) is the recommended option for second-line therapy of metastatic GIST that develop resistance to imatinib (*Lancet.* 2006;368:1329–1338). The role of resecting isolated pulmonary or hepatic lesions is unclear, but appears beneficial. Selected patients with metastatic GIST who have responsive disease or focal resistance (only one tumor has radiological evidence of growth) to tyrosine kinase inhibitor therapy appear to benefit from elective surgical resection (*Ann Surg.* 2007;245(3):347–352). Histologic grade and tumor size are the most important predictors of survival. After complete resection, the overall 5-year survival rate is 50%. In low-grade tumors [<10 mitotic figures/high power field (mf/hpf)], the survival rate is 60% to 80%, whereas in high-grade tumors (>10 mf/hpf), the survival rate is less than 20%. With local recurrence, the median length of survival is 9 to 12 months. With metastatic disease, the median length of survival is 20 months (*Br J Surg.* 2003;90:1178). However, imatinib mesylate treatment extends the 2-year survival rate to 78% for patients with metastatic disease (*Eur J Cancer.* 2004;40:689).

3. **Primary small-bowel lymphomas** are most common in the ileum because this area has the largest amount of gut-associated lymphoid tissue. Virtually all small-bowel lymphomas are non-Hodgkin, *B-cell lymphomas* that arise either *de novo* or in association with a preexisting systemic condition such as celiac disease, Crohn's disease, or immunosuppression (iatrogenic, HIV, etc.). The presentation of these patients is highly variable. Imaging can help make a diagnosis, but operation is frequently required for histologic confirmation. Treatment of lymphoma localized to the SI involves wide resection of the affected segment of intestine and its associated mesentery. To stage the tumor accurately, the liver should be biopsied and the periaortic lymph nodes sampled. For widespread disease, resection of the affected intestine should be performed to prevent complications such as obstruction or bleeding. The role of adjuvant chemotherapy and radiotherapy remains controversial. The 5-year survival for patients with fully resected disease approaches 80%, but individuals with more advanced disease usually die within 1 year of surgery.

4. **Carcinoid tumors** arise from the Kulchitsky or enterochromaffin cells of the intestinal crypts. Most intestinal carcinoids occur within 2 feet of the ileocecal valve. Small-bowel carcinoid tumors tend to be much more aggressive than their appendiceal or rectal counterparts. Patients rarely manifest signs or symptoms of the tumor until late in the course, such as the local complications of GI obstruction, pain, or bleeding, or the systemic symptoms of the carcinoid syndrome. Metastases are rare in tumors smaller than 1 cm in size, while half of tumors between 1 and 2 cm metastasize, and almost all tumors larger than 2 cm spread.

   a. *Carcinoid syndrome* presence implies hepatic metastatic spread. Normally, hormones released by carcinoid tumors are metabolized by the liver and produce no symptoms. However, hepatic metastases drain into the systemic circulation and classic symptoms including *diarrhea* and transient *flushing* of the face, neck, and upper chest occur. Tachycardia, hypotension, bronchospasm, and even coma can also be observed. In long-standing carcinoid syndrome, patients develop right heart endocardial and valvular fibrosis. Classically, diagnosis of GI carcinoid tumors has been made by measuring a 24 hour urinary 5-hydroxyindoleacetic acid (5-HIAA), the breakdown product of serotonin that is secreted by the tumor. In patients with symptoms of the carcinoid syndrome, the sensitivity and specificity of this test nears 100%. Serum chromogranin A measurement is another commonly used test for diagnosis of GI carcinoids and has a similarly high sensitivity (80% to 100%), but is less specific than urine 5-HIAA levels (*Surg Oncol Clin N Am.* 2006;15:463–478).

   b. The **treatment** of carcinoid tumors is operative. The entire SI should be inspected because in 30% of cases synchronous lesions are present. Jejunal and ileal tumors should be treated with segmental resection including the adjacent mesentery. Small tumors (<1 cm) located in the third or fourth portions of the duodenum can be either locally excised or included in a segmental resection. For large duodenal tumors and periampullary tumors, a pancreaticoduodenectomy should be performed. In the presence of locally advanced disease with involvement of adjacent organs or peritoneum, aggressive resection should be undertaken to delay the occurrence of mesenteric desmoplastic reaction, hepatic metastases, and carcinoid syndrome. Solitary and accessible liver lesions should be resected. Adjuvant cytotoxic chemotherapy and radiotherapy are of little benefit. The somatostatin analog **octreotide** offers excellent palliation of carcinoid syndrome in patients with unresectable disease. Octreotide decreases the concentration of circulating serotonin and urinary 5-HIAA, and can relieve diarrhea and flushing in 90% of patients.

   c. Carcinoids are slow-growing tumors, and **prognosis** depends on the stage of the tumor. The overall 5-year survival rate is 60%. Patients with local disease that is completely resected have a normal life expectancy. For patients with resectable node-positive disease, the median length of survival is 15 years. The median length of survival drops to 5 years with unresectable intra-abdominal disease and is 3 years for those with hepatic metastases.

5. **Carcinomatosis** is diffuse studding of the peritoneal, mesenteric, and bowel surfaces by tumor nodules. Many tumors can cause peritoneal carcinomatosis, including cancer of the pancreas, stomach, ovaries, appendix, and colon. Carcinomatosis has an extremely poor prognosis, and surgical treatment is palliative, usually for obstruction. The only exception is pseudomyxoma peritonei, a low-grade malignancy, where patients may benefit from resection and intraperitoneal chemotherapy.

6. **Metastases** can spread to the small bowel and palliative resection may be appropriate if required for symptom relief. Several primary cancers are known to metastasize to the SI including melanoma, colorectal, gynecologic, breast, stomach, lung, prostate, and renal cancers among others. In patients who undergo laparotomy with or without small-bowel resection, complication rates are high (35%) and mortality significant (10%). Furthermore, median survival is poor (5 months), though patients with a history of colorectal cancer have been to shown to have better survival than patients other cancers. The extent of recurrent disease may be the primary factor that affects overall survival (*World J Surg Onc.* 2007;5:122). Cases should be considered individually and discussion made with patients over their poor prognosis. Palliative gastrostomy tubes to relieve obstruction with or without TPN may be appropriate in advanced cases where nonoperative management is chosen.

Acute Abdominal Pain and Appendicitis

William Symons and Alicia Kieninger

ACUTE ABDOMINAL PAIN

Acute abdomen is defined as the recent or sudden onset of severe abdominal pain. This can be new pain or an increase in chronic pain. Evaluation of the patient with acute abdominal pain requires a careful history and physical examination by a skilled physician in conjunction with selective diagnostic testing. Acute abdominal pain is the most common general surgical problem presenting to the emergency department. It has a vast **differential diagnosis,** including both intra- and extraperitoneal processes. The acute abdomen **does not always** signify the need for surgical intervention; however, surgical evaluation is warranted.

I. **PATHOPHYSIOLOGY.** This chapter focuses on intra-abdominal causes of abdominal pain. However, one must be cognizant of the fact that pathology on the surface of the abdomen (e.g., rectus sheath hematoma) or even outside the abdomen (e.g., testicular torsion) can present as abdominal pain. Abdominal pain arising from intra-abdominal pathophysiology originates in the peritoneum, which is a membrane comprising two layers. These layers, the visceral and parietal peritoneum, are developmentally distinct areas with separate nerve supplies.

A. Visceral pain

1. **Visceral peritoneum** is innervated bilaterally by the autonomic nervous system. The bilateral innervation causes visceral pain to be midline, vague, deep, dull, and poorly localized (e.g., vague periumbilical pain of the midgut).

2. Visceral pain is **triggered by inflammation, ischemia, and geometric changes** such as distention, traction, and pressure.

3. Visceral pain signifies **intra-abdominal disease** but not necessarily the need for surgical intervention.

4. **Embryologic origin** of the affected organ determines the location of visceral pain in the abdominal midline. **Foregut-derived structures** (stomach to the second portion of the duodenum, liver and biliary tract, pancreas, spleen) present with epigastric pain. **Midgut-derived structures** (second portion of the duodenum to the proximal two thirds of the transverse colon) present with periumbilical pain. **Hindgut-derived structures** (distal transverse colon to the anal verge) present with suprapubic pain.

B. **Parietal pain**

1. **Parietal peritoneum** is innervated unilaterally via the spinal somatic nerves that also supply the abdominal wall. Unilateral innervation causes parietal pain to localize to one or more abdominal quadrants (e.g., inflamed appendix producing parietal peritoneal irritation).

2. Parietal pain is **sharp, severe, and well localized.**

3. Parietal pain is **triggered by irritation of the parietal peritoneum** by an inflammatory process (e.g., chemical peritonitis from perforated peptic ulcer or bacterial peritonitis from acute appendicitis). It may also be triggered by mechanical stimulation, such as a surgical incision.

4. Parietal pain is **associated with physical examination findings of local or diffuse peritonitis** and frequently, but not always, signifies the need for surgical treatment.

C. **Referred pain** arises from a deep visceral structure but is superficial at the presenting site (Fig. 11-1).

1. It results from **central neural pathways** that are common to the somatic nerves and visceral organs.

2. Examples include **biliary tract pain** (referred to the right inferior scapular area) and **diaphragmatic irritation** from any source, such as subphrenic abscess (referred to the ipsilateral shoulder).

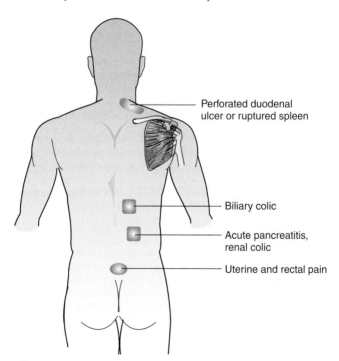

Perforated duodenal ulcer or ruptured spleen

Biliary colic

Acute pancreatitis, renal colic

Uterine and rectal pain

Figure 11-1. Frequent sites of referred pain and common causes.

II. **EVALUATION** of the acute abdomen remains heavily influenced by patient history and physical exam findings. Ancillary imaging and lab tests can help to complete the diagnosis and guide treatment decisions.

A. **History of present illness**

1. **Onset and duration of pain**

a. **Sudden onset of pain** (within seconds) suggests perforation or rupture [e.g., perforated peptic ulcer or ruptured abdominal aortic aneurysm (AAA)]. Infarction, such as myocardial infarction or acute mesenteric occlusion, can also present with sudden onset of pain.

b. **Rapidly accelerating pain** (within minutes) may result from several sources.

(1) **Colic syndromes,** such as biliary colic, ureteral colic, and small-bowel obstruction.

(2) **Inflammatory processes,** such as acute appendicitis, pancreatitis, and diverticulitis.

(3) **Ischemic processes,** such as mesenteric ischemia, strangulated intestinal obstruction, and volvulus.

c. **Gradual onset of pain** (over several hours) increasing in intensity may be caused by one of the following:

(1) **Inflammatory conditions,** such as appendicitis and cholecystitis.

(2) **Obstructive processes,** such as nonstrangulated bowel obstruction and urinary retention.

(3) **Other mechanical processes,** such as ectopic pregnancy and penetrating or perforating tumors.

2. **Character of pain**

a. **Colicky pain** waxes and wanes. It usually occurs **secondary to hyperperistalsis of smooth muscle** against a mechanical site of obstruction (e.g., small-bowel obstruction and renal stone). An important exception is **biliary colic,** in which pain tends to be constant, intense and lasts at least 30 minutes and up to several hours.

b. **Pain that is sharp, severe, persistent, and steadily increases in intensity** over time suggests an infectious or inflammatory process (e.g., appendicitis).

3. **Location of pain**

a. Pain caused by **inflammation of specific organs** may be localized [e.g., right upper quadrant (RUQ) pain caused by acute cholecystitis].

b. Careful attention must be given to the **radiation of pain.** The pain of renal colic, for example, may begin in the patient's back or flank and radiate to the ipsilateral groin, whereas the pain of a ruptured aortic aneurysm or pancreatitis may radiate to the patient's back.

4. **Alleviating and aggravating factors**

a. Patients with **diffuse peritonitis** describe worsening of pain with movement (i.e., parietal pain); the pain is ameliorated by lying still. This is in contrast to the patient with renal colic who is usually writhing in pain unable to sit still.

b. Patients with **intestinal obstruction** have visceral pain and usually experience a transient relief from symptoms after vomiting.

5. **Associated symptoms**
   a. **Nausea and vomiting** frequently accompany abdominal pain and may hint at its etiology. Vomiting that occurs after the onset of pain may suggest appendicitis, whereas vomiting before the onset of pain is more consistent with the diagnosis of gastroenteritis or food poisoning. The sequence as well as the character of the emesis should be documented. Bilious emesis suggests a process distal to the duodenum. Hematemesis may suggest a peptic ulcer or gastritis.
   b. **Fever or chills** suggests an inflammatory or an infectious process, or both.
   c. **Anorexia** is present in the vast majority of patients with acute abdominal pain.

B. **Past medical history, surgical history, and organ-system review**
   1. **Medical conditions** may precipitate intra-abdominal pathology.
      a. Patients with **peripheral vascular disease or coronary artery disease** may have abdominal vascular disease (e.g., AAA or mesenteric ischemia).
      b. Patients with a history of **cancer** may present with bowel obstruction or perforation from recurrence.
      c. **Major medical problems** are important to recognize early in the patient and may call for urgent surgical exploration.
   2. A **thorough medical history and organ-system review** must be carried out to exclude various extra-abdominal causes of abdominal pain.
      a. **Diabetic** patients or patients with known **coronary artery disease or peripheral vascular disease** who present with vague epigastric symptoms may have myocardial ischemia as the cause of the abdominal symptoms.
      b. **Right lower lobe pneumonia** may present as RUQ pain in association with cough and fever.
      c. A thorough gynecologic history is essential in women. Problems such as ruptured ovarian cysts, ectopic pregnancy, and pelvic inflammatory disease (PID) must be considered.

C. **Medications**
   1. **Nonsteroidal anti-inflammatory medications,** such as aspirin or ibuprofen, place patients at risk for the complications of peptic ulcer disease, including bleeding, obstruction, and perforation.
   2. **Corticosteroids** may mask classic signs of inflammation, such as fever and peritoneal irritation, making the abdominal examination less reliable.
   3. **Antibiotics** consumed by patients may aid or hinder diagnosis.
      a. Patients with **peritonitis** may have decreased pain due to a partial treatment of their disease process.
      b. Patients who have diarrhea and abdominal pain may have **antibiotic-induced pseudomembranous colitis** caused by *Clostridium difficile.*

D. Physical examination

1. **Overall appearance** should be assessed.

   a. **Patients with diffuse peritonitis appear acutely ill** and tend to lie quietly on their side with their knees drawn toward their chest.

   b. **Patients with colic tend to be restless** and unable to find a comfortable position. Patients with ureteral colic may writhe in pain or walk around the examination room.

2. **Vital signs** are important indicators of a patient's overall condition.

   a. **Fever** suggests the presence of inflammation or infection. Marked fever (>39°C) suggests an abscess, cholangitis, or pneumonia.

   b. **Hypotension and/or tachycardia** may indicate hypovolemia or sepsis.

3. The **abdominal examination** should be carried out thoroughly and systematically. Although opioid analgesia administered prior to physical examination may alter physical exam findings, this is not associated with a decrease in diagnostic accuracy (*Ann Emerg Med.* 2006;48:150) or an increase in management errors (*JAMA.* 2006;296:1764).

   a. The patient's abdomen should be inspected for **distention, surgical scars, bulging masses, and areas of erythema.**

   b. **Auscultation** may reveal the high-pitched, tinkling bowel sounds of obstruction or the absence of sounds due to ileus from diffuse peritonitis.

   c. **Percussion** may reveal the tympanitic sounds of distended bowel in intestinal obstruction or the fluid wave that is characteristic of ascites. Percussion is also useful in localizing tenderness and peritoneal irritation (deep palpation or rebound is usually unnecessary to determine peritoneal irritation).

   d. **Palpation** of the patient's abdomen should be performed with the patient in a supine position and with his or her knees flexed, if necessary, to relieve pain and relax the abdominal musculature.

      (1) **Begin the examination** at a point remote from the reported site of pain.

      (2) **Areas of tenderness and guarding** should be noted. Peritonitis may also be elicited by rocking the patient's pelvis or shaking the bed to create friction between the abdominal wall and the peritoneal viscera.

      (3) **Pain out of proportion to physical examination findings** suggests mesenteric ischemia.

      (4) Thoroughly search for **hernias** (incisional, ventral, umbilical, inguinal, femoral).

      (5) Any **palpable masses** should be noted.

      (6) Referred pain to the site of inflammation may be noted on palpation of areas remote from the disease process.

   e. Rectal examination should be performed routinely in all patients with symptoms suspicious for GI bleeding, obstruction, or lower abdominal/pelvic pathology.

      (1) A **mass in the rectum** may indicate obstructing cancer. Important details are the fraction of circumference involved, tumor mobility, and distance from the anal verge.

(2) The presence of **occult blood in the stool specimen** may indicate GI bleeding from peptic ulcer disease.

f. **Pelvic examination** must be performed in all women of childbearing age who present with lower abdominal pain.

(1) **Cervical discharge** and overall appearance of the cervix should be noted.

(2) **Bimanual examination** should be performed to assess cervical motion tenderness, adnexal tenderness, and the presence of adnexal masses.

g. **Testicular and scrotal examination** is essential in all males who complain of abdominal pain.

(1) **Testicular torsion** produces a painful, swollen, and tender testicle that is retracted upward in the scrotum.

(2) **Epididymitis** may coexist with urinary tract infection (UTI). The epididymis is swollen and tender, and the vas deferens may also be inflamed.

E. **Laboratory evaluation**

1. A **complete blood count** with cell count differential is important in the assessment of surgical conditions and should be obtained in every patient with acute abdominal pain.

a. **White blood cell (WBC) count elevation** may indicate the presence of an infectious source.

b. **Left shift on the differential** to more immature forms is often helpful because this may indicate the presence of an inflammatory source even if the WBC count is normal.

c. **Hematocrit elevation** may be due to volume contraction from dehydration. Conversely, a **low hematocrit** may be due to occult blood loss.

2. An **electrolyte profile** may reveal clues to the patient's overall condition.

a. **Hypokalemic, hypochloremic, and metabolic alkalosis** may be seen in patients with prolonged vomiting and severe volume depletion. The hypokalemia reflects the potassium–hydrogen ion exchange occurring at the cellular level in an effort to correct the alkalosis.

b. **Low serum bicarbonate** or **metabolic acidosis** suggests general tissue hypoperfusion. This may indicate intestinal ischemia.

c. **Elevation of the blood urea nitrogen or creatinine** is also indicative of volume depletion.

3. **Liver enzyme levels** may be obtained in the appropriate clinical setting.

a. A mild elevation of transaminases (<2 times normal), **alkaline phosphatase, and total bilirubin** is sometimes seen in patients with acute cholecystitis.

b. A **moderate elevation of transaminases** (>3 times normal) in the patient with acute onset of RUQ pain is most likely due to a common bile duct (CBD) stone. Elevation of the transaminases often precedes the rise in total bilirubin and alkaline phosphatase in patients with acute biliary obstruction.

c. **Markedly elevated transaminases** (i.e., >1,000 IU/L) in the patient are more likely due to acute hepatitis or ischemia.

4. **Pancreatic enzymes** (amylase and lipase) should be measured if the diagnosis of pancreatitis is considered. It is important to note that the degree of enzyme elevation does not correlate with the severity of the pancreatitis.

   a. **Mild degrees of hyperamylasemia** may be seen in several situations, such as intestinal obstruction.

   b. **Elevation of lipase** is more specific for pancreatic parenchymal damage.

5. **Lactic acid level** may be obtained when considering intestinal ischemia.

   a. **Serum lactate** is an indicator of tissue hypoxia.

   b. Mild lactic acidosis may be seen in patients with arterial hypotension.

   c. Ongoing elevation of serum lactate despite resuscitation is indicative of progression of tissue ischemia (e.g., mesenteric ischemia or worsening sepsis).

6. **Urinalysis** is helpful in assessing urologic causes of abdominal pain.

   a. **Bacteriuria, pyuria, and a positive leukocyte esterase** usually suggest a UTI. Recurrent UTI in males is unusual and should always elicit an evaluation.

   b. **Hematuria** is seen in nephrolithiasis and renal and urothelial cancer.

7. β-Human chorionic gonadotropin must be obtained in any woman of child-bearing age. A positive urine result should be quantitated by serum levels.

   a. A **low level** (<4,000 mIU) is seen in ectopic pregnancy.

   b. **Levels above 4,000 mIU** indicate intrauterine pregnancy [i.e., one that should be seen on ultrasonography (US)].

F. **Radiologic evaluation** of the patient with abdominal pain is a key element in the workup. However, its use should be very selective to avoid unnecessary cost and possible morbidity associated with some modalities.

1. **Plain abdominal X-rays** often serve as the initial radiologic evaluation.

   a. The acute abdominal series consists of three X-rays: upright chest X-ray, and supine and upright abdominal X-rays.

   b. Free intraperitoneal air is best visualized on an **upright chest X-ray** with both hemidiaphragms exposed.

      (1) If the patient is unable to assume an upright position, a **left lateral decubitus X-ray** should be obtained.

      (2) Free air may not be detectable in up to 50% of cases of **perforated viscus** (*AJS*. 1983;146:830–836).

   c. The **bowel gas pattern** is assessed for dilation, air-fluid levels, and the presence of gas throughout the small and large intestine.

      (1) In **small-bowel obstruction,** one sees small-bowel dilation (valvulae conniventes) and **air-fluid levels** in the bowel proximal to the obstruction. There is a paucity of gas in the segment of bowel distal to the obstruction. The absence of air in

the rectum suggests complete obstruction (beware of the presence of colonic gas following rectal examination, or the colon that has not yet completely evacuated, despite the proximal obstruction).

(2) A **sentinel loop** (i.e., a single, dilated loop of bowel) may be seen adjacent to an inflamed organ (as in pancreatitis) and is due to localized ileus.

(3) **The "bent inner tube"** and **"omega"** signs are indicative of possible sigmoid and cecal volvulus, respectively.

d. **Calcifications** should be noted.

(1) The vast majority of **urinary stones** (90%) contain calcium and are visible on plain X-rays, whereas only 15% of **gallstones** are calcified.

(2) **Calcifications in the region of the pancreas** may indicate chronic pancreatitis.

(3) **Calcification in the wall of the aorta** may suggest an AAA.

(4) The most common calcifications seen in the abdomen are **"phleboliths"** (benign calcifications of the pelvic veins). Phleboliths can be distinguished from renal stones by their central lucency, which represents the lumen.

e. Intramural gas in the GI tract **(pneumatosis)** or gas in the biliary tree **(pneumobilia)** (in the absence of a surgical enteric anastomosis, or prior sphincterotomy) is suggestive of bowel ischemia. The **presence of gas** in the portal or mesenteric venous systems is an ominous finding when associated with intestinal ischemia and carries a mortality of >75%. However, portal venous gas can be associated with benign infectious processes that can be managed conservatively (*Arch Surg.* 2009;144(6):575–581).

2. **Ultrasonography (US)** may provide diagnostic information in some conditions. US is portable, relatively inexpensive, and free of radiation exposure. It is particularly useful in biliary tract disease and in evaluating ovarian pathology. US visibility is limited in settings of obesity, bowel gas, and subcutaneous air.

a. US can detect up to 95% of gallstones. Findings suggestive of **acute cholecystitis** include gallbladder wall thickening of greater than 3 mm, pericholecystic fluid, a stone impacted at the neck of the gallbladder, or a sonographic Murphy's sign. **Murphy's sign** is inspiratory arrest, while continuous pressure is maintained in the RUQ. Murphy's sign reflects the descent of an inflamed gallbladder with inspiration. When the inflamed gallbladder makes contact with the examiner's hand, the patient experiences pain, causing the inspiratory arrest. **Dilation of the CBD** (>8 mm, or larger in elderly patients) indicates biliary obstruction.

b. **Pelvic or transvaginal US** is particularly useful in women in whom ovarian pathology or an ectopic pregnancy is suspected.

c. **Testicular US** is adjunctive to physical exam in diagnosing testicular pathology (e.g., testicular torsion, epididymitis, and orchitis).

3. **Contrast studies,** although rarely indicated in the acute setting, may be helpful in some situations.
   a. **Contrast enema** is particularly useful in differentiating adynamic ileus from distal colonic obstruction.
   b. In most instances, a **water-soluble contrast agent** (e.g., Hypaque) should be used to avoid possible barium peritonitis in the event of bowel perforation.

4. **Computed tomographic (CT) scanning** may provide a thorough evaluation of the patient's abdomen and pelvis relatively quickly. Oral and intravenous contrast should be administered if not specifically contraindicated by allergy, renal insufficiency, or patient hemodynamic instability. CT scanning is the best radiographic study in the patient with unexplained abdominal pain. It is of particular benefit in certain situations, including the following:
   a. When **an accurate history cannot be obtained** (e.g., the patient is demented or obtunded or has an atypical history).
   b. When a patient has **abdominal pain and leukocytosis and examination findings are worrisome but not definitive for peritoneal irritation.**
   c. When a patient with a chronic illness (e.g., Crohn's disease) experiences **acute abdominal pain.**
   d. When **evaluating retroperitoneal structures** (e.g., suspected leaking AAA or nephrolithiasis).
   e. When evaluating patients with a history of **intra-abdominal malignancy.**
   f. Evaluation for acute mesenteric ischemia with **CT angiography.**
   g. Differentiating sources of pelvic and lower abdominal pain in women.

5. **Magnetic resonance imaging (MRI)** provides cross-sectional imaging while **avoiding ionizing radiation.**
   a. Image acquisition **takes longer** than for CT scan; patients must be able to lie on their backs for a prolonged period of time and cannot be claustrophobic.
   b. MRI has its greatest application in **pregnant women** with acute abdominal and pelvic pain (*AJR.* 2005;184:452; *J Magn Reson Imaging.* 2008;428–433).

6. **Radionuclide imaging studies** have few indications in the acute setting.
   a. **Biliary radiopharmaceuticals,** such as hepatic 2,6-dimethylaminodiacetic acid or di-diisopropyliminodiacetic acid, evaluate filling and emptying of the gallbladder. Nonfilling implies cystic duct obstruction and may indicate acute cholecystitis. This test is especially valuable in the diagnosis of acalculous cholecystitis and biliary dyskinesia.
   b. **Radioisotope-labeled red blood cell (RBC) or WBC scans** are sometimes helpful in localizing sites of bleeding or inflammation, respectively.

TABLE 11-1	Differential Diagnosis for Acute Abdominal Pain	
Upper abdominal		Perforated peptic ulcer
		Acute cholecystitis
Mid and lower abdominal		Acute appendicitis
		Acute diverticulitis
		Intestinal obstruction
		Mesenteric ischemia
		Ruptured AAA
Other	OB/GYN	PID
		Ectopic pregnancy
		Ruptured ovarian cyst
	Urologic	Nephrolithiasis
		Pyelonephritis/cystitis
	Nonsurgical	Acute MI
		Gastroenteritis
		Pneumonia
		DKA
		Acute pancreatitis
		Hepatitis

AAA, abdominal aortic aneurysm; DKA, diabetic ketoacidosis; MI, myocardial infarction; OB/GYN, obstetric/gynecologic; PID, pelvic inflammatory disease.

c. **Technetium-99m pertechnetate** may be used to detect a Meckel diverticulum because this isotope is concentrated in the ectopic gastric mucosa that frequently lines the diverticulum. This diagnostic test is most frequently ordered in a child with lower GI bleeding.

7. **Invasive radiologic techniques** may have a role in some situations, including angiographic diagnosis and therapeutic intervention for **mesenteric arterial occlusion and acute GI bleeding.**

III. **DIFFERENTIAL DIAGNOSES.** See Table 11-1.

APPENDICITIS

I. **EPIDEMIOLOGY**

A. **Appendectomy** is the most common urgently performed surgical procedure.

B. **Lifetime risk** of undergoing appendectomy is between 7% and 12%.

C. The **maximal incidence** occurs in the second and third decades of life.

D. The **male:female ratio** of approximately 2:1 gradually shifts after age 25 years toward a 1:1 ratio (*Am Fam Physician.* 1999;60(7):2027–2034).

II. PATHOPHYSIOLOGY

A. **Appendiceal obstruction** is the most common initiating event of appendicitis.

   1. **Hyperplasia** of the submucosal lymphoid follicles of the appendix and appendiceal **fecalith** are the most common etiologies of obstruction (*Ann Surg.* 1985;202(1):80–82).

B. **Intraluminal pressure** of the obstructed appendiceal lumen increases secondary to continued mucosal secretion and bacterial overgrowth; the appendiceal wall thins, and lymphatic and venous obstruction occurs.

C. **Necrosis and perforation** develop when the arterial flow is compromised.

III. DIAGNOSIS. The diagnosis of acute appendicitis is made by clinical evaluation. Although laboratory tests and imaging procedures can be helpful, they are of secondary importance.

A. Clinical presentation

   1. **Classic presentation.** Appendicitis typically begins with progressive, persistent midabdominal discomfort caused by obstruction and distention of the appendix, stimulating the visceral afferent autonomic nerves (levels T8 to T10). Anorexia and a low-grade fever (<38.5°C) follow. As distention of the appendix increases, venous congestion stimulates intestinal peristalsis, causing a cramping sensation that is soon followed by nausea and vomiting. Symptoms include anorexia (90%), nausea and vomiting (70%), and diarrhea (10%). Once the inflammation extends transmurally to the parietal peritoneum, the somatic pain fibers are stimulated and the pain localizes to the right lower quadrant (RLQ). Peritoneal irritation is associated with pain on movement, mild fever, and tachycardia. One-fourth of patients present with localized pain and no visceral symptoms (*Br J Surg.* 2004;91(1):28–37). The onset of symptoms to time of presentation is usually less than 24 hours for acute appendicitis and averages several hours.

   2. **Unusual presentations**
      a. When the appendix is **retrocecal or behind the ileum,** it may be separated from the anterior abdominal peritoneum, and abdominal localizing signs may be absent. Irritation of adjacent structures can cause diarrhea, urinary frequency, pyuria, or microscopic hematuria depending on location.
      b. When the appendix is **located in the pelvis,** it may simulate acute gastroenteritis, with diffuse pain, nausea, vomiting, and diarrhea.

B. Physical examination

   1. The examination begins by **assessing the patient's abdomen** in areas other than the area of suspected tenderness. Location of the appendix is variable. However, the base is usually found at the level of the S1 vertebral body, lateral to the right midclavicular line at **McBurney's point** (two thirds of the distance from the umbilicus to the anterosuperior iliac spine).

2. **Rectal examination** is performed to evaluate the presence of localized tenderness or an inflammatory mass in the pararectal area. It is most useful for atypical presentations suggestive of a pelvic or retrocecal appendix.

3. In women, a **pelvic examination** is performed to assess for cervical motion tenderness and adnexal pain or masses.

4. A **palpable mass in the RLQ** is uncommon, but may suggest a periappendiceal abscess or phlegmon.

5. Specific physical examination findings for appendicitis include the following:

   a. The **obturator sign** reflects inflammation adjacent to the internal obturator muscle (as is sometimes seen in appendicitis). It may also be present within an obturator hernia. While the patient is supine with the knee and hip flexed, the hip is internally and externally rotated. The test is positive if the patient experiences hypogastric pain during this maneuver.

   b. The **iliopsoas sign** is seen when an adjacent inflammatory process irritates the iliopsoas muscle. It is classically observed in retrocecal appendicitis. The patient's thigh is usually already drawn into a flexed position for relief. The test is best performed with the patient lying on the left side. With the knee flexed, the thigh is hyperextended. The test is positive if the patient experiences pain on the right side with this maneuver.

   c. **Rovsing's sign** may also be seen in acute appendicitis. Indicative of an inflammatory process in the RLQ, Rovsing's sign is RLQ pain resulting from palpation in the left lower quadrant (LLQ).

C. **Differential diagnosis for RLQ abdominal pain is very broad**

   1. **Gynecologic diseases must always be considered in the female patient with RLQ pain.**

      a. **PID** can present with symptoms and signs indistinguishable from those of acute appendicitis, but the two often can be differentiated on the basis of several factors. Cervical motion tenderness and milky vaginal discharge strengthen a diagnosis of PID. In patients with PID, the pain is usually bilateral, with intense guarding on abdominal and pelvic examinations. Transvaginal US can be used to visualize the ovaries and to identify tubo-ovarian abscesses.

      b. **Ectopic pregnancy** needs to be ruled out in all female patients of child-bearing age presenting with abdominal complaints. A positive pregnancy test should prompt US investigation.

      c. **Ovarian cysts** are best detected by transvaginal or transabdominal US.

      d. **Ovarian torsion produces** inflammation around the ischemic ovary that can often be palpated on bimanual pelvic examination. These patients can have a fever, leukocytosis, and RLQ pain consistent with appendicitis. A twisted viscus, however, differs in that it produces sudden, acute intense pain with simultaneous frequent and persistent emesis. Ovarian torsion may be confirmed by Doppler US.

2. **Urologic diseases are also often confused with appendicitis**
   a. **Pyelonephritis** causes high fevers, rigors, costovertebral pain, and tenderness. Diagnosis is confirmed by urinalysis with culture.
   b. **Ureteral colic.** Passage of renal stones causes flank pain radiating into the groin but little localized tenderness. Hematuria suggests the diagnosis, which is confirmed by intravenous pyelography or noncontrast CT. Abdominal plain films frequently show renal stones.

3. **Other causes of RLQ tenderness**
   a. **Gastroenteritis** is characterized by nausea and emesis before the onset of abdominal pain, along with generalized malaise, high fever, diarrhea, and poorly localized abdominal pain and tenderness. Although diarrhea is one of the cardinal signs of gastroenteritis, it can occur in patients with appendicitis. In addition, WBC count is often normal in patients with gastroenteritis.
   b. **Meckel diverticulitis** presents with symptoms and signs indistinguishable from those of appendicitis, but it characteristically occurs in infants.
   c. **Peptic ulcer disease, diverticulitis, and cholecystitis** can present clinical pictures similar to those of appendicitis.
   d. **Mesenteric lymphadenitis** usually occurs in patients younger than 20 years old and presents with middle, followed by RLQ, abdominal pain but without rebound tenderness or muscular rigidity. Nodal histology and cultures obtained at operation can identify etiology, most notably *Yersinia* and *Shigella* species and *Mycobacterium tuberculosis.* Mesenteric lymphadenitis is known to be associated with upper respiratory tract infections.
   e. **Typhlitis,** characterized by inflammation of the wall of the cecum or terminal ileum, is managed nonoperatively. It is most commonly seen in immunosuppressed patients undergoing chemotherapy for leukemia and in HIV-positive patients. It is difficult to distinguish preoperatively between typhlitis and appendicitis.

D. **Laboratory evaluation.** The following tests should be obtained preoperatively for patients with suspected appendicitis.
   1. **Complete blood cell count.** A leukocyte count of greater than 10,000 cells/μL, with polymorphonuclear cell predominance (>75%), carries a 77% sensitivity and 63% specificity for appendicitis (*Radiology.* 2004;230:472). The total number of WBCs and the proportion of immature forms increase if there is appendiceal perforation. In older adults, the leukocyte count and differential are normal more frequently than in younger adults. Pregnant women normally have an elevated WBC count that can reach 15,000 to 20,000 as their pregnancy progresses.
   2. **Urinalysis** is frequently abnormal in patients with appendicitis. Pyuria, albuminuria, and hematuria are common. Large quantities of bacteria suggest UTI as the cause of abdominal pain. A urinalysis showing more than 20 WBCs per high-power field or more than 30 RBCs per high-power field suggests UTI. Significant hematuria should prompt consideration of urolithiasis.

3. Serum electrolytes, blood urea nitrogen, and serum creatinine are obtained to identify and correct electrolyte abnormalities caused by dehydration secondary to vomiting or poor oral intake.

4. A serum pregnancy test must be performed on all ovulating women.

E. **Radiologic evaluation.** Diagnosis of appendicitis can usually be made without radiologic evaluation, particularly in young, thin males. In complex cases, however, the following can be helpful.

1. **X-rays** are rarely helpful in diagnosing appendicitis. An appendicolith can rarely be seen on plain films. However, suggestive radiologic findings include a distended cecum with adjacent small-bowel air-fluid levels, loss of the right psoas shadow, scoliosis to the right, and gas in the lumen of the appendix. A perforated appendix rarely causes pneumoperitoneum (*Can Assoc Radiol J.* 1988;39(4):254–256).

2. **Ultrasound** is most useful in women of child-bearing age and in children because this diagnostic modality avoids ionizing radiation. US also allows for evaluation of gynecologic pathology. Findings associated with acute appendicitis include an appendiceal diameter greater than 6 mm, lack of luminal compressibility, and presence of an appendicolith. An enlarged appendix seen on US has a sensitivity of 86% and specificity of 81% (*Radiology.* 2004;230:472). The sensitivity is better in thin patients. The perforated appendix is more difficult to diagnose and is characterized by loss of the echogenic submucosa and the presence of loculated periappendiceal or pelvic fluid collection. The quality and accuracy of US are highly operator dependent.

3. **CT scan,** originally recommended only in cases that were clinically complex or diagnostically uncertain, has emerged as the most commonly used radiographic diagnostic test. It is superior to US in diagnosing appendicitis, with a sensitivity of 94% and specificity of 95% (*Ann Intern Med.* 2004;141:537). CT findings of appendicitis include a distended, thick-walled appendix with inflammatory streaking of surrounding fat, a pericecal phlegmon or abscess, an appendicolith, or RLQ intra-abdominal free air that signals perforation. CT scan is particularly useful in distinguishing between periappendiceal abscesses and phlegmon.

4. **MRI** is an alternative when one needs cross-sectional imaging that avoids ionizing radiation. It is particularly useful in a pregnant patient whose appendix is not visualized on US (*Radiology.* 2006;238:891).

IV. TREATMENT

A. **Preoperative preparation.** Intravenous isotonic fluid replacement should be initiated to achieve a brisk urinary output and to correct electrolyte abnormalities. Nasogastric suction is helpful, especially in patients with peritonitis. Temperature elevations are treated with acetaminophen and a cooling blanket.

B. **Antibiotic therapy.** Antibiotic prophylaxis is generally effective in the prevention of postoperative infectious complications (wound infection, intra-abdominal abscess). Preoperative initiation is preferred. Coverage typically consists of a second-generation cephalosporin. In patients with acute nonperforated appendicitis, a single dose of antibiotics is adequate. Antibiotic therapy in perforated or gangrenous appendicitis should be continued for 3 to 5 days.

C. **Appendectomy.** With very few exceptions, the treatment of appendicitis is appendectomy. The decision to perform an open appendectomy via a transverse incision (e.g., Rockey-Davis and Fowler-Weir) or a laparoscopic appendectomy is surgeon preference.

1. **Laparoscopic appendectomy** is associated with marginally briefer postoperative lengths of stay, reduced postoperative pain, quicker return to full function, and lower risk of wound infection (*Surg Endosc.* 2006;20:495). However, these benefits have to balanced with the higher cost and longer operative time required for a laparoscopic appendectomy. Regardless of the technique, most patients undergoing routine appendectomy can be safely discharged from the hospital on the first postoperative day. Laparoscopic appendectomy is most useful when the diagnosis is uncertain or when the size of the patient would necessitate a large incision. Laparoscopy is useful in ovulating woman to evaluate for gynecologic pathology if the appendix is normal.

   a. **Patient positioning** during laparoscopic appendectomy is surgeon specific, but most surgeons place a Foley and tuck the left arm. Three ports are typically placed; a 10-mm port at the umbilicus, a 5-mm LLQ port, and a-5 mm supra pubic midline port. Some surgeons use a RUQ port instead of a LLQ port. The patient is then placed in Trendelenburg with the right side up so that gravity can assist in moving the small bowel out of the operating field.

   b. **The details of the procedure** will vary slightly according to surgeon preference. However, removal of the appendix begins by splaying out the mesoappendix. A window is made in the mesoappendix at the base of the appendix. The mesoappendix is divided using a vascular stapler or vascular sealing device. The appendix is then divided at its base using the endoscopic stapler. If a normal appearing appendix is identified upon entering the abdomen with the videoscope, another etiology of the acute abdomen such as a Meckel's diverticulitis, tubo-ovarian abscess, or Crohn's disease is sought. Some have advocated that there is no need to remove a normal appendix during a laparoscopic appendectomy (*Br J Surg.* 2001;88:251). However, most surgeons will remove the appendix if no other clear etiology of the abdominal pain is found.

2. **Open appendectomy** begins with a transverse incision lateral to the rectus at McBurney's point (one-third of the distance from the anterior superior iliac spine [ASIS] to the umbilicus). If a preoperative CT scan has been obtained, the location of the incision can be adjusted based on the location of the base of the appendix. The external and internal oblique and transversus abdominis muscle layers may be split in the direction of their fibers. After entering the peritoneal cavity, if purulent fluid is encountered it is sent for Gram stain and culture. Once the

cecum is identified, the anterior taenia can be followed to the base of the appendix. The appendix is gently delivered into the wound and any surrounding adhesions carefully disrupted. If the appendix is normal on inspection (5% to 20% of explorations), it is removed and appropriate alternative diagnoses are entertained.

D. **Drainage of periappendiceal abscess.** Management of appendiceal abscesses remains controversial. Patients with appendiceal abscesses who undergo immediate-appendectomy have a higher complication rate and longer hospital stay than patient who are treated nonoperatively (*Am Surg.* 2003;69:829). Patients who have a well-localized periappendiceal abscess can be treated with systemic antibiotics and considered for percutaneous US- or CT-guided catheter drainage, followed by elective appendectomy 6 to 12 weeks later (*Radiology.* 1987;163:23). This strategy is successful in more than 80% of patients. Many surgeons will argue that an interval appendectomy is not necessary (*Ann Surg.* 2007;246(5):741–748).

E. **Incidental appendectomy** is removal of the normal appendix at laparotomy for another condition. The appendix must be easily accessible through the present abdominal incision, and the patient must be clinically stable enough to tolerate the extra time needed to complete the procedure. Because most cases of appendicitis occur early in life, the benefit of incidental appendectomy decreases substantially once a person is older than 30 years. Crohn's disease involving the cecum, radiation treatment to the cecum, immunosuppression, and vascular grafts or other bioprosthesis are all contraindications for incidental appendectomy because of the increased risk of infectious complications or appendiceal stump leak.

V. APPENDICITIS IN PREGNANCY

A. The **incidence of appendicitis during pregnancy** is 1/1,500 pregnancies. Appendicitis is the most common nongynecologic surgical emergency during pregnancy (*Can Fam Physician.* 2004;50:355).

B. **The evaluation of a pregnant woman with appendicitis** can be quite confusing. Appendicitis must be suspected in any pregnant woman with abdominal pain.

1. Nausea and vomiting can be incorrectly attributed to the morning sickness that is common in the first trimester.

2. Tachycardia is a normal finding in pregnancy.

3. Fever a common finding in appendicitis is often not present in pregnancy.

4. Leukocytosis is common in pregnancy. A WBC of 12,000 cell/mL is a normal finding in pregnancy. However, a left shift is always abnormal and requires further investigation.

5. The most common location for pain in the pregnant woman is RLQ pain. It is frequently sited that the location of the appendix shifts during pregnancy due to displacement by the gravid uterus. However, when pregnant females at 19 to 26 weeks who underwent appendectomy were compared to nonpregnant females undergoing appendectomy, there

was no statistical difference in the location of the appendix (*Int J Gyn & OB.* 2003;81:3).

C. **Appendectomy during pregnancy** is indicated in a pregnant patient as soon as the diagnosis of appendicitis is suspected. A negative laparotomy carries a risk of fetal loss of up to 3%, but fetal demise rates reach 35% in the setting of perforation and diffuse peritonitis (*Southern Med J.* 1976;69:1161–1163). The choice to perform open versus laparoscopic appendectomy is still debated. Multiple retrospective studies have shown a laparoscopic approach to be as safe as open appendectomy. Some alteration in technique is required; insufflation pressure is set lower usually at 8 mm Hg and no higher than 12 mm Hg; the umbilical port is placed 6 cm above the uterine fundus. Prophylactic intraoperative tocolytic therapy has not been shown to be effective (*J Am Coll Surg.* 2007;205(1):37–42).

VI. APPENDICITIS IN CHILDREN

A. The **annual incidence of appendicitis in children** increases with age until a peak in the second decade of life (*Pediatr Emerg Care.* 1992;8:126–128). Appendicitis is the most common indication for emergent abdominal surgery in childhood. Delayed diagnosis is common, particularly in young children, and has been reported in as many as 57% of cases in children less than 6 years (*Ann Emerg Med.* 2000;36(1):39–51).

B. Appendicitis in young children can be a difficult diagnosis because of children's inability to articulate their symptoms and their increased rate of atypical presentation.

1. **Physical exam findings** may be absent or unusual. As many as 50% of children lack of migration of pain to RLQ, 40% will not have anorexia and 52% will not have rebound tenderness (*Acad Emerg Med.* 2007;14(2):124–129). Although the classic signs of appendicitis (RLQ tenderness, guarding, and rebound tenderness) are noted less frequently, they may still be elicited and a complete exam should be performed.

2. **Laboratory findings.** The WBC or the percentage of neutrophils is elevated in up to 96% of children with appendicitis (*Ann Emerg Med.* 2000;36(1):39–51). Pyuria may be noted in 7% to 25% of patients with appendicitis (*Ann Emerg Med.* 1991;20(1):45–50), although bacteria are not typically present in a clean catch specimen.

3. **Imaging.** Despite increased utilization of CT and improved accuracy of imaging for acute appendicitis since the mid 1990s, substantially lower rates of negative appendectomy have not been achieved, and the perforation rate remains as high as 33% (*J Pediatr Surg.* 2004;39(6):886–890; discussion 886–890). In addition, the lifetime cancer mortality risk attributable to the radiation exposure from a single abdominal CT examination in a 1-year-old child is approximately one in 550. Currently, over 600,000 abdominal and head CT examinations are performed on children under 15 years of age per year. If these estimates are correct, approximately 500 individuals will ultimately die

from a cancer attributable to the radiation from CT scans (*Am J Roentgenol.* 2001;176:289–296). Given this increasing concern over ionizing radiation and its negative health effects, greater emphasis is being placed on US as the initial imaging modality of choice. The absence of nausea, lack of maximal tenderness in the RLQ, and absolute neutrophil count less than 6.7 had a negative predictive value of 98% for identifying children who could be safely observed or discharged without any imaging studies (*Pediatrics.* 2005;116(3):709–716).

VII. COMPLICATIONS OF ACUTE APPENDICITIS

A. **Perforation** is accompanied by severe pain and fever. It is unusual within the first 12 hours of appendicitis but is present in 50% of appendicitis patients younger than 10 years and older than 50 years. Acute consequences of perforation include fever, tachycardia, and generalized peritonitis. Treatment is appendectomy, peritoneal irrigation, and broad-spectrum intravenous antibiotics for 3 to 5 days, or until fever and leukocytosis resolve.

B. **Postoperative wound infection risk** can be decreased by appropriate intravenous antibiotics administered before skin incision. The incidence of wound infection increases from 3% in cases of nonperforated appendicitis to 4.7% in patients with a perforated or gangrenous appendix. Primary closure is not recommended in the setting of perforation (*Surgery.* 2000;127:136). Wound infections are managed by opening, draining, and packing the wound to allow healing by secondary intention. Intravenous antibiotics are indicated for associated cellulitis or systemic sepsis.

C. **Intra-abdominal and pelvic abscesses** occur most frequently with perforation of the appendix. Postoperative intra-abdominal and pelvic abscesses are best treated by percutaneous CT- or US-guided drainage. If the abscess is inaccessible or resistant to percutaneous drainage, operative drainage is indicated. Antibiotic therapy can mask but does not treat or prevent a significant abscess. Patients that continue to have fever and elevated white count beyond post-op day number 7 should have a CT to evaluate for abscess (*Cochrane Database Syst Rev.* 2005;20:CD001439).

D. Other complications

1. **Small-bowel obstruction** is four times more common after surgery in cases of perforated appendicitis than in uncomplicated appendicitis.

2. **Enterocutaneous fistulae** may result from a leak at the appendiceal stump closure. They occasionally require surgical closure, but most close spontaneously.

3. **Pylephlebitis** is septic portal vein thrombosis caused by *Escherichia coli* and presents with high fevers, jaundice, and eventually hepatic abscesses. CT scan demonstrates thrombus and gas in the portal vein. Prompt treatment (operative or percutaneous) of the primary infection is critical, along with broad-spectrum intravenous antibiotics.

Colon, Rectum, and Anus

Nicholas A. Hamilton and James W. Fleshman

COLORECTAL PHYSIOLOGY

I. NORMAL COLON FUNCTION

A. **Water absorption.** Normal ileal effluent totals 900 to 1,500 mL/day, with stool water loss typically less than 200 mL/day. The right colon maximally can absorb 6 L of fluid/day, and only when large-bowel absorption is less than 2 L/day does an increase in fecal water content result in diarrhea.

B. **Electrolyte transport.** Sodium and chloride absorption occur by active processes in exchange for potassium and bicarbonate in the right colon.

C. **Nutrition.** Although absorption of nutrients is minimal in the colon, mucosal utilization of short-chain fatty acids (SCFAs) produced by colonic bacteria can account for up to 540 kcal/day. Chronic absence of SCFAs such as butyrate and propionate results in "diversion colitis," a condition characterized by rectal bleeding and rare stricture formation. Subclinical diversion colitis occurs in almost all diverted patients and uniformly resolves following stomal closure.

D. **Motility patterns of the colon** allow for mixing and elimination of intestinal contents. Factors influencing motility include emotional state, amount of exercise and sleep, amount of colonic distention, and hormonal variations.

   1. **Retrograde movements** occur mainly in the right colon. These contractions prolong the exposure of luminal contents to the mucosa and thereby increase the absorption of fluids and electrolytes.

   2. **Segmental contractions,** the most commonly observed motility pattern, represent localized simultaneous contractions of the longitudinal and circular colonic musculature in short colonic segments.

   3. **Mass movements** occur three to four times a day and are characterized by an antegrade, propulsive contractile wave involving a long segment of colon.

E. **Microflora.** One-third of the dry weight of feces is normally composed of bacteria. Anaerobic *Bacteroides* species are most prevalent (10^{11}/mL), whereas *Escherichia coli* has a titer of 10^9/mL. Bacteria produce much of the body's vitamin K. Endogenous colonic bacteria also suppress the emergence of pathogenic microorganisms. Antibiotic therapy can alter the endogenous microflora, resulting in changes in drug sensitivity (warfarin) or infectious colitides due to pathogenic microbial overgrowth (*Clostridium difficile* colitis).

F. **Colonic gas** (200 to 2,000 mL/day) is composed of (1) swallowed oxygen and nitrogen and (2) hydrogen, carbon dioxide, and methane produced during fermentation by colonic bacteria. Because hydrogen and methane are combustible gases that may explode when electrocautery is used for biopsy, adequate bowel cleansing is mandatory before using hot-snare techniques during colonoscopy.

II. DISORDERS OF COLONIC PHYSIOLOGY

A. **Constipation** is generally defined clinically **as one or fewer spontaneous bowel movements or stools per week,** though patients may use the term to describe a number of different defecatory symptoms.

1. **Etiologies** include medications (narcotics, anticholinergics, antidepressants, calcium channel blockers), hypothyroidism, hypercalcemia, dietary factors (low fluid or fiber intake), decreased exercise, neoplasia, and neurologic disorders (e.g., Parkinson disease and multiple sclerosis). Abnormalities of pelvic floor function (obstructed defecation), such as paradoxical puborectalis muscle function or intussusception of the rectum (internal or external rectal prolapse), may result in constipation, as may idiopathic delayed transit of feces through the colon (dysfunction of the intrinsic colonic nerves or colonic inertia).

2. **Evaluation.** Change in bowel habits is a common presentation of colorectal neoplasia. The initial evaluation of constipation should include digital rectal exam and colonoscopy. If this workup is negative and the patient fails to respond to a trial of fiber supplementation and increased fluid intake, the next step is a **colonic transit time study.** The patient is given a standard amount of fiber (12 g of psyllium per day) for a week prior to the test and continued throughout the study. On day 0, the patient ingests an enteric-coated capsule containing 24 radiopaque rings. Abdominal plain X-rays are obtained on days 3 and 5. Normal transit results in 80% of the rings in the left colon by day 3 and 80% of all the rings expelled by day 5. The persistence of rings throughout the colon on day 5 indicates colonic inertia. When the rings stall in the rectosigmoid region, functional anorectal obstruction (obstructed defecation) may be present. This may be evaluated with cine defecography, anorectal manometry, or both; the task is to look for nonrelaxation of the puborectalis muscle or internal intussusception of the rectum.

3. **Treatment** of colonic inertia initially includes increased water intake, laxatives (polyethylene glycol, 12 oz/day), fiber (psyllium 12 g/day), increased exercise, and avoidance of predisposing factors. In patients with long-standing, debilitating symptoms refractory to nonoperative measures, **total abdominal colectomy with ileorectal anastomosis** may prove curative. The risk of total intestinal inertia after surgery is significant, and the patient should understand this.

B. **Colonic pseudo-obstruction** (Ogilvie syndrome) is a profound colonic ileus without evidence of mechanical obstruction. It most commonly occurs in critically ill or institutionalized patients. Colonic obstruction or volvulus must be ruled out; Hypaque enema is often therapeutic as well as diagnostic. The initial management consists of nasogastric decompression, rectal tube placement, an aggressive enema regimen (e.g., cottonseed and docusate sodium enema), correction of metabolic disorders, and discontinuation of medications that decrease colonic motility (including narcotics). Neostigmine intravenous infusion (2 mg/hour) in a monitored setting has been shown to be useful in resistant cases (*N Engl J Med.* 1999;341:137). Rapid cecal dilation or a cecal diameter greater than 12 cm on plain abdominal X-rays requires prompt colonoscopic decompression. This is successful in 70% to 90% of cases, with a recurrence rate of 10% to 30% (recurrence is usually amenable to repeat colonoscopic decompression). Laparotomy is reserved for patients with peritonitis, at which time a total abdominal colectomy with end-ileostomy should be performed.

C. **Volvulus** is the twisting of an air-filled segment of bowel about its mesentery and accounts for nearly 10% of bowel obstruction in the United States.

1. **Sigmoid volvulus** accounts for 80% to 90% of all volvulus and is most common in elderly or institutionalized patients and in patients with a variety of neurologic disorders. It is an acquired condition resulting from sigmoid redundancy with narrowing of the mesenteric pedicle.

   a. **Diagnosis** is suspected when there is abdominal pain, distention, cramping, and obstipation. **Plain films** often show a characteristic **inverted-U,** sausage-like shape of air-filled sigmoid pointing to the right upper quadrant. If the diagnosis is still in question and gangrene is not suspected, water-soluble **contrast enema** usually shows a **bird's-beak deformity** at the obstructed rectosigmoid junction.

   b. In the absence of peritoneal signs, **treatment** involves **sigmoidoscopy,** with the placement of a rectal tube beyond the point of obstruction. The recurrence rate after decompressive sigmoidoscopy approaches 40%; therefore, elective sigmoid colectomy should be performed in acceptable operative candidates. If peritonitis is present, the patient should undergo laparotomy and **Hartmann procedure** (sigmoid colectomy, end-descending colostomy, and defunctionalized rectal pouch). An alternative in the stable patient without significant fecal soilage of the peritoneal cavity is sigmoidectomy, on-table colonic lavage, and colorectal anastomosis with or without proximal fecal diversion (loop ileostomy).

2. **Cecal volvulus** occurs in a younger population than does sigmoid volvulus, likely due to congenital failure of retroperitonealization of the cecum (in axial volvulus) or a very redundant pelvic cecum that flops into the left upper quadrant to kink the right colon (in bascule volvulus).

   a. **Diagnosis.** Presentation is similar to that of distal small-bowel obstruction, with nausea, vomiting, abdominal pain, and distention. Plain films show a **coffee bean-shaped,** air-filled cecum with the convex aspect extending into the left upper quadrant. A **Hypaque enema** may be performed, which shows a tapered (in axial volvulus) or linear cutoff (in bascule volvulus) of the ascending colon.

   b. **Management** involves urgent laparotomy and right hemicolectomy. Cecopexy has an unacceptably high rate of recurrent volvulus, and although cecectomy will prevent recurrence, it is technically more challenging than formal right hemicolectomy. Colonoscopic decompression **is not** an option.

3. **Transverse volvulus** is rare and has a clinical presentation similar to that of sigmoid volvulus. Diagnosis is made based on the results of plain films (which show a dilated right colon and an upright, U-shaped, dilated transverse colon) and contrast enema or computed tomography (CT). Endoscopic decompression has been reported, but operative resection is usually required.

D. Diverticular disease

1. **General considerations.** Colonic diverticula are **false diverticula** in which mucosa and submucosa protrude through the muscularis propria. Outpouchings occur along the mesenteric aspect of the antimesenteric taenia where arterioles penetrate the muscularis. The **sigmoid colon** is most commonly affected, perhaps owing to decreased luminal diameter and increased luminal pressure. Diverticula are associated with a low-fiber diet and are rare before age 30 years (<2%), but the **incidence increases with age** to a 75% prevalence after the age of 80 years.

2. **Complications**

a. **Infection (diverticulitis).** Microperforations can develop in long-standing diverticula, leading to fecal extravasation and subsequent peridiverticulitis. Diverticulitis develops in 10% to 25% of patients with diverticula (90% left-sided, 10% right-sided).

(1) **Presentation** is notable for left-lower-quadrant pain (which may radiate to the suprapubic area, left groin, or back), fever, altered bowel habit, and urinary urgency. Physical examination varies with severity of the disease, but the most common finding is localized left-lower-quadrant tenderness. The finding of a mass suggests an abscess or phlegmon.

(2) **Evaluation** by CT scan and complete blood count (CBC) is the standard of care. CT findings may include segmental colonic thickening, focal extraluminal gas, and abscess formation. Neither sigmoidoscopy nor contrast enema is recommended in the initial workup of diverticulitis because of the risk of perforation or barium or fecal peritonitis, respectively.

(3) **Treatment** is tailored to symptom severity.

(a) **Mild diverticulitis** can be treated on an outpatient basis with a clear liquid diet and broad-spectrum oral antibiotics for 10 days.

(b) **Severe diverticulitis** is treated with complete bowel rest, intravenous fluids, narcotic analgesics, and broad-spectrum parenteral antibiotics (e.g., ciprofloxacin and metronidazole). If symptoms improve within 48 hours, a clear liquid diet is resumed, and antibiotics are given orally when the fever and leukocytosis resolve. A high-fiber, low-residue diet is resumed after 1 week of pain-free tolerance of a liquid diet. Fiber supplements and stool softeners should be given to prevent constipation. A colonoscopy or water-soluble contrast study must be performed after 4 to

6 weeks to rule out colon cancer, inflammatory bowel disease (IBD), or ischemia as a cause of the segmental inflammatory mass.

(4) The lifetime likelihood of **recurrence** is 30% after the first episode and more than 50% after the second episode of diverticulitis. Young patients (<50 years) have the same risk of recurrent diverticulitis following an uncomplicated attack as their older counterparts (*Dis Colon Rectum.* 2006;49:1341). Resection of contained, nonfistulizing diverticulitis should be individualized according to patient lifestyle, tolerance of recurrent episodes and progression to complicated disease with stricture, fistula, or recurrent abscess.

(5) **Elective resection** for diverticulitis usually consists of a sigmoid colectomy. The proximal resection margin is through uninflamed, nonthickened bowel, but there is no need to resect all diverticula in the colon. The distal margin extends to normal, pliable rectum, even if this means dissection beyond the anterior peritoneal reflection. Recurrent diverticulitis after resection is most frequently related to inadequate distal margin of resection.

b. **Diverticular abscess** is usually identified on CT scan. A **percutaneous drain** should be placed under **radiologic guidance.** This avoids immediate operative drainage, allows time for the inflammatory phlegmon to be treated with intravenous antibiotics, and turns a two- or three-stage procedure into a one-stage procedure.

c. **Generalized peritonitis** is rare and results if diverticular perforation leads to widespread fecal contamination. In most cases, resection of the diseased segment is possible **(two-stage procedure),** and a Hartmann procedure is performed. The colostomy can then be reversed in the future. An alternative in the management of the stable patient undergoing urgent operation for acute diverticulitis without significant fecal contamination is sigmoidectomy, on-table colonic lavage (in the setting of a large fecal load), and colorectal anastomosis with or without proximal fecal diversion (loop ileostomy).

d. **Fistulization** secondary to diverticulitis may occur between the colon and other organs, including the bladder, vagina, small intestine, and skin. Diverticulitis is the most common etiology of colovesical fistulas. Colovaginal and colovesical fistulas usually occur in women who have previously undergone hysterectomy. Colocutaneous fistulas are uncommon and are usually easy to identify. Coloenteric fistulas are likewise uncommon and may be entirely asymptomatic or result in corrosive diarrhea.

(1) The presentation of **enterovesical fistula** includes frequent urinary tract infections and often is unsuspected until **fecaluria** or **pneumaturia** is noted. CT findings of air and solid material in a noninstrumented bladder confirm the diagnosis. Lower endoscopy, barium enema, intravenous pyelography, and cystoscopy often fail to demonstrate the fistula.

(2) A **colovaginal fistula** is usually suspected based on the passage of air per vagina. The fistula may be difficult to identify

on physical examination or the previously mentioned tests. The presence of methylene blue staining on a tampon inserted in the vagina following dye instillation in the rectum is diagnostic.

(3) **Definitive treatment.** Colonoscopy is performed after 6 weeks to rule out other possible etiologies, including cancer or IBD. Elective sigmoid resection is performed after preoperative placement of temporary ureteral catheters. Ureteral catheters can be very helpful in identifying the distal ureter in the inflammatory pericolonic mass, thereby shortening the operative time. Usually, the fistula tract can be broken using finger fracture, and the bladder defect can be repaired in a single layer. A Foley catheter is left in place for 7 to 10 days to allow this defect to heal. A colovaginal fistula is managed in a similar fashion. It may be helpful to interpose omentum between the colorectal anastomosis and the bladder or vaginal defect.

E. **Acquired vascular abnormalities and lower gastrointestinal (GI) bleeding** are more common in elderly patients than in younger individuals. Most cases of massive lower GI hemorrhage stop spontaneously, but surgery is required in 10% to 25% of cases.

1. **Etiologies** (with relative approximate incidence) of lower GI bleeding in industrialized nations include the following:

a. **Diverticulosis (60%).** The media of the perforating artery adjacent to the colonic diverticulum may become attenuated and eventually erode. This arterial bleeding usually is bright red and is not associated with previous melena or chronic blood loss. Bleeding most commonly occurs from the left colon. Urgent resection of the affected colonic segment should be considered in patients with active ongoing bleeding (>6 units packed red blood cells (RBCs)/24 hours). Elective resection of the affected colonic segment should be performed in patients with recurrent bleeding or need for long-term anticoagulation or in those in whom excessive blood loss may be poorly tolerated.

b. **IBD (13%).** Bleeding due to IBD tends to occur in a younger population; it is more commonly due to ulcerative colitis than Crohn's disease.

c. **Benign anorectal disease (11%)** is discussed later in this chapter.

d. **Neoplasia (10%)** of the colon and rectum rarely presents with massive blood loss, but rather with chronic microcytic anemia and possible syncope.

e. Hemorrhage following **polypectomy** can occur up to 1 month postprocedure and has an incidence of 3% in some series.

f. **Angiodysplasias (<5%)** are small arteriovenous malformations composed of small clusters of dilated vessels in the mucosa and submucosa. An acquired condition, they rarely occur before age 40 years and are more common in the right colon (80%). Diagnosis can be made by colonoscopy or angiographic features (delayed filling of a dilated venule).

2. **Massive lower GI bleeding** is defined as hemorrhage distal to the ligament of Treitz that requires more than **3 units of blood in 24 hours. Management** consists of simultaneously restoring intravascular volume and identifying the site of bleeding so that treatment may be instituted.

   a. **Resuscitation** is performed using a combination of isotonic crystalloid solutions and packed RBCs as needed, administered via short, large-bore peripheral intravenous catheters.

   b. **Diagnosing the site of bleeding** is more important initially than identifying the cause. Gastric lavage via a nasogastric tube must be performed to rule out an upper GI source of bleeding. Digital rectal exam can eliminate hemorrhoidal bleeding. The choice of localizing study depends on the estimate of bleeding rate.

      (1) **Nuclear scan** using technetium-99m sulfur colloid or tagged RBCs can identify bleeding sources with rates as low as 0.1 to 0.5 mL/minute. Tagged RBC scan can identify bleeding up to 24 hours after isotope injection, but they do not definitively identify the anatomic source of bleeding; hence, planning a segmental GI resection based on this study is not reliable. A rapidly positive scan indicates that angiography has a high likelihood of identifying the source.

      (2) **Mesenteric angiography** should be performed in the patient with a positive nuclear medicine bleeding scan to identify the anatomic source of bleeding. Angiography can localize bleeding exceeding 1 mL/minute and allows either therapeutic vasopressin infusion (0.2 unit/minute) or embolization, which together are successful in stopping the bleeding in 85% of cases. The advantage is that this can convert an emergent operation in an unstable patient with unprepared bowel to an elective one-stage procedure.

      (3) **Colonoscopy** frequently fails to identify the source of massive lower GI bleeds. With slower bleeding after the administration of an adequate bowel preparation over 2 hours, colonoscopy offers the therapeutic advantages of injecting vasoconstrictive agents (epinephrine) or vasodestructive agents (alcohol, morrhuate, sodium tetradecyl sulfate) or applying thermal therapy (laser photocoagulation, electrocoagulation, heater probe coagulation) to control bleeding.

      (4) In the rare **patients who continue to bleed with no source identified,** laparotomy should be considered. Intraoperative small-bowel enteroscopy may be performed if the source is not obvious at the time of exploration. If the source is still not identified, **total colectomy with ileorectal anastomosis or end-ileostomy** is performed. This is associated with an incidence of recurrent bleeding of less than 10%, but the mortality rate for patients who rebleed is 20% to 40%.

3. **Ischemic colitis** results from many causes, including venous or arterial thrombosis, embolization, iatrogenic inferior mesenteric artery (IMA) ligation after abdominal aortic aneurysm repair, and from acquired

or autoimmune vasculopathies. It is **idiopathic** in the majority of patients. Patients are usually elderly and present with lower abdominal pain localizing to the left and melena or hematochezia. The rectum often is normal on proctoscopy owing to its dual vascular supply. Contrast enema may show **thumbprinting** that corresponds to submucosal hemorrhage and edema. Diagnosis depends on the appearance of the mucosa on colonoscopy. Although it may occur anywhere in the colon, disease is present most frequently at the watershed areas of the splenic flexure and sigmoid colon. In the presence of full-thickness necrosis or peritonitis, emergent resection with diversion is recommended. Patients without peritonitis or free air but with fever or an elevated white blood cell (WBC) count may be treated with bowel rest, close observation, and intravenous antibiotics. Up to 50% of patients develop focal colonic strictures eventually. These are treated with serial dilations or segmental resection once neoplasm is ruled out.

4. **Radiation proctocolitis** results from pelvic irradiation for uterine, cervical, bladder, prostate, or rectal cancers. Risk factors include a dose of greater than 6,000 cGy, vascular disease, diabetes mellitus, hypertension, prior low anterior resection, and advanced age. The early phase occurs within days to weeks; mucosal injury, edema, and ulceration develop, with associated nausea, vomiting, diarrhea, and tenesmus. The late phase occurs within weeks to years, is associated with tenesmus and hematochezia, and consists of arteriolitis and thrombosis, with subsequent bowel thickening and fibrosis. Ulceration with bleeding, stricture, and fistula formation may occur. Medical treatment may be successful in mild cases, with the use of stool softeners, steroid enemas, and topical 5-aminosalicylic acid products. If these measures fail, transanal application of formalin 4% to affected mucosa may be efficacious in patients with transfusion-dependent rectal bleeding. Patients with stricture or fistula require proctoscopy and biopsy to rule out locally recurrent disease or primary neoplasm. Strictures may be treated by endoscopic dilation but often recur. Surgical treatment consists of a diverting colostomy and is reserved for medical failures, recurrent strictures, and fistulas. Proctectomy is rarely required and is usually associated with unacceptable morbidity and mortality.

ANORECTAL PHYSIOLOGY

I. NORMAL ANORECTAL FUNCTION

A. The **rectum functions as a capacitance organ,** with a reservoir of 650 to 1,200 mL compared to an average daily stool output of 250 to 750 mL.

B. The **anal sphincter mechanism** allows defecation and maintains continence. The internal sphincter (involuntary) accounts for 80% of resting pressure, whereas the external sphincter (voluntary) accounts for 20% of resting pressure and 100% of squeeze pressure. The external anal sphincter contracts in response to sensed rectal contents and relaxes during defecation.

C. **Defecation** has four components: (1) mass movement of feces into the rectal vault; (2) rectal–anal inhibitory reflex, by which distal rectal distention causes involuntary relaxation of the internal sphincter; (3) voluntary relaxation of the external sphincter mechanism and puborectalis muscle; and (4) increased intra-abdominal pressure.

D. **Continence** requires normal capacitance, normal sensation at the anorectal transition zone, puborectalis function for solid stool, external sphincter function for fine control, and internal sphincter function for resting pressure.

II. **INCONTINENCE** is the inability to prevent elimination of rectal contents.

A. **Etiologies** include (1) **mechanical defects,** such as sphincter damage from obstetric trauma, fistulotomy, and scleroderma affecting the external sphincter; (2) **neurogenic defects,** including spinal cord injuries, pudendal nerve injury due to birth trauma or lifelong straining, and systemic neuropathies such as multiple sclerosis; and (3) **stool content-related causes,** such as diarrhea and radiation proctitis.

B. **Evaluation** includes visual and digital examination observing for gross tone or squeeze abnormalities. **Anal manometry** quantitatively measures parameters of anal function, including resting and squeeze pressure (normal mean >40 and >80 mm Hg, respectively), sphincter length (4 cm in men, 3 cm in women), and minimal sensory volume of the rectum. Pudendal nerve terminal motor latency (**PNTML**) testing and endoanal ultrasound provide neural and anatomic information.

C. **Treatment** depends on the type and severity of the defect. Neurogenic and minor mechanical anal sphincter defects are treated using dietary fiber to increase stool bulk and **biofeedback** to strengthen muscle and improve early sensation. Major defects require **anal sphincter reconstruction,** in which the anatomic sphincter defect is repaired. Artificial anal sphincters may be used in patients without a reconstructible native anal sphincter. Severe denervations of an intact anal sphincter may be managed with sacral nerve stimulation, artificial sphincters, or palliative diverting colostomy.

III. **OBSTRUCTED DEFECATION** (pelvic floor outlet obstruction) presents with symptoms of chronic constipation and straining with bowel movements. Problems may include **fecal impaction** and **stercoral ulcer** (mucosal ulceration due to pressure necrosis from impacted stool); both are treated with enemas, increased dietary fiber, and stool softeners. Attempts at surgical correction of any of the following conditions without addressing the underlying pathology are doomed to failure.

A. **Physiologic evaluation** includes (1) **defecography** to evaluate fixation of the posterior rectum to the sacrum and relaxation of the puborectalis and (2) **colonic transit study.**

B. **Anal stenosis** is a rare cause of obstructed defecation and presents with frequent thin stools and bloating. The most common etiologies include scarring after anorectal surgery (rare), chronic laxative abuse, radiation, recurrent anal ulcer, inflammation, and trauma. Initial treatment is anal dilation, although advanced cases are treated with advancement flaps of normal perianal skin.

C. **Nonrelaxation of puborectalis** results in straining and incomplete evacuation. Colonic transit time reveals outlet obstruction. Persistent puborectalis distortion is seen on defecography. Biofeedback is the treatment of choice.

D. **Descending perineum syndrome** occurs when chronic straining causes pudendal nerve stretch and subsequent neurogenic defect. **Rectocele** results from a weak, distorted rectovaginal septum that allows the anterior rectal wall to bulge into the vagina due to failure of the pelvic floor to relax during defecation.

IV. **ABNORMAL RECTAL FIXATION** leads to internal or external prolapse of the full thickness of the rectum.

A. **Internal intussusception (internal rectal prolapse)** causes outlet obstruction with mucus discharge, hematochezia, tenesmus, and constipation. Proctoscopy demonstrates a **solitary rectal ulcer** at the lead point of the internal prolapse. **Treatment** consists of increased bulk, stool softeners, and glycerin suppositories. **Indications for surgery** are chronic bleeding, impending incontinence, and lifestyle-changing symptoms. Surgical options are controversial. The most frequent procedure is transabdominal rectopexy (suture fixation of the rectum to the presacral fascia) and anterior resection of the sigmoid colon if constipation is prominent among the patient's complaints. Chronic ischemia of the solitary rectal ulcer causes entrapment of mucin-producing cells, eventually resulting in **colitis cystica profunda.** Treatment is low anterior resection and rectopexy.

B. **External rectal prolapse** is protrusion of full-thickness rectum through the anus. Symptoms include pain, bleeding, mucous discharge, and incontinence. Physical examination can distinguish rectal prolapse (concentric mucosal rings) from prolapsing internal hemorrhoids (deep radial grooves). **Risk factors** include increased age, female gender, institutionalization, antipsychotic medication, previous hysterectomy, and spinal cord injury. Evaluation includes **barium enema or colonoscopy** to rule out malignancy. In general, abdominal procedures trade higher operative morbidity with lower recurrence rates relative to perineal-only operations. Continence improves in almost all patients, regardless of procedure.

1. **Sigmoid resection and rectopexy** (Frykman–Goldberg procedure) shortens the redundant rectosigmoid colon with posterior sacral fixation. Prolapse recurs in less than 10% of patients following rectopexy with or without resection.

2. **Perineal proctectomy** (modified Altemeier procedure) is an alternative for patients with severe anal incontinence due to complete eversion and stretch of the anal canal. Recurrence rate is generally around 20%, although lower rates have been reported in retrospective, single-institution studies (*Dis Colon Rectum.* 2006;49:1052).

V. **HEMORRHOIDS** are vascular and connective tissue cushions that exist in three columns in the anal canal: right anterolateral, right posterolateral, and left

TABLE 12-1	Classification and Treatment of Symptomatic Internal Hemorrhoids	
Grade	Description	Treatments
I	Palpable, nonprolapsing enlarged venous cushions	Dietary fiber, stool softeners
II	Prolapse with straining and defecation, spontaneously reduce	Dietary fiber, stool softeners, elastic ligation
III	Protrude spontaneously or with straining, require manual reduction	Dietary fiber, stool softeners, elastic ligation, excisional hemorrhoidectomy, stapled hemorrhoidectomy
IV	Chronically prolapsed and cannot be reduced, often with dentate line released from internal position	Dietary fiber, stool softeners, excisional hemorrhoidectomy, stapled hemorrhoidectomy

lateral. **Internal hemorrhoids** are above the dentate line and thus covered with mucosa. These may bleed and prolapse, but they do not cause pain. **External hemorrhoids** are below the dentate line and covered with anoderm. These do not bleed but may thrombose, which causes pain and itching, and secondary scarring may lead to skin tag formation. Hard stools, prolonged straining, increased abdominal pressure, and prolonged lack of support to the pelvic floor all contribute to the abnormal enlargement of hemorrhoidal tissue. **Treatments** are based on grading and patient symptoms (Table 12-1); options include the following:

A. **Medical treatment** of first-degree and most second-degree hemorrhoids includes increased dietary fiber and water, stool softeners, and avoidance of straining during defecation. Refractory second- and third-degree hemorrhoids may be treated in the office by **elastic ligation.** The ligation must be 1 to 2 cm above the dentate line to avoid pain and infection. One quadrant is ligated every 2 weeks in the office, and the patient is warned that the necrotic hemorrhoid may slough in 7 to 10 days with bleeding occurring at that time. Patients on anticoagulation should have their anticoagulation stopped for a full 7 to 10 days after banding. Severe sepsis may occur after banding in immunocompromised patients or those who have had full-thickness rectal prolapse ligated by mistake. Patients present with severe pain, fever, and urinary retention within 12 hours of ligation. Patients with this life-threatening disorder should undergo examination under anesthesia, immediate removal of rubber bands, and debridement of any necrotic tissue, accompanied by broad-spectrum intravenous antibiotics.

B. **Excisional hemorrhoidectomy** is reserved for large third- and fourth-degree hemorrhoids, mixed internal and external hemorrhoids, and thrombosed, incarcerated hemorrhoids with impending gangrene. The procedure is performed with the patient in the **prone flexed position,** and the resulting elliptical defects are completely closed with chromic suture (Ferguson hemorrhoidectomy). Complications include a 10% to 50% incidence of urinary retention, bleeding, infection, sphincter injury, and anal stenosis from taking too much mucosa at the dentate line.

C. **Stapled hemorrhoidectomy** is an alternative to traditional excisional hemorrhoidectomy for large prolapsing, bleeding third-degree hemorrhoids with minimal external disease. This procedure is performed by a circumferential excision of redundant rectal mucosa approximately 5 cm superior to the dentate line using a specially designed circular stapler. (*Dis Colon Rectum.* 2004;47:1824). Stapled hemorrhoidectomy results in significantly less perioperative discomfort. There is significantly greater recurrence rate following stapled hemorrhoidectomy (*Cochrane Database Syst Rev.* 2006;4:5393).

D. **Acutely thrombosed external hemorrhoids** are treated by excision of the thrombosed vein outside the mucocutaneous junction, which can be done in the office or emergency room with the wound left open. If the thrombosis is more than 48 hours old, the patient is treated with nonsurgical management.

VI. **ANAL FISSURE** is a split in the anoderm. Ninety percent of anal fissures occur posteriorly and 10% occur anteriorly; location elsewhere should prompt exam under anesthesia and biopsy. Symptoms include tearing pain with defecation and severe anal spasm that lasts for hours afterward and blood (usually on the toilet paper). Manometry and digital rectal examination demonstrate increased sphincter tone and muscular hypertrophy in the distal one-third of the internal sphincter. An external skin tag or "sentinel pile" may also be present. Differential diagnosis includes Crohn's disease (fissure often in the lateral location), tuberculosis, anal cancer, abscess or fistula, cytomegalovirus, herpes simplex virus, chlamydia, and syphilis. **Ninety percent of patients heal with medical treatment** that includes increased fiber, sitz baths, and topical nifedipine ointment (0.2%) TID. If surgery is required, **lateral internal sphincterotomy** is 90% successful. Recurrence and minor incontinence occur in fewer than 10% of patients.

INFECTIONS

I. COLITIS

A. **Pseudomembranous colitis** is an acute diarrheal illness resulting from toxins produced by overgrowth of *Clostridia difficile* after antibiotic treatment (especially the use of clindamycin, ampicillin, or cephalosporins). Antibiotics already have been discontinued in one-fourth of cases, and symptoms can occur up to 6 weeks after even a single dose. **Diagnosis** is made by detection of **toxin A** in one of at least three stool samples or stool culture if toxin A is not found but symptoms are present. Proctoscopy demonstrates sloughing colonic mucosa or pseudomembranes, and CT often shows transmural colonic thickening. **Treatment** begins with stopping unnecessary antibiotics and starting oral or intravenous metronidazole. Oral (not intravenous) vancomycin is an alternative but more expensive therapy. For severe cases in patients unable to take oral medications, vancomycin enemas (500 mg in 250 mL saline) may be useful. Rarely, pseudomembranous colitis presents with severe peritoneal irritation and colonic distention with **toxic megacolon** or **perforation.** Emergency laparotomy with total colectomy and end-ileostomy is required.

B. **Amebic colitis** results from invasive infection by the protozoan *Entamoeba histolytica,* which is spread by the fecal-oral route. It is most commonly encountered in patients who have traveled abroad. The cecum usually is affected with small ulcers that may perforate or form an inflammatory mass or **ameboma. Diagnosis** is made by examining stool for ova and parasites, which is 90% sensitive in identifying the trophozoites. **Treatment** is oral metronidazole and iodoquinol. Surgical treatment is reserved for perforation or for ameboma refractory to treatment.

C. **Actinomycosis** is an abdominal infection that most commonly occurs around the cecum after appendectomy owing to the anaerobic Gram-positive *Actinomyces israelii.* An inflammatory mass often is present with sinuses to the skin that can drain **sulfur granules. Diagnosis** is confirmed by anaerobic culture (the organism may take up to 1 week to isolate), and **surgical drainage** combined with penicillin or tetracycline is required.

D. **Neutropenic enterocolitis** after chemotherapy occurs most commonly in the setting of acute myelogenous leukemia after cytosine arabinoside therapy. It is also seen frequently in patients undergoing chemotherapy for stage III or IV colon cancer. Patients present with abdominal pain, fever, bloody diarrhea, distention, and sepsis. The cecum often dilates, and there may be pneumatosis. **Initial treatment** includes bowel rest, total parenteral nutrition, granulocyte colony-stimulating factor (G-CSF), and broad-spectrum intravenous antibiotics. Laparotomy with total colectomy and ileostomy is required only if peritonitis develops.

E. **Cytomegalovirus colitis** presents with bloody diarrhea, fever, and weight loss. It affects 10% of patients with acquired immunodeficiency syndrome (AIDS) and is the most common cause for emergent abdominal surgery in patients with AIDS. Ganciclovir is the treatment of choice; emergent colectomy with ileostomy is reserved for toxic megacolon.

II. INFECTION OF THE ANORECTUM

A. **Anorectal abscess**

1. **Cryptoglandular abscess** results from infection of the anal glands in the crypts at the dentate line. The initial abscess occurs in the intersphincteric space. Infection then can spread (1) superficial to the external sphincter into the **perianal** space, (2) through the external sphincter into the **ischiorectal** space (which in turn may connect posteriorly via the deep postanal space, resulting in a horseshoe abscess), or (3) deep to the external sphincter into the **supralevator** space.

a. **Diagnosis** usually is obvious, with severe anal pain and a palpable, tender, fluctuant mass. An intersphincteric abscess yields only a painful bulge in the rectal wall and no external manifestations.

b. **Treatment** is surgical drainage, with the skin incision kept close to the anal verge to avoid the possible creation of a long fistula tract. Intersphincteric abscesses are drained by an internal sphincterotomy over the entire length of the abscess. Perianal and ischiorectal abscesses are drained through the perianal skin with a small mushroom-shaped catheter placed to keep the abscess unroofed. Antibiotic therapy is not necessary unless the patient (1) is immunocompromised, (2) is diabetic, (3) has extensive cellulitis, or (4) has valvular heart disease. Immunocompromised patients may present with anal pain without fluctuance because of the paucity of leukocytes. The painful indurated region must still be drained, and the underlying tissue must undergo biopsy and culture.

c. **Outcome from drainage alone** shows that 40% of patients develop a chronic fistula. We do not advocate fistulotomy at the initial operation because the internal opening may not be evident and a complicated fistulotomy may result in sphincter injury.

2. **Fistula-in-ano** represents the chronic stage of cryptoglandular abscess but also may be due to trauma, Crohn's disease, tuberculosis, cancer, or radiation.

a. Patients present with persistent fecopurulent **perianal drainage** from the external opening of the fistula. The location of the internal opening along the dentate line is approximated by using **Goodsall's rule:** fistulas with external openings anterior to a transverse plane through the anal canal penetrate toward the dentate line in a radial direction, whereas fistulas posterior to that plane curve so that the internal opening is in the posterior midline (see Fig. 12-1), and may involve the sphincters in one of four configurations (see Fig. 12-2).

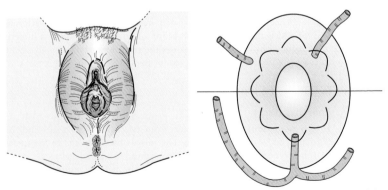

Figure 12-1. Goodsall's rule. The anterior–posterior location of the external opening of the fistula helps to identify the internal opening of the fistula.

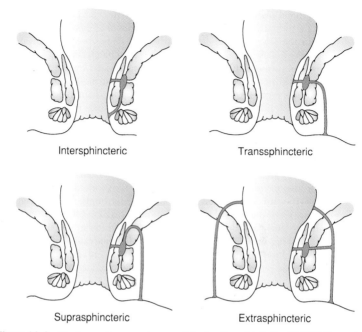

Intersphincteric

Transsphincteric

Suprasphincteric

Extrasphincteric

Figure 12-2. The four main anatomic types of fistula. (From Mulholland MW, Lillemoe KD, Doherty GM, et al. *Greenfield's Surgery: Scientific Principles and Practice,* 4th ed. New York: Lippincott Williams and Wilkins, 2005, with permission.)

   b. Treatment depends on the level of the fistula and preexisting sphincter function. Placement of a soft, noncutting seton permits resolution of surrounding inflammation while preserving sphincter musculature. **Fistulotomy,** dividing the overlying internal sphincter, may be performed for intersphincteric fistulas, which necessitates incision to the anal verge without transversing any external sphincter (trans-sphincteric). **Fibrin glue injection** of the tract has a high failure rate but does not limit future options. A newer alternative is insertion of an **anal fistula plug** composed of lyophilized porcine submucosa to create a collagen scaffold to allow tract healing with variable results (*Dis Colon Rectum.* 2006;49:1817). Definitive treatment of a posterior midline fistula is fistulotomy, whereas anterior fistulas require sliding flap repairs if less invasive options fail.

B. Necrotizing anorectal infection (Fournier gangrene) can result in massive, life-threatening tissue destruction. Patients present with systemic toxicity and perianal pain. There may be crepitance and extensive necrosis under relatively normal skin. Synergistic flora (including clostridial and streptococcal species) of anorectal and urogenital origin may be involved. Immediate wide surgical debridement of all nonviable tissue and intravenous antibiotics are mandatory. Early treatment is critical, but mortality still approximates 50%.

C. **Pilonidal disease** occurs secondary to infection of a hair-containing sinus in the postsacral intergluteal fold 5 cm superior to the anus. Patients present with pain, swelling, and drainage when the sinuses become infected. The disease is most prevalent in men in the second and third decades of life. Symptoms are distinguished from perianal abscess by the lack of anal pain, the more superior location of the fluctuant mass, and the presence of midline cutaneous pits. Treatment is incision, drainage, and curettage, with allowance for secondary closure when the sinus is acutely inflamed. The disease tends to recur, however, and once the active inflammation has resolved, the sinus can be excised electively, with primary closure and a higher chance of cure.

D. **Hidradenitis suppurativa** is an infection of the apocrine sweat glands and mimics fistula-in-ano except that involvement is external to the anal verge. The treatment of choice is wide incision of the involved skin.

E. **Pruritus ani** is a common symptom of hemorrhoids, fissure, rectal prolapse, rectal polyp, anal warts and intraepithelial dysplasia of squamous or apocrine gland origin. Treatment is directed toward resolution of the underlying cause. Failure to find an underlying cause should prompt investigation of dietary factors (e.g., coffee and alcohol). Children should be evaluated for pinworms, which, if found, are treated with piperazine citrate.

F. **Condyloma acuminatum** is an anorectal and urogenital wart caused by infection with human papilloma virus. The disease is most commonly transmitted through anal intercourse and presents with visible perianal growth, often accompanied by pruritus, anal discharge, bleeding, and pain. Common treatments include topical trichloroacetic acid, Aldara (imiquimod), or excision with electrocoagulation under local anesthesia. Smoke generated by coagulation contains viable organisms and must be completely evacuated. Anal canal warts must be destroyed at the same time as external warts. Biopsies should be obtained looking for high-grade squamous intraepithelial lesions.

INFLAMMATORY BOWEL DISEASE

I. GENERAL CONSIDERATIONS

A. **Ulcerative colitis** is an inflammatory process of the colonic mucosa characterized by alterations in bowel function, most commonly bloody diarrhea with tenesmus. It has a male predominance. The disease **always involves the rectum** and extends continuously variable distances in the proximal colon. Patients often have abdominal pain, fever, and weight loss. As the duration of the inflammation increases, pathologic changes progress. Initially, mucosal ulcers and crypt abscesses are seen. Later, mucosal edema and pseudopolyps (islands of normal mucosa surrounded by deep ulcers) develop, and the end-stage pathologic changes show a flattened, dysplastic mucosa. The lumen is normal in diameter. Cancer must be considered in any colonic stricture in a patient with ulcerative colitis.

B. **Crohn's disease** is a transmural inflammatory process that can affect any area of the GI tract, from the mouth to the anus. It has a female predominance.

The disease has a segmental distribution, with **normal mucosa interspersed between areas of diseased bowel.** Common symptoms include diarrhea, abdominal pain, nausea and vomiting, weight loss, and fever. There can be signs of an abdominal mass or perianal fistulas on physical examination. The **terminal ileum** is involved in up to 45% of patients at presentation. Common pathologic changes include fissures, fistulas, transmural inflammation, and granulomas. Grossly, the mucosa shows aphthoid ulcers that often deepen over time and are associated with fat wrapping and bowel wall thickening. As the disease progresses, the bowel lumen narrows, and obstruction or perforation may result. Over time, the areas of stricture may develop dysplastic or even neoplastic changes.

C. **"Indeterminate colitis"** is a term used for cases in which the pathologic pattern does not fall clearly into one or the other of the aforementioned patterns (10% to 15% of patients with IBD). The indeterminacy can be due either to inadequate tissue biopsy or to a truly indeterminate form of disease.

D. **Extraintestinal manifestations** of IBD are common with ulcerative colitis and with Crohn's disease. Patients with either disease can develop dermatologic conditions such as erythema nodosum and pyoderma gangrenosum, ocular inflammatory diseases, and arthritis/synovitis. These typically correlate with the degree of colonic inflammation. Ulcerative colitis patients also can develop sclerosing cholangitis.

II. ULCERATIVE COLITIS

A. **Indications for surgery**

1. **Failure to respond to medical treatment.** Inability to wean from high-dose steroids after two successive tapers prompts evaluation for surgery.

2. The **risk of malignancy** is related to the extent and duration of the disease but not the intensity of the disease. Colitis-associated cancer usually infiltrates submucosally and has signet-ring histology. The risk increases by 1% per year after 10 years of disease. Colonoscopy is performed 7 to 10 years after the diagnosis and every 1 to 2 years thereafter, with random biopsies every 10 cm and directed biopsies of mass lesions. Resection is recommended for dysplasia or stricture.

3. **Severe bleeding** that does not respond adequately to medical therapy requires resection for control.

4. **Acute severe fulminant colitis** [white blood cell (WBC) count >16,000, fever, abdominal pain, distention] initially is treated with bowel rest, antibiotics, steroids, and avoidance of contrast enemas, antidiarrheals, and morphine. If the patient develops worsening sepsis or peritonitis, abdominal colectomy with end-ileostomy is performed.

B. **Surgical management** aims at removing the colorectal mucosa while maintaining bowel function as much as possible. Because the disease is localized to the rectum and colon, curative resection is possible. Sphincter-sparing procedures are preferred to preserve the functions of continence and defecation. However, they are associated with higher postoperative complication risk. Anal sphincter function is assessed with manometry to ensure normal function before contemplation of a sphincter-sparing procedure in a patient medically able to undergo the operation.

1. **Restorative proctocolectomy (ileal pouch–anal anastomosis, IPAA)** maintains enteral continuity through the anal sphincter mechanism and is the operation of choice in most patients. A total proctocolectomy is carried out to the anal transition zone. The rectum is transected, leaving the sphincters and levators intact. A distal ileal pouch is constructed over a distance of 15 cm in a J configuration, pulled through the sphincters, and stapled or sutured to the rectal cuff. Stapled anastomoses leaving a 2-cm cuff of anal canal mucosa technically are easier but require long-term surveillance of the residual mucosa. A diverting loop ileostomy is constructed, then reversed 3 months later after healing of the distal anastomosis. **Complications** include increased stool frequency (five to seven times daily), nocturnal soiling (20%), pouch fistula (<10%), and pouchitis (28%), an intermittent inflammatory process that typically responds to metronidazole. Pouch capacity increases over time; eventually, the patient needs to empty the pouch an average of four to five times daily. The pouch procedure can be performed laparoscopically.

2. **Total proctocolectomy with end-ileostomy** is performed in patients who have perioperative sphincter dysfunction or incontinence and in high-risk patients who would not tolerate potential postoperative complications. Most patients do well with a well-placed **Brooke ileostomy** that has a spigot configuration and empties into a bag appliance in an uncontrolled fashion. A **Kock pouch** or continent ileostomy does not empty spontaneously, does not require a permanent appliance, and requires cannulation six to eight times daily. These are more difficult to construct and prone to obstruction. This alternative is occasionally offered to patients who desire continence or who have severe skin allergies, which make ileostomy appliances problematic.

III. **CROHN'S DISEASE** is a chronic disease that is not surgically curable. Surgery should be performed only for complications of the acute disease, such as perforation, fistulas, and phlegmon or when chronic disease results in stricture formation. When a patient presents with a complication requiring surgery, all attempts should be made to prepare the patient so that a single operation will suffice and as much intestine as possible can be preserved. Preparations often include parenteral nutrition, antibiotics, anti-inflammatory medications, and percutaneous drainage of abscesses.

A. **Surgical management** of Crohn's disease is limited to resection of the diseased segment of intestine responsible for the complication. Resection is bounded by grossly normal margins; no attempt is made to obtain microscopically negative margins because outcome and recurrence are unaffected by this. If significant intra-abdominal infection or inflammation is encountered during surgery, a proximal ostomy is created to allow complete diversion of intestinal contents and resolution of the initial process. If no infection or inflammation is encountered, normal-appearing bowel can be primarily anastomosed. **Stricturoplasty** to preserve small-bowel length is favored by some groups, with single-institution retrospective reviews demonstrating comparable recurrence rates to resectional treatment (*J Am Coll Surg.* 2001;192:330).

B. **Small-intestinal Crohn's disease is covered in Chapter 10.**

C. **Colonic Crohn's disease** often requires operation after a shorter duration of symptoms than is typical for patients with either small-intestinal or ileocolic Crohn's disease. Perforation can occur without dilation of the colon secondary to thickening of the colonic wall. Surgical options include total abdominal colectomy with ileorectal anastomosis, total abdominal colectomy with an end-ileostomy, and maintenance of the rectum as a Hartmann pouch, or total proctocolectomy with permanent end-ileostomy. Rarely, colonic strictures can occur in an isolated segment, causing obstruction. The risk of colon cancer with Crohn's disease is 7% at 20 years; thus, any colonic stricture should be biopsied. Segmental resection is the treatment of choice for isolated segmental colonic Crohn's disease; stricturoplasty has no role in colonic strictures. All efforts should be directed to preserving the rectum in colonic Crohn's disease because restorative proctocolectomy is not an option.

D. **Rectal Crohn's disease** rarely occurs in isolation. Once the rectum has become so fibrotic that it loses its reservoir capacity, proctectomy should be considered. Precise **intersphincteric** dissection along the rectal wall beginning at the anal verge should minimize complications.

E. **Anal disease** occurs in 35% of patients with Crohn's disease, but only 2% present with disease confined exclusively to the perineum. Treatment of acute disease entails surgical drainage of perianal sepsis followed by medical therapy (steroids, bowel rest, antibiotics). Antitumor necrosis factor-α (TNF-α) antibody (infliximab) also has a role in acute and chronic perianal fistulas to reduce local disease activity and allow for subsequent surgical therapy. The ACCENT II (A Crohn's disease Clinical study Evaluating infliximab in a New long-term Treatment regimen) study was a landmark multicenter, double-blind, randomized trial of more than 300 patients with fistulizing Crohn's disease that demonstrated improved outcomes with anti-TNF-α therapy (*N Engl J Med.* 2004;350:876). Prolonged treatment with azathioprine is necessary to maintain remission. Ultimately, proctectomy or diversion may be the only way to return quality of life to the patient.

NEOPLASTIC DISEASE

I. The **etiology** of colorectal neoplasia has genetic and environmental components.

A. **Familial cancer syndromes** account for 10% to 15% of colorectal cancers (Table 12-2).

B. **Sporadic cancers** account for approximately 85% of colorectal neoplasia. First-degree relatives of patients with colorectal cancer have a three- to ninefold increase in the risk of developing the disease despite no identifiable inherited genetic mutation. Overwhelming evidence suggests that colorectal carcinomas develop from precursor adenomas and are associated with an

TABLE 12-2 Hereditary Colorectal Cancer (CRC) Syndromes

Syndrome	Percentage of Total RC Burden	Genetic Basis	Phenotype	Extracolonic Manifestations	Treatment	Notes
Familial adenomatous polyposis (FAP)	<1%	Mutations in tumor suppressor gene *APC* (5q21)	<100 adenomatous polyps; near 100% with CRC by age 40 yr	CHRPE, osteomas, epidermal cysts, periampullary neoplasms	TPC with end-ileostomy or IPAA or TAC with IRA and lifelong surveillance	Variants include Turcot (CNS tumors) and Gardener (desmoids) syndromes
Hereditary nonpolyposis colorectal cancer (HNPCC)	5%–7%	Defective mismatch repair: *MSH2* and *MLH1* (90%), *MSH6* (10%)	Few polyps, predominantly right-sided CRC, 80% lifetime risk of CRC	At risk for uterine, ovarian, small intestinal, pancreatic malignancies	Genetic counseling; consider prophylactic resections, including TAH/BSO	High microsatellite instability (MSI-H) tumors, better prognosis than sporadic CRC

					Surveillance	
Peutz–Jeghers (PJS)	<1%	Loss of tumor suppressor gene *LKB1/STK11* (19p13)	Hamartomas throughout GI tract	Mucocutaneous pigmentation, risk for pancreatic cancer	EGD and colonoscopy q3 yr; resect polyps >1.5 cm	Majority present with SBO due to intussuscepting polyp
Familial juvenile polyposis (FJP)	<1%	Mutated *SMAD4/DPC* (18q21)	Hamartomas throughout GI tract; >3 juvenile polyps; 15% with CRC by age 35 yr	Gastric, duodenal, and pancreatic neoplasms; pulmonary AVMs	Genetic counseling; consider prophylactic TAC with IRA for diffuse disease	Presents with rectal bleeding or diarrhea

AVM, arteriovenous malformation; CHRPE, congenital hypertrophy of retinal pigmented epithelium; CNS, central nervous system; EGD, esophagogastroduodenoscopy; GI, gastrointestinal; IPAA, ileal pouch–anal anastomosis; IRA, ileal–rectal anastomosis; TAC, total abdominal colectomy; TAH/BSO, total abdominal hysterectomy and bilateral salpingo-oophorectomy; TPC, total proctocolectomy.

increasing number of genetic mutations (the so-called **Vogel stein progression**). A single genetic mutation in the germline of a patient may cause an adenoma to develop. Further mutations in either tumor-suppressor genes or oncogenes are responsible for further development of the adenoma and eventually transformation to neoplasia. Genes implicated in this journey from normal epithelium to carcinoma include *K-ras, DCC,* and *p53.*

C. **Environmental factors** have also been proposed to play a significant role in the etiology of colorectal neoplasia. Dietary factors shown to increase cancer risk include a diet high in unsaturated animal fats and highly saturated vegetable oils. Increased fiber decreases cancer risk in those on a high-fat diet. Epidemiologic studies indicate that people from less-industrialized countries have a lower risk of colorectal cancer, likely due to dietary differences. This survival benefit disappears in people who immigrate to the United States.

II. **DETECTION. Surveillance** is the periodic complete examination of a patient with known increased risk. **Screening** is the limited examination of a population with the goal of detecting patients with increased risk.

A. **Screening** of the general population is recommended starting at **age 50** years by the American Cancer Society, the American College of Gastroenterology, and the American Society of Colon and Rectal Surgeons. Screening entails either dual-contrast barium enema with sigmoidoscopy or total colonoscopy, and these should be repeated every 10 years if normal or if the patient is not at high risk for colorectal neoplasia. Colonoscopy has a perforation risk of 0.1%, hemorrhage incidence of 0.3%, and mortality of 0.01%. It offers the advantages of obtaining a tissue diagnosis of any abnormality (potentially therapeutic) and greater sensitivity over barium enema. CT colonography is available for those patients unfit or unable to undergo endoscopic evaluation. Individuals over 40 should have yearly fecal occult blood testing.

B. **High-risk individuals** should be in a surveillance program. Previous cancer or polypectomy increases the risk of metachronous cancer by a factor of 2.7 to 7.7. Routine surveillance has been shown to reduce the incidence of metachronous cancer, although its influence on survival is unknown. High-risk patients are those with (1) ulcerative colitis of more than 10 years' duration, (2) Crohn's or ulcerative colitis with stricture, (3) a history or family history of polyps or cancer, or (4) a family history of adenomatous polyposis (FAP) or hereditary nonpolyposis colorectal cancer (HNPCC). Our surveillance algorithm calls for initial or perioperative colonoscopy followed by yearly examination until no lesions are detected, followed by examination every 3 years until no lesions are detected, and then examination every 5 years.

III. **POLYPS**

A. **Nonadenomatous polyps**

1. **Peutz–Jeghers syndrome** is an autosomal-dominant condition characterized by **hamartomatous polyps** of smooth muscle throughout

the GI tract and mucocutaneous pigmentation. Symptoms include bleeding or obstruction secondary to intussusception. Although hamartomas are benign, patients with Peutz–Jeghers syndrome are at increased risk for GI adenocarcinoma as well. Therefore, treatment of polyps greater than 1.5 cm in diameter is polypectomy. Surveillance colonoscopy and esophagogastroduodenoscopy (EGD) are recommended every 2 years, as well as periodic screening for breast, cervical, testicular, ovarian, and pancreatic cancer.

2. **Juvenile polyps** are cystic dilations of glandular structures in the lamina propria without malignant potential that may result in bleeding or obstruction. There are two peaks in incidence of isolated juvenile polyps: in infants and at age 25 years. They are the most common cause of GI bleeding in children and should be treated with polypectomy. **Multiple polyposis coli** (diffuse juvenile polyps) is an autosomal-dominant syndrome characterized by multiple juvenile polyps and increased risk for GI malignancy. These patients are considered for total abdominal colectomy or proctocolectomy with IPAA.

3. **Hyperplastic polyps** show epithelial dysmaturity and hyperplasia and are the most common colorectal neoplasm (10 times more common than adenomas). They have limited malignant potential and may serve as a marker for more aggressive diseases when >1 cm in size. We do not have strong data regarding long-term outcome. Most are less than 0.5 cm in diameter and rarely need treatment. However, those showing mixed adenoma/hyperplastic histology carry the same risks as adenomatous polyps.

B. **Adenomas** are benign neoplasms with unrestricted proliferation of glandular epithelium within the colonic mucosa but with no invasion of the basement membrane. The degree of differentiation decreases as a polyp becomes more like a cancer. *Severe atypia* refers to malignant cells in a polyp that have not invaded the muscularis mucosae (formerly known as *carcinoma in situ*). Adenomatous polyps fall into three broad categories, based on the percentage of villous composition:

1. **Tubular adenomas** are usually pedunculated and account for roughly 85% of adenomas. They have a 5% risk of containing malignant cells.

2. **Tubulovillous adenomas** account for 10% of adenomas. They have a 22% risk of containing cancer.

3. **Villous adenomas** are usually sessile and account for 5% of adenomas. Both size and induration of the polyp reflect cancer risk. For example, a 4-cm sessile villous adenoma has a 40% risk of cancer, whereas the same polyp with induration has a 90% risk.

C. **Treatment** consists of colonoscopic removal. Pedunculated polyps have a stalk and can be removed using the cautery snare. Semisessile and sessile polyps may require piecemeal extraction or endoscopic mucosal lift resection. The site of incomplete removal should be marked with 0.1 mL of India ink for possible later intraoperative or repeat colonoscopic identification. For sessile or large polyps (>3 cm) that cannot be removed endoscopically, surgical resection is required.

1. **The risk of metastatic cancer** in regional lymph nodes is 1% in a completely excised, pedunculated polyp in which cancer invades only the head of the polyp, unless there is lymphatic or vascular invasion. These cases may be treated with either colectomy or polypectomy with close follow-up. Invasion of the cancer down the stalk to the lower third requires colectomy.

2. **Sessile polyps** containing cancer require colectomy, even if completely excised, as the risk of local recurrence and lymph node metastasis is greater than 10% to 20%.

D. **Villous adenoma of the rectum** can present with watery diarrhea and hypokalemia. The risk of cancer in lesions greater than 4 cm with induration is 90%, and transrectal ultrasonography should be used to determine the depth of invasion before excision. Treatment of favorable lesions is by transanal, full-thickness local excision followed by closure of the defect with suture. The role of **transanal endoscopic microsurgery (TEM)** continues to evolve and has become an accepted approach to rectal villous adenomas. Accurate interpretation of the existing small series of patients with early rectal cancer undergoing TEM is difficult due to heterogeneous inclusion criteria, misstaging of rectal cancer, and varying surgeon experience. If the adenoma is large (>4 cm), circumferential, contains invasive cancer, or is located above the peritoneal reflection (generally 10 cm above the anal verge), a transabdominal proctectomy should be performed.

IV. COLON CANCER

A. The **incidence** of colorectal cancer in the United States has been stable since the 1950s, with 145,000 new cases (105,000 colon and 40,000 rectal) each year and 58,000 deaths each year. It is the third-most lethal cancer in men and women, with a slight female predominance in colon cancer and male predominance in rectal cancer. There is a 5% lifetime risk; 6% to 8% of cases occur before age 40 years, and the incidence increases steadily after age 50 years.

B. **Clinical presentation** of colon cancer depends on the location of the lesion. Many tumors are asymptomatic and discovered on routine screening colonoscopy. **Right-colon** lesions occasionally cause hematochezia, but more often bleeding is occult, causing anemia and fatigue. **Left-colon** lesions more often cause crampy abdominal pain, altered bowel habit, or hematochezia. In less than 10% of cases, left-colon cancer presents as large-bowel obstruction with inability to pass flatus or feces, abdominal pain, and distention. Approximately 50% of patients with other symptoms complain of weight loss, but weight loss is almost never the sole manifestation of a colorectal tumor. Rarely, colon cancer presents as perforation with focal or diffuse peritonitis or as a fistula with pneumaturia or feculent vaginal discharge. These symptoms may be difficult to distinguish from those of diverticulitis. Metastatic disease is usually asymptomatic but may present with jaundice, pruritus, and ascites or with cough and hemoptysis.

C. **Diagnosis and staging**

1. **Once the diagnosis is suspected based on history, physical examination, or screening tests,** every attempt should be made to obtain biopsy of the primary lesion and rule out synchronous cancer (3% to 5%). Colonoscopy to the cecum or flexible sigmoidoscopy and barium enema are acceptable. In patients presenting with obstructive symptoms, water-soluble contrast enema is performed to assess the degree and level of obstruction and to "clear" the colon proximal to the obstruction.

2. **Staging studies** to look for distant metastases include chest X-ray and abdominal CT scan. CT identifies liver metastases as well as adrenal, ovarian, pelvic, and lymph node metastases. Serum carcinoembryonic antigen (CEA) is a useful prognostic and surveillance tumor marker in colorectal cancer. CEA should be obtained preoperatively as part of the staging evaluation. Recently, positron emission tomography (PET)-CT has been shown to have greater sensitivity for detecting metastatic disease than CT alone. It is routinely performed prior to concurrent colectomy and liver resection for hepatic metastases.

D. **Surgical treatment**

1. **Bowel preparation.** Mechanical bowel preparation has been shown to be unnecessary in patients undergoing proximal colectomy (right, transverse, or splenic flexure). A modified mechanical prep may be used with Phospho Soda enemas to empty the rectum in patients undergoing left and sigmoid colectomy. A complete mechanical prep is currently recommended for patients undergoing restorative procto-colectomy but not abdominoperineal resection. All patients undergoing laparoscopic procedures may benefit from complete or modified prep to reduce stool volume and facilitate colonic manipulation. The choice of preparation varies by surgeon. All patients undergoing colectomy should receive preoperative intravenous antibiotics (typically cefoxitin or ciprofloxacin and metronidazole) within 1 hour of skin incision. We routinely administer prophylactic enoxaparin preoperatively to reduce the risk of deep venous thrombosis.

2. **Open operative technique** begins with a thorough exploration that includes palpation of the liver. After mobilization of the involved segment, the main segmental vessels are then ligated and divided, and *en bloc* resection of colon and any adherent structure is carried out. If curative resection is not possible, palliative resection should be attempted; if this cannot be done, bypass should be performed. For right-colon cancer, resection includes the distal 10 cm of terminal ileum to the transverse colon, taking the ileocolic, right colic, and right branch of the middle colic vessels. A transverse colon lesion is resected with either an extended right colectomy or a transverse colectomy, taking only the middle colic vessels. Left-colon lesions require dividing the IMA at its origin. If multiple carcinomas are present, or if a colon carcinoma with multiple neoplastic polyps is present, then a subtotal colectomy is performed. The specimen margin is inspected in the operating room to ensure at least a

2-cm margin (5 cm for poorly differentiated tumors). Pathologic evaluation should produce 12 lymph nodes in the mesenteric specimen.

3. **Laparoscopic colectomy** offers a shorter hospital stay and faster recovery for patients with colon cancer. Oncologically, it is guided by the same principles as open resection. The Clinical Outcomes of Surgical Therapy (COST) trial demonstrated noninferiority of the laparoscopic approach as compared to open surgery, with statistically similar times to tumor recurrence, wound implantation, and overall survival at 5 years (*Ann Surg.* 2007;246(4):655–662).

4. **Emergency operations** are undertaken without bowel preparation and have a higher incidence of wound infection. For obstruction, right colectomy still can be performed with primary anastomosis and no diversion. Options with a left-colon cancer include (1) resection with colostomy and either mucous fistula or Hartmann pouch, (2) resection with primary anastomosis, (3) resection with primary anastomosis and proximal diverting ileostomy, (4) subtotal colectomy and ileosigmoidostomy, and (5) colostomy with staged resection of the tumor in an unstable patient with markedly dilated colon. In all but the subtotal colectomy, the proximal colon must be evaluated in the postoperative period for synchronous cancer.

E. **Staging and prognosis.** The American Joint Committee on Cancer (AJCC) TNM staging identifies the depth of invasion of the tumor (T), regional lymph node status (N), and presence of distant metastases (M) (see Table 12-3). Stage I tumors do not involve the muscularis and have a 90% 5-year survival. Stage II tumors penetrate the muscularis and have a 60% to 80% 5-year survival. Stage III tumors involve lymph nodes and have a 60% 5-year survival. Stage IV tumors have distant metastases and a 5-year survival of 10% (see Table 12-4 for staging definitions). Unfavorable characteristics include poor differentiation, multiple lymph node involvement with tumor, mucinous or signet-ring pathology, venous or perineural invasion, bowel perforation, aneuploid nuclei, and elevated CEA.

F. **Adjuvant chemotherapy** remains a standard treatment of stage III and IV colon cancer or patients with stage II cancer in whom less than 12 lymph nodes have been harvested. Current therapy involves the combination of 5-fluorouracil/leucovorin with either irinotecan (FOLFIRI) or oxaliplatin (FOLFOX). The role of targeted therapy using vascular endothelial growth factor (VEGF) inhibitors (bevacizumab) or epidermal growth factor receptor (EGFR) inhibitors (cetuximab) in patients with k-ras mutations in the tumor may be beneficial. Patients with stage IIb tumors with poor prognostic factors may also benefit from adjuvant chemotherapy, although the risk-to-benefit ratio is not as great.

G. **Follow-up** is crucial in the first 2 years after surgery, when 90% of recurrences occur. Surveillance colonoscopy is recommended the first year after resection and then every 3 years until negative, at which time every 5 years is recommended. CEA should be checked every 3 months in the first year and every 6 months in the next 4 years, and rising levels should prompt a CT scan, a chest X-ray, and a PET scan to detect and stage recurrence. A yearly CT scan is recommended in patients with greater than stage I disease.

TABLE 12-3	TNM Categories for Colorectal Cancer
T	Local tumor spread
T0	No tumor
Tis	Tumor only involves mucosa and has not grown beyond muscularis mucosa
T1	Tumor extends into the submucosa
T2	Tumor extends into muscularis propria
T3	Tumor extends through muscularis propria but not beyond outermost layer of colon
T4	Tumor extends through other organs or structures or penetrates the visceral peritoneum
N	Nodal involvement
N0	No lymph node involvement
N1	Cancer cells in 1–3 nearby lymph nodes
N2	Cancer cells in 4 or more nearby lymph nodes
M	Distant spread
M0	No distant organ spread
M1	Spread to a distant organ or distant set of lymph nodes

V. RECTAL CANCER

A. The **pathophysiology** of rectal cancer differs from that of colon cancer because of several anatomic factors: (1) confinement of pelvis and sphincters, making wide excision impossible; (2) proximity to urogenital structures and nerves, resulting in high levels of impotency in men; (3) dual blood supply and lymphatic drainage; and (4) transanal accessibility. The rectum is defined by the NCI as within 12 cm above the anal verge on rigid proctoscopy.

B. **Diagnosis and staging**

1. **Local aspects.** Digital rectal examination can give information on the size, fixation, ulceration, local invasion, and lymph node status. Rigid sigmoidoscopy and biopsy are crucial for precisely measuring the

TABLE 12-4	AJCC/Dukes Colorectal Cancer Staging	
AJCC	TNM	Dukes
0	Tis, N0, M0	—
I	T1–2, N0, M0	A
IIA	T3, N0, M0	B
IIB	T4, N0, M0	B
IIIA	T1–3, N1, M0	C
IIIB	T3–4, N1, M0	C
IIIC	Any T, N2, M0	C
IV	Any T, Any N, M1	—

distance to the anal verge and dentate line and for obtaining a tissue diagnosis. Flexible sigmoidoscopy cannot accurately assess the height of the tumor. **Transrectal ultrasonography** or **rectal protocol magnetic resonance imaging (MRI)** should be an integral part of staging rectal tumors.

2. **Regional aspects.** Pelvic CT, magnetic resonance (MR) scan, and transrectal ultrasound can yield information on the local extension of the tumor toward the bony pelvis and the proximity to the mesorectal envelope. Pelvic examination is necessary to assess the possible fixation of the tumor to adjacent genitourinary structures. Cystoscopy may be required in some men to evaluate extension into the prostate or bladder.

3. **Distant spread** is evaluated (as with colon cancer) with chest X-ray, abdominal CT, and serum CEA. PET scanning is frequently helpful in identifying recurrent disease or disease outside of the liver or lung.

C. **Surgical treatment goals** are to remove cancer with adequate margins, complete mesorectal package (total mesorectal excision, TME) and perform an anastomosis only if there is good blood supply, absence of tension, and normal anal sphincters. If any of these conditions cannot be met, the entire rectum must be removed and the patient left with a permanent colostomy.

1. **Bowel preparation** should be performed for planned restorative proctectomy or laparoscopic procedure. It is not necessary before abdominoperineal resection.

2. The **stoma sites on the abdominal wall should be marked** for possible colostomy on the left side, avoiding bony prominences, belt lines, and scars and staying medial to the rectus muscle at the summit of a fat

fold. The right lower quadrant should also be marked in the event that a temporary loop ileostomy is necessary. Stoma sites should be marked even if the surgeon is anticipating performing an anastomosis.

3. **Positioning and preparation.** If the patient has had previous pelvic surgery or the cancer is suspected to involve the bladder or ureter, ureteral stents should be placed after induction of anesthesia. The patient is placed in the dorsal lithotomy position, which gives access to the abdomen and perineum. A nasogastric tube, Foley catheter, and 34-French mushroom rectal catheter are placed, and the rectum is irrigated until clear with warm saline before instilling 100 mL of povidone–iodine (Betadine).

4. **Operative technique.** Operative goals include high ligation of the IMA at the aorta, careful attention to preserving gonadal vessels and the ureter, and transection of the colon at the descending/sigmoid junction with a purse-string suture around an end-to-end anastomosis stapler anvil in the remaining end of the proximal colon. Rectal dissection then proceeds posteriorly along the avascular presacral plane, laterally through the vascular lateral ligaments, and finally anteriorly, with preservation of the seminal vesicles or vagina. Dissection continues distally well beyond the tumor so that transection allows at least a 2-cm distal margin and a full removal of the rectal mesentery transected at a right angle at the level of the distal intestinal margin. The Dutch Rectal Cancer Trial demonstrated the value of this standardized surgical approach, **the TME,** reporting a local recurrence rate of only 2.4% at 2-year follow-up in patients receiving preoperative short-course radiation and TME (*N Engl J Med.* 2001;345:638).

5. **Surgical options** at this point depend on the height of the lesion, the condition of the sphincters, and the condition of the patient. An abdominoperineal resection is performed for tumors that cannot be resected with a 2-cm distal margin or if sphincter function is questionable. Low anterior resection using an intraluminal stapler is the operation of choice for tumors that can be resected with an adequate distal margin. A colonic J-pouch or coloplasty may also be constructed to recreate the reservoir function of the rectum. Generally, ultralow resections or those with marginal blood supply should be protected with a temporary diverting ileostomy. A hand-sewn coloanal anastomosis is required when the distal margin includes the anal transition zone.

6. **Complications**
   a. **Impotence** occurs in 50% of men and must be discussed preoperatively. The sites of nerve injury are the IMA origin, the presacral fascia, the lateral ligaments, and anteriorly at the level of the seminal vesicles. Prosthesis may be considered 1 year after surgery, once the pelvis is shown to be free of recurrence and the patient has had appropriate time to adapt to changes in body image.
   b. **Leakage** at the anastomosis occurs in up to 20% of patients, typically between postoperative days 4 and 7. Fever, elevated WBC count, increased or changed drain output, or abdominal pain during this period should prompt in-depth physical examination and CT scan evaluation. Intravenous antibiotics and bowel rest are usually

sufficient, but laparotomy and fecal diversion are necessary for large leaks. Patients at high risk for anastomotic leak and, therefore, candidates for diversion for loop ileostomy are those with low colorectal or coloanal anastomoses or recipients of neoadjuvant therapy.

c. **Massive presacral venous bleeding** can occur at the time of resection. This is controlled either with a pledget of abdominal wall muscle sutured to the sacrum or by packing the pelvis for 24 to 48 hours.

7. **Obstructive rectal cancer** requires emergent laparotomy on an unprepared bowel. The type of procedure depends on whether presurgical adjuvant therapy is considered. A decompressing transverse colostomy can be made through a small upper midline incision. This may be a blowhole type if the colon is massively dilated, or it may be a loop colostomy over a rod. If preoperative radiotherapy is not given, options include Hartmann resection, total colectomy with ileorectostomy, and low anterior resection protected by proximal diversion. Intraluminal stenting as a bridge to definitive therapy may preclude diversion.

D. **Adjuvant therapy** for rectal cancer should routinely be considered to reduce local recurrence and possibly improve overall survival.

E. **Neoadjuvant chemoradiation,** including chemotherapy with a 5-fluorouracil–based regimen, results in a modest survival benefit and decreased local recurrence over radiation therapy alone. It is generally reserved for patients with large, bulky tumors or evidence of nodal metastases (stage II/III, especially T4 lesions) in mid and low rectal tumors.

F. **Nonresectional therapy** is indicated in some early-stage cancers, patients with poor operative risk, and patients with widespread metastases. Options include transanal endoscopic microsurgical resection and endocavitary radiation in conjunction with external-beam radiation as the definitive treatment of favorable, but invasive rectal cancers.

G. If the patient has **incurable cancer** and a life expectancy of less than 6 months, external-beam radiation, with or without chemotherapy, combined with laser destruction or stenting the rectum can prevent obstruction. If the life expectancy exceeds 6 months, resectional therapy is attempted.

H. The major cause of **locally recurrent rectal cancer** is a positive margin on the pelvic side wall (radial margin). Recurrences tend to occur within 18 months and grow back into the lumen, presenting with pelvic pain, mass and rectal bleeding, or a rising CEA level. Diagnosis is confirmed by examination and biopsy as well as CT or PET scan. Treatment is not highly satisfactory, and there is a 10% to 20% palliation rate. If chemoradiation has not been given previously, it is given at this point using intensity-modulated radiation therapy (IMRT). Low anterior resection, abdominoperineal resection, or pelvic exenteration (resection of rectum and urinary bladder) is performed based on whether the sphincters and the genitourinary organs are involved in patients without distant disease.

VI. OTHER COLORECTAL TUMORS

A. **Lymphoma** is most often metastatic to the colorectum, but primary non-Hodgkin colonic lymphoma accounts for 10% of all GI lymphomas. The

GI tract is also a common site of non-Hodgkin lymphoma associated with human immunodeficiency virus. The most common presenting symptoms include abdominal pain, altered bowel habit, weight loss, and hematochezia. Biopsies are often not diagnostic because the lesion is submucosal. The workup is similar to that for colon cancer but should include a bone marrow biopsy and a thorough search for other adenopathy. Treatment is resection with postoperative chemotherapy. Intestinal bypass, biopsy, and postoperative chemotherapy should be considered for locally advanced tumors.

B. **Retrorectal tumors** usually present with postural pain and a posterior rectal mass on physical examination and CT scan (*Dis Colon Rectum.* 2005;48:1581).

   1. The **differential diagnosis** includes congenital, neurogenic, osseous, and inflammatory masses. Chordomas are the most common malignant retrorectal tumor; they typically are slow growing but difficult to resect for cure.

   2. **Diagnosis** is suspected based on CT scan and physical findings. Biopsy should not be performed. Formal resection should be undertaken.

C. Carcinoid tumor

   1. **Colonic carcinoids** account for 2% of GI carcinoids. Lesions less than 2 cm in diameter rarely metastasize, but 80% of lesions greater than 2 cm in diameter have local or distant metastases, with a median length of survival of less than 12 months. These lesions are treated with local excision if small and with formal resection if greater than 2 cm.

   2. **Rectal carcinoid** accounts for 15% of GI carcinoids. As with colonic carcinoids, lesions less than 1 cm in diameter have low malignant potential and are well treated with transanal or endoscopic resection. Rectal carcinoids greater than 2 cm in diameter are malignant in 90% of cases. Treatment of large rectal carcinoids is controversial, but low anterior resection or abdominoperineal resection is probably warranted.

VII. ANAL NEOPLASMS

A. Tumors of the anal margin

   1. **Squamous cell carcinoma** behaves like cutaneous squamous cell carcinoma, is well differentiated and keratinizing, and is treated with wide local excision and chemoradiation if large.

   2. **Basal cell carcinoma** is a rare, male-predominant cancer, and is treated with local excision.

   3. **High-grade squamous intraepithelial lesions** are becoming common in HIV-positive patients. Local excision or destruction of identified lesions during high-resolution anal mapping with 9% acetic acid can prevent progression to cancer.

B. Anal canal tumors

   1. **Epidermoid carcinoma** is nonkeratinizing and derives from the anal canal up to 6 to 12 mm above the dentate line.

     a. **Epidermoid cancer** usually presents with an indurated, bleeding mass. On examination, the inguinal lymph nodes should be examined specifically because spread below the dentate line passes to the inguinal nodes. Diagnosis is made by biopsy, and 30% to 40% are metastatic at the time of diagnosis.

b. **Treatment** involves chemoradiation according to the **Nigro protocol:** 3,000-cGy external-beam radiation, mitomycin C, and 5-fluorouracil. Surgical treatment is reserved for locally persistent or recurrent disease only. The procedure of choice is abdominoperineal resection; perineal wound complications are frequent.

2. **Adenocarcinoma** is usually an extension of a low rectal cancer but may arise from anal glands and has a poor prognosis.

3. **Melanoma** accounts for 1% to 3% of anal cancers and is more common in the fifth and sixth decades of life. Symptoms include bleeding, pain, and a mass, and the diagnosis is often confused with that of a thrombosed hemorrhoid. At the time of diagnosis, 38% of patients have metastases. Treatment is wide local excision, although the 5-year survival rate is less than 20%.

INTESTINAL STOMAS

A. **Ileostomy** creation and care was revolutionized with the description of the eversion technique by **Brooke** in 1952. Eversion eliminates the serositis reaction commonly observed from the proteolytic ileal effluent. Another advance has occurred with the widespread employment of trained nurse enterostomal therapists to educate and care for patients with ostomies.

1. **Physiology.** The small intestine adapts to ileostomy formation within 10 days postoperatively, with ileostomy output typically reaching a plateau between 200 and 700 mL/day. Because the effluent is highly caustic, it is crucial to maintain a stoma appliance that protects the surrounding skin and seals to the base of the ileostomy.

2. **Stoma construction** of either a loop ileostomy or end-ileostomy should include eversion of the functioning end to create a 2.5-cm spigot configuration. Stoma creation lateral to the rectus abdominis increases the risk of peristomal herniation. Precise apposition of mucosa and skin prevents serositis and obstruction. Preoperative marking of the planned stoma prevents improper placement near bony prominences, belt/pant lines, abdominal creases, and scars.

3. **Ileostomy care** requires special attention to avoid dehydration and obstruction. The patient is encouraged to drink plenty of fluids and to use antidiarrheal agents as needed to decrease output volume. Patients should be warned to avoid fibrous foods, such as whole vegetables and citrus fruits because these may form a bolus of indigestible solid matter that can obstruct the stoma. Irrigating the stoma with 50 mL of warm saline from a Foley catheter inserted beneath the fascia, in combination with intravenous fluids and nasogastric decompression, may relieve obstruction and dehydration. Alternatively, water-soluble contrast enema may be diagnostic as well as therapeutic.

4. **Reversal** of a loop ileostomy is relatively straightforward and rarely requires laparotomy. A side-to-side, functional end-to-end technique with a GIA stapler is utilized. Alternatively, the enterostomy is closed with sutures in two layers.

B. The **colostomy** construction technique depends on whether the goal is decompression or diversion. Ongoing surveillance of the remaining colon is necessary but often overlooked in patients with colostomies.

1. A **decompressing loop colostomy** vents the distal and proximal bowel limbs while maintaining continuity between the limbs.

2. **Diverting colostomies,** such as loop end-colostomy, are used following distal resection or perforation so that the distal limb is diverted from the fecal stream. All colostomies are matured in the operating room. If a stoma rod is used, it is removed 1 week after surgery.

3. **Complications** of colostomies include necrosis, stricture, and herniation. If necrosis (seen on endoscopy performed at bedside) does not extend below the fascia, it can be observed safely; otherwise, urgent revision is performed. **Parastomal hernias** are repaired only if they prevent application of a stomal appliance or cause small-bowel obstruction; these can be approached locally, although definitive treatment generally entails relocation of the stoma to a different site. Laparoscopic parastomal hernia repair has also been described.

4. **Hartmann reversal** is not a trivial procedure, with a reported morbidity rate of 20% to 30% (bleeding, anastomotic leak, abscess) and a mortality rate of 3%. Tagging the rectal stump with long, nonabsorbable sutures, mobilizing the splenic flexure during the initial resection and placing preoperative ureteral stents can facilitate reanastomosis. Placement of adhesion barriers at the time of initial exploratory laparotomy may reduce adhesions enough to allow laparoscopic colostomy closure.

13 Pancreas

Jonathan B. Mitchem and David C. Linehan

The pancreas is an entirely **retroperitoneal** structure. It is divided into four regions: the head/uncinate, neck, body, and tail. The head of the pancreas abuts the C loop of the duodenum and extends obliquely to the neck, anterior to the mesenteric vessels and portal vein. The neck then extends laterally into the body, which is generally accepted to begin at the left border of the superior mesenteric vein (SMV), lying posterior to the stomach and anterior to the splenic vessels. The pancreas then culminates in the tail that is associated with the splenic hilum anterior to the left adrenal gland. The pancreas receives its blood supply from both the celiac trunk and the superior mesenteric artery (SMA). The arterial supply of the pancreatic head is provided by the **inferior pancreaticoduodenal arteries** (from the SMA) and the superior pancreaticoduodenal arteries (from the gastroduodenal artery). The tail receives its arterial supply from branches of the splenic artery. Venous drainage is primarily by the pancreaticoduodenal veins, which drain into the portal vein. The pancreas has two ducts: the main pancreatic duct, called the **Duct of Wirsung,** which arises in the tail and traverses the length of the pancreas to terminate at the **papilla of Vater** within the wall of the duodenum; and the **Duct of Santorini,** which is much smaller and arises from the lower part of the head, terminating separately at the **lesser papilla.**

BENIGN PANCREATIC DISEASE

I. **ACUTE PANCREATITIS** is an inflammatory process of variable severity. Approximately 80% of cases of acute pancreatitis are self-limited and associated with mild transitory symptoms that do not cause fulminant morbidity or mortality. By contrast, 20% of patients develop a severe form of acute pancreatitis that is associated with a mortality rate as high as 40% (*Nat Clin Pract Gastroenterol Hepatol.* 2005;2:473). The exact mechanism by which various etiologic factors induce acute pancreatitis is unclear. However, most agree that the initial insult is **unregulated activation of trypsin within pancreatic acinar cells,** leading to autodigestion and an inflammatory cascade that may progress to SIRS (*Lancet.* 2008;371(9607):143–152).

A. **Etiology.** The two most common causes of acute pancreatitis in the United States are **gallstones** and **alcoholism,** collectively accounting for nearly 80% of cases. Endoscopic retrograde cholangiopancreatography (ERCP) accounts for another 2% to 5% of cases. Other causes include the following:

1. **Drugs** (1% to 2%):
   a. **Class I** (>20 reported cases, with at least 1 re-exposure case): azathioprine, steroids, sulfamethoxazole–trimethoprim, furosemide, opiates, valproic acid.
   b. **Class II** (10 to 20 reported cases with or without reexposure): hydrochlorothiazide, enalapril, octreotide, cisplatin, carbamazepine.
   c. **Class III** (<10 reported cases): statins.

2. **Metabolic:** hypercalcemia, hypertriglyceridemia (especially types I and V).

3. **Toxins:** scorpion bite, organophosphates.

4. **Infectious diseases** (mumps; orchitis; coxsackie virus B; Epstein–Barr virus; cytomegalovirus; rubella; hepatitis A, B, non-A, non-B; *Ascaris* species; *Mycoplasma pneumonia; Legionella sp.; Salmonella sp.*).

5. **Neoplasm:** intraductal papillary mucinous neoplasm of the pancreas (IPMN), pancreatic adenocarcinoma, etc.

6. **Trauma.**

7. **Autoimmune:** Sjogren syndrome, systemic lupus erythematosus (SLE), primary biliary cirrhosis (PBC), primary sclerosing cholangitis (PSC).

8. **Idiopathic.**

B. Diagnosis

1. Patients typically present with **epigastric pain,** often radiating to the back. Tenderness is usually limited to the upper abdomen but may manifest signs of diffuse peritonitis in more advanced cases. Occasionally, irritation from intraperitoneal pancreatic enzymes results in impressive peritoneal signs, simulating other causes of an acute abdomen. Nausea, vomiting, and low-grade fever are common, as are tachycardia and hypotension secondary to hypovolemia. Asymptomatic hypoxemia, renal failure, hypocalcemia, and hyperglycemia are evidence of severe systemic effects. Flank ecchymosis **(Gray-Turner sign)** or periumbilical ecchymosis **(Cullen sign)** is almost always manifestations of severe pancreatitis and have been associated with a 40% mortality rate. However, these signs are present in only 1% to 3% of cases and do not usually develop until 48 hours after the onset of symptoms.

2. **Laboratory studies**

   a. **Serum amylase** is the most useful test. Levels rise within a few hours of the onset of symptoms and may return to normal over the following 3 to 5 days. Persistent elevations of levels for longer than 10 days indicate complications, such as pseudocyst formation. Normal levels may indicate resolution of acute pancreatitis; however, there is no correlation between amylase level and etiology, prognosis, or severity. In addition, hyperamylasemia can be found in a variety of other clinical conditions including renal failure, intestinal obstruction, appendicitis, gynecologic disorders, sialoadenitis, and malignancy.

   b. **Serum lipase** generally is considered more sensitive for pancreatic disease (95%), and remains elevated for a longer period of time, which can be useful in patients with a delayed presentation.

   c. **Acute phase proteins** such as C-reactive protein (CRP), tumor necrosis factor-alpha (TNF-a), and interleukin-6 (IL-6) may be measured as a marker of severity.

   d. **Serum calcium** levels may fall as a result of complexing with fatty acids (saponification) produced by activated lipases.

   e. **Hepatic function panel** [aspartate aminotransferase (AST), alanine aminotransferase (ALT), bilirubin, alkaline phosphatase] should be checked to assess for concomitant biliary disease, or as an etiology of pancreatitis (gallstone disease) although normal values do not rule out biliary etiologies.

3. **Radiologic imaging** complements clinical history and exam because no single modality provides a perfect diagnostic index of severity.

a. The specificity of **ultrasonography** (US) in pancreatitis can be greater than 95%, yet its sensitivity ranges between 62% and 95%, and both are highly user dependant. The pancreas is not visualized in up to 40% of patients due to overlying bowel gas and body habitus. The primary utility of US in acute pancreatitis is to evaluate for biliary etiology.

b. **Computed tomography (CT)** is superior to US in evaluating the pancreas. The sensitivity and specificity of CT are 90% and 100%, respectively. Iodinated contrast enhancement is essential to detect the presence of pancreatic necrosis. CT may also be helpful in differentiating acute pancreatitis from conditions such as malignancy, small-bowel obstruction, or acute cholecystitis. CT findings include parenchymal enlargement and edema, necrosis, blurring of fat planes, peripancreatic fluid collections, bowel distention, and mesenteric edema. CT imaging may be useful in predicting the severity and course of disease using the modified CT severity index (CTSI, see below, *Am J Roent.* 2004;183:1261–1265). Every patient with a presumed diagnosis of acute pancreatitis does not require a CT scan. In general, patients who warrant further imaging include those in whom the diagnosis is not conclusive, any severely ill patient in whom necrosis is more likely (only after aggressive resuscitation so as to diminish risk of contrast-associated nephropathy), and any patient who exhibits a deterioration in clinical course or fails to improve after 4 days of medical management.

c. **Magnetic resonance imaging (MRI)** is a useful substitute for CT scan in patients allergic to iodinated contrast or in acute renal failure with sensitivity 83% and specificity 91%. In addition, MRI/MR cholangiopancreatography (MRCP) is better than CT at visualizing cholelithiasis, choledocholithiasis, and anomalies of the pancreatic and common bile ducts.

4. **ERCP** is not routinely indicated for the evaluation of patients during an attack of acute pancreatitis, and is a subject of some controversy. **Indications for ERCP** are as follows:

a. **Preoperative evaluation** of patients with suspected traumatic pancreatitis to determine whether the pancreatic duct is disrupted.

b. Patients with **jaundice, suspected biliary pancreatitis, and possible cholangitis** who are not clinically improving by 24 hours after admission should undergo endoscopic sphincterotomy and stone extraction. However, the literature is clear that early endoscopic intervention for gallstone pancreatitis does not beneficially influence morbidity or mortality (*Ann Surg.* 2008;247(2):250–257).

c. **Patients older than age 40 years with no identifiable cause** to rule out occult common bile duct stones, pancreatic, or ampullary carcinoma or other causes of obstruction.

TABLE 13-1	Ranson Criteria

Admission

Age	>55 y
White blood cell count	>16,000/μL
Blood glucose	>200 mg/dL
Serum lactate dehydrogenase	>350 IU/L
Aspartate aminotransferase	>250 IU/L

Initial 48 hr

Hematocrit decrease	>10%
Blood urea nitrogen elevation	>5 mg/dL
Serum calcium	<8 mg/dL
Arterial Po_2	<60 mm Hg
Base deficit	>4 mEq/L
Estimated fluid sequestration	>6 L

Mortality	
Number of Ranson Signs	**Approximate Mortality (%)**
0–2	0
3–4	15
5–6	50
>6	70–90

    d. Patients younger than age 40 years who have had cholecystectomy or have experienced more than one attack of unexplained pancreatitis.

C. **Prognosis.** Because the associated mortality of fulminant acute pancreatitis approaches 40% and randomized studies have shown that early aggressive supportive care improves outcomes, attempts have been made to identify clinical parameters that predict patients at higher risk of developing severe outcomes.

    1. **Ranson criteria** (Table 13-1) constitute the most frequently utilized predictor of mortality associated with acute pancreatitis. The limitation of this assessment tool is that a score cannot be calculated until 48 hours after admission.

    2. **CTSI** is a prognostic scale based on CT findings, including peripancreatic fluid collections, fat inflammation, and extent of pancreatic necrosis was originally described by Balthazar et al. (*Radiology.* 1994;174:331–336) and then modified to a simpler model (*Am J Roent.* 2004;183:1261–1265). The usefulness of this criterion is limited to patients with normal renal function able to undergo contrast-enhanced CT, and by the fact that many patients with limited disease do not undergo CT imaging, potentially skewing study results (see Tables 13-2 and 13-3).

    3. The **Glasgow** scoring, like Ranson criteria, requires 48 hours to prognosticate patients and is based on clinical and laboratory values.

TABLE 13-2	CT Severity Grading Index (CTSI) Scoring Based on Imaging Characteristics

Scoring for Pancreatic Necrosis

0 Points	No pancreatic necrosis
2 Points	≤30% pancreatic necrosis
4 Points	>30% necrosis

Evaluation of Pancreatic Morphology, Not Including Necrosis

0 Points (grade A)	Normal pancreas
2 Points (grade B/C)	Focal or diffuse enlargement of the gland, including contour irregularities and inhomogeneous attenuation with or without peripancreatic inflammation
4 Points (grade D/E)	Pancreatic or peripancreatic fluid collection or peripancreatic fat necrosis
Additional 2 points	Extra pancreatic complications including one or more of the following: pleural effusion, ascites, vascular complications, parenchymal complications, or gastrointestinal tract involvement

4. The **Acute Physiology and Chronic Health Evaluation (APACHE) II** score was developed in 1985 for assessing critically ill patients and incorporates physiology, age, and chronic health. The major benefit of the APACHE II score is that it can be calculated at admission and updated daily to allow continual reassessment. However, the APACHE II score is somewhat cumbersome and difficult to calculate that limits its everyday use.

5. **Multiple Organ Dysfunction Score (MODS) and Sequential Organ Failure Assessment (SOFA)** have been shown to be important predictors of disease severity in critically ill patients and have been extended to patients with severe acute pancreatitis and are predictive of mortality and development of complications (*Br J Surg.* 2009; 96(2):137–150).

TABLE 13-3	Prognosis Based on CTSI Score	
Index	Predicted Morbidity	Predicted Mortality
0–3	8%	3%
4–6	35%	6%
7–10	92%	17%

D. Complications

1. **Necrotizing pancreatitis** occurs in about 10% to 20% of acute pancreatitis cases, and its presence correlates with prognosis (see CTSI above). It can be present at initial presentation or develop later in the clinical course. Necrosis is diagnosed on CT as failure to enhance with intravenous contrast.

2. **Infected pancreatic necrosis** occurs in 5% to 10% of cases and is associated with mortality as high as 80%, and is the cause of most late deaths (>14 days). Whether pancreatic necrosis visualized on CT scan is infected cannot be determined by imaging; however, some signs such as gas in the areas of necrosis can be suggestive. The gold standard for diagnosing infected pancreatic necrosis is fine needle aspiration (FNA), but this is rarely used in our practice, so infected pancreatic necrosis is more commonly a clinical diagnosis. Gram-negative organisms are more common than Gram-positive organisms (typically *Pseudomonas, Escherichia coli, Klebsiella, Proteus, Enterobacter*, and *Staphylococcus* species).

3. **Acute pseudocyst** (see Section V).

4. **Visceral pseudoaneurysm** is a rare complication in pancreatitis, but is most common among patients with necrotizing pancreatitis. Visceral pseudoaneurysm is believed to result from exposure of visceral arteries to the proteolytic pancreatic enzymes frequently extravasated during bouts of acute pancreatitis. The most common arteries involved are the splenic and left gastric arteries. Detection of pseudoaneurysms usually occurs 3 to 5 weeks following the onset of acute pancreatitis, but hemorrhage can occur at any time. A ruptured pseudoaneurysm can be a surgical emergency and often presents with signs and symptoms associated with upper gastrointestinal bleeding. Therapeutic angiography is the most appropriate first step in management as this can be both diagnostic and therapeutic (*Am J Surg*. 2005;190(3):489–495). For patients with lesions in the tail of the pancreas, distal pancreatectomy after stabilization may provide improved long-term hemorrhage control.

5. Because of the proximity of the splenic, superior mesenteric, and portal veins, **venous thrombosis** is not uncommon in patients with acute pancreatitis, and patients with severe disease are at higher risk. Although thromboses can be temporary, progression can lead to collateralization and gastroesophageal varices, but there is a low risk of bleeding (<10%) associated with venous thrombosis.

E. Treatment.
Many predictors of poor outcome in acute pancreatitis are associated with end-organ dysfunction, and end-organ failure is highly associated with poorer outcomes. Therefore, the initial approach to managing acute pancreatitis focuses on supporting patients with aggressive fluid resuscitation and close monitoring.

1. **Supportive care**
   a. **Volume resuscitation** with isotonic fluids is crucial; urinary output is monitored with a Foley catheter targeting greater than 0.5 mL/kg/hr. If patients do not respond to initial resuscitation appropriately, central venous monitoring (CVP) may help direct further

resuscitation. During the course of resuscitation, patients should be maintained on continuous pulse oximetry as patients often require large volume fluid resuscitation and frequent monitoring of electrolytes, including **calcium,** is mandatory (at least every 6 to 8 hours initially).

b. Gastric rest with nutritional support. Nasogastric decompression is performed to decrease neurohormonal stimulation of pancreatic secretion. Acute pancreatitis is a hypercatabolic state, and nutritional support has been shown to have a significant impact on outcomes in critically ill patients. Enteral feeding is generally preferred to parenteral nutrition. Early enteral feeding in patients with severe acute pancreatitis is associated with lower rates of infection, surgical intervention, and length of stay (*BMJ.* 2004;328:1407). An ongoing randomized clinical trial (RCT) to investigate further the benefits of early versus normal initiation of enteral feeding is open in the Netherlands (*Trials.* 2011;12(1):73).

c. Analgesics are required for pain relief.

d. Respiratory monitoring and arterial blood gases should be done at least every 12 hours for the first 3 days in severe pancreatitis to assess oxygenation and acid–base status. Hypoxemia is extremely common, even in mild cases of acute pancreatitis given the volume of fluid resuscitation and the potential for development of sympathetic effusions. Pulmonary complications occur in up to 50% of patients.

e. Antibiotics. The routine use of antibiotic prophylaxis in acute pancreatitis, especially in mild-to-moderate cases, is not supported in the literature. Conflicting data exist regarding antibiotics in severe cases, as there are small prospective, randomized trials demonstrating significantly lower rates of septic complications in patients receiving antibiotics (*Ann Surg.* 2006;243:154) and subsequent data from a RCT that found differences in infection or surgical intervention (*Ann Surg.* 2007;245:674). A recent meta-analysis demonstrated no difference in mortality, infected necrosis or overall infections with antibiotic therapy; however, most data is anecdotal and a large multi-institutional RCT may be indicated to further evaluate this issue (*Cochrane Database Syst Rev.* 2010 May 12;(5):CD002941). When infection is confirmed or suspected, patients should be treated with broad-spectrum systemic antibiotics that cover Gram-negative bacteria and, depending on length of hospitalization, common hospital-acquired pathogens, including fungal organisms, as super infection can be seen commonly.

2. Surgical treatment must be entertained for the small percentage of patients who continue to deteriorate despite aggressive supportive therapy. Although there is no clear consensus of the indications for operative intervention, most surgeons advocate operative intervention in the setting of severe systemic illness refractory to medical management, diagnostic uncertainty, or life-threatening complications unable to be treated via endoscopic or angiographic means (intra-abdominal hemorrhage, visceral perforation, etc). The long-held belief that patients with infected pancreatic necrosis must undergo surgery has become somewhat controversial, with some groups advocating an initial approach using percutaneous intervention and treating only those patients who fail to improve with surgical debridement (*NEJM.* 2010;362(16):1491–1502; *Br J Surg.* 2011;98(1):18–27). Additionally, patients with gallstone pancreatitis should undergo cholecystectomy as soon as medically feasible.

a. Wide debridement **(necrosectomy),** supplemented by either open packing or closed drainage, is the standard operative approach for managing infected necrotizing pancreatitis. At our institution, the preference is for wide debridement; drain placement and packing often with serial repeated debridement in the operating room. A positive correlation exists between repeated surgical interventions and morbidity, including fistula, gastric outlet obstruction, local bleeding, and incisional hernia. Marsupialization of the lesser sac allows rapid access to the pancreatic bed and can facilitate daily dressing changes (usually done in the intensive care unit).

b. **Pancreatic resection.** Because severe pancreatitis often leads to necrosis in large areas of the pancreas and peripancreatic fat, some have attempted to gain control of fulminant disease by resecting much or even the entire pancreas (partial or total pancreaticoduodenectomy, PD). Radical resection procedures place greater stress on already severely ill patients; PD or total pancreatectomy is associated with very high mortality and is not recommended in the acute setting.

c. **Gallstone-induced pancreatitis.** Ongoing choledocholithiasis is found in only 25% of biliary acute pancreatitis cases. Nonetheless, all patients with pancreatitis should be evaluated for the presence of gallstones because the etiology has specific therapeutic implications. Cholecystectomy should be carried out as soon as possible after recovery to prevent recurrent attacks of pancreatitis, as patients with biliary pancreatitis who do not undergo cholecystectomy have a 30% 6-week recurrence rate. During open or laparoscopic cholecystectomy, intraoperative cholangiography is recommended.

II. CHRONIC PANCREATITIS

A. **Etiology.** Alcohol (EtOH) abuse is the most common cause (70%); however, other etiologies include idiopathic, metabolic (hypercalcemia, hypertriglyceridemia, hypercholesterolemia, hyperparathyroidism), drugs, trauma, genetic (SPINK1, cystic fibrosis), and congenital abnormalities (sphincter of Oddi dysfunction or pancreas divisum). It also appears that tobacco abuse plays an important role in the development of chronic pancreatitis and particularly in patients with EtOH-related disease (*Arch Intern Med.* 2009;169:1035–1045). A history of recurrent acute pancreatitis (RAP) is present in some but not all patients with chronic pancreatitis.

B. **Pathophysiology.** Chronic pancreatitis is characterized by diffuse scarring and strictures in the pancreatic duct and commonly leads to endocrine or exocrine insufficiency, although substantial glandular destruction must occur before secretory function is lost. The islets of Langerhans have a greater resistance to injury than do the exocrine tissues; most patients who develop diabetes already have pancreatic exocrine insufficiency and steatorrhea. There are several theories to describe the pathogenesis of this disease; however, no consensus has been reached as to the specific inciting events (*Lancet.* 2011; Mar 10, epub ahead of print), and further work is necessary to discover the interplay between genetic, metabolic, immuno- logic, and structural factors in disease development.

C. **Diagnosis** is based on history and examination, complemented by appro- priate investigative studies. **Upper midepigastric pain radiating to the back** is the cardinal symptom and is present in 85 to 90% of cases, and becomes progressively worse over time. Changes in bowel habits and bloating are other common early symptoms, followed later by steatorrhea and diabetes as the disease progresses. Physical findings include weight loss relating to anorexia and malabsorption. Tenderness of the upper abdomen may be present. An enlarged pancreas is occasionally palpable, especially in a thin person, but a mass suggests the presence of a pseudocyst. Occasional findings include jaundice secondary to stricture of the common bile duct, enlarged spleen secondary to thrombosis of the splenic vein, or ascites sec- ondary to a pancreatic peritoneal fistula.

1. **Laboratory tests**
   a. **Amylase and lipase levels** are elevated in acute pancreatitis but rarely are useful in chronic pancreatitis and are **commonly normal** due to "burn out" of the pancreas.
   b. **Pancreatic secretin stimulation tests** have proven to be highly sensitive (90% to 100%) and specific (>90%) test for the diagnosis of chronic pancreatitis, and is considered the "gold-standard" of diagnosis of pancreatic insufficiency.
   c. **Pancreatic endocrine function.** Fasting and 2-hour postprandial blood glucose levels or glucose tolerance tests may be abnormal in 14% to 65% of patients with early chronic pancreatitis and in up to 90% of patients when calcifications are present.
   d. **A 72-hour fecal collection for estimation of daily fecal fat** is relatively simple and cheap, but plays a limited role in the definitive diagnosis of chronic pancreatitis as patients must have a high degree of pancreatic insufficiency to have a positive test.

2. **Radiologic studies**
   a. **Plain films** of the abdomen may show diffuse calcification of the pancreas in 30% to 40% of patients.
   b. **Ultrasound.** Transabdominal ultrasound is a noninvasive, cheap, and well-tolerated procedure but has low sensitivity and is subject to limitations related to user, body habitus, and overlying bowel gas, so plays a limited role in diagnosis of chronic pancreatitis.
   c. **CT** is 80% sensitive and 75% to 90% specific for the diagnosis of parenchymal or ductal disease. Common findings include ductal dilatation, calcifications, atrophy, and cystic lesions. CT is also use- ful to evaluate for mass lesions and sequelae of chronic pancreatitis.
   d. **MRI** is less sensitive than CT for detection of calcification. MR pancreatography is more sensitive in visualizing a dilated duct and strictures but loses sensitivity relative to ERCP in evaluating side

branch disease (i.e., small duct disease). MR pancreatography can be useful in patients whose postsurgical anatomy makes ERCP technically unfeasible. As technology improves, this may play a more important role.

e. **ERCP is the current gold standard imaging test** for the diagnosis of chronic pancreatitis (*Gut.* 1984;25:1107–1112) and correlates with pancreatic function. ERCP is also beneficial for evaluation of pancreatic mass lesions, cytology, delineation of ductal anatomy prior to surgery, and can be therapeutic. The characteristic character is a "chain of lakes" appearance of ductal anatomy. There are drawbacks, however, in that images must be interpreted by specialized individuals, and there is a 3% to 7% risk of causing acute pancreatitis.

f. **Endoscopic ultrasound (EUS).** EUS has come to play a more important role in the diagnosis of biliary disease. Criteria for the diagnosis of chronic pancreatitis based on EUS characteristics, referred to as the Rosemont criteria, have been proposed (*Gastrointest Endosc.* 2009;69(7):1251–1261); however, these criteria have yet to be validated in a multicenter trial and warrant further evaluation before acceptance as the new gold standard.

D. Complications

1. **Common bile duct obstruction** may result from transient obstruction from pancreatic inflammation and edema or from stricture of the intrapancreatic common bile duct. When present, **strictures** are often **long and smooth** (2 to 4 cm in length) and must be distinguished from pancreatic carcinoma.

2. **Duodenal obstruction** can occur due to acute pancreatic inflammation, chronic fibrotic reaction, pancreatic pseudocyst, or neoplasm.

3. **Pancreaticoenteric fistulas** result from spontaneous drainage of a pancreatic abscess cavity or pseudocyst into the stomach, duodenum, transverse colon, or biliary tract. They are often asymptomatic but may become infected or result in hemorrhage.

4. **Pancreaticopleural fistulas** often have communication from the distal duct traversing the esophageal hiatus.

5. **Pseudocyst** (see Section V.A).

6. **Splenic vein thrombosis** (see Section I.D.5).

7. **Pancreatic carcinoma.** Chronic pancreatitis has been suggested in some studies to increase the risk of pancreatic carcinoma by two- to threefold.

E. Treatment

1. **Medical management**

   a. **Malabsorption or steatorrhea.** Most patients will make improvement in steatorrhea and fat absorption with enzymatic supplementation. Additionally, there is some evidence that adequate oral pancreatic enzyme supplementation improves pain control.

   b. **Diabetes** initially is responsive to careful attention to overall good nutrition and dietary control; however, use of oral hypoglycemic agents or insulin therapy often is required. There is some propensity for hypoglycemic attacks, but diabetic ketoacidosis is rare.

   c. **Narcotics** are often required for pain relief. In selected patients, tricyclic antidepressants and gabapentin may be effective.

   d. **Abstinence** from alcohol results in improved pain control in approximately 50% of patients.

   e. **Cholecystokinin antagonists and somatostatin analogs** have been considered for treatment of chronic pancreatitis, but have yet to show improvements in pain control.

   f. **Tube thoracostomy or repeated paracentesis** may be required for pancreatic pleural effusions or pancreatic ascites. Approximately 40% to 65% of patients respond to nonsurgical management within 2 to 3 weeks.

2. **Endoscopic therapy.** Endoscopic sphincterotomy, stenting, stone retrieval, and lithotripsy have all been used with moderate success in the management of patients with ductal complications from chronic pancreatitis. There is no consensus on the usefulness of these interventions and further study is warranted. In addition to pancreatic-directed therapy, endoscopic celiac plexus block may improve symptoms in patients with severe pain. See Section V.A for the discussion of pancreatic pseudocysts.

3. **Surgical principles**
   a. **Indications for surgery.** By far the most common indication is unremitting pain, but others include the inability to rule out neoplasm and management of complications (pseudocyst, aneurysm, and fistula).

   b. **Choice of procedure.** The goals of surgical therapy are drainage and/or resection of the diseased pancreas to alleviate pain and complications associated with chronic pancreatitis. Procedures are classified as drainage, resectional, or a combination of both. Initially, drainage procedures were preferred due to the high morbidity and mortality associated with resection, as it is preferable for patients with low functioning glands to retain as much tissue as possible; however, drainage procedures are often only possible in patients with dilated ducts. As modern surgical techniques have developed, resection has become safer permitting the development of combination procedures (*Ann Surg.* 2010;251(1):18–32).

   c. **Drainage only procedures** at our institution are uncommon because of poor relief of symptoms postoperatively.

      (1) **Puestow** procedure includes a distal pancreatectomy with a distal pancreaticojejunostomy for drainage, with reported success in postoperative pain relief ranging between 61% and 90% (*Am J Surg.* 1987;153:207); success is strongly associated with a minimum duct size of 7 mm or greater, restricting this operation to a small number of patients (*Gastrointest Surg.* 1998;2:223). Because of poor results with the Puestow procedure, we more commonly use the Frey procedure (see below).

      (2) **Longitudinal side-to-side pancreaticojejunostomy (Partington-Rochelle)** is a modification of the Puestow procedure,

eliminating the distal pancreatectomy portion. This procedure, as with the Puestow, can provide effective symptom relief, but achieves consistent success best in patients with large, dilated ducts.

d. Combined duct drainage-resection

(1) The Beger procedure is a duodenum-preserving resection of a portion of the pancreatic head. This operation preserves a small amount of pancreatic tissue within the C-loop of the duodenum and also in front of the portal vein. The pancreas is then transected at the pancreatic neck. Reconstruction requires two pancreaticojejunostomies. A Roux jejunal loop is anastomosed to both the proximal (duodenal) stump and the larger distal stump of the remaining pancreas. This procedure has shown excellent long-term results in altering the course of disease, controlling pain and safety (*Ann Surg.* 1999;230(4):512–519); however, since pancreatic neck transaction is often impossible or unsafe, the Beger procedure is rarely performed at our institution.

(2) The Frey procedure is a modification of the Beger procedure consisting of a duodenum-sparing limited pancreatic head resection combined with a lateral pancreaticojejunostomy. In the Frey procedure, the pancreatic neck is not transected, but the pancreatic parenchyma is extensively cored out from the head to the extent of diseased segment distally. This is the most common procedure performed at our institution as postoperative morbidity has been shown to be lower in Frey patients than in those undergoing a pylorus-sparing Whipple procedure (19% vs. 53%). In addition, patient satisfaction indices were increased by 71% versus 43% in Whipple patients (*Ann Surg.* 1998;228:771).

e. Pancreatectomy

(1) PD (Whipple procedure) is indicated in cases in which the pancreatitis disproportionately involves the head of the pancreas, the pancreatic duct is of small diameter, or cancer cannot be ruled out in the head of the pancreas. For chronic pancreatitis, the pylorus-preserving technique is advocated. The use of vagotomy is controversial. For chronic pancreatitis, the Whipple has been shown to be inferior to both the Beger (*Int J Pancreatol.* 2000;27(2):131–142) and Frey (*Ann Surg.* 1998;228:771) procedures.

(2) Distal subtotal pancreatectomy is used for disease in the tail of the gland and in patients with previous ductal injury from blunt abdominal trauma with fracture of the pancreas and stenosis of the duct at the midbody level.

(3) Total pancreatectomy is performed only as a last resort in patients whose previous operations have failed and who appear to be capable of managing a pancreatic state. Some centers have combined this procedure with islet cell transplantation.

f. Celiac plexus block can be achieved surgically by either ganglionectomy or direct injection of sclerosing agents.

III. EXOCRINE PANCREATIC CANCER

A. **Incidence and epidemiology.** Pancreatic cancer is the fourth-leading cause of cancer-related mortality in the United States. Most patients have incurable disease at the time of diagnosis, and the overall 5-year survival is approximately 5%. The median age at diagnosis is 65 years (*Cancer Statistics.* 2010;60(5):277–300).

B. **Risk factors.** An increased risk of pancreatic cancer has been associated with smoking, alcoholism, family history, hereditary disorders [hereditary nonpolyposis colon cancer (HNPCC), von Hippel–Lindau disease (VHL), Peutz–Jeghers syndrome, familial breast cancer (BRCA2), familial atypical multiple mole melanoma (FAMMM)], and chronic pancreatitis. Inherited pancreatic cancers represent approximately 5% to 10% of all diagnoses of the disease.

C. **Pathology.** Approximately 90% of pancreatic carcinoma is ductal adenocarcinoma. Seventy percent of pancreatic cancers occur at the head, 20% in the body, and 10% in the tail. Other periampullary tumors, such as carcinomas of the distal bile duct, duodenum, and ampulla of Vater, are less common and constitute approximately one-third of resectable periampullary cancers.

D. **Diagnosis.** The symptoms associated with pancreas cancer are almost always gradual in onset and are nonspecific.

1. **History and examination.** Patients complain of dull midepigastric pain, malaise, nausea, fatigue, and weight loss. Classically, the report of new-onset "painless jaundice" is believed to be pancreas cancer until proven otherwise. Pruritus may accompany obstructive jaundice. If obstructive jaundice is present, patients will also note darkening of the urine and "light-colored" stools. New-onset diabetes within the year prior to diagnosis is found in 15% of patients with pancreatic cancer, but the correlation is yet unclear. *Trousseau sign* (migratory thrombophlebitis) has been associated with pancreas cancer.

2. **Laboratory tests.**
   a. Elevated serum bilirubin.
   b. Elevated alkaline phosphatase.
   c. Prolonged obstruction may lead to mild increase in AST and ALT.
   d. **Tumor markers. CA19-9** is a useful marker to follow in patients with elevated levels prior to initiation of therapy; however, it is often low in patients with resectable disease and can be elevated in nonmalignant biliary obstructive disease. CA19-9 levels pretreatment may also have some role in prognosis (*Cancer.* 2009;115(12):2630–2639). Carcinoembryonic antigen (**CEA**) is a common tumor marker in a variety of gastrointestinal malignances but has been found to be elevated in only 40% to 50% of patients with pancreas cancer.

3. **Radiologic studies**
   a. **Plain films** of the abdomen are of little benefit. **Chest X-ray** is used to screen for pulmonary metastasis.
   b. Pancreatic cancer on **CT** appears as hypoattenuating indistinct mass that distorts the normal architecture of the gland, often paired with findings of a dilated pancreatic or biliary ductal system (the

so-called "double-duct" sign). If there is pancreatic ductal obstruction, it is also possible that the remainder of the gland will be atrophied. CT imaging should be a fine-cut, "pancreatic protocol CT" including 3-phases (arterial, venous, and portal venous) and thin slices (≤3 mm) to allow for assessment of the relationship of the mass to vascular structures as this is crucial to determine resectability. The use of CT to determine resectable versus borderline resectable disease is imperative as some advocate borderline resectable disease is a marker of worse biology and that these patients should undergo neoadjuvant therapy. The CT criteria used to define resectability were recently outlined in an expert consensus statement (*Ann Surg Oncol.* 2009;16(7):1727–1733):

(1) **Local resectable disease:** no distant metastases; no radiographic evidence of SMV and portal vein abutment, distortion, tumor thrombus, or venous encasement; clear fat planes around the celiac axis, hepatic artery, and SMA.

(2) **Borderline resectable:** no distant metastases; venous involvement of SMV/portal vein demonstrating tumor abutment with or without impingement and narrowing of the lumen, encasement of the SMV/portal vein but without encasement of the nearby arteries, or short segment venous occlusion resulting from either tumor thrombus or encasement but with adequate vessel to allow for safe resection and reconstruction; Gastroduodenal artery encasement up to the hepatic artery with either short segment encasement or direct abutment of the hepatic artery, without extension to the celiac axis; tumor abutment of the SMA not to exceed greater than 180° of the vessel circumference.

(3) **Unresectable:** Distant metastases; major venous thrombosis of the SMV or portal vein for several centimeters; encasement of SMA, celiac axis, or hepatic artery.

c. **Positron emission tomography (PET)** is limited to investigating for occult metastatic disease and has limited utility in primary diagnosis. A relatively high false-positive rate has been reported in pancreatitis when evaluating the pancreas for the diagnosis of cancer.

d. **Percutaneous (CT- or US-guided) needle biopsies** have a limited role, and are used only in unresectable patients who cannot undergo EUS-guided biopsy. If the patient has a pancreatic mass with disseminated lesions (e.g., liver lesions), these may be more accessible for tissue sampling.

e. **EUS** and **ERCP** play an important role in patients in which a mass is not seen on CT, obtaining tissue diagnosis when necessary (e.g., to determine candidacy for neoadjuvant therapy). Additionally, ERCP can be performed for drainage of biliary obstruction; however, this plays a minimal role in the treatment of patients with resectable disease as it is clear that preoperative stenting increases postoperative complications (*NEJM.* 2010;362(2):129–137). Preoperative stenting should only be undertaken in patients with an anticipated prolonged time to surgery (significant liver dysfunction, other medical comorbidities, neoadjuvant therapy).

    f. MRI and MRCP have improved over time and can provide information similar to that in conventional CT; however, MR technology is not the same across institutions, which results in differential quality in imaging.

    g. Staging laparoscopy historically has been undertaken to diagnose disease unable to visualize on CT. We recommend staging laparoscopy in patients with pancreatic adenocarcinoma (*Ann Surg.* 2002;235(1):1–7).

E. Treatment

  1. Resection

    a. PD (Whipple procedure) consists of *en bloc* resection of the head of the pancreas, distal common bile duct, duodenum, jejunum, and gastric antrum. Pylorus-sparing PD has been advocated by some, but there are no data demonstrating improved survival or lower morbidity (*Cochrane Database Syst Rev.* 2011;2:CD006053). Extended lymphadenectomy, including nodes from the celiac axis to the iliac bifurcation and nodes from the portal vein and SMA, has not been shown to affect survival but does increase morbidity (*Surg Oncol Clin North Am.* 2007;16:157). There has been a sharp decline in morbidity and mortality in specialized centers, with a 30-day mortality of less than 5%.

    b. Distal pancreatectomy. The procedure of choice for lesions of the body and tail of the pancreas is distal pancreatectomy. Distal pancreatectomy consists of resection of the pancreas, generally at the SMV laterally to include the spleen. Currently, distal pancreatectomy is undergoing considerable study. Some groups have published similar survival rates for open and laparoscopic resections (*J Am Coll Surg.* 2010;210(5):779–785), but only a trend toward lower postoperative stay, leading to considerable discussion regarding the appropriate method of approach. Additionally, we have recently described a technique that provides a more radical resection with improved R0 resection rates, the radical antegrade modular pancreatosplenectomy (RAMPS), when compared to traditional series (*J Am Coll Surg.* 2007;204(2):244–249), which is the procedure of choice for malignant tumors of the distal pancreas at our institution.

  2. Postoperative considerations. Delayed gastric emptying, pancreatic fistula, and wound infection are the three most common complications of PD. Up to 10% of patients require a nasogastric tube for longer than 10 days, but delayed gastric emptying almost always subsides with conservative treatment. The rate of pancreatic fistula has been demonstrated to be reduced to less than 2% by meticulous attention to the blood supply of the pancreaticoenteric duct-to-mucosa anastomosis (*J Am Coll Surg.* 2002;194:746). Most surgeons routinely place abdominal drains, although there no consensus has been reached regarding the utility and there may be potential harm that warrants further study. Distal pancreatectomy has a higher morbidity and leak rates than PD with an approximately 20% pancreatic leak rate in most series;

however, this is usually amenable to percutaneous treatment, and distal pancreatectomy has a similar mortality to PD.

3. Radiotherapy and chemotherapy.

a. Neoadjuvant therapy. Some groups have shown an improvement in survival with neoadjuvant chemoradiation therapy (*J Clin Oncol.* 2008;26(21):3496–3502); however, this has yet to be validated in a RCT and is felt to be related to stage migration.

b. Adjuvant therapy. There is a clear benefit to adjuvant therapy in pancreatic cancer (*J Gastrointest Surg.* 2008;12(4):657–661); however, the choice between chemoradiation and chemotherapy is less clear as there are conflicting studies (*Lancet.* 2001;358(9293):1576–1585; *Cancer.* 1987;59:2006–2010). The role of radiation therapy in pancreatic cancer and what role clinic-pathologic factors may play in selecting patients for radiation therapy has yet to be fully elucidated.

4. Prognosis. Surgical resection increases survival over patients with similar stage disease that do not undergo resection. Overall 5-year survival rates are approximately 20% for patients after resection. In patients with small tumors, negative resection margins, and no evidence of nodal metastases, the 5-year survival rate is as high as 40%. Median survival for unresectable locally advanced disease is 9 to 12 months, and for hepatic metastatic disease it is 3 to 6 months.

F. Pseudotumors of the pancreas

1. Inflammatory and fibrosing conditions of the pancreas such as chronic pancreatitis or mycobacterial infection may form dense, fibrotic masses, and segmental fibrosis that are difficult to differentiate from carcinoma preoperatively. Additionally, given the lethality of pancreatic cancer, lesions where malignancy cannot be ruled out should be resected.

a. Lymphoplasmacytic sclerosing pancreatitis is often misdiagnosed as pancreatic cancer. Patients are typically young (30s to 50s) and may be associated with other autoimmune disorders (Sjogren's, ulcerative colitis, sclerosing cholangitis). When compared to patients with pancreatic cancer of all stages, these patients have increased levels of serum IgG4, which can aid in making this diagnosis (*Ann Surg Oncol.* 2008;15(4):1147–1154).

IV. CONGENITAL ABNORMALITIES

A. Failure of the ventral and dorsal pancreatic buds to fuse during the 6th week of development results in **pancreatic divisum.** In this condition, the normally minor duct of Santorini becomes the primary means of pancreatic drainage from the larger mass of pancreatic tissue. The condition is detected by either ERCP or MRCP, and the incidence is estimated to be as high 11% in autopsy studies, and there is the suggestion that this increases the risk of pancreatitis (*Gut.* 2011;Feb 15, epub ahead of print). Minor papilla endotherapy (MPE) may improve outcomes in patients with RAP, but has less of an effect on patients with chronic pancreatitis and often requires multiple interventions (*Gastrointest Endo.* 2008;68(4):667–673). Patients with severe symptomatic pancreas divisum may require surgical therapy.

B. Typical locations for **ectopic pancreatic tissues** include the stomach, duodenal or ileal wall, Meckel diverticulum, and umbilicus. Less common sites are the colon, appendix, gallbladder, omentum, and mesentery. Most ectopic pancreatic tissue is functional; islet tissue is most often present in the stomach and duodenum. Heterotopic pancreas may result in pyloric stenosis, disruption of peristalsis, peptic ulcers, or neoplasms.

C. Malrotation of the ventral primordium during the 5th week results in **annular pancreas:** a thin, flat band of normal pancreatic tissue surrounding the second part of the duodenum. The annular pancreas usually contains a duct that connects to the main pancreatic duct. Annular pancreas may cause duodenal obstruction and the treatment of choice is duodenoduodenostomy as opposed to resection for symptomatic patients.

V. CYSTIC DISEASES

A. **Pancreatic pseudocysts.** It is important to distinguish pseudocysts from tumors, cystic pancreatic neoplasms (CPN) and other fluid collections. An acute pancreatic fluid collection follows in approximately 25% of patients with acute pancreatitis. It is characterized by acute inflammation, cloudy fluid, a poorly defined cyst wall, and necrotic but sterile debris, and many resolve spontaneously. Pseudocysts differ from true cysts in that the have no epithelial lining. By definition, a fluid collection in the first 4 weeks is an *acute fluid collection;* after 4 weeks, it becomes an *acute pseudocyst.*

1. **Causes.** Pseudocysts develop after disruption of the pancreatic duct with or without proximal obstruction, usually occurring after an episode of acute pancreatitis. In children, most pseudocysts arise as a complication of blunt abdominal trauma.

2. **Diagnosis**
   a. **Clinical presentation.** The most common complaint is recurrent or persistent upper abdominal pain. Other symptoms include nausea, vomiting, early satiety, anorexia, weight loss, back pain, and jaundice. Physical examination may reveal upper abdominal tenderness, a mass. Occasionally, patients may present with rupture into the abdomen or fistula formation.
   b. **Laboratory tests**
      (1) **Amylase.** Serum concentrations are elevated in approximately one-half of cases.
      (2) **Liver function tests** occasionally are elevated and may be useful if biliary obstruction is suspected.
      (3) **Cystic fluid analysis** is discussed in Section V.B.2.
   c. **Radiologic studies**
      (1) **CT** is the radiographic study of choice for initial evaluation of pancreatic pseudocysts and is twice as sensitive as US in detection of pseudocysts. CT scan findings that determine prognosis include the following:
         (a) Pseudocysts **smaller than 4 cm** usually resolve spontaneously.
         (b) Pseudocysts with **wall calcifications** generally do not resolve.

      (c) Pseudocysts with **thick walls** are resistant to spontaneous resolution.

  (2) US detects approximately 85% of pseudocysts. Its use is limited by obesity and bowel gases, and is not able to delineate pancreatic and adjacent anatomy as well as CT, but it may be used in follow-up studies once a pseudocyst has been identified by CT scan.

  (3) MRI and MRCP can be useful to delineate ductal anatomy and are not associated with the risks of pancreatitis and infection with ERCP. MRCP is not as sensitive for small duct involvement as ERCP.

  d. ERCP allows for the determination of pancreatic duct anatomy and influences therapeutic intervention. Approximately one-half of pseudocysts have ductal abnormalities identified by ERCP, such as proximal obstruction, stricture, or communications with the pseudocyst. ERCP itself risks infection of a communicating pseudocyst.

3. Complications

  a. Infection is reported in 5% to 20% of pseudocysts and requires external drainage.

  b. Hemorrhage results from erosion into surrounding visceral vessels and occurs in approximately 7% of cases. The most common arteries are the splenic (45%), gastroduodenal (18%), and pancreaticoduodenal (18%) arteries. Immediate angiography has emerged as the initial treatment of choice.

  c. Obstruction. Compression can occur anywhere from the stomach to the colon. The arteriovenous system also can be subject to compression, including the vena caval and portal venous system. Hydronephrosis can result from obstruction of the ureters. Biliary obstruction can present as jaundice, cholangitis, and biliary cirrhosis.

  d. Rupture occurs in fewer than 3% of cases. Approximately one-half of patients can be treated nonsurgically, with total parenteral nutrition and symptomatic paracentesis or thoracentesis. Rupture is occasionally associated with severe abdominal pain and presents as a surgical emergency.

  e. Enteric fistula can occur spontaneously and usually results in resolution of the cyst.

4. Treatment depends on symptoms, age, pseudocyst size, and the presence of complications. **Pseudocysts smaller than 6 cm and present for less than 6 weeks have low complication rates.** The chance of spontaneous resolution after 6 weeks is low, and the risk of complications rises significantly after 6 weeks.

  a. Nonoperative. If the pseudocyst is new, asymptomatic, and without complications, the patient can be followed with serial CT scans or US to evaluate size and maturation.

  b. Percutaneous drainage can be considered for patients in whom the pseudocyst does not communicate with the pancreatic duct and for those who cannot tolerate surgery or endoscopy. External drainage is indicated when the pseudocyst is infected and without a mature wall. The results are variable, and the rate of complications (e.g., fistulas) may be high.

c. **Excision,** including resection is only performed in unusual settings including bleeding, systemic sepsis, and concern for malignancy.

d. **Internal drainage.** Cystoenteric drainage is the procedure of choice in uncomplicated pseudocysts requiring intervention. Drainage can be undertaken by either surgical or endoscopic means. Endoscopic cystogastrostomy or cystoduodenostomy has a 60% to 90% success rate, has been improved with improvements in EUS, and is the initial treatment of choice at our center. Endoscopic therapy also allows transsphincteric stenting in the case of duct-cyst communication. Characteristics that are relative contraindications to endoscopic drainage are high degree of necrotic debris and structural impediments (e.g., pseudoaneurysm). In the event drainage cannot be accomplished by endoscopic methods, surgical methods include Roux-en-Y cystojejunostomy, loop cystojejunostomy, cystogastrostomy, and cystoduodenostomy. A biopsy of the cyst wall should be obtained to rule out cystic neoplasm. At our institution, we favor the Roux-en-Y cystojejunostomy or cystogastrostomy in most patients.

B. **True pancreatic cysts**

1. **Serous cystadenoma** are benign lesions and are usually asymptomatic. Symptoms correlate with size (>4 cm). They are more common in women, are most commonly located in the head of the pancreas, and account for 30% of all CPNs. Lesions are characterized by cuboidal epithelial cells, nonviscous fluid and low CEA and amylase on cyst fluid analysis. Asymptomatic serous cystadenomas should not be resected.

2. **Mucinous cystic neoplasms (MCNs)** are considered premalignant lesions and account for approximately 50% of all CPNs. At presentation they are most likely to be asymptomatic, are twice as likely to present in women, and anatomically are more commonly located in the body or tail. The cystic lesions do not communicate with the pancreatic ductal system and are characterized by rests of ovarian stroma on pathologic analysis. A recent study showed invasive cancer in 17.5% of resected MCN, and this was associated with larger size (>4.0 cm) and advanced age (>55), indicating that noninvasive MCN are likely precursor lesions. Five-year survival was 100% for noninvasive MCN and 57% for patients with malignant lesions (*Ann Surg.* 2008;247(4):571–579). As there is a clear survival advantage for those patients who undergo resection prior to the development of invasive cancer, and it is felt that there is an adenoma-adenocarcinoma sequence, it is recommended that all patients with MCN undergo resection, although those with less risk of invasive cancer may undergo nonradical resection.

3. **IPMNs** account for 25% of all CPNs and have a slight male predominance. They can be symptomatic and do communicate with the pancreatic ductal system. Characteristics of IPMN on ERCP include diffuse gland involvement, ductal dilation and thick, viscous fluid within the cyst. **IPMN are separated into three subgroups based on ductal involvement: main duct, side branch, and mixed;** and therapy is

different depending on subgroup. Main duct IPMN carries a malignant potential, up to 50% in some series (*Ann Surg.* 2004;239(6):788–799) and require resection. Given the risk of carcinoma associated with main duct involvement, it is recommended that mixed-type IPMN also be resected. Side branch IPMN represents a more controversial topic with evolving guidelines for resection, as 70% of patients with pure side branch IPMN had no invasive component in the same series (*Ann Surg.* 2004;239(6):788–799). Currently accepted criteria for resection of side-branch IPMN include symptomatic, size greater than 3 cm, and mural nodules. High cyst fluid CA19-9 has also been shown to be predictive of malignancy. Patients with IPMN requiring resection should undergo a standard oncologic resection (Whipple or distal pancreatectomy). Currently, there are mixed thoughts regarding the role of margin status and extending resection in IPMN, as this is a multifocal disease. The current recommendation is to extend resection based on invasive component or high-grade dysplasia only, and should be tailored to clinical situation (*World J Gastrointest Surg.* 2010;2(10):352–358). Additionally, there is no defined role for adjuvant therapy in cases of invasive cancer (*HPB(Oxford).* 2010;12(7):447–455), but this topic warrants further study.

4. **Other rare CPNs** (remaining 10%) include cystadenocarcinoma, acinar cell cystadenocarcinoma, cystic choriocarcinoma, cystic teratoma, and angiomatous neoplasms. All lesions with carcinoma noted on preoperative biopsy or with a concern for malignancy should undergo resection if tolerated.

14 Surgical Diseases of the Liver

Matthew R. Porembka and William C. Chapman

SURGICAL ANATOMY OF THE LIVER

I. **ANATOMIC NOMENCLATURE.** The standardized nomenclature for hepatic anatomy and resection is based on divisions delineated by the arterial and biliary anatomy (Figure 14-1; *HPB.* 2000;2:333).

A. **Internal anatomy: first division.** The liver is divided into two almost equally sized *hemilivers.* The plane between the hemilivers is the *midplane* of the liver that runs from the gallbladder fossa to the inferior vena cava (IVC) (Cantlie's line). Each hemiliver is usually supplied by one hepatic arterial branch, one bile duct, and one portal vein. A resection of a hemiliver is termed a *hepatectomy* or *hemihepatectomy* (e.g., right hepatectomy).

B. **Internal anatomy: second division.** Further divisions of the liver are based on the internal course of the hepatic artery and bile duct. These structures retain a high order of bilateral symmetry, whereas the portal vein does not. Its asymmetry results from retained portions from the fetal circulation. The liver is thus divided into four nearly equal **sections:** the right anterior and posterior sections and the left medial and lateral sections. A vessel supplying a section is a sectional vessel (e.g., the right anterior sectional artery).

C. **Internal anatomy: third division.** The liver is further subdivided into **segments** numbered I to VIII. These are the same as originally described by Couinaud. Resection of a segment is termed a *segmentectomy.*

II. OPERATIVE CONDUCT

A. **Open liver resection.** Optimal exposure for major liver resection can be achieved with a bilateral subcostal incision, with a midline extension to the xiphoid process as needed ("Mercedes Benz" **incision**). The ipsilateral vascular pedicles are isolated. The hepatic vein(s) draining the part of the liver to be resected are similarly isolated. During transection, maintenance of a low central venous pressure (<5 mm Hg) and placement of the patient in the Trendelenburg position reduce blood loss. A small amount of positive end-expiratory pressure (5 cm H_2O) is used to prevent air embolism. Vascular control can be augmented by intermittent occlusion of all hepatic inflow **(Pringle maneuver)** or total vascular exclusion. Postoperatively, frequent blood sugar measurements should be obtained. Monitoring and supplementation of phosphorous levels is important to support liver regeneration. Hyperbilirubinemia is unusual but may occur and persist for

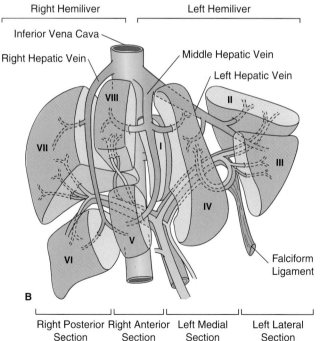

Figure 14-1. Anatomic divisions of the liver according to IHPBA/AHPBA-sanctioned terminology. Panel A depicts the segmental anatomy of the liver *in situ*. The first-order divisions (hemilivers), second-order divisions (sections), and third-order divisions (segments) are illustrated in Panel B. (From Greenfield's Surgery: Scientific Principles and Practice, LWW.)

days to weeks. Prolongation of the International Normalized Ratio (INR) may develop but usually is not severe; if necessary, fresh-frozen plasma is infused to keep the INR less than 2. Because of decreased clearance of hepatically metabolized drugs posthepatectomy, the dose of pain medications should be adjusted and monitored. The most common complication from liver resection is intra-abdominal abscess. Bile leaks from the cut surface of the liver or a damaged biliary duct may also occur. These manifest as a bile fistula or a *biloma,* a localized collection of bile. This can usually be managed by percutaneous drainage. Liver failure may result from insufficient residual functional hepatic parenchyma after extensive resections.

B. **Laparoscopic liver resection** has recently emerged as an option for hepatic resection. Types of minimally invasive resection can be classified as pure laparoscopic, hand-assisted, or hybrid procedures (which entail a combination of laparoscopic and open techniques). Although multiple case series have demonstrated similar mortality (0.3%) and morbidity (10.5%) for laparoscopic liver resection when compared to open procedures, no randomized controlled trial has compared both surgical approaches (*Ann Surg.* 2009;250(5):831–841). The learning curve is steep with these procedures with studies estimating 60 cases are required to develop proficiency (*Ann Surg.* 2009;250(5):772–782). Conversion to an open procedure occurs in about 4% of patients. Laparoscopic resection of malignant tumors (colorectal metastasis and hepatocellular carcinoma, HCC) has been demonstrated to be oncologically effective in carefully selected patients (*Ann Surg.* 2009;250(5):842–848; *Br J Surg.* 2009;96(9):1041–1048).

DISEASES OF THE LIVER

I. HEPATIC NEOPLASMS

A. Benign neoplasms of the liver

1. **Hemangioma is the most common benign liver tumor,** with the prevalence ranging from 3% to 20%. The majority are diagnosed in middle-aged women, and there is a female-to-male ratio of 5 to 6:1. The pathogenesis of hemangiomas is poorly understood. They are thought to represent hamartomatous outgrowths of endothelium rather than true neoplasms. Some of these tumors express estrogen receptors, and accelerated growth has been associated with high-estrogen states, such as puberty, pregnancy, and when oral contraceptives (OCPs) and androgens are used.

a. **Pathology.** Hemangiomas are usually less than 5 cm in diameter, but they can reach 20 cm or larger. Their blood supply is derived from the hepatic artery. Macroscopically, they are spherical, well circumscribed, soft, and easily compressible. Microscopically, the tumor consists of multiple large vascular channels lined by a single layer of endothelial cells supported by collagenous walls. Malignant degeneration does not occur, and spontaneous rupture is exceedingly rare.

b. Most hemangiomas are **asymptomatic** and are identified incidentally during imaging examinations for unrelated reasons. Patients with large lesions (>5 cm) occasionally complain of nonspecific abdominal symptoms such as upper abdominal fullness or vague abdominal pain. Intermittent symptoms may occur when there is necrosis, infarction, or thrombosis of the tumor. Life-threatening hemorrhage is extremely uncommon, even in large tumors, but can be precipitated by needle biopsy. **Kasabach–Merritt syndrome** is a rare consumptive coagulopathy resulting from sequestration of platelets and clotting factors in a giant hemangioma, and this is usually treated with urgent resection.

c. **Diagnosis.** Laboratory abnormalities are rare. Because of the possibility of severe hemorrhage from attempts at biopsy, diagnosis relies on imaging investigations. On ultrasound, hemangiomas appear as well-defined, lobulated, homogeneous, hyperechoic masses, although there may be hypoechoic regions representing hemorrhage, fibrosis, and/or calcification. Compressibility of the lesion is pathognomonic. Ultrasound is highly sensitive but not specific, with an estimated overall accuracy of 70% to 80%. Multiphasic (contrast) computed tomography (CT) scans reveal a low-density area with characteristic peripheral enhancement in the early phase. Subsequently, contrast enhancement progresses toward the center of the lesion until, in the delayed enhanced images, the tumor appears uniformly enhanced. The best imaging study is gadolinium-enhanced magnetic resonance imaging (MRI), with specificity and sensitivity approximately 90% and 95%, respectively. These tumors appear bright on T2-weighted images, with a similar pattern of enhancement as seen with multiphasic CT.

d. Most hemangiomas are treated safely with **observation.** Indications for intervention include symptoms, complications, and inability to exclude malignancy. In these select patients, the preferred treatment is surgical removal. Hemangiomas can usually be enucleated under vascular control (intermittent Pringle maneuver). Formal anatomic resection (e.g., right hepatectomy) is used when the tumor has largely replaced a distinct anatomic unit. Regression after low-dose radiation therapy or embolization in select cases has been described but should be reserved for large, unresectable lesions or for a patient unfit for surgery. In the very rare case of spontaneous hemorrhage, control with vascular embolization provides temporary help until a definitive operative approach can be safely implemented.

2. **Focal nodular hyperplasia (FNH)** is the second most common benign hepatic tumor, constituting about 8% of cases. The pathogenesis of FNH is a matter of debate. Currently, it is thought to represent a non-neoplastic, hyperplastic response to a congenital vascular malformation. FNH is found predominantly in women of child-bearing age, with a female-to-male ratio of 6 to 8:1. Although an association with OCPs has been suggested, the correlations are much lower than are those for hepatic adenomas (HAs).

a. **Pathology.** The lesions usually are solitary and small and often are located near the edge of the liver. Grossly, they are well circumscribed and lobulated but unencapsulated. Histologically, they are classically characterized by a dense, central stellate scar with septa radiating outward, thereby dividing the tumor into nodules. The parenchyma between the septa has the appearance of normal hepatic cords composed of hepatocytes, sinusoids, and Kupffer cells.

b. **Clinical manifestations** of FNH are rare. Epigastric or right-upper-quadrant pain with a palpable mass is present only in a small minority of patients. Spontaneous rupture with hemorrhage is extremely rare. Malignant degeneration has not been reported, but it is critical to distinguish FNH from the **fibrolamellar variant of HCC,** a malignant lesion that may have a similar central scar. It is important to note that the latter's scar is usually large and eccentric, with broad fibrous bands and calcifications.

c. **Diagnostic studies.** Although ultrasound is often the imaging study that first detects focal hepatic lesions, it does not discriminate FNH from other pathology well. FNH lesions have an echogenicity very similar to that of surrounding normal liver. However, distinguishing characteristics on multiphasic CT can be readily identified. In the late arterial phase, FNH has a bright homogeneous enhancement with a **hypodense central scar.** Delayed-phase images may show hyperattenuation of the central scar. Occasionally, the radiating septa may also be visualized. When MRI is employed, the central scar appears hyperintense on T2-weighted images, and when contrast is used, the enhancement pattern is similar to that seen on CT. Superparamagnetic iron oxide (SPIO) is an MR contrast agent that undergoes phagocytosis by the reticuloendothelial system (RES) (the Kupffer cells in the liver). On SPIO-enhanced T2-weighted images, FNH is hypointense but with a bright central scar. On hepatic scintigraphy with 99 m Tc-sulfur colloid, FNH has variable colloid uptake compared with the normal liver. However, intense colloid uptake (10% of cases, related to the number of Kupffer cells present) is a very specific finding for FNH. In combination, use of different imaging modalities, especially MRI, yields a precise diagnosis of FNH in 70% to 90% of cases. When the diagnosis remains in doubt, histologic examination is indicated.

d. **Treatment.** Elective resection is not indicated in asymptomatic patients when studies differentiate FNH from adenoma or malignant lesions. When the lesion is unresectable, it can be treated with transarterial embolization. OCPs should be stopped. There is no contraindication to pregnancy with this lesion, but close observation for tumor growth during pregnancy and the postpartum period is prudent.

3. **HA** is the benign proliferation of hepatocytes. It is not to be confused with the term "hepatoma," which refers to HCC. HA is found in young women and has a 10:1 female-to-male ratio. There is a strong association with all synthetic estrogen and progesterone preparations; however, the incidence has stabilized due to the decreased estrogen content found in OCPs. In addition, anabolic steroids may drive the growth of these lesions.

a. **Pathology.** Adenomas are usually solitary (70% to 80%), round, well-circumscribed lesions. Although they are unencapsulated, there is often a pseudocapsule formed by compression of normal surrounding tissue. Microscopically, they are made up of monotonous sheets of hepatocytes separated by dilated sinusoids. HA does not contain bile ductules, a key histologic finding distinguishing it from FNH where these are present.

b. HA is of clinical importance because of its tendency to **spontaneous rupture and hemorrhage.** The rate of rupture has been estimated between 25% and 35% with nearly 100% of all spontaneous ruptures occurring in lesions greater than 5 cm (*Ann Surg Oncol.* 2009;16(3):640–648). About one-third of patients with symptoms present with intraperitoneal bleeding, and others present with abdominal pain without rupture. More often, these lesions present with vague symptoms such as fullness or discomfort in the right upper quadrant or are detected incidentally. These lesions are potentially premalignant, with large or multiple tumors carrying a greater risk of malignant degeneration. Spontaneous rupture occurs more often in men, especially in steroid users. It may also occur during pregnancy due to rapid growth under the influence of estrogens.

c. **Diagnostic studies.** Ultrasonography can identify lesions but cannot differentiate an adenoma from a malignant lesion. Unlike FNH, HA frequently appears heterogeneous on CT due to intratumor hemorrhage, necrosis, and fat. On multiphasic CT, HA demonstrates **early enhancement,** often first in the periphery with centripetal progression. The relative lack of Kupffer cells in HA compared to FNH allows SPIO-enhanced MRI and scintigraphy with 99 m Tc-sulfur colloid to distinguish between these two entities.

d. Because of the risk of spontaneous rupture and malignant transformation, HA must be identified and treated promptly. Operative intervention after HA rupture is mandatory. Small (<5 cm), asymptomatic lesions occasionally regress with cessation of OCPs. Although radio frequency ablation (RFA) may be an option when there are multiple adenomas, resection of HA remains the standard therapy. **Indications** for operative intervention include the following:

(1) Patients with lesions that are 5 cm or greater in diameter.

(2) Tumors that do not shrink after discontinuation of OCPs.

(3) Patients who medically cannot stop OCP use with HA greater than 5 cm.

4. **Bile duct hamartomas** are the most common liver lesions seen at laparotomy. They are usually peripherally located and firm, smooth, and white in appearance. Typically, lesions are 1 to 5 mm in diameter, but they may be larger. Distinguishing them from miliary metastatic lesions (especially those from colorectal cancer or cholangiocarcinoma) may be difficult. Where there is uncertainty, biopsy should be performed.

B. **Malignant neoplasms of the liver** are either primary (such as HCC and cholangiocarcinoma) or secondary. The latter are far more common in Western countries.

1. **HCC, also known as hepatoma**

   a. **Demographics.** The annual incidence in the United States is approximately 2.4 per 100,000. The incidence is rising rapidly due in large part to the hepatitis C epidemic. There is a 2 to 3:1 male-to-female predominance. The incidence in African American men is almost twice that in white men. HCC is diagnosed mainly in the fifth and sixth decades.

   b. **Major risk factors** for cirrhosis in the United States include hepatitis C, alcohol abuse, autoimmune phenomena such as primary biliary cirrhosis and autoimmune hepatitis, and hereditary metabolic disorders. From 70% to 85% of HCC arises in the setting of cirrhosis. Malignant tumors of the liver occur in 4.5% of cirrhotic patients and in up to 10% when hemochromatosis is the inciting factor.

   c. **Pathology.** Gross patterns of HCC include the nodular type (aggregate of clusters of nodules), the massive type (single large mass), and the diffuse type (widespread fine nodular pattern). The right hemiliver is involved more frequently than the left. Microscopically, the formation of giant cells is a feature of HCC. HCC cells frequently invade venous branches (portal venous and hepatic venous), causing vascular dilation, which contributes to the nodular appearance of the liver.

   d. **Clinical manifestations.** Eighty percent of patients experience weight loss and weakness. Approximately 50% have abdominal pain that is dull, persistent, and occurs in the epigastrium or right upper quadrant. Acute severe abdominal pain infrequently has been associated with intraperitoneal hemorrhage due to rupture of a necrotic nodule or erosion of a blood vessel.

   e. **Diagnostic studies**

      (1) In cirrhotic patients, HCC may be associated with abnormal liver function tests due to hepatitis. Elevated **serum α-fetoprotein** (AFP) occurs in 75% of affected African patients but in only 30% of patients in the United States. AFP is also often elevated in chronic hepatitis and cirrhosis. A level greater than 200 ng/mL (normal <20 ng/mL) is suggestive of HCC, even in the cirrhotic patient.

      (2) **Radiologic studies**

         (a) **Ultrasonography** can be highly accurate in the detection of HCC, especially when coupled with concomitant AFP elevations.

         (b) **MR scan** can be useful in differentiating other small nodular masses from HCC. This is the most accurate imaging modality for distinguishing HCC from dysplastic or regenerative nodules in the cirrhotic patient.

         (c) **Multiphasic CT scan** with arterial and portal venous phase contrast imaging can distinguish among different types of liver masses. **HCC enhances in the arterial**

and not usually in the portal venous phase. Washout of contrast in the delayed (portal venous) phases of enhancement is an additional characteristic of HCC. Washout is defined as hypointensity of a nodule in the delayed phase compared with surrounding liver parenchyma. A mass in a cirrhotic liver that manifests arterial enhancement with washout has a sensitivity of about 80% with specificity of 95% to 100%.

(3) When required, laparoscopic or image-guided percutaneous biopsies may be used to obtain a tissue diagnosis. However, **a tissue diagnosis is *not* required before therapeutic intervention** (including surgical resection and liver transplantation) if other diagnostic modalities favor HCC as the diagnosis. Unresectable tumors likewise usually do not require biopsy to confirm the diagnosis because imaging and laboratory studies allow a definitive diagnosis in the majority of cases.

f. **Staging.** Several staging systems for HCC have been proposed. The most commonly used in the United States is the AJCC TNM (tumor, nodes, and metastases) classification. The individual TNM stages are grouped into overall stages: T1 to T4 with N0M0 correspond to stages I, II, IIIA, and IIIB, respectively, whereas N1M0 with any T stage is stage IIIC, and M1 disease is designated stage IV. Another commonly used system is the American Liver Tumor Study Group (ALTSG) staging system; this system uses a modified TNM staging system that provides T staging according to nodule size and number and is used as the basis for liver transplantation in patients with HCC. Other liver cancer staging systems like the Barcelona Clinic Liver Cancer (BCLC) system, the Cancer of the Liver Italian Program (CLIP) system, and the Okuda system expand on the TNM system by including tumor extent and assessment of liver function.

g. **Treatment**

(1) **Surgical resection** with anatomic resection is the treatment of choice for noncirrhotic patients who have HCC. However, this constitutes only 5% of HCC patients in the United States and up to 40% of those in Asian countries. A macroscopic margin of 1 cm generally is regarded as adequate. Overall 5-year survival rates for patients with HCC treated with resection is 40% to 50%, with recurrence rates of around 40% to 50%. The most important predictors of recurrence are microvascular invasion and multinodular tumors. Repeat hepatic resection for recurrence has been demonstrated to be safe and effective in selected lesions.

(2) **Orthotopic liver transplantation (OLT)** is theoretically the best treatment option for HCC because it removes the tumor together with the entire diseased liver, thus eliminating the risk of *de novo* or recurrent disease. Initial results of OLT for HCC were dismal. However, Mazzaferro and colleagues (*N Engl J Med.* 1996;334:693) demonstrated that when OLT is restricted to patients with a single tumor 5 cm or less or

patients with up to three tumors with the largest less than 3 cm in size (with no vascular invasion on imaging and absence of nodal and distant metastases), the 4-year actuarial survival rate was 75%, with recurrence-free survival of 83%. These so-called "Milan criteria" have subsequently been adopted by the United Network for Organ Sharing (UNOS). Recent reports (*Ann Surg*. 2008;248(4):617–625) suggest that even more-advanced stage III patients who are downstaged with pretransplant therapy have results similar to those with stages I and II HCC.

(3) **Local ablation** is the best treatment option for patients who have early-stage HCC and are not suitable for resection or OLT. In addition, these therapies may serve as bridges to OLT for those on the transplant waiting list. Indeed, downstaging tumors improve survival of HCC patients who subsequently undergo OLT. Today ablation is most frequently accomplished by physical ablation (radio frequency, microwave, or cryoablation) or with transarterial approaches. **RFA** has emerged as the procedure of choice in most centers. A needle electrode is placed into the tumor, destroying tissue by heating it to temperatures of 60°C to 100°C. RFA may be performed intraoperatively or percutaneously under imaging guidance. Extendable electrodes within the needle allow larger tumors to be ablated compared to ethanol injection, as well as allow the specific volume of tissue for ablation to be varied. **Transarterial chemoembolization (TACE)** involves selective intra-arterial administration of chemotherapeutic agents followed by embolization of the major tumor artery. HCC preferentially derives its blood supply from the hepatic artery rather than from a combination of the hepatic artery and portal vein as for normal hepatic parenchyma. TACE has a survival benefit for select patients with unresectable tumors, Child class A cirrhosis and tumors less than 5 cm. The procedure rarely may be complicated by hepatic failure due to infarction of adjacent normal liver. For this reason, it should not be used in decompensated (Child class C) cirrhosis.

(4) **Systemic chemotherapy and external beam radiation** have had poor results. Chemotherapy with conventional cytotoxic agents is ineffective and does not seem to modify the natural history of disease. Recent identification of signaling pathways in HCC has resulted in the development of drugs directed at specific therapeutic targets. One such drug is Sorafenib, a kinase inhibitor with antiangiogenic and antiproliferative properties that has shown modest efficacy in patients with advanced HCC. Toxicity may lead to decompensation of liver disease. Combining chemotherapy with surgical resection preoperatively or postoperatively has no benefit in terms of patient survival.

h. Without treatment, HCC has a very poor prognosis, with a median length of survival of 3 to 6 months after the diagnosis.

i. **Fibrolamellar hepatocellular carcinoma (FLC)** is a rare histologic variant of HCC. However, there is considerable evidence that FLC is distinct from HCC in its epidemiology, biology, and prognosis. Males and females are equally affected, commonly at a younger age (20 to 40 years old). It is uncommon for FLC to be associated with underlying liver disease such as cirrhosis. The histology of FLC strongly resembles that of focal nodular hyperplasia, but any etiologic association between them remains unproven. FLC appears as a hypoattenuated, well-defined, solitary mass on nonenhanced CT scan. On contrast-enhanced CT, the cellular portion enhances homogeneously; the central scar usually does not enhance, unlike the scar of FNH. FLC is best treated with complete surgical resection, which is possible in 80% of patients. Compared with standard HCC, FLC is associated with a better prognosis: Patients with resectable FLC have a greater 5-year survival rate (>70%) than noncirrhotic patients who have resectable nonfibrolamellar HCC. Late recurrence is common (more than two thirds of cases), and repeat resection of local disease should be considered (*Cancer.* 2006;106:1331). Liver transplantation is an option for unresectable but nonmetastatic lesions.

2. **Metastatic disease to the liver** represents the most common malignancy of the liver in the United States. The liver is a common site of metastasis from gastrointestinal (GI) cancers because it is the first organ drainage site of venous blood from the GI tract.

a. **Colorectal cancer metastatic to the liver** is the prototype disease treated by partial hepatectomy. Approximately 50% of all patients with colorectal cancer develop metastases, and of these, about one-third have disease limited to the liver. Without treatment, hepatic metastasis has a dismal prognosis, with a median survival of 6 to 12 months. In contrast, numerous studies have shown that resection of hepatic metastases is associated with a 25% to 45% 5-year survival rate and a 20% 10-year survival rate. As a result, operative resection has been established as the most effective therapy for patients with isolated colorectal liver metastases.

(1) **Staging.** The purpose of preoperative evaluation is to exclude the presence of extrahepatic disease and to identify all the metastatic lesions in the liver that require treatment. An abdominal/pelvic CT scan with oral and intravenous contrast is performed, along with chest X-ray. There should be a colonoscopy within the last 6 months to document absence of anastomotic recurrence or a metachronous colorectal cancer. Whole-body positron emission tomography (PET) after administration of ^{18}F-fluorodeoxyglucose (FDG) is valuable for the detection of occult metastases, both intra- and extrahepatic. On MRI, hepatic metastases appear as low-intensity lesions on T1-weighted images and intermediate intensity on T2-weighted images. MRI also provides greater visualization of vascular structures such as the hepatic veins and the IVC.

(2) **Partial hepatectomy.** The main objective in the resection of colorectal metastasis is removal of all disease with gross negative margins. Formal anatomic resection has not been demonstrated to improve survival (*Ann Surg Oncol.* 2009;16(2):379–384). Resection type should be based on the number and location of tumors, rather than on segmental anatomy. In the case of synchronous liver metastasis, the primary colonic tumor and the secondary liver tumor may be resected simultaneously or sequentially. Combined resection avoids a second laparotomy and reduces the overall complication rate without changing operative mortality. When the colorectal and liver resections are both extensive (e.g., extended hepatic lobectomy and low anterior resection), then a staged approach may be preferable. Factors predictive of poor prognosis after resection of hepatic colorectal metastases include node positivity of the primary tumor, multiple metastases, and size of the largest metastasis greater than 5 cm. An emphasis on the preservation of hepatic parenchyma may be of increasing importance in the setting of chemotherapy-associated steatohepatitis, and the growing number of patients undergoing repeated metastasectomy.

(3) **Postoperative follow-up** consists of serial physical examination, serum CEA level, and abdominal/pelvic CT scans every 3 to 4 months for the first 2 years, then every 6 months for the subsequent 3 years. Unfortunately, disease recurrence is common, but when cancer is isolated to the liver, repeat resection can provide additional survival benefit.

(4) For **unresectable hepatic colorectal metastases,** multidrug systemic chemotherapy (e.g., oxaliplatin plus infusional 5-fluorouracil/leucovorin, also known as FOLFOX) with or without bevacizumab, an anti-VEGF antibody, is offered to patients with adequate performance status. Hepatic arterial infusion (HAI) of the 5-fluorouracil derivative fluorodeoxyuridine (FUDR) has not been shown to offer better survival than systemic therapy, but may have greater response rates.

(5) **Local ablation** with RFA should be considered in patients unfit for operative resection or who have unresectable disease. In those patients with multiple scattered tumors, a combined approach of resection of the dominant or larger tumors with RFA of the remaining lesions may be feasible.

b. **Other liver metastases**

(1) **GI neuroendocrine tumors.** There are a number of reasons supporting resection of neuroendocrine hepatic metastases. These include their relatively long tumor doubling time, lack of effective chemotherapy, and the ability of metastasectomy to provide symptom palliation and long-term survival. For those patients with unresectable disease, hepatic artery embolization may provide symptom relief.

(2) There is limited experience with liver resection for **noncolorectal and nonneuroendocrine metastasis.** Liver resection may

provide the only chance for long-term survival. In a study at Memorial Sloan-Kettering Cancer Center of 96 patients with noncolorectal, nonneuroendocrine metastatic tumors of the liver, liver resection was associated with an overall actuarial survival of 37% at 5 years, with a median survival of 32 months (*Surgery.* 1997;121:625). The presence of liver metastasis from melanoma or cancer of the breast or stomach should be viewed as a marker of disseminated disease, and liver resection in these contexts is not recommended (*Annu Rev Med.* 2005;56:139).

II. **HEPATIC ABSCESS.** Liver abscesses may originate from bacterial, parasitic, or fungal pathogens. Bacterial abscesses predominate in the United States, whereas amebic (parasitic) abscesses are more common in younger age groups and in endemic areas.

A. **Pyogenic abscesses** in the liver occur secondary to other sources of bacterial sepsis. Up to 60% of cases arise from direct spread of bacteria from biliary infections such as empyema of the gallbladder or cholangitis. Ruptured appendicitis or diverticulitis is other potential sources for bacterial seeding to the liver.

1. **Pathogenesis.** For liver abscesses arising from an intra-abdominal infection, it is important to note that hematogenous seeding is *not* the usual pathway for the development of the abscess; rather, the mechanism of spread of infection to the liver is along channels within the peritoneal cavity. For unknown reasons, liver abscesses are usually found in the right lobe of the liver.

2. **Microbiology.** The bacteria cultured from pyogenic liver abscesses reflect the origin of the infectious process. Most commonly, **mixed species** are isolated, with one-third of cultures containing anaerobes. When the biliary tree is the source, enteric Gram-negative bacilli and enterococci are common isolates. When the abscess develops from hematogenous seeding, there is most likely a single organism responsible, such as *Staphylococcus aureus* or *Streptococcus milleri.* Fungal abscesses have been associated with patients who are recovering from chemotherapy. There should be suspicion of amebic abscesses in patients who are from or have recently traveled to an endemic area in the last 6 months.

3. **Fever and abdominal pain** are the most common symptoms, whereas nonspecific symptoms such as anorexia, weight loss, chills, and malaise may also be present.

4. **Laboratory findings** are usually nonspecific, such as leukocytosis and elevated serum alkaline phosphatase. A chest X-ray may demonstrate new elevation of the right hemidiaphragm, an infiltrate at the right lung base, or a right-sided pleural effusion. Definitive diagnosis is by CT scanning.

5. Treatment consists in identifying the infectious source as well as managing the liver abscess. **Pyogenic liver abscesses require drainage and systemic antibiotic therapy.** Drainage can be performed percutaneously in

most cases, but an operative procedure is recommended when there are multiple, large, loculated abscesses and in patients who otherwise require laparotomy for the underlying cause of the abscess. Drains are usually left in place until drainage becomes minimal, typically 7 days. Empirical antibiotic treatment should include coverage for bowel flora (e.g., metronidazole plus ciprofloxacin or monotherapy with piperacillin/tazobactam). Once identification has been made of the causative organism(s), antibiotic therapy should be modified to reflect their sensitivities. Aggressive antibiotic therapy should continue for at least 1 week beyond clinical recovery and resolution of the abscess on follow-up imaging.

B. **Amebic abscess** should be considered in *every* case of solitary hepatic abscess. Amebiasis is caused by the protozoan *Entamoeba histolytica*. This parasite exists in two forms: an infective cyst stage and a trophozoite stage, which is the form that causes invasive disease. Amebic liver abscess is the most common extraintestinal manifestation of amebiasis. Infection occurs by hematogenous spread from the gut via the portal venous system.

1. **Epidemiology.** Amebic liver abscesses are 7 to 10 times more frequent in adult men, despite an equal sex distribution of intestinal amebic disease. An abscess can develop after travel exposures of just 4 days.

2. Clinical symptoms are classically **persistent fever and right-upper-quadrant pain.** The presence of diarrhea (reflecting concurrent intestinal amebiasis) is more variable. Presentation usually occurs with 4 months after return from endemic areas. On examination, patients have hepatomegaly and point tenderness over the liver. Rupture of the abscess may cause peritonitis.

3. **Diagnosis.** Serologic tests for amebic infestation are positive in nearly 100% of affected patients. Ultrasound and CT are the most useful imaging modalities.

4. Treatment requires systemic **metronidazole** (750 mg orally three times a day, or 500 mg intravenously every 6 hours, for 7 to 10 days). Needle aspiration should be considered if there is no response to initial therapy or if there is doubt about the diagnosis. The material aspirated contains proteinaceous debris and an "anchovy paste" fluid of necrotic hepatocytes. After completion of the course of metronidazole, the patient should be treated with an intraluminal agent, even if stools are negative for amebae. Intraluminal agents include paromomycin, iodoquinol, and diloxanide furoate. Complications can include bacterial superinfection, erosion into surrounding structures, or free rupture into the peritoneal cavity. Although mortality is infrequent in uncomplicated cases, complicated cases may carry a considerable mortality (as high as 20%).

III. **HEPATIC CYSTS** can be divided into nonparasitic cysts and echinococcal cysts.

A. **Nonparasitic cysts** generally are benign. They can be solitary or multiple and often are identified incidentally on imaging for other symptoms.

1. Asymptomatic cysts require no treatment regardless of size. Large cysts may be symptomatic because of increased abdominal girth or compression of adjacent structures. Bleeding, infection, or obstructive jaundice can occur but are infrequent.

2. Symptomatic cysts can be unroofed operatively by either an open approach or, more recently, by laparoscopy. Infected cysts are treated in a similar manner to hepatic abscesses. If the cyst contains bile, communication with the biliary tree is assumed. It should be excised, enucleated, or drained, with closure of the biliary communication.

3. Polycystic kidney disease sometimes is accompanied by **polycystic liver disease,** which usually is asymptomatic. Symptoms generally are attributable to hepatomegaly from numerous cysts. Liver function is rarely impaired by the gross displacement of parenchyma by these massive cystic cavities. Symptomatic polycystic liver disease has been treated by drainage of the superficial cysts into the abdominal cavity and fenestration of deeper cysts into the superficial cyst cavities. Liver resection and retention of the least-cystic areas of hepatic parenchyma may be more effective. Neoplastic cystic lesions such as cystadenoma or cystadenocarcinoma rarely occur in the liver. These lesions are distinguished from simple cysts by the presence of a mass or septa. They are treated by resection or enucleation (in the case of cystadenoma) to completely remove cyst epithelium.

B. **Echinococcal cysts** are the most common hepatic cystic lesions in areas outside the United States. Approximately 80% of hydatid cysts are single and in the right liver. The most common presenting symptoms and signs are right-upper-quadrant abdominal pain and palpable hepatomegaly. Imaging by nuclear medicine scan, ultrasonography, CT scan, or MR scan can demonstrate the abnormality. The **cyst should not be aspirated** as an initial test because aspiration can cause spillage of the organisms and spread the disease throughout the abdominal compartment. A peripheral **eosinophilia** is often detected. Serologic tests include indirect hemagglutination and Casoni skin test, each of which is 85% sensitive. **Treatment** is primarily operative consisting of cyst aspiration, scolicidal treatment (hypertonic saline, 80% alcohol, or 0.5% cetrimide), and pericystectomy. Formal hepatectomy is rarely necessary except for large and/or multiple cysts. Postoperative therapy with mebendazole or albendazole has been advocated to prevent recurrence. Percutaneous treatment after antihelminthic treatment is increasingly utilized for treatment with acceptable results.

IV. **PORTAL HYPERTENSION (PH)** is defined as a chronic increase in portal pressure due to mechanical obstruction of the portal venous system. It is an almost unavoidable consequence of cirrhosis and is responsible for many of the lethal complications of chronic liver disease, including bleeding from gastroesophageal varices, ascites, and hepatic encephalopathy (HE).

A. The most common cause of PH in the United States is *intrahepatic* obstruction of portal venous flow from **cirrhosis** (most commonly due to alcohol and/or hepatitis C); intrahepatic portal venous obstruction can also be due to hepatic fibrosis from hemochromatosis, Wilson disease, and congenital fibrosis. *Prehepatic* portal venous obstruction due to congenital atresia or portal vein thrombosis is far less common. Posthepatic obstruction may occur at any level between the liver and the right heart. This includes thrombosis of the hepatic veins (Budd–Chiari syndrome), congenital IVC malformations (web, diaphragm), IVC thrombosis, and constrictive pericarditis.

B. **The clinical manifestations of liver disease with PH result from hepatic insufficiency and the mechanical effects of portal venous hypertension.**

1. **HE** is the spectrum of neuropsychiatric abnormalities in patients with advanced chronic liver disease. It results from portosystemic shunting of neurotoxins usually cleared by the liver. In addition to the usual signs of severe hepatic dysfunction (jaundice, ascites, spider telangiectasias, etc.), manifestations characteristic of encephalopathy include disrupted sleep–wake cycles (insomnia and hypersomnia), asterixis, and hyperreflexia. There are a number of conditions that can precipitate HE, including hypovolemia, hypoxia, GI bleeding, electrolyte and acid–base disorders, sedatives, hypoglycemia, and infection. An elevated ammonia level is the best-described neurotoxin associated with HE, but other agents not adequately cleared by the diseased liver have also been implicated, such as γ-aminobutyric acid, mercaptans, and short-chain fatty acids. HE is a clinical diagnosis, and the utility of measuring ammonia levels remains controversial. Treatment is directed at the precipitating cause and reduction in ammoniagenic substrates using lactulose, with second-line therapy including oral antibiotics such as neomycin and rifaximin.

2. **Portosystemic shunting.** Increased blood flow through the portal vein leads to increased flow through collateral venous beds that bypass the liver, thereby connecting the portal circulation directly to the systemic circulation. The most clinically significant sites are those at the gastroesophageal junction connecting the left gastric vein (a part of the portal circulation) to the esophageal veins (systemic circulation). Other common collaterals develop when a recanalized umbilical vein collateralizes to the abdominal wall veins or a superior hemorrhoidal vein collateralizes to middle and inferior hemorrhoidal veins. Left-sided **(sinistral)** PH can be caused by isolated splenic vein thrombosis. This is most often caused by adjacent pancreatitis. Thrombosis results in increased pressure in the splenic vein at the distal end of the pancreas and the development of collaterals through the short gastric vessels and gastric mucosa back to the liver. This segmental area of PH typically causes gastric varices without esophageal varices.

3. The **mechanisms of ascites and edema** are salt and water retention by the kidneys, decreased plasma oncotic pressure, and increased lymphatic flow from increased portal venous hydrostatic pressure. Although the ascites can be massive, it is rarely life-threatening unless complications occur, such as erosion or incarceration of an umbilical hernia, respiratory compromise, and spontaneous bacterial peritonitis (SBP). The diagnosis of SBP is made by paracentesis and is likely when

ascitic fluid contains more than 250 polymorphonuclear leukocytes per microliter and if a single organism is cultured. The most common organisms are *Escherichia coli,* pneumococci, and streptococci. Frequently, however, it is not possible to obtain a positive culture, and so the diagnosis relies on ascitic fluid cell count and differential.

C. **Diagnosis.** Formal measurement of portal pressure by catheterization of the portal vein is seldom performed. Indirect evaluation by measurement of the hepatic wedge pressure after hepatic vein catheterization is considered the gold standard for diagnosis and monitoring PH. The hepatic venous pressure gradient (HVPG) is the difference between the wedged and free hepatic venous pressures. **PH is considered present when the HPVG is 8 mm Hg or greater.** Varices do not develop until the HVPG reaches 10 to 12 mm Hg. Reduction in the HVPG below 12 mm Hg is accepted as the therapeutic target for treating PH.

D. **Management of PH**

1. **Prophylaxis of variceal bleeding** includes both the prevention of variceal hemorrhage in patients who have never bled (primary prophylaxis) and preventing rebleeding in patients who have survived a bleeding episode (secondary prophylaxis). Every cirrhotic patient should be screened endoscopically for varices at time of diagnosis. Those without varices at this time should have endoscopy repeated after 2 to 3 years, whereas monitoring every 1 to 2 years is recommended when varices are present. **Propranolol** or nadolol therapy has been shown to markedly reduce risk of variceal bleeding, as well as slow the progression of small varices into larger ones. The dose should be titrated to the maximal tolerable dose and maintained indefinitely. For prevention of recurrent bleeding, endoscopic band ligation versus combination pharmacologic therapy (beta-blocker plus isosorbide mononitrate) have equivalent results. Transjugular intrahepatic portosystemic shunting **(TIPS)** has been shown to be superior to either endoscopic or pharmacologic therapies at reducing the rate of rebleeding. However, its use does not improve mortality, has been associated with a greater risk of encephalopathy, and is more costly than endoscopic procedures. Thus, it is limited to situations in which endoscopic therapy has failed or in patients who would not tolerate a rebleed such as those with Child class C cirrhosis (*Eur J Gastroenterol Hepatol.* 2006;18:1167).

2. **Management of active variceal hemorrhage.** Up to one-third of patients with hemorrhage from gastroesophageal varices die during the initial hospitalization for GI bleeding. All patients with known or suspected esophageal varices and active GI bleeding should be admitted immediately to an intensive care unit for resuscitation and monitoring. Endotracheal intubation to protect the airway, prevent aspiration, and facilitate the safe performance of endoscopy and other procedures is nearly always indicated. Vascular access via short, large-bore peripheral lines should be secured. Recombinant activated factor VII (rFVIIa) may be useful for correcting the prothrombin time in cirrhotics. Infection is a strong prognostic indicator in acute variceal hemorrhage, and use of antibiotics has been shown to reduce both the risk of rebleeding

and mortality. Once stabilized, the patient should have emergent upper endoscopy to document the source of hemorrhage. Because up to 50% of patients with known esophageal varices have upper GI hemorrhage from an alternative source, such as a gastric or duodenal ulcer, a thorough endoscopy is required. Recommendations for specific therapy are (1) early administration of vasoactive drugs, even if active bleeding is only suspected, and (2) endoscopic band ligation after initial resuscitation.

a. The pharmacologic treatment of choice for active variceal bleeding in the United States is **octreotide** (intravenous bolus, then infusion for 5 days). It has been shown to be more effective for controlling bleeding than placebo or vasopressin, as well as have fewer side effects than vasopressin. Terlipressin is not available in the United States but is the only pharmacologic treatment associated with a reduction in mortality.

b. **Endoscopic therapy** is the definitive therapy for active variceal hemorrhage. Two forms of treatment are available: sclerotherapy and variceal band ligation (EBL). A meta-analysis found that EBL is superior to sclerotherapy in the initial control of bleeding and is associated with fewer adverse events and improved mortality (*Semin Liver Dis.* 1999;19:439). Emergent endoscopic therapy fails to control bleeding in 10% to 20% of patients. If a second attempt at endoscopic hemostasis fails, then more definitive therapy must be enacted immediately.

c. **Balloon tamponade** is useful as a temporary remedy for severe variceal bleeding while more definitive therapy is planned. The specially designed balloon catheters include the Sengstaken-Blakemore tube, the Minnesota tube, and the Linton-Nachlas tube. Each has a gastric balloon; the Sengstaken-Blakemore and Minnesota tubes also have an esophageal balloon. For safe and effective use of these devices, the balloons must be carefully placed according to the manufacturer's directions. The position of the gastric balloon in the stomach must always be confirmed radiographically before inflation because inflation of the larger gastric balloon in the esophagus can be disastrous. The pressure of the esophageal balloon must be maintained as directed by the manufacturer to avoid the complications of mucosal ulceration and necrosis. Balloon tamponade achieves bleeding control in 60% to 90% of cases, but should be used only when there is massive bleeding and for a short period of time (<24 hours) until definitive therapy is instituted.

d. **TIPS** can be used in the acute management of patients with variceal bleeding. It involves the intrahepatic placement of a stent between branches of the hepatic and portal venous circulation. Technical success rates approach 95%, with short-term success in controlling acute variceal hemorrhage observed in more than 80% of patients. The TIPS procedure can provide acute decompression of portal pressure and thus control refractory variceal bleeding. TIPS stenosis requires careful follow-up and revision procedures in a significant percentage of patients. Use of polytetrafluoroethylene (PTFE) stents rather than bare metal stents has dramatically decreased the rate of TIPS dysfunction, clinical relapses, and the need for interventions.

e. **Emergency portacaval shunt** generally is reserved for patients in whom other measures have failed and is almost never performed today. This operation carries significant in-hospital mortality and risk of HE, particularly because the patients undergoing the operation typically have failed other measures and have advanced liver disease. Only the technically simpler central portacaval shunts (end to side or side to side) should be used in the emergency setting because other shunts require more dissection and operative time.

3. **Management of ascites** must be gradual to avoid sudden changes in systemic volume status that can precipitate HE, renal failure, or death.

   a. **Salt restriction** is the initial treatment. Sodium intake should be limited to 1,000 mg/day. Stricter limitations are unpalatable.

   b. **Diuretic therapy** should be gradually applied in patients in whom ascites is not controlled by salt restriction. Weight loss should rarely be more than 500 g/day to avoid significant side effects. **Spironol-actone** is the initial diuretic of choice at 25 mg orally twice per day. This dose may be increased to a maximum of 400 mg/day in divided doses. Furosemide (20 mg orally/day initially) may be added if spironolactone fails to initiate diuresis. Volume status must be monitored closely by daily weight check and frequent examinations during initial furosemide treatment.

   c. **Paracentesis** is useful in the initial evaluation of ascites, when SBP is included in the differential diagnosis, and to provide acute decompression of tense ascites. Up to 10 L of ascites can be removed safely if the patient has peripheral edema, the fluid is removed over 30 to 90 minutes, and oral fluid restriction is instituted to avoid hyponatremia. Paracentesis can be used to provide acute relief of symptoms of tense ascites, including respiratory compromise, impending peritoneal rupture through an ulcerated umbilical hernia, or severe abdominal discomfort.

   d. **TIPS** can be used for refractory ascites. Complete resolution of ascites has been reported in 57% to 74% of patients and partial response in another 9% to 22%.

   e. A **peritoneovenous shunt,** which reinfuses ascites into the vascular space, is now rarely used for ascites refractory to medical therapy. The main complication of peritoneal venous shunting is disseminated intravascular coagulation, which can be fulminant after shunt placement and requires shunt occlusion. Shunts are **contraindicated** in patients with bacterial peritonitis, recent variceal hemorrhage, liver failure, advanced hepatorenal syndrome, or existing severe coagulopathy. The shunts tend to occlude with time and are used very rarely today.

4. **Control of HE** requires the limitation of dietary protein intake and the use of lactulose and oral antibiotics.

   a. **Dietary changes** should be initiated first. Dietary protein should be eliminated while adequate nonprotein calories are administered. After clinical improvement, a 20-g/day protein diet may be administered, with increasing protein allowances of 10 g/day every 3 to 5 days if encephalopathy does not recur.

b. If the encephalopathy is not controlled by diet alone, oral agents can be added.

  (1) Lactulose is a nonabsorbed synthetic disaccharide that produces an osmotic diarrhea, thus altering intestinal flora. The oral dosage is 15 to 45 mL two to four times a day. The dose then is adjusted to produce two to three soft stools daily. Alternatively, a lactulose enema can be prepared with 300 mL of lactulose and 700 mL of tap water administered two to four times a day.

  (2) Useful oral antibiotic preparations include neomycin (1 g orally every 4 to 6 hours or 1% retention enema every 6 to 12 hours) and metronidazole (250 mg orally every 8 hours). The oral antibiotics are used as second-line agents to lactulose because, although they are equally effective, neomycin carries some risk of ototoxicity and nephrotoxicity, and metronidazole carries some risk of neurotoxicity.

15 Biliary Surgery

Marcus C.B. Tan and Steven M. Strasberg

I. CHOLELITHIASIS

A. The **incidence** of cholelithiasis increases with age. At the age of 60 years, approximately 25% of women and 12% of men in the United States have gallstones. In some countries (e.g., Sweden and Chile) and ethnic groups (e.g., Pima Indians), the incidence of gallstones may approach 50%.

B. **Pathogenesis and natural history.** Patients can be divided into three clinical stages: asymptomatic, symptomatic, and those with complications of cholelithiasis. There is generally a stepwise progression from stage to stage. Annually, only 1% to 2% of those with asymptomatic disease progress to the symptomatic stage. It is unusual (<0.5% per year) for an asymptomatic patient to develop complicated gallstone disease without first suffering symptoms.

1. **Cholesterol gallstones** (85% of stones, radiolucent) are associated with increasing age, obesity, female gender, and Western diet. The female-to-male ratio is 2:1, and the increased incidence among women is in part related to pregnancy and/or oral contraceptive use. Obesity is an independent risk factor, increasing the prevalence of cholesterol gallstones by a factor of 3. Western diet is closely related, and these stones are rare in vegetarians.

2. **Pigment gallstones** (15% of stones, radiopaque, two distinct types):
   a. **Black gallstones** are hard, spiculated, and brittle, and are composed of calcium bilirubinate, calcium phosphate, and calcium carbonate. Risk factors include hemolytic disorders, cirrhosis, and ileal resection.
   b. **Brown gallstones** are soft, associated with biliary stasis and infection (especially *Klebsiella* species), and are composed of bacterial cell bodies, calcium bilirubinate, and calcium palmitate.

C. Asymptomatic gallstones
1. **Diagnosis.** Asymptomatic gallstones are usually discovered on routine imaging studies or incidentally at laparotomy for unrelated problems. Common abdominal symptoms such as dyspepsia, bloating, eructation, or flatulence *without associated pain* are probably not caused by gallstones.

2. **Management.** There is no role for prophylactic cholecystectomy in most patients with asymptomatic gallstones, with a few exceptions.
   a. Patients with a **porcelain gallbladder** should undergo cholecystectomy due to a high risk of malignancy. Prophylactic cholecystectomy may be warranted in patients with asymptomatic gallstones who have other risk factors for gallbladder cancer as outlined in Section VI.C.1.

b. **Children with gallstones** have a relative indication for cholecystectomy due to the general difficulty of declaring and interpreting symptoms in this population.

c. In adult patients with **diabetes mellitus, spinal cord trauma,** and **sickle cell anemia,** prophylactic cholecystectomy is generally *not* indicated for *asymptomatic* or uncomplicated gallstone disease. Even after cholecystectomy, sickle cell patients may still develop bile duct stones.

d. Management of **gallstones discovered at laparotomy** remains controversial because the literature is conflicting with regard to the incidence of biliary symptoms after surgery in patients in whom the gallbladder is not removed.

D. **Symptomatic gallstones (biliary colic)**

1. **Diagnosis** largely depends on correlating symptoms with the presence of stones on imaging. Differential diagnosis includes acute cholecystitis, liver diseases, peptic ulcer disease, renal colic, gastroesophageal reflux, irritable bowel syndrome, and diseases based in the chest, including inferior wall myocardial ischemia/infarct or right-lower-lobe pneumonia. Appropriate testing is dictated by clinical suspicion of these entities.

a. **Symptoms.** Biliary colic is the main symptom and is initiated by impaction of a gallstone in the outlet of the gallbladder, as characterized by the following:

(1) **Periodicity.** The pain comes in distinct attacks lasting 30 minutes to several hours.

(2) **Location.** The pain occurs in the epigastrium or right upper quadrant.

(3) **Severity.** The pain is steady and intense and may cause the patient to restrict breathing. Frequently, it is so severe that immediate care is sought and narcotics are necessary for control.

(4) **Timing.** The pain occurs within hours of eating a meal, often awakening the patient from sleep.

(5) **Other symptoms** include back pain, left-upper-quadrant pain, nausea, and vomiting. These *usually* occur in addition to, rather than in place of, the pain as described.

b. **Physical signs** include mild right-upper-quadrant tenderness, although there may be few abdominal findings during an attack. Jaundice is not caused by impaction of a stone in the cystic duct without inflammation. If jaundice is present, another cause should be sought.

c. **Diagnostic imaging.** Ultrasound diagnosis is based on the presence of echogenic structures having posterior acoustic shadows. There is usually little or no associated gallbladder wall thickening or other evidence of cholecystitis. The bile ducts must be assessed for evidence of dilation or choledocholithiasis (gallstones in the common bile duct, CBD).

2. **Laparoscopic cholecystectomy (LC)** is the appropriate treatment of the vast majority of patients with symptomatic gallstones (see Section I.F.1).

E. **Complications of cholelithiasis**

1. **Acute calculous cholecystitis** is initiated by obstruction of the cystic duct by an impacted gallstone. Persistence of stone impaction leads to inflammation of the gallbladder. Although the onset and character of the resulting pain resemble those of biliary colic, the pain is unremitting. Severe complications include empyema, gangrene, or contained or free gallbladder perforation. Abscess formation may develop in some cases.

   a. **Diagnosis** depends on the constellation of symptoms and signs and the demonstration of characteristic findings with diagnostic imaging.

      (1) The **symptoms** of acute cholecystitis are similar to but more severe and persistent than those of biliary colic. As the inflammatory process spreads to the parietal peritoneum, tenderness develops in the right upper quadrant or even more diffusely, and movement becomes painful. Systemic complaints such as anorexia, nausea, and vomiting are common. Fever may or may not be present. Elderly patients tend to have mild symptoms and may present only with reduced food intake. **Murphy's sign** (inspiratory arrest during deep palpation of the right upper quadrant) is characteristic of acute cholecystitis and is most informative when the acute inflammation has subsided and direct tenderness is absent. Mild jaundice may be present, but severe jaundice is rare and suggests the presence of CBD stones, cholangitis, or obstruction of the CBD caused by external compression from a stone impacted in an inflamed Hartmann's pouch **(Mirizzi syndrome).**

      (2) **Laboratory abnormalities** may include leukocytosis (typically 12,000 to 15,000 cells/μL), although often the white blood cell count is normal. Complications, such as gangrene, perforation, or cholangitis, are suggested by an extremely high white blood cell count (>20,000 cells/μL). Liver function tests (LFTs), including serum bilirubin, alkaline phosphatase, alanine transaminase (ALT), aspartate transaminase (AST), and serum amylase, also may be abnormal.

      (3) **Diagnostic imaging**

         (a) **Ultrasonography** is the most commonly used test for diagnosing acute cholecystitis and any associated cholelithiasis. Findings indicative of acute cholecystitis include gallbladder wall thickening, pericholecystic fluid, and a **sonographic Murphy sign** (tenderness over the gallbladder when compressed by the ultrasound probe). In one meta-analysis, the sensitivity and specificity of ultrasonography for diagnosing gallstones were 0.84 and 0.99, respectively. For the diagnosis of acute cholecystitis, the sensitivity was 0.88 and the specificity was 0.80 (*Arch Int Med.* 1994;154:2573).

         (b) **Radionuclide cholescintigraphy** can be useful as an adjunct in the diagnosis of acute cholecystitis; although its sensitivity and specificity for gallstones are lower than those for ultrasound. Scintigraphic scanning with hepatic 2,6-dimethyliminodiacetic acid (HIDA) enables visualization of the biliary system. The radionuclide is concentrated and secreted by the liver, allowing visualization of the bile ducts and the gallbladder normally within 30 minutes. Since the test depends on hepatic excretion of bile, it may not be useful in jaundiced patients. Nonfilling of the gallbladder after 4 hours is deemed evidence of acute cholecystitis. Administration of morphine may enhance the test by causing spasm of the sphincter of Oddi and thereby stimulating gallbladder filling.

(c) **Computed tomographic (CT) scanning** is now frequently performed to evaluate the patient with acute abdominal pain. CT can demonstrate gallstones, although it is less sensitive for these than ultrasonography. Other signs of acute cholecystitis on CT include gallbladder wall thickening, pericholecystic fluid, edema, and emphysematous cholecystitis (air in the gallbladder wall).

b. **Management**

(1) **Initial management** for patients with acute cholecystitis includes hospitalization, intravenous (IV) fluid resuscitation, and parenteral antibiotics (e.g., piperacillin/tazobactam). Separate coverage for enterococci is not necessary because they are rarely the solitary pathogen.

(2) The **Tokyo guidelines** (*J Hepatobiliary Pancreat Surg.* 2007; 14:91) provide further recommendations depending on the severity of acute cholecystitis (see Table 15-1). For mild acute

TABLE 15-1	Severity Grading for Acute Cholecystitis (According to the Tokyo Guidelines)
Grade	Criteria
Mild (grade 1)	Acute cholecystitis that does not meet the criteria for a more severe grade Mild gallbladder inflammation, no organ dysfunction
Moderate (grade 2)	The presence of one or more of the following: – Leucocytosis >18,000 cells per cubic millimeter – Palpable tender mass in the right upper quadrant – Duration >72 hr – Marked local inflammation including biliary peritonitis, pericholecystitis abscess, hepatic abscess, gangrenous cholecystitis, emphysematous cholecystitis
Severe (grade 3)	Presence of multiorgan dysfunction (e.g., hypotension, mental status changes, respiratory failure, and acute renal failure)

Miura F, Takada T, Kawarada Y, et al: Flowcharts from the diagnosis and treatment of acute cholangitis and cholecystitis: Tokyo Guidelines. Modified from *J Hepatobiliary Pancreat Surg.* 2007;14:78.

cholecystitis, early LC is recommended. For moderate acute cholecystitis, either early or delayed cholecystectomy may be performed. Early LC should be performed only by an experienced surgeon with conversion to open cholecystostomy if operative conditions make identification of critical structures difficult. In the small minority of patients with severe acute cholecystitis or with severe concomitant medical illness, **percutaneous cholecystostomy** can be performed. Drainage of the gallbladder in this manner almost always allows the episode of acute cholecystitis to resolve. Subsequently, the patient can undergo either cholecystectomy or percutaneous stone extraction and removal of the cholecystostomy tube. Such nonoperative stone removal as definitive treatment is reasonable in very elderly or debilitated patients who cannot tolerate general anesthetic.

(3) **Several prospective, randomized trials** have compared early versus delayed (6 weeks) LC for acute cholecystitis. Five recent meta-analyses of the existing literature showed no significant differences in early versus delayed procedures with regard to mortality, conversion rate, bile duct injury, and perioperative complications. However, these studies almost universally showed, in the early group, significantly fewer readmissions for interval complications (due to failure of conservative therapy in ~20% of patients) and a significantly reduced hospital length of stay (*Br J Surg.* 2010;97:141; *Cochrane Database Syst Rev.* 2006;4:CD005440; *Surg Endosc.* 2006;20:82; *Surg Today.* 2005;35:553; *Am J Gastroenterol.* 2004;99:147). Nonetheless, controversy still exists about the relationship between operation in the acute phase of inflammation and bile duct injury. A large registry series from Connecticut reported that when LC is performed for acute cholecystitis, the incidence of injury is three times higher (0.51%) than for elective LC and twice as high as for open cholecystectomy (*Arch Surg.* 1996;131:382).

2. **Choledocholithiasis** generally is due to gallstones that originate in the gallbladder and pass through the cystic duct into the common duct. In Western countries, stones rarely originate in the hepatic or common ducts, although these "primary" stones, usually brown pigment stones, are more prevalent in Asia.

a. **Diagnosis.** The most common manifestation of uncomplicated choledocholithiasis is **jaundice,** with bilirubin typically between 3 and 10 mg/dL. Biliary colic is common. The only finding on physical examination may be icterus. Ultrasonography usually demonstrates gallbladder stones and bile duct dilation. Because of obscuring gas in the duodenum, ductal stones are visible in only about 50% of cases. The diagnosis may be confirmed by endoscopic retrograde cholangiopancreatography (ERCP) or percutaneous transhepatic cholangiography (PTC), which can opacify the biliary tree and demonstrate the intraductal stones. Occasionally, the diagnosis of choledocholithiasis is confirmed by intraoperative cholangiography (IOC) at the time of cholecystectomy.

b. **Management** depends on available expertise and clinical situation.

   (1) In patients with choledocholithiasis who also have cholelithiasis, standard management consists of LC and IOC, possibly followed by laparoscopic CBD exploration if stones are seen. Intraoperative measures to clear the CBD of stones include administration of IV glucagon, use of irrigation, blind passage of balloon catheters or stone baskets, or passage of these devices via choledochoscope. If the bile duct cannot be cleared of stones by laparoscopic exploration, open bile duct exploration or postoperative ERCP may be required, but this is uncommon.

   (2) In some cases, choledocholithiasis should be handled by ERCP or PTC. **ERCP with sphincterotomy and stone removal** is used in patients who are not surgical candidates or have had prior cholecystectomy. It is also used in patients who are jaundiced (these patients may have tumors as opposed to choledocholithiasis), including all patients with acute cholangitis. Patients with intrahepatic stones and those with many CBD stones are also usually treated with ERCP. ERCP with sphincterotomy carries a less than 1% risk of mortality and a 5% to 10% risk of morbidity, principally acute pancreatitis. An intraoperative cholangiogram should be performed at the time of surgery even when preoperative ERCP has been done because residual stones may be present in a small percentage of patients.

3. **Biliary pancreatitis** is caused by blockage of pancreatic secretions by passage of a gallstone into the common biliary-pancreatic channel. The greatest risk is carried by small (~2 mm) stones. Once the acute episode of pancreatitis has resolved, the gallbladder should be removed as expeditiously as possible to avoid recurrent pancreatitis. A longer delay may be justified in patients who have had severe pancreatitis and in whom local inflammation or systemic illness contraindicates surgery. An IOC should *always* be done at the time of the cholecystectomy to confirm that the bile duct is free of stones. In patients in whom cholecystectomy is contraindicated, endoscopic sphincterotomy (ES) may be protective against further attacks of pancreatitis.

4. **Cholangitis is often caused by choledocholithiasis (see Section II.B).**

5. **Gallstone ileus (bowel obstruction caused by a gallstone)** is an uncommon complication that results from a gallstone eroding through the wall of the gallbladder into the adjacent bowel (usually duodenum). Usually the stone migrates until it lodges in the narrowest portion of the small bowel, just proximal to the ileocecal valve. Patients present with symptoms of bowel obstruction and air in the biliary tree (from the cholecystenteric fistula). Treatment is exploratory laparotomy and removal of the obstructing gallstone by milking it back to an enterotomy made in healthy intestine. The entire bowel should be searched diligently for other stones, and cholecystectomy should be performed if the patient is stable and the inflammation is not too severe.

F. **Surgical management of symptomatic cholelithiasis and acute chole-cystitis**

1. **LC** has a low complication rate, and the patient's recovery and return-to-work times are excellent.

   a. **Indications.** Approximately 95% of patients with cholelithiasis are candidates for the laparoscopic approach. Contraindications include generalized peritonitis, cholangitis, concomitant diseases that prevent use of a general anesthetic, and the patient's refusal of open chole-cystectomy should urgent conversion be required. Local inflammation in the triangle of Calot can prevent complete visualization of the appropriate structures and increases the risk of injury to the bile ducts or hepatic arteries.

   b. **Technique.** Because misidentification of the cystic duct is the commonest cause of biliary injury, the surgeon must use a technique to provide conclusive identification of the cystic duct and artery.

      (1) In the **Critical View of Safety Technique** pioneered at our institution, the triangle of Calot is dissected free of fat, fibrous, and areolar tissue. Importantly, the lower end of the gallbladder must be dissected off of the liver bed (*J Am Coll Surg.* 2010;211:132). A complete dissection demonstrates two and *only* two structures (the cystic duct and artery) entering the gallbladder, constituting the "critical view of safety."

      (2) **IOC** may be used as the sole method of ductal identification. In addition, an absolute indication is the need to confirm the ductal anatomy during LC whenever the critical view is not achieved. IOC is also indicated in patients with known choledocholithiasis, a history of jaundice, a history of pancreatitis, a large cystic duct and small gallstones, any abnormality in preoperative LFTs, or dilated biliary ducts on ultrasonography. **Laparoscopic ultrasound** as an alternative method for the detection of CBD stones is highly accurate and has decreased operative time and cost in experienced hands (*Surg Clin North Am.* 2000;80:1151).

   c. **Complications.** LC appears to be associated with a higher incidence (~2.5/1,000) of major bile duct injury than open chole-cystectomy. The serious problems include both misidentification injuries and technical problems such as cautery-induced damage (*Surg Clin North Am.* 2010;90:787). In addition, there are also risks to other structures, including the hepatic artery and the bowel. Unretrieved gallstone spillage can be the source of infrequent but serious long-term complications such as abscess and fistula formation. Factors associated with an increased rate of conversion to an open procedure include emergent cholecystectomy, male sex, age greater than 60 years, obesity, gallbladder inflammation (acute cholecystitis), choledocholithiasis, and prior upper abdominal surgery.

2. **Open cholecystectomy** is performed in the minority of patients who have contraindications to LC, in patients who require conversion from

LC because of inability to complete the laparoscopic procedure, or when necessary in conjunction with a laparotomy for another operation (e.g., pancreaticoduodenectomy).

3. **Medical dissolution** of gallstones can sometimes be achieved with oral bile acid therapy, but given the proven effectiveness of LC, there is virtually no current application of medical dissolution. Development of gallstones after gastric bypass for morbid obesity is very common and may largely be prevented by bile acid therapy. The current optimal bile acid therapy for dissolution of gallstones is ursodeoxycholic acid (10 to 15 mg/kg/day).

II. ACALCULOUS CHOLECYSTITIS AND OTHER BILIARY TRACT INFLAMMATIONS

A. **Acalculous cholecystitis** typically occurs in severely ill hospitalized [i.e., intensive care unit (ICU)] patients, especially those with a history of hypotension. It is also associated with prolonged nothing-by-mouth (NPO) status and dependence on parenteral nutrition, with episodes of systemic sepsis, or during multiple-organ-system failure. Mortality rate is high, at around 30% (*Clin Gastroenterol Hepatol.* 2010;8:15).

1. A high index of suspicion is required to make the **diagnosis.**
   a. **Presentation** depends largely on the patient's concurrent medical conditions. Alert patients typically complain of right-upper-quadrant or diffuse upper abdominal pain and tenderness. However, many of these patients may not be alert, and therefore pain and tenderness are absent in up to 75% of patients. Unexplained deterioration in severely ill patients should lead to suspicion of this diagnosis.
   b. In sedated patients, **leukocytosis and abnormal LFTs,** although variable, may be the only indication of acalculous cholecystitis.
   c. Diagnostic **imaging** is essential for establishing the diagnosis because a false-positive result may lead to an unnecessary intervention in a critically ill patient.
      (1) **Ultrasonography** can be done at the bedside in the critically ill patient. Typical findings are similar to those of acute calculous cholecystitis. Limitations include overlying bowel gas, concomitant abdominal wounds or dressings, and the fact that gallbladder abnormalities are often seen in the ICU population (e.g., congestive heart failure may lead to gallbladder wall thickening), even in those patients not suspected of having acute cholecystitis.
      (2) **Hepatobiliary scintigraphy** (HIDA) can also be done at the bedside and has been demonstrated to be superior to ultrasonography in terms of sensitivity, specificity, and positive and negative predictive value (PPV and NPV) for the diagnosis of acute acalculous cholecystitis.
      (3) **CT scan** is as sensitive as ultrasonography for acalculous cholecystitis and has the advantage of providing more complete imaging of the abdominal cavity from the lung bases to the pelvis. However, CT requires transfer of the patient to the

radiology suite, which may be a prohibitive risk in the critically ill.

(4) In difficult cases, **percutaneous cholecystostomy** may be both diagnostic and therapeutic because an infected gallbladder can be decompressed and inciting stones extracted via the tube.

(5) **The choice of imaging** depends largely on the clinical picture, and a high index of suspicion is often necessary to make the diagnosis in sedated or unresponsive ICU patients. Because of its portability and low cost, ultrasound is almost universally the first test of choice, but if the diagnosis is in doubt, then scintigraphy can be added significantly to improve the diagnostic index. CT can be used to evaluate other potential sources of abdominal pathology, whereas percutaneous cholecystostomy may avoid a trip to the operating room for patients who are unable to tolerate surgery.

2. **Management** of acalculous cholecystitis must be tailored to the individual patient, but at the minimum involves systemic antibiotics, NPO status, and treatment of any comorbidities. Primary treatment involves decompression of the gallbladder, typically with a percutaneously placed tube. The definitive treatment is interval cholecystectomy.

B. **Acute cholangitis** is a potentially life-threatening bacterial infection of the biliary tree typically associated with partial or complete obstruction of the ductal system. Although acute cholangitis is often associated with cholelithiasis and choledocholithiasis, other causes of biliary tract obstruction and infection, including benign and malignant strictures of the bile ducts or at biliary-enteric anastomoses, parasites, and indwelling tubes or stents, also have a causative relationship. ERCP without concomitant stenting in the presence of a stricture may lead to cholangitis above the stricture. Therefore, patients should routinely be pretreated with antibiotics in case a stent cannot be placed.

1. **Diagnosis**
   a. Patients present with a spectrum of disease severity, ranging from subclinical illness to acute toxic cholangitis. Greater than 90% of patients with cholangitis present with fever. **Charcot's triad** (fever, jaundice, and right-upper-quadrant pain) remains the hallmark of this disease but is present in only 50% to 70% of patients. The advanced symptoms of **Reynold's pentad** (Charcot's triad with hemodynamic instability and mental status changes) are seen in less than 10% of patients, are more prevalent in the elderly, and suggest a more toxic or suppurative course of cholangitis (*J Hepatobiliary Pancreat Surg.* 2007;14:52).
   b. **Laboratory data** supportive of acute cholangitis include elevations of the white blood cell count and LFTs.
   c. Investigation of the biliary tree is mandatory to demonstrate and relieve the underlying etiology of the obstruction. Ultrasonography or CT scan may reveal gallstones and biliary dilatation, but **definitive diagnosis is made by ERCP or PTC.** These studies are both diagnostic and therapeutic because they demonstrate the level of

obstruction and allow culture of bile, removal of stones or indwelling foreign bodies, and placement of drainage catheters if necessary.

2. Management

    a. Initial management of cholangitis includes **IV antibiotics** appropriate for the coverage of the most commonly cultured organisms: *Escherichia coli, Klebsiella pneumoniae,* enterococci, and *Bacteroides fragilis.* In patients with acute toxic cholangitis or in patients who fail to respond to antibiotic therapy, **emergent decompression of the biliary tree** via ERCP or PTC is required. If decompression by these means is not available or possible, operative intervention to decompress the biliary tree is indicated, though it should usually be limited to extraction of obvious stones and insertion of a T tube in the CBD.

    b. Cholangitis in patients with indwelling tubes or stents generally requires **stent removal and replacement.**

    c. **Definitive operative therapy** for benign or malignant biliary tract strictures should be deferred until a later date.

C. **Oriental cholangiohepatitis,** also known as **recurrent pyogenic cholangitis,** is endemic to the Far East. It is usually due to infestation of the biliary tree with parasites such as *Opisthorchis* species (Thailand) and *Clonorchis* species (China) that cause stasis, bacterial overgrowth, and brown stone formation. Typical findings include multiple intrahepatic and extrahepatic biliary ductal stones, strictures, and repeated bacterial infections of the biliary tract. **Management** involves palliation of biliary strictures and the provision of wide biliary drainage, usually using a choledochoduodenostomy or Roux-en-Y hepaticojejunostomy above the level of the strictured CBD.

III. BILIARY DYSKINESIA is seen in patients with *typical* symptoms of biliary colic but without evidence of gallstones. These patients require extensive workup to exclude other causes of right-upper-quadrant pain. Cholecystokinin-technetium-HIDA scan is useful in evaluation. After the gallbladder has filled with the labeled radionuclide, cholecystokinin is administered, and a gallbladder ejection fraction is calculated 20 minutes later. An ejection fraction of less than 35% is suggestive of biliary dyskinesia. The definitive treatment is cholecystectomy, and greater than 85% of patients report postoperative improvement or relief of symptoms.

IV. PRIMARY SCLEROSING CHOLANGITIS (PSC) is an autoimmune cholestatic disorder characterized by a progressive fibrous obliteration of the bile ducts. It has an estimated incidence of 1 per 100,000, and is predominantly a disease of young and middle-aged men, with a mean age at diagnosis of 40 years. An association with inflammatory bowel disease (IBD) exists; PSC is present in 1% to 5% of those with IBD and approximately 75% of patients with PSC have or will ultimately develop IBD. PSC is a risk factor for cholangiocarcinoma, which may occur in approximately 10% to 20% of patients.

A. **Pathology.** Liver biopsy most commonly shows periductal concentric fibrosis around the macroscopic bile ducts. Obliterative fibrous cholangitis, or concentric fibrosis with obliteration of the small ducts, is virtually diagnostic but is seen in less than 10% of cases. Additional findings may include cholestasis, inflammation (with accumulation of plasma cells, lymphocytes, and polymorphonuclear leukocytes), and secondary biliary sclerosis. Findings may be either diffuse or segmental, and both intrahepatic and extrahepatic ductal segments are generally involved. The hepatic duct bifurcation is typically the area most severely involved.

B. **Diagnosis** is based on a combination of findings.

1. There are **no pathognomonic signs** of PSC. Although patients can be asymptomatic for up to 15 years, prolonged disease ultimately leads to progressive hepatic failure. The condition is characterized by relapses and remissions, with quiescent periods. Jaundice with pale (acholic) stools and dark urine forms the initial clinical picture. With advanced disease, pain in the right upper quadrant, pruritus, fatigue, and weight loss often accompany the jaundice. Cholangitis may ultimately occur. Physical exam commonly reveals jaundice and hepatosplenomegaly.

2. **Laboratory data.** The alkaline phosphatase level is almost always elevated, usually out of proportion to the bilirubin. Serum transaminases may be mildly elevated. Screening for hepatitis viruses is negative. Perinuclear antineutrophil cytoplasmic antibodies (pANCA) are present in the serum of 80% of patients who have PSC, and are highly suggestive but not specific.

3. **Diagnostic imaging.** The procedure of choice is ERCP; PTC may be complementary if the intrahepatic biliary tree is not well visualized. The most common finding is diffuse and irregular narrowing of the entire biliary tree, with short, annular strictures giving a beaded appearance. In progressive disease, the strictures become confluent, and diverticula of the ducts appear. Although cholangiography is the gold standard, sonography and axial imaging [including CT scan, magnetic resonance imaging (MRI), and magnetic resonance cholangiopancreatography (MRCP)] also are useful in making the diagnosis.

C. **Management.** Symptomatic improvements have been reported with the use of various drugs aimed at reversing the presumed autoimmune etiology, including corticosteroids, azathioprine, cyclosporine, and methotrexate. However, none of these alters the natural history of the disease. PSC has been effectively palliated with endoscopic or percutaneous dilation of strictures. Although operative intervention is required for most patients, placement of stents after dilation can be a valuable preoperative adjunct.

1. **Resection or bypass of localized strictures.** The role of nontransplant surgery in this disease is limited. Rarely, surgery is indicated when the disease is located only in the extrahepatic bile ducts and a dominant stricture exists that can be excised or bypassed by hepaticojejunostomy.

2. Extensive, diffuse stricture disease with end-stage cirrhosis is an indication for orthotopic **liver transplantation (OLT).** If the patient has undergone a previous decompressive operation, transplantation is technically more challenging but not contraindicated.

3. Because PSC is a risk factor for cholangiocarcinoma, **close surveillance** of patients is needed. The diagnosis is difficult because cholangiocarcinomas also masquerade as strictures. A dominant biliary stricture or elevated carbohydrate antigen 19-9 level should raise the suspicion of cholangiocarcinoma in a PSC patient and suggests the need for further evaluation.

D. **Prognosis.** Many patients have a course that progresses to cirrhosis and liver failure despite early palliative interventions. Liver transplantation likely improves survival and quality of life, and early referral for liver transplantation is indicated to decrease the risk of developing cholangiocarcinoma. Overall, the median length of survival from diagnosis to death or liver transplantation is 10 to 12 years.

E. **IgG4-associated cholangitis** (IAC) is a newly described entity that shares a number of clinical and radiologic features with PSC. However, in contrast to PSC, IAC mainly affects elderly men (typically older than 60 years), is not associated with IBD, and, most importantly, does respond to immunosuppressive treatment. IAC is considered a variant of IgG4-related systemic disease (*Digestion.* 2009;79:220).

V. CHOLEDOCHAL CYSTS are congenital dilations of the biliary tree that may occur in any bile duct but characteristically involve the common hepatic and CBDs. They are more frequently identified in women (3:1 ratio) and those of Asian descent. Sixty percent are diagnosed in patients under the age of 10 years. Diagnosis and treatment are essential because the cysts predispose to choledocholithiasis, cholangitis, portal hypertension, and cholangiocarcinoma, which develop in up to 30% of cysts and usually present in the fourth decade of life.

A. **An anatomic classification scheme** has identified five distinct types. Type I cysts are fusiform dilations of the CBD and are the most common (65% to 90%). Type II cysts are rare, isolated saccular diverticula of the CBD. Type III cysts, also termed *choledochoceles*, are localized dilations within the intraduodenal part of the CBD. Most lesions thought to be choledochoceles are in fact duodenal duplications. Type IV cysts are characterized by multiple cystic areas of the biliary tract, both inside and outside of the liver. Type V cysts are single or multiple lesions based only in the intrahepatic portion of the tract (Caroli disease).

B. **Diagnosis.** The classic triad of jaundice, a palpable abdominal mass, and right-upper-quadrant pain mimicking biliary colic is present only a minority of the time. Neonates frequently present with biliary obstruction, whereas older children suffer from jaundice and abdominal pain. Rarely, pancreatitis or duodenal obstruction can be caused by a choledochocele. Initial diagnosis is often made with ultrasonography and/or CT. Further evaluation of the cyst should be obtained with specific biliary imaging such as ERCP or MRCP.

C. **Treatment** is primarily surgical. Cyst excision with a Roux-en-Y hepatico-jejunostomy is the treatment of choice for types I and IV. Simple excision of the rare type II cyst has been performed. Local endoscopic cyst unroofing plus sphincteroplasty is usually effective for type III disease. Caroli disease can be treated with hemihepatectomy when it is confined to one side of the liver. More often, bilateral disease is present with associated liver damage and mandates OLT.

VI. TUMORS OF THE BILE DUCTS

A. **Benign tumors of the bile ducts,** usually adenomas, are rare and arise from the ductal glandular epithelium. They are characteristically polypoid and rarely are larger than 2 cm. Most are found adjacent to the ampulla, with the CBD being the next-most-common site. The malignant potential of these uncommon lesions is unclear.

1. Most patients present with **intermittent obstructive jaundice,** often accompanied by right-upper-quadrant pain. This presentation may be confused with choledocholithiasis.

2. **Treatment** should involve complete resection of the tumor with a margin of duct wall. High recurrence rates have been reported after simple curettage of the polyps. Lesions situated at the ampulla can usually be managed by transduodenal papillotomy or wide local excision.

B. **Cholangiocarcinoma** arises from the bile duct epithelium and can occur anywhere along the course of the biliary tree. Cholangiocarcinoma is an uncommon malignancy, with an incidence in the United States of approximately 0.85/100,000 population and representing about 2% of all cancers (approximately 5,000 new cases per year). Tumors tend to be locally invasive, and when they metastasize, they usually involve the liver and the peritoneum. They characteristically spread along the bile ducts microscopically for long distances beyond the palpable end of the tumor. The median age of onset is approximately 65 years. Predisposing conditions include male gender, PSC, choledochal cysts, intrahepatic stones, parasitic infestations such as *Opisthorchis* and *Clonorchis* species, and exposure to the radiocontrast agent Thorotrast (historical).

1. **Classification.** Cholangiocarcinoma has been classified according to anatomic location and growth pattern. The anatomic location classification includes three main types: intrahepatic (20%), extrahepatic upper duct (also called *hilar* or *Klatskin tumor*, 40%), and extrahepatic lower duct (40%). Tumor morphology is also divided in three primary types: (1) a mass-forming (or MF) type that grows in a nodular fashion and projects into both the bile duct lumen and the surrounding tissues; (2) a periductal infiltrating (PI) type characterized by a cicatrizing growth pattern that infiltrates the walls of the bile ducts and grows both within them and along their exterior surfaces; and (3) an intraductal growing (IG) type that displays a polypoid or sessile pattern that forms intraductal excrescences of tumor that may grow along the inside of, but do not penetrate, the wall of the duct (also commonly

TABLE 15-2	Bismuth-Corlette Classification of Hilar Cholangiocarcinoma
Type I	Tumor remains below the confluence of the right and left hepatic ducts
Type II	Tumor involves the confluence of the right and left hepatic ducts
Type III	Tumor involves *either* the right *or* the left hepatic duct and extends to secondary radicals
Type IV	Tumor involves secondary radicals of *both* the right *and* left hepatic ducts

referred to as "papillary subtype"). The specific anatomic location and growth pattern of perihilar tumors are further described by the Bismuth-Corlette classification scheme as shown in Table 15-2.

2. **Staging** is currently based on the TNM (tumor, nodes, and metastases) system of the sixth edition of the American Joint Committee on Cancer (AJCC) guidelines. Intrahepatic malignancies are staged along with those of primary hepatic origin, whereas extrahepatic lesions have their own set of criteria (see Tables 15-3 and 15-4). Jarnagin and Blumgart developed a

TABLE 15-3	American Joint Committee on Cancer TNM (Tumor, Nodes, and Metastases) Staging for Extrahepatic Cholangiocarcinoma

Primary Tumor

TX	Primary tumor cannot be assessed
T0	No evidence of primary tumor
Tis	Carcinoma *in situ*
T1	Tumor confined to the bile duct histologically
T2	Tumor invades beyond the wall of the bile duct
T3	Tumor invades the liver, gallbladder, pancreas, and/or ipsilateral branches of the portal vein or hepatic artery
T4	Invades any of the following: main portal vein or bilateral branches, common hepatic artery, adjacent structures such as colon, stomach, duodenum, or abdominal wall

Regional Lymph Nodes

NX	Regional lymph nodes cannot be assessed
N0	No regional lymph node metastasis
N1	Regional lymph node metastasis

Distant Metastasis

MX	Distant metastasis cannot be assessed
M0	No distant metastasis
M1	Distant metastasis

TABLE 15-4	Staging of Extrahepatic Cholangiocarcinoma and Gallbladder Cancer		
Stage	TNM Status		
Stage 0	Tis	N0	M0
Stage IA	T1	N0	M0
Stage IB	T2	N0	M0
Stage IIA	T3	N0	M0
Stage IIB	T1–3	N1	M0
Stage III	T4	Any N	M0
Stage IV	Any T	Any N	M1

preoperative clinical T staging system for hilar cholangiocarcinoma (*Ann Surg.* 2001;234:507) that defines both radial and longitudinal tumor spread, which are critical determinants of resectability. It incorporates three factors based on preoperative imaging studies: (1) location and extent of ductal involvement, (2) presence or absence of portal vein invasion, and (3) presence or absence of hepatic lobar atrophy. This staging system has been shown to correlate well with resectability and survival (Table 15-5).

3. **Diagnosis**
   a. **Jaundice,** followed by weight loss and pain, is the most frequently encountered clinical feature at presentation.
   b. **Serum markers.** Numerous serum tumor markers are currently in use and/or being evaluated for their utility in the diagnosis of cholangiocarcinoma.
      (1) **Carbohydrate antigen 19-9 (CA19-9)** is a carbohydrate antigen that is traditionally associated with pancreatic cancer but is also the most commonly used marker in the diagnosis of cholangiocarcinoma. Sensitivity and specificity vary depending on the threshold used and on coexisting conditions such as inflammation and cholestasis. For example, two large studies encompassing over 300 patients each showed sensitivities and specificities of 73% to 76% and 63% to 74%, respectively, when a cutoff value of 37 U/mL was applied in a patient population without cholangitis. However, the specificity dropped to approximately 42% when patients with cholangitis were included (*Am J Gastroenterol.* 1999;64:1941; *Br J Cancer.* 1991;63:636). In two other studies of 55 and 74 patients with PSC, higher CA19-9 cutoffs of 180 and 100 U/mL yielded improved specificities of 98% and 91%, respectively, whereas

TABLE 15-5	American Joint Committee on Cancer TNM Staging for Gallbladder Cancer

Primary Tumor

TX	Primary tumor cannot be assessed
T0	No evidence of primary tumor
Tis	Carcinoma *in situ*
T1a	Tumor invades lamina propria
T1b	Tumor invades muscle layer
T2	Tumor invades perimuscular connective tissue; no extension beyond serosa or into liver
T3	Tumor perforates serosa and/or directly invades the liver and/or one other adjacent organ or structure, e.g., stomach, duodenum, colon, and extrahepatic bile ducts
T4	Tumor invades the main portal vein or hepatic artery or invades multiple extrahepatic organs or structures

Regional Lymph Nodes

NX	Regional lymph nodes cannot be assessed
N0	No regional lymph node metastasis
N1	Regional lymph node metastasis

Distant Metastasis

MX	Distant metastasis cannot be assessed
M0	No distant metastasis
M1	Distant metastasis

sensitivities were comparable to those of other series – 67% and 60%, respectively (*Gastrointest Endosc.* 2002;56:40; *Gastroenterology.* 1995;108:865). Thus, whereas a CA19-9 cutoff of around 40 U/mL is likely to be adequate in patients without any evidence of cholangitis or cholestasis, a higher value (probably in the 150 U/mL range) should be used for those patients with either of these concurrent conditions.

(2) **Carcinoembryonic antigen (CEA).** Although most commonly used for the diagnosis of colorectal cancer, CEA has also demonstrated some elevation in patients with malignancies of biliary origin.

c. **Diagnostic imaging**

(1) **MRCP** can be used for an all-purpose investigation of cholangiocarcinoma. It provides cholangiography, demonstrates the tumor and its relationship to key vessels, and detects intrahepatic metastases.

(2) **Ultrasonography** can demonstrate bile duct masses and dilation and provide rudimentary information on the extent of tumor involvement within the liver. Reports indicate that ultrasonography is more than 80% accurate in predicting portal vein involvement.

(3) **CT** may be helpful in delineating the mass and defining its relation to the liver, especially when MRI is contraindicated or cannot be tolerated.

(4) **Positron emission tomography (PET)** may be helpful in the diagnosis of cholangiocarcinoma; however, it is currently incompletely studied and not yet part of the standard diagnostic workup.

(5) **ERCP** is the most valuable diagnostic tool for cholangiography of lower duct tumors. Distal lesions may be indistinguishable from small pancreatic carcinomas on preoperative evaluation, and the distinction is often not made until final pathologic analysis. It is also valuable for upper duct tumors, but if obstruction is complete, the upper limit of the tumor cannot be delineated. Since the advent of MR cholangiography, ERCP is increasingly being used for preoperative **therapeutic decompression** of the biliary tree. Preoperative decompression of the biliary tree has the advantage of improving liver function prior to resection but has the risk of cholangitis and increased postoperative infection. It is not usually performed unless the bilirubin is greater than 10 mg/dL. When used, only the less-affected hemiliver should be decompressed so that it will hypertrophy while the undrained side (the side to be resected) atrophies. The side to be resected should be drained only if cholangitis is present. ERCP carries the potential added benefit of obtaining cellular material for **cytologic analysis,** either via ductal brushing, fine needle aspiration (FNA), or forceps biopsy. In an attempt to increase diagnostic yields, new molecular techniques have been applied to biopsy samples, including digital image analysis (DIA) and fluorescence *in situ* hybridization (FISH). These tests can detect genetic aneuploidy and chromosomal rearrangements as indicators of malignancy.

(6) **PTC** has been used when ERCP and MRI cannot precisely delineate the upper limit of a tumor. Under PTC guidance, FNA cytology can also provide a tissue diagnosis in many of patients. If a tumor is resectable, extensive efforts to obtain a tissue diagnosis before resection are inappropriate.

(7) **Endoscopic ultrasound (EUS)** with FNA represents an important development in the investigation of *lower* bile duct strictures and masses. It is useful as an alternative to ERCP for obtaining tissue to establish a cytologic diagnosis, especially if a primary pancreatic mass is suspected. A recent study demonstrated that EUS-FNA has a sensitivity, specificity, PPV, NPV, and accuracy of 86%, 100%, 100%, 57%, and 88%, respectively, for the diagnosis of extrahepatic cholangiocarcinoma (both hilar and distal CBD), and the test results positively changed the management of 84% of the study participants (*Clin Gastroenterol Hepatol.* 2004;2:209). The potential value of such a biopsy needs to be weighed against risks such as bleeding and potentially seeding the traversed peritoneal cavity with malignant cells (*Am J Gastroenterol.* 2004;99:45).

4. **Assessment of tumor resectability and treatment.** Resection remains the primary treatment of cholangiocarcinoma, although only 15% to 20% are resectable at presentation. Adjuvant radiation and chemotherapy have been attempted, but clinical trials are limited by the paucity of eligible patients.

   a. **Intrahepatic tumors** are best treated with hepatic resection. Resectability is assessed as for other types of intrahepatic tumors, with a goal of 1-cm tumor-free margins and retention of at least 30% of functioning liver mass. If resection of more than 60% of the hepatic parenchyma is required, preoperative portal vein embolization can be used to cause atrophy of the affected hemiliver and hypertrophy of the unaffected liver segments (future liver remnant).

   b. **Extrahepatic upper duct (hilar) tumors.** Because hilar lesions are generally not as easily biopsied, resection is often undertaken based on clinical assessment and radiographic demonstration of a mass lesion at the ductal bifurcation. With the rare exception of low-lying Bismuth I tumors in which a negative common hepatic duct margin may be obtained, resection of hilar tumors includes the bile duct bifurcation and the caudate lobe; ipsilateral hemihepatectomy is often required to obtain an R0 resection. Biliary reconstruction is performed as a Roux-en-Y hepaticojejunostomy. Pancreaticoduodenectomy may be necessary in some cases to obtain negative lower margins of the CBD. Vascular involvement is not an absolute contraindication to resection because portal venous resection and reconstruction may be possible. Contraindications to resection are as follows:

      (1) Bilateral intrahepatic ductal spread.
      (2) Extensive involvement of the main trunk of the portal vein.
      (3) Bilateral involvement of hepatic arterial and/or portal venous branches.
      (4) A combination of vascular involvement with evidence of contralateral ductal spread.
      (5) Lymph node involvement or distant spread.

      At select centers, patients with locally unresectable hilar cholangiocarcinoma are treated with neoadjuvant chemoradiation followed by OLT (*Transplant Proc.* 2009;41:4023).

   c. Some lesions situated in the **middle of the extrahepatic bile duct** may be approached with an excision of the supraduodenal extrahepatic bile duct, cholecystectomy, and portal lymphadenectomy. However, most malignant strictures in the mid-CBD are due to local invasion of a gallbladder cancer rather than cholangiocarcinoma.

   d. **Extrahepatic lower duct tumors.** The considerations are the same as for carcinoma of the head of the pancreas, although vascular involvement is much less common. In contrast to more-proximal tumors, approximately 80% of lower duct tumors are resectable by pancreaticoduodenectomy, and 5-year survival rates range from 17% to 39%. Tumors derived from the bile duct have a slightly better prognosis than those of pancreatic origin in the same region, probably reflecting a more favorable biologic behavior.

    e. Adjuvant therapy. There is a lack of level 1 evidence supporting use of adjuvant therapy for resectable extrahepatic cholangiocarcinoma. Retrospective cohort studies comparing resection alone to resection plus adjuvant chemoradiation, and have suggested a slight survival advantage (*Am Surg.* 2001;67:839). The current NCCN guidelines recommend consideration of 5-FU or gemcitabine-based chemoradiation, especially in the setting of positive margins or lymph nodes.

  5. Palliation for patients with unresectable disease involves surgical, radiologic, or endoscopic biliary decompression. When unresectability is demonstrated preoperatively or at staging laparoscopy, the first choice for biliary decompression is via endoscopic or percutaneous internal stenting. When encountered at laparotomy, internal biliary drainage is best achieved by choledochojejunostomy for lower duct lesions.

  6. Prognosis is highly dependent on resectability of the tumor at presentation. Patients with resectable cholangiocarcinoma with microscopically negative margins and negative lymph nodes have a 5-year survival of approximately 35%, whereas median survival for patients with unresectable cholangiocarcinoma is only 3 to 6 months. An R0 resection is necessary for any chance of a cure because recurrence is almost universal within 5 years in patients with R1 resections. Other factors associated with increased survival include papillary phenotype, lower tumor grade, unaffected local lymph nodes, and a lack of vascular involvement.

C. Gallbladder cancer is the most common cancer of the biliary tract and the sixth-most-common cancer of the gastrointestinal (GI) tract, representing about 9,000 new cases per year in the United States. It is more aggressive than cholangiocarcinoma, has a poor prognosis, and accounts for approximately 6,000 deaths yearly. The incidence peaks at 70 to 75 years, with a 3:1 female-to-male ratio. There is a strong correlation with gallstones (95%). Histologically, nearly all gallbladder cancers are adenocarcinomas, and concomitant cholecystitis is frequently present. Tumors spread primarily by direct extension into liver segments IV and V adjacent to the gallbladder fossa, but also via lymphatics along the cystic duct to the CBD. Because of its generally late stage at presentation, only a small percentage of patients with a preoperative diagnosis of gallbladder cancer are resectable for potential cure.

  1. Risk factors

    a. The presence of gallstones is the most common risk factor. Longer duration of cholelithiasis and larger stone size seem to further increase the risk, with reported cancer development odds ratios (ORs) of up to 10 for stones 3 cm or greater (*JAMA.* 1983;250:2323).

    b. Polyps 1.5 cm or greater in diameter have a 46% to 70% prevalence of cancer, whereas those in the 1- to 1.5-cm range have an 11% to 13% incidence. For polyps smaller than 1 cm, the risk of malignancy is <5%. Malignant polyps also tend to be sessile in nature and echopenic on ultrasound. Prophylactic cholecystectomy should be considered for polyps >1 cm in size or meeting morphologic criteria.

c. **Anomalous junction of the pancreatobiliary duct (AJPBD)** has been noted in approximately 10% of patients with gallbladder cancer, and up to 40% of patients with this anomaly develop a biliary tract malignancy. The anomaly represents a union of the pancreatic and biliary ducts outside of the duodenal wall, resulting in a long common channel. Subsequent reflux of pancreatic juice into the biliary system is thought to be the initiator of carcinogenesis.

d. **Porcelain gallbladder** is a condition characterized by calcification of the gallbladder wall. Although the overall incidence of carcinoma associated with porcelain gallbladder has been estimated at approximately 20%, studies have shown that gallbladders with diffuse intramural calcification rarely harbor cancer. Conversely, the selective mucosal calcification variant has been associated with malignancy in 7% to 42% of cases. Regardless, prophylactic cholecystectomy is generally recommended for any finding of gallbladder wall calcification on imaging studies.

e. **Other risk factors** include PSC, gallbladder infection with *E. coli* and/or *Salmonella* species, and exposure to certain industrial solvents and toxins.

2. **Diagnosis.** Approximately one-third of these tumors are diagnosed incidentally during cholecystectomy, and **cancer is found in 0.3% to 1%** of all cholecystectomy specimens. Symptoms of stage I and II gallbladder cancer are often directly caused by gallstones rather than the cancer, whereas stage III and IV cancers present with weight loss and symptoms typical of CBD obstruction. Suggestive ultrasound findings include thickening or irregularity of the gallbladder, a polypoid mass, or diffuse wall calcification indicative of porcelain gallbladder.

3. **Staging** is similar to that of cholangiocarcinoma, as shown in Tables 15-3 and 15-4. At present, there is insufficient data to determine the usefulness of FDG-PET.

4. **Treatment**
   a. **Mucosal disease** confined to the gallbladder wall (Tis and T1a tumors) is often identified after routine LC. Because the overall 5-year survival rate is as high as 80%, cholecystectomy alone with negative resection margins (including the cystic duct margin) is adequate therapy. Patients with a preoperative suspicion of gallbladder cancer should undergo open cholecystectomy because port site recurrences and late peritoneal metastases (associated with bile spillage) have been reported even with *in situ* disease.

   b. **Early disease** (T1b and T2 tumors) may be treated by radical cholecystectomy that includes the gallbladder, the gallbladder bed of the liver, as well as the hepatoduodenal ligament, periduodenal, peripancreatic, hepatic artery, and celiac lymph nodes.

   c. **Stage II or III disease** (invasion of adjacent organs or the presence of lymph node metastases) requires more radical resection. Depending on the extent of local invasion, extirpation may range from wedge resection of the liver adjacent to the gallbladder bed to resection of 75% of the liver. Dissection of the portal, paraduodenal, and hepatic artery lymph nodes should accompany the liver resection. Improvement in survival has been demonstrated after radical resection. Because of the aggressive nature of this malignancy, adjuvant chemoradiation is often recommended, but little proof of efficacy is available.

   d. Most gallbladder cancers have invaded adjacent organs, extend into the porta hepatis, or distantly metastasized before clinical diagnosis. **Extensive liver involvement or discontiguous metastases** preclude surgical resection. Jaundice may be palliated by percutaneous or endoscopically placed biliary stents. Duodenal obstruction can be surgically bypassed if present. Palliative chemotherapy (5-FU or gemcitabine-based) is recommended but has poor efficacy.

  5. Prognosis is stage dependent, and the respective 5-year survival rates are shown in Table 15-3. The median survival for stage IB cancers is less than 2 years, and for stage II lesions, it is less than 1 year. With stage II disease or higher, fewer than 20% of patients are alive at 2 years.

VII. BENIGN STRICTURES AND BILE DUCT INJURIES occur in association with a number of conditions, including pancreatitis, choledocholithiasis, Oriental cholangiohepatitis, PSC, prior hepatic transplantation, trauma, or iatrogenic injury after instrumentation or surgery. LC is the leading cause of iatrogenic bile duct injuries and subsequent benign strictures. Biliary malignancy may masquerade as a benign stricture. Attempts to differentiate between the two etiologies should be made prior to surgery because the patient may not be a candidate for a curative resection if an advanced stage of cancer is found.

  A. Risk factors for intraoperative bile duct injury have been divided into three categories: (1) patient-related factors, (2) procedure-related factors, and (3) surgeon/hospital-related factors (*J Hepatobiliary Pancreat Surg.* 2002;9:543).

    1. Patient-related factors

      a. Inflammation

        (1) Acute inflammation, such as that seen in acute cholecystitis, may cause the gallbladder, cystic duct, and CBD to appear as a single mass (*J Am Coll Surg.* 2000;191:661). This can lead to misidentification of the CBD as the cystic duct with subsequent clipping and transection.

        (2) Severe chronic inflammation and dense scarring may result from repeated bouts of cholecystitis and/or choledocholithiasis, effectively obliterating the triangle of Calot and leaving a shrunken, contracted gallbladder densely adherent to the common hepatic duct and/or right hepatic artery.

      b. Congenital anomalies including aberrant right hepatic ducts and aberrant course or insertion of the cyst duct can complicate LC and lead to CBD injury.

      c. Large, impacted gallstones may prevent proper retraction of the gallbladder and can obscure the anatomic relationships between the cystic duct and surrounding structures.

   d. **Obesity** can contribute to a difficult operation due to both intra-abdominal and extra-abdominal fat and loss of intra-abdominal domain during laparoscopy.

2. **Procedure-related factors**
   a. **Operative technique** likely represents the most important factor contributing to the risk of inadvertent bile duct injury.
   b. **IOC** can be extremely helpful in the avoidance of potentially devastating bile duct injury.
   c. **Technical problems** frequently arise secondary to other risk factors such as inflammation but may also occur even in the absence of a specific predisposing condition.
      (1) **Inadvertent injury** to a bile duct during the course of dissection most commonly results form the injudicious use of electrocautery, although sharp dissection and excessive traction on the gallbladder or adjacent structures may also contribute to this type of injury.
      (2) **Failure to securely close the cystic duct** may be due to a poorly placed or incompletely closed surgical clip, usually in the setting of a thickened fibrotic cystic duct or increased biliary pressure secondary to retained CBD stones. If there is any concern for incomplete closure, a **laparoscopic loop ligature** should be used.
      (3) **Tenting injuries** occur when the CBD or common hepatic duct is clipped after being elevated due to excessive traction on the gallbladder and cystic duct.

3. **Surgeon/hospital-related factors**
   a. **The learning-curve effect** may be due to a lack of sufficient operator experience with safe techniques for performing cholecystectomy, either laparoscopically or open.
   b. **Surgeon mindset,** often characterized by a sense of infallibility even when faced with adversity, may result in biliary injury.
   c. **Laparoscopic equipment** must be regularly maintained in excellent working condition. Loss of insulation from electrocautery instruments may be particularly hazardous, and preventative systems should be employed.

4. **The difficult cholecystectomy.** In an attempt to preoperatively identify what factors might contribute to a "difficult cholecystectomy," 22,953 cases of LC performed in Switzerland were studied. Those factors associated with an increase in all intraoperative complications (not limited to only bile duct injury) included the presence of acute cholecystitis (OR = 1.86), male gender (OR = 1.18), patient age (OR = 1.12 per 10 years), increased body weight (OR = 1.34 for >90 kg vs. <60 kg), and surgeon experience (OR = 1.36 for 11 to 100 cases vs. >100 cases). Multivariate analysis also showed an increase in complications for each additional 30 minutes of operative time, with OR = 1.68 (*J Am Coll Surg.* 2006;203:723). Conversion to an open operation in the face of a difficult laparoscopic procedure should never be viewed as a surgical failure or complication but rather as a way to avoid potential injury to the patient.

B. **Classification.** A widely accepted classification scheme has been developed at this institution (*Surg Clin North Am.* 2010;90:787). Type A injuries are cystic duct leaks or leaks from small ducts in the liver bed. Type B and C injuries involve an aberrant right hepatic duct. Type B represents an occluded segment, whereas type C involves open drainage from the proximal draining duct not in continuity with the common duct. Type D injuries are *lateral* injuries to the extrahepatic bile ducts. Type E injuries (subtypes 1 to 5) are derived from the Bismuth classification and represent circumferential transections or occlusions at various levels of the CBD.

C. **Diagnosis**

1. **Presentation** depends on the type of injury. Approximately 25% of major bile duct injuries are recognized at the time of the initial procedure. Intraoperative signs of a major ductal injury include unexpected bile leakage, abnormal IOC, and delayed recognition of the anatomy after transection of important structures. If an injury is not recognized intraoperatively, the patient usually presents with symptoms within 1 week and almost always within 3 to 4 weeks after the initial procedure. Patients with a bile leak often present with right-upper-quadrant pain, fever, and sepsis secondary to biloma and may have bile drainage from a surgical incision. Patients with occlusion of the CBD without a bile leak present with jaundice. Occasionally, a delayed presentation of months or years is seen.

2. **Diagnostic imaging.** Axial imaging with CT scan or MRI is useful for detecting abdominal bile collections that require percutaneous drainage. MRCP with angiography is now often the initial imaging test of choice because of its ability to define the vascular as well as the biliary anatomy, as biliary injuries are frequently associated with vascular injuries. Ongoing bile leaks can also be diagnosed by HIDA scan. ERCP is also useful to demonstrate biliary anatomy, and therapeutic stent placement is often possible for ductal leaks. In the case of occlusion of the CBD, PTC can demonstrate the proximal biliary anatomy, define the proximal extent of the injury, and be used for therapeutic decompression of the biliary tree.

D. **Management** depends on the type and timing of the presentation.

1. If the injury is identified at the time of the initial procedure, the surgeon should proceed directly to open exploration and repair only if qualified and comfortable with complex techniques in hepatobiliary surgery or to control life-threatening hemorrhage. If the surgeon is not prepared to perform a definitive repair, a drain should be placed in the right upper quadrant and the patient immediately **referred to a specialist hepatobiliary center.**

2. **Immediate management.** Many of the simpler injuries can be successfully managed with ERCP and sphincterotomy, stenting, or both. Occlusive lesions require decompression of the proximal system via PTC. In general, if an injury requires operative repair and the patient is stable, the repair should be done within the first few days after the initial procedure while inflammation is at a minimum. If this is not

possible due to delayed diagnosis, longer-term temporization (at least 8 weeks) is required to allow the acute inflammation to resolve. In addition, if there is a concern about a vascular injury along with the bile duct injury, definitive repair should be delayed to more easily identify areas of ductal ischemia, which should not be incorporated in the repair.

3. Control of sepsis, percutaneous drainage, and adequate nutrition should be **optimized before definitive repair.**

4. **Operative repair,** when indicated, is best achieved by means of a Roux-en-Y hepaticojejunostomy, in which the bile duct is debrided back to viable tissue. All bile ducts must be accounted for, and an adequate blood supply must be apparent for each. A tension-free mucosa-to-mucosa anastomosis constructed with fine absorbable suture is desired. Excellent long-term outcomes have been described, with anastomotic stricture the most common, yet infrequent, complication (*Ann Surg.* 2009;249:426).

16 Spleen

Malcolm MacConmara and L. Michael Brunt

SPLENIC ANATOMY AND PHYSIOLOGY

I. SPLENIC ANATOMY

A. **Macroscopic Anatomy.** The spleen develops from mesoderm within the dorsal mesogastrium and following rotation of the gut becomes located in the **left upper quadrant of the abdomen** beneath the 9th to 11th ribs. It is approximately 12 cm long, 7 cm wide, and 4 cm thick and weighs 100 to 150 g. The costodiaphragmatic recess of the left pleural cavity extends as far as the inferior border of a normal spleen. It is **intimately related** to the splenic flexure of the colon, the greater curvature of the stomach, the left kidney, and the pancreatic tail. The tail of the pancreas extends laterally to within 1 cm of the splenic hilum in most patients and is in direct contact with the spleen in up to 30% of patients (Fig. 16-1).

Peritoneal reflections in the region surrounding the spleen form the fibrous suspensory "ligaments" through which most of the principal vascular structures course. These ligaments are splenocolic, splenorenal, gastrosplenic, and splenophrenic. Their division is one of the keys to splenectomy. The pancreas is partially invested in the leaves of the splenorenal ligament, just inferior to the contained splenic artery and its branches.

The **splenic artery** is a branch of the celiac trunk and follows a serpiginous path along the superior border of the pancreas. The terminal branching pattern into the spleen is most commonly distributive in which the main trunk arborizes into multiple arterial branches that enter the hilum broadly over its surface. Less commonly, the arterial supply has a magistral configuration, with one dominant splenic artery entering over a narrow and compact area (Fig. 16-2).

Accessory spleens occur in 10% to 20% of patients and are most commonly found at the splenic hilum, the gastrosplenic omentum, along the tail of the pancreas, and in the retroperitoneum posterior to the spleen. However, accessory splenic tissue can be found throughout the abdomen and pelvis (Fig. 16-3).

B. **Microscopic Anatomy.** The **spleen consists** of red pulp with interspersed areas of white pulp. The red pulp is highly vascular and is composed of large, branching, thin-walled sinuses, with intervening areas filled with phagocytic cells and blood cells, known as splenic cords. The white pulp has three components: periarteriolar lymphoid sheaths (T cells), lymphoid nodules (B cells), and the marginal zone.

II. SPLENIC FUNCTION.

The spleen has two major functions: (1) mechanical filtration of erythrocytes as part of the reticuloendothelial system and (2) a component of the immune system.

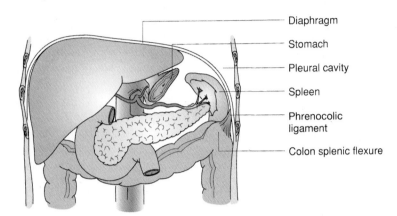

Figure 16-1. Relationships of the spleen. Anatomic relation of the spleen to the liver, diaphragm, pancreas, colon, and kidney. The stomach is sectioned to illustrate the anatomic relation *in situ.* (Adapted from splenic disorders *Greenfields Surgery: Scientific Principles and Practice.* 4th ed., 2006.)

A. **Reticuloendothelial/Filtration System.** The spleen is highly vascular receiving 5% of the cardiac output. The red pulp serves as a mechanical filter for the removal of senescent erythrocytes (*culling*) and the remodeling of healthy red cells, including removal of nuclear remnants, denatured hemoglobin, and iron granules (*pitting*). A minor hematologic function of the spleen is to serve as a reservoir for platelets. In certain disease states (e.g., myelofibrosis), the adult spleen becomes a major site of extramedullary hematopoiesis.

B. **Immune System.** The white pulp is a nonspecific filter and removes blood-borne pathogens (e.g., bacteria and viruses) that are coated with complement. Encapsulated bacteria are also effectively removed from the circulation, likely via prolonged contact with macrophages in the splenic parenchymal cords. The spleen also participates in the specific immune responses. The white pulp architecture provides a platform for cytokine-regulated T

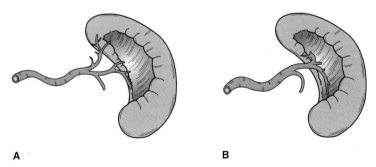

A   **B**

Figure 16-2. Variations in the splenic artery. The two most common variations of blood supply are illustrated: **(A)** Early branching characteristic of distributive and **(B)** magistral where the splenic artery branches close to the hilum of the spleen

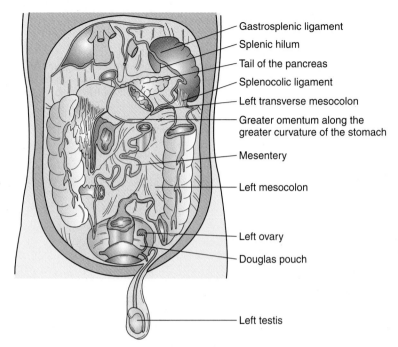

Gastrosplenic ligament

Splenic hilum

Tail of the pancreas

Splenocolic ligament

Left transverse mesocolon

Greater omentum along the greater curvature of the stomach

Mesentery

Left mesocolon

Left ovary

Douglas pouch

Left testis

Figure 16-3. Location of accessory spleens. Usual location of accessory spleens: *(1)* gastrosplenic ligament, *(2)* splenic hilum, *(3)* tail of the pancreas, *(4)* splenocolic ligament, *(5)* left transverse mesocolon, *(6)* greater omentum along the greater curvature of the stomach, *(7)* mesentery, *(8)* left mesocolon, *(9)* left ovary, *(10)* Douglas pouch, and *(11)* left testis.

and B cell interaction with antigen-presenting cells leading to specific cellular and antibody responses. The spleen also manufactures opsonins, namely, properdin, and tuftsin.

INDICATIONS FOR SPLENECTOMY

I. **GENERAL INDICATIONS.** The initial therapy for most hematologic disorders of the spleen is medical. In general, splenectomy is warranted only after the failure of medical therapy, as an adjunct to medical therapy, for diagnostic reasons, or in some cases as primary therapy for an underlying malignancy (see Table 16-1).

II. **SPECIFIC INDICATIONS**

  A. Hematologic splenic pathology

   1. **Thrombocytopenias**

     a. **Idiopathic (immune) thrombocytopenic purpura (ITP)** is the most common indication for elective splenectomy. It is an acquired

TABLE 16.1	General Indications for Splenectomy

1. **Cure or palliation of hematologic disease.** Idiopathic (immune) thrombocytopenic purpura and hemolytic anemias are the most common indications for splenectomy. Splenectomy may also be used to palliate other disease states (e.g., chronic lymphocytic leukemia, hairy cell leukemia, Felty syndrome), primarily via the control of cytopenias.

2. **Palliation of hypersplenism.** Patients with refractory cytopenias due to hypersplenism that require frequent transfusion or significantly limit the delivery of cytotoxic therapy may benefit from splenectomy.

3. **Relief from symptomatic splenomegaly.** Patients with a massively enlarged spleen can develop early satiety, abdominal pain, and weight loss from mass effect.

4. **Diagnosis of splenic pathology.** Solid mass lesions in the spleen can be an indication for splenectomy, particularly if a malignant diagnosis is suspected. Splenectomy may be used to establish a diagnosis of lymphoma in the absence of more easily accessible tissue but is no longer indicated for staging lymphomas.

5. **Control of splenic hemorrhage.** Although splenic injury is increasingly managed nonoperatively, splenectomy is the definitive treatment for patients with ongoing traumatic splenic hemorrhage. Splenic hemorrhage may also rarely occur spontaneously in disease states such as infectious mononucleosis.

disorder in which autoantibodies are produced against a platelet glycoprotein. The spleen is the major site for the production of antiplatelet antibodies and also serves as the principal site of platelet destruction (see Table 16-2).

(1) **Children** usually present with acute ITP, often associated with a recent viral syndrome. In 90% of cases, the disease spontaneously remits. Only refractory cases require splenectomy, and a waiting period of at least 12 months is recommended where possible (*Blood.* 1996;88:3–40). In younger children under 5 years where the risk of infection postsplenectomy is higher, temporizing therapies are especially important (*Br J Haematol.* 1999;105:871–875). Adolescent females have a disease course similar to that seen in adults (*Blood.* 2010;115:168–186).

(2) **Adults** typically present with a more chronic form of ITP that is much less likely to spontaneously remit. Asymptomatic patients with platelet counts greater than 50,000/mm^3 may simply be followed. Symptomatic patients or those with counts less than 30,000/mm^3 should be treated with oral glucocorticoids. More than 50% of patients respond to glu-

TABLE 16.2 Clinical Conditions that May Require Splenectomy

	Common	Uncommon
Thrombocytopenias	Immune thrombocytopenic purpura	Thrombotic thrombocytopenic purpura
Anemias	Hereditary hemolytic anemias (hereditary spherocytosis) Autoimmune hemolytic anemias Congenital hemoglobinopathies (sickle cell anemia)	Thalassemias Hereditary elliptocytosis
Myeloproliferative and myelodysplastic disorders	—	Chronic myelogenous leukemia Polycythemia vera Myelofibrosis or myeloid metaplasia Essential thrombocytosis Myeloproliferative disorder not otherwise specified
Lymphoproliferative disorders	—	Chronic lymphocytic leukemia Hairy-cell leukemia Non-Hodgkin lymphoma (e.g., splenic marginal zone lymphoma) Hodgkin lymphoma
Neutropenias	—	Felty syndrome
Nonhematologic splenic disorders	Trauma Incidental splenectomy Vascular problems (splenic artery aneurysm, splenic vein thrombosis)	Splenic abscess Splenic cyst/pseudocyst Storage diseases

cocorticoids although many will not maintain normal counts after steroid discontinuation (*Am J Med.* 1995;98:436–442, *N Engl J Med.* 2003;349:831–836). In refractory cases, or in patients with bleeding, intravenous immunoglobulin (IVIG) is used, although the effects are transient (*Mayo Clin Proc.*

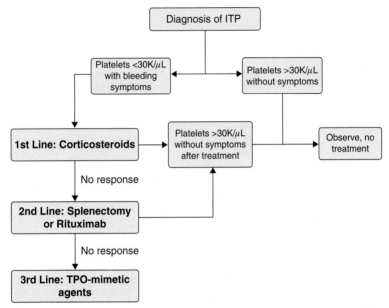

Figure 16-4. Treatment approach in ITP in adults. This diagram represents a simplified approach to the treatment of patients with ITP. A threshold platelet count of 30,000/µL for clinical decisions, rather than a range of platelet counts, is presented, but clinical symptoms and patients' concerns are more important for treatment decisions. (Adapted from George J, Leung LLP. Treatment and prognosis of immune (idiopathic) thrombocytopenic purpura in adults, *UpToDate*, 2011.)

2004;79:504–522). Newer second- line agents include rituximab (anti-CD20 monoclonal antibody) and thrombopoiesis-stimulating agents have demonstrated short-term effectiveness and may be used where splenectomy is refused (*Ann Intern Med.* 2007;146:25–33). Indications for splenectomy are failure to respond to medical therapy and intolerable side effects from steroid administration (Fig. 16-4). Indications for more urgent splenectomy in patients with ITP include need for other emergency surgery or a life-threatening bleed, including central nervous system hemorrhage. Most patients who respond to splenectomy do so within the first 10 postoperative days (*Am J Surg.* 2004;187:720–723).

(3) A systematic review of 135 case series spanning 58 years found a complete remission in two-thirds of patients. Either a complete or partial response was observed in 88% of patients. Complete response was defined as achievement of a platelet count of at least 100×10^9/L. A partial response included a platelet count response of at least 30×10^9/L. Variables associated with a response to splenectomy include younger age and response

to IVIG therapy. Mortality rates of 0.2% to 1% are similar to mortality due to medically treated severe ITP over 5 to 10 years (0.4% to 1.6%). Surgical complication rates range from 10% to 13% (*Blood.* 2004;104:2623–2634).

(4) Patients who fail splenectomy or relapse after an initial response should be investigated for **accessory splenic tissue.** A peripheral smear and magnetic resonance imaging or nuclear medicine studies with technetium (Tc)-99 m–labeled heat-damaged red cells are indicated. If accessory splenic tissue is found, re-exploration should be considered, although long-term response to removal of an accessory spleen is uncommon (*N Engl J Med.* 2002;346:995–1008). Rituximab has been of benefit to patients who fail to respond to splenectomy (*Am J Hematol.* 2005;78:275–280).

b. **Thrombotic thrombocytopenic purpura (TTP)** is characterized by the pentad of hemolytic anemia, consumptive thrombocytopenia, mental status changes, renal failure, and fever, although only hemolytic anemia and thrombocytopenia (without other obvious cause) are required to initiate therapy. Symptoms result from multiorgan microvascular thrombosis.

(1) **First-line therapy** for TTP is medical, with plasmapheresis. A randomized, controlled trial with 102 patients demonstrated significantly improved initial response (47% vs. 25%) and 6-month survival (78% vs. 63%) for plasmapheresis as compared with plasma infusion (*N Engl J Med.* 1991;325:393–397). Glucocorticoids, in addition to plasmapheresis, are prescribed in the rare case of relapse. Second-line medical treatment for relapsing or refractory cases includes rituximab, cyclosporin, and increased plasma exchange frequency.

(2) **Splenectomy** has limited indication in patients who do not respond to medical therapy or those with chronically relapsing disease and has shown benefit only when used in conjunction with plasmapheresis. Severe deficiency of ADAMTS-13, a von Willebrand factor-cleaving protein has been found in many TTP patients, and reports suggest splenectomy may restore ADAMTS-13 levels. A retrospective review of 33 patients found that those who were continuously dependent on plasmapheresis and underwent splenectomy had a postoperative relapse rate of 0.07 per patient-year. In those patients who were not continuously dependent on plasmapheresis, splenectomy reduced the relapse rate from 0.74 to 0.10 per patient-year (*Br J Haematol.* 2005;130:768–776).

2. **Anemias**

a. **Hemolytic anemias** constitute a group of disorders in which splenectomy is almost universally curative.

(1) **Hereditary spherocytosis** is an autosomal dominant disorder characterized by a defect in *spectrin*, a red blood cell (RBC) membrane protein. This defect results in small, spherical, relatively rigid erythrocytes that fail to deform adequately to

traverse the splenic microcirculation leading to sequestration and destruction in the splenic red pulp. In addition to anemia, patients may have jaundice from the hemolytic process and splenomegaly from RBC destruction in the spleen. Splenectomy is indicated in nearly all cases, but should be delayed to age 6 years in children to minimize the risk of overwhelming postsplenectomy sepsis. An exception is if the child is transfusion dependent. Prior to splenectomy, patients should have a right-upper-quadrant ultrasound, and if gallstones are present (usually pigment stones from hemolysis), a cholecystectomy can be performed concomitantly. The recently described technique of subtotal splenectomy (leaving a 10 cm^3 remnant) may reduce the risks of infection and sepsis (*Br J Haematol.* 2006;132:791–793).

(2) **Hereditary elliptocytosis** is an autosomal dominant disorder in which an intrinsic cytoskeletal defect causes the RBCs to be elliptical. Most patients have an asymptomatic and mild anemia that does not need specific treatment. Patients with symptomatic anemia should undergo splenectomy to prolong RBC survival.

b. Acquired autoimmune hemolytic anemias are characterized as either warm or cold, depending on the temperature at which they interact with antibody.

(1) **Warm autoimmune hemolytic anemia** results from splenic sequestration and destruction of RBCs coated with autoantibodies that interact optimally with their antigens at 37°C. Anti-immunoglobulin IgG antiserum causes agglutination of the patient's RBCs (positive direct Coombs test). Etiologies include chronic lymphocytic leukemia (CLL), non-Hodgkin lymphoma, collagen vascular disease, and drugs, although most cases are idiopathic. Primary treatment is directed against the underlying disease. If this is unsuccessful, therapy is corticosteroids. Nonresponders or patients requiring high steroid doses respond to splenectomy in 60% to 80% of cases (*Ann Surg.* 1998;228:568–578). Immunosuppressive and cytotoxic agents have a role in patients unable or unwilling to undergo splenectomy or in relapsed patients

(2) **Cold autoimmune hemolytic anemia** is characterized by fixation of C3 to IgM antibodies that bind RBCs with greater affinity at temperatures approaching 0°C and cause Raynaud-like symptoms combined with anemia. Hemolysis occurs either immediately by intravascular complement–mediated mechanisms or via removal of C3-coated RBCs by the spleen. Treatment is usually successful with use of increased protective clothing. Severe cases may benefit from treatment with low-dose alkylating agents, rituximab or interferon. Splenectomy has no therapeutic benefit.

c. Congenital hemoglobinopathies

1. **Sickle cell anemia** is due to the homozygous inheritance of the S variant of the hemoglobin β chain. The disease is usually

associated with autosplenectomy due to repeated vaso-occlusive crises, but splenectomy may be required for those patients with acute splenic sequestration crisis, evidence of hypersplenism, splenic abscess, and symptomatic splenomegaly.

2. **Thalassemias** are hereditary anemias caused by a defect in hemoglobin synthesis. β-Thalassemia major is primarily treated with iron chelation therapy, but splenectomy may be required to treat symptomatic splenomegaly or pain from splenic infarcts.

3. **Myeloproliferative and myelodysplastic disorders**
   a. **Chronic myelogenous leukemia (CML)** is a myelodysplastic disorder characterized by the *bcr-abl* fusion oncogene, known as the *Philadelphia chromosome.* This oncogene results in a constitutive activation of tyrosine kinase.
      (1) First-line therapy utilizes the tyrosine kinase inhibitor (TKI) imatinib mesylate (Gleevec). Alternative TKI treatments (*dasatinib* and *nilotinib*) are used in cases of intolerance or suboptimal response. Stem cell transplantation is used for cases of treatment failure in eligible patients (*Blood.* 2006;108:1809–1820)
      (2) A large prospectively randomized trial compared splenectomy plus chemotherapy or chemotherapy alone in the treatment of early phase of CML. Splenectomy had no effect on survival or disease progression, but it did increase the rate of thrombosis and vascular accidents (*Cancer.* 1984;54:333–338). Splenectomy is indicated only for palliation of symptomatic splenomegaly or hypersplenism that significantly limits therapy.
   b. **Polycythemia vera and essential thrombocytosis** are chronic diseases of uncontrolled RBC and platelet production, respectively. These diseases are treated medically, but splenectomy can be required to treat symptomatic splenomegaly or pain from splenic infarcts. Splenectomy can result in severe thrombocytosis, causing thrombosis or hemorrhage, which requires perioperative antiplatelet, anticoagulation, and myelosuppressive treatment.
   c. **Myelofibrosis and myeloid metaplasia** are incurable myeloproliferative disorders that usually present in patients older than 60 years. The condition is characterized by bone marrow fibrosis, leukoerythroblastosis, and extramedullary hematopoiesis, which can result in massive splenomegaly. Indications for splenectomy include symptomatic splenomegaly and transfusion-dependent anemias. Although the compressive symptoms are effectively palliated with splenectomy, the cytopenias frequently recur. In addition, these patients are at increased risk for postoperative hemorrhage and thrombotic complications after splenectomy.

4. **Lymphoproliferative disorders**
   a. **Chronic lymphocytic leukemia,** a B-cell leukemia, is the most common of the chronic leukemias and is characterized by the accumulation of mature but nonfunctional lymphocytes. Primary therapy is medical, with splenectomy reserved for those patients with symptomatic splenomegaly and severe hypersplenism.

  b. The **non-Hodgkin lymphomas** are a diverse group of disorders with a wide range of clinical behaviors, ranging from indolent to highly aggressive. As with other malignant processes, splenectomy is indicated for palliation of hypersplenism and cytopenias or for diagnosis in patients with suspected persistent or recurrent disease after systemic therapy. Splenectomy plays an important role in the diagnosis and staging of patients with isolated splenic lymphoma (known as *malignant lymphoma with prominent splenic involvement*). In these cases, improved survival has been shown in patients undergoing splenectomy (*Cancer.* 1993;71:207–215).

  c. **Hodgkin lymphoma.** Splenectomy has a limited role in the diagnosis and treatment of Hodgkin lymphoma due to refinements in imaging techniques and progress in the methods of treatment. Indications for surgery are similar to those for non-Hodgkin lymphoma.

  d. **Hairy cell leukemia** is a rare disease of elderly men that is characterized by B lymphocytes with membrane ruffling. Splenectomy was previously regarded as the primary therapy for this disease, but improvements in systemic chemotherapy have reduced the role of splenectomy, which is now reserved for patients with massive splenomegaly or refractory disease.

5. **Neutropenias**

  a. Felty syndrome is characterized by rheumatoid arthritis, splenomegaly, and neutropenia. The primary treatment is steroids, but refractory cases may require splenectomy to reverse the neutropenia. Patients with recurrent infections and significant anemia may benefit from splenectomy. Granulocytopenia is improved in approximately 80% of patients (*Arch Intern Med.* 1978;138:597–602). The clinical course of the arthritis is not affected.

B. **Nonhematologic splenic disorders**

1. **Splenic cysts** are uncommon and can be parasitic or nonparasitic. Most are located in the lower pole in a subcapsular position.

  a. **Parasitic cysts** make up more than two-thirds of splenic cysts worldwide but are rare in the United States. The majority are hydatid cysts caused by *Echinococcus* species. They are typically asymptomatic but may rupture or cause symptoms due to splenomegaly. The primary treatment is splenectomy, with careful attention not to spill the cyst contents. The cyst may be aspirated and injected with hypertonic saline prior to mobilization if concern about rupture exists.

  b. **Nonparasitic cysts** can be true cysts or pseudocysts, but this differentiation is difficult to make preoperatively.

    (1) **True cysts** (or primary cysts) have an epithelial lining and are most often congenital. Other rare true cysts include epidermoid and dermoid cysts.

    (2) **Pseudocysts** (or secondary cysts) lack an epithelial lining and make up more than two-thirds of nonparasitic cysts. They typically result from traumatic hematoma formation and subsequently resorb.

       (3) Treatment. Splenic cysts are typically asymptomatic, but they may present with left upper abdominal or shoulder pain. Those smaller than 5 cm can be followed with ultrasonography and often resolve spontaneously. Larger cysts risk rupture and require cyst unroofing or splenectomy. Percutaneous aspiration is associated with infection and reaccumulation and is not indicated. Laparoscopic management of splenic cysts yields shorter hospital length of stay and fewer complications with no adverse effects (*Surg Endosc.* 2007;21:206–208).

  2. Splenic abscesses are rare but potentially lethal if untreated. Approximately two-thirds are due to seeding from a distant bacteremic focus, most commonly endocarditis or urinary tract infection. Fever is present in nearly all cases, and abdominal discomfort and splenomegaly occur in one half of patients. Associated conditions include sickle cell anemia. Computed tomography (CT) scanning and ultrasonography are the best diagnostic modalities for splenic abscess. CT scanning typically shows an area of low homogeneous density with edges that do not intensify with intravenous contrast. Antibiotic therapy should be instituted immediately after blood cultures are obtained. More than 60% of identified infectious agents are aerobes, with one half being *Staphylococcus* and *Streptococcus* species. A minority of splenic abscesses involve fungal organisms, which can be cured with antifungal agents alone. Unilocular abscesses may be amenable to treatment by percutaneous drainage. Splenectomy, open or laparoscopic, in combination with postoperative antibiotics is the definitive therapy. Laparoscopic unroofing and open partial splenectomy are alternative spleen-preserving options.

C. Other forms of splenic pathology

  1. Trauma to the adult spleen has historically been managed with laparotomy (most children have been successfully managed nonoperatively). With imaging advances, grading of this solid organ injury and conservative management in the stable adult patient have become standard therapy. The common grading system for splenic injury is listed in Table 16-3. Management depends on stability and age (adult vs. child) of the patient and associated injuries (Fig. 16-5).

  2. Incidental splenectomy occurs when the spleen is injured iatrogenically during another abdominal operation. This can occur either by damage from a retractor in the left upper quadrant or from mobilization of the splenic flexure in colon resection. Capsular tears can often be treated with topical hemostatic agents or even with use of the argon beam coagulator, but if significant hemorrhage results and cannot be controlled expeditiously, splenectomy is indicated.

  3. Splenic artery aneurysm is the most common visceral artery aneurysm and has a particular tendency to affect women, with increased incidence of rupture during pregnancy. Asymptomatic aneurysms less than 2 cm in size in patients in whom pregnancy is not anticipated can be followed closely with serial imaging. Operative management is

TABLE 16.3	American Association for the Surgery of Trauma Spleen Injury Scale (2008 Version)	
	Grade[a]	**Injury description**
I	Hematoma	Subcapsular, <10% surface area
	Laceration	Capsular tear, <1 cm parenchymal depth
II	Hematoma	Subcapsular, 10%–50% surface area; intraparenchymal, <5 cm in diameter
	Laceration	1–3 cm parenchymal depth that does not involve a trabecular vessel
III	Hematoma	Subcapsular, >50% surface area or expanding ruptured subcapsular or parenchymal hematoma
		Intraparenchymal hematoma >5 cm or expanding
	Laceration	3 cm parenchymal depth or involving trabecular vessels
IV	Laceration	Laceration involving segmental or hilar vessels producing major devascularization (>25% of spleen)
V	Laceration	Completely shattered spleen
	Vascular	Hilar vascular injury that devascularizes spleen

[a]Advance one grade for multiple injuries up to grade III.
With permission from Tinkoff G, Esposito TJ, Reed J, et al. American Association for the Surgery of Trauma Organ Injury Scale 1: spleen, liver and kidney. *J Trauma* 2008;207(5):646–655.

warranted for (1) larger (≥ 2 cm) or symptomatic aneurysms, (2) those in whom pregnancy is anticipated, and (3) pseudoaneurysms associated with inflammation. Endovascular management such as transcatheter embolization and laparoscopic excision has been used in selected patients. However, pain from splenic infarcts may occur as a result. For proximal and middle-third aneurysms, the aneurysms may simply be excluded by proximal and distal ligation, with the splenic blood supply then coming predominantly from the short gastric vessels. For distal-third aneurysms, resection with splenectomy is usually performed.

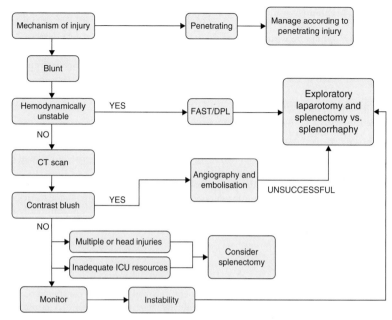

Figure 16-5. Treatment algorithm for splenic trauma. Algorithm for the diagnosis and management of traumatic splenic injury. (Adapted from Esposito TJ, Gamelli RL. Injury to the spleen. In: Feliciano DV, Mattox KL, Moore EE, eds: *Trauma.* 6th ed. Stamford, CT: Appleton & Lange.)

PREOPERATIVE CONSIDERATIONS IN SPLENECTOMY

I. VACCINATIONS

A. **Polyvalent pneumococcal vaccine (Pneumovax)** covers 85% to 90% of pneumococcal types and should be administered at least 2 to 3 weeks before splenectomy, or at least 14 days post-operatively, to all patients older than 2 years. The vaccine should be repeated every 5 to 7 years.

B. **Meningococcal vaccine** is a one-time vaccination for patients older than 2 years.

C. *Haemophilus influenzae* **type B** conjugate vaccine should be considered if the patient was not vaccinated in infancy.

II. CONSIDERATIONS FOR TRANSFUSION

A. **Patients with hematologic disease,** particularly those with autoimmune disorders, often have autoantibodies and are difficult to cross-match. Thus, blood should be typed and screened at least 24 hours prior to the scheduled operative time. Patients with splenomegaly should have 2 to 4 units of packed RBCs cross-matched and available for surgery.

B. **Patients with severe thrombocytopenia** (particularly those with counts <10,000/μL) should have platelets available for transfusion, but these should be withheld until the splenic artery is ligated so they will not be quickly consumed by the spleen. Most patients with thrombocytopenia from ITP can undergo splenectomy safely without platelet transfusion even in the setting of very low platelet counts.

III. PREOPERATIVE IMAGING

A. Either **ultrasound or CT** may be necessary in patients with malignancy or suspected splenomegaly to determine spleen size and to evaluate splenic hilar adenopathy that may complicate a laparoscopic approach. Imaging is not usually indicated in patients with ITP.

B. **Right-upper-quadrant ultrasound** is indicated preoperatively for those who are at high risk for developing gallstones (hemolytic anemias, sickle cell anemia) so that cholecystectomy may be performed concomitantly if indicated.

VI. OTHER CONSIDERATIONS

A. Perioperative stress-dose steroids treatment should be considered for patients receiving steroids pre-operatively and should be continued orally postoperatively and tapered gradually once a hematologic response to splenectomy has occurred.

B. Patients who are to undergo a laparoscopic splenectomy should be counseled preoperatively about the possibility of **conversion to open splenectomy or a hand-assisted approach** and should be prepared identically to those patients for whom an open procedure is planned.

OPERATIVE APPROACH

I. **LAPAROSCOPIC SPLENECTOMY** has become the preferred method for elective splenectomy for all but the most difficult or largest spleens. It is now increasingly used for selected patients with splenomegaly. **Contraindications** to laparoscopic splenectomy are presented in Table 16-4.

A. **Splenomegaly** increases the complexity of the laparoscopic approach because of the difficulty of manipulating the organ atraumatically and achieving adequate exposure of the ligaments and hilum. Large spleens are also more difficult to place in an entrapment bag using a strictly laparoscopic approach. Although the size limits for attempting laparoscopic or laparoscopic-assisted splenectomy are evolving, most moderately enlarged spleens (<1,000 g weight or 15 to 20 cm in length) can be removed in a minimally invasive fashion, often without a hand-port device. For spleens larger than 20 cm in longitudinal length or those that weigh between 1,000 and 3,000 g, the use of a hand port should be considered. The use of a hand port in this setting has been associated with reduced operative times, less blood loss, and lower rates of conversion to open operation (*Arch Surg.* 2006;141:755–761; discussion 61–62). In general, spleens

TABLE 16.4	Contraindications to Laparoscopic Splenectomy
Absolute contraindications	**Difficult cases**
Massive splenomegaly (>30 cm length)	Moderate splenomegaly (>20–25 cm)
Portal hypertension	Severe uncorrectable cytopenia
Splenic trauma, unstable patient	Splenic vein thrombosis
—	Splenic trauma, stable patient
—	Bulky hilar adenopathy
—	Morbid obesity

greater than 30 cm in craniocaudal length (and weighing >3,000 g) should be approached in an open fashion because of the reduced working space and increased difficulty in manipulating the spleen. A search for **accessory splenic tissue** should always be conducted, particularly if the patient has a hematologic indication for splenectomy.

B. **Outcomes of laparoscopic splenectomy.** Several large series of laparoscopic splenectomy have been published with excellent results. In a meta-analysis of 51 reports including 2,940 patients, laparoscopic splenectomy was associated with significantly fewer complications overall, primarily as a result of fewer wound and pulmonary complications.

II. **OPEN SPLENECTOMY.** The incision used is either an upper midline or a left subcostal incision. When significant splenomegaly is present, a midline incision is usually preferred. A drain is not routinely required unless it is suspected that the pancreatic tail may have been injured during the hilar dissection.

COMPLICATIONS OF SPLENECTOMY

I. INTRAOPERATIVE COMPLICATIONS

A. **Hemorrhage.** The most common intraoperative complication of splenectomy is hemorrhage, which can occur during the hilar dissection or from a capsular tear during retraction. The incidence of this complication is 2% to 3% during open splenectomy but is nearly 5% using the laparoscopic approach. Bleeding during laparoscopic splenectomy may necessitate conversion to a hand-assisted or open procedure.

B. Clinical evidence of **pancreatic injury** occurs in 0% to 6% of splenectomies, whether done open or laparoscopically. A retrospective review of one center's experience with laparoscopic splenectomy found pancreatic injury in 16% of patients; half of these were isolated instances of hyperamylasemia. If one suspects that the pancreatic parenchyma has been violated during laparoscopic splenectomy, a closed suction drain should be placed adjacent to the pancreas, and a drain amylase obtained prior to removal after the patient is eating a regular diet.

C. **Bowel injury**

1. **Colon.** Because of the close proximity of the splenic flexure to the lower pole of the spleen, it is possible to injure the colon during mobilization, but this complication is rare. Mechanical bowel preparation is not indicated pre-operatively.

2. **Stomach.** Gastric injuries can occur by direct trauma or can result from thermal injury during division of the short gastric vessels. Use of energy devices too close to the greater curvature of the stomach can result in a delayed gastric necrosis and perforation.

D. **Diaphragmatic injury** has been described during the mobilization of the superior pole, especially with perisplenitis, and is of no consequence if recognized and repaired. In laparoscopic splenectomies, it may be more difficult to recognize the injury given the pneumoperitoneum, but careful dissection of the splenophrenic ligament can minimize its occurrence. The pleural space should be evacuated under positive-pressure ventilation prior to closure to minimize the pneumothorax.

II. EARLY POSTOPERATIVE COMPLICATIONS

A. **Pulmonary complications** develop in nearly 10% of patients after open splenectomy, and these range from atelectasis to pneumonia and pleural effusion. Pulmonary complications are significantly less common with the laparoscopic approach.

B. **Subphrenic abscess** occurs in 2% to 3% of patients after open splenectomy but is uncommon after laparoscopic splenectomy (0.7%). Treatment usually consists of percutaneous drainage and the intravenous antibiotics.

C. **Wound problems** such as hematomas, seromas, and wound infections occur commonly (4% to 5%) after open splenectomy because of the underlying hematologic disorders. Wound complications after laparoscopic splenectomy are usually minor and occur less frequently (1.5%).

D. **Thrombocytosis and thrombotic complications** can occur after either open or laparoscopic splenectomy. The presumed causes of thrombosis after splenectomy may relate to the occurrence of thrombocytosis, alterations in platelet function, and a low-flow stasis phenomenon in the ligated splenic vein. As a result, splenomegaly is a major risk factor for splenic/portal vein thrombosis. Symptomatic portal vein thrombosis occurs more commonly than expected (8% to 10%) and can result in extensive mesenteric thrombosis if not recognized promptly and treated expeditiously. Symptoms of portal vein thrombosis may be subtle and include abdominal pain and low-grade fever. Massive splenomegaly and myelofibrosis are the two main risk factors for portal vein thrombosis.

E. **Ileus** can occur after open splenectomy, but a prolonged postoperative ileus should prompt the surgeon to search for concomitant problems such as a subphrenic abscess or portal vein thrombosis (*Surgery.* 2003;134:647–553; discussion 54–55).

III. LATE POSTOPERATIVE COMPLICATIONS

A. **Overwhelming postsplenectomy infection (OPSI)** is an uncommon complication of splenectomy that may occur at any point in an asplenic or hyposplenic patient's lifetime. The risk of overwhelming infection is very small with an estimated mortality of 0.73 per 1,000 patient years (*Ann Intern Med.* 1995;122:187–188). Patients present with nonspecific flu-like symptoms rapidly progressing to fulminant sepsis, consumptive coagulopathy, bacteremia, and ultimately death within 12 hours to 48 hours. Encapsulated bacteria, especially *Streptococcus pneumoniae, H. influenzae* type B, and *Neisseria meningitidis,* are the most commonly involved organisms. Successful treatment of OPSI requires early supportive care and high-dose third-generation cephalosporins. OPSI appears to have a higher incidence in children, particularly under the age of five. Daily prophylactic antibiotics have been recommended after operation in all children younger than 5 years and in immunocompromised patients because these patients are unlikely to produce adequate antibody in response to pneumococcal vaccination. All patients who have had splenectomy should be educated about the risk of OPSI, and the need for early physician consultation in the event that fever or other prodromal symptoms should occur.

B. **Splenosis** is the presence of disseminated intra-abdominal splenic tissue, which usually occurs after splenic rupture. Splenosis does not appear to be more common after laparoscopic splenectomy, but care should be taken during splenic morcellation to avoid bag rupture and spillage of splenic tissue.

17 Cerebrovascular Disease and Vascular Access

Abdulhameed Aziz and Gregorio A. Sicard

EXTRACRANIAL CEREBROVASCULAR DISEASE

Atherosclerotic occlusive disease of the extracranial carotid artery is a major risk factor for stroke, the primary cause of disability, and the third-most-common cause of death in the United States. More than 700,000 new strokes occur annually, with an estimated total cost of more than $40 billion. The initial mortality from stroke is approximately 30%. Of patients who survive the initial event, 10% recover almost completely, 30% recover with mild deficits, and 60% recover with significant deficits. Furthermore, 25% of survivors have stroke within 5 years. Carotid bifurcation disease is responsible for 25% to 35% of ipsilateral cerebrovascular events.

I. PRESENTATION

A. The clinical presentation of patients with symptomatic occlusive disease is a **neurologic deficit.** However, many patients have an asymptomatic stenosis that is identified by a health-care provider based on auscultation of carotid bruits or screening Doppler study.

B. **Lateralizing ischemic events** can result in aphasia (expressive or receptive), combined sensory and motor deficits, and various visual disturbances. Deficits such as these are usually associated with the anterior cerebral circulation [i.e., the internal carotid artery (ICA) and its branches].

1. Transient ischemic attacks (TIAs) are transient hemispheric neurologic deficits that may last from several seconds to hours but fewer than 24 hours. TIAs that occur in rapid succession, interspersed with complete recovery but with progressively smaller intervals between attacks, are termed **crescendo TIAs** and carry a high risk of progression to a permanent neurologic deficit; emergent evaluation is mandatory.

2. **Amaurosis fugax** (temporary monocular blindness), often described as a shade coming down over one eye, results from emboli lodging in the ophthalmic artery. Fundoscopic examination demonstrates Hollenhorst plaques.

3. If the neurologic deficit persists beyond 24 hours, it is considered a **stroke.** In addition, some patients may present with a neurologic deficit that fluctuates, gradually worsening over a period of hours or days while the patient is under observation. This situation is considered a stroke in evolution and, like crescendo TIAs, needs prompt treatment.

C. **Global ischemic events** are manifested by symptoms such as vertigo, dizziness, perioral numbness, ataxia, or drop attacks. These are usually associated with interruption of posterior circulation supplying the brain stem (i.e., the vertebrobasilar system).

II. **PATHOPHYSIOLOGY AND EPIDEMIOLOGY.** Ischemic events in patients with extracranial vascular disease can be the result of emboli or a low-flow state. Although it can cause clinical symptoms, disease of the vertebral arteries typically remains asymptomatic. On the other hand, even when it is asymptomatic, significant occlusive carotid arterial disease carries with it a doubling of baseline stroke risk. Once a significant carotid lesion results in an ipsilateral lateralizing cerebral event, the risk of stroke may be as high as 26% over 2 years.

III. **DIAGNOSIS.** A careful neurologic examination is performed before obtaining any diagnostic studies. The presence of a carotid bruit warrants diagnostic evaluation. Imaging of the carotid arterial system attempts to classify the degree of stenosis, which is useful for determining prognosis. Because of methodologic differences in calculating the percentage of stenosis encountered in different studies, there is some disagreement about exact cutoff percentages. However, four levels of stenosis are typically described: mild (<50%), moderate (50% to 79%), severe (80% to 99%), and occluded (100%). A variety of noninvasive and invasive diagnostic studies are available.

A. **Color-flow duplex scanning** uses real-time B-mode ultrasound and color-enhanced pulsed Doppler flow measurements to determine the extent of the carotid stenosis. **This is the initial screening test for carotid disease.** The reliability of this study depends in large part on the abilities of the vascular technicians. When using an accredited vascular laboratory, treatment of most carotid lesions can be instituted based on ultrasound duplex scanning alone.

B. **Arteriography** remains the gold standard for the diagnosis of cerebrovascular disease. Unlike duplex scanning, however, arteriography is an invasive procedure with inherent risks, such as contrast allergy, renal toxicity, and stroke (2% to 4% of patients). Because of these risks and improvements in duplex ultrasonography, carotid arteriography is generally limited to patients with technically inadequate duplex ultrasonography, planning for carotid artery stenting (CAS), or for verification of carotid occlusion.

C. **Magnetic resonance angiography (MRA)** and **Computed tomographic angiography (CTA)** are reliable means of supplementary imaging but remain inferior to conventional angiography. Both have advantages of being noninvasive. Limitations of MRA include the appearance of lumen smaller than actual diameter, but with improvement after administration of gadolinium. CTA can be performed with excellent three-dimensional reconstructions but carries the risk of contrast-induced nephropathy. For patients with complete occlusion and contralateral high-grade occlusion, results of duplex ultrasound are often confirmed by CTA or angiography.

IV. MANAGEMENT

A. **Medical therapy.** It is important to make every effort to modify risk factors to prevent progression of carotid occlusive disease. Control of hypertension, cessation of smoking, management of lipid disorders, attainment of ideal body weight, and regular exercise should be undertaken. No drug therapy has been shown to reduce the risk of stroke in patients with asymptomatic carotid disease. Medical management in symptomatic patients is focused primarily on the use of antiplatelet agents, specifically aspirin. Aspirin is effective in reducing stroke and stroke-related deaths. In a meta-analysis of more than 8,000 patients, the risk of major vascular events was reduced by 22% in patients receiving aspirin (*Br Med J.* 1988;296:320). Low doses (81 mg/day) are as efficacious as higher doses (325 mg/day). Clopidogrel (Plavix) is a potent antiplatelet agent, but it has not been evaluated as part of medical therapy compared to carotid endarterectomy (CEA). Anticoagulation with heparin sodium is beneficial in patients who have cardiac emboli. In addition, heparin may be useful in preventing progression of thrombus in evolving nonhemorrhagic strokes. The major contraindication to heparinization is a recent hemorrhagic brain infarct; therefore, a CT scan of the brain should be obtained before heparin is given.

B. **Surgical/endovascular management** is the treatment of choice for extracranial cerebrovascular disease and has been documented to reduce stroke.

1. **Indications** for CEA have been extensively studied in both asymptomatic and symptomatic patients, comparing surgical treatment to best medical therapy. Two commonly cited studies include the Asymptomatic Carotid Atherosclerosis Study (ACAS) (*JAMA.* 1995;273:1421) and the North American Symptomatic Carotid Endarterectomy Trial (NASCET) (*NEJM.* 1991;325:445). In the ACAS trial, the ipsilateral 5-year stroke rate in asymptomatic patients with at least 60% stenosis was 5.1% in patients undergoing a CEA versus 11% receiving best medical therapy. For symptomatic patients with at least 70% stenosis in the NASCET trial, the 2-year ipsilateral stroke rate was 9% versus 26% in the CEA and best medical therapy groups, respectively. Based largely on these two definitive trials, current indications for CEA include the following:

a. **Asymptomatic patients with greater than 70% stenosis.**

b. **Symptomatic patients with greater than 50% stenosis.**

c. **Symptomatic patients with greater than 50% stenosis** who have an **ulcerated lesion** or whose **symptoms persist** while they are on **aspirin** or other antiplatelet therapy.

d. **Selected patients with stroke in evolution.** Surgery is performed to restore normal blood flow to allow recovery of ischemic brain tissue that is nonfunctional yet metabolically alive. Surgical candidates have mild-to-moderate neurologic defects and no evidence of hemorrhage on CT scan. The timing of surgery in these cases is controversial.

e. **Selected patients with completed strokes.** Interventions in these patients are performed in the hope of reducing stroke recurrence, which is 7% to 8% per year with nonsurgical therapy. Candidates for surgery include patients with a mild deficit and (1) greater than 70% stenosis or (2) greater than 50% stenosis and an ulcerated plaque, and patients with a moderate deficit and a lesion greater than 70% with an occluded contralateral carotid artery. The timing of surgery in these cases is debatable; however, surgery traditionally has been delayed to reduce the risk of perioperative hemorrhagic stroke. A prudent approach is to wait 4 to 6 weeks postinfarction to minimize the risk of intracranial hemorrhage.

   f. Rarely, endarterectomy is performed on patients with **completely occluded carotid arteries.** Candidates for surgery include those who have:

      (1) Recent endarterectomy with immediate postoperative thrombosis.

      (2) Bruit disappears under observation while remaining asymptomatic.

      (3) Recent occlusion with fluctuating or progressive symptoms.

      (4) New internal carotid occlusion that can be operated on within 2 to 4 hours of the onset of symptoms.

2. CEA has been performed for more than 50 years and is the most commonly performed vascular operation. A beneficial outcome depends on meticulous technique. The use of such technique can keep the perioperative adverse event rate (stroke and death) below 3%.

   a. Anesthesia for CEA can be general endotracheal anesthesia, regional cervical block, or local anesthesia. The choice of anesthesia depends on a combination of patient factors and surgeon expertise. No single method of anesthesia has been demonstrated superior.

   b. During **exposure and mobilization** of the common carotid artery (CCA) and its branches, it is important to proceed with gentle dissection and minimal manipulation of the carotid bulb to prevent embolization from the atherosclerotic plaque.

   c. After **systemic heparinization** of the patient, the internal, external, and common carotid arteries are clamped, and a longitudinal arteriotomy is made from just proximal to the plaque in the CCA to just beyond the distal extent of the plaque in the ICA.

   d. Placement of tubing to **shunt** blood from the CCA around the operative field to the ICA during endarterectomy is a controversial practice. Adequate cerebral perfusion without shunting occurs in 85% to 90% of patients. Intraoperative neurologic assessment of the awake patient under local anesthesia can be as simple as having the patient squeeze a noise toy in the contralateral hand and answering a few simple questions after carotid occlusion. **Awake assessment** is the most sensitive and specific method of determining the need for shunt placement (*J Vasc Surg.* 2007;45:511). Patients who develop weakness or changes in mental status should be shunted. For patients under general anesthesia, an alternative method of cerebral perfusion is required, although some surgeons simply choose routinely to shunt these patients. Stump pressure and intraoperative electroencephalogram (EEG) monitoring are commonly used alternative methods for the determination of cerebral perfusion and subsequent need for shunting. Shunting can be performed safely without an increased risk of stroke (*Ann Vasc Surg.* 2006;20:482).

   e. The **plaque** is carefully separated from the media and removed. The CEA is closed using a running suture. A Cochrane review of patch angioplasty (venous or synthetic) shows that it is associated with a significantly reduced risk for perioperative ipsilateral arterial occlusion and decreased restenosis during long-term follow-up (*Cochrane Database Syst Rev.* 2009 Oct 7;(4) CD000160) Determining differences in the material for patch angioplasty requires further study.

f. Postoperative care

(1) Immediately after endarterectomy, **neurologic function and blood pressure (BP) alterations** should be monitored. Hypertension and hypotension are common after endarterectomy and may cause neurologic complications. The extremes of BP should be treated with either sodium nitroprusside or phenylephrine (Neo-Synephrine) to keep the systolic BP between 140 and 160 mm Hg (slightly higher in chronically hypertensive patients). The wound should be examined for hematoma formation. Aspirin is resumed in the immediate postoperative period. Some advocate the use of dextran-40 (up to 20 mL/kg/day for up to 72 hours) as an additional antithrombotic agent, which can be started intraoperatively and continued into the early postoperative period.

(2) Patient follow-up. A baseline duplex scan is obtained 3 months after the procedure and again at 12 months. Patients can then be followed yearly. Patients who can tolerate aspirin are given 325 mg/day.

g. Complications

(1) Stroke rates must be low (3%) to make operative management of cerebrovascular disease reasonable, especially in asymptomatic patients.

(2) Myocardial infarction (MI) remains the most common cause of death in the early postoperative period. As many as 25% of patients who undergo endarterectomy have severe, correctable coronary artery lesions. The timing of coronary intervention relative to CEA is under debate.

(3) Cranial nerve injuries occur in 5% to 10% of patients who undergo CEA. The most commonly injured nerve is the marginal mandibular, followed by the recurrent laryngeal, superior laryngeal, and hypoglossal nerves.

(4) Recurrent carotid stenosis has been reported to occur in 5% to 10% of cases, although symptoms are present in fewer than 3%. Two types of lesions have been characterized. Neointimal hyperplasia may occur early (within 2 to 3 years). Recurrent atherosclerosis also may cause restenosis (typically after 3 years at the bifurcation site). The presence of symptoms is an indication for treatment of a recurrent lesion. Frequently, these lesions do not lend themselves to endarterectomy and are best treated by CAS.

3. Carotid artery stenting

a. The **indications** for CAS are the same as those for a CEA; however, this technique is under intense investigation. Several studies have been completed or are underway to examine the efficacy of CAS compared to CEA, particularly in high-risk patients. Outcomes have varied, especially as device technology and operator experience has improved. The CREST (Carotid Revascularization Endarterectomy v. Stenting Trial) randomly assigned patients with symptomatic or asymptomatic carotid stenosis to undergo carotid artery stenting or CEA. This trial showed the risk of stroke, MI, or death did not differ significantly in the group undergoing CAS and the group undergoing CEA. During the periprocedural period, there was a higher risk of stroke with stenting and a higher risk of MI with endarterectomy (*NEJM.* 2010;363:11–23).

(1) Because CEA is well tolerated and has a very low risk of complications, CAS is commonly reserved for **high-risk patients,** including patients with the following conditions:

  (a) Severe cardiac disease.

  (b) Severe chronic obstructive pulmonary disease (COPD).

  (c) Severe renal insufficiency or end-stage renal disease (ESRD) requiring hemodialysis.

  (d) Prior ipsilateral neck surgery.

  (e) Prior neck radiation.

  (f) Contralateral vocal cord paralysis.

  (g) Surgically inaccessible lesion.

(2) **Relative contraindications** to CAS include the following:

  (a) Severe tortuosity of common and ICA.

  (b) Complex aortic arch anatomy (increasing difficulty as great vessels arise from ascending rather than transverse aortic arch).

  (c) Severe calcification or extensive thrombus formation.

  (d) Near-complete or complete occlusion.

b. **CAS** has evolved and is commonly performed in the following basic steps. Meticulous technique is critical for reducing the incidence of stroke. Special attention must be taken to avoid catheter and wire manipulation of the lesion prior to cerebral protection device deployment and to ensuring removal of all air bubbles within the angiography tubing.

c. Embolization of plaque debris has been shown to occur with almost any endovascular manipulation of a carotid artery lesion. Consequently, **embolic protection devices** have been developed that significantly reduce the risk of stroke during CAS. The typical device used today is a filter-like device that is advanced across the lesion and then opened in the distal ICA prior to angioplasty and stent deployment. Flow reversal is created after balloon occlusion of the external carotid artery (ECA) and CCA, thus eliminating the need to cross the lesion and possibly decreasing the risk of stroke.

d. **Complications**

(1) **Embolic stroke** is the most common complication of CAS. Risk factors include lack of a cerebral protection device, long or multiple lesions, and age older than 80 years. Thrombolysis may be a successful treatment option, especially if the source of emboli is an acute thrombus. When an embolus is composed of atheroma or chronic thrombus, however, mechanical removal of emboli may become necessary to restore flow.

(2) **Hemodynamic instability** may occur during manipulation and angioplasty of the carotid bifurcation. Bradycardia should be anticipated and treated with atropine prior to dilation of the carotid bifurcation. Postoperatively, as with CEA, patients should be monitored to avoid extremes of BP.

(3) **Restenosis** occurs in approximately 5% of patients at 12 to 24 months and is typically secondary to intimal hyperplasia. These lesions are often amenable to repeat angioplasty.

e. Follow-up using duplex ultrasound is important to identify patients with restenosis and is usually performed at baseline following CAS and then at 3, 6, and 12 months and every year thereafter. Significant elevation of peak systolic velocity from baseline should prompt further evaluation with angiography.

VASCULAR ACCESS FOR DIALYSIS

The success of hemodialysis depends on the rate of blood flow through the dialyzer. Flow rates of between 350 and 450 mL/minute are required to provide adequate dialysis within a reasonable time frame (3 to 4 hours). The dialysis access is a port or site in the body that provides the necessary blood flow for dialysis. The access should be easy to cannulate and last for years with minimal maintenance. The incidence of complications, such as infection, stenosis, pseudoaneurysm formation, thrombosis, and outflow deterioration, should also be low. To date, no vascular access fulfills all of these criteria.

I. INDICATIONS

A. **Temporary hemodialysis access** provided with short- or intermediate-term central venous access device (CVAD) is indicated when acute short-term dialysis is needed, as in (1) acute renal failure, (2) overdose or intoxication, (3) ESRD needing urgent hemodialysis without available mature access, (4) peritoneal dialysis patients with peritonitis, and (5) transplant recipients needing temporary hemodialysis during severe rejection episodes.

B. **Permanent hemodialysis access** is created using subcutaneous conduits having high blood flows when long-term hemodialysis is needed, as in (1) long-term treatment of chronic renal failure and (2) patients awaiting renal transplantation.

II. DIALYSIS ACCESS CATHETERS

A. **Nontunneled central venous catheters.** Short-term dialysis access includes percutaneous catheters in internal jugular, subclavian, or femoral veins. The **Quinton catheter** provides access for short-term hemodialysis in acute renal failure. Noncuffed, double-lumen catheters can be percutaneously inserted at the bedside and provide acceptable blood flow rates (250 mL/minute) for temporary hemodialysis – no more than 3 weeks for internal jugular or 5 days for femoral catheters due to considerations of infection and dislodgement.

B. **Tunneled central venous silicone dialysis catheters.** Tunneled catheters [e.g., **Tesio, Ash Split** (Bard Access Systems) and **Duraflow catheters** (AngioDynamics)] have cuffs that anchor them to the subcutaneous tissues. Tunneled, cuffed venous catheters should be placed preferentially in the right internal jugular vein because this site offers a more direct route to the cavoatrial junction and a lower risk of complications than other potential catheter insertion sites. Advantages of tunneled catheters include the ability to insert into a variety of sites, no maturation time requirement, no hemodynamic consequences, ease and cost of catheter placement and replacement, and a life span of the access of months to years. Disadvantages of tunneled, cuffed venous catheters include potential morbidity due to thrombosis, infection, risk of permanent central venous stenosis or occlusion, and lower blood flow rates than for atrioventricular grafts and fistulas.

C. **Catheter complications**
   1. **Early dysfunction** usually occurs secondary to either malposition or intracatheter thrombosis. Almost all catheters inserted into a central vein develop a fibrin sleeve after insertion, resulting in **late dysfunction.** They are usually clinically silent until they obstruct the ports at the distal end of the catheter. They also serve as a nidus for infection.
   2. **Central vein stenosis, thrombosis, or stricture.** Central vein stenosis arises from endothelial injury at the site of catheter–endothelial contact. Incidence increases with the use of nonsilicone catheters, with the use of a subclavian approach, and with a history of prior catheter-related infections. Removal of the CVAD may not improve the underlying problem and, by definition, sacrifices the access. Systemic anticoagulation remains the primary therapy.

III. ARTERIOVENOUS (AV) ACCESS NOMENCLATURE

A. **Conduit.** An **autogenous AV access** (also known as an **AV fistula,** a **native vein fistula,** and a **primary fistula**) is an access created by connecting a native vein to an adjacent artery. A **nonautogenous AV access** (also known as an **AV graft** or a **graft fistula**) uses grafts that are either synthetic or biologic. **Synthetic grafts** include expanded polytetrafluoroethylene (ePTFE, e.g., Gore-Tex or Impra) and polyester (e.g., Dacron) grafts. **Biologic grafts** include bovine heterografts, human umbilical veins, and cryopreserved allogeneic human vein grafts.

B. **Configuration.** A **direct access** often connects a native vein to an adjacent artery. An **indirect access** uses an autogenous or prosthetic material placed subcutaneously between the artery and vein. The course of the subcutaneous prosthesis may be **looped** (loop graft) or **straight** (straight graft).

IV. PREOPERATIVE EVALUATION

A. **Timing.** Ideally, any patient with renal insufficiency should be referred for surgical evaluation approximately 1 year before the anticipated need for dialysis. This point is reached when the creatinine clearance is less than

25 mL/minute or the serum creatinine rises above 4 mg/dL. This allows ample opportunity for appropriate access planning, and efforts can be instituted to ensure preservation of the native veins for later AV fistula creation.

B. **Preservation of access sites.** All ESRD patients should protect their forearm veins from venipuncture and intravenous catheters. Likewise, hospital staff should be instructed to avoid damaging these essential veins. The nondominant arm is preferred for initial access creation. Subclavian vein cannulation should be avoided at all costs because this may induce central venous stenosis, which could preclude later use of an entire arm.

C. **History.** A detailed assessment for the presence of peripheral vascular disease, diabetes mellitus, cardiopulmonary disease, and coagulation disorders best determines the type of vascular access needed for a particular patient. Any conditions that suggest stenosis or occlusion of the venous or arterial system should be elicited because these may limit options for dialysis access. These include prior central venous line; transvenous pacemaker; previous surgery; trauma; or radiation treatment to the chest, neck, or arm. Evidence of early cardiac dysfunction or volume overload indicates a patient at risk for congestive heart failure following fistula creation due to increased preload. Comorbid conditions that limit life expectancy, such as severe coronary artery disease or malignancy, may render a cuffed catheter the best option.

D. **Physical examination**
  1. **Pulse examination.** The axillary, brachial, radial, and ulnar artery pulses are carefully palpated in both upper extremities, and, when indicated, the femoral, popliteal, and pedal arteries are palpated. Residual scars from previous central venous catheters or surgery should also be carefully assessed.

  2. **Cardiovascular status.** Evaluation involves determining capillary refill, the presence of edema, unequal extremity size, and collateral veins on the chest wall. A tourniquet, gravity, and gentle percussion are used to distend the forearm and upper arm veins. Their patency and continuity can be addressed by palpation and detection of a fluid thrill.

  3. **Segmental BP measurements.** Discrepancies between the two upper extremities should be noted.

  4. **Allen test.** This is intended to assess the integrity of the palmar circulatory arches and allow assessment of the dominant blood supply to the hand.

E. **Duplex ultrasound scanning** can determine the diameter of the artery and the adequacy of the superficial and deep veins. For venous evaluation, tourniquets are placed on the patient's midforearm and upper arm. Details of the venous lumen, such as webs, sclerosis, and occlusion, can be visualized. Doppler venous studies may also identify suitable veins for AV fistula creation that are not readily visible on the surface anatomy, especially in heavier patients.

F. **Diagnostic imaging.** History or physical findings suggestive of central venous stenosis or previous complicated vascular access warrant further diagnostic imaging.

1. **Contrast venography** is the gold standard for determining the patency and adequacy of the superficial and deep venous systems, particularly the central veins.

2. **Conventional arteriography** also remains the gold standard for the evaluation of a suspected arterial inflow stenosis or occlusion. When in doubt as to the adequacy of the donor artery or the runoff, it is advisable to obtain an arteriogram that shows the entire arterial system from the origin of the subclavian artery to the distal branches. **MRA** can also be used for the same purpose and is particularly useful when severe contrast allergy, vascular disease, or poor renal function precludes arteriography.

G. **Laboratory studies.** Hyperkalemia and acidosis are the most common electrolyte abnormalities seen in ESRD patients. Therefore, preoperative testing should include evaluation of serum electrolytes and glucose to avoid possible procedural or anesthesia-related complications.

V. NATIVE VEIN AV FISTULAS

A. **Characteristics.** Native vein fistulas are created by connecting a vein to the adjacent artery, usually the radial or brachial artery. These are the safest and longest-lasting permanent means of vascular access, with the highest 5-year patency rates and minimum requirements for intervention. Disadvantages include a long maturation time of weeks to months to provide a flow state adequate to sustain dialysis. Revision of the outflow vein and hand exercises to increase flow to the extremity can accelerate fistula maturation. The patient's arterial and venous anatomy remains the most significant limitation because diseased vessels (e.g., due to diabetes or atherosclerosis) can hinder normal maturation or may preclude the creation of a fistula altogether. Of the ESRD population in the United States, approximately 30% have AV fistulas as their permanent dialysis access (*Kidney Int.* 2000;58:2178). The Kidney Disease Outcomes Quality Initiative (K/DOQI) guidelines recommend a 50% fistula placement rate for first-time access in ESRD patients.

B. **Location.** The Brescia–Cimino fistula at the wrist (creating an end-to-side anastomosis between the cephalic vein and radial artery) and the Gratz fistula at the elbow (i.e., anastomosing the cephalic vein to the brachial artery) are the two most commonly performed autogenous AV fistulas. Flow of arterial blood under pressure distends the outflow vein to produce the subcutaneous conduit. Peripheral sites should be used first, moving to more-central sites as the former sites fail.

C. **Construction.** Most procedures can be performed on an outpatient basis, using only conscious sedation administered intravenously and local anesthetics. The end of a superficial vein, usually the cephalic, is anastomosed to the side of the artery. A side-to-side anastomosis can result in venous hypertension and swelling in the distal extremity due to higher venous pressures. An end-to-end anastomosis performed in a radial artery fistula has the advantage of providing limited flow, thereby reducing a hypercirculatory state. The disadvantage is that the anastomosis is technically challenging and carries the risk of hand ischemia. This risk is particularly high in elderly and diabetic patients. The length (diameter) of the anastomosis dictates the blood flow in fistulas based on larger arteries (e.g., the brachial artery), making it an important determinant in the development of vascular steal symptoms in distal extremity.

VI. AV GRAFT

A. **Characteristics.** AV grafts consist of biologic or synthetic conduits that connect an artery and a vein and are tunneled under the skin and placed in a subcutaneous location. PTFE allows ingrowth of host tissue and formation of a pseudointimal lining, which resists infection and self-seals after needle puncture. The advantages of AV grafts over AV fistulas include (1) large surface area, (2) easy cannulation, (3) short maturation time, and (4) easy surgical handling. However, the long-term patency of AV grafts remains inferior to that of AV fistulas, despite a fourfold increase in salvage procedures. Synthetic grafts require 3 to 6 weeks before they can be used; this period allows sufficient time for the material to incorporate into the surrounding subcutaneous tissues and for the inflammation and edema to subside.

B. **Location.** AV grafts are typically placed between the brachial artery and the cephalic or brachial vein in the antecubital fossa and arranged in a loop configuration in the forearm. Upper-arm grafts can also be created between the brachial artery and basilic or axillary veins. When all upper-extremity sites are exhausted, attention is turned to the lower extremity, where loop grafts typically connect the superficial femoral artery and femoral or saphenous veins.

C. **Placement.** AV grafts are placed under local anesthesia with conscious sedation. Prophylactic antibiotics (e.g., second-generation cephalosporins) are commonly administered immediately prior to the surgery.

VII. COMPLICATIONS OF AV ACCESS

A. **Stenosis.** Pseudointimal hyperplasia within a synthetic graft or neointimal hyperplasia in a native AV fistula or outflow vein of a graft constitutes the most common cause of dysfunction. Approximately 85% of graft thromboses result from hemodynamically significant stenosis (*J Vasc Surg.* 1997;26:373). Arterial inflow lesions are less common but can lead to low flow as well as elevated recirculation, making it more difficult to distinguish them from outflow lesions. Elevated venous pressures, increased recirculation, or recurrent thrombosis necessitate a fistulogram and treatment of any underlying lesion(s) by angioplasty or surgical revision. Stenoses in long segments (>30% after angioplasty) or those that recur within a short interval require surgical intervention.

B. **Thrombosis.** Thrombosis occurring within a month of placement is often due to anatomic or technical factors, such as a narrow outflow vein, misplaced suture, or graft kinking. Early thrombosis of native vein fistulas often results in permanent loss of the access. Prolonged hypotension during and after dialysis occasionally precipitates thrombosis, as can trauma from needle puncture or excessive compression after needle removal following hemostasis.

By 24 months, 96% of grafts require thrombectomy, angioplasty, or surgical revision. Prosthetic AV shunt thrombosis can be managed by pharmacologic thrombolysis, mechanical maceration, or surgical thrombectomy, either separately or in combination. Fistulography at the time of treatment usually reveals the precipitating cause, allowing immediate intervention. Surgical thrombectomy should be followed by fistulography to detect stenosis not fully appreciable during standard balloon thrombectomy. The rate of secondary graft patency after intervention reaches only 65% at 1 year and 51% at 2 years (*Am J Kidney Dis.* 2000;36:68).

C. **Infection.** Infection and bacteremia in dialysis patients are usually caused by *Staphylococcus aureus.* The type of access constitutes the major risk factor for infection. AV fistula infections usually respond to a prolonged course (6 weeks) of antibiotic therapy. If septic embolization occurs, the fistula should be revised or taken down. AV graft infections occur in approximately 5% to 20% prosthetics placed and present a more challenging problem. Antibiotic treatment should cover Gram-positive organisms (including enterococci) as well as Gram-negative organisms (e.g., *Escherichia coli*). A superficial skin infection not involving the graft may respond to antibiotics alone. Focal graft infections can be salvaged with resection of the infected portion of the graft, but extensive infections and those that involve newly constructed, unincorporated grafts should be managed with complete excision. Evidence of bacteremia, pseudoaneurysm formation, or local hemorrhage should prompt graft removal, with placement of a new access at a different site.

D. **Pseudoaneurysm formation.** Pseudoaneurysms result from destruction of the vessel wall and replacement by biophysically inferior collagenous tissue, usually after repetitive puncture of the same vessel segment. A downstream stenosis predisposes to upstream aneurysm formation. Major complications include rupture, infection (which is promoted by intra-aneurysmal thrombus), and, rarely, antegrade or retrograde embolization. Prior to any intervention, imaging is indispensable for identification of thrombus and assessment of the venous anastomosis and outflow. Aneurysmal dilations of AV fistulae often can be treated by surgical correction, including partial or complete resection of the aneurysmal sac, repair of accompanying stenoses, and reconstruction of an adequate lumen. Aneurysm in an AV graft calls for replacement of the weakened graft segment.

E. **Arterial "steal" syndrome.** All AV accesses divert or "steal" blood from the distal circulation to a certain extent. A clinical syndrome resulting from this decrease in distal circulation occurs when the various local compensatory mechanisms fail; this syndrome is reported to occur in approximately 1% to 4% of patients with distal AV accesses (*Ann Vasc Surg.* 2000;14(2):138–144). The clinical presentations of arterial insufficiency in the tissues distal to the fistula may include ischemic pain, neuropathy, ulceration, and gangrene. Patients with diabetes, prior AV access, or atherosclerotic disease are at a higher risk. Patients with mild ischemia complain of subjective coldness and paresthesias without sensory or motor loss and can be managed expectantly with increasing exercise tolerance. Failure of these symptoms to improve may require surgical correction with banding or ligation. Severe ischemia requires immediate surgical intervention to avoid irreversible nerve injury.

F. **Venous hypertension.** Venous hypertension can be caused by the presence or development of outflow vein obstruction. It manifests as swelling, skin discoloration, and hyperpigmentation in the access limb. In chronic cases, ulceration and pain may develop. Management consists of correction of stenosis and disconnecting the veins that are responsible for retrograde flow and pressure transmission.

G. **Congestive heart failure.** Venous return to the heart, cardiac output, and myocardial work can significantly increase after AV fistula or graft placement, leading to cardiomegaly and congestive heart failure in some patients. Hypercirculation ensues if the outflow resistance is too low and the anastomosis is too wide. This problem is more common with ePTFE grafts and brachial artery fistulas. Correction involves narrowing the proximal shunt or graft with either a prosthetic band or suture ligature. Occasionally, a new access must be constructed using a smaller-diameter conduit or tapered prosthetic material.

VIII. VASCULAR ACCESS MONITORING

A. **Angiography** (fistulogram) remains the gold standard for the evaluation of access problems. However, the need for frequent evaluations and the invasive nature of angiography prevent it from being a practical option for routine surveillance.

B. **Doppler ultrasound** measures access flow and correlates with the presence and severity of stenoses detected by angiography. Blood flow below a critical level (350 mL/minute) or a reduction in flow over time (>15%) predicts the presence of stenosis and the development of thrombosis.

18 Thoracoabdominal Vascular Diseases

Enjae Jung, Jeffrey Jim, and Luis A. Sanchez

The vast majority of vascular diseases are secondary to atherosclerotic changes of the arterial wall, influenced to a degree by genetic predisposition and age. However, the evolution of the disease for most individuals can be modified by changes in environmental factors, particularly diet, smoking, and exercise. The arterial wall is comprised of the intimal, medial, and adventitial layers. Endothelium lines the intima. The media contains layers of smooth muscle cells and an extracellular matrix (ECM) of elastin, collagen, and proteoglycans. The adventitia is made of loose connective tissue and fibroblasts. An arterial aneurysm is a weakness of the arterial wall resulting in a permanent localized dilation greater than 50% of the normal vessel diameter. All three layers are dilated, but the majority of degeneration occurs in the media. Occlusive arterial disease, on the other hand, is caused by atherosclerotic change of the intima.

I. **ABDOMINAL AORTIC ANEURYSMS (AAAs)** are the most common type of arterial aneurysm, occurring in 3 to 9% of people older than 50 years of age in the Western world (*Br J Surg.* 1998;85:155). They are five times more common in men than in women and 3.5 times more common in whites than in African Americans. In the United States, ruptured AAAs are the 15th leading cause of death overall and the 10th leading cause of death in men older than 55 years, a rate that has held steady for the past two decades despite improvements in operative technique and perioperative management.

A. **Pathophysiology.** Ninety percent of AAAs are believed to be degenerative in origin, whereas 5% are inflammatory and the remainder are idiopathic (*J Vasc Surg.* 2003;38:584). AAAs are strongly associated with older age, smoking, white race, positive family history, hypertension (HTN), hyperlipidemia, and emphysema. Familial clustering of AAAs has been noted in 15% to 25% of patients undergoing aneurysm surgery. The risk of rupture correlates with wall tension in accordance with Laplace's law, such that the risk of aneurysm rupture increases exponentially with aneurysm diameter. Majority of AAAs are infrarenal; 25% involve the iliac arteries, and 2% involve the renal or other visceral arteries (*J Cardiovasc Surg.* 1991;32:636). Fourteen percent are associated with peripheral (e.g., femoral or popliteal) aneurysms (*J Vasc Surg.* 2000;31:863).

B. **Diagnosis**

1. **Clinical manifestations.** Seventy-five percent of AAAs are asymptomatic and are found incidentally. Aneurysm expansion or rupture may cause severe back, flank, or abdominal pain and varying degrees of

shock. Distal embolization, thrombosis, and duodenal or ureteral compression can produce symptoms. Fifty percent of AAAs are identifiable on physical examination as a pulsatile mass at or above the umbilicus. AAA rupture may mimic renal colic, peritonitis, duodenal perforation, pancreatitis, degenerative spine disease, acute disk herniation, or myocardial infarction.

2. **Radiologic evaluation**
   a. **Abdominal radiographs.** In 75% of patients with an AAA, arterial wall calcification suggests the presence of an aneurysm and permits a gross estimation of aneurysm diameter.
   b. **Ultrasonography and computed tomography (CT) scanning** demonstrate AAAs with an accuracy of 95% and 100%, respectively, and are useful for serial examinations of small aneurysms. **CT angiography** (CTA) is rapidly becoming the gold standard for evaluating AAAs because it allows operative planning for endovascular approaches.
   c. **Magnetic resonance (MR) scan** is comparable to CT but avoids radiation exposure and is useful in patients with intravenous contrast contraindications.
   d. **Aortography** is **not** sensitive for the diagnosis of AAA because it may underestimate the aneurysm size or fail to reveal the aneurysm owing to the presence of mural thrombus. However, aortography is indicated to evaluate suspected renal or mesenteric artery stenosis and lower-extremity occlusive disease (*Ann Vasc Surg.* 1990; 4:419).

C. **Elective management of AAA.** The risk of aneurysm rupture correlates best with aneurysm size (*Ann Surg.* 1966;164:678). However, even small aneurysms can rupture.

1. **Medical management.** Patients with small aneurysms (<4.5 cm in diameter) without risk factors for rupture can be followed using ultrasound or CT scan yearly, and patients with larger ones are followed more frequently. Smoking cessation, exercise, control of HTN, and treatment of chronic pulmonary obstructive disease are very important (*J Vasc Surg.* 2002;35:72).

2. **Elective surgical treatment.** Operative mortality ranges from less than 5% for uncomplicated AAA to greater than 50% for ruptured AAA (*Br J Surg.* 1998;85:1624). Five-year survival after elective repair of AAA is no different from that for age-matched patients without AAA. Associated cardiovascular disease, HTN, decreased renal function, chronic obstructive lung disease, and morbid obesity increase operative risk (*Arch Intern Med.* 1995;155:1998). Indications for **surgical management** for AAAs include the following:
   a. Symptomatic aneurysms of any size.
   b. Aneurysms exceeding 5.5 cm diameter (may consider greater than or equal to 5 cm for females).
   c. Increase in diameter by more than 0.5 cm/year (*J Vasc Surg.* 2003;37:1106).
   d. Saccular aneurysms (due to potential for active infection).

       e. Relative indications for repair of smaller AAAs include poorly controlled HTN (diastolic blood pressure ≥100 mm Hg) and significant chronic obstructive pulmonary disease (1-second forced expiratory volume <50% of predicted value) (*Ann Surg.* 1999;230:289).

       f. Relative contraindications to elective repair include recent myocardial infarction, intractable congestive heart failure, unreconstructable coronary artery disease, life expectancy of less than 2 years, and incapacitating neurologic deficits after a stroke.

  3. Operative technique. In the transabdominal repair, the aneurysm is approached through a midline abdominal incision and exposed by incising the retroperitoneum. Next, the duodenum and left renal vein are dissected off the aorta. After systemic heparinization, the aorta and iliac arteries are cross-clamped. An aortotomy is then made and extended longitudinally to the aneurysm "neck," where the aorta is either transected or cut in a T fashion. The thrombus is removed, and any bleeding lumbar arteries are suture ligated. The proximal anastomosis is performed to nonaneurysmal aorta using a graft. The distal anastomosis is completed at the aortic bifurcation (tube graft) or at the iliac or femoral arteries (bifurcated graft), as the extent of the aneurysmal disease dictates. After the clamps have been removed and hemostasis is ensured, the aneurysm wall is closed over the graft. An alternative approach is through a left retroperitoneal incision. This approach is advantageous in obese patients, those with chronic pulmonary obstructive disease, and patients with previous intra-abdominal surgery. In addition, more proximal suprarenal or supraceliac control of the aorta is more easily achieved via this latter approach.

D. Management of ruptured AAA

  1. Preoperative management. Unstable patients with a presumed diagnosis of a ruptured aneurysm (hypotension, abdominal or back pain, and a pulsatile abdominal mass or history of aneurysmal disease) are gently resuscitated with fluids (crystalloid, colloid, or blood) to maintain organ perfusion pressure. HTN is avoided to lessen further bleeding. Unstable patients are transferred immediately to the operating room for exploration, whereas those who are stable should undergo emergent CT scanning to confirm the diagnosis.

  2. Operative management is aimed at rapidly controlling the aorta. Anesthetic induction is delayed until the surgeon is ready to make the abdominal incision. Through a midline incision, the supraceliac aorta is cross-clamped or compressed at the diaphragmatic hiatus. The retroperitoneal hematoma is opened, and the proximal neck of the aneurysm is identified and cross-clamped. Distal vessel dissection continues, and management is similar to repair of an elective AAA. The use of bifurcated grafts should be avoided in favor of the more expeditious tube graft reconstruction if possible. Heparin should also be avoided in these patients who are likely to already be coagulopathic due to the high risk of intraoperative and postoperative bleeding. Some centers are now approaching ruptured AAAs with endovascular techniques by deploying an occlusive balloon inserted through the femoral artery as a means of controlling the aorta above the aneurysm.

3. **Complications** from open AAA repair
   a. **Arrhythmia, myocardial ischemia, or infarction** may occur.
   b. **Intraoperative hemorrhage** can be reduced by clamping the aorta proximal to the aneurysm and the iliac arteries distally. Once the aneurysm is opened, retrograde bleeding from lumbar arteries must be controlled rapidly with transfixing ligatures. Blood should be salvaged in the operating room and autotransfused to the patient.
   c. **Aortic unclamping** is often associated with hypotension initially due to a sudden decrease in systemic vascular resistance, as well as release of previously sequestered vasodilatory metabolites back into the systemic circulation from the recently reperfused tissues. Thus, management of resuscitation, electrolytes, and pressors is critically important during this step.
   d. **Renal insufficiency** may be related to the use of intravenous contrast, inadequate hydration, hypotension, renal ischemic from a period of aortic clamping above the renal arteries, or embolization of the renal arteries.
   e. **Lower-extremity ischemia** may result from embolism or thrombosis, especially in emergency operations for which heparin might not be used. Embolism to the lower extremities can be prevented by minimizing manipulation of the aneurysm prior to clamping and by reperfusing the hypogastric arteries prior to reperfusion of external iliac arteries at the time of unclamping. Use of a Fogarty balloon catheter to remove distal emboli from lower-extremity vessels is indicated when leg ischemia is identified in the operating room.
   f. **Microemboli** arising from atherosclerotic debris can cause cutaneous ischemia (trash foot), which is usually treated expectantly as long as the major vessels are patent. Amputation may be required if significant necrosis results.
   g. **Gastrointestinal complications** consist of prolonged paralytic ileus, anorexia, periodic constipation, or diarrhea. This problem is diminished by using the left retroperitoneal approach. A more serious complication, ischemic colitis of the sigmoid colon, is related to ligation of the inferior mesenteric artery (IMA) in the absence of adequate collateral circulation. Symptoms include leukocytosis, significant fluid requirement in the first 8 to 12 hours postoperatively, fever, and peritoneal irritation. Diagnosis is confirmed by flexible sigmoidoscopy to 20 cm above the anal verge. Necrosis that is limited to the mucosa may be treated expectantly with intravenous antibiotics and bowel rest. Necrosis of the muscularis causes segmental strictures, which may require delayed segmental resection. Transmural necrosis requires immediate resection of necrotic colon and construction of an end colostomy.
   h. **Paraplegia,** a rare complication of infrarenal aneurysm surgery, may occur after repair of a ruptured AAA due to spinal cord ischemia. Supraceliac cross-clamping and prolonged hypotension increase the risk of paraplegia. Obliteration or embolization of important collateral flow to the spinal artery via the internal iliac arteries or an abnormally low origin of the accessory spinal artery (artery of Adamkiewicz) can result in paraplegia.

    i. Sexual dysfunction and retrograde ejaculation result from damage to the sympathetic plexus during dissection near the aortic bifurcation, especially around the proximal left common iliac artery.

E. **Endovascular management** of AAAs has dramatically decreased the acute morbidity of aneurysm surgery. It is important to note that the **indications** for endovascular treatment of AAA are no different than those for traditional open repair.

  1. The most important **selection criterion** for endovascular treatment of an AAA is appropriate aortoiliac anatomy. Preoperative CT assessment includes the following factors:

    a. Length and diameter of nondilated and healthy infrarenal aorta (the neck). Commercially available devices allow treatment of a proximal neck between 10 and 15 mm long. The maximal aneurysm neck diameter that can be treated with standard devices is 32 mm.

    b. Angle between the neck and aneurysm. Significant angulation between the neck and adjacent aneurysm ($\geq$60 degrees) makes proximal graft deployment technically difficult and is associated with a higher risk of treatment failure.

    c. Presence of intraluminal thrombus or significant calcification. Significant mural thrombus or atheroma in the proximal neck can prevent adequate sealing of an endograft and therefore represents a relative contraindication for endovascular treatment. Similarly, extensive calcification of the aortic neck also remains a relative contraindication.

    d. Shape of the aortic neck. The proximal neck segment geometry is also important in that a cone-shaped neck or reverse taper (i.e., widens more distally) may preclude adequate apposition of the endograft to the aortic wall.

    e. The most commonly used devices for endovascular repair are bifurcated endografts with limbs that extend into the bilateral iliac arteries. Iliac artery tortuosity, calcification, and luminal narrowing, in combination with the profile of the delivery system, are critical factors that play an important role in successful endograft delivery and deployment without complication.

    f. Patent aortic branches may influence the decision as to whether to proceed with endograft placement. A renal artery or large accessory renal artery arising from the proximal neck or the presence of a horseshoe kidney with multiple renal arteries is often a contraindication for endograft placement. Patent lumbar arteries arising from the aneurysm do not preclude endograft placement. A patent IMA associated with large mesenteric collaterals (e.g., meandering mesenteric artery) or a large patent IMA suggests abnormal mesenteric blood supply and risk of large-bowel ischemia with endograft coverage of the IMA orifice. Therefore, these vascular patterns are contraindications to endograft placement.

  2. **Technique.** Endovascular devices are introduced retrograde through femoral arterial access. The most commonly utilized devices are

bifurcated and modular (consisting of two or more components) in design. Endografts typically have a full-length stent skeleton that maintains structural integrity and prevents graft kinking. Appropriate oversizing of stent grafts (by 10% to 15%) is based on preoperative assessment of arterial diameter to ensure adequate graft apposition to the aortic wall. If necessary, graft length can be tailored by means of overlapping extension segments in modular devices. The distal end of the iliac limbs is typically positioned proximal to the hypogastric orifices to maintain pelvic perfusion. Advanced endovascular (catheter and wire handling) skills are paramount to the success of endovascular aneurysm repair.

3. **Complications of endograft repairs of AAAs**
   a. Early complications include **branch occlusion, distal embolization, graft thrombosis, and arterial injury** (especially iliac artery avulsion at the iliac bifurcation in patients with small, calcified, diseased iliac arteries). These complications can often be corrected using endovascular techniques but may require emergent conversion to open repair.
   b. **Arterial dissection** may occur but this may not require additional treatment if the endograft spans the segment of dissection. Additional stents can be used to treat the dissected vessel if necessary.
   c. **Bowel ischemia** may occur postoperatively secondary to embolization or hypoperfusion, but this is rare compared to open surgical repair. **Renal dysfunction** may occur because of the nephrotoxicity of the contrast agent used for intraoperative angiography or because of direct injury due to embolization or renal artery occlusion.
   d. **Graft migration** occurs in 1% to 6% of patients, and is associated with challenging arterial anatomy and poor graft placement. This complication can typically be treated with secondary endovascular procedures.
   e. **Endoleak** is defined as failure to exclude the aneurysmal sac fully from arterial blood flow, potentially predisposing to rupture of the aneurysm sac (*J Endovasc Surg.* 1997;4:152). Management strategies for endoleaks discovered on follow-up imaging studies are evolving. For any endoleak that is associated with aneurysm sac enlargement, intervention is required. Endoleaks are usually corrected by endovascular means but may require conversion to open surgical repair.
      (1) In general, endoleaks from the proximal or distal attachment sites **(type I)** warrant intervention because these are frequently associated with increasing aneurysm sac size. Type I endoleaks may be sealed with angioplasty, or placement of a stent or endovascular graft component.
      (2) **Type II** endoleaks are due to collateral flow (IMA, lumbar arteries) and may be closely observed in the absence of aneurysm expansion. Type II endoleaks may be treated with embolization through collateral vessels (via the hypogastric artery for lumbar branch bleeding, via the superior mesenteric artery (SMA) for IMA bleeding) or directly through injection of the aneurysm sac via a translumbar approach, which is usually the most successful strategy.

(3) Type III endoleaks are caused by inadequate seal between graft components. They should be corrected as soon as they are diagnosed.

(4) Type IV endoleaks are due to porosity of the graft material. This is rare with newer generations of endografts.

4. **Results.** Relative to open surgical repair, endovascular treatment of AAA is associated with a reduction in perioperative morbidity, shorter duration of hospitalization (*J Vasc Surg.* 2003;37:262), and reduction in perioperative mortality (EVAR 1; *Lancet.* 2004;364:843–848; DREAM; *NEJM.* 2005;352:2398–2405). However, studies of long-term outcome comparing open versus endovascular repair have demonstrated similar rates of survival after 4 years (DREAM; *NEJM.* 2010;362:1881–1889; UK EVAR; *NEJM.* 2010;362:1863–1871). Close follow-up with CT scanning every 6 months initially and yearly after the first year is essential to maintaining long-term clinical success using this technique. Further advances in fenestrated and branched devices are allowing treatment of pararenal and other more complex AAAs.

II. THORACIC AORTIC ANEURYSMS (TAAs) are primarily a disease of the elderly. Ascending aortic aneurysms are most common (~60%) followed by aneurysms of the descending aorta (~35%) and of the transverse aortic arch (<10%). Most descending TAAs begin just distal to the orifice of left subclavian artery.

A. **Pathophysiology.** TAAs are divided into five main types: ascending, transverse, descending, thoracoabdominal, and traumatic. Ascending aortic aneurysms are usually caused by medial degeneration. Transverse, descending, and thoracoabdominal aortic aneurysms are related to atherosclerosis with HTN contributing to their expansion. Traumatic aneurysms are usually due to blunt injury to the chest.

B. **Diagnosis**

1. **Clinical manifestations** are usually absent; most nontraumatic TAAs are detected as incidental findings on chest imaging obtained for other purposes. A minority of patients may present with chest discomfort or pain that intensifies with aneurysm expansion or rupture, aortic valvular regurgitation, congestive heart failure, compression of adjacent structures (recurrent laryngeal nerve, left main-stem bronchus, esophagus, superior vena cava), erosion into adjacent structures (esophagus, lung, airway), or distal embolization.

2. **Radiologic evaluation. Chest x-ray** may reveal a widened mediastinum or an enlarged calcific aortic shadow. Traumatic aneurysms may be associated with skeletal fractures. **MR or CT imaging** with intravenous contrast provides precise estimation of the size and extent of aneurysms and facilitates surgical planning. **Echocardiography** may be useful in evaluating aneurysms involving the aortic arch. **Aortography** demonstrates the proximal and distal extent of the aneurysm and its relationship with aortic branch vessels arising from it.

C. **Surgical management** varies by type and location of the TAA. Repair of proximal arch aneurysms requires cardiopulmonary bypass and circulatory arrest. Preclotted woven polyethylene terephthalate **(Dacron)** is the graft of choice. Ascending and transverse arches are repaired through a median sternotomy incision. Descending and thoracoabdominal aneurysms are approached through a left posterolateral thoracotomy or thoracoabdominal incision. Intraoperative management of patients undergoing thoracotomy is facilitated by selective ventilation of the right lung using a double-lumen endobronchial tube. Cerebrospinal fluid drainage during and after surgery for descending and thoracoabdominal aneurysms can lower the incidence of postoperative paraplegia.

1. **Ascending aortic arch aneurysms**
   a. Size criteria for TAA repair are not as clearly defined as for infrarenal AAAs. **Indications** for surgical repair include symptomatic or rapidly expanding aneurysms, aneurysms greater than or equal to 6 cm in diameter, ascending (type A) aortic dissections, mycotic aneurysms, and asymptomatic aneurysms greater than or equal to 5.5 cm in diameter in patients with Marfan syndrome (*Coron Artery Dis.* 2002;13:85).
   b. **Operative management.** An aneurysm arising distal to the coronary ostia is replaced with an interposition graft. An aneurysm resulting in aortic valve incompetence is replaced with a composite valved conduit **(Bentall procedure)** or a supracoronary graft with separate aortic valve replacement. All ascending arch aneurysms due to Marfan syndrome or cystic medial necrosis are repaired with aortic valve replacement owing to the high incidence of valvular incompetence associated with aneurysmal dilation of the native aortic root. When a composite graft is used, the coronary arteries are anastomosed directly to the conduit.

2. **Transverse aortic arch aneurysms**
   a. **Indications** for repair include aneurysms greater than or equal to 6 cm in diameter, aortic arch dissections, and ascending arch aneurysms that extend into the transverse arch.
   b. **Operative management.** After opening the aorta under hypothermic circulatory arrest, the distal anastomosis is performed using a beveled graft, followed by anastomosis of a patch that incorporates the orifices of the brachiocephalic vessels to the superior aspect of the graft. The proximal anastomosis is constructed to the supracoronary aorta (if the aortic valve is not involved) or to a segment of the composite valved conduit interposed to complete the arch reconstruction. Involvement of the transverse arch and its branch vessels requires interposition grafting to the involved vessels.

3. **Descending thoracic aortic aneurysms**
   a. **Indications** for repair include asymptomatic aneurysms greater than or equal to 6 cm in diameter and any symptomatic aneurysms.
   b. **Operative management.** After the distal clamp is applied, a proximal clamp is placed just distal to the left subclavian artery or between

the left common carotid and left subclavian arteries. Selected intercostal branches are reattached to the aortic interposition graft. Left heart (atriofemoral) bypass is often used, both to protect the heart from overdistention and to provide distal blood flow while the aorta is clamped. Sodium nitroprusside may be given before cross-clamping to reduce proximal blood pressure, and cerebrospinal fluid drainage is used as an adjunct to decrease the incidence of postoperative paraplegia.

4. **Thoracoabdominal aneurysms**
   a. **Indications** for repair include aneurysms greater than or equal to 6 cm in diameter and any symptomatic aneurysms.
   b. **Operative management** consists of tube graft replacement along with anastomosis of the major visceral branches to the graft. Aneurysms involving the thoracic and proximal abdominal aortic segments may be approached through a left posterolateral thoracotomy extended to the umbilicus. Use of left heart (atriofemoral) bypass is a valuable adjunct, and drainage of cerebrospinal fluid may reduce the incidence of postoperative paraplegia. The thoracic aorta is clamped and opened to perform the proximal anastomosis, while visceral perfusion is maintained retrograde. The aorta is clamped distally opening the remaining aneurysm. The orifices of all major aortic branches are occluded with balloon catheters or vascular clamps. Temporary perfusion can be maintained to those branches during aneurysm repair by using balloon catheters connected to the atriofemoral bypass. The anastomoses of significant aortic branches to the graft are performed as a patch or with separate bypasses. The clamp is moved to the graft below the renal arteries to reperfuse all visceral vessels in a prograde fashion. The distal anastomosis is made either to the uninvolved aorta or to the iliac arteries.

5. **Traumatic aortic aneurysms**
   a. **Indications.** Urgent repair is indicated, except when precluded by more compelling life-threatening injuries or major central nervous system trauma.
   b. **Operative management.** These aneurysms may be repaired by primary aortorrhaphy, aneurysmectomy, and end-to-end reanastomosis or by interposition grafting. Endovascular techniques have also been reported.

D. Possible **complications** of thoracic aortic surgery include arrhythmia, myocardial infarction, intraoperative hemorrhage, stroke, aortic cross-clamp shock, renal insufficiency, lower-extremity ischemia, microemboli, and disseminated intravascular coagulopathy. The incidence of paraplegia may be as high as 30% with some types of TAAs (*Ann Thorac Surg.* 2007;83:S856). This risk can be reduced by multimodal therapies used to minimize spinal cord ischemia: distal aortic perfusion, intercostal and lumbar artery reimplantation, pre- or intraoperative localization of spinal cord blood supply, hypothermia, cerebrospinal fluid drainage, and pharmacotherapy.

E. **Endovascular management of thoracic aortic aneurysm**

1. **Indications and technique.** Because of the considerable morbidity and mortality associated with surgical repair of descending thoracic aneurysms, the endovascular approach to aneurysm exclusion is particularly attractive. Treatment with endovascular stent graft placement requires specific anatomic criteria: adequate length (2 cm) and diameter (20 to 45 mm) of the proximal and distal aneurysm necks, absence of significant mural thrombus within the sealing zones, and aortic and iliofemoral anatomy amenable to device introduction. In situations in which the proximal neck length is too short, coverage of the left subclavian artery with placement of the graft over the origin of the left subclavian artery can be performed with or without an adjunctive left carotid-left subclavian transposition or bypass. Over the past decade, multiple devices have been developed for the use of treating descending TAAs.

2. **Results and complications.** Reported results for the use of endovascular devices are encouraging. Various studies have suggested low morbidity and mortality with high rates of aneurysm exclusion (*J Vasc Surg.* 2008;47:1094–1098; *J Vasc Surg.* 2006;43(suppl A):12A-19A; *J Vasc Surg.* 2008;47:247–257; *J Vasc Surg.* 2008;48:546–554). Fenestrated and branched grafts along with hybrid techniques using extra-anatomic bypass procedures are being used to approach more complex aneurysm anatomy.

III. OTHER ARTERIAL ANEURYSMS

A. **Renal artery aneurysms** occur in approximately 0.1% of the general population and constitute approximately 1% of all aneurysms (*Semin Vasc Surg.* 2005;18:202).

1. **Pathophysiology.** These aneurysms can be either extrarenal (85%) or intrarenal (15%). Extrarenal renal artery aneurysms are subdivided into saccular (most common), fusiform, and dissecting. Saccular aneurysms classically occur near the bifurcation of the renal artery (*Semin Vasc Surg.* 1996;9:236). Fusiform aneurysms are poststenotic dilations associated with renal artery stenosis. Renal artery dissections are associated with renal artery fibroplasias. Intrarenal aneurysms may be congenital, traumatic, or related to collagen vascular disease.

2. **Diagnosis**

a. Most are asymptomatic and are found incidentally on imaging studies performed for other intra-abdominal pathology. Rupture and dissection may produce flank pain or hematuria (intrarenal aneurysms).

b. Physical examination commonly reveals **HTN and an abdominal bruit.** A palpable mass occurs in fewer than 10% of cases.

c. Laboratory tests may reveal anemia or hematuria.

d. Abdominal films may demonstrate **ring-shaped calcifications** in the renal hilum in patients with calcific saccular aneurysms. CT scan may reveal an incidental renal artery aneurysm. Arteriography confirms the diagnosis and details the anatomy of the renal branches.

3. Operative management is indicated for aneurysms greater than 2 cm, which rupture, are associated with dissection, or produce renal artery stenosis leading to HTN. Saccular aneurysms are repaired in women of childbearing age owing to an increased risk of rupture during pregnancy. Small aneurysms at the bifurcation can be treated with aneurysmectomy and reconstruction of the bifurcation. Aneurysmectomy with aortorenal or splenorenal bypass is advised for large aneurysms or stenotic lesions. Polar renal artery aneurysms can be excised with end-to-end arterial reanastomosis. *Ex vivo* renal artery reconstruction with renal autotransplantation is useful in patients with complex lesions that require microvascular techniques and for whom exposure *in situ* is inadequate. These procedures are time consuming, and adequate hypothermic protection from ischemic renal injury may be difficult with the kidney *in situ*. In general, operations requiring more than two branch artery reconstructions or anastomoses should be considered for *ex vivo* repair. Once repair is accomplished, the kidney can be transplanted orthotopically or heterotopically to the ipsilateral iliac fossa. Ruptured renal artery aneurysms are usually treated with nephrectomy as salvage of renal function is unlikely.

B. **Infected aneurysms** have risen in incidence with the increased prevalence of immunocompromised patients and invasive transarterial procedures.

1. **Pathophysiology.** Infected aneurysms can be divided in to four types: mycotic aneurysm, microbial arteritis with aneurysm, infection of preexisting aneurysm, and posttraumatic infected false aneurysm. *Staphylococcus aureus* is the most common pathogen, although *Salmonella* species (arteritis), *Streptococcus* species, and *Staphylococcus epidermidis* (preexisting aneurysms) also may occur. The risk of rupture for Gram-negative exceeds that for Gram-positive infections.

2. **Diagnosis**
   a. Clinical manifestations may be absent or include fever, tenderness, or sepsis. Physical examination may demonstrate a **tender, warm, palpable mass** in an infected peripheral aneurysm. Laboratory tests may reveal leukocytosis. Aerobic and anaerobic blood cultures should be obtained, but are positive in only 50% of patients.
   b. **MRI or CTA** can demonstrate an aneurysm and verify its rupture. **Angiography** delineates the characteristics of the aneurysm. Aneurysms that are saccular, multilobed, or eccentric with a narrow neck are more likely a result of infection.

C. Management
   a. **Preoperative.** Broad-spectrum antibiotics should be administered intravenously after aerobic and anaerobic blood cultures have been obtained.
   b. **Intraoperative.** Goals of surgery include (1) controlling hemorrhage; (2) obtaining arterial specimens for Gram's stain, aerobic and anaerobic cultures, and drug sensitivities; (3) resecting the aneurysm with wide debridement and drainage; and (4) reconstructing major arteries through uninfected tissue planes. Extra-anatomic bypass may be nec-

essary to avoid contamination of the graft. Inline reconstructions with antibiotic-impregnated grafts, cryopreserved homografts, or native veins are alternatives that can be used for arterial reconstructions depending on the location of the aneurysm and the extent of the infection.

c. **Postoperative.** Adequate drainage of the aneurysm cavity and long-term antibiotic therapy for at least 6 weeks typically are required.

IV. **RENOVASCULAR DISEASE.** Stenosis or occlusion of the renal arteries may result in HTN, ischemic nephropathy, or both. **Renovascular HTN is the most common form of surgically correctable secondary HTN.** However, because of the predominance of primary HTN and difficulties in clinical diagnosis of renovascular HTN, its exact prevalence is difficult to assess.

A. A high index of suspicion is necessary to distinguish patients with renovascular HTN from the majority of patients with primary HTN. There are several clinical features that may be used to identify patients with potential renovascular HTN (ACC/AHA practice guideline; 2005):

1. The onset of **HTN** in a child/young adult or an adult older than the age of 55.
2. **Accelerated, resistant, or malignant HTN.**
3. HTN and unexplained impairment of renal function.
4. HTN that is **refractory** to appropriate multidrug therapy.
5. HTN in a patient with extensive coronary disease, cerebral vascular disease, or peripheral vascular disease.

B. On **physical examination,** these patients may have an epigastric, subcostal, or flank bruit. However, majority of the patients have a normal physical exam. The finding of a unilateral small kidney on any imaging study is a possible indicator.

C. Pathophysiology

1. Renal arterial stenosis (RAS) is perceived by the ipsilateral kidney as a hypovolemic state, and activation of the **renin-angiotensin-aldosterone system** results in volume expansion due to angiotensin-II mediated sodium retention and severe HTN results from the combined effects of volume expansion and peripheral vasoconstriction. Even in the **absence of HTN,** a significant RAS may be present and may lead to renal failure.

a. In **acute renal failure,** RAS should be considered in the differential diagnosis if the urinary sediment is unremarkable and there are no signs of acute tubular necrosis, glomerulonephritis, or interstitial nephritis. Acute ischemic nephropathy may occur within 2 weeks of starting an angiotensin-converting enzyme (ACE) inhibitor or other antihypertensive or diuretic.

b. RAS may account for up to 20% of **unexplained chronic renal failure** in patients older than 50 years of age. The diagnosis is more likely in those with generalized atherosclerosis or uncontrolled HTN.

c. Isolated unilateral RAS generally **do not** cause rise in serum creatinine.

2. **Atherosclerosis** accounts for nearly 90% of cases of renovascular HTN and usually affects the ostia and proximal 2 cm of the renal artery. Associated extrarenal atherosclerosis occurs in 15% to 20% of patients.

3. The second-most-common renovascular lesion is **fibromuscular dysplasia,** most commonly medial fibroplasia. These lesions are multifocal, have a characteristic **string-of-beads** appearance on angiography, and typically occur in young women.

D. **Diagnosis.** Testing for clinically significant renal artery disease must evaluate the **anatomic and physiologic changes.** Anatomic lesions of the renal arteries by themselves correlate poorly with physiologic effect. More important, they also correlate poorly with treatment response.

1. **Arteriography** remains the "gold standard" for the diagnosis of anatomic RAS. However, the usual risks of arteriography, especially the nephrotoxic effects of the contrast agent, are important caveats to consider.

2. In patients with a relative contraindication to arteriography, **duplex scanning** is useful for screening. However, this procedure is highly technician dependent.

3. **MR angiography** with gadolinium-based intravenous contrast is an excellent test for evaluating kidney and main renal artery morphology without the use of nephrotoxic agents.

4. Two commonly used tests to determine the functional significance of a renal artery lesion are **captopril renal scintigraphy** and **selective renal vein renin measurement.** These tests can be complicated to perform and interpret, especially in patients with bilateral disease or in those taking ACE inhibitors or beta-blockers.

E. Management of fibromuscular disease

1. RAS resulting from fibromuscular dysplasia rarely causes renal failure, and endovascular treatment of the lesions is frequently successful in treating the HTN.

2. **Endovascular techniques (balloon angioplasty) have a high success rate for the treatment of this arterial pathology.** For failure of endovascular treatment (see Section F.3), surgical therapy may be employed.

F. **Management of atherosclerotic disease** has a dual purpose: to control target organ damage from HTN and to avoid progressive ischemic renal failure. However, even with preoperative functional studies, response to therapy is difficult to predict because the HTN may be primarily essential and the renal failure due to hypertensive glomerulosclerosis.

1. **Medical therapy** with antihypertensive drugs is often successful in the management of patients with renovascular HTN and remains the cornerstone of treatment. A combination of beta-blockers and a calcium channel blocker, an ACE inhibitor, or an angiotensin II–receptor inhibitor is commonly used as first-line therapy.

2. **Surgical therapy**
   a. The recently published ASTRAL trial (*NEJM.* 2009;361:20) was a multicenter, randomized trial that compared medical management alone to medical management with endovascular revascularization. The investigators **did not** find a significant difference in rate of progression of renal impairment, blood pressure, or survival. However, they included patients with clinically insignificant lesions and excluded any patients whose doctors felt would benefit from revascularization. Until further clinical trials and guidelines can better identify those who might benefit from surgery, interventions should be offered only to those with severe disease who fail medical management. In patients undergoing aortic surgery for aneurysmal or occlusive disease with concomitant renal stenoses, consideration should also be given to renal revascularization.
   b. **Procedures**
      (1) **Aortorenal bypass** is the classic treatment of renal revascularization. The stenotic renal artery is isolated with a segment of infrarenal aorta, and bypass is accomplished using saphenous vein, autologous hypogastric artery (in children), or prosthetic graft.
      (2) **Renal endarterectomy** is another option and is often used for bilateral orificial lesions. Most commonly, a transverse arteriotomy is made over the orifices of both renal arteries.
      (3) **Alternative bypass procedures** are available for patients who are not good candidates for aortorenal bypass due to prior aortic surgery, the presence of severe aortic disease, or unfavorable anatomy. Grafts can be taken from the supraceliac aorta or the superior mesenteric, common hepatic, gastroduodenal, splenic, or iliac arteries. Results for these procedures are comparable to those for direct aortic reconstruction but with less morbidity and mortality.
      (4) **Nephrectomy** may be required in patients who have renal infarction, severe nephrosclerosis, severe renal atrophy, noncorrectable renal vascular lesions, failed revascularizations, or a normal contralateral kidney and who are high-risk surgical candidates.
   c. **Postoperative care**
      (1) **Immediately after operation,** patients should be kept well hydrated to maintain adequate urine output. Concern about the patency of the reconstruction may be addressed by a renal or duplex scan.
      (2) **Patient follow-up** should consist of routine blood pressure monitoring, a renal scan, and creatinine determination at 3 months, 12 months, and then yearly. Any recurrence of HTN or deterioration in renal function should prompt diagnostic imaging. Duplex scanning often serves as a useful surveillance test.
   d. **Complications** of surgery include persistent HTN, acute renal failure, renal artery restenosis, thrombosis, aneurysm formation, and distal embolization.

3. Endovascular management of renal artery stenosis

a. **Indications** for angioplasty of RAS include failure of medical management of renovascular HTN in the absence of any clear indications for open aortic surgery. Balloon angioplasty is the treatment of choice for clinically significant fibromuscular dysplastic lesions. Angioplasty for atherosclerotic lesions has less favorable results but entails significantly less procedure-related morbidity than surgical bypass or endarterectomy. Surgical therapy may be preferred in cases of long-segment disease or occlusions or when atherosclerosis is severe and widespread (i.e., to avoid the risk of atheroembolic complications with intra-arterial instrumentation). Renal artery stents are routinely used for restenosis after previous angioplasty, treatment of procedural complications (e.g., dissection), and the treatment of atherosclerotic ostial lesions.

b. **Technique.** Intravascular access to the renal artery may be obtained from the femoral, brachial, or axillary arteries (access from the upper extremity may be preferable in cases of caudally angled renal arteries). In patients at high risk for renal failure (e.g., type II diabetes and preexisting renal insufficiency), nephrotoxic contrast may be avoided and angiography can be performed using gadolinium or carbon dioxide (CO_2). Technical success for renal artery angioplasty is defined as a less than 30% residual stenosis and a pressure gradient across the lesion of less than 10 mm Hg.

c. **Results.** Patients with fibromuscular dysplasia respond favorably to percutaneous transluminal angioplasty, with cure rates of greater than 50%. Patients with atherosclerotic disease respond less favorably in the long term, although immediate technical success is seen in almost all patients. Improvements in blood pressure are observed in approximately two thirds of patients; however, only 15% of patients with renal insufficiency demonstrate improved excretory renal function. In addition, up to 15% of patients exhibit decreased renal excretory function following intervention. Angiographic restenosis occurs in 15% to 20% of patients within 1 year of treatment, most commonly in small renal arteries (<4 mm). Based on these data, percutaneous angioplasty with stenting of atherosclerotic disease of the renal artery yields blood pressure, renal function, and anatomic results that are slightly inferior but comparable to contemporary surgical results. Percutaneous intervention is, however, associated with lower morbidity and mortality rates than open surgical procedures.

V. **MESENTERIC ISCHEMIA** can be a difficult diagnosis to make because most patients are asymptomatic until late in the disease process. Although considerable advances have been made in the perioperative care as well as the diagnosis and treatment of intestinal ischemia, mortality remains 60% to 80% (*Langenbecks Arch Surg.* 2008;393:163).

A. **Acute mesenteric ischemia (AMI)**

1. **Pathophysiology.** The most common cause of acute mesenteric ischemia (AMI) is embolization to the SMA, but other causes include

thrombosis of the SMA or portomesenteric venous thrombosis. Patients with AMI often have multiple **risk factors,** including significant cardiac disease (frequently atrial fibrillation) and severe atherosclerotic disease of nonmesenteric vessels, and may have a history consistent with chronic intestinal ischemia (CMI).

  a. Abdominal pain usually is sudden in onset and intermittent at first, progressing to continuous severe pain. It is often described as **pain out-of-proportion to exam.** These patients may also have bloody diarrhea before or after the onset of pain.

  b. Mesenteric venous thrombosis presents with varying manifestations, ranging from an asymptomatic state to catastrophic illness. Patients usually complain of prolonged, generalized abdominal pain that develops somewhat less rapidly than with acute mesenteric arterial occlusion. These patients may have occult gastrointestinal bleeding but no frank hemorrhage.

2. **Diagnosis**

  a. Angiography of the mesenteric circulation, including lateral views of the celiac axis and SMA, remains the "gold standard." However, most centers use **CT angiography** especially for the diagnosis of AMI.

  b. Other laboratory findings can include elevated white blood cell count with a left shift, persistent metabolic acidosis, and possibly lactic acidosis in more advanced cases, but are insensitive and nonspecific for the diagnosis of mesenteric ischemia (*Langenbeck's Arch of Surg.* 2011;396:3–11).

  c. Abdominal plain radiographs are of limited utility. After acute arterial occlusion, the abdominal plain x-ray appears relatively normal. After venous thrombosis, x-rays may show small-bowel wall thickening or air in the portal venous system.

3. **Surgical therapy**

  a. Patients with AMI frequently require intestinal resection; therefore, laparotomy with open revascularization is the preferred method of treatment.

   (1) Assessment of bowel viability at laparotomy is made based on the gross characteristics of the bowel. The bowel is likely viable if it appears pink and if arterial pulsations are present in the adjacent vascular arcades. A number of other techniques have been described, including the use of fluorescein dye, Doppler studies, and tissue oximetry, but these are not substitutes for experienced clinical judgment.

   (2) Second-look procedures are prudent when bowel viability is questionable. Whether to perform a second operation 24 to 48 hours after initial exploration is decided at the time of initial laparotomy, and that decision should not be changed even if the patient's condition improves. This approach is especially important in patients who have extensive bowel involvement and in whom resection of all questionable areas could result in short-bowel syndrome.

  b. For **venous occlusion,** surgical intervention rarely is helpful, although anecdotal reports suggest that portomesenteric venous thrombectomy may be beneficial. Similarly, the role of lytic therapy in the treatment of this disorder is unclear. It is imperative to begin systemic anticoagulation as soon as the diagnosis is made to limit progression of the thrombotic process. Frequently, the diagnosis is made at laparotomy. If the diagnosis is made before exploration, however, operation should be reserved until evidence of bowel infarction exists.

    c. Nonocclusive mesenteric ischemia (NOMI) is intestinal ischemia in the absence of thromboembolic occlusion. It occurs in patients with a low-cardiac-output state and chronic intestinal angina. Mortality associated with NOMI is high and treatment is directed toward improving circulatory support and increasing cardiac output.

  4. Perioperative care usually requires maximal medical support; these patients frequently are hemodynamically unstable and develop multiple organ system failure. Admission to the intensive care unit, prolonged endotracheal intubation, parenteral nutrition, and broad-spectrum antibiotic therapy are typically required.

B. Chronic mesenteric ischemia (CMI)

  1. Patients with CMI present with **intestinal angina,** which is pain related to eating, usually beginning within an hour after eating and abating within 4 hours (postprandial pain). Such patients experience significant weight loss related to the decreased intake secondary to recurrent pain (food fear). The diagnosis usually is made from obtaining a thorough history alone because physical finding are usually lacking.

  2. Surgical therapy. Elective revascularization of the SMA and celiac artery using autologous or prosthetic grafts from the aorta or iliac arteries is the treatment of choice. Aortic endarterectomy is an alternative in patients with aortic and orificial disease. Advances in endovascular techniques have greatly expanded the use of percutaneous interventions for patients with CMI with excellent technical results.

  3. Perioperative care. These patients often are malnourished. Some advocate parenteral nutrition for 1 to 2 weeks before surgery, which is continued postoperatively. Some patients develop a revascularization syndrome consisting of abdominal pain, tachycardia, leukocytosis, and intestinal edema. Concern about the adequacy of revascularization should prompt diagnostic imaging.

19 Peripheral Arterial Occlusive Disease

Jeremy Leidenfrost and Patrick J. Geraghty

The majority of occlusive disease is secondary to atherosclerotic change of the arterial intima. Major risk factors for developing atherosclerosis include cigarette smoking, diabetes, dyslipidemia, hypertension, and hyperhomocysteinemia. Some of these risk factors may be influenced to a degree by genetic predisposition. However, the evolution of the disease for most individuals can be modified by changes in environmental factors, particularly diet and exercise. Atherosclerotic disease is a systemic illness, and although symptomatic disease may predominate in one organ, subclinical disease, particularly of the coronary arteries, is generally present. In fact, 50% of the mortality associated with peripheral arterial reconstructions for atherosclerotic disease is cardiac in nature. Other, less common causes of occlusive disease include fibromuscular dysplasia, radiation-induced vascular injury, and the vasculitides (e.g., Takayasu arteritis and Buerger disease).

ACUTE ARTERIAL OCCLUSION OF THE EXTREMITY

Symptoms of acute arterial insufficiency occur abruptly. The presentation generally includes the **five Ps** of acute ischemia: **pain, pallor, pulselessness, paresthesias, and paralysis;** patients may also develop poikilothermy, the inability to thermoregulate. The level of occlusion may be localized by the absence of pulses and the level of coolness of the limb. If adequate collateral circulation is not present, irreversible changes may appear as early as 4 to 6 hours after onset. Therefore, priority must be given to restoration of blood flow within this time period. Once the occlusive process has begun, regardless of its cause, vasospasm and propagation of thrombus distal to the site of initial occlusion can contribute to further ischemia.

I. ETIOLOGY

A. The most common cause of acute arterial insufficiency is **embolization.**

1. **Cardiac sources** account for more than 70% of emboli and are usually the result of mural thrombi that develop due to cardiac aneurysms following myocardial infarction or arrhythmias such as atrial fibrillation. Other cardiac sources of emboli include valvular heart disease, prosthetic heart valves, bacterial endocarditis, and atrial myxoma.

2. **Arterial–arterial emboli** can result from ulcerated atheroma or aneurysms, although embolization from abdominal aortic aneurysms is distinctly rare. The *blue toe syndrome* occurs in patients with microemboli from unstable proximal arterial plaques and is characterized by intact pulses and painful ischemic lesions in the distal extremity. Atheroemboli

in the lower extremity secondary to plaque disruption by catheters can occur. The severely diseased distal aorta in some of these patients is evident on computed tomography (CT) scan and arteriography and has been termed *shaggy aorta.*

3. Venous–arterial emboli (paradoxical emboli) can result from an intracardiac shunt (e.g., patent foramen ovale) or intrapulmonary arteriovenous malformations (e.g., Osler–Weber–Rendu syndrome).

4. Occasionally, it is difficult to discern whether a person with advanced atherosclerotic disease has had an embolus or whether an already compromised vessel has undergone acute thrombosis. This is particularly true in patients without arrhythmias or prior myocardial infarction. The presence of contralateral pulses and the absence of a history of claudication may help in making this differentiation.

B. Direct arterial trauma is frequently obvious but may initially be occult. Arterial stenosis or occlusion occurs only after an intimal flap or arterial wall hematoma progresses sufficiently to cause symptoms. Arterial compromise can also occur in the setting of compression by joint dislocations (e.g., knee), bone fragments (e.g., tibial plateau fracture), or compartment syndrome.

C. Other causes of acute ischemia include arterial thrombosis, aortic dissection, venous outflow occlusion, and low-flow state.

II. DIAGNOSIS AND EVALUATION

A. If history and physical examination demonstrate clear evidence of embolization, **definitive therapy** should not be delayed. If there is a concern that the occlusive process may be thrombotic, however, **arteriography** may be indicated. Angiographically, embolic occlusions can be distinguished from thrombotic occlusions by their occurrence just distal to vascular bifurcations and by the concave shadow formed at the interface with the contrast. In select cases, thrombolysis may be a useful adjunct for defining underlying occlusive disease. In general, patients with acute ischemia unrelated to trauma should be considered to have coexistent cardiac disease. All patients should have an electrocardiogram and chest x-ray performed. After limb revascularization, a transesophageal echocardiogram can be useful in diagnosing a cardiac source.

B. Patients who present with penetrating **trauma,** long-bone fractures, or joint dislocations may have vascular injuries. In certain situations, duplex scan of the injured area can be useful in the diagnosis of intimal flap, pseudoaneurysm, or arterial or venous thrombi. Patients with penetrating injuries who display "hard" signs of arterial injury need urgent surgical intervention without preoperative angiography. **Hard signs** of arterial injury include the following:

1. Diminished or absent pulses distal to an injury

2. Ischemia distal to an injury

3. Visible arterial bleeding from a wound

4. A bruit at or distal to the site of injury

5. Large, expanding, or pulsatile hematomas

Soft signs of injury include the anatomic proximity of a wound to a major vessel, injury to an anatomically related nerve, unexplained hemorrhagic shock, or a moderately sized hematoma. In those with only soft signs, a careful documentation of pulses by **Doppler pressure** distal to the injury should be undertaken, along with comparison with the contralateral limb. A difference of greater than 10% to 20% suggests the need for arteriography or exploration.

III. MANAGEMENT

A. Once a diagnosis of acute arterial ischemia due to emboli or thrombi is made, **heparin** should be administered immediately. An intravenous bolus of 80 units/kg followed by an intravenous infusion of 18 units/kg/hour is usually satisfactory. Partial thromboplastin time (PTT) should be maintained between 60 and 80 seconds.

1. **Surgical therapy,** such as embolectomy, should be performed urgently in patients with an obvious embolus and acute ischemia. Embolectomy can be done under local anesthesia if the patient cannot tolerate general anesthesia. Once the artery is isolated, a Fogarty catheter is passed proximally and distally to extract the embolus and associated thrombus. In some cases, intraoperative thrombolysis may be necessary because distal vessels may be thrombosed beyond the reach of the Fogarty catheter. Distal patency can be proved with an intraoperative arteriogram, depending on the status of distal vessels and pulses after embolectomy. In the leg, if adequate distal perfusion is not established and an angiogram demonstrates distal thrombus, the distal popliteal artery and tibial arteries may be explored via angiographic or surgical approach. In conjunction with steerable guidewires, Fogarty catheters can be used to select the anterior tibial, posterior tibial, and peroneal arteries to retrieve distal thrombus. When angiographic approaches fail, popliteal artery cutdown can allow direct access to these vessels. The arteriotomy can be closed with a patch graft if there is arterial narrowing. Bypass grafting may also be required if significant preexisting arterial disease in the affected segment is discovered.

2. **Thrombolytic therapy** may be useful in patients with clearly viable extremities in whom thrombosis is the likely underlying cause of their acute ischemia. In general, the fresher the thrombus, the more successful thrombolysis can be. Thrombolysis and follow-up angiography frequently identify an underlying stenosis that may be treated by balloon angioplasty/stent or by surgical means.

   a. Lytic agents are instilled through an intra-arterial catheter placed as close to the thrombus as possible. Current agents in use include alteplase, urokinase, and reteplase. These agents are also commonly used in conjunction with percutaneous mechanical thrombectomy for large clot burdens.

   b. During thrombolysis, the patient is usually monitored in the **intensive care unit (ICU).** Thrombin time, fibrinogen level, fibrin degradation product level, PTT, and complete blood count are followed closely to limit the risk of hemorrhage. In general, the likelihood of serious hemorrhagic complications increases when fibrinogen levels drop below 100 mg/dL and the PTT rises above three to five times normal. Once the artery is open, the patient can be managed either with systemic anticoagulation or with surgical intervention (i.e., operative arterial reconstruction, balloon angioplasty).

3. Mechanical thrombectomy devices such as the AngioJet Thrombectomy system (Possis Medical, Minneapolis, MN) and the Trellis system (Bacchus Vascular, Santa Clara, CA) allow prompt debulking of acute thrombotic lesions, but are less effective at treating older adherent thrombus. These systems can be used with or without tPA. The Trellis system is designed for use with tPA which is contained between balloons and withdrawn after treatment to reduce systemic spread of lytic agent.

B. In the setting of **trauma,** operative exploration should be performed in any limb that is ischemic or if arteriography demonstrates a significant intimal flap or other pathology. In the presence of coexistent neurologic or orthopedic injuries, it is essential to reestablish arterial flow first, by direct repair, bypass grafting, or temporary shunting. At the conclusion of the orthopedic repair, the arterial repair should be reexamined to ensure that it has not been disrupted and has been correctly fashioned to the final bone length. In cases of joint dislocation, reduction of the dislocation should be accomplished first because this may alleviate the need for arterial reconstruction.

1. Intraoperatively it is essential to **obtain proximal and distal control** of the injured artery before exploring the hematoma or wound. When repairing an artery, an end-to-end anastomosis is preferable. A few centimeters of the artery can usually be mobilized proximally and distally to accomplish reapproximation. However, the uninjured leg or other potential vein harvest site should be prepared in case a conduit is required. It is preferable to use autologous tissue in this setting. In most stable patients, concomitant vein injuries are also repaired. A completion angiogram can help to document distal flow. This is especially important if significant spasm is present and distal pulses are not readily palpable.

2. In general, injuries to the subclavian, axillary, brachial, femoral, superficial femoral, profunda femoral, and popliteal arteries should be repaired. The radial or ulnar artery may be ligated if the other vessel is intact and functioning. Similarly, isolated injuries to the tibial arteries may be ligated if one or more of the tibial arteries remain intact.

IV. COMPLICATIONS

A. Reperfusion injury occurs after reestablishment of arterial flow to an ischemic tissue bed and may lead to further tissue death. It results from the formation of oxygen free radicals that directly damage the tissue and cause white blood cell accumulation and sequestration in the microcirculation.

This process prolongs the ischemic interval because it impairs adequate nutrient flow to the tissue, despite the restoration of axial blood flow. There is no proven therapy that limits reperfusion injury.

B. **Rhabdomyolysis** following reperfusion releases the by-products of ischemic muscle, including potassium, lactic acid, myoglobin, and creatinine phosphokinase. The electrolyte and pH changes that occur can trigger dangerous arrhythmias, and precipitation of myoglobin in the renal tubules can cause pigment nephropathy and ultimately acute renal failure. The likelihood that a patient will develop these complications relates to the duration of ischemia and the muscle mass at risk. **Aggressive hydration,** diuresis promotion with mannitol (25 g intravenously), and intravenous infusion of bicarbonate to alkalinize the urine are accepted methods of mitigating renal impairment secondary to rhabdomyolysis.

C. **Compartment syndrome** results when prolonged ischemia and delayed reperfusion cause cell membrane damage and leakage of fluid into the interstitium. The edema can result in extremely high intracompartmental pressures, particularly in the lower extremity. Additional muscle and nerve necrosis occurs when the intracompartmental pressures exceed capillary perfusion (generally >30 mm Hg). A four-compartment fasciotomy should be performed when there is concern about the possible development of leg compartment syndrome. **Fasciotomy should be routinely considered** in any patient with more than 6 hours of lower-extremity ischemia or in the presence of combined arterial and venous injuries.

D. Follow-up care is usually directed at treating the underlying cause of the obstruction. Patients with mural thrombi or arrhythmias require long-term anticoagulation. The in-hospital mortality rate associated with embolectomy is as high as 30%, mostly due to coexistent cardiac disease.

CHRONIC ARTERIAL OCCLUSIVE DISEASE OF THE EXTREMITY

The lower extremities are most frequently affected by chronic occlusive disease, although upper-extremity disease can occur. The principal early symptom of arterial occlusive disease is **claudication,** which is usually described as a cramping pain or heaviness in the affected extremity that occurs after physical exertion. Claudication is relieved by rest but recurs predictably with exercise. Lower-extremity occlusive disease may be subdivided into three anatomic sections on the basis of symptoms and treatment options. Aortoiliac occlusive disease, or "inflow disease," affects the infrarenal aorta and the common and external iliac arteries. Femoral–popliteal occlusive disease, or "outflow disease," affects the common femoral, superficial femoral, and popliteal arteries. Finally, tibial–peroneal disease, or "runoff disease," affects the vessels distal to the popliteal artery.

I. CLINICAL PRESENTATION

A. **Aortoiliac disease** presents with **symptoms of lower-extremity claudication,** usually of the **hip, thigh, or buttock.** It may coexist with femoral–popliteal disease, contributing to more distal symptoms as well. The symptoms usually develop gradually, although sudden worsening of symptoms suggests acute thrombosis of a diseased vessel. Patients ultimately develop incapacitating claudication but not rest pain unless distal disease is present as well. *Leriche syndrome* (sexual impotence, buttock and leg claudication, leg musculature atrophy, trophic changes of the feet, and leg pallor) is a constellation of symptoms that results from the gradual occlusion of the terminal aorta.

B. Patients with **femoral–popliteal** and **tibial–peroneal disease** present with claudication of the lower extremity, usually most prominent in the **calves.** More severe impairment of arterial flow can present as rest pain. **Rest pain** is a burning pain in the distal foot, usually worse at night or when the leg is elevated and often relieved by placing the leg in a dependent position. Examination findings of the chronically ischemic extremity include the following:

1. Decreased or absent distal pulses

2. Dependent rubor

3. Trophic changes that include thickening of the nails, loss of leg hair, shiny skin, and ulceration at the tips of the toes.

C. Symptomatic arterial occlusive disease of the **upper extremity** is relatively rare.

1. The proximal subclavian artery is most commonly affected by **atherosclerotic disease,** followed by axillary and brachial arteries. These patients typically present with arm claudication or finger–hand ischemia or necrosis. Occasionally, ulcerated plaques of the innominate or subclavian arteries can be a source of embolization to the hand.

2. Most patients with proximal subclavian lesions are completely asymptomatic. **Subclavian steal** can result when an occlusive subclavian artery lesion is located proximal to the origin of the vertebral artery. With exercise of the affected limb, the arm's demand for blood is supplied by retrograde flow in the ipsilateral vertebral artery, shunting blood from the posterior cerebral circulation and resulting in drop attacks, ataxia, sensory loss, or diplopia.

II. **DIAGNOSIS** of chronic arterial occlusive disease is concerned with determining the presence of **significant flow-limiting lesions** and distinguishing the disease from those that may mimic it, such as arthritis, gout, and neuromuscular disorders.

A. For patients presenting with **lower-extremity symptoms,** it is essential to examine the femoral and distal pulses at rest and after exercise. The absence of femoral pulses is indicative of aortoiliac disease, although some patients with aortoiliac disease have palpable pulses at rest that are lost after exercise. Bruits may also be appreciated over the lower abdomen or femoral vessels. It is also important to differentiate ulcers that arise from arterial insufficiency versus those generated by venous insufficiency and neuropathy.

1. Arterial insufficiency ulcers are usually painful and have an irregular appearance.

2. Neuropathic ulcers are painless and usually occur over bony prominences, particularly the plantar aspect of the metatarsophalangeal joints.

3. Venous stasis ulcers are located on the malleolar surface ("gaiter" distribution) and are dark and irregular in shape.

B. **Noninvasive testing** can quantify flow through larger vessels and tissue perfusion.

1. **Segmental arterial Doppler** readings with waveforms should be performed in all patients with suspected symptomatic arterial disease. The **ankle-brachial index (ABI)** (the ratio of the systolic blood pressure in the leg to that in the arm) allows one to quantify the degree of ischemia. In general, patients without vascular disease have an ABI of greater than 1, patients with claudication have an ABI of less than 0.8, and patients with rest pain and severe ischemia have an ABI of less than 0.4. Waveform changes help to localize the site of significant disease. Patients with history of claudication and normal resting waveforms require postexercise ABI measurements.

2. Transcutaneous measurement of **local tissue oxygenation** has been developed to attempt to quantify the physiologic derangements of ischemia. However, the usefulness of this test in the general vascular patient has not been validated.

C. **Digital subtraction arteriography** is the **gold standard** for evaluating the arterial tree before planned revascularization. Typical digital subtraction arteriography of the lower extremities includes images of the infrarenal aorta and the renal, iliac, femoral, tibial, and pedal vessels. Noninvasive angiography using imaging modalities such as magnetic resonance or CT has been gaining widespread use as the technology improves for both. **Magnetic resonance angiography (MRA)** is an excellent imaging modality for assessing PAD and is useful for selecting patients who are endoluminal candidates. However, MRA does have a tendency to overestimate the degree of stenosis and may be inaccurate in stented arteries. **CT angiography** produces high-resolution images of the vascular tree and gives other information about soft tissues that may be associated with PAD, such as aneurysms, popliteal entrapment, or cystic adventitial disease. However, diffuse calcifications may make interpretation of CT angiography images difficult. In addition, CT angiography does require iodinated contrast, which may adversely affect patients with renal insufficiency.

III. MANAGEMENT

A. With adequate control of risk factors, intermittent claudication follows a benign course in most patients. In patients presenting with claudication alone, 70% to 80% remain stable or improve and 10% to 20% worsen over the ensuing 5-year period. Only 5% to 10% of patients develop gangrene and are at risk for limb loss. Therefore, first-line treatment for patients with claudication should be medical therapy, with emphasis on risk factor modification. **Indications for surgical intervention include the following:**

1. **Limb salvage** is the goal of surgery in patients with ischemic rest pain or tissue loss (critical limb ischemia). These patients typically display multilevel occlusive disease. When significant aortoiliac disease and distal disease are jointly present in a patient with a threatened limb, however, an inflow (aortoiliac) procedure should be performed first.

2. **Prevention of further peripheral atheroembolization** from aortoiliac ulcerated plaques, even if there is little or no history of claudication, is an indication for exclusion and bypass or endarterectomy of the culprit lesion.

3. **Incapacitating claudication** that jeopardizes a patient's livelihood or severely influences his or her quality of life may be considered for revascularization after failure of risk factor modification and exercise therapy.

B. **Medical therapy** is available for those patients with symptoms who are not candidates for surgical intervention. However, no medical therapy is available to significantly reverse the changes of advanced atherosclerotic disease.

1. **Risk factor modification** is the most important intervention for reducing the impact of advanced atherosclerotic disease. Control of hypertension and serum glucose, cessation of smoking, management of lipid disorders, attainment of ideal body weight, and regular exercise should be the goals.

   a. **Lipid reduction** is imperative in patients with PAD because majority of the morbidity associated with PAD is related to cardiac events. On the basis of the Heart Protection Study involving statins, it is recommended to keep the low-density-lipoprotein level of patients with PAD less than a 100 mg/dL to help reduce the likelihood of morbidity associated with cardiac events (*J Vasc Surg.* 2007;45:645).

   b. **Antihypertensives** should be administered to normalize blood pressure. Medications such as beta-blockers or angiotensin-converting enzyme inhibitors have been shown in several studies to help reduce mortality-associated cardiovascular disease.

2. Because many of these patients have concomitant coronary artery or cerebrovascular disease, daily **aspirin** therapy (81 or 325 mg) is indicated to reduce the risk of myocardial infarction or stroke.

3. **Clopidogrel** is an **antiplatelet agent** that has been shown to reduce cardiac and cerebral events in patients with systemic atherosclerosis. Although rigorous proof of its utility following peripheral arterial interventions is lacking, clopidogrel is frequently prescribed following these procedures.

4. **Cilostazol** is a type III **phosphodiesterase inhibitor** and the newest agent available for treatment of claudication. Cilostazol inhibits platelet aggregation and causes vasodilation. Given at 50 mg or 100 mg twice daily, it increases walking distances when compared with placebo

and pentoxifylline. Early studies suggest that the drug is safe in most patients, although **its use is contraindicated in those with class III or IV heart failure** due to the toxicity of phosphodiesterase inhibitors in these patients.

C. **Preoperative care** of patients with PVD includes a complete arterial evaluation. In addition to angiographic evaluation of the symptomatic arterial tree, patients generally undergo screening for associated cardiac, renal, cerebrovascular, and pulmonary disease, so that any correctable lesions can be addressed. Myocardial complications account for the majority of early and late deaths; therefore, patients with questionable myocardial function may require more extensive cardiac evaluation. Screening for carotid disease should also be performed, including a history of stroke or transient ischemic attack and carotid auscultation.

D. **Open surgical therapy**

1. Aortoiliac occlusive disease

   a. **Aortobifemoral grafting** is the treatment of choice in low-risk patients with diffuse aortoiliac stenoses and occlusions. Aortobifemoral bypass may be performed through a transperitoneal or a retroperitoneal approach. Distal endarterectomy may be performed in conjunction with a bypass to improve outflow. Results are excellent, with reported patency rates of up to 95% at 5 years.

   b. **Femorofemoral, ilioiliac, or iliofemoral bypasses** are alternatives in high-risk patients with unilateral iliac disease. The patency rates are lower than those achieved with aortobifemoral grafts.

   c. **Axillobifemoral bypass** is an alternative for high-risk patients who need revascularization. This bypass avoids an intra-abdominal procedure and the need for cross-clamping the aorta. The patency rates are poorer than those achieved with aortobifemoral bypass.

   d. **Aortoiliac endarterectomy** may be considered for patients who have disease localized to the distal aorta and common iliac vessels, although its use is now uncommon. Advantages include the avoidance of prosthetic material and preservation of antegrade flow into the hypogastric arteries.

2. Femoral, popliteal, and tibial occlusive disease

   a. In patients with above-knee occlusion, an **above-knee femoral–popliteal bypass** may be constructed. In patients who have disease below the knee, a distal bypass may be performed to the below-knee popliteal, posterior tibial, anterior tibial, or peroneal arteries. If all tibial vessels are occluded, pedal vessels may serve as suitable outflow vessels. These grafts usually originate from the common femoral artery, although a more distal vessel may be used if the inflow into that vessel is unobstructed.

   b. The best results are obtained with the use of **autologous vein** as a conduit. The greater saphenous is the vein of choice, but the lesser saphenous vein or the arm veins provide suitable alternatives. These autologous grafts can be used either in situ or reversed. The advantages of the in situ bypass are that (1) the vein's nutrient supply is left intact and (2) the vein orientation allows for a better size match (the large end of the vein is sewn to the large common femoral artery, and the small end is sewn to the distal vessel). The advantage of the reversed-vein bypass is that endothelial trauma is minimized because valve lysis is not necessary.

c. When autologous vein is not available, polytetrafluoroethylene (PTFE) grafts and cryopreserved vein grafts can be used. Patency rates for PTFE above-knee grafts approach those achieved with venous conduit, but use of PTFE for more distal bypass procedures is associated with substantially lower patency and is reserved for patients with critical limb ischemia who lack venous conduit. An alternative technique when performing PTFE bypass is the use of a small cuff of vein (Miller cuff) or patch angioplasty (Taylor patch) at the distal anastomosis. These modifications are believed to improve prosthetic graft patency by improving compliance match at the distal anastomosis. Cryopreserved vein graft patency also fares poorly in comparison to native autologous conduit, but it may prove useful when bypass is required in an infected field.

d. Endarterectomy is most commonly used to address severe stenosis or occlusion of the common femoral and profunda femoris arteries.

e. Amputation is reserved for patients with gangrene or persistent painful ischemia not amenable to vascular reconstruction. These patients often have severe coexistent vascular and cardiovascular disease, and the survival rate for patients undergoing major amputations is approximately 50% at 3 years and 30% at 5 years.

 (1) The level of amputation is determined clinically. Important factors include the necessity of removing all the infected tissue and the adequacy of the blood supply to heal the amputation. A general principle is to preserve as much length of the extremity as safely possible, as this improves the patient's opportunity for rehabilitation. Revascularization before amputation may enable a more distal amputation to heal adequately.

 (2) Digital amputations are performed commonly in diabetic patients who develop osteomyelitis or severe foot infections.

 (3) Transmetatarsal amputations are usually performed when several toes are involved in the ischemic process or after previous single-digit amputations.

 (4) Syme amputation involves the removal of the entire foot and calcaneus while preserving the entire tibia. It is rarely appropriate for PVD.

 (5) Below-knee amputation (BKA) is the most common type of amputation performed for patients with severe occlusive disease.

 (6) Above-knee amputation (AKA) heals more easily than BKA and is useful in older patients who do not ambulate.

 (7) Hip disarticulation is rarely performed for PVD.

3. Upper-extremity occlusive disease
 a. For proximal subclavian disease, the choice of bypass procedure depends primarily on the patency of the ipsilateral common carotid artery.

   b. If the ipsilateral common carotid artery is patent, carotid–subclavian bypass is performed through a supraclavicular approach using a prosthetic graft (vein grafts are to be avoided). Subclavian artery transposition to ipsilateral carotid artery is an excellent alternative if anatomically feasible.

   c. If the ipsilateral carotid artery is occluded, subclavian–subclavian bypass may be performed. This is an extra-anatomic approach using a longer segment prosthetic graft, with reduced patency.

4. Intraoperative anticoagulation is employed during most vascular reconstructions. Generally, unfractionated heparin (100 to 150 units/kg) is administered intravenously shortly before cross-clamping and supplemented as necessary until the cross-clamps are removed. Anticoagulation can be monitored intraoperatively by following activated clotting time levels. The anticoagulant effect of heparin can be reversed with protamine administration.

E. Postoperative care

1. For open aortic procedures, early postoperative care is usually administered in the ICU, where frequent hemodynamic and hematologic measurements are performed. Assessment of distal pulses should be done intraoperatively, immediately after reconstruction and regularly thereafter. In uncomplicated cases, the patients are usually extubated on the day of surgery or on postoperative day 1. Patients are kept well hydrated for the first 2 postoperative days, after which third-space fluid begins to mobilize and diuresis ensues. Fluid management may be guided by central pressure monitoring. Antibiotics are continued for 24 hours postoperatively. A nasogastric tube is kept in place until return of bowel function. Patients are instructed not to sit with the hips flexed at greater than 60 degrees for the first 72 hours after graft placement, although ambulation as early as possible is encouraged.

2. For distal bypass grafts, **pulses should be assessed frequently.** Antibiotics are continued for 24 hours postoperatively or longer if infected ulcers warrant such treatment. Early ambulation is encouraged in patients without tissue necrosis. In patients who are unable to ambulate immediately, physical therapy can help to increase strength in the limb and prevent contracture. Sitting with the hips flexed to 90 degrees is discouraged in any patient with a femoral anastomosis. Patients should be instructed to elevate their legs while resting because this will mitigate the edema that develops in the revascularized extremity. Staples are left in place for 2 to 3 weeks because these patients frequently have delayed wound healing.

3. **Perioperative antithrombotic therapy** should include aspirin (81 to 325 mg/day) for all infrainguinal reconstructions. In patients sensitive to aspirin, clopidogrel (75 mg/day) may be substituted.

4. Postoperative oral anticoagulation has a more limited role. Owing in part to the increased risk of hemorrhage, anticoagulation with warfarin (international normalized ratio 2:3) is generally limited to grafts considered to be at a high risk for thrombosis.

5. Following major amputations, weight bearing is delayed for 4 to 6 weeks. Some advocate the use of compressive wraps to aid in the maturation of the stump. In all cases, early consultation with a physical therapist is recommended. Physical therapy is essential for maintaining strength in the limb, preventing contractures, and rehabilitating the patient once a prosthesis is fitted. In addition, as soon as the patient is ready, he or she should be fitted with a prosthetic limb and ambulation training should begin. Rehabilitation rates (ability to walk without assistance) for patients undergoing unilateral BKA or AKA are 60% and 30%, respectively. For those with bilateral amputations, rehabilitation rates drop to 40% for patients with bilateral BKA and 10% for patients with bilateral AKA.

6. **Long-term follow-up** for distal bypass grafts consists of serial evaluations of graft patency by clinical examination and duplex ultrasound. Less frequent follow-up is necessary for aortoiliac bypasses. Detection of severe stenosis predicts pending graft failure, and such grafts should be studied further by arteriography. Intervention to repair or revise stenosed grafts results in much higher long-term patency than repairing or replacing occluded grafts.

F. **Complications**

1. Early complications occur in approximately 5% to 10% of patients after aortic surgery and frequently relate to preoperative comorbid disease. Myocardial infarction, congestive heart failure, pulmonary insufficiency, and renal insufficiency are most common. Complications related directly to aortic reconstruction include hemorrhage, embolization or thrombosis of the distal arterial tree, microembolization, ischemic colitis, ureteral injuries, impotence, paraplegia, and wound infection. Late complications include anastomotic pseudoaneurysm or graft dilation, graft limb occlusion, aortoenteric erosion or fistula, and graft infections.

2. In distal revascularizations, most of the early complications are also related to comorbid conditions. Early graft thrombosis (within 30 days of surgery) most often results from technical errors, hypercoagulability, inadequate distal runoff, and postoperative hypotension. **Technical errors** are responsible for more than 50% of early graft failures and include graft kinks, retained valve leaflets, valvulotome trauma, intimal flaps, significant residual arteriovenous fistulas, and the use of poor quality conduit.

G. **Endovascular options**

1. Aortoiliac occlusive disease
   a. Indications. Balloon angioplasty and intravascular stent placement for aortoiliac occlusive lesions produce excellent results. These procedures are indicated for symptomatic stenotic or occlusive lesions. Short-segment stenoses (less than 3 cm in length) of the common and external iliac arteries display excellent long-term patency rates when treated with angioplasty alone, or with stent placement. Angioplasty failure (defined as residual stenosis of ≥30%, residual

mean translesional pressure gradient of ≥10 mm Hg, or flow-limiting dissection) is an indication for stent deployment.

b. Technique. Access for iliac artery angioplasty and stenting is generally via the femoral arterial approach. When the occlusive lesion is in the distal aorta or ostial common iliac artery, angioplasty should be performed using two balloons, one in each iliac artery and both partially projecting into the distal aorta ("kissing balloons"). The rationale for this technique is that lesions in proximity to the aortic bifurcation typically involve the distal aorta and both common iliac arteries. Unilateral balloon dilation may cause plaque shifting with compromise of the contralateral iliac artery lumen. Stenting may produce a more favorable result if postangioplasty dissection or lesion recoil is noted. Balloon-expandable and self-expanding stents are generally oversized 10% to 15% relative to the adjacent normal artery to ensure satisfactory stent apposition to the vessel wall. If stent deployment is required in proximity to the aortic bifurcation, "kissing stents" are utilized in a fashion similar to that described above.

c. Complications. Procedural complications of iliac angioplasty and stenting include bleeding, arterial dissection, vessel occlusion, arterial rupture, and distal embolization, which may result in the need for surgical intervention or amputation.

d. Results. Early balloon angioplasty failure can result from elastic recoil of atherosclerotic plaque or arterial wall dissection. These complications are potentially amenable to stent placement. Late failure is usually due to intimal hyperplasia or progressive atherosclerosis. Iliac artery balloon angioplasty 2-year patency rates between 60% and 70% have been reported. Reports of iliac artery stenting demonstrate 4-year patency rates as high as 85%. In general, the results of angioplasty and stenting are better for common iliac artery lesions than for external iliac artery lesions, and are better for short-segment disease than for long-segment disease.

2. Infrainguinal occlusive disease

a. Indications. Balloon angioplasty and stenting of infrainguinal occlusive lesions has been widely applied for the treatment of claudication and critical limb ischemia. Aggressive modification of risk factors, institution of antiplatelet and statin medications, and a trial of exercise therapy are recommended prior to intervention, particularly in the setting of claudication. The Trans-Atlantic Inter-Society Consensus (TASC) group has provided recommendations regarding the characteristics of femoropopliteal and infrapopliteal lesions that are best addressed by either endovascular or surgical therapy. See Table 19-1. Short, focal stenoses (TASC A) are felt to be amenable to endovascular therapy, whereas long-segment occlusions (TASC D) are best addressed by surgical bypass.

b. Technique. Arterial access for infrainguinal intervention is usually accomplished via retrograde contralateral femoral artery approach or ipsilateral antegrade femoral artery approach. The most frequent cause of treatment failure is the inability to negotiate across the stenosis or occlusion and into the distal outflow target vessel. In general,

TABLE 19-1	TASC Classification
TASC Classification	Lesion Characteristics
A	Single stenosis <10 cm Single occlusion <5 cm
B	Multiple lesions <5 cm Single or multiple lesions in the absence of continuous tibial vessels Single stenosis/occlusion <15 cm Heavily calcified occlusion <5 cm Single popliteal stenosis
C	Multiple stenoses/occlusions totaling >15 cm Recurrent stenoses/occlusions needing intervention after two prior interventions
D	Chronic total occlusions of CFA or SFA Chronic total occlusion of popliteal and proximal trifurcation vessels

CFA, common femoral artery; SFA, superficial femoral artery; TASC, The Trans-Atlantic Inter-Society Consensus.

once guidewire access to the distal target vessel has been established, technical success rates are excellent. Hydrophilic guidewires and catheters, occlusion crossing devices, lumen reentry devices, and specialized sheaths have been developed to facilitate this process.

c. **Complications.** Procedural complications of infrainguinal endovascular intervention include bleeding, arterial thrombosis, vessel perforation, flow-limiting dissection, arteriovenous fistula formation, and distal embolization. Severe complications may require surgical intervention or, rarely, amputation.

d. **Results.** Unfortunately, midterm and long-term outcomes data for endovascular intervention in the treatment of claudication and critical limb ischemia remain relatively scarce. For moderate severity lesions of the femoropopliteal distribution, the ABSOLUTE trial demonstrated that primary nitinol stenting may provide a patency advantage over plain balloon angioplasty, and that this may be sustained through 2 years of follow-up (*NEJM*. 2006;354:1879). Perhaps the most compelling data regarding endovascular versus surgical intervention have been derived from the Bypass versus Angioplasty in Severe Ischemia of the Leg (BASIL) trial from the United Kingdom (*J Vasc Surg*. 2010;51:52S). Although the initial results reported from the trial were widely interpreted as demonstrating equivalency between angioplasty and bypass surgery for this patient cohort, longer term follow-up has shown an advantage in both overall survival and amputation-free survival in those patients who underwent bypass surgery and survived beyond 2 years. Interestingly, the BASIL investigators noted that outcomes were worse for patients who underwent angioplasty followed by salvage bypass surgery, rather than a bypass-first approach. Good surgical candidates—in particular, those possessing good venous conduit—should be considered for surgical reconstruction. Endovascular intervention is the preferred approach for the medically compromised patient, particularly those lacking autologous venous conduit. Finally, hybrid open surgical/endovascular procedures are also utilized in the treatment of critical limb ischemia. Vascular surgeons who are skilled in both open surgical reconstruction and endovascular interventions will therefore tailor their therapeutic approach based on each patient's unique risk factors and arterial anatomy.

20 Venous Disease, Thromboembolism, and Lymphedema

Wande Pratt and Brian Rubin

VENOUS ANATOMY

Venous anatomy is divided into three compartments: the superficial, the perforating veins, and the deep compartment. In general, blood flows from superficial to deep through the perforating system. In the lower extremity, the major superficial veins are the *greater saphenous vein*, formed from the union of the dorsal vein of the great toe and the dorsal venous arch; the *lesser saphenous vein*, formed from the joining of the dorsal vein of the fifth toe and the dorsal venous arch; and the *posterior arch vein*, also called *Leonardo's vein*, beginning in the medial ankle and joining the greater saphenous vein below the knee. The deep veins in the leg are named according to their paired arteries. The deep veins of the calf typically are duplicated as venae comitantes with numerous communicating branches. The posterior tibial and peroneal veins also communicate with the soleal sinusoids. In the thigh, the deep venous system includes the superficial and deep femoral veins that join approximately 4 cm below the inguinal ligament. Perforating veins connect the superficial and deep systems through both direct and indirect mechanisms. Venous return from the lower extremities depends largely on compression of the deep veins by the muscles of the calf (gastrocnemius, soleus) during walking. Flow is unidirectional due to a series of one-way valves, which prevent reflux during this cycle of compression. Failure of these valves to close leads to pooling, stasis, and congestion of veins in the lower extremities, and subsequent distention of the superficial veins.

CHRONIC VENOUS INSUFFICIENCY

Chronic venous disease includes cosmetically undesirable telangiectasias, varicose veins, venous ulceration, and claudication. Advances in duplex scanning and minimally invasive surgical techniques such as subfascial endoscopic perforating vein surgery (SEPS) and thermal ablation techniques are used to tailor medical and surgical therapies, resulting in marked improvement in clinical outcomes and patient satisfaction.

I. PATHOPHYSIOLOGY

A. Etiology

1. Congenital (may present later in life).

2. Primary (cause undetermined).

3. Secondary (postthrombotic, posttraumatic, or other).

B. Risk factors

1. Obesity.

2. Tobacco use.

3. Multiparity.

4. Hormone therapy.

5. Obstruction within a proximal segment (e.g., from adenopathy, arterial compression, or pregnancy).

6. History of deep venous thrombosis (DVT). DVT accounts for most secondary cases and may be responsible for a significant number of other cases because many deep vein thrombi are asymptomatic.

C. Reflux disease from venous valvular incompetence accounts for most (>80%) chronic venous disease.

1. Valve malfunction can be inherited or acquired through sclerosis or elongation of valve cusps.

2. May also result from dilation of the valve annulus despite normal valve cusps.

3. Varicose veins may represent superficial venous insufficiency in the presence of competent deep and perforator systems, or they may be a manifestation of perforator or deep disease.

4. Valvular disease below the knee appears to be more critical in the pathophysiology of severe disease than the disease above the knee.

5. The perforator veins are frequently implicated when venous ulcers exist, but any component of the venous system, either alone or in combination, may be incompetent.

6. All of the above components need evaluation in the workup of chronic venous insufficiency (CVI) (*Am Surg.* 2010;76:125).

D. Obstructive physiology is a less common cause of venous pathology, with reflux often being present simultaneously.

II. DIFFERENTIAL DIAGNOSIS

A. Arterial disease

1. Ulcers with discrete edges and pale bases; more painful than venous ulcers.

2. Poor or absent pulses on exam.

3. Dependent rubor.

4. Pallor with elevation.

5. Claudication.

B. Lymphedema

1. Pitting edema without pigmentation and ulceration.

2. Less responsive to elevation, usually requiring several days to improve.

C. Squamous cell carcinoma

D. Trauma

E. Arteriovenous malformation
F. Orthostatic edema

III. NOMENCLATURE

A. **CEAP classification**

1. Based on the conclusions of an international consensus committee.

2. Standardized nomenclature of chronic venous disease (*J Vasc Surg.* 2004;40:1248; *Eur J Vasc Endovasc Surg.* 1996;12:487).

3. CEAP: **C**linical signs, **E**tiology, **A**natomic distribution, and **P**athophysiology (Table 20-1).

4. Useful in defining clinical severity of disease and subsequent management strategies.

5. Assessing response to therapy over time with the system proves difficult.

B. **Venous clinical severity score (VCSS)**

1. Developed by the American Venous Forum in 2000, and revised in 2010; expands the existing system.

2. Ten clinical descriptors: pain, varicose veins, venous edema, skin pigmentation, inflammation, induration, number of active ulcers, duration of active ulceration, size of ulcer, and compressive therapy use.

3. Better assesses ongoing response to therapy.

4. The revised VCSS, in conjunction with the CEAP classification system, provides a standard clinical language to describe and compare management approaches to chronic venous disease (*J Vasc Surg.* 2010;52:1387).

IV. DIAGNOSIS

A. **History**

1. A history of any DVT or trauma.

2. Family history of varicose veins or CVI.

3. Complaint of lower-extremity edema, aching, skin irritation, or varicose veins. Leg pain is described as a dull ache, worsening at the end of the day, and often relieved with exercise or elevation.

4. In rare instances, individuals can experience acute, bursting pain with ambulation (*venous claudication*). Prolonged rest and leg elevation (20 minutes) are needed to obtain relief.

B. **Physical examination**

1. Ankle edema.

2. Subcutaneous fibrosis.

3. Hyperpigmentation (brownish discoloration secondary to hemosiderin deposition).

4. Lipodermatosclerosis.

5. Venous eczema.

TABLE 20-1	Classification of Chronic Lower-Extremity Venous Disease
Classification	**Definition**
C	Clinical classification C_0: No visible or palpable signs of venous disease C_1: Telangiectasias or reticular veins C_2: Varicose veins; distinguished from reticular veins by a diameter of 3 mm or more C_3: Edema C_4: Changes in skin and subcutaneous tissue secondary to CVD C_{4a}: Pigmentation or eczema C_{4b}: Lipodermatosclerosis or atrophie blanche C_5: Healed venous ulcer C_6: Active venous ulcer *S: Symptomatic (includes aching, pain, tightness, skin irritation, heaviness, muscle cramps, and other complaints attributable to venous dysfunction)* *A: Asymptomatic*
E	Etiologic classification E_c: Congenital E_p: Primary E_s: Secondary (i.e., postthrombotic) E_n: No venous cause identified
A	Anatomic distribution A_s: Superficial veins involved A_p: Perforator veins involved A_d: Deep veins involved A_n: No venous location identified
P	Pathophysiologic dysfunction P_r: Reflux P_o: Obstruction $P_{r,o}$: Reflux and obstruction P_n: No venous pathophysiology identified

CVD, chronic venous disease.

6. Dilation of subcutaneous veins, including telangiectasias (0.1 to 1 mm), reticular veins (1 to 4 mm), and varicose veins (>4 mm).

7. Ultimately, ulcers develop, typically proximal to the medial malleolus.

8. Any signs of infection should be noted.

9. Arterial pulses should be examined and are usually adequate.

C. Noninvasive studies

1. Duplex scanning

   a. B-mode ultrasound imaging combined with Doppler frequency shift display.

   b. Used in assessing valvular incompetence and obstruction, presence of acute or chronic DVT.

   c. With the leg in a dependant position, cuffs are placed on the thigh, calf, and foot and inflated; then the cuffs are rapidly deflated in an attempt to create retrograde venous blood flow in segments of valvular incompetence.

   d. Competent valves generally take no more than 0.5 to 1 second to close.

   e. Detailed mapping of valve competence of each segment of the venous system is possible, including the common femoral, superficial femoral, greater saphenous, lesser saphenous, popliteal, posterior tibial, and perforator veins.

   f. Has a predictive value of 77% for diagnosing reflux leading to severe symptoms.

2. Descending phlebography has a predictive value of 44%, previously considered the gold standard (*J Vasc Surg.* 1992;16:687). Descending phlebography is limited by its inability to study valves distal to a competent proximal valve.

3. Continuous wave Doppler

   a. Easily performed in the office using a handheld probe.

   b. Helpful for screening for reflux at the saphenofemoral and saphenopopliteal junctions.

   c. Limited due to inability to quantitate reflux and to provide precise anatomic information.

4. Trendelenburg test

   a. Largely replaced by the much more accurate duplex imaging studies.

   b. Patient's leg is elevated to drain venous blood. An elastic tourniquet is applied at the saphenofemoral junction, and the patient then stands.

   c. Rapid filling (<30 seconds) of the saphenous system from the deep system indicates perforator valve incompetence.

   d. When tourniquet is released, additional filling of the saphenous system occurs if the saphenofemoral valve is also incompetent.

V. NONSURGICAL TREATMENT

A. Infected ulcers

   1. Necessitate treatment of the infection first.

   2. *Staphylococcus aureus*, *Streptococcus pyogenes*, and *Pseudomonas* species are responsible for most infections.

   3. Usually treated with local wound care, wet-to-dry dressings, and oral antibiotics.

   4. Topical antiseptics should be avoided.

   5. Severe infections require intravenous antibiotics.

B. Leg elevation can temporarily decrease edema and should be instituted when swelling occurs. This should be done before a patient is fitted for stockings or boots.

C. Compression therapy is the primary treatment for CVI.

1. **Elastic compression stockings**
   a. Fitted to provide a compression gradient from 30 to 40 mm Hg, with the greatest compression at the ankle.
   b. Donned on arising from bed and removed at bedtime.
   c. Effective in healing ulcers, *but can take months* to obtain good results.
   d. Study of 113 patients treated with initial bed rest, local wound care, and elastic compression stockings demonstrated a 93% ulcer healing rate in a mean of 5.3 months (*Surgery.* 1991;109:575).
   e. Stockings do not correct the abnormal venous hemodynamics and must be worn after the ulcer has healed to prevent recurrence.
   f. Principal drawback is patient compliance.
   g. Recurrence for compliant patients in the same study was 16% at a mean follow-up of 30 months.

2. **Unna boots**
   a. Paste gauze compression dressings that contain zinc oxide, calamine, and glycerin.
   b. Used to help prevent further skin breakdown.
   c. Provide nonelastic compression therapy.
   d. Changed once or twice a week.

3. **Pneumatic compression devices**
   a. Provide dynamic sequential compression.
   b. Used primarily in the prevention of deep vein thrombi in hospitalized patients.
   c. Also used successfully to treat venous insufficiency.

D. Topical medications

1. Largely ineffective as a stand-alone therapy for venous stasis ulcers.
2. Topical therapy is directed at absorbing wound drainage and avoiding desiccation of the wound.
3. Antiseptics can be counterproductive. Hydrogen peroxide, povidone-iodine, acetic acid, and sodium hypochlorite are toxic to cultured fibroblasts and should be used for the shortest duration necessary to control ulcer infection.

VI. SURGICAL THERAPY is indicated for severe disease refractory to medical treatment and for patients who cannot comply with the lifelong regimen of compression therapy. Surgical therapy includes sclerotherapy, saphenous vein stripping, endovenous laser ablation of the saphenous vein, SEPS, and varicose vein stab avulsion.

A. Preoperative evaluation. All patients should undergo a thorough history and physical examination with special attention to symptoms of chronic venous disease, including aching pain, sense of heaviness in the legs, and fatigability with ambulation. Patients often describe their symptoms as worsening throughout the course of the day, particularly if they are required to stand for long periods. Diagnostic evaluation consists primarily of duplex imaging (including vein mapping, reflux studies, and assessment for DVT) in a reliable vascular laboratory. This allows for visualization of the affected venous segments and for determination of points of reflux. Valve closure time should be assessed, usually within the great saphenous vein, with times greater than 500 milliseconds considered abnormal.

B. Sclerotherapy

1. Effective in treating telangiectasias, reticular varicosities, and small varicose veins.

2. If saphenous reflux is present, it should be corrected first.

3. Contraindications include arterial occlusive disease, immobility, acute thrombophlebitis, and hypersensitivity to the drug.

4. **Sclerosing agents**
   a. 1% or 3% sodium tetradecyl sulfate.
   b. Sodium morrhuate (rarely used because of anaphylactic reactions).
   c. Hypertonic saline.
   d. Polidocanol (approved in March 2010, by the U.S. Food and Drug Administration).

5. Varices are marked while the patient is standing. A 25-gauge needle is used to inject 0.25 to 0.50 mL of sclerosant slowly into the lumen of larger veins. A 30-gauge needle is used for sclerosing reticular veins and telangiectasias in supine patients.

6. Compression stockings are applied at the end of the procedure and are worn for several days to 6 weeks. Patients should walk for 30 minutes after the procedure.

7. Complications include cutaneous necrosis, hyperpigmentation, telangiectatic matting (new, fine, red telangiectasias), thrombophlebitis, anaphylaxis, allergic reaction, visual disturbances, venous thromboembolism (VTE), and even death (*J Vasc Surg.* 2010;52:939; *Dermatol Surg.* 1995;21:19).

C. **Saphenous vein stripping,** once considered the gold standard for superficial venous surgery, has since been replaced by the use of minimally invasive techniques in many practices by the US surgeons treating CVI; however, the surgeons should be familiar with this technique. Stripping of the entire length of the saphenous vein is usually unnecessary. Typically, the vein is stripped from mid-calf or knee level to the saphenofemoral junction. If the entire vein is involved, one incision is made anterior to the medial malleolus and another just below the inguinal crease. A standard vein stripper is inserted into the vein lumen at one site and advanced through the lumen to the other site. High ligation of the vein is performed at the saphenofemoral junction, including all venous tributaries. Reconnection of the saphenous to the femoral system via multiple tributaries near the saphenofemoral junction is thought to be the major cause of recurrent varices. At the completion of the procedure, compressive bandages are applied to reduce hematoma formation, and compression stockings are worn for several weeks. Complications include ecchymosis, DVT, and saphenous nerve injury. Stripping only the thigh portion is probably the most important aspect of the procedure, and eliminates much of the risk to the saphenous nerve because this nerve is closely associated with the saphenous vein from the knee to the ankle. In addition, this preserves the portion of the vein below the knee to be used for arterial bypass if needed in the future (*Lancet.* 1996;348:210). Because the goal of stripping is to prevent reflux of the involved venous segment, removal of a limited portion of the saphenous system is now widely accepted. Ligation alone, however, is associated with high rates of recanalization and is therefore not adequate therapy.

D. **Endovenous ablation of the saphenous vein**

1. This was shown to effectively treat saphenous reflux and associated varicose veins with less morbidity than saphenectomy (*J Vasc Surg.* 2003;38:207).

2. A probe is inserted into the greater saphenous vein under ultrasound guidance. The probe emits either laser or radiofrequency energy, which coagulates and coapts the vein walls, causing complete obliteration of the lumen.

3. Potential complications
   a. Skin burns.
   b. DVT.
   c. Pulmonary thromboembolism.
   d. Vein perforation and hematoma.
   e. Paresthesias.
   f. Phlebitis.

4. Reported outcomes achieved with endovenous radiofrequency and laser obliteration are comparable to those resulting from saphenectomy (*Ann Vasc Surg.* 2010;24:360; *J Vasc Interv Radiol.* 2009;20:752; *J Vasc Surg.* 2008;47:151). Incomplete obliteration and recanalization occur in a small percentage of patients.

5. A contraindication to endovenous obliteration is saphenous vein thrombosis.

E. **Subfascial Endoscopic Perforating Vein Surgery**

1. This is associated with decreased morbidity and has gained recognition as an alternative treatment option.

2. Performed by making small port incisions in unaffected skin in the calf and fascia of the posterior superficial compartment. Various types of endoscopes (laparoscopic, arthroplastic, or bronchoscopic) can be used for visualization. Carbon dioxide insufflation in the subfascial space may or may not be used. A balloon expander can expand the subfascial space to improve visualization. Typically, 3 to 14 perforators are identified and ligated.

3. Most patients are discharged within 24 hours of surgery.

F. **Varicose vein stab avulsion**

1. Preoperatively, the patient's varicose veins are carefully marked with indelible ink while the patient is standing. Some authors consider this to be the most important technical step.

2. Small incisions (2 to 3 mm) are made next to the markings. The vein is pulled out of the incision with a small vein hook, and the two arms of the vein are pulled taut and avulsed. This can be repeated many times to remove large clusters of veins. The small incisions can be closed with Steri-Strips. The patient's leg is covered with compression stockings for several days to weeks. This technique is often used in conjunction with saphenous stripping to provide optimal results. Alternatively, the greater saphenous vein can be removed by sequential avulsion instead of stripping.

VENOUS THROMBOEMBOLISM

I. **EPIDEMIOLOGY.** VTE, which includes DVT and pulmonary embolism (PE), is a common cause of death. The true incidence of DVT is difficult to determine because its clinical diagnosis can be inaccurate and often occurring in the setting of other critical illnesses. Venous thromboembolic disease represents a significant problem, with 250,000 hospitalizations for DVT/PE annually. Approximately 50% to 60% of DVT episodes are asymptomatic. Of those patients with DVTs, 30% will have a symptomatic PE with a mortality of 17.5% if untreated. DVT and PE occur in approximately 10% to 40% of general surgical patients without perioperative prophylaxis, and 40% to 60% following major orthopedic surgery (*Chest.* 2008;133:381S–453S).

II. **PATHOPHYSIOLOGY.** DVT starts as a platelet nidus, usually in the venous valves of the calf. The thrombogenic nature of the nidus activates the clotting cascade, leading to platelet and fibrin accumulation. The fibrinolytic system is subsequently activated, with thrombus growth if thrombogenesis predominates over thrombolysis. A thrombus can detach from the endothelium and migrate into the pulmonary system, becoming a PE; alternatively, it can also organize and grow into the endothelium, resulting in venous incompetency and phlebitis. Thrombi localized to the calf have less tendency to embolize than thrombi that extend to the thigh veins (*Am Rev Respir Dis.* 1990;141:1). Approximately 20% of cases of calf DVT propagate to the thigh, and 50% of cases of thigh or proximal DVT embolize.

III. **RISK FACTORS FOR VENOUS THROMBOEMBOLISM**

A. **Malignancy**

1. Tumor cell activation of the clotting cascade can occur directly through interactions with factors VIIa, X, and tissue factor (TF).

2. Indirect clotting activation can occur through stimulation of mononuclear cells to produce TF or factor X activators and stimulation of macrophages to produce TF activators.

3. Reactive thrombocytosis can occur in patients, especially those with advanced disease of the lung, colon, stomach, or breast; it is caused by spontaneous clumping of platelets or increased levels of thrombopoietin, a glycoprotein regulating the maturation of megakaryocytes.

B. Endothelial injury

1. Adhesion of tumor cells to endothelium can lead to disruption of endothelial intracellular junctions and expose the highly thrombogenic subendothelial surface.

2. Chemotherapeutic drugs, such as bleomycin, carmustine, vincristine, and doxorubicin (Adriamycin), can also cause vascular endothelial cell damage.

C. Venous stasis

1. This is caused by immobility, venous obstruction, increased venous pressure, and increased blood viscosity.

2. Venous stasis promotes thrombus formation by reducing clearance of activated coagulation factors and by causing endothelial hypoxia, leading to reduced levels of surface-bound thrombomodulin and increased expression of TF.

3. Two very common causes of immobility leading to DVT formation are surgery and critical illness. Major chest surgery, abdominal/pelvic surgery, and lower-extremity surgery have all been associated with increased risk of DVT development. Similarly, a prolonged non-ambulatory state, such as fracture of the hip, pelvis, or leg; multisystem trauma; neurologic injury; or other critical injury requiring bed rest can increase DVT risk.

D. Oral contraceptives (OCPs) and estrogen hormone replacement therapy

1. These have been linked to increased risk of venous thrombus formation. Many studies have found an odds ratio of 3 to 5 for risk of DVT in patients taking OCPs compared to non–OCP-using patients.

2. An increased risk is still found with patients using third-generation OCPs containing new progestins.

E. Hypercoagulable states

1. Primary hypercoagulable states are inherited conditions that can lead to abnormal endothelial cell thromboregulation.
    a. Decreased thrombomodulin-dependent activation of protein C (factor V Leiden mutation).
    b. Impaired heparin binding of antithrombin III.
    c. Downregulation of membrane-associated plasmin production.
    d. Increased serum prothrombin levels (G20210A prothrombin gene mutation).
    e. Decreased thrombogenic inhibitors (e.g., antithrombin III, protein C, protein S).

2. Secondary hypercoagulable states are states in which endothelial activation by cytokines leads to an inflammatory, thrombogenic vessel wall.
    a. Antiphospholipid syndrome.
    b. Venous trauma.
    c. Surgery.
    d. Hyperhomocysteinemia.

    e. Heparin-induced thrombopathy.

    f. Myeloproliferative syndromes.

    g. Cancer.

    h. Chemotherapy agents: cyclophosphamide, methotrexate, and 5-fluorouracil, cause a decrease in the plasma levels of proteins C and S.

IV. DIAGNOSIS

A. Initial evaluation

1. Approximately 75% of patients with suspected DVT or PE turn out not to have these conditions.

2. Assessment of risk factors (see Section III).

3. Clinical presentation

    a. Extremity pain.

    b. Increased circumference with respect to contralateral extremity.

    c. Dilation of superficial veins of the suspected extremity only.

    d. Calf pain on dorsiflexion of the ankle.

    e. Phlegmasia alba dolens represents a more severe manifestation of DVT in which the deep venous channels of the extremity are affected *while sparing collateral veins* and therefore maintaining some degree of venous return. Patients present with blanching of the extremity, edema, and discomfort.

    f. Phlegmasia cerulea dolens occurs with extension of thrombus into the collateral venous system, resulting in limb pain and swelling, accompanied by cyanosis, a sign of arterial ischemia.

B. Suspected DVT

1. Compression ultrasonography of the femoral, popliteal, and calf trifurcation veins is highly sensitive (>90%) in detecting thrombosis of the proximal veins (femoral and popliteal) but less sensitive (50%) in detecting calf vein thrombosis.

2. It represents the preferred diagnostic modality because it is less invasive than the reference standard of venography and is more sensitive than impedance plethysmography.

3. Approximately 2% of patients with initial normal ultrasound results have positive results on repeat tests performed 7 days later. Delayed detection rate is attributed to extension of calf vein thrombi or small, nonocclusive proximal vein thrombi.

C. Assessment of PE

1. **Contrast-enhanced spiral computed tomography (CT)** has sensitivity (70% to 90%) comparable to that of pulmonary angiography. Spiral CT is preferable to angiography (less invasive and less expensive).

2. Chest CT can be combined with CT angiography of pelvic and deep thigh veins to detect DVT as well as PE.

3. Patients with significant contrast allergy or renal insufficiency are not candidates for CT scanning.

4. Radionucleotide ventilation and perfusion lung imaging (V/Q scan) has been replaced by chest CT as the initial imaging test for suspected PE. V/Q scanning is used in situations in which CT is deemed not feasible. A V/Q scan result of "high probability" strongly suggests the presence of PE. However, more than 50% of patients have "intermediate probability" results. Because approximately 25% of these patients have PE, further evaluation or initiation of empiric treatment must be considered.

5. **Pulmonary angiography,** the reference test, is reserved for patients whose diagnosis is still uncertain.

V. PREVENTION AND TREATMENT OF VENOUS THROMBOEMBOLISM. For anticoagulation treatments following specific procedures, please see the recent guidelines published by the American College of Chest Physicians (*Chest.* 2008;133:381S).

A. **Low-dose unfractionated heparin (LDUH)**

1. This is given subcutaneously at 5,000 units 1 to 2 hours before surgery, and every 8 or 12 hours postoperatively (*N Engl J Med.* 1988;318:18).

2. LDUH reduces the risk of VTE by 50% to 70% (*N Engl J Med.* 1988;318:18) and does not require laboratory monitoring. Because of the potential for minor bleeding, it should not be used for patients undergoing cerebral, ocular, or spinal surgery.

B. **Graduated compression stockings**

1. These are effective in preventing DVT formation by reducing venous stasis.

2. In surgery patients, the use of graduated compression stockings appears to augment the protective benefit of low-dose heparin by nearly 75%. The combination of graduated compression stockings and LDUH is significantly more effective than LDUH alone, with DVT rates of 4% and 15%, respectively (*Cochrane Database Syst Rev.* 2000;1:CD001484; *Br J Surg.* 1985;72:7).

3. Graduated compression stockings are relatively inexpensive and should be considered for all high-risk patients, even when other forms of prophylaxis are used. Furthermore, the early use of either over-the-counter or custom-fit stockings following diagnosis of DVT results in a reduction in the incidence of postthrombotic syndromes (*Lancet.* 1997;349:759; *Ann Intern Med.* 2004;141:249).

C. **Intermittent pneumatic compression of the extremities**

1. Enhances blood flow in the deep veins, and increases blood fibrinolytic activity through upregulation of thrombomodulin, fibrinolysin, t-PA and endothelial nitric oxide synthase expression (*Acta Anaesthesiologica Scandinavica.* 2005;49:660).

2. For patients with significant bleeding risk with anticoagulation, pneumatic compression is an effective alternative.

3. Compression devices should not be placed on an extremity with known DVT.

4. In the case of known bilateral lower-extremity DVT, the compression devices can be placed on the upper extremity.

5. Pedal compression devices are also effective in patients whose body habitus does not allow conventionally sized devices to fit around the thighs or calves.

D. Low–molecular-weight heparins (LMWHs)

1. Several advantages over unfractionated heparin, with longer half-lives, a more predictable dose–response curve, a lower risk of heparin-induced thrombocytopenia (HIT), the possibility of ambulatory treatment at home and in laboratory animals, fewer bleeding complications with equivalent anticoagulation effects.

2. In large randomized trials of patients with DVT, outpatient treatment with a LMWH was as safe and effective as inpatient treatment with intravenous unfractionated heparin.

E. Other medications such as the direct thrombin inhibitors (DTIs) and fondaparinux represent a possible alternative to the unfractionated and LMWHs in the prevention of thromboembolic disease. The univalent DTI Argatroban as well as the bivalent DTIs (binding to both the active site and an additional accessory site on the thrombin molecule) lepirudin, bivalirudin, hirudin, and desirudin, administered by intravenous, intramuscular, or subcutaneous injection, offer an alternative to the heparins, particularly in situations in which heparin is contraindicated, such as HIT. These medications, however, are less suitable for long-term treatment (*N Engl J Med.* 2005;353:2827). Fondaparinux, the first synthetic pentasaccharide, blocks thrombin generation by accelerating the rate of factors IIa, VIIa, IXa, Xa, XIa, and XIIa inactivation by antithrombin. The agent possesses almost complete bioavailability after subcutaneous injection, with clearance by the kidneys in unaltered form (*Curr Opin Anaes.* 2006;19:52).

F. Caval interruption with intracaval filters. The American College of Chest Physicians recommends inferior vena cava (IVC) filter placement only in those patients with proven VTE with a contraindication for anticoagulation, a complication of anticoagulation, or recurrent VTE despite adequate anticoagulation. No randomized trials have examined the prophylactic use of IVC filters in any patient population. In fact, several meta-analyses found no difference in the rates of PE among patients with and without prophylactic IVC filters (*J Trauma.* 2000;49:140; *J Am Coll Surg.* 1999;189:314). Absolute and relative indications for caval interruption are listed in Table 20-2 (*Chest.* 2008;133:381S; *Am J Med.* 2007;120:S13; *Prog Cardiovasc Dis.* 2006;49:98; *J Am Coll Surg.* 2005;201:957; *Chest.* 2004;126:401S; *J Vasc Interv Radiol.* 2003;14:425; *Blood.* 2000;95:3669). Complications related to filter insertion occur in 4% to 11% of patients. The most common complications are related to thrombotic complications: insertion site thrombosis (2% to 28%); IVC thrombosis (3% to 11%); and recurrent DVT (6% to 35%). Other complications include filter migration, penetration of the IVC, filter fracture, vena caval obstruction, and guidewire entrapment. The specific types of

TABLE 20-2   Use of Inferior Vena Cava Filters

Absolute indications (*strongly* recommended according to evidence-based guidelines)
Proven VTE with contraindication for anticoagulation.
Proven VTE with complication of anticoagulation treatment.
Recurrent VTE despite anticoagulation treatment ("failure of anticoagulation").

Relative indications (*expanded* use; not guideline recommended)
Recurrent PE complicated by pulmonary hypertension.
Patients with DVT and limited cardiopulmonary reserve or chronic obstructive pulmonary disease.
Patients with large, free-floating ileofemoral thrombus.
Following thrombectomy, embolectomy, or thrombolysis of DVT.
High-risk trauma patients (head and spinal cord injury, pelvic or lower extremity fractures) with a contraindication for anticoagulation.
Patients with DVT who have cancer or burns, or are pregnant.

Contraindications for filter placement
Chronically thrombosed IVC.
Anatomical abnormalities preventing access to the IVC for filter placement.

VTE, venous thromboembolism; PE, pulmonary embolism; DVT, deep venous thrombosis; IVC, inferior vena cava.

retrievable and permanent filters are beyond the scope of this chapter, but the use of retrievable filters can reduce the incidence of thrombotic complications (*Am J Med.* 2007;120:S13).

G. The **choice of prophylaxis method** depends on the risk of VTE compared with the risk of anticoagulation. See Chapter 1 for a detailed description.

H. **Catheter-directed thrombolysis** of acute DVT with or without mechanical thrombectomy devices has been advocated to avoid sequelae of DVT. The goals are to restore venous flow, preserve venous valve function, and eliminate the possibility of thromboembolism. Technical success and early clinical benefit have been reported, but long-term data are unavailable. In patients with migration of DVT resulting in severe PE and hemodynamic instability, potentially life-saving thrombolytics should be considered (*Curr Opin Anaes.* 2006;19:52).

LYMPHEDEMA

I. PATHOPHYSIOLOGY

A. **Primary lymphedema** is the result of congenital aplasia, hypoplasia, or hyperplasia of lymphatic vessels and nodes that causes the accumulation of a protein-rich fluid in the interstitial space. Swelling of the patient's leg initially produces pitting edema, which progresses to a nonpitting form and may lead to dermal fibrosis and disfigurement.

1. Primary lymphedema is classified according to age at presentation.

    a. Congenital primary lymphedema (present at birth) represents 10% to 15% of all cases, which can be hereditary (Milroy disease) or nonhereditary.

    b. Praecox (early in life) or Meige disease represents 70% to 80% of cases.

        (1) It is seen in female patients 80% to 90% of the time.

        (2) It presents during the second and third decades of life, typically with localized swelling of the foot and ankle. Such swelling is worsened by prolonged standing.

        (3) A single lower extremity is affected in 70% of patients.

    c. Tarda (late in life) primary lymphedema, representing 10% to 15% of cases, is seen equally in men and women and presents after the third or fourth decade of life.

B. Secondary lymphedema results from impaired lymphatic drainage secondary to a known cause. Surgical or traumatic interruption of lymphatic vessels (often from an axillary or groin lymph node dissection), carcinoma, infection, venous thrombosis, and radiation are causes of secondary lymphedema. Secondary lymphedema in the context of filariasis, caused by the parasite *Wuchereria bancrofti*, represents the most common worldwide presentation of the disease.

II. DIAGNOSIS

A. Clinical presentation

  1. Symptoms

    a. Early lymphedema is characterized by unilateral or bilateral arm or pedal swelling that resolves overnight. With disease progression, the swelling increases and extends up the extremity, producing discomfort and thickened skin. With more advanced disease, swelling is not relieved overnight. Significant pain is unusual.

    b. Secondary lymphedema patients commonly present with repeated episodes of cellulitis secondary to high interstitial protein content.

  2. Physical examination

    a. Edema of the affected extremity is present.

    b. When a lower extremity is involved, the toes are often spared.

    c. With advanced disease, the extremity becomes tense, with nonpitting edema.

    d. Dermal fibrosis results in skin thickening, hair loss, and generalized keratosis.

B. Imaging studies

  1. Lymphoscintigraphy is the injection of radiolabeled (technetium-99m) colloid into the web space between the patient's second and third toes or fingers. The patient's limb is exercised periodically, and images are taken of the involved extremity and the whole body. Lymphedema is seen as an abnormal accumulation of tracer or as slow tracer clearance along with the presence of collaterals. For the diagnosis of lymphedema, the study has a sensitivity and specificity of 92% and 100%, respectively (*J Vasc Surg.* 1989;9:683).

2. **CT and magnetic resonance (MR) scan** are able to exclude any mass obstructing the lymphatic system. MR scan has been able to differentiate lymphedema from chronic venous edema and lipedema (excessive subcutaneous fat and fluid).

3. **Lymphangiography** involves catheter placement and injection of radiopaque dye directly into lymphatic channels; it has largely been replaced by lymphoscintigraphy and CT. A decreased total number of lymphatic channels and structural abnormalities can be seen. Lymphangiography can demonstrate the site of a lymphatic leak in postsurgical or traumatic situations. Complications include lymphangitis and hypersensitivity reaction to the dye.

III. DIFFERENTIAL DIAGNOSIS includes all other causes of a swollen extremity.

A. Trauma.
B. Infection.
C. Arterial disease.
D. CVI.
E. Lipedema.
F. Neoplasm.
G. Radiation effects.
H. Systemic diseases, such as right ventricular failure, myxedema, nephrosis, nephritis, and protein deficiency. These causes must be excluded before invasive study.

IV. TREATMENT

A. **Medical management** is limited by the physiologic and anatomic nature of the disease. The use of diuretics to remove fluid is not effective because of the high interstitial protein concentration. Development of fibrosis and irreversible changes in the subcutaneous tissue further limit options. The objectives of conservative treatment are to control edema, maintain healthy skin, and avoid cellulitis and lymphangitis.

1. **Combination of physical therapies (CPT)** is the primary approach recommended in a consensus document by the International Society of Lymphology Executive Committee (*Lymphology.* 2009;42:51). CPT consists of a two-stage treatment program, beginning with skin care, followed by the application of compression bandages. Phase 1 involves gentle manual manipulation of tissues to direct lymph flow (manual lymph drainage), range of motion exercises, and multilayered compression bandage wrapping. Phase 2 conserves and optimizes results obtained in Phase 1; patients wear custom-made compression garments. In a study of 119 patients with 3-year follow-up, CPT reduced lymphedema by 63% (*Oncology.* 1997;11:99).

2. **Sequential pneumatic compression** has been shown to improve lymphedema. Several designs have been used with various degrees of

success. Elastic stockings or sleeves should be fitted and worn afterward to maintain results. Extremity elevation may also help.

3. **Skin care and good hygiene** are important. Topical hydrocortisone cream may be needed for eczema.

4. **Benzopyrones** (such as warfarin) have been effective in reducing lymphedema due to filariasis. Their action is believed to derive from enhanced macrophage activity and extralymphatic absorption of interstitial proteins.

5. **Cellulitis and lymphangitis** should be suspected when sudden onset of pain, swelling, or erythema of the leg occurs. Intravenous antibiotics should be initiated to cover staphylococci and β-hemolytic streptococci. Broad-spectrum penicillins, cephalosporins, or vancomycin usually are adequate. Limb elevation and immobilization should be initiated, and warm compresses can be used for symptomatic relief. Topical antifungal cream may be needed for chronic infections.

B. **Surgical options.** Surgical intervention is an alternative approach for patients whose lymphedema has been refractory to nonoperative therapies. Only 10% of patients with lymphedema are surgical candidates, and surgery is directed at reducing limb size. Indications for operation are related to function because cosmetic deformities persist postoperatively. Results are best when surgery is performed for severely impaired movement and recurrent cellulitis. Surgical therapies for lymphatic disease are not without consequence, and have largely been abandoned (*Cancer.* 2001;92:980).

1. **Total subcutaneous excision** is performed for extensive swelling and skin changes. Circumferential excision of the skin and subcutaneous tissue from the tibial tuberosity to the malleoli is performed. The defect is closed with a split- or full-thickness skin graft from the resected specimen or a split-thickness skin graft from an uninvolved site. Recurrent lymphedema and hyperpigmentation occur more frequently when split-thickness skin grafts are used.

2. Closure of disrupted lymphatic channels.

3. Omental transposition.

4. Lymphatic transposition includes direct (lymphovenous bypass, lymphatic grafting) and indirect (mesenteric bridge, omental flap) procedures. Lymphatic grafting is performed for upper-extremity or unilateral lower-extremity lymphedema. Good results have been reported in 80% of patients (*Plast Reconstr Surg.* 1990;85:64). A mesenteric bridge is formed by suturing a segment of mucosa-stripped ileum with intact blood supply to transected distal iliac or inguinal nodes. An omental flap placed in a swollen limb is believed to improve lymphatic drainage through spontaneous lympholymphatic anastomoses. Because of their complexity and associated complications, indirect procedures are not widely used.

5. Microsurgical lymphovenous anastomoses bypass the obstructed lymphatic system in patients with chronic lymphedema. With improved microvascular techniques, patency rates of 50% to 70% can be expected many months after surgery (*J Vasc Surg.* 1986;4:148).

21 Endocrine Surgery

Brian T. Bucher and Jeffrey F. Moley

THYROID

I. EMBRYOLOGY, ANATOMY, AND PHYSIOLOGY

A. **Embryology.** The thyroid gland develops from the endoderm of the primitive foregut and arises in the ventral pharynx in the region of the base of the tongue (later indicated by the foramen cecum). With further development, the thyroid descends into the neck anterior to the hyoid bone and laryngeal cartilages. Certain congenital anomalies such as ectopic thyroid tissue or thyroglossal duct cysts are directly related to this embryologic descent. The parafollicular cells, or C cells, are derived from the neural crest, migrate to the thyroid, and produce calcitonin.

B. **Anatomy.** The adult thyroid is a bilobar structure connected by an isthmus that lies anterior to the junction of the larynx and trachea. The blood supply to the thyroid arises from two pairs of main arteries: the superior thyroid artery (branch of the external carotid) and the inferior thyroid artery (branch of the thyrocervical trunk). The recurrent laryngeal nerve (RLN) usually courses 1 cm anterior or posterior to the inferior thyroid artery. Careful dissection around this artery is necessary to avoid injury to the RLN.

C. **Physiology.** The thyroid is stimulated to release thyroid hormone in response to thyroid-stimulating hormone (TSH) secreted from the anterior pituitary gland. TSH secretion is stimulated by thyrotropin-releasing hormone (TRH) from the hypothalamus. Thyroid hormone synthesis begins when dietary iodide is ingested, actively transported into the thyroid gland, and then oxidized by thyroid peroxidase into iodine. Iodination of tyrosine results in monoiodotyrosine (MIT) and diiodotyrosine (DIT). Iodine coupling of MIT and DIT results in the formation of triiodothyronine (T_3) and thyroxine (T_4), which are bound to thyroglobulin while in the thyroid. On release into plasma, 80% of T_3 and T_4 are bound to thyroxine-binding globulin (TBG). Only the unbound or "free" hormones are active (i.e., available to tissues) with T_3 being much more potent than T_4.

II. BIOCHEMICAL. **Evaluation of thyroid disorders** confirms clinically suspected abnormalities in thyroid function; however, test results must be interpreted in the context of clinical findings.

A. Measurement of TSH (0.3 to 5 mIU/L) is the most useful biochemical test in the diagnosis of thyroid illness. In most patients without pituitary disease, increased TSH signifies hypothyroidism, suppressed TSH suggests hyperthyroidism, and normal TSH reflects a euthyroid state.

B. Assessment of free T_4 (4.5 to 11.2 µg/dL) concentration supports identified abnormalities in TSH and provides an index of severity of thyroid dysfunction. Total T_4 (3 to 12 μg/dL) is affected by changes in hormone product or binding and does not directly reflect the small "free" or active T_4 fractions.

C. An indirect measurement of free T_4 can be obtained using the resin T_3 uptake (RT_3U). This assay measures unoccupied thyroid hormone-binding sites on TBG by allowing radiolabeled T_3 to compete for binding between TBG. The RT_3U is directly related to the FT_4 fraction and inversely related to the TBG-binding sites. The FT_4 index [FT_4I = total $T_4 \times RT_3U$] (0.85 to 3.5) correlates more closely with the level of FT_4, eliminates ambiguity introduced by altered thyroglobulin levels, and is the preferred test for estimating FT_4.

D. Measurement of T_3 (80 to 200 ng/dL) is unreliable as a test for hypothyroidism. This test is useful in the occasional patient with suspected hyperthyroidism, suppressed TSH, and normal FT_4I (T_3 thyrotoxicosis).

E. Antithyroid microsomal antibodies are found in the serum of patients with autoimmune thyroiditis (Hashimoto thyroiditis). Anti-TSH receptor antibodies, which stimulate the TSH receptor, are detectable in more than 90% of patients with autoimmune hyperthyroidism (Graves' disease).

F. The American Thyroid Association has published evidence-based guidelines on the detection of thyroid dysfunction (*Arch Intern Med.* 2000;160(11):1573–1575). These guidelines recommend serum TSH as an initial screen test for thyroid dysfunction.

III. BENIGN THYROID DISORDERS

A. Hyperthyroidism reflects increased catabolism and excessive sympathetic activity caused by excess circulating thyroid hormones. Symptoms of hyperthyroidism include weight loss despite normal or increased appetite, heat intolerance, excessive perspiration, anxiety, irritability, palpitations, fatigue, muscle weakness, and oligomenorrhea. Signs of hyperthyroidism include goiter, sinus tachycardia or atrial fibrillation, tremor, hyperreflexia, fine or thinning hair, thyroid bruit, muscle wasting, and weakness, particularly of the proximal thigh musculature.

1. Autoimmune diffuse toxic goiter (Graves' disease) is the most common cause of hyperthyroidism and is caused by stimulating immunoglobulins directed against the TSH receptor. Diagnosis is made by history and physical exam, depressed TSH levels and detection of anti-TSH-R antibodies. Graves' disease may be treated with antithyroid drugs, ablation with radioactive iodine (RAI), or surgery.

   a. Ablation with RAI is the treatment of choice for most patients with Graves' disease. An initial dose given orally is 75% effective after 8 to 12 weeks. The initial dose is repeated in the 25% of patients with persistent thyrotoxicosis. Cure rates approach 90%, and hypothyroidism will eventually develop. Contraindications to radiotherapy include pregnant women, newborns, patients who refuse, and patients with low RAI uptake (<20%) in the thyroid. Treatment of children or young adults (<30 years) with RAI is controversial because of presumed long-term oncogenic risks.

  b. Thyroidectomy for Graves' disease may be indicated for people whom RAI is contraindicated, have an obstructive goiter, or refuse RAI. Total thyroidectomy is the procedure of choice in patients with Graves' due to the unacceptable high recurrence rate in patients treated with subtotal thyroidectomy (10% to 30%). Patients with recurrent hyperthyroidism after thyroidectomy should be considered for treatment with RAI because reoperation carries a higher complication rate.

  c. Thioamide drugs, such as propylthiouracil (PTU) or methimazole, are used for antithyroid drug therapy. However, long-term remission is achieved in less than 20% to 30% of patients. Antithyroid drugs are also used to prepare thyrotoxic patients for surgery or ablative therapy.

 2. Toxic adenoma (Plummer's disease) is an autonomously functioning thyroid nodule that produces thyroid hormone independent of TSH stimulation. A radioactive ^{131}I scan is diagnostic with one or two "hot" areas with the rest of the gland suppressed. These lesions are treated with either RAI or by surgical excision (thyroid lobectomy).

 3. Rare causes of hyperthyroidism include self-administration of excessive thyroid hormone (factitious hyperthyroidism), iodine-induced hyperthyroidism, pituitary TSH-secreting adenoma, trophoblastic tumors secreting chorionic gonadotropin, struma ovarii, and thyroiditis.

B. Hypothyroidism is caused by decreased production of thyroid hormone due to a lack of sufficient dietary iodine intake, surgical removal, or radioactive ablation of the thyroid. Clinical features of hypothyroidism include cold intolerance, weight gain, constipation, edema (especially of the eyelids, hands, and feet), dry skin, dry and thinning hair, weakness, somnolence, and menorrhagia. Diagnosis is made by an increased serum TSH level and decreased free T_4 levels. Treatment consists of oral thyroid hormone replacement.

C. Thyroiditis is a group of autoimmune and inflammatory disorders characterized by infiltration of the thyroid with inflammatory cells and subsequent fibrosis of the gland.

 1. Hashimoto thyroiditis is a chronic autoimmune disorder characterized by destructive lymphocytic infiltration of the thyroid. The disease is 15 times more common in women, and more than 90% of patients have circulating antibodies directed against thyroid microsomes and thyroglobulin. Although patients initially are euthyroid, hyperthyroidism and hypothyroidism may occur later. Thyroid hormone is given to hypothyroid patients both as replacement therapy and to suppress TSH. Thyroidectomy is indicated for compressive symptoms, a dominant nodule suspicious for malignancy, or cosmetic preference.

 2. Acute suppurative thyroiditis is rare and caused by pyogenic infection with *Streptococcus* or *Staphylococcus* species. Treatment consists of appropriate antibiotic therapy and surgical drainage of abscesses. Long-term effects on thyroid function are uncommon.

 3. Subacute (de Quervain) thyroiditis is a rare condition that occurs in young women, often after a viral upper respiratory tract infection.

Symptoms include fatigue, weakness, and painful thyroid enlargement radiating to the patient's jaw or ear. Fine needle aspiration (FNA) can be diagnostic with the identification of giant cells. Treatment with nonsteroidal anti-inflammatory drugs or steroids can alleviate symptoms. The condition almost always remits spontaneously within a few weeks.

   4. Riedel's thyroiditis (struma) is a rare, progressive inflammatory condition of the entire thyroid gland, strap muscles, and other neck structures. Its cause is unknown, and it can be associated with other fibrotic processes, including retroperitoneal fibrosis, sclerosing cholangitis, and fibrosing mediastinitis. Riedel's thyroiditis may require surgical excision to exclude malignancy or relieve compressive symptoms on the trachea or esophagus.

   D. Nontoxic goiter. In multinodular goiter, a large goiter or retrosternal extension can compress the trachea. The cause is typically iodine deficiency. Subtotal or total thyroidectomy is the treatment of choice if there are symptoms of compression, suspicion of malignancy, or questionable nodules or if the gland is cosmetically bothersome.

IV. A SOLITARY THYROID NODULE is defined as a discrete lesion that is distinct from the surrounding thyroid parenchyma. These lesions commonly occur in 4% to 7% of adults, and are usually benign. However, the malignant potential of the newly discovered thyroid nodule is of justifiable concern to both physician and patient. The goal of diagnostic testing is to separate the relatively few patients with thyroid malignancy from the larger group of patients with benign thyroid nodules. The frequency of cancer in surgically excised nodules is 8% to 17% (*N Engl J Med.* 1993;328:553). The American Thyroid Association Guidelines Taskforce has issued a management guideline for the diagnosis and work-up of thyroid nodules (*Thyroid.* 2009;19(11):1167–1214).

   A. History and physical examination are invaluable in the management of the thyroid nodule. Nodules in the very young and very old (especially men) are more likely to be malignant. Exposure to ionizing radiation is a well-recognized risk factor for the development of thyroid carcinoma. A family history of thyroid malignancy, familial polyposis, or other endocrine disease also increases the risk of cancer. Rapid nodule growth, pain, compressive symptoms, or hoarseness of voice increase the likelihood of malignancy but are nonspecific. Physical findings of a solitary nodule with firm or irregular texture or with fixation to surrounding structures suggest malignancy. Generally, only nodules greater than 1 cm should undergo further work-up. Similarly, the presence of enlarged cervical lymph nodes is extremely important because this finding is associated with thyroid cancer.

   B. The next step is determination of the patient's thyroid state by determination of the serum TSH level. Malignancy is uncommon in hyperfunctioning nodules. In patients with a suppressed TSH, a ^{131}I radionucleotide scan may identify hyperfunctioning nodules versus Graves' disease. Patients with "cold" nodules should undergo a diagnostic ultrasound and subsequent FNA of suspicious nodules.

C. FNA is the most accurate and cost-effective diagnostic modality for evaluating thyroid nodules. FNA can be performed at the bedside or under ultrasound guidance. The latter modality is preferred for small or difficult to palpate nodules. The cytologic results of FNA are divided into four categories:

1. Nondiagnostic cytology fails to meet the criteria for an adequate specimen. These patients should undergo repeat FNA under ultrasound guidance. Nodules that continue to yield nondiagnostic FNA specimens require either close observation or surgical excision.

2. Benign cytology requires no further diagnostic testing and can be clinically followed with serial ultrasounds for 6 to 18 months with gradually longer periods between ultrasounds if the lesion remains stable.

3. Cytology noting "follicular lesion of undetermined significance" or "atypia of undetermined significance" carries a 5% to 10% risk of malignancy. These patients should undergo repeat FNA (*CytoJournal.* 2008;5:6).

4. Intermediate or suspicious cytology is typically reported as "follicular" or "Hürthle cell" neoplasms. These lesions carry a 20% to 30% risk of malignancy (*Diagn Cytopathol.* 2008;36(6):425–437). Given the risk of malignancy, these lesions are typically treated with surgical excision (thyroid lobectomy). If the final pathology reveals thyroid cancer, no further treatment is necessary for small (<1 cm) low-risk tumors. For patients with large (>1 cm) or high-risk tumors, a completion thyroidectomy should be performed along with a lymph node dissection if clinically indicated (*Thyroid.* 2009;19(11):1167–1214).

5. Suspicious for malignancy and malignant are treated as thyroid cancer.

D. **Thyroid imaging**

1. Thyroid ultrasonography accurately determines gland volume, as well as the number and character of thyroid nodules (*Am J Med.* 1995;99:642). Features suggestive of malignancy on ultrasound include hypoechoic pattern, incomplete peripheral halo, irregular margins, and microcalcifications. Ultrasound is useful for guiding FNA biopsy and cyst aspiration. Cysts seen on ultrasound, especially those larger than 3 cm, are malignant in up to 14% of cases.

2. Technetium thyroid scanning can be useful in differentiating solitary functioning nodules from multinodular goiter or Graves' disease. Hypofunctioning areas (cyst, neoplasm, or suppressed tissue adjacent to autonomous nodules) are "cold," whereas areas of increased synthesis are "hot." Thyroid scans cannot differentiate benign from malignant lesions and therefore are not generally useful in the routine work-up of a thyroid nodule. Radioactive iodine scanning 4 to 24 hours after administration of oral iodine-131 (^{131}I) is useful for identifying metastatic differentiated thyroid tumors, confirming a diagnosis of Graves' disease, and predicting a response to ^{131}I radioablation.

3. CT scan and MR scan of the thyroid are costly and generally reserved for assessing substernal or retrosternal masses suspected to be goiters or for staging known malignancy.

E. In summary, thyroid lobectomy is indicated for (1) nodules with malignant or indeterminate aspiration cytology, (2) nodules in children, (3) nodules in patients with either a history of neck irradiation or a family history of thyroid cancer, and (4) symptomatic or cosmetically bothersome nodules.

V. THYROID NEOPLASMS

A. Differentiated (papillary and follicular) thyroid cancer is an indolent cancer (*N Engl J Med.* 1998;338:297). These tumors arise from thyroid follicular epithelial cells and are by far the most common thyroid cancer. Childhood exposure to radiation is the best documented etiologic factor. These cancers are rare in children and increase in frequency with age; the female-to-male ratio is approximately 2.5:1. The prognosis of thyroid cancer depends mostly on the patient's age as well as the extent and histologic subtype of the disease. In all, 85% to 90% of patients fall into a low-risk category with favorable prognosis. The American Thyroid Association Guidelines Taskforce has issued a management guideline for the work-up and treatment of differentiated thyroid cancers (*Thyroid.* 2009;19(11):1167–1214).

1. Papillary thyroid carcinoma (PTC) represents 85% of thyroid carcinomas. PTC is often multifocal and frequently metastasizes to cervical lymph nodes. Occult, clinically insignificant foci of microscopic PTC are found in 4% to 28% of autopsies or in thyroidectomy specimens for benign diseases. Despite its nonaggressive nature, PTC has metastasized to cervical lymph nodes in 20% to 50% of patient at the time of diagnosis. Therefore, preoperative neck ultrasound with subsequent FNA of suspicious nodes is recommended prior to surgical excision.

   a. Total thyroidectomy is recommended for the following conditions: tumors greater than 1 cm, presence of bilateral nodules, regional or metastatic disease, patients with a history of radiation therapy or first-degree relatives with PTC.

   b. Thyroid lobectomy is appropriate for patients with small (less than 1 cm), low risk, unifocal tumors without evidence of regional or metastatic disease.

   c. Lymph node dissection of the central neck compartment (level VI) and the lateral neck compartment (levels II, III, IV) should be performed in all patients with biopsy-proven lymph node metastases. Given 20% to 50% of patients with PTC have cervical lymph node metastases at the time of surgery, and neck ultrasound of the central compartment may miss occult metastasis, prophylactic central neck dissection (level VI) is recommended in high-risk patients (large tumors, bilateral tumors, radiation exposure).

   d. Radioablation of metastatic or residual cancer and residual thyroid tissue is performed with 75 to 100 mCi of ^{131}I at 4 weeks after total thyroidectomy while the patient is hypothyroid (i.e., TSH 30 μIU/mL on no replacement of T_4). Ablation may be repeated at higher doses if residual disease is detected on follow-up surveillance.

  e. Lifelong long-term suppression of TSH therapy with thyroid hormone replacement decreases recurrences and may improve survival.

 2. Follicular thyroid carcinoma (10% of thyroid carcinomas) is rare before age 30 years and has a slightly worse prognosis than PTC. Unlike PTC, follicular thyroid cancer has a propensity to spread hematogenously to bone, lung, or liver. Small (<1 cm), unilateral follicular carcinomas with limited invasion of the tumor capsule may be treated with thyroid lobectomy, whereas larger tumors (>1 cm), multicentric tumors, and tumors with more extensive capsular and vascular invasion or distant metastases are treated with total thyroidectomy. Radioablation is indicated after total thyroidectomy, followed by lifelong thyroid hormone suppression.

B. Medullary thyroid carcinoma (MTC) arises from the thyroid parafollicular C cells that derive from the neural crest and secrete calcitonin. MTC accounts for 5% to 10% of all thyroid cancers in the United States. MTC may occur sporadically (75% to 80%) or may be inherited, either alone or as a component of multiple endocrine neoplasia (MEN) type 2A or 2B (20% to 25%). Sporadic MTC usually is detected as a firm, palpable, unilateral nodule with or without involved cervical lymph nodes. Patients with hereditary MTC develop bilateral, multifocal tumors and often are diagnosed on the basis of family screening. MTC spreads early to cervical lymph nodes and may metastasize to liver, lungs, or bone. All patients with suspected or known MTC should be genetically tested for DNA mutations in the tyrosine kinase receptor *RET* proto-oncogene to exclude MEN 2A or MEN 2B syndromes. Similar to all thyroid malignancies, diagnosis is best made with an FNA of suspicious thyroid nodules. In addition, elevated basal serum calcitonin levels are elevated (>20 to 100 pg/mL). Neck ultrasound can identify regional metastases usually present prior to surgical resection. In addition, screening for a pheochromocytoma with serum or urine metanephrines/normetanephrines should be performed in all patients undergoing surgical resection of MTC. Total thyroidectomy alone is only indicated for patients with MEN 2 syndromes detected by genetic screening, who also have calcitonin levels less than 40 pg/mL. Otherwise, treatment of MTC is total thyroidectomy with removal of the lymph nodes in the central neck compartment (Level VI). A modified neck dissection is indicated for clinically involved ipsilateral cervical lymph nodes. There are no proven systemic chemotherapy options for MTC; however, clinical trials using multiple new agents are being carried out. The use of external beam radiation is controversial. The American Thyroid Association Guidelines Taskforce has issued a management guideline for the management of medullary thyroid cancer (*Thyroid* 2009;19(6):565–612).

C. Undifferentiated or anaplastic thyroid carcinoma (1% to 2% of thyroid carcinomas) carries an extremely poor prognosis, usually presents as a fixed, sometimes painful goiter, and usually occurs in patients older than 50 years. Invasion of local structures, with resultant dysphagia, respiratory compromise, or hoarseness due to RLN involvement can preclude curative resection. External irradiation or chemotherapy may provide limited palliation.

D. Primary malignant lymphoma of the thyroid often is associated with Hashimoto thyroiditis. Surgical resection is usually not indicated once a diagnosis is made.

VI. POSTOPERATIVE THYROID HORMONE REPLACEMENT is necessary after total or near total thyroidectomy or ablation with radioiodine. Oral levothyroxine is started before discharge at an average dose of 100 μg/day (0.8 μg/lb/day). Adequacy of thyroid hormone replacement is assessed by measuring T_4 and TSH at 6 to 12 weeks after surgery. Adjustments to the dose should not be more frequent than monthly in the absence of symptoms and should be cautious (12.5 to 25 μg increments).

VII. MANAGEMENT OF COMPLICATIONS AFTER THYROIDECTOMY

A. Hemorrhage is a rare but serious complication of thyroidectomy that usually occurs within 6 hours of surgery. Management can require control of the airway by endotracheal intubation and, rarely, can require urgent opening of the incision and evacuation of hematoma with creation of a surgical airway before return to the operating room for wound irrigation and control of bleeding.

B. Transient hypocalcemia commonly occurs 24 to 48 hours after thyroidectomy. Patients are started on oral calcium carbonate (1 gram TID) for 2 weeks after total thyroidectomy. Intravenous replacement is achieved by mixing six ampules of 10% calcium gluconate (540 mg of elemental calcium) in 500 mL of 5% dextrose in water (D5W), for infusion at 1 mL/kg/hour. Permanent hypoparathyroidism is uncommon after total thyroidectomy. Normal parathyroid tissue removed or devascularized at the time of total thyroidectomy must be minced into 1 × 3-mm fragments and autotransplanted into individual muscle pockets in the sternocleidomastoid muscle to maximize the chances that the patient will not develop postoperative hypoparathyroidism (*Ann Surg.* 1996;223:472). Normal parathyroid tissue should never be discarded.

C. RLN injury is a devastating complication of thyroidectomy that should occur rarely (<1%). Unilateral RLN injury causes hoarseness, and bilateral injury compromises the airway, necessitating tracheostomy. Repeat neck exploration, thyroidectomy for extensive goiter or Graves' disease, and thyroidectomy for fixed, locally invasive cancers are procedures particularly prone to RLN injury. Intentional (as with locally invasive cancer) or inadvertent transection of the RLN can be repaired primarily or with a nerve graft, although the efficacy of these repairs is not known. Temporary RLN palsies can occur during thyroidectomy, and these usually resolve over a period of 1 to 6 weeks.

PARATHYROID

I. EMBRYOLOGY, ANATOMY, AND PHYSIOLOGY

A. **Embryology.** The inferior and superior parathyroid glands are derived from the endoderm of the third and fourth pharyngeal pouches, respectively. The inferior parathyroid glands are intimately associated with the thymus as it descends into the chest, which also develops from the third pharyngeal pouch. Therefore, ectopic parathyroid glands can be found anywhere along this tract as the thymus descends. The superior glands have a limited descent from the neck and are thus rarely found in ectopic locations.

B. Anatomy. Typically, the inferior glands are found inferior, lateral or posterior to the inferior pole of the thyroid, and anterior to the RLN. The superior glands are usually found at the posterior aspect of the thyroid lobe superior to the inferior thyroid artery, posterior to the RLN. Because the embryologic descent of the inferior parathyroid crosses that of the superior gland, they can rarely be found at the same level, above or below the crossing of the inferior thyroid artery and RLN.

C. Physiology. Serum calcium levels are maintained between 8.2 and 10.2 mg/dL by the interplay of parathyroid hormone (PTH), vitamin D, and calcitonin. Upon stimulation, chief cells of the parathyroid glands secrete PTH that (1) acts on the bones to stimulate the resorption of calcium and phosphate, (2) stimulates the kidneys to increase calcium resorption and inhibit phosphate resorption. Together these actions aim to increase the serum calcium concentrations and decrease the serum phosphate concentration. Vitamin D is absorbed through the small intestine and undergoes hydroxylation in the liver to $25(OH)D_3$. A second hydroxylation is performed in the kidney, under the control of PTH, to the active form of vitamin D, $1,25(OH)D_3$. Vitamin D stimulates bone and intestine calcium resorption to increase serum calcium levels. Calcitonin is synthesized by the parafollicular cells of the thyroid gland. Its actions antagonize those of PTH by inhibiting bone and kidney resorption of calcium. The net result is a decrease in serum calcium concentration.

II. BENIGN PARATHYROID DISORDERS

A. Primary Hyperparathyroidism (HPT)

1. Incidence. Primary HPT has an incidence of 0.25 to 1 per 1,000 population in the United States and is especially common in postmenopausal women. It most often occurs sporadically, but it can be inherited alone or as a component of familial endocrinopathies, including MEN types 1 and 2A.

2. Clinical findings. The more common clinical findings associated with HPT include nephrolithiasis, osteoporosis, hypertension, and emotional disturbances. In addition, patients can have very subtle symptoms such as muscle weakness, polyuria, anorexia, and nausea.

3. Laboratory assessment. The diagnosis of HPT is biochemical and requires demonstration of hypercalcemia (serum calcium 10.5 mg/dL) and an elevated PTH level. Patients with hypercalcemia and suspected HPT should have their serum calcium, phosphate, creatinine, and PTH measured. The assay of choice for PTH is the highly sensitive and specific intact PTH-level radioimmunoassay. Ionized calcium is a more sensitive test of physiologically active calcium. Hypercalcemia without an elevated PTH can be due to a variety of causes (especially malignancy, Paget disease, sarcoidosis, and milk-alkali syndrome) that must be excluded. Familial hypocalciuric hypercalcemia (FHH) commonly causes a mild hypercalcemia and elevated PTH, as seen in HPT. FHH is caused by loss-of-function mutations in the calcium-sensing

receptors expressed in the kidney and parathyroid gland. This leads to a loss of feedback inhibition of PTH secretion by the parathyroids and inadequate clearance of calcium in to the urine. FHH can generally be distinguished from HPT by a 24-hour measurement of urinary calcium. It can also be distinguished by measuring the renal calcium/creatinine clearance ratio. A ratio less than 0.01 suggests FHH; the ratios seen in HPT are generally much higher. Parathyroidectomy is ineffective for FHH.

4. Radiography. Parathyroid imaging has no role in the diagnosis of HPT, but does have a role in operative planning in patients diagnosed with HPT. Current practice makes use of several techniques to facilitate limited neck exploration to ensure a high success rate in the outpatient setting. These techniques include radio- and/or image-guided exploration (sestamibi or ultrasound guided), videoscopic exploration, and intraoperative intact PTH-level monitoring. The most frequently applied approach is preoperative sestamibi scanning, followed by direct excision of the identified gland and confirmation of cure by intraoperative PTH measurement. This intraoperative test requires the availability of a rapid assay of intact PTH, which confirms the success of the surgery immediately if the PTH level falls more than 50% at 10 minutes after the apparent source of PTH has been removed. If the preoperative localization scan is not informative, then a standard four-gland exploration is appropriate.

5. Parathyroidectomy
   a. Indications. Parathyroidectomy is indicated for all patients with symptomatic primary HPT. Nephrolithiasis, bone disease, and neuromuscular symptoms are improved more often than renal insufficiency, hypertension, and psychiatric symptoms. Parathyroidectomy for asymptomatic HPT is somewhat controversial. Recent guidelines by the AACE/AAES Taskforce on primary HPT recommend parathyroidectomy for the following patients: (1) those younger than 50 years of age; (2) those who cannot participate in appropriate follow-up; (3) those with a serum calcium level greater than 1 mg/dL above the normal range; (4) those with urinary calcium greater than 400 mg per 24 hours; (5) those with a 30% decrease in renal function; and (6) those with complications of primary HPT, including nephrocalcinosis, osteoporosis [T score <2.5 standard deviations (SD) at the lumbar spine, hip, or wrist], or a severe psychoneurologic disorder (*J Bone Miner Res.* 2002;17(suppl 2):N57).
   b. Neck exploration and parathyroidectomy for HPT result in normocalcemia in more than 95% of patients when performed by an experienced surgeon without any preoperative or intraoperative localization studies. A thorough, orderly search and identification of all four parathyroid glands are the cornerstones of the standard surgical management of HPT. In the current era, preoperative localization studies are used in conjunction with rapid intraoperative PTH measurement to enable "minimally invasive parathyroidectomy," which generally means directed unilateral neck exploration and/or local/monitored anesthesia care (MAC) anesthesia. Most often, a

single adenomatous gland is found and resected; normal parathyroid glands should be left in place. Intraoperative measurement of PTH at 10 minutes demonstrating a 50% decrease and return to the normal level after resection of the adenoma is highly indicative of cure. In the event that an abnormally enlarged parathyroid or all four parathyroids cannot be found, a thorough exploration for ectopic or supernumerary glands should be performed. Ectopic superior glands may be found posterior and deep to the thyroid, in the tracheoesophageal groove, posterior to the inferior thyroid vessels, between the carotid artery and the esophagus. Undescended or incompletely descended glands may be found cranial to the superior thyroid pole, and excessive caudal migration may result in a gland residing in the middle mediastinum. Ectopic inferior glands are most likely found embedded in the thymus in the anterior mediastinum. Undescended inferior glands may be found in the superior neck between the carotid and the larynx. Occasionally, multiple parathyroid adenomas are found and should be removed, leaving at least one normal parathyroid behind. Four-gland parathyroid hyperplasia is rare, and its management is controversial. Acceptable options include total parathyroidectomy with parathyroid autotransplantation or 3.5-gland parathyroidectomy. The dictation of a clear, factual operative note detailing the identification and position of each parathyroid gland is essential as is pathologic verification of each parathyroid. This information is invaluable in the unlikely event of reoperation for persistent or recurrent HPT.

B. Recurrent or Persistent Primary HPT

  1. Diagnosis. In all cases of postparathyroidectomy hypercalcemia, HPT must be reconfirmed biochemically, and 24-hour urinary calcium should be obtained to exclude FHH.

  a. Imaging. Preoperative localization is mandatory and includes careful review of the operative note from the initial surgery and concordant noninvasive studies. Approximately 70% to 80% of patients undergoing re-exploration after an initial failed operation have a missed gland that is accessible through a cervical incision. Reoperative parathyroid surgery carries a substantially higher risk of injury to the RLN and of hypocalcemia due to postoperative scarring and disruption of normal tissue planes. Preoperative localization should include ^{99m}Tc-sestamibi scintigraphy and ultrasound or CT scanning. These noninvasive studies are successful in localizing the missed gland in 25% to 75% of cases (*Radiology.* 1987;162:133). With combined use of CT scan, ultrasonography, and scintigraphy, at least one imaging study identifies the tumor in more than 75% of patients. For patients with discordant or negative noninvasive studies, invasive localization via venous sampling with rapid PTH can be used to identify adenomas.

  b. Operative strategy. The goal of re-exploration is to perform an orderly search based on the information gained from the initial operation and from localization studies.

(1) Missed parathyroid glands are found either in the usual position or in ectopic sites, as determined by the embryology of parathyroid development. Rarely, a parathyroid gland is intrathyroidal (especially in patients with multinodular goiter), and intraoperative thyroid ultrasound or thyroid lobectomy can be performed if an exhaustive search fails to identify the parathyroid adenoma. If four normal glands have been located, the adenoma is likely to represent a supernumerary (fifth) gland. Intraoperative ultrasound is an effective tool for localizing parathyroid glands in the neck.

(2) Mediastinal adenomas within the thymus are managed by resecting the cranial portion of the thymus by gentle traction on the thyrothymic ligament or by a complete transcervical thymectomy using a specialized substernal retractor (*Ann Surg.* 1991;214:555). Median sternotomy carries a higher morbidity and increased postoperative pain, and the possibility of these should be discussed with the patient preoperatively.

C. **Parathyroid Autotransplantation**

1. Indications for total parathyroidectomy and heterotopic parathyroid autotransplantation include HPT in patients with renal failure, in patients with four-gland parathyroid hyperplasia, and in patients undergoing neck re-exploration in which the adenoma is the only remaining parathyroid tissue. The site of parathyroid autotransplantation may be the sternocleidomastoid muscle or the brachioradialis muscle of the patient's nondominant forearm. Parathyroid grafting into the patient's forearm is advantageous if recurrent HPT is possible (e.g., MEN type 1 or 2A). If HPT recurs, localization is simplified, and the hyperplastic parathyroid tissue may be excised from the patient's forearm under local anesthesia.

2. Technique. Freshly removed parathyroid gland tissue is cut into fine pieces approximately 1 mm × 1 mm × 2 mm and placed in sterile iced saline. An incision is made in the patient's nondominant forearm, and separate intramuscular beds are created by spreading the fibers of the brachioradialis with a fine forceps. Approximately four to five pieces are placed in each site, and a total of approximately 100 mg of parathyroid tissue are transplanted. The beds are closed with a silk suture to mark the site of the transplanted tissue. Transplanted parathyroid tissue begins to function within 14 to 21 days of surgery.

3. Cryopreservation of parathyroid glands is performed in MEN patients and all patients who may become aparathyroid after repeat exploration. Cryopreservation may be performed by freezing approximately 200 mg of finely cut parathyroid tissue in vials containing 10% dimethyl sulfoxide, 10% autologous serum, and 80% Waymouth medium. Cryopreserved parathyroid tissue can be used for autotransplantation in patients who become aparathyroid or in patients with failure of the initial grafted parathyroid tissue. Viable cryopreservation and subsequent thawing must be performed in a Food and Drug Administration (FDA)-approved GMP (good medical practice) facility.

D. Postoperative Hypocalcemia

1. Transient hypocalcemia commonly occurs after total thyroidectomy or parathyroidectomy and requires treatment if it is severe (total serum calcium <7.5 mg/dL) or if the patient is symptomatic. Chvostek's sign (twitching of the facial muscles when the examiner percusses over the facial nerve anterior to the patient's ear) is a sign of relative hypocalcemia but is present in up to 15% of the normal population. This sign is not necessarily an indication for calcium replacement.

2. Patients with persistent hypocalcemia after total thyroidectomy or after parathyroid autotransplantation can require continued supplementation for 6 to 8 weeks postoperatively. Usually, patients are given calcium carbonate, 500 to 1,000 mg orally three times per day, and 1,25-dihydroxyvitamin D_3, 0.25 μg orally per day.

3. Hypocalcemic tetany is a medical emergency that is treated with rapid intravenous administration of 10% calcium gluconate or calcium chloride until the patient recovers. Specifically, one to two ampules (10 to 20 mL) of 10% calcium gluconate are given intravenously over 10 minutes, and the dose may be repeated every 15 to 20 minutes, as required. Subsequently, a continuous infusion of six ampules of calcium gluconate in 500 mL of 5% dextrose water is initiated at 50 mL per hour. Patients with severe hypocalcemia must also have correction of hypomagnesemia.

   Hypercalcemia from secondary and tertiary HPT is treated initially with dietary phosphate restriction, phosphate binders, and vitamin D supplementation. Patients with medically unresponsive, symptomatic HPT (e.g., bone pain and osteopenia, ectopic calcification, or pruritus) may be surgically treated with total parathyroidectomy and heterotopic autotransplantation, or subtotal parathyroidectomy. Controversy exists as to what type of surgery is best and what postoperative level of parathyroid hormone is necessary to prevent adynamic bone disease after such procedures.

III. PARATHYROID CARCINOMA is rare and accounts for less than 1% of patients with HPT. Approximately 50% of these patients have a palpable neck mass, and serum calcium levels may exceed 15 mg/dL.

A. Diagnosis is made by the histologic finding of vascular or capsular invasion, lymph node or distant metastases, or gross invasion of local structures.

B. Surgical treatment is radical local excision of the tumor, surrounding soft tissue, lymph nodes, and ipsilateral thyroid lobe when the disease is recognized preoperatively or intraoperatively. Reoperation is indicated for local recurrence in an attempt to control malignant hypercalcemia.

C. Patients with parathyroid carcinoma and some patients with benign HPT may develop hyperparathyroid crisis. Symptoms of this acute, sometimes fatal illness include profound muscular weakness, nausea and vomiting, drowsiness, and confusion. Hypercalcemia (16 to 20 mg/dL) and azotemia are usually present. Ultimate treatment of "parathyroid crisis" is parathyroidectomy; however, hypercalcemia and volume and electrolyte abnormalities should be addressed first. Treatment is warranted for symptoms or a serum calcium level greater than 12 mg/dL. First-line therapy is infusion of 300 to 500 mL/hour of 0.9% sodium chloride (5 to 10 L/day intravenously) to restore intravascular volume and to promote renal excretion of calcium. After urinary output exceeds 100 mL/hour, furosemide (80 to 100 mg intravenously every 2 to 6 hours) may be given to promote further renal sodium and calcium excretion. Thiazide diuretics impair calcium excretion and should be avoided. Hypokalemia and hypomagnesemia are complications of forced saline diuresis and should be corrected. If diuresis alone is unsuccessful in lowering the serum calcium, other calcium-lowering agents may be used. These include the bisphosphonates pamidronate (60 to 90 mg in 1 L of 0.9% saline infused over 24 hours) and etidronate (7.5 mg/kg intravenously over 2 to 4 hours daily for 3 days); mithramycin [25 μg/kg intravenously over 4 to 6 hours daily for 3 to 4 days (malignant hypercalcemia only)]; and salmon calcitonin (initial dose, 4 IU/kg subcutaneously or intramuscularly every 12 hours, increasing as necessary to a maximum dose of 8 IU/kg subcutaneously or intramuscularly every 6 hours). Orthophosphate, gallium nitrate, and glucocorticoids also have calcium-lowering effects.

ENDOCRINE PANCREAS

I. EMBRYOLOGY, ANATOMY, AND PHYSIOLOGY

A. Embryology. The pancreas originates from two diverticula in the foregut to develop the final adult form around the fifth and sixth weeks of gestation. The endocrine cells that form the pancreatic islets also originate from the foregut endoderm.

B. Anatomy. In the adult, the pancreatic islets are scattered throughout the pancreas and are composed of four major cell types: A, B, D, PP cells. Beta cells occupy the center of the islets with the remainder of the cells scattered in the periphery.

C. Physiology. Each of the various pancreatic endocrine cells produces different hormones with a variety of local and systemic actions

    1. A cells produce glucagon that is a polypeptide whose main function is to promote the conversion of hepatic glycogen to glucose and increase the systemic glucose levels.

    2. B cells produce insulin whose main function is to promote glucose transport into cells and therefore decrease systemic glucose levels.

    3. D cells produce somatostatin that functions to inhibit the release of other gastrointestinal hormones, gastric acid secretion, and small bowel electrolyte secretions.

    4. D_2 cells produce vasoactive interstitial peptide that serves as an enteric vasodilator.

    5. G cells produce gastrin whose actions increase the secretion of gastric acid and pepsinogen.

II. PANCREATIC ISLET CELL TUMORS are rare tumors that produce clinical syndromes related to the specific hormone secreted. Insulinomas are the most

common of these tumors, followed by gastrinoma, then the rarer VIPoma, glucagonoma, and somatostatinoma. Islet cell tumors are often occult, and their localization may be difficult, especially for small, multifocal, or extrapancreatic tumors. Islet cell tumors may occur sporadically or as a component of MEN type 1 or von Hippel–Lindau disease (nearly always multifocal) and may be benign or malignant, although prediction may be based on the hormone produced rather than the tumor size.

A. **Insulinoma**

1. **Clinical features.** Patients with insulinoma develop profound hypoglycemia during fasting or after exercise. The clinical picture includes the signs and symptoms of neuroglycopenia (anxiety, tremor, confusion, and obtundation) and the sympathetic response to hypoglycemia (hunger, sweating, and tachycardia). These bizarre complaints initially may be attributed to malingering or a psychosomatic etiology unless the association with fasting is recognized. Many patients eat excessively to avoid symptoms, causing significant weight gain. *Whipple's triad* refers to the clinical criteria for the diagnosis of insulinoma: (1) hypoglycemic symptoms during monitored fasting, (2) blood glucose levels less than 50 mg/dL, and (3) relief of symptoms after administration of intravenous glucose. Factitious hypoglycemia (excess exogenous insulin administration) and postprandial reactive hypoglycemia must be excluded.

2. **Diagnosis.** A supervised, in-hospital 72-hour fast is required to diagnose insulinoma. Patients are observed for hypoglycemic episodes and have 6-hour measurement of plasma glucose, insulin, proinsulin, and C peptide. The fast is terminated when symptoms of neuroglycopenia develop. Nearly all patients with insulinoma develop neuroglycopenic symptoms and have inappropriately elevated plasma insulin (>5 µU/mL) associated with hypoglycemia (glucose <50 mg/dL). Elevated levels of C peptide and proinsulin are usually present as well (*Curr Probl Surg.* 1994;31:79).

3. **Localization.** Insulinomas typically are small (<2 cm), solitary, benign tumors that may occur anywhere in the pancreas. Rarely, an insulinoma may develop in extrapancreatic rests of pancreatic tissue. Dynamic CT scanning at 5-mm intervals with oral and intravenous contrast is the initial localizing test for insulinoma, with success in 35% to 85% of cases. Endoscopic ultrasound is also effective but is operator dependent (*N Engl J Med.* 1992;326:1721). The effectiveness of indium-111 (^{111}In)-octreotide scintigraphy for localizing insulinoma (approximately 50%) is less than for other islet cell tumors because insulinomas typically have few somatostatin receptors. Selective arteriography with observation of a tumor "blush" is the best diagnostic study for the primary tumor and hepatic metastases. If a tumor is still not identified, regional localization to the head, body, or tail of the pancreas can be accomplished by portal venous sampling for insulin or by calcium angiography. Calcium angiography involves injection of calcium into selectively catheterized pancreatic arteries and measurement of plasma insulin through a catheter positioned in a hepatic vein.

4. Treatment of insulinoma is surgical in nearly all cases. Surgical management of insulinomas consists in localization of the tumor by careful inspection and palpation of the gland after mobilization of the duodenum and the inferior border of the pancreas. Use of intraoperative ultrasonography greatly facilitates identification of small tumors, especially those located in the pancreatic head or uncinate process. Most insulinomas can be enucleated from surrounding pancreas, although those in the body or tail may require resection. In general, blind pancreatectomy should not be performed when the tumor cannot be identified. Approximately 5% of insulinomas are malignant and 10% are multiple (usually in association with MEN type 1). Medical treatment of insulinoma with diazoxide, verapamil, or octreotide has limited effectiveness but may be used in preparation for surgery or for patients unfit for surgery.

B. Gastrinoma

1. Patients with gastrinoma and the Zollinger–Ellison syndrome (ZES) have severe peptic ulcer disease (PUD) due to gastrin-mediated gastric acid hypersecretion. Most patients present with epigastric pain, and 80% have active duodenal ulceration at the time of diagnosis. Diarrhea and weight loss are common (40% of patients). ZES is uncommon (0.1% to 1% of PUD cases), and most patients present with typical duodenal ulceration. Gastrinoma and ZES should be considered in any patient with (1) PUD refractory to treatment of *Helicobacter pylori* and conventional doses of H_2 blockers or omeprazole; (2) recurrent, multiple, or atypically located (e.g., distal duodenum or jejunum) peptic ulcers; (3) complications of PUD (i.e., bleeding, perforation, or obstruction); (4) PUD with significant diarrhea; and (5) PUD with HPT, nephrolithiasis, or familial endocrinopathy. All patients considered for elective surgery for PUD should have ZES excluded preoperatively.

2. Diagnosis of ZES requires demonstration of fasting hypergastrinemia and basal gastric acid hypersecretion. A fasting serum gastrin level of 100 pg/mL or greater and a basal gastric acid output (BAO) of 15 mEq/hour or more (>5 mEq/hour in patients with previous ulcer surgery) secure the diagnosis of ZES in nearly all cases. Fasting hypergastrinemia without elevated BAO is seen in atrophic gastritis, in renal failure, and in patients taking H_2-receptor antagonists or omeprazole. Fasting hypergastrinemia with elevated BAO is seen in retained gastric antrum syndrome, gastric outlet obstruction, and antral G-cell hyperplasia. A secretin stimulation test is used to distinguish ZES from these conditions. This test is performed by measuring fasting serum gastrin levels before and 2, 5, 10, and 15 minutes after the intravenous administration of secretin (2 units/kg). Eighty-five percent of patients with ZES have an increase in gastrin levels (>200 pg/mL over baseline) in response to a secretin stimulation test, whereas patients with other conditions do not. This test is most useful when ZES is suspected in patients who have had prior gastric surgery and in patients with moderately increased fasting gastrin levels (100 to 1,000 pg/mL).

3. Localization of gastrinoma should be performed in all patients considered for surgery. Approximately 80% of gastrinomas are located within the "gastrinoma triangle," which is an area contained by a triangle formed by the junction of the cystic and common bile ducts, junction of the 2nd and 3rd portion of the duodenum, and the junction of head and neck of the pancreas. Gastrinomas are often malignant, with spread to lymph nodes or liver occurring in up to 60% of cases. Approximately 20% of patients with ZES have familial MEN type 1; these patients often have multiple, concurrent islet cell tumors. Dynamic CT scanning, ^{111}In-octreotide scintigraphy, endoscopic ultrasound, and MR scan are useful noninvasive tests for localizing gastrinoma; however, preoperative localization is unsuccessful up to 50% of the time. Selective angiography with or without secretin injection of the gastroduodenal, superior mesenteric, and splenic arteries and measurement of hepatic vein gastrin can localize occult gastrinoma in up to 70% to 90% of cases.

4. In cases of ZES, the primary goal of medical treatment is acid suppression with reduction in basal acid output to less than 15 mEq/h. Medical treatment with proton pump inhibitors (PPIs) is highly effective at reducing basal acid output. These medications are indicated preoperatively in patients undergoing operation for cure and in patients with unresectable or metastatic gastrinoma. Omeprazole (60 mg/day) is initiated and titrated with a basal acid output less than 15 mEq/h. Other PPIs such as pantoprazole, lansoprazole, or esomeprazole have also been used to medically treat ZES.

5. Surgical management of ZES is indicated in all fit patients with non-metastatic, sporadic gastrinoma. Goals of surgery include precise localization and curative resection of the tumor. Resection of primary gastrinoma alters the malignant progression of tumor and decreases hepatic metastases in patients with ZES. Intraoperative localization of gastrinomas is facilitated by extended duodenotomy and palpation, intraoperative ultrasonography, or endoscopic duodenal transillumination. Gastrinomas within the duodenum, pancreatic head, or uncinate process are treated by enucleation, whereas tumors in the body or tail of the pancreas can be removed by distal or subtotal pancreatectomy. Immediate cure rates are 40% to 90% for resections by experienced surgeons; however, half of patients initially cured according to biochemical tests experience recurrence within 5 years. Gastric acid hypersecretion is controllable with H_2 blockers or omeprazole in most patients with ZES, rendering gastrectomy unnecessary. If a gastrinoma cannot be localized intraoperatively, a parietal cell vagotomy may be performed. Surgical debulking of metastatic or unresectable primary gastrinoma facilitates medical treatment and prolongs life expectancy in select patients. Patients with ZES and MEN-1 most often cannot be cured surgically and usually are treated medically.

C. **Unusual Islet Cell Tumors**

1. VIPomas secrete vasoactive intestinal peptide and cause profuse secretory diarrhea (fasting stool output of >1 L/day), hypokalemia, and

either achlorhydria or hypochlorhydria (watery diarrhea, hypokalemia, and achlorhydria are the symptoms of Verner–Morrison syndrome). Hyperglycemia, hypercalcemia, and cutaneous flushing may be seen. Other, more common causes of diarrhea and malabsorption must be excluded. A diagnosis of VIPoma is established by the finding of elevated fasting serum vasoactive intestinal peptide levels (>190 pg/mL) and secretory diarrhea in association with an islet cell tumor. Octreotide (150 g subcutaneously every 8 hours) is highly effective as a means of controlling the diarrhea and correcting electrolyte abnormalities before resection. Most VIPomas occur in the distal pancreas and are amenable to distal pancreatectomy. Metastatic disease is commonly encountered (50%); nevertheless, surgical debulking is indicated to alleviate symptoms.

2. Glucagonomas secrete excess glucagon and result in type II diabetes, hypoaminoacidemia, anemia, weight loss, and a characteristic skin rash, necrolytic migratory erythema. Diagnosis is suggested by symptoms and by biopsy of the skin rash but is confirmed by elevated plasma glucagon levels (usually >1,000 pg/mL). Tumors are large and are readily seen on CT scan. Resection is indicated in fit patients after nutritional support, even if metastases are present.

3. Somatostatinomas are the rarest of the islet cell tumors and cause a syndrome of diabetes, steatorrhea, and cholelithiasis. These tumors are frequently located in the head of the pancreas and are often metastatic at the time of presentation.

4. Other rare islet cell tumors include pancreatic polypeptide-secreting, neurotensin-secreting, and adrenocorticotropic hormone (ACTH)-secreting tumors, as well as nonfunctioning islet cell tumors. These tumors usually are large and often are malignant. Treatment is surgical resection.

ADRENAL–PITUITARY AXIS

I. EMBRYOLOGY, ANATOMY, AND PHYSIOLOGY

A. Embryology. The adrenal cortex arises from the coelomic mesoderm around the fifth week of gestation. Steroidogenesis begins soon after and peaks during the third trimester. The adrenal medulla is populated by the neural crest cells originating from the neural ectoderm. The consequence of this migration is evident by the existence of paragangliomas (extra-adrenal pheochromocytomas) all along the paraspinal axis.

B. Anatomy. The adrenal glands are located in the retroperitoneum located superior to the kidney and lateral to the vena cava (right) and aorta (left). This relationship is important in determining the vascular supply to the adrenals. Each adrenal is supplied by three arteries: superior adrenal artery (arise from the inferior phrenic artery), middle adrenal artery (branch of the aorta), and inferior adrenal artery (branch of the renal artery). The right adrenal vein drains directly into the vena cava. The left adrenal vein drains into the left renal vein.

C. **Physiology.** The adrenal gland is histologically composed of four layers, each with their own biosynthetic products.

1. Adrenal Cortex

   a. Zona glomerulosa is responsible for mineralocorticoid production, of which aldosterone is the primary product. Aldosterone production is stimulated by angiotensin II and decreases in serum potassium levels. Aldosterone acts to increase circulating blood volume by increasing sodium and chloride reabsorption in the distal tubule of the kidney.

   b. Zona fasciculata produces the glucocorticoids of the adrenal glands, which cortisol is the primary product. Cortisol production is stimulated by the release of ACTH by the anterior pituitary. ACTH itself is stimulated by the release of corticotropin-releasing factor (CRF) by the hypothalamus. Glucocorticoids have extremely broad effects with the overall goal of inducing a catabolic state in the body in response to stress. Glucocorticoids increase blood glucose concentrations, stimulate lipolysis, enhance adrenergic stimulation of the cardiovascular system, and reduce the inflammatory response of the immune system.

   c. Zona reticularis produces the adrenal sex hormone androstenedione and DHEA. These hormones support the gonadal production of the same hormones.

2. The adrenal medulla produces catecholamines norepinephrine and epinephrine that act on peripheral alpha and beta adrenergic receptors. Alpha receptor stimulation produces peripheral vasoconstriction. Beta simulation of the myocardium via β_1 receptors increases heart rate and contractility. Stimulation of peripheral β_2 receptors causes relaxation of smooth muscles.

II. ADRENAL CORTEX

A. **Cushing Syndrome**

1. The clinical manifestations of Cushing syndrome include hypertension, edema, muscle weakness, glucose intolerance, osteoporosis, easy bruising, cutaneous striae, and truncal obesity (buffalo hump, moon facies). Women may develop acne, hirsutism, and amenorrhea as a result of adrenal androgen excess.

2. Pathophysiology of excess circulating glucocorticoids.

   a. Iatrogenic. The most common cause of Cushing syndrome is iatrogenic, namely, the administration of exogenous glucocorticoids or ACTH.

   b. Hypersecretion of ACTH from the anterior pituitary gland (Cushing disease) is the most common pathologic cause (65% to 70% of cases) of endogenous hypercortisolism. The adrenal glands respond normally to the elevated ACTH, and the result is bilateral adrenal hyperplasia. Excessive release of corticotropin-releasing factor by the hypothalamus is a rare cause of hypercortisolism.

   c. Hypersecreting adrenal adenoma. Abnormal secretion of cortisol from a primary adrenal adenoma or carcinoma is the cause of hypercortisolism in 10% to 20% of cases. Primary adrenal neoplasms secrete corticosteroids independent of ACTH and usually result in suppressed plasma ACTH levels and atrophy of the adjacent and contralateral adrenocortical tissue.

   d. Ectopic ACTH production. In approximately 15% of cases, Cushing syndrome is caused by ectopic secretion of ACTH or an ACTH-like substance from a small-cell bronchogenic carcinoma, carcinoid tumor, pancreatic carcinoma, thymic carcinoma, medullary thyroid cancer, or other neuroendocrine neoplasm. Patients with ectopic ACTH-secreting neoplasms can present primarily with hypokalemia, glucose intolerance, and hyperpigmentation but with few other chronic signs of Cushing syndrome.

3. Diagnosis of Cushing syndrome is biochemical. The goals are to first establish hypercortisolism and then identify the source.

   a. Establishing the presence of hypercortisolism

      (1) The best screening test for hypercortisolism is a 24-hour measurement of the urinary excretion of free cortisol. Urinary excretion of more than 100 μg/day of free cortisol in two independent collections is virtually diagnostic of Cushing syndrome. Measurement of plasma cortisol level alone is not a reliable method of diagnosing Cushing syndrome due to overlap of the levels in normal and abnormal patients.

      (2) An overnight dexamethasone suppression test (dexamethasone, 1 mg orally at 11 PM and measurement of plasma cortisol at 8 AM) is used to confirm Cushing syndrome, especially in obese or depressed patients who may have marginally elevated urinary cortisol. Patients with true hypercortisolism have lost normal adrenal-pituitary feedback and usually fail to suppress the morning plasma cortisol level to less than 5 μg/dL.

   b. Localization of the cause of hypercortisolism

      (1) Determination of basal ACTH by immunoradiometric assay is the best method of determining the cause of hypercortisolism. Suppression of the absolute level of ACTH below 5 pg/mL is nearly diagnostic of adrenocortical neoplasms. ACTH levels in Cushing disease may range from the upper limits of normal (15 pg/mL to 500 pg/mL). The highest plasma levels of ACTH (1,000 pg/mL) have been observed in patients with ectopic ACTH syndrome.

      (2) Standard high-dose dexamethasone suppression testing is used to distinguish a pituitary from an ectopic source of ACTH. Normal individuals and most patients with a pituitary ACTH-producing neoplasm respond to a high-dose dexamethasone suppression test (2 mg orally every 6 hours for 48 hours) with a reduction in urinary free cortisol and urinary 17-hydroxysteroids to less than 50% of basal values. Most patients with a primary adrenal tumor or an ectopic source of ACTH production fail to suppress to this level. However, this test does not separate clearly pituitary and ectopic ACTH hypersecretion because 25% of patients with the ectopic ACTH syndrome also have suppressible tumors.

(3) Additional tests that may be useful include the metyrapone test (an inhibitor of the final step of cortisol synthesis) and the corticotropin-releasing factor infusion test. Patients with pituitary hypersecretion of ACTH respond to these tests with a compensatory rise in ACTH and urinary 17-hydroxysteroids, whereas patients with a suppressed hypothalamic-pituitary axis (primary adrenal tumor, ectopic ACTH syndrome) usually do not have a compensatory rise.

c. Imaging tests are useful for identifying lesions suspected on the basis of biochemical testing.

(1) Patients with ACTH-independent hypercortisolism require thin-section CT scan or MRI scan of the adrenal gland, both of which identify adrenal abnormalities with more than 95% sensitivity. Patients with ACTH-dependent hypercortisolism and either markedly elevated ACTH or a negative pituitary MRI scan should have CT scan of the chest to identify a tumor producing ectopic ACTH.

(2) Gadolinium-enhanced MRI scan of the sella turcica is the best imaging test for pituitary adenomas suspected of causing ACTH-dependent hypercortisolism.

(3) Bilateral inferior petrosal sinus sampling can delineate unclear cases of Cushing disease from other causes of hypercortisolism. Simultaneous bilateral petrosal sinus and peripheral blood samples are obtained before and after peripheral intravenous injection of 1 μg/kg of corticotropin-releasing hormone. A ratio of inferior petrosal sinus to peripheral plasma ACTH of 2 at basal or of 3 after corticotropin-releasing hormone administration is 100% sensitive and specific for pituitary adenoma.

4 Surgical treatment of Cushing syndrome involves removing the cause of cortisol excess (a primary adrenal lesion or pituitary or ectopic tumors secreting excessive ACTH).

a. Transsphenoidal resection of an ACTH-producing pituitary tumor is successful in 80% or more of cases of Cushing disease.

b. Treatment of ectopic ACTH syndrome involves resection of the primary lesion, if possible.

c. Primary adrenal causes of Cushing syndrome are treated by removal of the adrenal gland containing the tumor. All patients who undergo adrenalectomy for primary adrenal causes of Cushing syndrome require perioperative and postoperative glucocorticoid replacement because the pituitary-adrenal axis is suppressed.

B. Hyperaldosteronism

1. Primary hyperaldosteronism (Conn syndrome) is a syndrome of hypertension and hypokalemia caused by hypersecretion of the mineralocorticoid aldosterone.

  a. Pathophysiology of hyperaldosteronism

    (1) An aldosterone-producing adrenal adenoma (APA) is the cause of primary aldosteronism in two thirds of cases and is one of the few surgically correctable causes of hypertension.

    (2) Idiopathic bilateral adrenal hyperplasia (IHA) causes 30% to 40% of cases of primary aldosteronism.

    (3) Adrenocortical carcinoma and autosomal dominant glucocorticoid-suppressible aldosteronism are rare causes of primary aldosteronism.

  b. Diagnosis

    (1) Given the prevalence of essential hypertension, it is not cost-effective to screen all adults with hypertension for primary hyperaldosteronism. Adults who should be evaluated include those with new onset severe hypertension, those with absence of contributing factor, and those whose blood pressure is labile or poorly controlled with several antihypertensives.

    (2) Laboratory diagnosis of primary aldosteronism begins with the demonstration of hypokalemia (<3.5 mEq/L), inappropriate kaliuresis (>30 mEq/day), and elevated aldosterone (>15 ng/dL) with normal cortisol. The upright plasma renin activity (PRA) of less than 3 ng/mL/hour corroborates the diagnosis. A ratio of plasma aldosterone concentration (PAC) (ng/dL) to PRA (ng/mL/hour) of greater than 20 to 25 further suggests primary hyperaldosteronism. Confirmation of primary aldosteronism involves determination of serum potassium and PRA and a 24-hour urine collection for sodium, cortisol, and aldosterone after 5 days of a high-sodium diet. Patients with primary hyperaldosteronism do not demonstrate aldosterone suppressibility (>14 μg/24 hours) after salt loading. Before biochemical studies, all diuretics and antihypertensives are discontinued for 2 to 4 weeks, and a daily sodium intake of at least 100 mEq is provided.

    (3) Differentiation between adrenal adenoma and IHA is important because unilateral adenomas are treated by surgical excision, whereas bilateral hyperplasia is treated medically. Because suppression of the renin-angiotensin system is more complete in APA than in IHA, these two disorders can be distinguished imperfectly (with approximately 85% accuracy) by measuring plasma aldosterone and PRA after overnight recumbency and then after 4 hours of upright posture. Patients with IHA usually have an increase in PRA and aldosterone in response to upright posture, but patients with adenoma usually show continued suppression of PRA, and their level of aldosterone does not change or falls paradoxically. In practice, this test usually is not necessary because, after a biochemical diagnosis of primary hyperaldosteronism, sensitive imaging tests are used to localize the lesion or lesions.

  c. Localization. High-resolution adrenal CT scan should be the initial step in localization of an adrenal tumor. CT scanning localizes an adrenal adenoma in 90% of cases overall, and the presence of a unilateral adenoma larger than 1 cm on CT scan and supportive biochemical evidence of an aldosteronoma are generally all that is needed to make the diagnosis of Conn syndrome. Uncertainty regarding APA versus IHA after biochemical testing and noninvasive localization may be definitively resolved by bilateral adrenal venous sampling for aldosterone and cortisol. Simultaneous adrenal vein blood samples for aldosterone and cortisol are taken. The ratio of aldosterone to cortisol is greater than 4:1 for a diagnosis of aldosteronoma and less than 4:1 for a diagnosis of IHA.

    d. Treatment. Surgical removal of an APA through a posterior or laparoscopic approach results in immediate cure or substantial improvement in hypertension and hypokalemia in more than 90% of patients with Conn syndrome. The patient should be treated with spironolactone (200 to 400 mg/day) preoperatively for 2 to 3 weeks to control blood pressure and to correct hypokalemia. Patients with IHA should be treated medically with spironolactone (200 to 400 mg/day). A potassium-sparing diuretic, such as amiloride (5 to 20 mg/day), and calcium channel blockers have also been used. Surgical excision rarely cures bilateral hyperplasia.

  2. Secondary aldosteronism is a physiologic response of the renin-angiotensin system to renal artery stenosis, cirrhosis, congestive heart failure, and normal pregnancy. In these conditions, the adrenal gland functions normally.

C. Acute adrenal insufficiency is an emergency and should be suspected in stressed patients with a history of either adrenal insufficiency or exogenous steroid use. Adrenocortical insufficiency is most often caused by acute withdrawal of chronic corticosteroid therapy but can result from autoimmune destruction of the adrenal cortex, adrenal hemorrhage (Waterhouse–Friderichsen syndrome), or, rarely, infiltration with metastatic carcinoma. The diagnosis and treatment of acute adrenal insufficiency in the treatment of patients in septic shock is very controversial. Two prospective randomized trials have shown different effects in the use of hydrocortisone in patients with septic shock (*N Engl J Med.* 2003;348:727; *N Engl J Med.* 2008;358:111–124).

  1. Signs and symptoms include fever, nausea, vomiting, severe hypotension, and lethargy. Characteristic laboratory findings of adrenal insufficiency include hyponatremia, hyperkalemia, azotemia, and fasting or reactive hypoglycemia.

  2. Diagnosis. A rapid ACTH stimulation test is used to test for adrenal insufficiency. Corticotropin (250 μg), synthetic ACTH, is administered intravenously, and plasma cortisol levels are measured on completion of the administration and then 30 and 60 minutes later. Normal peak cortisol response should exceed 20 μg/dL.

  3. Treatment of adrenal crisis must be immediate, based on clinical suspicion, before laboratory confirmation is available. Intravenous volume replacement with normal or hypertonic saline and dextrose is essential, as is immediate intravenous steroid replacement therapy with 4 mg of dexamethasone. Thereafter, 50 mg of hydrocortisone is administered intravenously every 8 hours and is tapered to standard replacement doses as the patient's condition stabilizes. Subsequent recognition and treatment of the underlying cause, particularly if it is infectious, usually resolves the crisis. Mineralocorticoid replacement is not required until intravenous fluids are discontinued and oral intake resumes.

4. Prevention. Patients who have known adrenal insufficiency or have received supraphysiologic doses of steroid for at least 1 week in the year preceding surgery should receive 100 mg of hydrocortisone the evening before and the morning of major surgery, followed by 100 mg of hydrocortisone every 8 hours during the first postoperative 24 hours.

III. ADRENAL MEDULLA: PHEOCHROMOCYTOMA

A. **Pathophysiology.** Pheochromocytomas are neoplasms derived from the chromaffin cells of the sympathoadrenal system that result in unregulated, episodic oversecretion of catecholamines.

B. **Clinical features.** Approximately 80% to 85% of pheochromocytomas in adults arise in the adrenal medulla, whereas 10% to 15% arise in the extra-adrenal chromaffin tissue, including the paravertebral ganglia, posterior mediastinum, organ of Zuckerkandl, and urinary bladder. Symptoms of pheochromocytoma are related to excess sympathetic stimulation from catecholamines and include paroxysms of pounding frontal headache, diaphoresis, palpitations, flushing, or anxiety. The most common sign is episodic or sustained hypertension, but pheochromocytoma accounts for only 0.1% to 0.2% of patients with sustained diastolic hypertension. Uncommonly, patients present with complications of prolonged uncontrolled hypertension (e.g., myocardial infarction, cerebrovascular accident, or renal disease). Pheochromocytomas can occur in association with several hereditary syndromes, including MEN types 2A and 2B and von Hippel–Lindau syndrome. Tumors that arise in familial settings frequently are bilateral.

C. The biochemical diagnosis of pheochromocytoma is made by demonstrating elevated plasma metanephrines or 24-hour urinary excretion of catecholamines and their metabolites (metanephrines, vanillylmandelic acid). If possible, antihypertensive medications (especially monoamine oxidase inhibitors) should be discontinued before the 24-hour urine collection, and creatinine excretion should be measured simultaneously to assess the adequacy of the sample.

D. Radiographic tests are used to demonstrate the presence of an adrenal mass.

1. CT scanning is the imaging test of choice and identifies 90% to 95% of pheochromocytomas larger than 1 cm. MR scan can also be useful because T2-weighted images have a characteristic high intensity in patients with pheochromocytoma and metastatic tumor compared with adenomas.

2. Scintigraphic scanning after the administration of ^{131}I-meta-iodobenzylguanidine (MIBG) provides a functional and anatomic test of hyperfunctioning chromaffin tissue. MIBG scanning is very specific for both intra- and extra-adrenal pheochromocytomas.

E. The treatment of benign and malignant pheochromocytomas is surgical excision.

1. Preoperative preparation includes administration of an α-adrenergic blocker to control hypertension and to permit re-expansion of intra-vascular volume. Phenoxybenzamine, 10 mg orally twice a day, is initiated and increased to 20 to 40 mg orally twice a day until the desired effect or prohibitive side effects are encountered. Postural hypertension is expected and is the desired end point. β-Adrenergic blockade (e.g., propranolol) may be added if tachycardia or arrhyth-mias develop but only after complete α-adrenergic blockade. Patients with cardiopulmonary dysfunction may require a pulmonary artery (Swan–Ganz) catheter perioperatively, and all patients should be monitored in the surgical intensive care unit in the immediate post-operative period.

2. The classic operative approach for familial pheochromocytomas is exploration of both adrenal glands, the preaortic and paravertebral areas, and the organ of Zuckerkandl through a midline or bilateral subcostal incision. In patients with MEN type 2A or 2B and a unilat-eral pheochromocytoma, it is acceptable to remove only the involved gland (*Ann Surg.* 1993;217:595). In patients with a sporadic, uni-lateral pheochromocytoma localized by preoperative imaging stud-ies, adrenalectomy may be performed by an anterior or posterior approach or (increasingly) by laparoscopic adrenalectomy. Intra-operative labile hypertension can occur during resection of pheo-chromocytoma. This can be prevented by minimal manipulation of the tumor but can be controlled most effectively with intravenous sodium nitroprusside (0.5 to 10 μg/kg/minute) or phentolamine (5 mg).

IV. **ADRENOCORTICAL CARCINOMA** is a rare but aggressive malignancy. Most patients with this cancer present with locally advanced disease.

A. Syndromes of adrenal hormone overproduction may include rapidly pro-gressive hypercortisolism, hyperaldosteronism, or virilization. Large (>6 cm) adrenal masses that extend to nearby structures on CT scanning likely represent carcinoma.

B. Complete surgical resection of locally confined tumor is the only chance for cure of adrenocortical carcinoma. Definitive diagnosis of adrenocorti-cal carcinoma requires operative and pathologic demonstration of nodal or distant metastases. Any adrenal neoplasm weighing more than 50 g should be considered malignant.

C. Often, patients with adrenocortical carcinoma present with metastatic disease, most often involving the lung, lymph nodes, liver, or bone. Pal-liative surgical debulking of locally advanced or metastatic adrenocortical carcinoma may provide these patients with symptomatic relief from some slow-growing, hormone-producing cancers. Chemotherapy with mitotane may be somewhat effective. Overall, the prognosis for patients with adren-ocortical carcinoma is poor.

V. INCIDENTAL ADRENAL MASSES are detected in 0.6% to 1.5% of abdominal CT scans obtained for other reasons. Most incidentally discovered adrenal masses are benign, nonfunctioning cortical adenomas of no clinical significance. The AACE and AAES recommend all adrenal masses be evaluated with a 1-mg dexamethasone suppression test and a measurement of plasma-free metanephrines (*Endocr Pract.* 2009;15(suppl 1):1–20). Patients with coexisting hypertension should also be evaluated for primary aldosteronism. Surgery should be considered in all patients with clinically apparent functional adrenal cortical tumors and pheochromocytomas. Tumors greater than 6 cm should be surgically removed. Tumors less than 4 cm should be monitored clinically and radiologically in 3 to 6 months followed by annually for 2 years. Either open or laparoscopic adrenalectomy is acceptable. Laparoscopic adrenalectomy has been associated with shorter hospitalization and faster recovery. Its use is generally limited to malignant lesions less than 5 cm in diameter and benign-appearing lesions up to 8 to 10 cm in diameter.

CARCINOID TUMORS

I. Carcinoid tumors are classified according to their embryologic origin: foregut (bronchial, thymic, gastroduodenal, and pancreatic), midgut (jejunal, ileal, appendiceal, right colic), and hindgut (distal colic, rectal).

A. **Biochemical Diagnosis.** In general, the diagnosis of carcinoid rests on the finding of elevated circulating serotonin or urinary metabolites [5-hydroxyindoleacetic acid (5-HIAA)] and localizing studies. The best biochemical test is an elevated urinary 5-HIAA (normal, 2 to 8 mg/day).

B. **Radiography.** Rectal or jejunoileal tumors may be visualized by contrast studies, whereas bronchial carcinoids can be identified on chest X-rays, CT scans, or bronchoscopy. Abdominal or hepatic metastases are best identified by CT scanning, ultrasonography, or angiography. As with other neuroendocrine tumors, some carcinoids can be detected with metaiodobenzylguanidine (^{131}I-MIBG) scanning, and most are detectable by ^{111}In-octreotide scintigraphy.

II. SPECIFIC CARCINOID TUMORS

A. **Carcinoid of the appendix** is by far the most common carcinoid tumor and is found in up to 1 in 300 appendectomies. The risk of lymph node metastases and the prognosis of appendiceal carcinoids depend on the size: tumors less than 1 cm never metastasize, tumors 1 to 2 cm have a 1% risk of metastasis, and tumors larger than 2 cm have a 30% risk of metastasis (*World J Surg.* 1996;20:183). Extent of surgery for appendiceal carcinoid is based on size: simple appendectomy for tumors less than 1 cm, right hemicolectomy for tumors larger than 2 cm, and selective right hemicolectomy for tumors 1 to 2 cm. Prognosis for completely resected appendiceal carcinoid is favorable, with 5-year survival of 90% to 100%.

B. **Small intestine carcinoid** tumors usually present with vague abdominal symptoms that uncommonly lead to preoperative diagnosis. Most patients are operated on for intestinal obstruction, which is caused by a desmoplastic reaction in the mesentery around the tumor rather than by the tumor itself. Extended resection, including the mesentery and lymph nodes, is required, even for small tumors. Meticulous examination of the remaining bowel is mandatory because tumors are multicentric in 20% to 40% of cases, and synchronous adenocarcinomas are found in up to 10% of cases. An almost linear relationship exists between size of tumor and risk of nodal metastases, with a risk of up to 85% for tumors larger than 2 cm. Prognosis depends on the size and extent of disease; overall survival is 50% to 60%, which is substantially decreased if liver metastases are present. Small-bowel carcinoids have the highest propensity to metastasize to the liver and produce the carcinoid syndrome.

C. Rectal carcinoids are typically small, submucosal nodules that are often asymptomatic or produce one or more of the nonspecific symptoms of bleeding, constipation, and tenesmus. These tumors are hormonally inactive and almost never produce the carcinoid syndrome, even with spread to the liver. Treatment of small (<1 cm) rectal carcinoids is endoscopic removal. Transmural excision of tumors 1 to 2 cm can be done locally. Treatment of 2-cm and larger tumors or invasive tumors is controversial but may include anterior or abdominoperineal resection for fit patients without metastases.

D. Foregut carcinoids include gastroduodenal, bronchial, and thymic carcinoids. These are a heterogeneous group of tumors with variable prognosis. They do not release serotonin and may produce atypical symptoms (e.g., violaceous flushing of the skin) related to release of histamine. Gastroduodenal carcinoids may produce gastrin and cause ZES. Resection is advocated for localized disease.

III. **THE CARCINOID SYNDROME** occurs in less than 10% of patients with a carcinoid and develops when venous drainage from the tumor gains access to the systemic circulation, as with hepatic metastases. The classic syndrome consists of flushing, diarrhea, bronchospasm, and right-sided cardiac valvular fibrosis. Symptoms are paroxysmal and may be provoked by alcohol, cheese, chocolate, or red wine. Diagnosis is made by 24-hour measurement of urinary 5-HIAA or of whole-blood 5-hydroxytryptamine. Surgical cure usually is not possible with extensive abdominal or hepatic metastases; however, debulking of the tumor may alleviate symptoms and improve survival when it can be performed safely. Hepatic metastases also have been treated with chemoembolization using doxorubicin, 5-fluorouracil, and cisplatin. Carcinoid crisis with severe bronchospasm and hemodynamic collapse may occur perioperatively in patients with an undiagnosed carcinoid. Prompt recognition is crucial because administration of octreotide (100 μg intravenously) can be lifesaving.

HEREDITARY ENDOCRINE TUMOR SYNDROMES

I. MULTIPLE ENDOCRINE NEOPLASIA SYNDROMES

A. MEN-1 is an autosomal-dominant syndrome characterized by tumors of the parathyroid glands, pancreatic islet cells, and pituitary gland. Hyperparathyroidism occurs in virtually all patients. Clinical evidence of pancreatic islet cell and pituitary tumors develops in 50% and 25% of patients, respectively. Lipomas, thymic or bronchial carcinoid tumors, and tumors of the thyroid, adrenal cortex, and central nervous system (CNS) may also develop. The gene responsible for MEN-1, *MENIN*, is located on chromosome 11q13 and appears to act through transcription factors (*Science.* 1997;276:404). Genetic testing is available in many centers, but if it is not available, screening of family members should begin in their early teens, including yearly determinations of plasma calcium, glucose, gastrin, fasting insulin, vasoactive intestinal polypeptide, pancreatic polypeptide, prolactin, growth hormone, and β-human gonadotropin hormone.

1. Hyperparathyroidism. Because HPT is frequently the first detectable abnormality in patients with MEN-1, yearly calcium screening of asymptomatic kindred members is recommended. Patients with HPT and MEN-1 usually have generalized (four-gland) parathyroid enlargement. Surgery should consist of 3.5-gland parathyroidectomy or a total parathyroidectomy with autotransplantation of parathyroid tissue to the forearm. This method achieves cure in more than 90% of cases and results in hypoparathyroidism in less than 5%. Graft-dependent recurrent HPT, however, is seen in up to 50% of cases. It is managed by resecting a portion of the autografted material (*Ann Surg.* 1980;192:451).

2. Pituitary tumors occur in up to 40% of MEN-1 patients and most commonly are benign prolactin-producing adenomas. Growth-hormone, ACTH-producing, and nonfunctioning tumors are also seen. Patients may present with headache, diplopia, or symptoms referable to hormone overproduction. Bromocriptine inhibits prolactin production and may reduce tumor bulk and obviate the need for surgical intervention. Transsphenoidal hypophysectomy may be necessary if medical treatment fails.

3. Pancreatic islet cell tumors pose the most difficult clinical challenge and account for most of the morbidity and mortality of the syndrome. Gastrinomas (ZES) are most common, but vasoactive intestinal polypeptide-secreting tumors, insulinomas, glucagonomas, and somatostatinomas, are also encountered. The pancreas is usually diffusely involved, with islet cell hyperplasia and multifocal tumors. Tumors may be found in the proximal duodenum and peripancreatic areas (gastrinoma triangle), and these are virtually always malignant. The treatment goal is relief of symptoms related to excessive hormone production and cure or palliation of the malignant process. Patients frequently require medical and surgical therapy. Before surgical exploration, the patient should be evaluated for an adrenal tumor by measuring urinary excretion rates of glucocorticoids, mineralocorticoid, sex hormones, and plasma metanephrines.

II. **MULTIPLE ENDOCRINE NEOPLASIA TYPE 2 (MEN-2)** is characterized by MTC and includes MEN-2A, MEN-2B, and familial, non-MEN MTC [familial MTC (FMTC)]. These autosomal-dominant syndromes are caused by gain-of-function mutations in the *RET* proto-oncogene, which encodes a transmembrane tyrosine kinase receptor. Mutations in *RET* lead to constitutive activation (tyrosine phosphorylation) of the RET protein, which drives tumorigenesis. Genetic testing should be performed on all suspected individuals. Because MTC occurs universally in all MEN-2 variants, prophylactic thyroidectomy is indicated for all RET-mutation carriers. Current guidelines call for thyroidectomy in the first year of life for MEN-2B-mutation carriers and thyroidectomy before age 5 years in MEN-2A-mutation carriers (*J Clin Endocrinol Metab.* 2001;86:5658). Genetic counseling for parents of affected children is crucial prior to prophylactic surgery. In more than 50% of patients with MTC, the cancer recurs after primary surgical resection. Although reoperation is advocated for local recurrence, there is no accepted adjuvant regimen for effectively treating metastatic disease. Investigational therapies and clinical trials with targeted inhibitors of RET tyrosine kinase activity are being evaluated (*Surgery.* 2002;132:960).

A. **MEN-2A.** All patients with MEN-2A will develop MTC, whereas pheochromocytomas arise in approximately 40% to 50% of patients, and hyperplasia of the parathyroid glands arises in approximately 25% to 35%. Patients with MEN-2A also develop gastrointestinal manifestations, including abdominal pain, distention, and constipation as well as Hirschsprung's disease (*Ann Surg.* 2002;235:648). On genetic analysis, patients with MEN-2A and Hirschsprung's disease (MEN-2A-HD) share common mutations in either codon 609, 618, or 620 of exon 10 of the *RET* proto-oncogene. MTC generally occurs earlier than pheochromocytoma or hyperparathyroidism. Nonetheless, biochemical testing to exclude pheochromocytoma is mandatory in all MEN-2 and MTC patients prior to thyroidectomy.

B. **MEN-2B** is a variant of MEN-2 in which patients develop MTC and pheochromocytomas but not hyperparathyroidism. Patients also develop ganglioneuromatosis and a characteristic physical appearance, with hypergnathism of the midface, marfanoid body habitus, and multiple mucosal neuromas. MTC is particularly aggressive in these patients. MEN-2B patients also demonstrate multiple gastrointestinal symptoms and megacolon.

C. **FMTC** is characterized only by the hereditary development of MTC without other endocrinopathies. MTC is generally more indolent in these patients.

22 Trauma Surgery

Jennifer A. Leinicke and Douglas J.E. Schuerer

Injury is a leading cause of death and disability around the world. This chapter outlines an overall approach to trauma care, provides a framework for therapy, and highlights critical aspects of decision making and interventions. The Eastern Association for the Surgery of Trauma (EAST) Web site (http://www.east.org) provides evidence-based clinical guidelines and can be referred to for additional detail.

TRAUMA CARE

I. **PREHOSPITAL CARE.** Field professionals are responsible for performing the three major functions of prehospital care: (1) assessment of the injury scene, (2) stabilization and monitoring of injured patients, and (3) safe and rapid transportation of critically ill patients to the appropriate trauma center. The observations and interventions performed are important in guiding the resuscitation of an injured patient. The MVIT (*m*echanism, *v*ital signs, *i*njury inventory, *t*reatment) system of reporting is one method of communicating data to the trauma team in an efficient, fast, and organized manner.

A. The **mechanism of a trauma** partially determines the pattern and severity of injuries sustained in the event. For instance, motor vehicle collisions can cause direct contact between the driver's knees and the dashboard resulting in patellar fracture, posterior knee dislocation (with popliteal artery injury), femoral shaft fracture, and posterior rim fracture of the acetabulum. Also, feet-first falls from significant heights cause axial loading and a possible combination of calcaneal fracture, lower-extremity long-bone fracture, acetabular injury, and lumbar spine compression fracture.

B. **Vital signs,** including level of consciousness and voluntary movement, give insight into the clinical trajectory of the patient and are a key element in leveling trauma. Emergency medical service (EMS) providers typically measure and report these values, often in less than ideal conditions. Deterioration of vital signs *en route* to the trauma center suggests life-threatening injuries requiring immediate intervention.

C. The **injury inventory** consists of the description of injuries as observed by EMS personnel. Important prehospital observations include whether the patient was trapped in a vehicle, was crushed under a heavy object, or suffered significant exposure secondary to prolonged extrication. Such findings alert the trauma team to critical secondary injuries, including rhabdomyolysis, traumatic asphyxia, and hypothermia.

D. **Prehospital treatment** is aimed at stabilization of the injured patient and involves securing an airway, providing adequate ventilation, assessing and supporting circulation, and stabilizing the spine. EMS caregivers fulfill these goals through various therapies that include (but are not limited to) administration of oxygen and intravenous (IV) fluids, prevention of heat loss, and immobilization of the spine with a backboard and properly fitting hard cervical collar. All such interventions need to be taken into account during the initial evaluation, including immediate confirmation of any prehospital airway.

II. **INITIAL HOSPITAL CARE.** Trauma deaths have a **trimodal distribution:** (1) immediate death occurring at the time of injury due to devastating wounds; (2) early death occurring within the first few hours of injury due to major intracranial, thoracic, abdominal, pelvic, and extremity injuries; and (3) late death occurring days to weeks after the initial injury due to secondary complications (sepsis, acute respiratory distress syndrome, systemic inflammatory response syndrome, or multiple organ dysfunction and failure). Initial hospital care usually takes place in the emergency department and has two main components: the primary and secondary surveys.

A. **Primary survey.** The primary survey is a systematic, rapid evaluation of the injured patient following the **ABCDE algorithm** (*a*irway, *b*reathing, *c*irculation, *d*isability, *e*xposure). On completion of the survey, the patient should have an established airway with cervical spine control, adequate ventilation and oxygenation, proper IV access and control of hemorrhage, and an inventory of the patient's neurologic status and disability. Additionally, the patient should be completely exposed (all clothing removed) with environmental control. During the survey, a rudimentary history is obtained, if possible. This history follows the acronym **AMPLE** (*a*llergies, *m*edications, *p*ast medical history, *l*ast meal, *e*vents surrounding the injury).

1. **Airway.** Establishing a patent airway is the highest priority in the care of a trauma patient because, without one, irreversible brain damage from hypoxia can occur within minutes. The airway should always be secured under cervical spine control. The quickest way to evaluate airway patency is to engage the patient in conversation. A patient who is able to respond verbally has a patent airway. A patient who cannot respond verbally must be assumed to have an obstructed airway until proven otherwise. Every trauma patient initially should have oxygen administered (via nasal cannula or bag valve facemask) and an oxygen saturation monitor (i.e., pulse oximeter) placed. An oximeter device is helpful, but it is important to remember that its output readings can be misleading in certain clinical situations (e.g., patients with severe anemia, carbon monoxide poisoning, insufficient pulse pressure, hypothermia, or burns with inhalation injury).

   a. **Basic maneuvers to alleviate obstruction**
      (1) **Simple suctioning.** This removes obstructions caused by vomitus, phlegm, or other debris in the oropharynx.
      (2) **Jaw-thrust maneuver.** The tongue itself can occlude the airway. A jaw thrust can successfully displace the tongue anteriorly from the pharyngeal inlet, relieving the obstruction.
      (3) **Nasopharyngeal airway.** In the semiconscious patient, this can provide a conduit for ventilation, but it may result in emesis if it is used in fully conscious patients.

(4) **Oropharyngeal airway.** Mechanically displace the tongue anteriorly, securing airway patency. Because of the strong induction of the gag reflex and emesis, these devices should be used only in unconscious patients.

b. **Tracheal intubation** is indicated in any patient in whom concern for airway integrity exists (unconscious or semiconscious patients, patients with mechanical obstruction secondary to facial trauma or debris, combative and hypoxic patients). The emergent tracheal intubation of an uncooperative trauma patient is a high-risk undertaking. The most skilled operator available should secure the airway by the most expeditious means possible. The preferred method of intubation is via the orotracheal route using **rapid-sequence induction (RSI).** Nasotracheal intubation should be discouraged. Rapid-sequence intubation follows a systematic protocol to ensure successful provision of an airway. The patient is first **spontaneously ventilated with 100% oxygen.** During this time, a team member provides in-line cervical spine stabilization to prevent unintentional manipulation as the hard cervical collar is removed anteriorly. A separate team member provides anterior pressure on the cricoid cartilage (Sellick maneuver) to occlude the esophagus and prevent aspiration during intubation. There is increasing controversy as to the utility of cricoid pressure due to concerns about its efficacy and potential for obscuring the view of the vocal cords. Therefore, cricoid pressure should be removed if its use results in difficulty with securing the airway (*Resuscitation.* 2010;81(7):810–816). Following preoxygenation, a **short-acting sedative or hypnotic medication is administered** via a functioning IV line with a stopcock. The choice of medication depends on the clinical situation. In general, etomidate, 0.3 mg/kg intravenously, or a short-acting benzodiazepine, such as midazolam, 1 to 2.5 mg intravenously, is used because these medications tend to have minimal effects on the cardiovascular status of the patient. In addition, midazolam provides anterograde amnesia. Opiates, such as fentanyl citrate, 2 μg/kg intravenously, should be used only in patients who are adequately perfused because their mild cardiac depressant activity can cause unexpected cardiovascular decompensation in hypoxic, hypoperfused patients. Sodium thiopental, 2 to 5 mg/kg intravenously, is exclusively reserved for the well-perfused patient with a seemingly isolated head injury because it diminishes the transient elevation in intracranial pressure (ICP) associated with tracheal intubation. A **paralytic agent is administered immediately after the sedative.** Succinylcholine, 1 to 1.25 mg/kg intravenously, is the paralytic of choice because, as a depolarizing muscle relaxant, it has a rapid onset (fasciculations within seconds) and a short half-life (recovery within 1 to 2 minutes). Contraindications in the acute trauma setting are limited to patients with known pseudocholinesterase deficiency or previous spinal injury. Succinylcholine can be used safely in patients with acute burns or spinal trauma. Rocuronium, 0.60 to 0.85 mg/kg intravenously, is an alternative paralytic, but as a nondepolarizing relaxant, it has a slower onset (up to 90 seconds) and a longer half-life (recovery after 40 minutes) than succinylcholine. **After onset of paralysis, the endotracheal tube (the largest for patient size and airway) is inserted through the vocal cords under direct vision** with the assistance of a laryngoscope and with the balloon deflated. The tube position is usually around 21 cm from the incisors in women and 23 cm from the incisors in men. Proper positioning of the tube in the trachea should be confirmed by exhalation of carbon dioxide over several breaths (using a litmus paper device or cap-nometer). **Adequacy of ventilation** should be verified by bilateral auscultation in each axilla. A chest X-ray should be taken within the next few minutes and checked to ensure proper endotracheal tube position. Tracheal intubation should secure an airway within 90 to 120 seconds (about three attempts). If it is unsuccessful, an airway placed directly through the cricoid membrane is often necessary.

c. **Cricothyrotomy** is the method of choice for establishing a surgical airway in adults, for instances, in which orotracheal intubation is not possible (unsuccessful orotracheal attempts or massive facial trauma). The cricoid membrane is easily palpated between the cricoid cartilage and the larynx. Because it is both superficial and relatively avascular, it provides rapid, easy access to the trachea. A 1.5-cm transverse skin incision is made over the trachea, and a scalpel is used to poke a hole through the membrane. Care is taken to avoid exiting through the trachea posteriorly, injuring the esophagus. Next, the scalpel handle, a tracheal spreader, or a similar surgical instrument is used to expand the hole. Finally, a 6-mm endotracheal or tracheostomy tube is inserted into the trachea through the cricothyrotomy. Historically, a cricothyrotomy would eventually require revision to a tracheostomy to decrease the risk of tracheal stenosis, but this has been challenged, and many institutions now use the cricothyrotomy site as a tracheostomy site. Cricothyrotomy is contraindicated in children younger than 12 years of age because of the anatomic difficulty in performing the procedure and risk of stenosis. In this situation, percutaneous transtracheal ventilation is an alternative. Laryngeal mask airway (LMA) and Combitube are appropriate alternatives to cricothyrotomy when expertise is limited (EAST guidelines 2002).

d. **Percutaneous transtracheal ventilation** can provide a temporary airway until a formal surgical airway can be supplied, especially in young children in whom cricothyrotomy is not possible. A small cannula (usually a 14-gauge IV catheter) is placed through the cricoid membrane. The cannula is connected to oxygen tubing containing a precut side hole. Temporary occlusion of the side hole provides passage of oxygen into the lungs via the cannula. Exhalation occurs passively through the vocal cords. Through this means, alveolar oxygen concentrations can be maintained for up to 30 to 45 minutes.

B. **Breathing.** Once an airway is established, attention is directed at assessing the patient's breathing (i.e., the oxygenation and ventilation of the lungs).

A patent airway does not ensure adequate breathing because the trachea can be ventilated without successfully ventilating the alveoli. One hundred percent oxygen is administered through the secured airway. The chest is then examined, and important life-threatening abnormalities involving the thorax are identified and treated. The following are potentially fatal conditions that require immediate attention and treatment. (See Chapter 37 for a description of the **technique of tube thoracostomy.**)

1. Tension pneumothorax
    a. Diagnosis. Absence of breath sounds, hyperresonance, tracheal deviation away from the side of the abnormality, and associated hypotension due to decreased venous return.
    b. Treatment. Immediate decompressive therapy (a chest X-ray should not delay treatment) via placement of a 14-gauge IV catheter in the second intercostal space in the midclavicular line, immediately followed by tube thoracostomy.

2. Pneumothorax or hemothorax
    a. Diagnosis. Absent or decreased breath sounds without tracheal deviation usually indicate a simple pneumothorax or hemothorax on the affected side. A chest X-ray can usually confirm these conditions.
    b. Treatment. Tube thoracostomy (32 Fr. or larger for hemothorax), connected to an underwater seal-suction device adjusted to –20 cm water suction.

3. Flail chest
    a. Diagnosis. Paradoxical chest wall motion with spontaneous respirations (three or more contiguous ribs with two or more fractures per rib). Pulmonary contusion often accompanies such an injury. Chest X-ray often reveals the extent of fractures and underlying lung injury.
    b. Treatment. Adequate pain control (often with epidural analgesia), aggressive pulmonary toilet, and respiratory support. Many patients require early mechanical ventilatory support.

4. Open pneumothorax
    a. Diagnosis. A chest wound communicating with the pleural space that is greater than two thirds the diameter of the trachea will preferentially draw air into the thorax ("sucking chest wound").
    b. Treatment. Cover with a partially occlusive bandage secured on three sides (securing all four sides can result in a tension pneumothorax and should be avoided), preventing air from entering the thorax but allowing it to exit via the wound if necessary. Prompt tube thoracostomy should follow placement of the partially occlusive dressing.

5. Tracheobronchial disruption
    a. Diagnosis. Severe subcutaneous emphysema with respiratory comprise is suggestive; bronchoscopy is diagnostic.
    b. Treatment. Tube thoracostomy placed on the affected side will reveal a large air leak, and the collapsed lung may fail to re-expand. The patient is stabilized by intubation of the unaffected bronchus until operative repair can be performed (see Section V.D.2).

C. **Circulation.** The goal of this portion of the primary survey is to identify and treat the presence of shock. Initially, all active external hemorrhage is controlled with direct pressure, and obvious fractures are stabilized. The pulse and blood pressure (BP) are obtained. The skin perfusion is determined by noting skin temperature and evaluating capillary refill. Over time, end-organ perfusion during a trauma resuscitation is estimated using mental status and urine output as markers. Shock is defined as the inadequate delivery of oxygen and nutrients to tissue. The etiologies of shock can be divided into three broad categories: hypovolemic, cardiogenic, and distributive. The trauma team must be familiar with the manifestations and therapy of each category of shock because any of the three may be encountered in the injured patient.

1. **Hypovolemic shock** is the most common type of shock seen in trauma patients and occurs as a result of decreased intravascular volume, most commonly secondary to acute blood loss. It is divided into four classes (Table 22-1). In its severe form, it can manifest as a rapid pulse, decreased pulse pressure, diminished capillary refill, and cool, clammy skin. Therapy is restoration of the intravascular volume. Thus, the patient should have **two large-bore IV lines placed (14 or 16 gauge). The antecubital veins are the preferred sites.** Increasingly, intraosseous access is being used as a rapid way to gain access for both fluid resuscitation and medication administration for patients in whom peripheral IV access is difficult to obtain (*J Trauma.* 2009;66(6):1739–1741). If a peripheral IV catheter cannot be placed secondary to venous collapse, an 8.5-French cannula (Cordis catheter) may also be placed via the Seldinger technique into the **femoral vein.** The subclavian and

TABLE 22-1	Estimated Blood Loss by Initial Hemodynamic Variables			
	Class I	Class II	Class III	Class IV
Blood loss (mL)	Up to 750	750–1,500	1,500–2,000	>2,000
Blood loss (% blood volume)	Up to 15%	15%–30%	30%–40%	>40%
Pulse rate	<100	>100	>120	>140
Blood pressure (mm Hg)	Normal	Normal	Decreased	Decreased
Pulse pressure (mm Hg)	Normal or increased	Decreased	Decreased	Decreased
Urinary output (mL/hr)	>30	20–30	5–15	Negligible

internal jugular veins should be reserved for those patients in whom major venous intra-abdominal injury or pelvic fractures prevent effective use of a femoral approach. Short, wide IV catheters are used to maximize the flow of resuscitation fluids into the circulation (the rate of fluid flow is proportional to the cross-sectional area of a conduit and inversely proportional to the fourth power of its radius). A blood specimen should be simultaneously obtained for cross-matching and for any other pertinent labs. Resuscitation should consist of an **initial bolus of 2 L of crystalloid solution** (children should receive an initial bolus of 20 mL/kg). All fluids administered should be warmed to prevent hypothermia. If the patient remains hypotensive despite the initial fluid bolus, type O blood should be administered and an additional 2 L of fluid should be given. Premenopausal women should receive Rh- blood. Men and postmenopausal women can receive either Rh– or Rh+ blood. Once the patient is blood-typed, type-specific blood should be used. If massive transfusion is required [>10 units of packed red blood cell (PRBCs)], attempts should be made at maintaining a 1:1 ratio of PRBCs and fresh-frozen plasma (FFP). In the setting of penetrating torso injury involving a large blood vessel, less aggressive resuscitation (keeping BP around 90 mm Hg) until formal surgical control of the bleeding site is obtained has been shown to have some benefit in diminishing blood loss (*N Engl J Med.* 1994;331:1105). Resuscitative thoracotomy is sometimes indicated for severe cardiopulmonary collapse (see Section VI.A.1).

2. **Cardiogenic shock** occurs when the heart is unable to provide adequate cardiac output to perfuse the peripheral tissues. In the trauma setting, such shock can occur in one of two ways: (1) **extrinsic compression** of the heart leading to decreased venous return and cardiac output or (2) **myocardial injury** causing inadequate myocardial contraction and decreased cardiac output. Patients in cardiogenic shock secondary to extrinsic compression of the heart usually present with cool, pale skin, decreased BP, and distended jugular veins. They often respond transiently to an initial fluid bolus, but more definite therapy is always needed. Tension pneumothorax is the most common etiology. Cardiac tamponade is a less common cause. It usually occurs in the setting of a penetrating injury near the heart. Rapid diagnosis can be obtained with the use of ultrasound. Therapy consists of pericardial drainage and repair of the injury, usually a proximal great vessel or cardiac wound (see Sections V.D.5.a and V.D.6.a). Resuscitative thoracotomy may be required. Patients in cardiogenic shock secondary to myocardial injury can also present with cool skin, decreased BP, and distended jugular veins. Acute myocardial infarction can manifest in this way. Often, it is responsible for the traumatic event, but it can also occur as a result of the stress following an injury. Diagnosis of a myocardial infarction is via electrocardiogram (ECG) and troponin levels. Therapy should follow Advanced Cardiac Life Support guidelines, keeping in mind that anticoagulants may need to be avoided early until active bleeding related to the trauma has been excluded. Severe blunt cardiac injury (BCI) is another manifestation. It usually occurs in the

setting of high-speed motor vehicle crashes. An ECG and possibly an echocardiogram are essential. Therapy ranges from close monitoring with pharmacologic support in an intensive care unit (ICU) to operative repair (see Section V.D.6.b).

3. **Distributive shock** occurs as a result of an increase in venous capacitance leading to decreased venous return. Neurogenic shock secondary to acute quadriplegia or paraplegia is one type. Loss of peripheral sympathetic tone is responsible for the increased venous capacitance and decreased venous return. These patients present with warm skin, absent rectal tone, and inappropriate bradycardia. They often respond to an initial fluid bolus but often require pharmacologic support. Phenylephrine or norepinephrine can be used to restore peripheral vascular resistance. Chronotropic agents such as dopamine are sometimes used for bradycardic patients. Of note, the leading cause of shock in a trauma patient is hypovolemia, and thus neurogenic shock is usually a diagnosis of exclusion.

D. **Disability.** The goal of this phase of the primary survey is to identify and treat life-threatening neurologic injuries. Priority is given to evaluating level of consciousness and looking for lateralizing neurologic signs. The level of consciousness is quickly assessed using the **AVPU system** (ascertaining whether the patient is *a*wake, opens eyes to *v*oice, opens eyes to *p*ainful stimulus, or is *u*narousable). The pupils are examined, and their size, symmetry, and responsiveness to light are noted. Focal neurologic deficits are noted. Signs of significant neurologic impairment include inability to follow simple commands, asymmetry of pupils or their response to light, and gross asymmetry of limb movement to painful stimuli. Both intracranial and spinal injuries require urgent evaluation.

1. **Intracranial injuries.** Head injury remains a leading cause of trauma fatality in the United States. **Herniation (either uncal or cerebellar)** is often the final common pathway leading to death. Vigilance on the part of the trauma team can sometimes trigger interventions before such an event becomes irreversible. Measures used to prevent increases in ICP and herniation include head elevation to 30 to 45 degrees, sedation, and prevention of jugular venous outflow obstruction. Pharmacologic diuretic therapy is used to decrease ICP by reducing the volume of both the cerebrospinal fluid (CSF) and the brain. **Mannitol, 0.25 to 1 g/kg,** is the preferred agent, but hypertonic saline is also used. Sedation and therapeutic paralysis can acutely lower ICP, but they have the disadvantage of obscuring ongoing clinical neurologic examination. Although once advocated as an initial means of lowering ICP, hyperventilation is no longer recommended as a first-line therapy because of its adverse ischemic effects (it decreases ICP by causing intracranial vasoconstriction secondary to inducing hypocarbic alkalosis). It may be used in an acute setting with impending herniation until pharmacologic agents are available, and if it is used, the partial pressure of carbon dioxide (P_{CO_2}) should be closely monitored and kept at a level of 30 to 35 mm Hg.

2. **Spinal cord injuries.** Acute injury to the spinal cord can result in neurogenic shock, which should be treated appropriately (see Section II.C.3).

In addition, spinal cord trauma produces debilitating neurologic loss of function. The appropriate acute management of such deficits remains controversial. Currently, the use of high dose corticosteroids is not routinely recommended due to increasing evidence that corticosteroids do not result in improved functional outcomes. Additionally, multiple trials have demonstrated an increase in mortality secondary to infection, specifically ventilator associated pneumonia, as well as increased hospital costs and length of stay [*Spine.* (Phila Pa 1976) 2009;34(20):2121–2124] (*J Trauma.* 2004;56(5):1076–1083).

3. Neurosurgical consultation. A neurosurgeon should be consulted immediately in all patients with severe neurologic injuries. Early radiologic evaluation of the central nervous system (CNS) to exclude evacuable intracranial mass lesions is also critical (see Section III.D.3).

E. **Exposure.** The last component of the primary survey is exposure with environmental control. Its purpose is to allow for complete visual inspection of the injured patient while preventing excessive heat loss. The patient is first completely disrobed, with clothing cut away so as not to disturb occult injuries. The patient then undergoes visual inspection, including logrolling to examine the back, splaying of the legs to examine the perineum, and elevation of the arms to inspect the axillae. The nude patient loses heat rapidly to the environment unless specific countermeasures are undertaken. The resuscitation room should be kept as warm as possible. Any cold backboard should be removed as quickly as possible and all soggy clothing should be taken off expeditiously. All resuscitation fluid should be warmed. Finally, the patient should be covered with warm blankets or a "hot air" heating blanket.

III. **COMPLETION OF THE PRIMARY SURVEY.** The completion of the primary survey should be followed by a brief assessment of the adequacy of the initial resuscitation efforts.

A. **Monitoring.** Appropriate monitoring is essential to determine the clinical trajectory of the injured patient. If not already in place, **ECG leads and a pulse oximeter** should be applied. A manual BP should be taken in all patients. An **automatic cuff** should be placed for subsequent serial BP measurements, although it should be kept in mind that such measurements can be inaccurate in a patient with a systolic BP less than 90 mm Hg. Finally, an **indwelling urinary catheter** should be placed. Before insertion of the catheter, however, the urethral meatus should be inspected and found free of blood (the labia and scrotum should not harbor a hematoma). In addition, all male patients require palpation of the prostate to ensure that it is in the normal position, not displaced superiorly ("high riding"). If any genitourinary structures are abnormal, a retrograde urethrogram is necessary. If it is normal, the catheter may be passed. If urethral injuries are present, immediate consultation with a urologist is required before attempting to pass the catheter.

B. **Laboratory values.** After placement of two IV catheters, blood should be sent for laboratory studies. The most important test to obtain is the cross-match. Other studies include blood chemistries, hematologic analysis, coagulation profile, blood gas with base deficit, toxicologic analysis (with ethanol level), urinalysis, and β-human chorionic gonadotropin level if the patient is a woman of child-bearing age. The hematocrit value is the most commonly misinterpreted measure because it is not immediately altered with acute hemorrhage. It should not, therefore, be considered to be an indicator of circulating blood volume in the trauma patient. Serial hematocrit values, however, may give an indication of ongoing blood loss.

C. **Adequacy of resuscitation.** The adequacy of resuscitation can best be determined by using urine output and blood pH. Resuscitation, therefore, should strive for a blood pH of 7.4 and a urinary output of 0.5 to 1 mL/kg/hour in adults (1 to 2 mL/kg/hour in children). Base deficit and lactic acid levels are also used as markers of adequate resuscitation and have been shown to have prognostic value.

D. **Radiographic investigations.** Essential radiographic investigations are ordered during this period. These tests can provide critical data regarding injuries sustained in a trauma, but their performance should not get in the way of ongoing physical examinations and interventions.

1. Plain radiography

   a. **Blunt trauma.** Patients who have sustained blunt trauma with major energy transfer require **chest and possibly pelvic radiographs.** If time permits and the patient is stable but unable to be clinically cleared, a formal three-view cervical spine series should be obtained if computed tomography (CT) is unavailable. The best screening exam to evaluate for cervical spine injuries is a CT extending from the occiput through T1 with coronal and sagittal reformats (see Section IV.C. for detailed description of cervical spine evaluation). If there is no evidence of spine or pelvic injury, an upright chest X-ray should be obtained because it provides crucial information with regard to hemothorax, pneumothorax, mediastinal widening, and subdiaphragmatic gas that sometimes cannot be gleaned from a supine film. Finally, plain radiographs should be obtained of any area of localized blunt trauma, especially if fractures are suspected on the basis of physical exam.

   b. **Penetrating trauma.** Patients who have sustained penetrating injuries require regional plane radiographs to localize foreign bodies and exclude perforation of gas-filled organs (e.g., intestines and lungs). When these films are being obtained, all entrance and exit sites should be identified with a radiopaque marker. This technique gives insight into the trajectory of the penetrating object and the potential organs injured.

2. **Trauma ultrasonography.** Many trauma centers now use **focused abdominal sonography for trauma (FAST)** as an initial radiographic screening evaluation for all trauma following the primary survey. As the name implies, it is a focused examination designed to identify free intraperitoneal fluid and/or pericardial fluid. An ultrasound machine is used to take multiple views of six standard areas on the torso: **(1) right paracolic gutter, (2) Morrison's pouch,**

(3) pericardium, (4) perisplenic region, (5) left paracolic gutter, and (6) suprapubic region. Free fluid in the abdomen and within the pericardium appears anechoic. FAST has many advantages: portable, rapid, inexpensive, accurate, noninvasive, and repeatable. Its disadvantages include operator variability as well as difficulty of use in morbidly obese patients or those with large amounts of subcutaneous air. It is most useful in evaluating patients with blunt abdominal trauma, especially those who are hypotensive. It may not be as useful in evaluating children or patients with penetrating trauma. It is important to note that if a FAST exam is negative, it does not exclude major intra-abdominal injury. Finally, some trauma centers use sonography to evaluate the thorax for traumatic effusions and pneumothoraces.

3. **CT.** The care of injured patients has been significantly changed by the use of CT scanning. Unnecessary laparotomy is associated with significant morbidity and cost. Because of CT, an increasing amount of both blunt and penetrating trauma has been safely managed nonoperatively. Triple-contrast CT (oral, IV, rectal) has been shown accurately to predict the need for laparotomy in patients with penetrating trauma, decreasing the incidence of unnecessary laparotomy. More recent evidence suggests that single-contrast CT scanning with a high-resolution, multislice scanner may obviate the need for oral and rectal contrast. In patients with an increased risk associated with radiation exposure (e.g., pregnant women and children), consideration should be given as to the risk of radiation exposure versus the potential benefit of any radiologic test ordered.

IV. **SECONDARY SURVEY.** The secondary survey follows the primary survey. It is a complete head-to-toe examination of the patient designed to inventory all injuries sustained in the trauma. Thoroughness is the key to finding all injuries, and a systematic approach is required. Only limited diagnostic evaluation is necessary for making decisions about subsequent interventions or evaluations. A review of important aspects of the secondary survey according to anatomic region follows. This review emphasizes only highlights and is not to be considered exhaustive.

A. **Head.** The patient should be evaluated for best motor and verbal responses to graded stimuli so that a **Glasgow Coma Score (GCS)** can be calculated. The GCS is highly reproducible and exhibits little interobserver variability. Severity of head trauma can be stratified according to the score obtained. Any patient with a GCS of 8 or below is considered to have severe neurologic depression and should be intubated to protect the airway. Inspection and palpation of the head are used to identify obvious lacerations and bony irregularities. All wounds require specific evaluation for evidence of depressed skull fractures or devitalized bone. Signs suggestive of basal skull fractures should be sought. These include periorbital hematomas ("raccoon eyes"), mastoid hematomas ("Battle's sign"), hemotympanum, and CSF rhinorrhea and otorrhea.

B. **The face** should be inspected for lacerations, hematomas, asymmetry, and deformities. The cranial nerves should be evaluated. The bones should be palpated in a systematic fashion to search for evidence of tenderness, crepitus, or bony discontinuity. In particular, the presence of a midfacial fracture should be sought by grasping the maxilla and attempting to move it. The nares should be examined for evidence of a septal hematoma. The oral cavity should be illuminated and inspected for evidence of mucosal violation (commonly seen in mandibular fractures). All dentures and/or displaced teeth should be removed to prevent airway occlusion. The conscious patient should be asked to bite down to determine whether abnormal dental occlusion is present (highly suggestive of a maxillary or mandibular fracture). The eyes should be examined for signs of orbital entrapment and the pupils reexamined. Finally, a nasogastric tube (contraindicated if there is a question of trauma to the midface) or orogastric tube (in patients who have midfacial fractures or are comatose) should be placed to decompress the stomach.

C. **The neck** should be inspected and palpated to exclude cervical spine, vascular, or aerodigestive tract injury.

1. **Cervical spine evaluation.** Assessing the status of the cervical spine is an important aspect of the secondary survey. Signs of cervical spine injury include midline cervical spine tenderness or vertebral step-off on palpation. Excluding the presence of a cervical injury can often be challenging. The proper algorithm is often dictated by the overall condition of the patient.

   a. **Awake, unimpaired patient without complaint of midline neck tenderness.** In the awake, alert, oriented, cooperative, unimpaired, neurologically intact patient, the cervical spine should be palpated for signs of injury (e.g., midline cervical spine tenderness, and vertebral step-off). If the physical examination is normal, the patient may be allowed, under supervision, to move the neck through the full range of motion. If there is not any cervical spine pain during this movement, the likelihood of a cervical spine injury is very low, and the stabilizing cervical collar can be removed. Imaging of the cervical spine may not be necessary. If any cervical spine pain is elicited during this movement, the stabilizing cervical collar should remain in place, and a CT scan of the cervical spine extending from the occiput through T1 with coronal and sagittal reformats should be obtained. Plain radiographs do not provide any additional information and are not as sensitive as CT scanning, but in situations where CT is unavailable may be an acceptable substitute in patients at low risk of cervical spine injury.

   b. **Awake, unimpaired patient with complaint of midline neck tenderness.** These patients should undergo a CT scan of the cervical spine extending from the occiput through T1 with coronal and sagittal reformats. If the CT is interpreted as normal, then the possibility of ligamentous injury should be entertained, and the patient should undergo MRI of the cervical spine. MRI should be performed within 48 hours when possible as nonspecific changes may occur after this time and make detection of ligamentous injury difficult. If these films are interpreted as normal, the likelihood of cervical spine injury is low, and the stabilizing cervical collar can be removed (a soft collar may be placed for comfort). The on call spine service (orthopedic or neurosurgery) should be consulted for any diagnosed injury.

c. **High-risk patients.** In patients who are awake, alert, and oriented but with multiple traumatic injuries or a high likelihood of cervical spine injury (pretest probability greater than 5%), a CT of the cervical spine should be obtained. Any suspicion for ligamentous injury should be followed immediately by MRI of the cervical spine. The on call spine service should be contacted for any injury.

d. **Unconscious or impaired patient.** In the unconscious or impaired patient, the cervical spine should be considered to be unstable until a reliable clinical examination can be performed because significant ligamentous instability can exist despite a normal CT scan. In patients with a short-term alteration of consciousness (e.g., chemically sedated or intoxicated), CT scan of the cervical spine should be obtained, and any suspicion of ligamentous injury followed up with an MRI. The stabilizing cervical collar should remain in place until the patient is fully awake and unimpaired. Patients with altered levels of consciousness of unknown duration (e.g., diffuse head injury patients) can be evaluated the same way. However, if the patient is unlikely to regain consciousness within 7 days, MRI should be obtained within 48 hours. If there is no evidence of injury on either the CT or MRI, a bedside upright lateral cervical spine film should be obtained, and the cervical collar can be removed if there is no evidence of misalignment. The film should be repeated with the collar off. If this again does not demonstrate misalignment, the cervical spine can be considered "cleared," although occult injury may still be present. If at any time in the above workup an injury is identified, a spine consult should be obtained. In the event that a patient who is likely to have altered consciousness for more than 7 days does not undergo MRI within 48 hours or injury, a spine consult should be obtained. The method used to clear the cervical spine is dependent on the consultant, but may include repeat plain films, CT, MRI, and/or flexion-extension studies under fluoroscopy (EAST guidelines 2009).

2. **Vascular/aerodigestive evaluation.** In addition to evaluating the cervical spine, the neck should be inspected for active hemorrhage and palpated for local tenderness, hematomas, and evidence of subcutaneous air. Wounds should be classified according to their depth and their location. A wound is considered superficial if it does not penetrate the platysma; it is considered deep if the platysma is penetrated. The neck is divided anatomically into three zones: **Zone I** covers the thoracic inlet (manubrium to cricoid cartilage), **zone II** encompasses the midneck (cricoid cartilage to angle of the mandible), and **zone III** spans the upper neck (angle of mandible to base of skull).

D. **Thorax.** Significant pulmonary, cardiac, or great-vessel injury may result from both penetrating and blunt trauma. In all cases, examination of the thorax includes inspection, palpation, percussion, and auscultation.

Particular attention should be directed at observing the position of the trachea, checking for symmetric excursion of the chest, palpating for fractures
and subcutaneous emphysema, and auscultating the quality and location
of breath sounds. Two points bear further comment. First, thoracic extra-
anatomic air (subcutaneous air, pneumomediastinum, or pneumopericar-
dium) is frequently noted on physical examination or chest radiography
in trauma patients (*Surg Clin North Am.* 1996;76:725). Such a finding
should alert the trauma team to four potential etiologies: (1) pulmonary
parenchymal injury with occult pneumothorax (most common cause), (2)
tracheobronchial injury, (3) esophageal perforation, and (4) cervicofacial
trauma (usually self-limiting). Second, symmetric breath sounds are not
a guarantee of adequate ventilation and oxygenation. End-tidal carbon
dioxide, oxygen saturation, and arterial blood gas values must be monitored to ensure that breathing is intact.

E. **The abdomen** extends from the diaphragm to the pelvic floor, corre-
sponding to the space **between the nipples and the inguinal creases** on
the anterior aspect of the torso. When examining the abdomen during
the secondary survey, the primary goal is to determine the presence of an
intra-abdominal injury rather than to characterize its exact nature. Detecting those patients with occult injuries of the abdomen requiring operative
intervention remains a diagnostic challenge. The mechanism of injury,
however, often provides important clues.

1. **Penetrating trauma.** Stab wounds to the anterior abdomen can be
divided into thirds: One third do not penetrate the peritoneal cavity, one third penetrate the peritoneal cavity but do not cause any significant intra-abdominal injury, and one third penetrate the peritoneal
cavity and do cause significant intra-abdominal damage. As a result,
the ability to exclude penetration of the peritoneal cavity in the patient
with a stab wound to the abdomen has important therapeutic implications. In the stable patient without obvious signs of intra-abdominal
injury (e.g., peritonitis), **local wound exploration** remains a viable
screening option. It is a well-defined procedure that entails preparing
and draping the area of the wound, infiltrating the wound with local
anesthetic, and extending the wound as necessary to follow its track.
If the track terminates without entering the anterior fascia, as occurs
in approximately one half of the patients who undergo the procedure,
the injury can be managed as a deep laceration. Otherwise, penetration
of the peritoneum is assumed, and significant injury must be excluded
by further diagnostic evaluation. Options include laparoscopy or celiotomy, CT, FAST, diagnostic peritoneal lavage (DPL), and admission
with observation. Gunshot wounds within the surface markings of
the abdomen have a high probability of causing a significant intra-
abdominal injury and have therefore been taken to require immediate
celiotomy, but this imperative has been challenged for those patients
with stable hemodynamics and no peritoneal signs on physical examination. In a large retrospective study of patients with abdominal gunshot wounds, selective nonoperative management was reported to result
in a significant decrease in the percentage of unnecessary laparotomies
(*Ann Surg.* 2001;234:395). Current recommendations for nonoperative

management of penetrating trauma include the use of triple-contrast CT (accurately predicts the need for laparotomy) and serial examination. The majority of these patients can be discharged after 24 hours of observation (EAST guidelines 2007).

2. **Blunt trauma.** In the patient sustaining blunt abdominal trauma, physical signs of significant organ involvement are often lacking. As a result, a number of algorithms have been proposed to exclude the presence of serious intra-abdominal injury.

   a. **In the awake, unimpaired patient** without abdominal complaints, combining hospital admission and serial abdominal examinations is a cost-effective strategy for excluding serious abdominal injury as long as the patient is not scheduled to undergo an anesthetic that would interfere with observation. However, such patients are rare in the trauma setting.

   b. **Unstable patient with abdominal injury.** An unstable patient with injuries confined to the abdomen requires immediate celiotomy.

   c. **Unstable patient with multiple injuries.** If an unstable patient has multiple injuries and there is uncertainty about whether the abdomen is the source of shock, a FAST exam may be useful. If a patient is fairly stable and access to CT is readily available, head and abdomen/pelvis CT scans can be obtained. DPL may be useful in patients with head injuries requiring immediate operative therapy. In many large centers, a CT scan can be obtained as readily as the performance of a DPL.

   d. **Stable patient with multiple injuries.** If a stable patient has multiple injuries and the abdomen may harbor occult organ involvement that is not immediately life threatening, a CT evaluation is necessary. In addition to identifying the presence of intra-abdominal injury, CT scanning can provide information helpful for determining the probability that a celiotomy will be therapeutic. Laparoscopy has also been proposed as an adjunct in this situation.

F. **The pelvis** should be assessed for stability by palpating (not rocking) the iliac wings. Signs of fracture include scrotal hematoma, unequal leg length, and iliac wing hematomas. Careful inspection for lacerations (and possible open fracture) is undertaken.

G. **The back** should be inspected for wounds and hematomas, and the spine should be palpated for vertebral step-off or tenderness. If there are positive signs of spinal injury, CT scan should be obtained.

H. **The genitalia and perineum** should be inspected closely for blood, hematoma, and lacerations. In particular, signs of urethral injury should be sought (see Section III.A). A vaginal examination is needed to rule out open pelvic fractures and laceration. A rectal examination is mandatory to assess rectal tone and to look for the presence of gross blood in the rectum.

I. **The extremities** should be inspected and palpated to exclude the presence of soft tissue and orthopedic, vascular, or neurologic injury. Inspection should look for gross deformity of the limb, active bleeding, open wounds, expanding hematomas, and evidence of ischemia. Obvious dislocations or displaced fractures should be reduced as soon as possible. All wounds should be examined for continuity with joint spaces or bone fractures. The limb should be palpated for subcutaneous air, hematomas, and the presence and character of peripheral pulses. A thorough neurologic examination should be undertaken to determine the presence of peripheral nerve deficits. Radiographs of suspected fracture sites should be obtained, and ankle-brachial indices (ABIs) should be measured in the setting of possible vascular injury even if pulses are normal.

J. **General.** During the secondary survey (and throughout the initial evaluation of the injured patient), any rapid decompensation by the patient should initiate a return to the primary survey in an attempt to identify the cause. Finally, in any penetrating trauma, all entrance and exit wounds must be accounted for during the secondary survey to avoid missing injuries.

V. DEFINITIVE HOSPITAL CARE. With the completion of the primary and secondary surveys, definitive hospital care is undertaken. During this phase of care for the trauma patient, extensive diagnostic evaluations are completed and therapeutic interventions performed. In this section, important therapeutic principles are discussed according to the anatomic location of the injury.

A. Head injuries

1. **Lacerations.** Active bleeding from scalp wounds can result in significant blood loss. Initial therapy involves application of direct pressure and inspection of the wound to exclude bone involvement (i.e., depressed skull fracture). If significant bone injury has been excluded, the wound may be irrigated and debrided. A snug mass closure incorporating all the layers of the scalp will effectively control any hemorrhage and should be done as soon as possible (i.e., before CT evaluations).

2. **Intracranial lesions.** Traumatic intracranial lesions are diverse. They include extraparenchymal lesions, such as epidural hematomas, subdural hematomas, and subarachnoid hemorrhages, as well as intraparenchymal injuries, such as contusions and hematomas. CT is the diagnostic modality of choice. Acute therapy is focused on controlling ICP and maximizing cerebral perfusion pressure (CPP) to provide an adequate supply of glucose and oxygen to the injured tissue. CPP is defined as the difference between mean arterial pressure (MAP) and ICP (CPP = MAP − ICP). Maximization of CPP therefore involves manipulating both MAP and ICP, and this is achieved when the BP is adequate (MAP >70 to 80 mm Hg) and the ICP is normal (<10 to 15 mm Hg in adults). A CPP of more than 60 to 70 mm Hg is the goal.

   a. **MAP.** Maintaining an adequate MAP is very important in the patient with head trauma because hypotension is a major risk factor for poor outcome. Pharmacologic support may be used as necessary to maintain an adequate BP. Extreme hypertension should be avoided. Hypoxia is especially detrimental in traumatic head injuries, and all efforts to maintain adequate oxygenation should be made during trauma resuscitations.

   b. **ICP** is defined according to the modified Monro–Kellie hypothesis, which states that the intracranial contents are contained in a rigid sphere (skull). The three major constituents—brain, blood, and CSF—are distributed in a constant volume. An increase in the volume occupied by one constituent therefore must be accompanied by a decrease in the volume occupied by one of the remaining constituents or there will be a rise in pressure. In the trauma setting, early and rapid delineation of intracranial injuries by CT scan is important because it allows decisions regarding the need for ICP monitoring to be made early. Usually reserved for the ICU or operating room, ICP monitoring is usually accomplished via the placement of a **subarachnoid pressure monitor ("bolt").** An **intraventricular catheter** placed in the nondominant lateral ventricle can also be used. This placement has the advantage of providing a means of draining CSF when necessary.

   3. For patients with severe traumatic brain injury (GCS less than or equal to 8) and no other contraindications (e.g., coagulopathy), prophylactic mild to moderate hypothermia (32 to 34 °C) has been shown to decrease mortality and increase the probability of good neurologic outcome. Hypothermia protocols should begin as early as possible (e.g., in the emergency department after CT scan) regardless of initial ICP or even before ICP is measured (*CJEM.* 2010;12(4):355–364). Patients with intracranial hemorrhage should be placed on seizure prophylaxis for 1 week. A neurosurgeon should be consulted early because emergent surgical intervention may be required.

B. **Maxillofacial injuries**

   1. **Lacerations.** All lacerations of the face should be meticulously irrigated, debrided, and closed primarily with fine suture. Alignment of anatomic landmarks is essential. Given the highly vascular nature of the face, primary closure can be performed up to 24 hours after an injury (except a bite wound) as long as it is accompanied by adequate irrigation and debridement. Any deep laceration in the region of the parotid or lacrimal ducts should be examined for ductal involvement and consultation with the appropriate specialist undertaken.

   2. **Fractures.** Patients with significant craniofacial soft-tissue injury or clinical signs of facial fractures require radiographic evaluation to determine bony integrity. Facial CT has supplanted most facial plain films other than the Panorex view (obtained for mandible fractures) and is often required in complex midface fractures to define fracture fragments in detail. Therapy is predicated on the type of fracture present.

      a. **Frontal sinus fractures.** Nondisplaced anterior table fractures are treated with observation. Displaced anterior table fractures and posterior table fractures require operative intervention by a specialist.

      b. **Nasal fractures.** Displaced fractures often need to be reduced operatively, with subsequent packing of the nasal cavity for stability. The presence of a septal hematoma requires immediate incision and drainage to prevent avascular necrosis and resultant saddle-nose deformity.

    c. **Maxillary fractures** are classified according to the LeFort system. These fractures often require complex open reduction and fixation by a surgical specialist.

    d. **Mandibular fractures.** Fractures of the mandible typically occur in areas of relative weakness, including the parasymphysial region, angle, and condyle. These injuries are often treated by maxillomandibular fixation, but such therapy requires a 4- to 6-week interval. Rigid fixation using plates is another option. Patients with open fractures should receive antibiotics covering mouth flora.

C. Neck injuries

    1. **Penetrating neck wounds.** The diagnostic evaluation of penetrating neck trauma is evolving but has traditionally been determined by both the depth and location of the wound. Lacerations superficial to the platysma should be irrigated, debrided, and closed primarily. Lacerations longer than 7 cm should be evaluated and closed in the operating room to decrease the risk of infection. The traditional approach to wounds deep to the platysma is an evaluation based on the anatomic zone of the injury but is transitioning to a multislice CT angiography-based general approach.

      a. **Zone I injuries.** Thoracic inlet injuries commonly involve the great vessels. Routine four-vessel arteriography had been advocated by many surgeons because of the difficulty of clinical evaluation and operative exposure of this region. In two prospective studies (*Br J Surg.* 1993;80:1534; *World J Surg.* 1997;21:41), only 5% of zone I injuries required operation for vascular trauma. Furthermore, routine arteriography did not identify any clinically significant vascular injuries that did not already possess "hard" evidence of vascular trauma (severe active hemorrhage, shock unresponsive to volume expansion, absent ipsilateral upper extremity pulse, neurologic deficit) or "soft" evidence (bruit, widened mediastinum, hematoma, decreased upper-extremity pulse, shock responsive to volume expansion). In addition, patients who lacked clinical evidence of vascular trauma and were managed conservatively did not have any morbidity or mortality as a result of missed vascular injuries (*J Trauma.* 2000;48:208). Evaluation of the aerodigestive tract can also be approached selectively. Patients with clinical evidence of aerodigestive tract injury (hemoptysis, hoarseness, odynophagia, subcutaneous emphysema, or hematemesis) should undergo dual evaluation with bronchoscopy and meglumine diatrizoate (Gastrografin) or thin barium swallow. Esophagoscopy may be substituted for obtunded patients or patients otherwise unable to participate in a swallow study.

      b. **Zone II injuries.** Patients with evidence of obvious vascular or aerodigestive tract injury or patients with hemodynamic instability require immediate operative exploration. In stable patients without obvious injury, both selective operative management and mandatory operative exploration are equally justified and safe. CT angiography or duplex ultrasonography of the neck can be used in lieu of formal angiography in order to rule out arterial injury. Even without contrast administration, a CT of the soft tissues of the neck has been shown to rule out significant vascular injury if it demonstrates that the trajectory of penetration is well away from the vasculature. However, if the trajectory of penetration lies in close proximity to the vasculature, minor vascular injuries (e.g., intimal flaps) may be missed. Physical exam alone is inadequate to rule out injury to the aerodigestive tract. A CT of the soft tissues of the neck can be used to rule out significant aerodigestive tract injuries if the trajectory of penetration avoids the trachea and esophagus. However, if injury cannot be conclusively ruled out by CT, further workup must be undertaken. Esophageal injury may be evaluated by either contrast esophagram or esophagoscopy. The evaluation to exclude esophageal injury should be expeditious as a delay in esophageal repair greater than 24 hours significantly increases the risk of morbidity and mortality (EAST guidelines 2008). The trachea may be evaluated by bronchoscopy.

c. **Zone III injuries.** Upper neck injuries with clinical evidence of vascular involvement require prompt CT angiography owing to the difficulty of gaining exposure and control of vessels in this region. Embolization can be used for temporary or definitive management, except for the internal carotid artery. An injury without clinical evidence of vascular trauma may be managed selectively, with further evaluation by CT. Direct pharyngoscopy suffices to exclude aerodigestive trauma. In neck vascular injuries, endovascular stenting and/or embolization, especially in zones I and III, may be beneficial and should be considered if available.

d. **Operative therapy.** Regardless of the location of the cervical injury, common operative principles apply once surgical exploration is undertaken. Adequate exposure, including proximal and distal control of vascular structures, is essential. The most common approach is through an incision along the anterior border of the sternocleidomastoid muscle. A collar incision is reserved for repair of isolated aerodigestive injuries or for bilateral explorations (e.g., transcervical injuries). The track of the wound must be followed to its termination. Arterial injuries are repaired primarily if possible. Otherwise, prosthetic vascular grafts can be used. Veins can be ligated, except in the case of bilateral internal jugular injury. Tracheal and esophageal injuries should be repaired primarily using synthetic absorbable sutures. If these injuries occur in tandem, a well-vascularized flap of muscle or fascia should be interposed between the repairs to decrease the incidence of posttraumatic tracheoesophageal fistula. Unexpected laryngeal injuries should be evaluated with endoscopy. A drain may be placed if there is any suspicion of aerodigestive tract violation. This maneuver will allow for controlled cutaneous drainage of any leak, thereby preventing lethal mediastinitis. In the case of combined aerodigestive and vascular injuries, the aerodigestive repair should be drained to the contralateral neck to prevent breakdown of the vascular repair from gastrointestinal (GI) secretions should the aerodigestive repair leak.

2. **Blunt neck trauma.** Severe blunt neck trauma can result in significant laryngeal and vascular injuries. In the patient with a stable airway, CT is the best modality for evaluation of a suspected laryngeal injury because it can help to determine the need for operative intervention. Minor laryngeal injuries can be treated expectantly with airway protection, head-of-bed elevation, and possibly antibiotics. Major laryngeal injuries require operative exploration and repair. Blunt vascular trauma usually involves the internal or common carotid artery, but there may also be injury to the vertebral vessels without symptomatology. These injuries can be devastating because they often are not diagnosed until the onset of neurologic deficits. CT angiography is rapidly becoming the diagnostic test of choice over formal four-vessel arteriography, although nondiagnostic scans require formal angiography. Because the severity of the deficit and the time to diagnosis are strongly associated with outcome, a high index of suspicion is needed. An evaluation for vascular trauma should be performed in patients with any neurologic abnormality unexplained by a diagnosed injury, patients with epistaxis from an arterial source, and asymptomatic patients with injury patterns or mechanisms suggestive of a blunt carotid or vertebral artery injury (e.g., severe hyperextension or flexion with rotation of the neck; direct blow to the neck; significant anterior neck soft-tissue injury; cervical spine fracture; displaced midface fractures or mandibular fractures; basilar skull fracture involving the sphenoid, mastoid, petrous, or foramen lacerum; a GCS less than or equal to 8; or diffuse axonal injury diagnosed by CT). The current recommendation is for operative repair of surgically accessible lesions. Systemic anticoagulation (unless contraindicated) with heparin and/or antiplatelet therapy appears to improve neurologic outcome and is therefore recommended for surgically inaccessible lesions. Other anticoagulants are under evaluation for use in this setting (EAST guidelines 2007).

D. **Thoracic injuries.** Rapid diagnosis and treatment of thoracic injuries are often necessary to prevent devastating complications.

1. **Chest wall injuries.** Lacerations of the chest without pleural space involvement require simple irrigation, debridement, and closure. A chest wound communicating with the pleural space constitutes an open pneumothorax and should be treated accordingly (see Section II.B.4). Significant soft-tissue loss may occasionally be encountered and can be initially repaired with a biologic mesh. Complex myocutaneous flap or prosthetic closure, however, is often required for definitive treatment. Rib fractures are common, especially in blunt trauma. They are readily identified on chest X-ray. Any rib fracture can trigger a progression of pain, splinting, atelectasis, and hypoxemia. Preventing this cascade through the use of adequate analgesia and pulmonary toilet is essential. Parenteral narcotics are often required. In the case of multiple rib fractures, intercostal regional blockade using local anesthetics or epidural analgesia. Flail chest often results in significant respiratory compromise and must be treated aggressively (see Section II.B.3).

2. **Tracheobronchial injuries** often present with massive subcutaneous emphysema. Prompt diagnosis and initial stabilization are essential. The operative approach is dictated by the location of the injury. Upper tracheal injuries require a median sternotomy. Distal tracheal or right bronchial injuries are repaired via a right thoracotomy. Left bronchial injuries mandate a left thoracotomy. Penetrating injuries can be debrided and repaired primarily. Transections resulting from blunt injuries usually require debridement of the tracheobronchial segment with reanastomosis. Tracheal defects involving up to two rings can usually be repaired primarily through adequate mobilization. Complex bronchoplastic procedures or pulmonary resections are rarely required.

3. **Esophageal injuries** are most commonly encountered after penetrating trauma, and they can pose difficult diagnostic and therapeutic challenges. These injuries require prompt recognition because, as aforementioned, delay in diagnosis is often lethal. CT can be helpful for delineating the trajectory of the missile and possible esophageal injury. Esophagoscopy combined with meglumine diatrizoate (Gastrografin) swallow can detect virtually all injuries, but either modality is probably adequate for evaluating the thoracic esophagus (*J Trauma.* 2001;50:289). As in the case of tracheobronchial injuries, the operative approach is determined by the location of the injury. A right thoracotomy provides excellent exposure for most thoracic esophageal injuries, particularly those in the midesophagus. A left thoracotomy is recommended for distal esophageal injuries. Primary repair should be undertaken whenever possible and consists of closure using an absorbable synthetic suture. The repair can be buttressed with a vascularized flap (i.e., pleural or pericardial) or fundoplication (for distal injuries). Drain placement near (but not adjacent to) the repair is recommended. Treatment options in late-recognized esophageal injuries include esophageal repair and wide pleural drainage, diversion with injury exclusion, complex flap closure, and esophageal resection (reserved for the esophagus with underlying pathology). Morbidity and mortality are high in this situation.

4. **Pulmonary injuries.** All pulmonary injuries can potentially have an associated pneumothorax (simple or tension). Prompt diagnosis and treatment can be lifesaving (see Section II.B).

   a. **Pulmonary contusion** can be associated with both blunt and penetrating thoracic trauma. These lesions often have adequate perfusion but decreased ventilation. The consequent ventilation–perfusion mismatch results in severe hypoxemia. Diagnosis is often made by chest X-ray. Therapy consists of aggressive pulmonary toilet and respiratory support. Severe contusions often require intubation and mechanical ventilatory support. The management of such patients is extremely challenging because nonstandard modes of ventilation (e.g., pressure-controlled inverse-ratio or high-frequency oscillating ventilation) may be needed. Consultation with a critical care specialist is recommended.

   b. **Hemothorax** is typically diagnosed as opacification on chest X-ray, and it commonly arises from penetrating chest injuries. In the majority of cases, tube thoracostomy is sufficient therapy. A chest X-ray obtained after placement of the tube should be inspected for both tube placement and adequacy of drainage of the hemothorax. A persistent hemothorax with a properly placed thoracostomy tube should raise the possibility of persistent hemorrhage within the hemithorax. Operative intervention is often based on the amount of initial sanguinous drainage and ongoing hemorrhage from the tube. Guidelines vary according to institution and should be individualized to the clinical situation. In general, patients who drain *more than 1.5 L of blood at tube insertion or who have an ongoing blood loss greater than 200 mL/hour over 6 hours* should undergo operative thoracotomy for control of hemorrhage. Significant intrathoracic bleeding can result from pulmonary hilar or great-vessel injury (see Section V.D.5). Pulmonary parenchymal hemorrhage can often be controlled with pulmonary tractotomy and oversewing of bleeding intrapulmonary vasculature. Pulmonary resection (lobectomy or pneumonectomy) may be considered for intractable pulmonary hemorrhage (usually from a hilar injury). Morbidity and mortality after pneumonectomy in the trauma setting, however, are significant, and it should therefore be considered a last resort. Air embolism can develop in the setting of significant pulmonary parenchymal injury, especially in the patient on positive-pressure mechanical ventilation. It usually presents as sudden cardiovascular collapse, and therapy consists in placing the patient in steep Trendelenburg, aspirating air from the right ventricle, and providing cardiovascular support. Chest wall intrathoracic hemorrhage usually originates from an intercostal or internal mammary artery and is best treated by ligation. Evaluation for persistent hemothorax usually requires a CT scan and should be done before 5 days to ensure time for appropriate operative intervention.

5. Great-vessel injury
   a. **Penetrating trauma.** Thoracic great-vessel injury most commonly occurs secondary to penetrating trauma. These patients often present in profound shock with an associated hemothorax. Occasionally, they present with pericardial tamponade due to a proximal aortic or vena caval injury. Often, diagnostic investigations are not performed because immediate operative intervention is indicated (e.g., massive hemothorax and pericardial tamponade). In certain circumstances, however, diagnostic evaluation is possible and can be rather extensive. For example, the stable patient suffering from a transmediastinal gunshot injury requires evaluation of the thoracic great vessels, esophagus, trachea, and heart unless the trajectory of the missile clearly avoids these structures. CT angiography with three-dimensional reconstruction of the great vessels is the diagnostic modality of choice.
   b. Formal angiography is now generally limited to patients in whom an endovascular repair will be performed. The operative approach depends on the vessel involved. Median sternotomy is ideal for access to the proximal aorta, superior vena cava, right subclavian

artery, and carotid artery. A left infraclavicular extension ("trap-door") to the median sternotomy provides exposure to the left sub-clavian artery, but a high left anterolateral thoracotomy is probably a better approach. Finally, rapid median sternotomy with either right or left infraclavicular extensions is most appropriate in the patient who has undergone resuscitative thoracotomy before arrival in the operating room. Whenever possible, primary repair should be performed for arterial and vena caval injuries. Prosthetic graft-ing may be necessary for complex reconstructions. Brachiocephalic and innominate venous injuries can be ligated. Endovascular approaches are increasingly used to repair these injuries.

c. **Blunt trauma** associated with rapid deceleration (e.g., motor vehi-cle crashes and falls) can result in thoracic great-vessel injury. The descending thoracic aorta just below the origin of the left subcla-vian artery is particularly prone to rupture from rapid deceleration because it is tethered by the ligamentum arteriosum. Often such a trauma results in complete transection of the aorta and immediate death from exsanguination. In some patients, however, only par-tial disruption of the aorta occurs, and there is tamponade of the hemorrhage. These patients can arrive at the trauma center alive. If their injury goes unrecognized, however, mortality is near uni-versal. All patients presenting with blunt trauma associated with rapid deceleration therefore must be screened with a chest X-ray. Those patients with positive findings on chest X-ray (widened mediastinum, obscured aortic knob, deviation of the left main-stem bronchus or nasogastric tube, and opacification of the aortop-ulmonary window) require further evaluation. A CT angiogram is then performed, and if it is interpreted as normal, the likelihood of a blunt aortic injury is near zero. Arteriographic evidence of an aor-tic injury mandates prompt operative intervention, depending on associated injuries. Transesophageal echocardiography is an alter-native diagnostic modality in patients who are unable to undergo helical CT or arteriography, but is not preferred because of its lim-ited views of the aortic arch. Endovascular repair is rapidly becom-ing the preferred operative intervention for blunt aortic injury and is associated with decreased postoperative mortality and ischemic spinal cord complications. However, there is minimal long-term outcomes data available on the durability of endovascular repair and associated late complications, such as endoleaks (*J Vasc Surg.* 2008;48(5):1345–1351). In addition, devices currently available may not be small enough for young trauma patients. A left anterolateral thoracotomy is the preferred open approach to this portion of the aorta. Often, a prosthetic interposition graft is inserted at the level of the injury, but primary repair can also be performed. Whether to use partial cardiopulmonary bypass as a circulatory adjunct or the "clamp-and-sew" technique remains controversial. Definitive studies demonstrating the superiority of one method or the other in terms of morbidity and mortality do not exist. However, sufficient pro-spective data do exist to recommend delaying operative repair in patients requiring other emergent interventions (e.g., laparotomy and craniotomy) for more immediately life-threatening injuries or in patients who are poor operative candidates due to age or comorbidities (*J Trauma.* 2000;48:1128). These patients require close pharmacologic control of their BP until surgical repair can be accomplished.

6. Cardiac injury
    a. **Penetrating trauma.** Cardiac injury is usually associated with penetrating anterior chest trauma between the midclavicular lines, but it can occur in the setting of penetrating trauma outside these anatomic landmarks. Pericardial tamponade should be suspected in the patient presenting in shock with distended neck veins and diminished heart sounds **(Beck triad).** Tension pneumothorax must be excluded, however, by auscultating the lung fields. In the hemodynamically stable patient with suspicion for an occult penetrating cardiac injury, echocardiography is the diagnostic modality of choice. Transesophageal examination is preferred. The presence of pericardial fluid warrants emergent operative exploration. Another diagnostic modality is immediate subxiphoid pericardial exploration, especially in the setting of multiple injuries requiring emergent interventions. This procedure is performed in the operating room under general anesthesia. The pericardium is exposed via a subxiphoid approach, and a 1-cm longitudinal incision is made along it. The presence of straw-colored fluid within the pericardium constitutes a negative examination. Blood within the pericardium mandates definitive exploration and cardiorrhaphy. In the hemodynamically unstable patient, resuscitative thoracotomy is often the means of diagnosis. The preferred operative approach to the repair of penetrating cardiac injuries is via median sternotomy. Atrial and ventricular cardiac wounds are repaired primarily using interrupted or running monofilament sutures. Skin staples may also be used (especially in the setting of resuscitative thoracotomy). A Foley may also be placed into the cardiac wound and the balloon inflated as a temporary measure until definitive management can be performed in the operating room. Care must be taken to avoid injury to coronary arteries during the repair. Wounds adjacent to major branches of the coronary circulation therefore require horizontal mattress sutures placed beneath the artery. Distal coronary artery branches may be ligated. Early consultation with a cardiothoracic surgeon is essential, especially in cases involving complex repairs or cardiopulmonary bypass.
    b. **Blunt trauma.** BCI should be suspected in all patients presenting with the appropriate mechanism of injury (e.g., motor vehicle crash with chest trauma) or in those manifesting an inappropriate cardiovascular response to the injury sustained. Presentations range from unexplained sinus tachycardia to cardiogenic shock with cardiovascular collapse. Cardiac enzymes have little to no *clinical* value in the diagnosis or treatment of BCI. ECG is the screening modality

of choice. A normal ECG excludes significant BCI, whereas the presence of an ECG abnormality (i.e., arrhythmia, ST changes, ischemia, heart block, and unexplained sinus tachycardia) in the stable patient warrants further evaluation. In the unstable patient, a transthoracic echocardiogram should be performed to identify any dyskinetic/akinetic myocardium or valvular damage. If the transthoracic evaluation is suboptimal, a transesophageal study is mandatory (EAST guidelines 2010). Patients with frank myocardial or valvular rupture require emergent operative repair. Otherwise, supportive therapy with continuous monitoring and appropriate pharmacologic support (i.e., inotropes and vaso-pressors) in an ICU setting is warranted. Any arrhythmias are managed according to standard Advanced Cardiac Life Support protocols. Rarely, invasive mechanical cardiac support is necessary. Aneurysmal degeneration can be a long-term complication of BCI.

E. **Abdominal injuries.** The management of abdominal injuries must often be individualized to meet the needs of each patient, but certain guidelines apply. All patients undergoing laparotomy for trauma should be prepared and draped from the sternal notch to the knees anteriorly and from each posterior axillary line laterally to have access to the thorax if needed and to the saphenous vein for any potential vascular reconstruction.

1. **Diaphragmatic injuries** occur most commonly as a result of penetrating thoracic or abdominal trauma. Blunt trauma, however, can produce rupture secondary to rapid elevation of intra-abdominal pressure. Frequently, diagnosis is made during celiotomy, but injury can occasionally be recognized on radiographic studies (e.g., chest X-ray or CT). Therapy entails primary repair using permanent sutures in a horizontal mattress fashion. Immediate repair prevents the long-term complications associated with diaphragmatic hernias.

2. **Abdominal esophageal injuries** are managed much like thoracic esophageal wounds (see Section V.D.3). In addition to primary repair and drain placement, the fundus of the stomach can be used to buttress the site via a 360-degree (Nissen) wrap. Exposure of this portion of the esophagus can be difficult. Often, the left lobe of the liver must be mobilized and the crus of the diaphragm partially divided. Finally, placement of a feeding tube should be considered to allow for enteral nutrition in the postoperative period.

3. **Gastric injuries.** Injuries to the stomach occur most often in the setting of penetrating trauma. Sanguinous drainage from a nasogastric (or orogastric) tube should raise the possibility of gastric injury. Diagnosis is usually made at laparotomy. Simple lacerations can be repaired in one layer using synthetic absorbable suture. Alternatively, a full-thickness closure can be reinforced with Lembert stitches. Massive devitalization may require formal resection with restoration of GI continuity via gastroenterostomy. In such cases, vagotomy is helpful in reducing the risk of marginal ulcer.

4. **Hepatic injuries.** The use of CT in blunt trauma has increased the diagnosis of occult liver injuries, making the liver the most commonly injured abdominal solid organ.

a. **Penetrating trauma.** The diagnosis of penetrating hepatic injury is usually made at exploratory laparotomy, although CT has been used to identify injuries. Hemorrhage in the setting of hepatic trauma can be massive, and familiarity with maneuvers to gain temporary and definitive control of such bleeding is essential.

(1) **Initial hemostasis.** Rapid mobilization of the injured lobe with bimanual compression can often provide initial hemostasis. Perihepatic packing with laparotomy pads placed over the bleeding site and on the anterior and superior aspects of the liver to compress the wound is an extremely effective alternative. Temporary occlusion of the contents of the hepatoduodenal ligament (Pringle maneuver) with a vascular clamp decreases hepatic vascular inflow and is successful in controlling most intraparenchymal bleeding. It is often employed to allow further mobilization of the liver and exposure and repair of injuries. Occlusion times should not exceed 30 to 60 minutes because longer intervals of warm ischemia are poorly tolerated by the liver. Failure of the Pringle maneuver significantly to decrease bleeding suggests major hepatic venous involvement, including juxtahepatic and retrohepatic inferior vena cava injuries. Prompt recognition and temporary vascular control of such injuries via the placement of an atrial-caval shunt (Schrock shunt) can be lifesaving. Another option in this setting is total hepatic vascular isolation achieved by placing vascular clamps on the hepatoduodenal ligament (if not already done), the descending aorta at the level of the diaphragm, and the suprahepatic and suprarenal vena cava. Finally, bleeding from deeply penetrating injuries (e.g., transhepatic gunshot wounds) can sometimes be temporarily controlled through placement of an occluding intrahepatic balloon catheter.

(2) **Definitive hemostasis** is attained via multiple techniques. Raw surface oozing can be controlled by electrocautery, argon beam coagulation, or parenchymal sutures [horizontal mattress stitches placed in a plane parallel to the injury using large absorbable (no. 2 chromic) sutures on a wide-sweep, blunt-tip needle]. Topical hemostatic agents are also useful (i.e., microcrystalline collagen, thrombin, and oxidized cellulose). Deeper wounds are usually managed by hepatotomy and with selective ligation of bleeding vessels. A finger-fracture technique is employed to separate overlying liver parenchyma within a wound until the injured vessel is identified, isolated, and controlled. Major venous injuries should be repaired primarily. Omental packing of open injuries can provide buttressing. Resectional debridement is limited to frankly devitalized tissue. Hepatic artery ligation is reserved for deep lobar arterial injuries where hepatotomy may result in significant blood loss.

Formal anatomic resection should be avoided because of its high associated morbidity and mortality. Finally, closed suction drains should be placed near the wound to help to identify and control biliary leaks.

(3) **Damage control** principles are frequently applied to complex hepatic injuries. Perihepatic packing with ICU admission and resuscitation, followed by return to the operating room in 24 to 48 hours, is common. Liberal use of this algorithm can decrease mortality.

b. **Blunt trauma.** The management of blunt hepatic trauma has undergone a dramatic change over the last decade, largely due to improvement in CT imaging. CT with IV contrast is the recommended diagnostic modality for evaluation of the stable patient suspected of having blunt hepatic trauma because it can reliably identify and characterize the degree of an injury. In the presence of hepatic trauma, therapy should be predicated on the hemodynamic status of the patient. The unstable patient requires operative exploration and control of hemorrhage as described (see Section V.E.4.a). The stable patient without an alternate indication for celiotomy should be admitted for close hemodynamic monitoring and serial hematocrit determinations. Operative intervention should be promptly undertaken for hemodynamic instability. Evidence of ongoing blood loss in the hemodynamically stable patient warrants angiographic evaluation and embolization of the bleeding source. Transfusions are administered as indicated. The frequency of follow-up CT evaluation of the lesion should be dictated by the clinical status of the patient. Resumption of normal activity should be based on evidence of healing of the injury. Stable patients therefore do not require strict bed rest. Complications of blunt hepatic trauma include biliary leak and abscess formation, both of which are readily amenable to endoscopic and percutaneous therapy. Delayed hemorrhage is rare, but pseudoaneurysm formation can occur with hemorrhage or hemobilia, requiring angiography and embolization. Nonoperative management is successful in the vast majority of blunt hepatic injuries and has even been reported in certain cases of penetrating hepatic wounds.

5. **Gallbladder injuries.** Injury to the gallbladder frequently coexists with hepatic, portal triad, and pancreaticoduodenal trauma. Treatment consists of cholecystectomy. The gallbladder also provides an effective means of assessing biliary tree integrity via cholangiography.

6. **Common bile duct injuries.** Penetrating trauma is most often responsible for common bile duct injuries. Like gallbladder injuries, they often occur in association with other right upper quadrant organ trauma. Most often, diagnosis is apparent at the time of laparotomy, but occult injuries can occur. Intraoperative cholangiography, therefore, is warranted when biliary involvement is suspected. Primary repair of the injured duct over a T tube is the preferred management, but Roux-en-Y choledochojejunostomy is sometimes required (i.e., when significant segmental loss

of the duct is present). Choledochoduodenostomy and cholecystojejunostomy are poor options and should be avoided.

7. **Duodenal injuries** frequently coexist with devastating GI and abdominal vascular trauma and, as a result, can represent a diagnostic and therapeutic challenge. The type and severity of duodenal injury determine management.

   a. **Duodenal hematoma.** Intramural duodenal hematomas usually occur after blunt trauma to the upper abdomen. Patients present with abdominal pain, nausea, and vomiting. Diagnosis is made with CT or upper GI fluoroscopy using Gastrografin. Therapy consists of long-term nasogastric decompression and nutritional support (parenteral or enteral distal to the level of injury). The majority of duodenal hematomas are effectively treated in this manner, but operative evacuation may be indicated if obstruction persists for more than 14 days and CT reimaging confirms persistent hematoma.

   b. **Duodenal perforation** can be difficult to diagnose. Patients often complain only of vague back or flank pain, and symptoms can evolve slowly. Plain radiographic signs suggestive of perforation include evidence of retroperitoneal gas, blurring of the right psoas muscle, and leftward scoliosis. Upper GI fluoroscopy using water-soluble contrast may also show evidence of a leak. The diagnostic modality of choice, however, is CT using oral and IV contrast, with the oral contrast administered in the trauma room. Operative therapy depends on the degree of injury, but complete mobilization of the duodenum (Kocher maneuver) is essential for proper visualization and repair. Most defects (approximately 80%) can be repaired primarily in two layers, with a transverse closure to avoid luminal narrowing. Closed suction drainage placed around the repair is strongly recommended to control any anastomotic leak. Nasoduodenal decompression should be instigated. Alternatively, antegrade or retrograde (preferred) tube duodenostomy can be performed in conjunction with tube gastrostomy and feeding jejunostomy, the so-called triple tube drainage (*J Trauma* .1979;19:334).

   c. **Complex duodenal injuries** are an operative challenge, and management remains controversial, especially in the presence of tissue devitalization. Whenever possible, debridement with primary repair should be performed. The repair should be protected via triple-tube drainage or pyloric exclusion with diverting gastrojejunostomy. For large defects not amenable to primary closure, a retrocolic Roux-en-Y duodenojejunostomy is an option. Finally, pancreaticoduodenectomy (Whipple procedure) should be reserved only for the most complex injuries, including duodenal devascularization or severe combined injuries involving the pancreatic head and bile duct. This procedure has a very high morbidity and mortality in the trauma setting.

8. **Pancreatic injuries.** Injury to the pancreas often occurs as a result of penetrating trauma, although a significant number of cases do involve blunt mechanisms. Associated morbidity and mortality remain

significant and increase with the number of associated injuries. However, isolated pancreatic trauma is rare. Typically, the liver or stomach is also involved, but concomitant duodenal-pancreatic or biliary-pancreatic injuries do happen. CT is the best diagnostic imaging modality available, but occasionally endoscopic retrograde cholangiopancreatography or MR cholangiopancreatography studies should be used to help clarify the presence or absence of pancreatic duct injury. *Pancreatic enzymes are not helpful in the diagnosis.* Treatment focuses on determining the presence and location of major ductal involvement. Commonly, such information is obtained during operative inspection of the gland, but occasionally intraoperative pancreatography (endoscopic or transduodenal) may be necessary. Adequate exploration entails performing a Kocher maneuver (to visualize the head of the pancreas) as well as transecting the gastrohepatic and gastrocolic ligaments (to inspect the body and tail of the pancreas). If necessary, the retroperitoneal attachments along the inferior border are divided (to view the posterior aspect of the pancreas). Injuries in which the pancreatic duct is intact (e.g., Grade I and II injuries) are treated with closed suction drainage. Transection of the pancreatic duct (e.g., Grade III injuries and higher) requires more extensive procedures involving debridement and/or resection combined with closed suction drainage of the pancreatic bed. Pancreatography is not recommended. For ductal injuries occurring to the right of the superior mesenteric vessels, treatment consists in closing the proximal end of the duct with a stapler or suture and draining the distal end via a Roux-en-Y pancreaticojejunostomy. Distal pancreatectomy (with or without splenectomy) should be used for transections occurring to the left of the superior mesenteric vessels. In addition, it is an option for more-proximal injuries in which resection would preserve greater than 10% of the pancreas. Whatever the procedure, the proximal end of the duct should be closed, and the pancreatic bed should be extensively drained. The liberal use of closed suction drainage helps to decrease morbidity by controlling pancreatic leaks. Finally, severe injury to the head of the pancreas, especially in conjunction with duodenal and biliary trauma, may require pancreaticoduodenectomy but usually not during the initial operation (EAST guidelines 2009).

9. **Splenic injuries.** The spleen is the second-most-common solid organ injured in abdominal trauma. Like hepatic trauma, the management of splenic injuries has undergone an evolution over the last two decades.

   a. **Penetrating trauma.** In general, penetrating splenic injuries are diagnosed at laparotomy, although they are sometimes identified on CT imaging. Management depends on complete mobilization of the spleen. Initial hemostasis is possible through manual compression. Minor injuries contained within the splenic capsule do not require any intervention. Bleeding from small capsular lacerations can be controlled with direct pressure or topical hemostatic agents. More-complex injuries are treated according to the hemodynamic status of the patient. In the stable patient, splenorrhaphy can be employed in an attempt to preserve immune function (requiring salvage of 40% of the splenic mass). Devitalized tissue should be debrided and the wound closed with absorbable horizontal mattress sutures (usually 2-0 chromic). Alternatively, the spleen can be wrapped in absorbable mesh. Partial resection is indicated for isolated superior or inferior pole injuries. In unstable patients or in patients in whom splenic salvage fails, splenectomy should be performed in an expeditious manner. Drainage of the splenic bed is not necessary unless pancreatic injury is suspected. All patients who undergo emergent splenectomy are at risk for overwhelming postsplenectomy sepsis infection. Although this complication is rare (maximum risk is 0.5% in prepubertal children), the mortality is up to 50%. Therefore, all patients undergoing emergent splenectomy require postoperative immunization against *Streptococcus pneumoniae, Haemophilus influenzae,* and *Neisseria meningitidis.* Some authors even recommend penicillin prophylaxis for children because they are at highest risk. Yearly viral influenza vaccines are also recommended for postsplenectomy patients.

b. **Blunt trauma.** Most blunt splenic injuries are initially treated with nonoperative observation. CT remains the diagnostic modality of choice. All hemodynamically stable patients without an alternate indication for laparotomy should undergo close observation with continuous monitoring of vital signs, initial bed rest, nasogastric decompression (unless contraindicated), and serial hematocrit determinations. Patients with CT evidence of a contrast "blush" or evidence of continuing blood loss who remain stable should undergo transfusion and selective angiographic embolization. Patients who are hemodynamically unstable or are failing nonoperative management (e.g., require continuing transfusion) should undergo operative exploration and therapy as described (see Section V.E.9.a). Most often, splenectomy is performed. CT reimaging should be performed as clinical status indicates, especially for high-grade injuries.

10. **Small-bowel injuries.** Given its large volume and anatomy (tethering at the duodenojejunal flexure), the small bowel is prone to both penetrating (e.g., gunshot) and blunt (e.g., lap belt) trauma. Diagnosis is made at laparotomy or via radiographic imaging (plain radiograph or CT). Treatment consists of primary repair or segmental resection with anastomosis. Mesenteric defects should be closed.

11. **Large-bowel injuries.** Colonic injuries typically occur secondary to penetrating trauma and are diagnosed at the time of laparotomy. A prospective multicenter study has demonstrated that the surgical management (primary repair vs. diversion) of penetrating colonic injuries did not affect the incidence of abdominal complications regardless of associated risk factors (*J Trauma.* 2001;50:765). The only independent risk factors for such complications were severe fecal contamination, large transfusion requirement (>4 units) in the first 24 hours, and single-agent antibiotic prophylaxis. *Primary repair, therefore, should be*

considered in all penetrating colonic injuries unless the patient experiences prolonged intraoperative hypotension.

12. **Rectal injuries.** Penetrating trauma is also responsible for most rectal injuries. They often occur in association with genitourinary or pelvic vascular trauma, and they can be diagnosed via proctoscopy, CT, or at laparotomy. Traditional management advocated rectal washout (debridement), diverting sigmoid colostomy creation, and presacral drain placement. However, a prospective, randomized trial showed that omission of presacral drains in the management of low-velocity penetrating rectal injuries did not increase infectious complications (*J Trauma.* 1998;45:656). Debridement (with primary repair of rectal wounds when possible) and diverting colostomy formation therefore seem sufficient management. The distal stump should be tagged with proline suture to facilitate identification at the time of reversal. Reversal can be undertaken after 6 weeks if barium enema reveals healing of the rectum and the patient is medically stable.

F. **Retroperitoneal vascular injuries.** Injuries to the major retroperitoneal vessels or their abdominal branches can be life threatening. These wounds usually present with frank intra-abdominal hemorrhage or retroperitoneal hematoma formation. Management is based on both mechanism of trauma and location of injury.

1. **Penetrating trauma.** The majority of retroperitoneal vascular injuries are the result of penetrating trauma. By definition, any hematoma formed by a penetrating mechanism is uncontained and requires prompt exploration.

   a. **Initial access and hemostasis.** At times, vascular injuries present with massive intra-abdominal bleeding, and familiarity with techniques to control such hemorrhage expeditiously and to obtain access to vessels efficiently can be lifesaving. Packing the site of injury with laparotomy pads is always a reliable temporizing option. Often, initial control requires occluding the supraceliac aorta at the level of the diaphragmatic hiatus using a vascular clamp, a T bar, or direct pressure. Division of the gastrohepatic ligament and mobilization of the stomach and esophagus can provide access to this section of the aorta. Occasionally, division of the diaphragmatic crus is necessary for more proximal control. Once the proximal aorta has been occluded, definitive identification and repair of vascular injuries require adequate exposure of the involved vessels. A left medial visceral rotation (Mattox maneuver) provides excellent access to the aorta, celiac axis, superior mesenteric artery (SMA), left renal artery, and iliac arteries. A right medial visceral rotation (Catell maneuver) readily exposes the vena cava (with a combined Kocher maneuver), right renal vessels, and iliac veins. The infrarenal aorta may also be approached via a transperitoneal incision at the base of the mesocolon.

   b. **Repair of vascular injuries.** Most aortic and iliac arterial injuries can be repaired directly by lateral arteriorrhaphy. On occasion, reconstruction with graft prosthesis or autologous venous graft is necessary for significant circumferential or segmental defects. If enteric contamination is extensive, extra-anatomic bypass with oversewing of the proximal stump is mandatory. Injuries to the celiac root or its branches (left gastric or splenic arteries) can often be ligated without adverse outcome, especially in young patients. Splenectomy must follow splenic artery ligation. Common hepatic artery injuries should be repaired when possible (via lateral arterior-rhaphy, resection and reanastomosis, or graft), but ligation can be tolerated at times. SMA defects must be repaired. Vena cava and iliac venous injuries are repaired by lateral venorrhaphy. Injuries to the superior mesenteric vein (SMV) and portal vein should undergo repair, but cases of successful outcome after ligation have been reported. Because of the risk of postoperative thrombosis leading to portal hypertension or superior mesenteric infarction, SMV and portal venous reconstructions must be closely followed, and anticoagulation is often administered. Finally, major renal arterial and venous injuries require primary repair, whereas partial nephrectomy is recommended for segmental vessel involvement. Endovascular treatment has an expanding role in the treatment of all vascular trauma and may be beneficial.

2. **Blunt trauma** can cause retroperitoneal vascular injury with resultant hematoma formation. Often, these hematomas are discovered at operative exploration, but they are sometimes seen on preoperative imaging. The character and location of the hematoma determine management.

a. **Central abdominal hematomas (zone I).** All central abdominal hematomas caused by blunt trauma require operative exploration. Supramesocolic hematomas are usually due to injuries to the suprarenal aorta, celiac axis, proximal SMA, or proximal renal artery. They should be approached via a left medial visceral rotation. Inframesocolic hematomas are secondary to infrarenal aortic or inferior vena cava injuries and are best exposed by a transperitoneal incision at the base of the mesocolon. As with any vascular repair, proximal and distal control of the involved vessel should be obtained prior to exploration if possible.

b. **Flank hematomas (zone II).** Flank hematomas are suggestive of renal artery, renal vein, or kidney parenchymal injury. Unless they are rapidly expanding, pulsatile, or ruptured, they should not be explored if they are discovered at the time of celiotomy. Radiographic evaluation of the ipsilateral kidney is necessary in this situation to assess its function, usually by means of CT imaging. Evidence of nonfunction should prompt arteriography of the renal artery because blunt abdominal trauma often causes intimal tears, with resulting thrombosis of the artery. If it is discovered within 6 hours of the injury, revascularization may be performed, although the success rate is only 20%. Otherwise, nonoperative management is preferred. Nephrectomy is sometimes indicated when laparotomy is performed for associated injuries in a stable patient. In this setting, removal of the nonfunctioning kidney will decrease long-term renal complications (e.g., urinoma, hypertension, and delayed bleeding). There is no proven benefit of obtaining proximal control of the renal vessels in terms of blood loss or renal salvage. Total or partial (to preserve renal mass) nephrectomy may be necessary for a shattered kidney.

   c. **Pelvic hematomas.** Central pelvic hematomas in the setting of blunt trauma are usually due to pelvic fractures. If they are discovered at celiotomy, they should not be explored unless iliac arterial injury is suspected (loss of ipsilateral groin pulse, rapidly expanding hematoma, or pulsatile hematoma) or rupture has occurred. Bleeding from pelvic fractures can be massive, and management should focus on nonoperative control. Unstable pelvic fractures in association with hypotension should undergo some form of external stabilization. In extreme circumstances, temporary control of hemorrhage can be achieved by wrapping a pelvic binder tightly around the pelvis. Formal external fixation should follow as soon as possible. It should also be considered in those patients with unstable pelvic fractures who require celiotomy or who are hemodynamically stable but have a need for continued resuscitation. Pelvic angiography with selective embolization is the preferred intervention for patients in whom major pelvic fractures are the suspected source of ongoing bleeding. It should also be considered in patients with major pelvic fractures when CT imaging reveals evidence of arterial extravasation in the pelvis or when bleeding in the pelvis cannot be controlled at laparotomy.

G. **Genitourinary injuries.** Injuries to the genitourinary tract are discussed in detail in Chapter 35. Three points, however, warrant discussion in the context of trauma. Urethral injuries complicate the placement of an indwelling catheter. Their diagnosis and management have been discussed (Section III.A). In blunt abdominal trauma, **gross hematuria *or* microscopic hematuria in the setting of hemodynamic instability** mandates urologic evaluation. The absence of hematuria, however, does not always exclude an injury to the urinary tract, especially in the setting of penetrating torso trauma. CT is the best imaging modality for demonstrating urologic injury in the trauma patient who does not require laparotomy for other reasons, and it provides information regarding kidney perfusion. Although once commonly used, excretory urography intravenous pyelogram (IVP) in the trauma patient is often unsatisfactory and is now rarely used. In patients with suspected bladder rupture, especially those with gross *hematuria or pelvic fluid on CT in the presence of pelvic fractures,* cystography should be performed. **CT cystography** has been demonstrated to be equivalent to conventional cystography in assessing bladder injury (EAST guidelines 2003).

H. **Orthopedic injuries** are discussed in detail in Chapter 34, but three important considerations bear mentioning.

   1. **Blood loss.** Fractures can produce large blood losses. A broken rib can be associated with a 125-mL blood loss, a forearm fracture with a 250-mL blood loss, a broken humerus with a 500-mL blood loss, a

femur fracture with a 1,000-mL blood loss, and a complex pelvic fracture with a blood loss of 2,000 mL or more. Stabilization of fractures can minimize the amount of bleeding. Although the Medical Anti-Shock Trouser (MAST) (pneumatic antishock device) has been largely discredited as a device for raising BP, it may afford transient pneumatic stabilization to lower-extremity and pelvis fractures, thereby attenuating further blood loss while the patient is being prepared for more specific interventions (e.g., traction, fixation, or arteriography and embolization).

2. **Spinal fractures.** Fractures of the spine are multiple in 10% of cases. Complete radiographic evaluation of the spine is necessary, therefore, when a single fracture is discovered.

3. **Joint involvement.** Two joints overlie single-access arteries: the elbow and the knee. Fractures or dislocations of either of these joints increase the risk of ischemic complications of the involved distal limb. The integrity of the underlying artery therefore must be confirmed by duplex ultrasound or arteriography.

I. **Extremity injuries.** Extremity trauma can result in devastating injuries requiring the coordination of multiple specialists to perform complex reconstructions. The goal of management is limb preservation and restoration of function, and it should focus on ensuring vascular continuity, maintaining skeletal integrity, and providing adequate soft-tissue coverage.

1. **Penetrating trauma.** Penetrating-extremity trauma typically occurs in males younger than 40 years old. Multiple injuries can occur in association with such trauma, and a high index of suspicion is necessary for diagnosing and repairing them expeditiously.

2. **Vascular injuries.** A wounded extremity can tolerate approximately 6 hours of ischemia before the onset of irreversible loss of function. Quickly identifying and repairing vascular injuries, therefore, is essential in any extremity trauma. Immediate operative exploration is indicated for obvious (hard) signs of vascular involvement (pulse deficit, pulsatile bleeding, bruit, thrill, or expanding hematoma) in gunshot or stab wounds without associated skeletal injury. Arteriography should be employed for those patients with hard vascular signs in the setting of associated skeletal injury (fracture, dislocation) or shotgun trauma. Patients with possible (soft) signs of vascular injury (nerve deficit, nonexpanding hematoma, associated fracture, significant soft-tissue injury, history of bleeding or hypotension) require evaluation of vascular integrity. A useful algorithm is to check the ABI initially. If the ABI for the affected limb is greater than 0.9, no further radiographic evaluation is necessary. If it is less than 0.9, noninvasive Doppler ultrasonography, if technically feasible, should follow to exclude vascular injury. If ultrasonography is equivocal, arteriography is indicated; if it is positive, either operative exploration or arteriography can follow. Patients without hard or soft signs do not require arteriography to exclude vascular involvement. Occult vascular injuries can be managed nonoperatively, with subsequent repair as indicated, without an increase in morbidity. Arterial injuries should be repaired within 6 hours to maximize limb

salvage rates. The operative approach is similar to elective vascular procedures, and endovascular therapy may be feasible if available. Proximal and distal control of the involved vessel is essential. Primary repair using monofilament suture should be performed for limited arterial lacerations. For complex injuries (large segmental or circumferential defects), resection with reanastomosis, patch angioplasty, or interposition grafting is preferred. Whenever possible, autologous vein should be used instead of polytetrafluoroethylene (PTFE) for patching or grafting because of its higher patency rates. Ligation of single-artery forearm and calf injuries is possible in the presence of normal counterparts. Restoration of blood flow (via temporary shunt or formal repair) should precede any skeletal reconstruction in cases of combined injuries. Completion arteriography should be performed after any arterial repair. Venous injuries should undergo lateral venorrhaphy or resection with end-to-end reanastomosis if the patient is hemodynamically stable. Ligation with postoperative leg elevation and compression stocking placement (to reduce edema) is indicated in all other cases. Multiple compartment fasciotomies should be liberally used, especially after prolonged ischemia or in the presence of associated injuries.

3. **Skeletal injuries** are diagnosed with plain radiography. Restoration of skeletal integrity is attained by means of either internal or external fixation. Temporary vascular shunting should be performed before stabilization of an unstable fracture in the setting of combined injuries. External fixation is preferred in the presence of gross contamination or tissue loss (see Chapter 34 for further details).

4. **Soft-tissue injuries.** Definitive closure of large soft-tissue defects rarely occurs at the initial operation for extremity trauma. Complex wounds are often thoroughly irrigated and debrided, dressed, and reviewed daily in the operating room. Delayed closure is then undertaken and may require advanced soft-tissue flaps (pedicle or free). On rare occasions, a so-called mangled extremity may require primary amputation if there are severe soft-tissue defects, major bone injury, or unreconstructable peripheral nerve injury and loss of limb function.

5. **Blunt trauma.** Blunt extremity trauma can result in debilitating crush or near-avulsion injuries. Diagnosis and management are the same as in penetrating trauma, but limb salvage and preservation of function tend to be worse due to the extent of injury. These wounds often require the coordinated involvement of multiple specialists.

6. **Extremity compartment syndromes.** Compartment syndromes are common in distal extremity trauma. They typically occur in association with prolonged limb ischemia or external pressure, fractures, crush or vascular injuries (especially combined arterial and venous injuries), and burns. **Increased tissue pressure (>30 mm Hg)** within the inelastic fascial compartment leads to occlusion of capillary flow and ischemia. Signs and symptoms of compartment syndrome include **pain (especially on passive motion), pressure, paralysis, paresthesia, pulselessness, and pallor (the so-called six *P*s).** A high index of suspicion is necessary for early diagnosis because signs often occur

late in the process, especially the loss of pulses. Serial compartment pressure measurements should therefore be undertaken in any patient with risk factors. Fasciotomy of all involved compartments is necessary when pressures are 30 to 40 mm Hg (or lower if evidence of ischemia exists). Fasciotomy of all involved compartments should also be performed after repair of traumatic vascular injuries (particularly those presenting with ischemia), in extremities with combined vascular and orthopedic injuries, and in extremities at risk for massive edema or continued ischemia. In addition, fasciotomy should be performed if pressures cannot be obtained.

J. **Damage control surgery.** The concept of damage control is well accepted among trauma surgeons as a valuable adjunct in the surgical care of severely injured patients (*Surg Clin North Am.* 1997;77:753). The damage control philosophy centers on coordinating staged operative interventions with periods of aggressive resuscitation to salvage trauma patients sustaining major injuries. These patients are often at the limits of their physiologic reserve when they present to the operating room, and persistent operative effort results in exacerbation of their underlying **hypothermia, coagulopathy, and acidosis,** initiating a vicious cycle that culminates in death. In these situations, abrupt termination of the procedure after control of surgical hemorrhage and contamination, followed by ICU resuscitation and staged reconstruction, can be lifesaving. Although often discussed in the context of abdominal trauma, the practice of damage control can be applied to all organ systems. It is divided into three phases: initial exploration, secondary resuscitation, and definitive operation.

1. **Phase I (initial exploration).** The first phase in the damage control algorithm consists of performing an initial operative exploration to attain rapid control of active hemorrhage and contamination. The decision to revert to a damage control approach should occur early in the course of such an exploration. In the setting of abdominal trauma, the patient is prepared and draped as previously described (see Section V.E), and the abdomen is entered via a midline incision. Any clot or debris present on entering the abdomen is promptly removed. If exsanguinating hemorrhage is encountered, four-quadrant packing should be performed. The packing is then removed sequentially, and all surgical hemorrhage within a particular quadrant is controlled. Following control of bleeding, attention is directed at containment of any enteric spillage. Any violations of the GI tract should be treated with suture closure or segmental stapled resection. Anastomosis and stoma formation should be deferred until later definitive reconstruction, and any stapled ends of the bowel should be returned to the abdomen. External drains are placed to control any major pancreatic or biliary injuries. Laparotomy packs are then reinserted, especially in the presence of coagulopathic bleeding. Often, primary abdominal fascial closure is not possible secondary to edematous bowel or hemodynamic instability. Alternative methods of closing the abdomen include skin closure via towel clips or running suture, Bogota bag placement, prosthetic mesh insertion, abdominal wall zipper creation, or vacuum closure. Of

all these techniques, the vacuum closure is the most commonly used. It is fashioned by placing a nonadherent material (cassette drape) between the bowel and abdominal wall, with gauze and a suction device on top, which is then sealed with an adherent dressing. Closed suction drains covered with a sterile adhesive dressing eases wound care in the ICU. Throughout the initial operative exploration, communication among the surgeons, anesthesia team, and nursing staff is essential for optimal outcome.

2. **Phase II (secondary resuscitation).** The second phase in the damage control approach focuses on secondary resuscitation to correct hypothermia, coagulopathy, and acidosis. Following completion of the initial exploration, the critically ill patient is rapidly transferred to the ICU. Invasive monitoring and complete ventilatory support are often needed. Rewarming is initiated by elevating the room temperature, placing warming blankets, and heating ventilator circuits. All IV fluids, blood, and blood products are prewarmed. As body temperature normalizes, coagulopathy improves, but rapid infusion of clotting factors (FFP, cryoprecipitate, and platelets) is often still required. Development of "Massive Transfusion Protocols" has resulted in improved outcomes and decreased mortality following massive blood losses. Most protocols focus on delivering a minimum ratio of 2 units of FFP for every 3 units of PRBC and 1 unit of platelets for every 5 units of PRBC (*J Trauma.* 2008;65(3):527–534). Use of recombinant factor VIIa in this setting has been shown to decrease the need for blood transfusion. Circulating blood volume is restored with aggressive fluid and blood product resuscitation, improving end-organ perfusion and correcting acidosis. With these interventions, hemodynamic stability returns, urinary output increases, invasive monitoring parameters improve, and serum lactate levels and blood pH analysis improve. In the setting of abdominal trauma, a potentially lethal complication that can occur during this phase is abdominal compartment syndrome. It is a form of intra-abdominal vascular insufficiency secondary to increased intra-abdominal pressure. Presentation includes abdominal distention, low urinary output, ventilatory insufficiency in association with high peak inspiratory pressures, and low cardiac output secondary to decreased venous return (preload). Diagnosis is made via measurement of urinary bladder pressure (25 to 30 cm H_2O). When present, prompt operative reexploration is mandated to relieve the increased pressure. Vacuum or Bogota bag closure helps to prevent this complication. If surgical bleeding is found to be the cause of the intra-abdominal hypertension, it should be controlled and the abdomen closed. If severe edema of the intra-abdominal contents is the source of the compartment syndrome, the abdomen should be closed by using a vacuum closure to reduce intra-abdominal pressure. Following correction of the problem, phase II resuscitation is continued.

3. **Phase III (definitive operation).** The third phase of damage control consists of planned reexploration and definitive repair of injuries. This phase typically occurs 48 to 72 hours following the initial operation and after successful secondary resuscitation. In the setting of abdominal

trauma, all complex injuries are repaired, with precedence going to those involving the vasculature. Conservative principles should be applied. Risky GI anastomoses or complex GI reconstructions should be avoided. The abdomen should be closed primarily if possible. Otherwise, biologic mesh or simple skin closure and staged repair of the resulting ventral hernia should be performed. Even though the damage control approach allows for salvage of many severely injured patients, it is still associated with substantial morbidity and mortality. Outcome is often determined by providing excellent supportive care (ventilation, nutrition, appropriate antibiotics, and physical therapy with rehabilitation services).

VI. MISCELLANEOUS ASPECTS OF GENERAL TRAUMA CARE

A. **Resuscitative thoracotomy** is performed in a final attempt to salvage a certain subset of patients presenting in extremis to the emergency department. The goals are to control intrathoracic hemorrhage, relieve cardiac tamponade, cross-clamp the thoracic aorta, and restore cardiac output.

1. **Indications.** The indications for resuscitative thoracotomy have been refined over time. It should be used in the management of penetrating chest trauma associated with significant hemodynamic deterioration (systolic BP of <60 mm Hg) or cardiopulmonary arrest occurring within the emergency department or shortly before arrival. In addition, it can be used in certain cases of penetrating abdominal trauma fulfilling the same criteria.

2. **Technique.** Resuscitative thoracotomy is performed via an anterolateral left thoracotomy in the fifth or sixth intercostal space. The skin, subcutaneous tissues, and intercostal musculature are opened sharply. A Finochietto retractor is placed to spread the ribs and aid in exposure. First, the pericardium is identified and incised vertically anterior to the phrenic nerve. Any clot or debris is removed from around the heart. Specific cardiac injury is then sought, and repair is undertaken as previously described (see Section V.D.6.a). After cardiorrhaphy, air is evacuated from the heart by needle aspiration, and the adequacy of cardiac filling is assessed to determine intravascular volume status. In the absence of associated pulmonary vascular or great-vessel injury, vigorous volume resuscitation is undertaken. If peripheral vascular access is insufficient, direct infusion into the right atrial appendage can be performed. In severely hypovolemic patients, the descending thoracic aorta may be exposed and cross-clamped to maintain coronary and cerebral perfusion. The aorta should also be clamped if any intra-abdominal hemorrhage is suspected. During volume resuscitation, open cardiac massage is employed to provide adequate circulation. After restoration of adequate circulatory volume, the underlying cardiac rhythm is assessed, and internal cardioversion is used when appropriate. The patient should be transported to the operating room for definitive injury management and wound closure after a successful resuscitation.

3. **Complications of resuscitative thoracotomy** are many. They include lung injury while gaining access to the heart, transection of the phrenic nerve while performing pericardotomy, injury to the coronary vessels during cardiorrhaphy, and esophageal trauma while clamping the descending thoracic aorta. Therefore, care must be taken during each step of the procedure to avoid causing additional injuries. In addition, a member of the trauma team sustains a needle-stick or other sharp injury in roughly 10% of resuscitative thoracotomies performed in the emergency department. As this procedure is most commonly performed in a patient population at high risk of carrying blood-borne disease, the risk to the trauma team is not insubstantial and must be considered.

B. **Diagnostic peritoneal lavage (DPL).** Since the advent of FAST and rapid helical CT imaging, DPL is now rarely used in the evaluation of patients with suspected intra-abdominal injuries. It remains, however, a useful diagnostic modality in certain situations.

1. **Indications.** DPL is useful in excluding the presence of significant intra-abdominal organ injury in the presence of blunt trauma or a stab wound to the abdomen. It should be employed when less invasive techniques (e.g., serial abdominal examinations, CT, or FAST) are unavailable or if the patient develops unexplained hemodynamic instability while in the operating room for another injury. The only absolute contraindication to DPL is a planned celiotomy. Pelvic fracture, pregnancy, and prior abdominal surgery often mandate a change in indication and technique. All patients undergoing DPL require prior evacuation of the stomach via a gastric tube as well as drainage of the bladder by indwelling catheter.

2. **Technique.** Aspiration of 10 mL of gross blood or any enteric contents is considered a positive DPL. In addition, the microscopic presence of 100,000 red blood cells/μL or 500 white blood cells/μL in the setting of blunt abdominal trauma and the presence of 10,000 red blood cells/μL or 50 white blood cells/μL in the setting of penetrating abdominal trauma is considered a positive finding on DPL.

3. **Complications.** DPL can produce false-positive results due to bleeding near the incision or from pelvic fractures hemorrhaging into the anterior preperitoneal space of Retzius. False-negative findings can occur from improper placement of the catheter and infusion of fluid into the space of Retzius. Puncture of viscera is also possible, especially in the setting of pregnancy or adhesions from prior abdominal operations. An open technique is essential in such circumstances. Although it is associated with certain complications, DPL is a safe, simple, and reliable procedure for detecting intra-abdominal injuries with excellent sensitivity (95%).

C. **Deep venous thrombosis** with pulmonary embolus is the leading cause of preventable morbidity and mortality in trauma patients. Some form of prophylaxis is required in all such patients. When neural injuries (i.e., CNS or spinal cord injuries) are absent, subcutaneous low-molecular-weight heparin should be administered. When lower-extremity injuries do not preclude their use, sequential pneumatic compression devices are beneficial. Therapy combining compression devices with subcutaneous heparin is thought to be synergistic. Therapy should be initiated early because delay in the initiation of prophylaxis is associated with a threefold increase in venous thromboembolism (*J Trauma.* 2007;62:557). When the preceding techniques are contraindicated, serious consideration should be given to early placement of a vena cava filter. Although such a filter does not prevent thrombosis, it may decrease the risk of a deadly pulmonary embolus.

D. **Gastroduodenal ulceration.** Injured patients remain at risk for stress gastroduodenal ulceration and concomitant hemorrhage. Prophylaxis is therefore recommended. Enteral feeding remains the most effective method. Parenteral histamine-receptor blockers also prevent posttraumatic GI bleeding in ventilated or coagulopathic patients. Finally, newer IV proton-pump inhibitors may find a role in prophylaxis, but their expense may prove prohibitive.

E. **Rehabilitation in trauma care.** Rehabilitation is a crucial aspect of trauma care, and its planning should begin at the time of admission. Contractures and pressure sores can begin within hours of injury, and as a result, standardized prevention must be initiated promptly on the arrival of the patient on the ward. Regular turning of the patient, placement of air mattresses, and elevation of distal extremities (especially the heel) off the bed can decrease the formation of debilitating pressure sores. Specially designed orthotic splints, braces, and stockings prevent joint and scar contractures that can inhibit return of function. Finally, early physical and occupational therapy initiates the recovery process and prepares the patient for the often difficult rehabilitation to daily activity.

VII. **CONCLUSION.** A chapter of this nature is brief by necessity, but a comprehensive strategy for the care of patients who have been involved with traumatic events will clearly improve outcomes. This care should be coordinated by dedicated general surgeons with an interest or special training in trauma and should ideally use surgical specialty services staffed by individuals with trauma expertise. Although not all institutions will be able to have dedicated trauma-oriented surgeons on staff, the development of statewide trauma systems facilitates the care of patients by directing care of these patients toward those institutions with appropriate resources. For these statewide trauma systems to survive and for the hospitals within the systems to remain financially intact, there needs to be ongoing governmental financial support for the care of trauma victims. Trauma care now costs more than any other disease in the United States and requires comprehensive public health and governmental strategies for managing the complex issues surrounding it.

Transplantation

Elizabeth A. Fialkowski and Jeffrey A. Lowell

TRANSPLANT ORGAN PROCUREMENT

I. **DONOR SELECTION.** The greatest obstacle to transplantation is the lack of suitable donor organs. Live donation has provided an important solution, especially in kidney transplantation (live donors represented 49% of total donor pool in 2009) (https://www.unos.org). Less frequently, live donation is being utilized in liver, lung, and intestinal transplantation. The waiting list for organs grows each year; in the United States as of 2010 more than 108,000 people await a solid-organ transplant (http://www.unos.org).

II. **DECEASED DONORS** (formerly known as *brain-dead* or *cadaveric donors*). Strict criteria for establishing brain death include irreversible coma and the absence of brain stem reflexes (i.e., pupillary, corneal, vestibulo-ocular, and gag reflexes). Other useful diagnostic tests include blood flow scan, arteriography, and an apnea test. **Consent** is required, and the donor's medical history is reviewed. Ideally, the donor should have stable hemodynamics, although the use of vasopressors is common. A history of cardiopulmonary resuscitation (CPR) does not preclude donation, particularly with prompt resuscitation and recovery of vital signs. The criteria for donor organ use are not absolute; therefore, all patients meeting brain death criteria should be considered as potential donors. Contraindications for donation include the presence of a malignancy (with the exception of a primary brain tumor). **Exclusion criteria** for specific organs also exist. Potential kidney donors ideally have normal renal function before brain death. Underlying medical disease (e.g., diabetes and hypertension) or vascular disease time may preclude the use of a donor kidney. Kidney biopsy may assist in the decision to use donors with existing medical disease or advanced age. Selection of a donor liver takes into account donor size, ABO blood type, age, liver function studies, hospital course, hemodynamics, and prior medical and social history. "Expanded-criteria" liver and kidney donor (e.g., those not meeting traditional inclusion criteria) have been used with increasing success. **Hypothermic machine perfusion** assesses flow and resistance of donor kidneys. Its use in deceased donor kidneys, compared to static cold storage, may reduce the incidence of delayed graft function (defined as the need for hemodialysis in the first week posttransplant) and improve graft survival in the first year, based on data from a recent international randomized control trial (*N Engl J Med.* 2009;360(1):7).

III. **DONATION FOLLOWING CARDIAC DEATH (DCD)** refers to those potential organ donors who do not meet strict brain death criteria but who are considered to have nonrecoverable devastating neurologic insults. Life support is discontinued in the operating room, and organ procurement is initiated after a specified interval following cardiac asystole.

IV. **DECEASED-DONOR ORGAN RECOVERY.** The initial dissection identifies hepatic hilar structures, including the common bile duct, portal vein, hepatic artery, and any aberrant arterial blood supply, such as a left hepatic artery branch arising from the left gastric artery or a right hepatic artery from the superior mesenteric artery (SMA). After this dissection, the liver is flushed and cooled with University of Wisconsin (UW) preservation solution (a cold-storage solution containing a high concentration of potassium, lactobionate, hydroxyethyl starch, and other antioxidants) or HTK (histidine-tryptophan-ketoglutarate, a cold-storage solution containing amino acids, potassium, magnesium, calcium, and mannitol) via cannulae placed in the portal vein and the aorta proximal to the iliac artery bifurcation. A clamp is applied to the supraceliac aorta, and the abdominal viscera are flushed with either UW or HTK cold solution. The organs are packed with ice, while the solution infuses. The donor liver is removed with its diaphragmatic attachments, a cuff of aorta surrounding the celiac axis and the SMA, and a portion of the supra- and infrahepatic vena cava. The liver is packaged in UW or HTK solution and surrounded by iced saline during transportation. The remainder of the liver dissection is performed in the recipient's operating room under cold-storage conditions. The donor kidneys are removed *en bloc* and then separated. The ureters are dissected widely to minimize devascularization and are divided near the bladder. This technique minimizes risk of injury to the arteries and allows identification of multiple renal arteries. The pancreas may also be removed for transplantation, with the pancreas, duodenum, and spleen removed *en bloc.* The blood supply for the pancreas allograft comes from the donor splenic and superior mesenteric arteries, and outflow is via the portal vein. The small intestine mesentery below the pancreas is divided with a stapling device. With the advent of modern preservation solutions, donor livers can be preserved for up to 12 hours before revascularization (kidneys up to 24 hours), with a low incidence of allograft dysfunction. Ideally, cold ischemia time is minimized to less than 6 hours.

V. **HISTOCOMPATIBILITY**

A. **Cross-matching.** Antibodies to human leukocyte antigen (HLA) do not occur naturally but are produced upon exposure to foreign histocompat-ibility antigens that may occur after pregnancy, blood transfusions, or previous transplants. The traditional test used for detecting sensitization against donor histocompatibility antigens is termed a **cross-match** or **complement-dependent lymphocytotoxicity assay.** Several cross-match methods are available, each involving the addition of recipient serum, donor cells (T cells, B cells, or monocytes), and complement. If spe-cific antidonor antibodies are present, antibody binding results in com-plement fixation and lysis of the donor lymphocytes. Flow cytometry can also be used, and permits the detection of noncytotoxic antibodies. Polymerase chain reaction (PCR) and enzyme-linked immunosorbent assay (ELISA) technology are being used increasingly for HLA typing, particularly for the major histocompatibility (MHC) class II HLA anti-gens. HLA matching is of practical clinical significance only in renal and pancreatic transplantation.

B. **Panel reactive antibodies (PRA).** The PRA assessment helps to predict the likelihood of a positive cross-match. It is determined by testing the potential recipient's serum against a panel of cells of various HLA specificities in a manner similar to the cross-match. The percentage of specificities in the panel with which the patient's sera react is the PRA. Most normal individuals do not have preformed anti-HLA antibodies and thus have a low PRA (0% to 5%). Patients who have been exposed to other HLAs or who have autoimmune diseases with antibodies recognizing HLAs may have a high PRA. These patients are more likely to have a positive cross-match.

IMMUNOSUPPRESSION

An increasing variety of immunosuppressive medications are available. The protocols outlined here are currently in use at Washington University and are intended only to serve as guidelines. Most protocols rely on the use of several drugs owing to the different mechanisms and synergies of these medications. In the first section below, a brief overview of the immunology involved in rejection will serve to introduce the roles of the various immunosuppressive medications.

I. IMMUNOLOGY OF REJECTION

A. **Immunologic response.** Organ procurement inevitably causes tissue injury and ischemia, leading to activation of interstitial immune cells (Dendritic cells, DCs) and release of reactive molecules called "Damage activated molecular pattern molecules (DAMPs)." Recipient endothelial, mesenchymal, and epithelial cells express surface and/or cytoplasmic receptors for these DAMPs. Presence of DAMPs induces cytokine and chemokine release, leading to an inflammatory response. The encounter between HLA on donor DCs and recipient T cells (via the T-cell receptor, TCR) is a key inciting event in cellular rejection, leading to activation and maturation of recipient T cells. These activated T cells secrete interleukin-2 (IL-2) and express IL-2 receptors, leading to division and proliferation.

B. **Immunosuppression. Corticosteroids** play the broadest role against rejection, targeting both the innate (e.g., DCs and DAMPs) and adaptive (e.g., T and B cells) responses, leading to inhibition of T cell proliferation. The initial encounter between donor DCs and recipient TCRs is blocked by the monoclonal antibody **OKT3.** Other antibodies target the signaling process that occurs with this encounter (e.g., **Alefacept**). Once the signaling events are underway, calcineurin inhibitors **(Cyclosporine, Tacrolimus)** block the early stages of T-cell activation. Autocrine stimulation of T-cells by IL-2 is blocked by monoclonal antibodies to the T-cell IL-2 receptor **(Daclizmab, Basiliximab).** Multiple signaling pathways are activated by IL-2 binding, including the MAP kinase, PI3 kinase, and JAK/STAT pathways, the last of which is blocked by a JAK3 inhibitor **CP-690 550,** currently in clinical trials. In addition to IL-2, the mammalian target of rapamycin (mTOR) molecule is a potent stimulus for T-cell division, and is targeted by **Sirolimus.** Later inhibitors of the cell cycle include **Azathioprine** (purine synthesis inhibitor) and **Mycophenolic** acid (**CellCept/Myfortic** inhibits RNA synthesis).

II. IMMUNOSUPPRESSIVE MEDICATIONS

A. **Prednisone or methylprednisolone (Solu-Medrol).** Corticosteroids are part of most immunosuppressive regimens and are the first-line drug in the treatment of rejection. Steroids modify antigen processing and presentation, inhibit lymphocyte proliferation, and inhibit cytokine and prostaglandin production. After surgery, patients are placed on a steroid taper and maintained on a low dose of prednisone or eventually withdrawn from the drug altogether. Steroid avoidance and early steroid-withdrawal protocols have demonstrated good short-term results. Long-term results are unknown. Acute and chronic side effects of steroids include diabetes mellitus (DM) (10% of patients), infections, cataracts, hypertension, weight gain, and bone disease (osteoporosis, and joint deterioration with avascular necrosis).

B. **Tacrolimus (FK506, Prograf)** is a macrolide that has a mechanism of action similar to that of cyclosporine but is approximately 100 times more potent. Tacrolimus doses are adjusted to maintain 12-hour trough levels between 5 and 10 ng/mL [fluorescence polarization immunoassay (FPIA)]. The side effect profile is similar to that of cyclosporine but does not include hirsutism and gingival hyperplasia. Alopecia and posttransplant diabetes mellitus (PTDM) are more common with tacrolimus.

C. **Cyclosporine (Sandimmune, Neoral, Gengraf).** Cyclosporine is a small fungal cyclic compound, in a class of medications termed calcineurin inhibitors. These block T-cell activation, thus inhibiting T-lymphocyte proliferation, IL-2 production, IL-2 receptor expression, and interferon-γ release. Two-hour peaks and/or 12-hour troughs are monitored and adjusted based on time from transplant. Side effects include nephrotoxicity, hypertension, tremors, seizures, hyperkalemia, hyperuricemia, hypercholesterolemia, gingival hyperplasia, and hirsutism. Cyclosporine is metabolized by the liver. Common medications that may increase cyclosporine levels include diltiazem, verapamil, erythromycin, fluconazole, ketoconazole, tetracycline, metoclopramide, and cimetidine. Medications that decrease levels include intravenous trimethoprim/sulfamethoxazole, isoniazid, rifampin, phenytoin, phenobarbital, carbamazepine, and omeprazole.

D. **Sirolimus (Rapamune)** is an anti-T-cell agent that inhibits the mTOR molecule, blocking T-cell signal transduction. Side effects include thrombocytopenia, hyperlipidemia, oral ulcers, anemia, proteinuria, and impairment of wound healing.

E. **Mycophenolic acid (CellCept, Myfortic)** inhibits inosine monophosphate dehydrogenase (rate-limiting enzyme in guanine monophosphate synthesis,) inhibiting RNA synthesis. In so doing, this drug selectively inhibits T- and B-cell proliferation, cytotoxic T-cell generation, and antibody formation. It is used as an alternative to azathioprine, and is the antimetabolite of choice in most transplant programs. Major toxicities include gastrointestinal (GI) disturbances and increased cytomegalovirus (CMV) infection.

F. **Azathioprine (Imuran)** is an antimetabolite that is a thioguanine derivative of mercaptopurine. This purine analog alters the function or synthesis of DNA and RNA, inhibiting T- and B-lymphocyte proliferation. One of the major side effects is bone marrow suppression, manifested as leukopenia and thrombocytopenia. An important drug interaction occurs with allopurinol, which blocks the metabolism of azathioprine and increases the degree of bone marrow suppression.

G. **Polyclonal antithymocyte antibodies.** Polyclonal antibodies are immunologic products with antibodies to a wide variety of T-cell antigens, adhesion molecules, costimulatory molecules, cytokines, the T-cell receptor, and class I and II MHC molecules. These agents are used as induction therapy in the perioperative period or as rescue therapy following acute rejection. The most commonly used antithymocyte immunoglobulin in the United States is **Thymoglobulin.** Thymoglobulin, a rabbit-derived product, was shown to decrease the incidence of acute rejection in deceased donor renal transplants compared to use of an IL-2 receptor antagonist, basiliximab (*N Engl J Med.* 2006;355:1967). Common side effects include fever, leukopenia, and thrombocytopenia.

H. **Monoclonal antibodies.** **OKT3** is a murine monoclonal antibody that recognizes the T-cell receptor and blocks antigen recognition, hindering T-cell effector functions and potentiating T-cell lysis. OKT3 is usually administered to patients with steroid-resistant, severe rejection. Immediate side effects can include fever, chills, hypotension, respiratory distress, and pulmonary edema, all of which are secondary to the cytokine release syndrome. **Daclizumab (Zenapax)** and **basiliximab (Simulect)** are IL-2 receptor-specific monoclonal antibodies increasingly being used as induction therapy, which are begun immediately prior to transplantation and continued in the immediate postoperative period.

I. **Other immunomodulators** are under investigation and are at varying stages of development.

III. COMPLICATIONS OF IMMUNOSUPPRESSION

A. **Bacterial infections.** Pneumonia and urinary tract infections (UTIs) occur fairly commonly after transplantation. Infectious complications from opportunistic organisms are now uncommon because of appropriate prophylactic strategies.

B. **Viral infections.** The most common viral infections after transplantation include **CMV, Epstein–Barr virus (EBV), herpes simplex virus (HSV),** and **BK virus.** See Table 23-1 for a summary of prophylaxis and treatment for common viral and fungal infections.

1. **CMV** infection can occur at any time but is most common 1 to 4 months posttransplant, in the absence of prophylaxis. CMV may infect the recipient's liver, lungs, or GI tract. Signs and symptoms include fever, chills, malaise, anorexia, nausea, vomiting, cough, abdominal pain, hypoxia, leukopenia, and elevation in liver transaminases. CMV peripheral blood PCR or serologic assays are the most common tools for diagnosis. CMV can be associated with significant morbidity and even mortality, but typically responds well to early diagnosis and treatment. There is also evidence that CMV contributes to allograft injury. Prophylaxis may be useful in any patient who receives a CMV-positive allograft because many of these patients develop a significant CMV

TABLE 23-1	Prophylaxis and Treatment of Infections in Immunosuppressed Patients

CMV
Prophylaxis
Ganciclovir, 1,000 mg PO TID (1 yr for D+/R–, 6 mo for D+R+, 3 mo for D–/R+,) *or*
Valganciclovir, 900 mg PO QD (reduce dose for renal insufficiency)
Treatment
Ganciclovir, 5 mg/kg IV q12 hr for 3 wk, *or*
Valganciclovir, 900 mg PO BID for minimum 3 wk and until virus cleared, in the absence of invasive disease
Consider unselected IgG, 500 mg/kg IV QID for 5 d for pneumonitis or colitis, *or*
Hyperimmune CMV IgG, 100 mg/kg IV QID for 5 doses for pneumonitis or colitis

Epstein–Barr virus
Prophylaxis
Acyclovir, 200 mg PO BID for life (D+/R–)
Treatment
Decrease immunosuppression
Ganciclovir, 5 mg/kg IV q12 hr for 3 wk
Chemotherapy for patients with lymphoproliferative disorders

Herpes simplex virus (HSV)
Prophylaxis
Acyclovir 200 mg PO BID for 3 mo [only D (donor)–/R (recipient)–; otherwise CMV treatment will also cover HSV]
For liver transplant patients, for 3–6 mo or until prednisone is <10 mg/d
Treatment
Decrease immunosuppression
Acyclovir, 5–10 mg IV q8 hr for 7–10 d

Candida
Prophylaxis of oral candidiasis
Nystatin, 5 mL (500,000 units) swish and swallow QID for 3 mo, *or*
Miconazole, troche suck and swallow QID for 3 mo, *or*
Fluconazole, 100 mg PO every week for 3 mo
Treatment of esophageal candidiasis
Fluconazole, 100 mg PO BID, *or*
Voriconazole, 200 mg PO BID

***Pneumocystis* pneumonia**
Prophylaxis
Trimethoprim/sulfamethoxazole, 1 single-strength tablet PO QD
Dapsone, 50 mg PO QD for sulfa allergy, *or*
Pentamidine, 300 mg per nebulizer every month for sulfa allergy and G6PD deficiency

BID, twice daily; CMV, cytomegalovirus; G6PD, glucose-6-phosphate dehydrogenase; IgG, immunoglobulin G; IV, intravenously; PO, orally; q12h, every 12 hr; QD, daily; QID, four times a day.

infection if left untreated. Treatment consists of decreasing immuno-suppression and administering ganciclovir, which inhibits DNA synthesis. Valganciclovir, intravenous ganciclovir, and, to a lesser extent, oral ganciclovir dosing must be adjusted for renal dysfunction. The most common side effects of valganciclovir and ganciclovir are anemia, neutropenia, and thrombocytopenia.

2. **EBV** can infect B cells at any time after transplantation and may be associated with the development of a type of lymphoma, termed post-transplant lymphoproliferative disorder (PTLD), usually of mono-clonal B-cell origin. Infiltration of the hematopoietic system, central nervous system (CNS), lungs, or other solid organs may occur. The patient usually presents with fever, chills, sweats, enlarged lymph nodes, and elevated uric acid. Diagnosis is made by physical examination; EBV serology; computed tomography (CT) scan of the head, chest, and abdomen (to evaluate lymph nodes or masses); and biopsy of potential sites or lesions. Treatment consists of reducing or with-drawing immunosuppression. Acyclovir prophylaxis for life may be considered in EBV donor$^+$/recipient$^-$ patients. In addition, **rituximab** (monoclonal antibody against the protein CD20 on the surface of B cells) with standard chemotherapy should be considered for resistant advanced disease or polyclonal tumors.

3. **HSV** causes characteristic ulcers on the oral mucosa, in the genital region, and in the esophagus. Renal transplant patients, if not on gan-ciclovir, are given prophylactic acyclovir. Active HSV infections are treated by decreasing the patient's immunosuppression and instituting acyclovir therapy. Side effects of acyclovir are rare but include nephro-toxicity, phlebitis, bone marrow suppression, and CNS toxicity.

4. **BK virus** is a member of the polyoma virus family. Approximately 90% of individuals are seropositive. BK viruria (detected by "decoy cell" shedding or PCR) develops in 30% of kidney transplant recipi-ents and progresses to viremia in 15% of recipients within the first year. Persistent viremia leads to BK nephropathy, which occurs in up to 10% of kidney transplant recipients during the first year. There is no known effective treatment, though low-dose cidofovir (0.25 mg/kg intravenously every 2 weeks) has been tried. Until recently, early graft loss occurred in 50% of patients with BK nephropathy, and the other 50% were left with chronic allograft dysfunction. Recently, prospective monitoring and preemptive reduction in immunosuppression has been associated with prevention of nephropathy and better outcomes when nephropathy is diagnosed early.

C. **Fungal infections** can range from asymptomatic colonization to lethal invasive infections. Oral **candidiasis** can be prevented and treated with oral nystatin or fluconazole. Esophageal candidiasis can be treated with a short course of intravenous amphotericin B or fluconazole. Serious fungal infections are treated with intravenous amphotericin B, although use of less nephrotoxic agents such as caspofungin and anidulafungin is increasing.

D. **Other opportunistic infections.** *Pneumocystis jiroveci* (formerly *carinii*) *pneumonia* is a potentially lethal pneumonia that occurs in 5% to 10% of renal transplant patients receiving no prophylactic treatment. Patients typically present with fever, dyspnea, nonproductive cough, hypoxia, and pulmonary infiltrates. Diagnosis is made by bronchoalveolar lavage or lung biopsy. It can be prevented by low-dose trimethoprim/sulfamethoxazole, dapsone, or inhaled pentamidine. Treatment involves much higher doses of these agents, with a concomitant decrease in immunosuppression.

E. **Malignancies.** Cancers that occur at a higher frequency in transplant recipients include squamous cell carcinoma, basal cell carcinoma, Kaposi sarcoma, lymphomas, hepatobiliary carcinoma, and cervical carcinoma.

KIDNEY TRANSPLANTATION

I. **INDICATIONS. End-Stage Renal Disease (ESRD)** results when the functioning renal mass deteriorates to less than 10% to 20% of normal. **Indications** for renal transplantation include the presence of ESRD with an irreversible glomerular filtration rate (GFR) of less than 20 mL/minute. ESRD may affect multiple organ systems, resulting in altered fluid and electrolyte homeostasis, accumulation of metabolic waste products, anemia, hypertension, and metabolic bone disease. Excellent short- and long-term results can be achieved regardless of the cause of renal failure (Table 23-2). Renal failure secondary to DM is the most common disease process in the United States requiring renal transplantation, comprising as many as 25% of all cases.

TABLE 23-2	Causes of Renal Failure Requiring Transplantation
Type	**Characteristics**
Congenital	Aplasia, obstructive uropathy
Hereditary	Alport syndrome (hereditary nephritis), polycystic kidney disease, tuberous sclerosis
Neoplastic	Renal cell carcinoma, Wilms tumor
Progressive	Diabetic neuropathy, chronic pyelonephritis, Goodpasture syndrome (antiglomerular basement membrane disease), hypertension, chronic glomerulonephritis, lupus nephritis, nephrotic syndrome, obstructive uropathy, scleroderma, amyloidosis
Traumatic	Vascular occlusion, parenchymal destruction

II. CONTRAINDICATIONS

A. **Recent or metastatic malignancy.** In general, most transplantation centers require a significant (2- to 5-year) disease-free interval after the treatment of a malignant tumor. Exceptions include early-stage skin cancers and *in situ* cancers.

B. **Chronic infection.** The presence of any active, life-threatening infection precludes transplantation and the use of immunosuppressive therapy. If the infection can be treated either medically or surgically, the patient should be reconsidered for transplantation after therapy. Infection with the human immunodeficiency virus (HIV) is a contraindication to renal transplantation at most centers.

C. **Severe extrarenal disease** may preclude transplantation in certain circumstances, either because the patient is not an operative candidate or because the transplantation and associated immunosuppression may accelerate disease progression (i.e., chronic liver disease, chronic lung disease, and advanced uncorrectable heart disease). Severe peripheral vascular disease may also be a contraindication.

D. **Noncompliance.** Any patient with a history of repeated noncompliance with medical therapy should be considered high risk. A period of compliance before being placed on the waiting list is generally advised.

III. PREOPERATIVE WORKUP AND EVALUATION.
Patients referred to a transplantation center are seen by a transplantation surgeon, nephrologist, social worker, and transplantation coordinator. Evaluation of a potential recipient is outlined in Table 23-3. The evaluation identifies coexisting problems or disease entities that must be addressed to improve the outcome of the transplantation. Family history is important because it may provide information about the patient's kidney disease and allows a discussion about potential living donors. When the evaluation is complete, the patient is presented at a multidisciplinary evaluation committee meeting, where a decision is made as to whether to accept the patient as a potential recipient. Allocation of a given organ to a specific patient is done using a computer-generated algorithm run by the United Network for Organ Sharing (UNOS) and is based on specific criteria, which are different for each organ [e.g., blood type, HLA matching, waiting time, prior sensitization (i.e., high PRA rating), and medical urgency for kidney allocation]. Once a patient is active on the waiting list, blood is sent monthly to the tissue-typing laboratory for cross-matching and to determine the PRA.

A. **Special considerations.** The lower urinary tract should be sterile, continent, and compliant before transplantation. In patients with a history of bladder dysfunction, DM, or recurrent UTIs, a voiding cystourethrogram may be obtained before transplantation. Transplant ureter implantation into the native bladder is preferred and usually can be achieved, even in small bladders and those that have been diverted previously.

B. **Pretransplantation native nephrectomy** has been avoided secondary to the anemia that develops following removal of endogenous erythropoietin production. It is only performed in patients with chronic renal parenchymal infection, infected renal calculi, heavy proteinuria, intractable hypertension,

TABLE 23-3	Pretransplantation Evaluation of Renal Transplant Recipients

Initial workup

History and physical examination

Laboratory analyses: complete blood count; partial thromboplastin time; prothrombin time; serum electrolytes; total protein, albumin, cholesterol, glucose, calcium, magnesium, and phosphorus; liver function tests; intact parathyroid hormone; prostate-specific antigen (men >40 yr); viral serologies (herpes simplex virus; Epstein–Barr virus; varicella-zoster virus; cytomegalovirus; hepatitis A, B, C; and human immunodeficiency virus); urinalysis and culture; purified protein derivative; panel reactive antibody; ABO and human leukocyte antigen typing; serum for frozen storage

Electrocardiography

Chest X-ray

Routine examinations

Dental

Stool guaiac (Hemoccult)

Pap smear

Mammogram (women >35 yr)

Ophthalmologic (diabetic patients)

Psychosocial
Secondary workup (based on preliminary finding)
Cardiac: exercise stress electrocardiography, dobutamine stress echocardiography, coronary angiography
Pulmonary: arterial blood gas, pulmonary function tests
Gastrointestinal tract: upper and lower endoscopy, right upper quadrant ultrasonography
Genitourinary: voiding cystourethrography, cystoscopy, retrograde ureterography

massive polycystic kidney disease with pain or bleeding, renal cystic disease that is suspicious for carcinoma, or infected reflux nephropathy. Erythropoietin renders pretransplantation nephrectomy more acceptable, especially in patients with intractable hypertension whose posttransplantation management can be difficult without nephrectomy.

C. **Living donors.** Living kidney donation has become an important part of renal transplant practice. Parent–child or sibling combinations are the most common, although biologically unrelated donors are increasingly being used. Advantages of living-donor transplantation include improved short- and long-term graft survival (1-year survival >95%), improved immediate allograft function, planned operative timing to allow for medical optimization (and, often, avoidance of dialysis), fewer rejection and infection episodes, and shorter hospital stays. Although expanded-criteria deceased donors (who tend to be older) have increased the donor pool, a living donor, if available, is preferred to a deceased donor. The primary goal in evaluating a potential living donor is to ensure the donor's well-being and safety. The donor must be in excellent health and must not have any illnesses, such as hypertension or diabetes, which may threaten his or her renal function in the future. The donor anatomy is evaluated with CT or magnetic resonance (MR) angiography. Donor kidneys are now commonly removed using laparoscopic or mininephrectomy techniques to minimize donor morbidity.

D. **Expanded-criteria donors (ECD).** These donors are usually over 60 years of age, or over 50 years of age with at least 2 of the following: hypertension, serum creatinine greater than 1.5 mg/dL, or death from a cerebrovascular accident. A recent retrospective study of more than 1,000 deceased donor renal transplants demonstrated higher rates of delayed graft function with ECD kidneys, but similar 5-year graft survival (*Transplantation.* 2010;89(1):88).

IV. **ABO INCOMPATIBLE TRANSPLANTATION.** Incompatibility due to blood type or HLA alloantibodies has historically been a barrier to living kidney donation. Since the 1980s, however, transplantation across this barrier has been accomplished – through ABO incompatible (ABOi) transplantation and paired exchange, which enables donors to be matched with compatible recipients.

A. **ABOi transplantation.** Isohemagglutinins are antibodies against blood group A and/or B. Production of these antibodies in a recipient leads to hyperacute rejection and graft loss. Using preoperative plasmapheresis to deplete these isohemagglutinins, as well as induction immunosuppression and pretransplant splenectomy, GP Alexander and colleagues in Belgium pioneered ABOi transplantation in the 1980s. Since this time, experience in Belgium, Japan, and the United States has included more than 1000 ABOi transplants, and long-term outcomes have been comparable to traditional living donor renal transplants (5-year graft survival approximately 79%). There remains a significant early risk of rejection in these transplants—approximately 10% to 30% develop acute antibody-mediated rejection (AAMR), and up to 10% have irreversible rejection within the first month. Isohemagglutinin levels inevitably return to baseline, and yet the majority of grafts survive this early high-risk period. These grafts undergo accommodation, whereby antidonor antibodies are present and yet there is no allograft injury. Animal models have suggested that upregulation of endothelial protective mechanisms may be involved in this process, but research is ongoing. Current protocols to optimize long-term ABOi graft survival include (1) preoperative plasmapheresis and immunoabsorption to reduce isohemagglutinin titers (goal ≤1:8), (2) induction with rituximab, and (3) immunosuppression regimens involving tacrolimus and mycophenolate (*Curr Opin Organ Transplant*. 2010;15:526).

B. **Paired exchange and chain donation.** A living kidney donor with an intended ABOi recipient, or living donor with no intended recipient (altruistic), can donate to an ABO compatible recipient through paired exchange and chain donation. This idea was started in New England in 2001, when UNOS created a network that matched appropriate living kidney donors to recipients, and led to the New England Program for Kidney Exchange in 2004. Complex computer algorithms now allow similar programs across the country, matching donor to recipient based on ABO blood type, HLA typing, and predicted cross-match results. The simplest example of a kidney-**paired exchange** occurs as a two-pair exchange – where Donor no. 1 is compatible with Recipient no. 2, and Donor no. 2 is compatible with Recipient no. 1. These matches can become more complicated with several pairs involved. **Chain donation** occurs when living donors are combined with deceased donor grafts to complete a set of compatible pairs. This includes nondirected or altruistic donors, who enable multiple recipients to undergo transplantation by their single gift. Extensive planning is required to coordinate these paired donations, and all centers must agree on the logistics in advance. Final cross-matches are conducted prior to surgery, and donor surgeons converse in the operating room prior to incision time. Ethical and legal concerns about donation across transplant centers led to an amendment of the National Organ Transplant Act (NOTA) in 2007, clarifying that interstate human organ paired donation is legal.

V. **PREOPERATIVE CONSIDERATIONS.** When a kidney becomes available, the recipient is admitted to the hospital, and the surgeon, nephrologist, and anesthesiologist perform a final preoperative evaluation. Routine laboratory studies and a final cross-match are performed. The need for preoperative dialysis depends on the patient's volume status and serum potassium. Generally, a patient with evidence of volume overload or serum potassium greater than 5.6 mEq/L (5.6 mmol/L) requires preoperative HD. Induction therapy with a polyclonal antibody preparation is given intraoperatively.

VI. **OPERATIVE CONSIDERATIONS**

A. **Technique.** In the operating room, a Foley catheter is inserted, and the patient's bladder is irrigated with antibiotic-containing solution. A central venous pressure (CVP) line is inserted, and a first-generation cephalosporin is administered. The transplant renal vein and artery typically are anastomosed to the external iliac vein and artery, respectively. A heparin bolus of 3,000 units is administered before clamping the iliac vessels. Before reperfusion of the kidney, mannitol (25 g) and furosemide (100 mg) are administered intravenously, and the patient's systolic blood pressure (BP) is maintained above 120 mm Hg, with a CVP of at least 10 mm Hg to ensure optimal perfusion of the transplanted kidney. The ureter can be anastomosed to either the recipient bladder or the ipsilateral ureter, although the bladder is preferred. Establishing an antireflux mechanism is essential for preventing posttransplantation reflux pyelonephritis. This is accomplished by performing an extravesical ureteroneocystostomy (Litch). A double-J ureteral stent is commonly used.

B. **Intraoperative fluid management.** The newly transplanted kidney is sensitive to volume contraction, and adequate perfusion is essential for immediate postoperative diuresis and acute tubular necrosis (ATN) prevention. Volume contraction should not occur, and volume status is constantly monitored by checking the patient's cardiac function, CVP, and BP. The initial posttransplantation urine outputs can vary dramatically based on many factors. It is imperative to know the patient's native urine volume to assess the contribution of the native and the transplanted kidney to posttransplantation urine output. Dopamine may be administered at a level of 2 to 5 μg/kg/minute intravenously to promote renal blood flow and support systemic BP.

VII. POSTOPERATIVE CONSIDERATIONS

A. **General care.** Many aspects of postoperative care are the same as those for any other general surgical patient. Early ambulation is encouraged, and the need for good pulmonary toilet and wound care is the same. The bladder catheter is left in place for 3 to 7 days.

B. **Intravenous fluid replacement.** In general, the patient should be kept euvolemic or mildly hypervolemic in the early posttransplantation period. Hourly urine output is replaced with one-half normal saline on a milliliter-for-milliliter basis because the sodium concentration of the urine from a newly transplanted kidney is 60 to 80 mEq/L (60 to 80 mmol/L). Insensible fluid losses during this period typically are 30 to 60 mL/hour and essentially are water losses that can be replaced by a solution of 5% dextrose in 0.45% normal saline at 30 mL/hour. Therefore, during the early posttransplantation period, the patient's intravenous fluid consists of one-half normal saline administered at a rate equal to the previous hour's urine output plus 30 mL of 5% dextrose in 0.45% normal saline. This formula requires the patient's volume status to be assessed repeatedly. If the posttransplantation urine output is low and the patient is thought to be hypovolemic (based on clinical and hemodynamic evaluation), isotonic saline boluses are given. Potassium chloride replacement usually is not required unless the urine output is very high, and even then it should be given with great care. Potassium chloride especially should be avoided in the oliguric posttransplantation patient.

C. **GI tract.** Gastritis and peptic ulcer disease occur secondary to steroid therapy in the transplantation patient. Therefore, patients are prophylactically treated with famotidine (20 mg/day orally or intravenously) or lansoprazole (30 mg/day orally).

D. **Renal allograft function or nonfunction.** If the patient's urine output is low in the early postoperative period (<50 mL/hour), volume status must be addressed first. If the patient is hypovolemic, 250 to 500 mL of isotonic saline should be given in bolus fashion and repeated once, if needed. If the patient is euvolemic, the bladder catheter should be irrigated to ensure patency. If clots are encountered, a larger catheter and/or continuous bladder irrigation may be needed. If the catheter is patent and the patient is euvolemic or hypervolemic, furosemide (100 to 200 mg intravenously for recipients of deceased-donor transplants, 20 to 40 mg intravenously for those with living-donor transplants) should be given. If diuresis follows these maneuvers, urine output is again replaced milliliter for milliliter with one-half normal saline. Early poor function of a transplanted kidney is most commonly due to reversible ATN. Immunologic and reperfusion injury also may play some role in the mechanism leading to ATN. Before the diagnosis of ATN can be made, however, noninvasive studies (renal Doppler ultrasonography or technetium-99 m renal scan) demonstrating vascular patency and good renal blood flow in the absence of hydronephrosis (renal ultrasonography) or urinary leak must be obtained. If flow is confirmed, dialysis can be continued until the transplanted kidney function recovers.

E. **Immunosuppression.** A variety of immunosuppressive protocols exist. The protocol in use at Washington University is discussed here and another is outlined in Table 23-5. Induction therapy with Thymoglobulin (1.5 mg/kg intravenously) is given intraoperatively and then daily during the first 2 posttransplantation days. Posttransplantation, patients receive tacrolimus (0.05 mg/kg orally twice a day to maintain trough 5 to 7 ng/mL), Myfortic (720 mg orally twice a day, reduced to 360 mg on day 5), and prednisone (1 mg/kg orally per day for days 1 to 3, 0.5 mg/kg orally per day for days 4 to 14, then 20 mg orally per day, decreasing by 2.5 to 5 mg each week to a goal of 5 mg/day by week 13). Methylprednisolone (7 mg/kg intravenously) is given in the operating room.

VIII. **REJECTION.** There are several different types of rejection. Some are preventable, whereas others can be treated with varying degrees of success.

A. **Hyperacute** rejection occurs when preformed anti-HLA antibodies bind the endothelium of the allograft and initiate a cascade of events culminating in vascular thrombosis and ischemic necrosis. Hyperacute rejection usually can be prevented by cross-matching donor lymphocytes with recipient serum. Hyperacute rejection usually occurs within minutes of cross-clamp release and is irreversible. Viability of the allograft can be assessed by intraoperative biopsy. The only therapeutic option is to remove the allograft immediately. This is extraordinarily uncommon in the modern era of cross-matching.

B. **Accelerated** rejection also appears to be antibody-mediated and usually occurs 12 to 72 hours after transplantation. The patient usually is anuric or oliguric and has fever and graft tenderness. Although treatment is not well defined, administration of an antilymphocyte preparation may salvage the graft. Accelerated rejection can lead to an immunologically mediated ATN from which good renal function recovery can occur.

C. **Acute** rejection is cell-mediated and involves T lymphocytes and soluble mediators called lymphokines. It happens in 10% to 40% of patients and typically occurs 1 to 6 weeks after transplantation. The development of a rising creatinine level should prompt the consideration of

TABLE 23-4	Treatment of Rejection
Corticosteroids	
Intravenous pulse, methylprednisolone	
7 mg/kg QD for 3 d	
Consider if rejection is early (<3 mo) or mild	
Oral pulse, prednisone	
3 mg/kg QD in 2–4 divided doses for 3–5 d	
After pulse, restart steroids at previous dose	
Use if patient is reliable and rejection is early or mild	
Tacrolimus	
Target 12-hr trough level 5–15 ng/mL	
Antilymphocyte preparations	
Thymoglobulin	
2–3 mg/kg IV for 3–4 d	
Myfortic	
720 mg PO BID	
Rapamycin	
4 mg PO QD, target level 8–20 ng/mL	
Plasmapheresis	
Consider for antibody-mediated rejection	

BID, twice a day; IV, intravenously; PO, orally, QD, daily.

rejection. Technetium-99m renal scan demonstrates decreased but persistent perfusion. Diagnosis is confirmed by percutaneous needle biopsy. There are two basic treatment modalities (Table 23-4): high-dose methylprednisolone and an antilymphocyte preparation. The latter generally is reserved for steroid-resistant rejection, although antilymphocyte therapy may be used as first-line therapy for moderate or severe rejections with arteritis. Maintenance immunosuppression may also be switched (i.e., from cyclosporine to tacrolimus). More than 90% of acute rejection episodes can be treated successfully.

D. **Chronic** rejection is a poorly understood phenomenon that can occur weeks to years after transplantation. Emerging evidence suggests that in addition to calcineurin toxicity, the humoral immune response is an important contributor. Detection of antidonor-specific antibodies, an elevated posttransplant PRA, or C4d staining on a biopsy is supportive of humoral or antibody-mediated rejection. Plasmapheresis, intravenous immunoglobulin, and rituximab have been used to treat antibody-mediated rejection.

IX. **SURGICAL COMPLICATIONS OF RENAL TRANSPLANTATION.** Wound seromas, hematomas, and infections are treated according to usual surgical principles. Other complications require special consideration.

A. **Lymphoceles** are lymph collections that occur because of lymphatic leaks in the retroperitoneum. They present one week to several weeks after transplantation and are best diagnosed by ultrasonography. Most are asymptomatic and are found incidentally. They may produce ureteral obstruction, deep venous thrombosis, leg swelling, or incontinence secondary to bladder compression. Most lymphoceles arise from leakage of lymph from the donor kidney. Treatment of symptomatic lymphoceles consists of percutaneous drainage. Open or laparoscopic internal drainage by marsupialization into the peritoneal cavity may be necessary because repeated percutaneous drainage is not advised and seldom leads to resolution of the lymphocele.

B. **Renal artery and vein thrombosis.** Arterial and venous thromboses most often occur in the first 1 to 3 days after transplantation. If the kidney had been functioning but a sudden cessation of urine output occurs, graft thrombosis should be suspected. A rapid rise in serum creatinine, graft swelling, and local pain ensues. If the allograft had not been functioning or if the native kidneys make a large amount of urine, there may be no signs of graft thrombosis. The transplanted kidney has no collateral circulation and has minimal tolerance for warm ischemia. The diagnosis is made by technetium-99m renal scan or Doppler ultrasonography. Unless the problem is diagnosed and repaired immediately, the graft will be lost and transplantation nephrectomy will be required.

C. **Urine leak.** The etiology is usually anastomotic leak or ureteral sloughing secondary to ureteral blood supply disruption. Urine leaks present with pain, rising creatinine, and possibly urine draining from the wound. Diagnosis is made by locating the fluid collection with ultrasonography and then aspirating the fluid and comparing its creatinine level to the serum creatinine level. A renal scan demonstrates radioisotope outside the urinary tract. Urine leaks are treated by placing a bladder catheter to reduce intravesical pressure and subsequent surgical exploration. If an anastomotic leak is found, the distal ureter can be resected and reimplanted. If the transplanted ureter is nonviable or if there is inadequate length, ureteroureterostomy over a double-J stent using the ipsilateral native ureter can be performed. The stent can be removed via cystoscopy several weeks later.

TABLE 23-5	Long-Term Maintenance Immunosuppression for Renal Transplantation
Myfortic	
720 mg PO BID	
Reduce to 360 mg PO BID when used with tacrolimus and for WBC <5,000/mm^3, diarrhea, first week posttransplant	
Prednisone	
1 mg/kg QD for days 1–3	
20 mg QD for days 4–14	
15 mg QD for week 3	
10 mg QD for week 4	
5 mg QD for week 5 and onward	
Tacrolimus	
5 mg PO BID, target level 5–7 ng/mL (FPIA)	
Levels >15 ng/mL are considered toxic	

BID, twice daily; FPIA fluorescence polarization immunoassay; PO, orally; WBC, white blood cell count; QD, daily.

X. **LONG-TERM FOLLOW-UP.** Immunosuppression (Table 23-5) and infection prophylaxis (Table 23-1) should be tapered with time. After the initial 3-month period, when acute rejection becomes less of a risk, tacrolimus and steroid doses are tapered. Chronic long-term immunosuppression can be maintained at lower levels than those required for induction. Rarely immunosuppression can be discontinued completely. Specific metabolic consequences of tacrolimus (including hypertension and nephrotoxicity) can be alleviated with dose reduction, but often specific therapy is needed. Dietary manipulation and gradual dose reduction are important to correct steroid-associated weight gain. Long-term complications of steroids can be minimized by using as low a dose of prednisone as possible. Antibiotic prophylaxis should be used before any surgical or dental procedure.

LIVER TRANSPLANTATION

I. **INDICATIONS FOR HEPATIC TRANSPLANTATION** include complications attributable to end-stage liver disease (ESLD). In the absence of other

TABLE 23-6	Most Common Indications for Orthotopic Liver Transplantation

Adults

Chronic hepatitis C	Primary biliary cirrhosis
Alcoholic liver disease	Primary sclerosing cholangitis
Chronic hepatitis B	Autoimmune hepatitis

Children

Extrahepatic biliary atresia	Primary hepatic tumors
α_1-Antitrypsin deficiency	Metabolic liver disease
Cystic fibrosis	

medical contraindications, virtually any disease resulting in ESLD is amenable to transplantation. The most common diseases for which orthotopic liver transplantation (OLT) is performed are listed in Table 23-6. Common indications for OLT in patients with ESLD include variceal hemorrhage, intractable ascites, encephalopathy, intractable pruritus, and poor synthetic function. Stage I or II hepatocellular carcinoma in a cirrhotic liver is an increasingly common indication for transplantation, within the Milan criteria (single lesions less than 5 cm or three lesions less than 3 cm). Improved long-term survival has been achieved in select patients undergoing transplantation for early-stage hilar cholangiocarcinoma, according to a protocol developed by the Mayo Clinic (*HPB* (Oxford) 2008;10(3):186). This protocol involves neoadjuvant chemotherapy, staging abdominal exploration, and subsequent transplantation.

II. **CONTRAINDICATIONS.** There are a few absolute contraindications to liver transplantation: multisystem organ failure, extrahepatic malignancy, poor cardiac or pulmonary reserve, refractory pulmonary artery hypertension, severe infection, and ongoing substance abuse. Renal insufficiency increases the morbidity of hepatic transplantation but is not a contraindication. Renal transplantation can be performed at the time of liver transplantation for patients with ESRD. Some degree of preoperative renal insufficiency is often reversible after successful liver transplantation.

III. **PULMONARY SYNDROMES IN LIVER DISEASE**

A. **Hepatopulmonary syndrome (HPS).** This syndrome has two defining characteristics: (1) intrapulmonary vasodilation in the presence of hepatic dysfunction or portal hypertension, with (2) a widened age-corrected alveolar-arterial oxygen gradient on room air (more than 15 to 20 mm Hg), with or without hypoxemia (PaO_2 less than 70 mm Hg). Increased pulmonary nitric oxide (NO) production in these patients leads to dilation of pre-capillary and postcapillary pulmonary vasculature, impairing oxygenation of venous blood. The mechanisms causing increased NO production, as well as the correlation between NO production and severity of liver disease, remain unclear. Ten to 20% of cirrhotic patients develop HPS, with increased mortality.

1. **Evaluation and diagnosis.** The most common complaint in patients with HPS is dyspnea, especially increased on standing (platypnea) because of increased blood shunting to lung bases where vasodilation predominates. Patients may have clubbing or cyanosis on physical exam. Chest X-ray may show interstitial changes in the lower lobes, and pulmonary function tests may demonstrate reduced diffusing capacity for carbon monoxide (DLCO)—but these findings are nonspecific. The diagnosis is established by documenting both arterial gas exchange abnormalities and intrapulmonary vasodilation. While pulse oximetry may be used as a screening tool, arterial blood gas measurements are necessary because in less-advanced disease, a patient may not be hypoxemic (normal PaO_2 but widened PAO_2-PaO_2). The most sensitive test for pulmonary vasodilation is two-dimensional transthoracic echocardiography with agitated saline contrast. In normal patients, contrast bubbles are trapped in the pulmonary microvasculature and not seen in the left heart (except with intracardiac shunting). Visualization of bubbles in the left heart after three cycles is a positive test for HPS. In patients with intrinsic lung disease, radionuclide lung perfusion scanning using labeled macroaggregated albumin particles (99mTC MAA scan) is more specific for HPS. Labeled particles are usually trapped in the pulmonary microvasculature, but passage into the arterial circulation can be evaluated with imaging of the lung and brain. A shunt fraction of greater than 6% is diagnostic for HPS. High-resolution chest CT may also be used, but its role is still being defined.

2. **Treatment.** While medical therapies may transiently alleviate HPS (e.g., NO inhibition with methylene blue), transplantation is the only definitive therapy. Exception points are granted to patients with HPS to increase their Model for End-Stage Liver Disease MELD score (see section VI) and facilitate earlier OLT. A resting PaO_2 less than 60 to 65 mm Hg identifies patients who may meet exception criteria. Liver transplantation has been shown to improve and/or normalize gas exchange in more than 85% of patients, but changes in gas exchange are not immediate. Mortality after OLT is increased in patients with HPS. Severe preoperative hypoxemia (PaO_2 less than 50 mm Hg) and/or an MAA shunt fraction of at least 20% are predictive of postoperative mortality. This increased mortality is partially attributable to HPS-related postoperative complications including pulmonary hypertension, cerebral embolic hemorrhages, and prolonged ventilator requirement. Median survival of patients with HPS without OLT is approximately 5 months, versus 35 months with transplantation.

B. **Portopulmonary hypertension (POPH).** This syndrome is defined in the presence of portal hypertension, with a mean pulmonary artery pressure (PAP) of more than 25 mm Hg and a pulmonary capillary wedge pressure (PCWP) of less than 15 mm Hg. Additional criteria include an elevated transpulmonary gradient (mean PAP minus PCWP more than 10 mm Hg) and/or elevated pulmonary vascular resistance (more than 240 dyne sec/cm-5). The prevalence of POPH among cirrhotics being evaluated for transplantation is approximately 6%, and the presence of POPH does not correlate with severity of liver disease. The pathophysiology remains unclear, but is thought to be related to a hyperdynamic state in the setting of portal hypertension, with vascular shear forces and endothelial injury leading to the release of vasoactive substances and hypertension. Patients may have POPH with or without HPS. Symptoms relate to the degree of pulmonary hypertension, with dyspnea on exertion, fatigue, and peripheral edema. Transthoracic Doppler echocardiography is the best screening tool, demonstrating an elevated pulmonary artery systolic (PAS) pressure and right ventricular (RV) hypertrophy or dysfunction. An estimated PAS pressure of more than 40 mm Hg should prompt cardiac catheterization to differentiate intrinsic cardiopulmonary disease from POPH. Survival correlates with degree of RV dysfunction, and progression leads to cor pulmonale. Vasodilators (primarily intravenous prostacyclin) have been shown to improve PAP, but no agents have demonstrated prolonged survival. Outcomes of liver transplantation in patients with mild POPH (PAP less than 35 mm Hg) compare to patients without POPH, with similar postoperative risk. Moderate-to-severe POPH (PAP more than 50 mm Hg) is a contraindication to transplantation, with a perioperative mortality rate of approximately 40% and irreversible pulmonary hypertension.

IV. **HEPATORENAL SYNDROME.** Hepatorenal syndrome (HRS) is characterized by renal vasoconstriction in the setting of portal hypertension. The mechanisms leading to HRS are complex, and begin with splanchnic arterial vasodilation in response to increased portal vascular resistance. Despite increased cardiac output, flow is redirected to the splanchnic circulation with peripheral artery underfilling. In an effort to maintain peripheral BP, the renin-angiotensin-aldosterone system (RAAS) and sympathetic nervous system are activated, leading to vasoconstriction and sodium retention. Water retention follows, leading to accumulation of extracellular fluid as ascites and/or edema. Renal solute-free water excretion becomes impaired, primarily due to increased secretion of the antidiuretic hormone arginine vasopressin (AVP), leading to dilutional hyponatremia (serum sodium less than 130 mEq/L). Local renal vasodilators (e.g., prostaglandins) work to counteract renal vasoconstriction. With disease progression, however, local vasodilators lose the ability to maintain renal perfusion and renal failure ensues.

The incidence of HRS among cirrhotic patients with ascites is approximately 10%. These patients are classified according to severity into two types of HRS. Type one is defined by a doubling of the initial serum creatinine more than 2.5 mg/dL, or a 50% reduction in the initial creatinine clearance to less than 20 mL/min in less than 2 weeks. Type one HRS is acute and progresses rapidly. The median survival for these patients is 1 month, with 100% mortality at 12 weeks. Type two HRS is defined by a serum creatinine more than 1.5 mg/dL, without rapid progression to type one. Type two HRS patients typically have diuretic-refractory ascites. Survival is longer than in patients with type one HRS, but shorter than in patients without renal failure.

A. **Evaluation and diagnosis.** Sodium retention is the earliest functional abnormality in the spectrum of renal dysfunction in cirrhosis. Patients may present with ascites, dilutional hyponatremia, and/or low urinary sodium excretion (urine sodium less than 10 mEq/L). Renal dysfunction may progress to HRS without any identifiable precipitating factor, or may be related to an episode of spontaneous bacterial peritonitis (SBP), acute alcoholic hepatitis, or an operation. As many as one-third of patients with SBP develop type one HRS despite appropriate antibiotic treatment. Large volume paracentesis (more than 5 L) without albumin administration may also precipitate type one HRS. The diagnosis of HRS is based on a reduced GFR without other cause for renal failure. Major criteria for the diagnosis of HRS have been established by the International Ascites Club, including (1) low GFR (serum creatinine more than 1.5 mg/dL or 24-hour creatinine clearance less than 40 mL/min), (2) absence of shock, nephrotoxic drugs, fluid losses, or ongoing infection, (3) no sustained improvement in renal function following plasma expansion and diuretic withdrawal, and (4) proteinuria more than 500 mg/day and no ultrasonographic evidence of renal parenchymal disease or obstructive uropathy.

B. **Treatment.** Every patient with dilutional hyponatremia should be evaluated for OLT, as treating the underlying liver disease is the only definitive therapy. Fluid restriction to less than 1 L per day may slow the progression of dilutional hyponatremia. Antagonists to the V2 receptor of AVP are being investigated, and may improve solute-free water excretion. Once patients develop HRS, medical therapy aims to constrict the splanchnic circulation while expanding volume to improve renal perfusion. Use of the vasopressin analog terlipressin with albumin expansion has been associated with improved GFR and reduction in serum creatinine below 1.5 in patients with type one HRS. Transjugular intrahepatic portosystemic shunt (TIPS) and dialysis have been used as temporizing measures, but further studies are needed to define their role in HRS. Liver transplantation is the best treatment for patients with HRS. Priority is given to these patients, but unfortunately a significant number of patients with type one HRS die waiting for transplantation. The long-term outcomes for patients who receive a liver compare similarly to patients without HRS, with 85% survival at 1 year and 73% at 3 years.

V. **PREOPERATIVE EVALUATION.** Referrals to transplantation centers are made on an elective or urgent basis. The evaluation determines the need and urgency for OLT as well as its technical feasibility.

A. **Elective transplantation.** Under elective conditions, the potential candidate is presented to a multidisciplinary committee for evaluation. The patient's evaluation is based on history, physical examination, laboratory evaluation, results of endoscopic procedures, cardiac and pulmonary evaluation, and radiologic examination (Table 23-7). Active infection should be treated promptly, and transplantation should be postponed until the

TABLE 23-7	Pretransplantation Evaluation of Liver Transplant Recipients

Initial workup

History

Etiology of liver disease

Duration of liver disease

Complications of liver disease

Previous surgical procedures

Additional medical problems

Access to transplant center

Social support

Physical examination

Stigmata of chronic liver disease

Jaundice

Fluid retention

Nutritional status

Abdominal mass

Asterixis or encephalopathy

Growth and development (pediatric patients)

Laboratory analysis

ABO blood type; complete blood count; prothrombin time; partial thromboplastin time; serum electrolytes; urinary electrolytes; total protein, albumin, calcium, magnesium, and phosphorus; total and direct bilirubin; aspartate aminotransferase; alanine aminotransferase; alkaline phosphatase; γ-glutamyl transpeptidase; cholesterol serum ammonia; viral serologies (human immunodeficiency virus; hepatitis A, B, and C; cytomegalovirus; Epstein–Barr virus; and herpes simplex virus); urinalysis and culture; cell count; and culture of ascitic fluid and purified protein derivative

TABLE 23-7	Pretransplantation Evaluation of Liver Transplant Recipients *(Continued)*

Electrocardiogram

Chest X-ray

Arterial blood gas

Dobutamine stress echocardiography

Pulmonary function tests

Computed tomography or magnetic resonance imaging scan of the abdomen with liver volume

Esophagogastroduodenoscopy

Doppler ultrasonography

Psychosocial evaluation

Optional examinations

Computed tomography scan of chest and bone scan for patient with malignancy

Visceral angiogram

Cardiac catheterization

Endoscopic retrograde cholangiogram or percutaneous transhepatic cholangiography with brush biopsy for patients with sclerosing cholangitis (10% coincidence of cholangiocarcinoma in these patients)

Colonoscopy for patients with inflammatory bowel disease, sclerosing cholangitis, Hemoccult-positive stools, family history of colon cancer, previous history of colonic polyps

infection resolves. Patients with a recent history of alcohol or other substance abuse should be evaluated by a specialist prior to transplantation.

B. **Urgent transplantation.** Acceptable results with OLT can be achieved in select patients with fulminant liver failure. The pretransplantation evaluation is performed in a manner similar to that for the elective patient; however, timing, neurologic status, and hemodynamic stability may limit the number of tests obtained. A careful neurologic examination must be done in this setting, and the grade of coma should be determined. Patients in grade IV (unresponsive) coma have been shown in some studies to benefit from continuous perioperative monitoring of intracranial pressure (ICP) because untreated severe elevations in ICP can result in permanent brain injury and death. An attempt is made to keep cerebral perfusion pressure (mean arterial BP minus ICP) above 60 mm Hg. Low mean arterial BP is treated with vasopressors after volume resuscitation. Elevation in ICP is treated with hyperventilation, mannitol, and elevation of the head of the bed more than 45 degrees. ICP monitor placement may be complicated by severe coagulopathy and thrombocytopenia, which is common in these patients. Patients with acute hepatic failure may develop acute renal failure (ARF) as well, which can require hemofiltration or hemodialysis. Sepsis also is seen in acute hepatic failure and requires broad-spectrum antibiotics and antifungals. Pulmonary insufficiency is also common, and may require intubation, high-concentration oxygen, and positive end-expiratory pressure.

VI. **ORGAN ALLOCATION.** Livers are allocated based on the **MELD** scoring system. The MELD score is derived from the values for bilirubin, serum creatinine, and the international normalized ratio (INR) and ranges from 6 to 40 (http://www.unos.org). Livers are allocated to appropriate patients with the highest MELD scores. Special exception points may be granted, such as in cases of hepatocellular carcinoma, HPS or HRS. Children receive a Pediatric End-Stage Liver Disease (PELD) score.

VII. **DONOR SELECTION.** Selection of an appropriate donor liver takes into account donor size, ABO blood type, age, presence of infection, history of malignancy, liver function studies, hospital course, hemodynamic stability, and prior alcohol or drug use. Absolute contraindications to the use of a donor liver include the presence of extrahepatic malignancy and HIV. The use of expanded donor criteria allows transplantation of organs from older patients, patients with steatotic livers, and patients with hepatitis B or C.

VIII. **HEPATIC TRANSPLANTATION PROCEDURE**

A. **Whole-organ liver transplantation.** Conceptually, OLT comprises three distinct sequential phases. The **first phase** involves the dissection and removal of the recipient's diseased liver. The **second phase,** known as the **anhepatic phase,** refers to the period starting with devascularization of the recipient's liver and ending with revascularization of the newly implanted liver. During the anhepatic phase, venovenous bypass (VVB) may be used. VVB shunts blood from the portal vein and infrahepatic inferior vena cava (IVC) to the axillary, subclavian, or jugular veins. Alternatively, many transplant surgeons will create a temporary portocaval shunt, which has the advantages of VVB with much less risk and cost. Maintenance of venous return from the kidneys and lower extremities results in a smoother hemodynamic course, allows time for a more deliberate approach to hemostasis, reduces visceral edema and splanchnic venous pooling, and lowers the incidence of postoperative renal dysfunction. The liver allograft is implanted by anastomosing first the suprahepatic vena cava and then the infrahepatic IVC. The portal vein anastomosis is performed, and blood flow to the liver is reestablished. Finally, the hepatic arterial anastomosis is performed. If the recipient hepatic artery is not suitable for anastomosis, a donor iliac arterial graft can be used as a conduit from the infra- or suprarenal aorta. The **third phase** includes biliary reconstruction and abdominal closure. Biliary continuity is established via a duct-to-duct anastomosis or a choledochojejunostomy. A duct-to-duct anastomosis is preferable, but may not be possible when there is a donor–recipient bile duct size discrepancy or a diseased recipient bile duct (e.g., with primary sclerosing cholangitis, biliary atresia, or secondary biliary cirrhosis). In a modification of the foregoing technique, the recipient's retrohepatic IVC is preserved, and the donor suprahepatic IVC is anastomosed to the confluence of the recipient's right, middle, and left hepatic veins. The donor infrahepatic IVC is then oversewn. The temporary end-to-side portacaval shunt is also created at the beginning of the hepatectomy.

B. **Reduced and split-liver transplantation** was developed to support the needs of pediatric patients awaiting appropriately sized transplants. Benefits include better size matching and using a single liver to provide grafts for multiple recipients. These benefits have translated to the adult population as well. The liver has a remarkable capacity for regeneration. It can be divided based on the anatomic segments of Couinaud into a left lateral section (segments 2 and 3), a left hemiliver graft (segments 2 to 4), or a right hemiliver graft (segments 5 to 8). The left lateral section is most commonly used in children. Comparison of the size of the donor and the recipient is used to determine the appropriate-sized graft. Yersiz and colleagues demonstrated that children receiving a left lateral section have similar survival outcomes and morbidity to pediatric recipients of similar live donor or whole-organ grafts (*Ann Surg.* 2003;238:496).

C. **Living-donor liver transplantation** has been developed as a result of the success of reduced liver transplantation. The left lateral section or left hepatic lobe is usually used as the donor graft for adult-to-child transplantation. Advantages similar to those observed with living related kidney donors have been observed, such as reduced ischemic time and the inherent benefits of an elective operation. Adult-to-adult living-donor liver transplantation necessitates the use of the larger right hemiliver. An amount of liver approximately equal to 0.1% of patient weight (e.g., 700 g for a 70-kg recipient) is required.

IX. POSTOPERATIVE CARE

A. **Hemodynamic.** Intravascular volume resuscitation usually is required in the immediate postoperative period secondary to third-space losses, increased body temperature, and vasodilatation. Adequate perfusion is assessed by left and right heart filling pressures, cardiac output, urine output, and the absence of metabolic acidosis. Hypertension is common and should be aggressively treated.

B. **Pulmonary.** Ventilatory support is required postoperatively until the patient is awake and alert, is able to follow commands and protect the airway, and is able to maintain adequate oxygenation and ventilation.

C. **Hepatic allograft function.** Monitoring of hepatic allograft function begins intraoperatively after revascularization. Signs of satisfactory graft function include hemodynamic stability and normalization of acid–base status, body temperature, coagulation studies, maintenance of glucose metabolism, and bile production. Reassessment of allograft function continues postoperatively, initially occurring every 12 hours. Satisfactory function is indicated by an improving coagulation profile, decreasing transaminase levels, normal blood glucose, hemodynamic stability, adequate urine output, bile production, and clearance of anesthesia. Early elevations of bilirubin and transaminase levels may be indicators of preservation injury. The peak levels of serum glutamic-oxaloacetic transaminase and serum glutamate-pyruvate transaminase usually are less than 2,000 units/L, and should decrease rapidly over the first 24 to 48 hours postoperatively. After the patient leaves the intensive care unit, liver function tests are obtained daily. If hepatic dysfunction becomes evident at any time, prompt evaluation must be undertaken and treatment must be initiated. It is important to correctly diagnose the cause of liver dysfunction because each cause has a unique treatment.

1. **Primary nonfunction and initial poor function.** The use of modern organ preservation solutions for organ preservation has decreased the incidence of primary nonfunction. For poorly understood reasons, however, 1% to 3% of transplanted livers fail immediately after the surgery. Primary nonfunction is characterized by hemodynamic instability, poor quantity and quality of bile, renal dysfunction, failure to regain consciousness, increasing coagulopathy, persistent hypothermia, and lactic acidosis in the face of patent vascular anastomosis (as demonstrated by Doppler ultrasonography). Without retransplantation, death ensues.

2. **Rejection.** Acute rejection is relatively common after liver transplantation, with 60% of recipients experiencing at least one cell-mediated or acute rejection episode. However, rejection is an extremely uncommon cause of graft loss. The most common causes of early graft loss include primary nonfunction and hepatic artery thrombosis.

3. **Technical complications.** A variety of technical problems can lead to liver allograft dysfunction, including hepatic artery stenosis or thrombosis, portal vein stenosis or thrombosis, biliary tract obstruction, bile duct leak, and hepatic vein or vena caval thrombosis. **Hepatic artery thrombosis** in the early posttransplantation period may lead to fever, hemodynamic instability, and rapid deterioration, with a marked elevation of the transaminases. An associated bile leak may be noted soon after liver transplantation due to the loss of the bile ducts' main vascular supply. Acute thrombosis may be treated by attempted thrombectomy. If this is unsuccessful, retransplantation is needed. Thrombosis long after liver transplantation may produce intra- and extrahepatic bile duct strictures and may be an indication for elective

retransplantation. Occasionally, hepatic artery thrombosis is completely asymptomatic.

   a. Portal vein stenosis or thrombosis is rare. When it occurs, the patient's condition may deteriorate rapidly, with profound hepatic dysfunction, massive ascites, renal failure, and hemodynamic instability. Although surgical thrombectomy may be successful, urgent retransplantation is often necessary. Late thrombosis may allow normal liver function but usually results in variceal bleeding and ascites.

   b. Bile duct obstruction is diagnosed by cholangiography. A single short bile duct stricture may be treated by either percutaneous or retrograde balloon dilation. A long stricture, ampullary dysfunction, or failed dilation necessitates revision of the biliary anastomosis. Fever and abdominal pain in the early posttransplantation period should raise the possibility of biliary anastomotic disruption, which requires urgent surgical revision.

4. Recurrent infection and neoplasm. CMV can cause hepatic allograft dysfunction and usually occurs within 8 weeks of transplantation. Diagnosis is made by liver biopsy, with CMV inclusion bodies on light microscopy, or by peripheral blood PCR. Treatment consists of decreasing immunosuppression and administering ganciclovir (see Table 23-1).

   a. Viral hepatitis and malignancy (e.g., hepatoma, cholangiocarcinoma, and neuroendocrine tumors) can recur in the hepatic allograft but are uncommon in the early posttransplantation period. The clinical presentation includes elevated liver function tests, and diagnosis is made by liver biopsy. Imaging studies (e.g., CT scan and liver ultrasonography) are important in posttransplant surveillance for neoplasms. Patients transplanted for HCC should have regular surveillance with CT imaging and tumor markers.

   b. Hepatitis C virus (HCV) will recur in essentially all patients, but in most this is a mild hepatitis that does not lead to significant clinical sequelae. Occasionally, HCV recurrence is severe, and may lead to early recurrence of cirrhosis and liver failure. In general, retransplantation for early HCV recurrence is not performed. Various protocols for antiviral therapy for posttransplant HCV recurrence are under development.

   c. Hepatitis B virus (HBV) also recurs posttransplantation. Protocols are under investigation using different combinations of hepatitis B immune globulin (IG), hepatitis B vaccines, lamivudine, retroviral agents, and monoclonal antibodies. Strategies to prevent hepatitis B recurrence include the use of lamivudine before transplant to arrest viral replication, and posttransplant high-dose hepatitis B IG and lamivudine.

D. Electrolytes and glucose. The use of diuretics may result in hypokalemia, whereas cyclosporine or tacrolimus toxicity may cause hyperkalemia. Magnesium levels are maintained above 2 mg/dL (0.82 mmol/L) because the seizure threshold is lowered by the combination of hypomagnesemia and cyclosporine or tacrolimus. Calcium should be measured as free ionized calcium and kept above 4.4 mg/dL (1.1 mmol/L). Phosphorus levels should be maintained above 2.5 mg/dL (0.81 mmol/L) to avoid respiratory muscle weakness and altered oxygen hemoglobin dissociation. Glucose homeostasis is necessary because steroid administration may result in hyperglycemia, which is best managed with intravenous insulin because it is short acting and easily absorbed. Cyclosporine and tacrolimus are diabetogenic immunosuppressants and may alter glucose homeostasis. Hypoglycemia is a complication of liver failure, and in the presence of liver dysfunction, glucose administration may be necessary.

E. **GI tract.** H_2 blockade, proton-pump inhibition, and/or antacids are used to prevent stress ulcers. Endoscopy is performed liberally for any GI bleeding. Nystatin and GI tract decontamination solution containing gentamicin and polymyxin B are used in the perioperative period to prevent esophageal candidiasis and translocation of bacterial pathogens.

F. **Nutrition.** Patients who are severely malnourished should be placed on nutritional supplementation as soon fluid and electrolyte status has stabilized and graft function is deemed adequate. Patients with sufficient preoperative nutrition can be maintained on routine intravenous fluids until GI tract function returns (usually 3 to 5 days). Enteral nutrition is used as soon as the postoperative ileus resolves. Total parenteral nutrition (TPN) is indicated when the GI tract is nonfunctional.

G. **Infection surveillance.** The most common causes of bacterial infection after liver transplantation include line sepsis, UTIs, infected ascites, cholangitis, pneumonia, biliary anastomotic leak, and intra-abdominal abscess. Prophylactic antibiotics covering biliary pathogens are administered for the first 48 hours after liver transplantation. If a fever develops in the liver transplant recipient, a thorough examination should be performed. A chest X-ray and cultures of blood, urine, indwelling lines, and bile are necessary. A cholangiogram and Doppler ultrasonography of the liver can be performed to rule out perihepatic fluid collection and to evaluate hepatic vasculature.

H. **Posttransplantation immunosuppression.** The immunosuppressive agents used to prevent rejection include corticosteroids and tacrolimus. Myfortic may be added to reduce tacrolimus doses, which may be particularly useful in patients with renal disease or autoimmune liver disease.

X. **REJECTION.** Many liver transplant recipients experience at least one acute rejection episode, and it commonly occurs between days 4 and 21 postoperatively. Rejection is characterized by fever, increased ascites, decreased bile quality and quantity, and elevation of total white blood cell and eosinophil count, bilirubin, and transaminase levels. Rejection is diagnosed by percutaneous liver biopsy. In the early posttransplantation period, technical causes of hepatic dysfunction are ruled out by Doppler ultrasonography to ensure vascular patency, and cholangiography to rule out a bile duct obstruction or leak. Typical biopsy findings consistent with acute rejection include the triad of portal lymphocytes, endothelitis (subendothelial deposits of mononuclear cells), and bile duct infiltration and damage. The first-line treatment for acute rejection is a bolus of corticosteroids (methylprednisolone, 1 g intravenously). If the rejection responds appropriately, the patient undergoes steroid recycling.

PANCREAS AND ISLET TRANSPLANTATION

I. **INDICATIONS.** DM affects 7.8% of Americans and is the seventh-leading cause of death (as of 2007, www.diabetes.org). It is the leading cause of renal failure and blindness in adults. Other long-term complications caused by diabetes include myocardial infarction, stroke, amputation, and neuropathy. Invasive methods for maintaining euglycemia and preventing the long-term complications of DM include the use of autoregulating insulin pumps, pancreatic islet cell transplants, and whole-organ pancreatic transplantation.

Pancreas transplantation is commonly performed in the setting of kidney transplantation (either simultaneously or afterward) for diabetes complicated by ESRD. Pancreas-only transplants are also performed. Approximately 1,800 pancreas and islet transplants are performed per year in the United States.

II. **CONTRAINDICATIONS** to pancreas transplantation are the same as those for kidney transplantation, including disabilities secondary to DM (e.g., peripheral gangrene), intractable cardiac decompensation, and incapacitating peripheral neuropathy. Continued tobacco use also is considered a relatively strong contraindication.

III. **PREOPERATIVE WORKUP AND EVALUATION.** Workup of the potential pancreas transplantation patient is similar to that of the kidney recipient and identifies coexisting diseases, as outlined in Table 23-3. To allow identification of beneficial effects of pancreas transplantation on the complications of DM, a careful preoperative evaluation of the patient's neurologic and ophthalmologic status should be performed. Contraindications to pancreas donation include the presence of diabetes, pancreatitis, pancreatic trauma, or significant intra-abdominal contamination.

IV. **DECEASED-DONOR PANCREAS TRANSPLANTATION OPERATION**

A. **Forms of pancreatic transplantation**

1. **Simultaneous kidney–pancreas transplantation** may be considered in insulin-dependent diabetic patients who are dialysis dependent or imminent and have a creatinine clearance of less than 30 mL/minute. Some of the advantages of combined transplantation include the ability to monitor pancreas rejection by monitoring renal rejection, and exposure to only one set of donor antigens.

2. **Isolated pancreas transplantation.** The most widely accepted technique of pancreatic transplantation in the United States uses whole-organ pancreas with venous drainage into the systemic circulation and enteric exocrine drainage. Some centers advocate portal venous drainage. Under cold-storage conditions, the portal vein is isolated. If it is too short to allow for a tension-free anastomosis, an extension autograft is placed using donor iliac vein. The SMA and splenic artery then are reconstructed with a donor iliac artery Y-bifurcation autograft. Only

the second portion of the duodenum is retained with the pancreas. Then the portal vein is anastomosed to the iliac vein or the superior mesenteric vein, and the donor common iliac artery graft is anastomosed to the recipient's external iliac artery. The duodenal segment of the transplant is then opened, and a duodenojejunostomy is created. Alternatively, the duodenal segment can be anastomosed to the bladder. The pancreas transplant is placed in the right paracolic gutter, and if kidney transplantation is to be performed, it is done on the left side.

3. **Pancreatic islet cell transplantation** is still investigational and has not received widespread acceptance. Pancreatic islet cells are isolated and injected into the portal vein for engraftment in the liver. The major problems have been in obtaining enough islet cells to attain glucose homeostasis and failing to achieve long-term insulin independence. A large multicenter trial supported the proof of concept of islet transplantation (*N Engl J Med.* 2006;355:1318). Although 58% of patients were able to achieve insulin independence at some time during the trial, only 31% of those achieving insulin independence and 15% of those initially enrolled were insulin independent 1 year after transplantation.

B. Exocrine drainage. Most programs now use **enteric drainage,** which avoids the acidosis, volume depletion, and urologic complications associated with bladder drainage. Enteric drainage involves anastomosis of the duodenal segment to small bowel in a side-to-side fashion or via a Roux-en-Y limb. Disadvantages of enteric drainage include the inability to monitor exocrine secretions and a higher rate of technical failure.

V. POSTOPERATIVE MANAGEMENT AND MONITORING

A. **Immunosuppression** consists of quadruple therapy with antibody induction, tacrolimus, prednisone, and mycophenolate mofetil.

B. **Serum glucose** is followed during and after the transplantation. Intravenous insulin infusions are stopped within the first few hours after pancreas transplantation.

C. **Rejection** of the pancreas transplant is suggested by a rise in serum amylase or a fall in urinary amylase. Rejection of pancreas and kidney transplants usually occurs in parallel but may be discordant. The diagnosis of kidney rejection is suggested by a rise in creatinine, which is then confirmed by biopsy. Biopsy of the pancreas transplant is performed percutaneously or via cystoscopy. Rejection is treated with corticosteroids or antilymphocyte preparations.

D. Graft-related complications. Besides rejection, complications of pancreas transplantation include metabolic acidosis and dehydration. These are due to the loss of sodium and bicarbonate into the urine from the transplanted duodenum. Other common complications include pancreatitis, UTIs, urethritis, and anastomotic leak from the duodenocystostomy. Infections with CMV also may occur.

VI. EFFECT ON SECONDARY COMPLICATIONS OF DIABETES. The full effect of pancreatic transplantation on secondary complications of diabetes is unknown. Pancreatic transplantation may prevent the development of diabetic nephropathy in the transplanted kidney. It also may stabilize diabetic retinopathy and improve diabetic neuropathy.

INTESTINAL TRANSPLANTATION

Intestinal failure occurs when the functioning GI tract mucosal surface area has been reduced below the minimal amount necessary for adequate digestion and absorption of food. This may be caused by intestinal loss or intestinal disease (Table 23-8). The development of TPN has led to the possibility of long-term survival for infants and adults with intestinal failure. However, TPN has limitations and associated morbidity.

I. **INDICATIONS.** Adults and children who have documented intestinal failure without the potential for long-term survival on TPN are candidates for intestinal transplantation. **Intestinal failure** is said to occur when any child younger than 1 year requires more than 50% of his or her caloric needs from TPN after neonatal small-bowel resection or when a child older than 4 years requires more than 30% of calories from TPN. Older children and adults receiving more than 50% of their nutritional requirements from TPN for more than 1 year also should be considered for intestinal transplantation. Other considerations include elevated hepatic enzymes, multiple line infections, thrombosis of two of the central veins, and frequent episodes of dehydration.

II. **DONOR INTESTINAL PROCUREMENT** generally uses multiorgan recovery techniques. The liver, stomach, duodenum, pancreas, and small intestine are removed *en bloc* and separated under cold-storage conditions. Alternatively, the intestine may be recovered alone or with the liver.

TABLE 23-8	Causes of Intestinal Failure	
Superior mesenteric artery thrombosis	Crohn's disease
Superior mesenteric artery embolization	Trauma
Necrotizing enterocolitis	Radiation
Volvulus	Malignancy (desmoid, polyposis)
Gastroschisis	Pseudoobstruction
Intestinal atresia	

III. **INTESTINAL TRANSPLANTATION OPERATION.** Patients who receive isolated intestinal allografts have vascular anastomoses created between the donor superior mesenteric vein and the recipient portal vein, and between the donor SMA and the recipient aorta. Vascular reconstruction for patients who receive combined liver–intestinal grafts parallels that for patients undergoing a standard OLT. Supra- and infrahepatic vena caval anastomoses are completed, and arterial inflow is accomplished after the portal vein anastomosis by using a patch of aorta that contains the SMA and celiac.

IV. **POSTOPERATIVE MANAGEMENT**

   A. **Immunosuppression and infection prophylaxis.** Posttransplantation immunosuppressive protocols have varied greatly over the last decade, and a universally accepted standard protocol does not exist. Recent studies have demonstrated encouraging results with induction therapy (Thymoglobulin or Campath) followed by maintenance therapy with tacrolimus. Because the allograft ileum is more susceptible to rejection, ileoscopic biopsies through a temporary loop ileostomy are common. Watery diarrhea may be a sign of either rejection or superinfection. With the return of intestinal function, feedings are begun with an elemental diet and then advanced as tolerated. Viral and fungal infection prophylaxis includes ganciclovir, oral antibiotic bowel preparation, low-dose amphotericin B, and early removal of central lines.

   B. **Potential complications.** Inherent risks with intestinal transplantation include up to 50% graft failure (rejection) at 3 years, although recent advances in immunosuppression and perioperative management have promising results (*Lancet.* 2003;361:1502). More than 1,900 intestinal transplants have been performed in the United States since 1990, with 180 transplants in 2009 (2 living donors, 178 deceased). For primary intestinal transplants, graft survival averages 78% at 1 year and 40% at 5 years (www.unos.org). Combined liver–intestine transplantation carries all the additional risks inherent in liver transplantation. Intestinal transplant recipients are at increased risk for the development of graft-versus-host disease and posttransplantation lymphoproliferative disease. Complications related to tacrolimus-based immunosuppression include DM, headaches, CNS neurotoxicity, peripheral neurotoxicity, and nephrotoxicity. As with any effective immunosuppressant, there is an increased risk of infection and malignancy.

ADDITIONAL REFERENCES

Abu-Elmagd KM. Intestinal transplantation for short bowel syndrome and gastrointestinal failure: current consensus, rewarding outcomes, and practical guidelines. *Gastroenterology.* 2006;130:S132–S137.

Everson GT, Trotter JF. *Liver Transplantation: Challenging Controversies and Topics.* Totowa, NJ: Humana Press; 2009.

McKay DB, Steinberg SM, eds. *Kidney Transplantation: A Guide to the Care of Kidney Transplant Recipients.* New York: Springer; 2010.

Norman DJ, Turka LA, eds. *Primer on Transplantation.* 2nd ed. Thorofare, NJ: American Society of Transplant Physicians; 2001.

Schiff ER, Sorrell, MF, Maddrey, WC. *Schiff's Diseases of the Liver,* 10th ed. Philadelphia: Lippincott Williams & Wilkins; 2007.

Schulak JA. What's new in general surgery: transplantation. *J Am Coll Surg.* 2005;200(3):409–417.

24 Burns

Derek Wakeman and Robert E. Southard

Burns are tissue injuries resulting from direct contact with flames, hot liquids, gases, surfaces, caustic chemicals, electricity, or radiation. Most commonly, the skin is injured, which compromises its function as a barrier to injury and infection and as a regulator of body temperature and fluid loss. More than 1.2 million persons in the United States sustain burns each year, of whom, 500,000 receive formal medical attention, more than 40,000 are hospitalized, and 4,000 die (www.ameriburn.org). Like trauma, mortality from burns occurs in a bimodal pattern: immediately after the injury or weeks later from sepsis and multiorgan failure. Recently, the focus on burn care as a subspecialty of surgery in dedicated patient care units has improved overall survival and quality of life. Finally, it should be emphasized that most burns are preventable and, thus, prevention strategies are of utmost importance.

ASSESSMENT AND MANAGEMENT OF BURN INJURIES

I. ASSESSMENT

A. **Mechanism of injury.** Identify burn source, duration of exposure, time of injury, and environment. Burns sustained in a closed environment, such as a structure fire, often produce inhalation injury in addition to thermal trauma. Explosions can cause barometric injury to the eardrums and lungs and may also cause blunt trauma.

B. **Associated injuries** can result from explosions, falls, or jumping during escape attempts.

C. **Patient age** is a major determinant on outcome. Infants and elderly patients are at highest risk. Burns are a common form of child abuse and need to be considered in every child. Suggestive physical examination findings include stocking/glove injury patterns, lack of splash marks, and dorsally located contact burns of the hands (*Forensic Sci Int.* 2009;187:81). Elderly patients often have comorbid medical problems and decreased physiologic reserve.

D. **State of health.** Preexisting medical problems should be noted, with particular attention paid to cardiac, pulmonary, renal, and gastrointestinal systems.

E. **Prehospital treatment** is recorded, including care provided by the patient and by the emergency response team. Administered fluids are documented and subtracted from estimated fluid requirements for the first 24 hours of injury. Hypothermia is a significant complication, particularly during transport, and should be addressed both in the field and at the receiving facility. Common effective precautions include preheating patient-receiving areas and minimizing the use of wet dressings in the prehospital setting.

F. **Primary survey** should follow the guidelines established by the American College of Surgeons' Advanced Trauma Life Support Course. Burned patients should be evaluated and treated as victims of multisystem trauma because there is significant morbidity associated from missed injuries secondary to an explosion, falls, etc.

1. **Airway** assessment and security are the foremost priority. Supraglottic tissue edema progresses over the first 12 hours and can obstruct the airway rapidly. The larynx protects subglottic tissue from direct thermal injury but not from injury due to inhaled toxic gases. Inhalation injury should be suspected if the patient was burned in an enclosed structure or explosion. Physical signs include hoarseness, stridor, facial burns, singed facial hair, expectoration of carbonaceous sputum, and presence of carbon in the oropharynx. The decision to intubate the trachea for airway protection should be made early and is preferable to cricothyroidotomy in the edematous and swollen neck. Awake intubation or intubation over a bronchoscope is the safest approach if there is any question about the ease or adequacy of airway exposure (*Curr Opin Anaesthesiol.* 2003;16:183).

2. **Breathing** is evaluated for effort, depth of respiration, and auscultation of breath sounds. Wheezing or rales suggest either inhalation injury or aspiration of gastric contents. Most severely burned patients develop early pulmonary insufficiency and respiratory failure. The etiology of this failure can be direct thermal injury to the upper airways or, more commonly, indirect acute lung injury secondary to activation of systemic inflammation. In addition, the decreased pulmonary compliance and chest wall rigidity of burn patients can lead to iatrogenic ventilator-induced lung injury. The use of lower tidal volumes, permissive hypercapnia, and the "open lung" approach to ventilation can significantly improve outcome (*N Engl J Med.* 2000;342:1301).

3. **Circulation.** Circulatory support in the form of **aggressive and prompt fluid resuscitation** is a cornerstone of early burn management. Burn injury causes a combination of hypovolemic and distributive shock characterized by the release of inflammatory mediators, dynamic fluid shifts from the intravascular compartment to the interstitium, and exudative and evaporative water loss from the burn injury. Full-thickness circumferential extremity or neck burns require escharotomy if circulation distal to the injury is impaired; however, escharotomies are rarely needed within the first 6 hours of injury.

4. **Exposure. Remove all clothing** to halt continued burn from melted synthetic compounds or chemicals and to assess the full extent of body surface involvement in the initial examination. Irrigate injuries with water or saline to remove harmful residues. **Remove jewelry** (particularly rings) to prevent injury resulting from increasing tissue edema.

G. **Burn-specific secondary survey**
   1. **Depth of burn** (Table 24-1)
      a. **First-degree burns** are limited to the epidermis. The skin is painful and red. There are no blisters. These burns should heal spontaneously in 3 to 4 days.
      b. **Second-degree burns,** which are subdivided into **superficial or deep partial-thickness burns,** are limited to the dermal layers of

TABLE 24-1 Treatment Algorithm for the Three Clinically Important Burn Depths[a]

Burn Depth[b]	Level of Injury	Clinical Features	Treatment	Usual Result
Superficial partial-thickness	Papillary dermis	Blisters Erythema Capillary refill Intact pain sensation	Tetanus prophylaxis Cleaning (e.g., with chlorhexidine gluconate) Topical agent (e.g., 1% silver sulfadiazine)[c] Sterile gauze dressing[c] Physical therapy Splints as necessary	Epithelialization in 7–21 days Hypertrophic scar rare Return of full function
Deep partial-thickness	Reticular dermis	Blisters pale white or yellow color Absent pain sensation	As for superficial partial-thickness burns Early surgical excision and skin grafting an option	Epithelialization in 21–60 days in the absence of surgery Hypertrophic scar common Earlier return of function with surgical therapy
Full-thickness	Subcutaneous fat, fascia, muscle, or bone	Blisters may be absent Leathery, in classic, wrinkled appearance over bony prominences No capillary refill Thrombosed subcutaneous vessels may be visible Absent pain sensation	As for superficial partial-thickness burns Wound excision and grafting at earliest feasible time	Functional limitation more frequent Hypertrophic scar mainly at graft margins

[a]Epidermal (first-degree) burns present clinically with cutaneous erythema, pain, and tenderness; they resolve rapidly and generally require only symptomatic treatment.
[b]No clinically useful objective method of measuring burn depth exists; classification depends on clinical judgment.
[c]Sterile gauze dressings are frequently omitted on the face and neck.
Reprinted with permission from Monafo WW. Initial management of burns. N Engl J Med. 1996;335:1581.

the skin. **Superficial** partial-thickness burns involve the papillary dermis. They appear red, warm, edematous, and blistered, often with denuded, moist, mottled red or pink epithelium. The injured tissue is very painful, especially when exposed to air. Such burns frequently arise from brief contact with hot surfaces, liquids, flames, or chemicals. **Deep** second-degree burns involve the reticular dermis and thus can damage dermal appendages (e.g., nerves, sweat glands, or hair follicles). Hence, such burns can be less sensitive or hairs may be easily plucked out. Nonetheless, the only definitive method of differentiating superficial and deep partial-thickness burns is by length of time to heal. Superficial burns heal in less than 2 weeks; deep burns require at least 3 weeks. Furthermore, any partial-thickness burn can convert to full-thickness injury over time, especially if early fluid resuscitation is inadequate or infection ensues.

c. **Full-thickness** (third- or fourth-degree) burns involve all layers of the skin and some subcutaneous tissue. In **third-degree** burns, all skin appendages and sensory fibers are destroyed. This results in an initially painless, insensate dry surface that may appear either white and leathery or charred and cracked. **Fourth-degree** burns also involve fascia, muscle, and bone. They often result from prolonged contact with thermal sources or high electrical current. All full-thickness burns are managed surgically, and immediate burn expertise should be sought.

H. **Percentage of body surface area (BSA) estimation.** The accurate and timely assessment of BSA is a critical aspect of the initial evaluation of burned patients. It will determine whether transfer to a specialized burn center is required as well as the magnitude of initial fluid resuscitation and nutritional requirements (*J Burn Care Res.* 2007;28:42).

1. **Small areas:** The area of patient's hand (including palm and extended fingers) equals 1% of BSA (*Burns.* 2001;27:591).

2. **Large areas:** "rule of nines": Regions of the body approximating 9% BSA or multiples thereof are shown in Table 24-2. Note that infants and babies have a proportionally greater percentage of BSA in the head and neck region and less in the lower extremities than adults (*Burns.* 2000;26:156).

TABLE 24-2   Rule-of-Nines Estimation of Percentage of Body Surface Area

| | Head and Neck | Trunk | | Extremity | | |
		Anterior	Posterior	Upper	Lower	Genital
Adult	9	18	18	9	18	1
Infant	18	18	18	9	14	—

II. MANAGEMENT

A. Emergency room

1. **Resuscitation.** A surgical consultation is initiated for all patients with major injury.

   a. **Oxygen** should be provided to patients with all but the most minor injuries. A 100% oxygen high-humidity facemask for those with possible inhalation injury assists the patient's expectoration from dry airways and treats carbon monoxide poisoning.

   b. **Intravenous access.** All patients with burns of 15% or greater BSA require intravenous fluids. Two 16-gauge or larger peripheral venous catheters should be started immediately to provide circulatory volume support. Peripheral access in the upper extremities is preferred over central venous access because of the risk of catheter-related infection. An intravenous catheter may be placed through the burn if other sites are unavailable. Avoid lower-extremity catheters, if possible, to prevent phlebitic complications.

   c. **Fluid.** Improved survival in the era of modern burn care is largely attributable to early and aggressive volume resuscitation. Intravenous fluid in excess of maintenance fluids is administered to all patients with burns of 15% or greater BSA in adults (≥10% BSA in children) and generally follows established guidelines and formulas. Although several formulas have been described, most burn surgeons adhere to crystalloid-based formulations. In particular, fluid resuscitation based on the Consensus formula is widely used and has decreased the occurrence of burn-induced shock (*J Burn Care Res.* 2008;29:257).

      (1) **Consensus formula.** The estimated crystalloid requirement for the first 24 hours after injury is calculated on the basis of patient weight and BSA burn percentage. Lactated Ringer's solution volume in the first 24 hours = 2 to 4 mL × %BSA (second-, third-, and fourth-degree burns only) × body weight (kg). One-half of the calculated volume is given in the first 8 hours after injury, and the remaining volume is infused over the next 16 hours. Fluid resuscitation calculations are based on the time of injury, not the time when the patient is evaluated. Prehospital intravenous hydration is subtracted from the total volume estimate. It should be emphasized that formulas are only estimates, and more or less fluid may be required to maintain adequate tissue perfusion as measured by rate of urine output. Patients with inhalational injury, associated mechanical trauma, electrical injury, escharotomies, or delayed resuscitation require more fluid than that based on the formula alone. Furthermore, for children weighing 30 kg or less, 5% dextrose in one-quarter normal saline maintenance fluids should supplement the Parkland formula to compensate for ongoing evaporative losses. Patient body weight is determined early after the burn as a baseline measurement for fluid calculations and as a daily reference for fluid management.

(2) **Colloid-containing solutions** should be held for intravenous therapy until after the first 12 to 24 hours postburn, at which time capillary leak diminishes. Although controversial, some burn specialists recommend starting colloid formulations after this initial period to decrease the required volume of fluid administered (*J Trauma.* 2005;58:1011). However, a recent study of 7,000 critically ill (nonburned) patients found that while colloid resuscitation resulted in less volume administered, it did not improve organ failure rates, ventilator days, or mortality (*N Engl J Med.* 2004;350:2247). Even more troubling, a Cochrane review found that the relative risk of death was 2.4 times higher in burned patients who received albumin than in those who were given only crystalloid fluids (*Cochrane Database Syst Rev.* 2002;4:CD001208).

d. A **Foley catheter** is used to monitor hourly urine production as an index of adequate tissue perfusion. In the absence of underlying renal disease, a minimum urine production rate of 1 mL/kg/hr in children (weighing ≤30 kg) and 0.5 mL/kg/hr in adults is the guideline for adequate intravenous infusion.

e. **Nasogastric tube** insertion with low suction is performed if patients are intubated or develop nausea, vomiting, and abdominal distention consistent with adynamic ileus. Virtually, all patients with burns of greater than 25% BSA will have ileus.

f. **Escharotomy** may be necessary in full-thickness circumferential burns of the neck, torso, or extremities when increasing tissue edema impairs peripheral circulation or when chest involvement restricts respiratory efforts. Full-thickness incisions through (but no deeper than) the insensate burn eschar provide immediate relief (Fig. 24-1). Longitudinal escharotomies are performed on the lateral or medial aspects of the extremities and the anterior axillary lines of the chest (*World J Surg.* 2003;27:1323). Usually, they are done at the bedside and require no anesthesia. However, if the digits were burned so severely that desiccation results, midlateral escharotomies have minimal benefit. Escharotomies are rarely required within the first 6 hours after injury. Indications for escharotomy rest on clinical grounds. Traditionally, to aid in assessing peripheral circulation, the documentation of palpable peripheral pulse or the presence of a Doppler signal has been used. However, studies have indicated that correlation of intramuscular pressure with signs and symptoms of extremity compression, including Doppler pulse, is poor (*Am J Surg.* 1980;140:825). Infrared photoplethysmography has been a useful adjunct in assessing the need of escharotomies because photoplethysmography correlates well with blood flow and direct measurement of compartment pressure (*J Hand Surg.* 1984;9:314). Laser Doppler flowmetry has been shown to be predictive of the need for escharotomy and grafting in deep dermal upper extremity burns (*J Trauma.* 1997;43:35). Furthermore, laser Doppler imaging has been repeatedly shown to predict burn wound outcome and has been approved by the

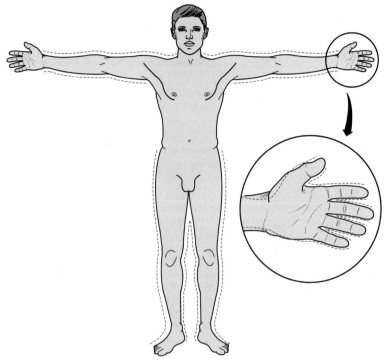

Figure 24-1. Placement of escharotomies. Midaxial escharotomies should be performed if vascular compromise occurs. Incisions should be performed through the dermis and subcutaneous tissue to allow maximal expansion of the underlying fascia.

Food and Drug Administration for assessing burn depth (*Burns.* 2008;34:761).

2. **Monitors.** Continuous pulse oximetry to measure oxygen saturation is useful. One caveat is that falsely elevated levels can be observed in carbon monoxide poisoning.

3. **Laboratory evaluation** includes a baseline complete blood cell count, type and crossmatch, electrolytes and renal panel, β-human chorionic gonadotropin (in women), arterial carboxyhemoglobin, arterial blood gas evaluation, and urinalysis. A toxicology screen and an alcohol level are obtained when suggested by history or mental status examination. A chest radiograph is obtained with the understanding that it rarely reflects early inhalation injury. Additional chest films should be obtained if endotracheal intubation or central catheter placement becomes necessary. An electrocardiogram is useful initially, particularly in elderly patients or those with electrical burns. Fluid and electrolyte fluxes during resuscitation and later mobilization of third-space edema can result in arrhythmias and interval electrocardiogram changes.

4. **Moist dressings** applied to partial-thickness burns provide pain relief from air exposure. Cool water applied to small partial-thickness burns can provide relief but must be avoided in patients with major burns (>25% BSA) and especially in infants, to avoid hypothermia. Cold water can also cause vasoconstriction and can extend the depth and surface area of injury.

5. **Analgesia** is given intravenously every 1 to 2 hours to manage pain but in small doses to guard against hypotension, oversedation, and respiratory depression.

6. Photographs or diagrams of the BSA involvement and thickness of burns are useful for documenting injuries. They also can facilitate communication between the various members of the team caring for the patient and serve medicolegal purposes in the case of assault or child abuse.

7. **Early irrigation** and debridement are performed using normal saline and sterile instruments to remove all loose epidermal skin layers, followed by the application of topical antimicrobial agents and sterile dressings. In general, it is safe to leave small blisters overlying superficial partial-thickness burns intact because they permit healing in a sterile environment and offer some protection to the underlying dermis. However, in larger and deeper partial-thickness burns, debridement of burn blisters should be done to relieve tension and purge inflammatory mediators. Nonviable tissue in the burn wound should be debrided early because the dead tissue provides a bacterial medium putting the patient at risk for both local and systemic infections. Early excision and grafting has been shown to benefit survival, blood loss, incidence of sepsis, and length of stay compared with serial debridement (*Burns.* 2006;32:145). If the burns resulted from liquid chemical exposure, they are irrigated continuously for 20 to 30 minutes. Dry chemicals are removed from the skin before irrigation to prevent them from dissolving into solution and causing further injury. Corneal burns of the eye require continuous irrigation for several hours and immediate ophthalmologic consultation.

8. **Topical antimicrobial agents** are the mainstay of local burn wound management. Prior to the use of topical antimicrobial agents, the most common organisms causing burn wound infections were *Staphylococcus aureus* and group A streptococci (*J Trauma.* 1982;22:11). Subsequent to the development of topical agents, gram-negative organisms, particularly *Pseudomonas aeruginosa,* and fungi are the most common causes of invasive burn wound sepsis (*J Burn Care Res.* 2011;32:324). Systemic antibiotics are not administered prophylactically but are reserved for documented infection. Bacterial proliferation may occur underneath the eschar at the viable–nonviable interface, resulting in subeschar suppuration and separation of the eschar. Microorganisms can invade the underlying tissue, producing invasive burn wound sepsis. The risk of invasive infection is higher in patients with multiorgan failure or burns greater than 30% BSA (*World J Surg.* 2004;22:135). When the identity of the specific organism is established, antibiotic

therapy is targeted to that organism. It may be useful on occasion to diagnose invasive infection. The technique requires a 500-mg biopsy of suspicious eschar and underlying unburned tissue. Wound infection is defined by more than 10^5 organisms per gram of tissue. Treatment requires infected eschar excision and appropriate topical/systemic antibiotic therapy.

a. **Silver sulfadiazine** (e.g., Silvadene): most commonly used agent. Advantages: broad spectrum (gram positive, most gram negative, some fungal), nonirritating, high patient acceptance, easy to use, fewest adverse side effects. It is formulated as a cream, which helps to minimize evaporative water and heat loss and thus diminishes caloric requirements. Disadvantages: some *Pseudomonas* resistance, poor eschar penetration, occasional transient leukopenia 3 to 5 days after use which is generally harmless and resolves regardless of cessation of treatment.

b. **Mafenide acetate** (Sulfamylon): advantages: broad spectrum, particularly against *Pseudomonas* and *Enterococcus* species, good eschar penetration. Disadvantages: painful, can cause allergic rash, readily absorbed systemically leading to metabolic acidosis via carbonic anhydrase inhibition. Therefore, its use is limited to small full-thickness burns.

c. **Polymyxin B sulfate** (Polysporin), neomycin, bacitracin: petroleum-based ointments. Advantages: painless, allow wound observation, tolerated well on facial burns, and do not discolor skin. Disadvantages: poor gram-negative coverage, poor eschar penetration. Mupirocin is an ointment with improved activity against methicillin-resistant *S. aureus* and gram-negative bacteria.

d. **Silver nitrate:** applied as a soak. Advantages: painless, complete antimicrobial coverage, useful for patients with sulfa allergy. Disadvantages: stains tissue gray to black making wound monitoring difficult. Also hypotonic and leaches electrolytes resulting in severe electrolyte abnormalities.

e. **Acticoat:** commercial dressing with impregnated silver ions. Advantages: easy application, excellent antimicrobial activity. Disadvantages: expensive, can only be left in place for 3 days.

f. **Dakin solution** (0.25% sodium hypochlorite): advantages: inexpensive, good antimicrobial activity. Disadvantages: cytotoxic (though less so at 0.025%) and can inhibit healing, must be changed frequently.

9. **Tetanus prophylaxis.** If last booster was administered greater than 5 years prior, tetanus toxoid 0.5 mL intramuscularly is given. If immunization status is unknown, 250 to 500 units of human tetanus immunoglobulin (Hyper-Tet) are given intramuscularly.

10. **Critical care issues with burns.** Issues include burn wound infection, pneumonia, sepsis, ileus, Curling's ulcer (gastroduodenal), acalculous cholecystitis, and superior mesenteric artery syndrome.

a. **Stress ulcer prophylaxis** (e.g., H_2 blockers or proton-pump inhibitors) should be provided for patients who have major burns and can receive nothing by mouth, especially those with coagulopathy (*Shock.* 1996;5:4).

b. **Deep venous thrombosis.** Burn patients are at increased risk for deep venous thrombosis and should receive pharmacologic prophylaxis (*Burns.* 2004;30:591).

c. **Sepsis.** In patients who survive the first 24 hours after injury, burn sepsis is the leading cause of mortality (*Burns.* 2006;32:545). The evidence-based recommendations of the Surviving Sepsis Campaign (*Crit Care Med.* 2008;36(1):296) include antibiotic therapy, source control, crystalloid resuscitation, vasopressor use, a hemoglobin transfusion trigger of 7 g/dL, an open-lung, low-tidal-volume ventilatory strategy, and maintenance of blood glucose less than 180 mg/dL.

B. **Outpatient.** Only minor first-degree or partial-thickness injuries should be considered for outpatient management. The decision to use outpatient management depends on many factors including patient reliability, opportunity for follow-up, and accessibility to health professionals. Surgical consultation is recommended at the time of initial evaluation in all but the most minor injuries.

1. **Dressings** are often managed by the patient when the injury is easily accessible. Home health nursing is a useful adjunct when self-application is suboptimal or wounds are in early healing stages and require close follow-up. Silver sulfadiazine is often applied as a light coating, followed by sterile dressings once or twice daily.

2. **Antibiotics** are not prescribed prophylactically. Their use is limited to documented wound infections.

3. Follow-up usually occurs once or twice a week during the initial healing of partial-thickness burns and split-thickness skin grafts until epithelialization is complete. Thereafter, patients are followed at 1- to 3-month intervals to evaluate and treat scar hypertrophy (application of foam tape or Jobst garments), hyperpigmentation (avoidance of direct sunlight, use of sunscreen), dry skin (unscented lotion massage), and pruritus (antihistamines). Rehabilitation potential and therapy (physical, occupational, social, and psychological) are also evaluated.

C. **Inpatient**

1. Transfer to a burn center should follow the guidelines of the American Burn Association (www.ameriburn.org). These criteria reflect multiple studies showing that age and BSA burn percentage remain the two most important prognostic factors.

a. Partial-thickness burns greater than 10% BSA.

b. Any full-thickness burn.

c. Burns that involve the face, hands, feet, genitalia, perineum, or major joints.

d. Any inhalation, chemical, or electrical injury (including lightning).

e. Burn injury in patients with preexisting medical conditions that could complicate management, prolong recovery, or affect mortality.

f. Burns in combination with significant associated mechanical trauma. Note, if the traumatic injury poses a greater threat to life, the patient should be stabilized at a trauma center before transfer to a burn unit.

    g. Burned children in hospitals without qualified personnel or equipment for the care of children.

    h. Patients requiring specialized rehabilitation, psychological support, or social services (including suspected neglect or child abuse).

2. Nutrition. Severe burns induce a hypermetabolic state proportional to the size of the burn up to 200% the normal metabolic rate. Early enteral feeding in burn patients helps to attenuate the catabolic response after burn injury and decrease the rate of infectious complications (*J Trauma.* 2003;54:755). The daily estimated metabolic requirement (EMR) in burn patients can be calculated from the Curreri formula: EMR = [25 kcal × body weight (kg)] + (40 kcal × %BSA). In children, formulas based on BSA are more appropriate. Protein losses in burn patients from both an increased oxidation rate and burn wound extravasation should be replaced by supplying 1.5 to 2 g/kg of protein/day (*Lancet.* 2004;363:1895). Therapeutic strategies should target prevention of body weight loss of more than 10% of the patient's baseline weight. Losses of more than 10% of lean body mass may lead to impaired immune function and delayed wound healing. Losses of more than 40% lead to imminent death (*Shock.* 1998;10:155).

    a. Enteral feedings are the preferred route when tolerated and can be administered through an enteral feeding tube positioned in the duodenum. For severe burns, early feeding within the first 24 hours has been shown to improve a number of outcome measures including overall mortality (*Burns.* 1997;23(Suppl 1):519). Increasing feedings beyond the EMR is associated with the development of fatty liver (*Ann Surg.* 2002;235:152) and hyperglycemia (*J Trauma.* 2001;51:540), which have a negative influence on outcome in burned patients.

    b. Total parenteral nutrition should be initiated after fluid resuscitation only if the patient is unable to tolerate enteral feeding.

    c. Daily vitamin supplementation in adults should include 1.5 g of ascorbic acid, 500 mg of nicotinamide, 50 mg of riboflavin, 50 mg of thiamine, and 220 mg of zinc. Although results from high-dose antioxidant therapy are promising, further clinical trials are needed to define its role in burn patients (*J Burn Care Rehabil.* 2005;26:207).

    d. Anabolic adjuncts, including growth hormone (*Ann Surg.* 2009 Sep 2, Epub), insulin-like growth factor, insulin, testosterone (*Crit Care Med.* 2001;29:1936), oxandrolone (*Pharmacotherapy* 2009;29:213), and propranolol (*N Engl J Med.* 2001;345:1223), have been shown to improve protein synthesis after severe injury. However, caution is advised as growth hormone therapy has been found to increase mortality in critically ill patients although patients with burns and sepsis were excluded from the study (*N Engl J Med.* 1999;341:785).

3. **Wound care**

    a. Analgesia and **sedation** for dressing changes are necessary for major burns. Benzodiazepines can be used with or without ketamine for sedation. Ketamine can cause tachycardia, hypotension, and arrhythmias. Alternatively, in patients with a secure airway, intravenous propofol has the desired effects of ease of titration and quick onset/offset of action. Either of these sedative regimens in concert with narcotic analgesia is well tolerated.

b. Daily dressing changes. While the wounds are exposed, the surgeon can properly assess the continued demarcation and healing of the injury. Physical therapy with active range of motion is performed at this time, before reapplying splints and dressings.

c. Debridement of all nonviable tissue should take place using sterile technique and instruments when demarcation occurs. Partial-thickness eschar can be abraded lightly using wet gauze. Enzymatic treatments can be useful in dissolving eschar to develop granulation tissue for tissue grafting. All full-thickness eschar should be identified early, excised, and closed or covered before the development of wound colonization and infection.

d. Temporary dressings for massive burns with limited donor sites give stable coverage without painful dressing changes.

(1) Biologic dressings include allograft (cadaver skin) and xenograft (pig skin). These dressings provide the advantages of ease of acquisition and application while providing barrier protection and a biologic bed under which dermis can granulate. After several days, the allograft can be removed, and a meshed autograft may be replaced for definitive coverage. The use of cultured autologous epithelium (keratinocytes) has shown encouraging results, particularly for patients with massive burns (>80% BSA) and limited donor sites (*J Cell Mol Med.* 2005;9:592). However, this technology is currently limited by the time needed to grow the autograft (2 to 3 weeks) and the relatively lower take rate (50% to 75%).

(2) Synthetic dressings have become an attractive alternative for early wound coverage. Biobrane is a collagen-coated silicone membrane that prevents moisture loss, but, therefore, can trap infection. It is relatively painless and can be easily peeled from the wound after epithelialization. It is useful for superficial partial-thickness burns and skin graft donor sites. Trancyte is similar to Biobrane, but also has growth factors from cultured fibroblasts to theoretically aid wound healing. Integra consists of an epidermal analogue (silastic film) and a dermal analogue (collagen matrix), making it useful for full-thickness burns. Once adequate vascularization is seen through the silicone layer, the film is removed, and an ultrathin autograft is placed onto the artificial dermis, which allows more rapid reharvesting from the donor site (*J Burn Care Rehabil.* 2003;24:42).

4. Operative management

a. Early tangential excision of burn eschar to the level of bleeding capillaries should follow the resuscitation phase. Debate persists as to the optimal timing of burn wound excision (range is 1 to 10 days), although evidence exists demonstrating benefit from early excision

Figure 24-2. Combined skin graft to cover burn wounds too extensive for other methods. The widely meshed autograft would allow continued fluid fluxes during the more extended time required for epithelialization. A more narrowly meshed allograft placed superficial to the autograft can accelerate the process by providing temporary coverage while the autograft fills in.

(*Burns.* 2006;32:145). Excision can be performed using a knife for small surfaces and a power- or gas-driven dermatome for larger surfaces. For each trip to the operating theater, consider limiting burn excision to less than 20% BSA or 2 hours of operating time. Even within such limits, aggressive debridement frequently produces profound blood loss and hypothermia (*Crit Care Clin.* 1999;15:333).

b. Split-thickness skin grafts are harvested at a thickness of 0.012 to 0.015 in. (*Clin Dermatol.* 2005;23:332). For cosmetically sensitive areas, autografts are not meshed, or, if necessary, meshed at a narrow ratio (≤2:1). Grafts are secured with absorbable sutures or staples. For very large wounds, split-thickness skin grafts can be meshed up to 4:1 and may be overlaid with meshed allograft tissue (Fig. 24-2). However, cosmesis is poor, and graft take rates may be compromised. Nonadherent dressings and bolsters are applied to minimize shear forces on the fresh grafts. Splints or pins may be required to improve graft survival at joints and to prevent contracture. Ideal point positions are extensions in the neck, knee, elbow, wrist, and interphalangeal joints, 15-degree flexion at metacarpophalangeal joints, and abduction at the shoulder (*Clin Plast Surg.* 1992;19:721).

c. Vacuum-assisted closure devices have gained popularity as a means of securing skin grafts with improved take rates compared with standard bolster dressing (*Arch Surg.* 2002;137:930).

III. BURN MECHANISMS: SPECIAL CONSIDERATIONS

A. Inhalational. Thermal injury to the airway generally is limited to the oropharynx or glottis. The glottis generally protects the subglottic airway from heat, unless the patient has been exposed to superheated steam. Edema formation can compromise the patency of the upper airway, mandating early assessment and constant reevaluation of the airway. **Gases** containing substances that have undergone incomplete combustion (particularly aldehydes), toxic fumes (hydrogen cyanide), and carbon monoxide can cause tracheobronchitis, pneumonitis, and edema. Mortality may be increased by as much as 20% in these patients. **Carbon monoxide** exposure is suggested by a history of exposure in a confined space with symptoms of nausea, vomiting, headache, mental status changes, and cherry-red lips. Carbon monoxide binds to hemoglobin with an affinity 249 times greater than that of oxygen, resulting in extremely slow dissociation (250-minute half-life with room air) unless the patient is administered supplemental oxygen (40-minute half-life with 100% oxygen via nonrebreathing mask). The arterial **carboxyhemoglobin** level is obtained as a baseline. If it is elevated (>5% in nonsmokers or >10% in smokers), oxygen therapy should continue until normal levels are achieved. The increased ventilation–perfusion gradient and the reduction in peak airway flow in distal airways and alveoli can be evaluated using a xenon-133 ventilation–perfusion lung scan. **Management** of minor inhalation injury is by delivery of humidified oxygen. Major injuries require endotracheal intubation for airway protection, preferably with a large-bore tube (7.5 to 8 mm) to facilitate pulmonary toilet of viscous secretions. As discussed earlier, decreased pulmonary compliance is often seen after inhalation injury and can lead to iatrogenic ventilator-associated lung injury. Inhaled bronchodilators can be given to treat bronchospasm whereas nebulized heparin and N-acetylcysteine can limit cast formation. It should be mentioned that inadequate fluid resuscitation actually worsens pulmonary injury, likely due to concentration of neutrophils, whose reactive mediators cause lung injury. Prophylactic antibiotic usage is not indicated. Extubation is performed as soon as possible to prevent pneumonia because coughing clears pulmonary secretions more effectively than suctioning.

B. Electrical

1. **Factors influencing severity** include the voltage (high is >1,000 V), resistance, type of current, current pathway through the body, and duration of contact with an electrical source (*Annu Rev Biomed Eng.* 2000;2:477). Electrical current passes in a straight line between points of body contact with the source and the ground. When current passes through the heart or brain, cardiopulmonary arrest can result. In most cases, these injuries respond to resuscitation and usually do not cause permanent damage (*Ann Intern Med.* 2006;145:531). **Severity of injury frequently is underestimated** when only the entrance and exit wounds are considered.

a. **Tissue resistance.** Heat and subsequent injury from thermal necrosis is directly proportional to resistance to current flow. Tissues that have a higher resistance to electricity, such as skin, bone, and fat, tend to increase in temperature and coagulate, causing deep thermal burns. Nerves and blood vessels have low resistance and readily conduct electricity (*Crit Care Clin.* 1999;15:319). In addition to direct tissue injury, thrombosis can occur with distal soft-tissue ischemia. Peripheral perfusion should be monitored closely because fasciotomy may become necessary to treat compartment syndrome. Fluid resuscitation requirements often are higher than calculated by published formulas.

  b. **Current**

   (1) **Alternating** current (household, power lines) can lead to repetitive, tetanic muscle contraction. In fact, when contact occurs between the palm and an electrical source, alternating current can cause a hand to grip the source of electricity (because of a stronger flexor than extensor tone) and lead to longer electrical exposure (*J Forensic Sci.* 1980;25:514). High-voltage injury, which is commonly seen in workers operating near power lines, can present with full-thickness, charred skin at the entrance and exit wounds, with full arrest, and with fractures sustained while current passed through the body or during a fall.

   (2) **Direct** current emanates from batteries and lightning and causes a single muscle contraction, often throwing the person receiving the electrical shock away from the source of electricity. With a voltage of at least 100 million V and a current of 200,000 A, lightning kills 150 to 300 people in the United States every year. Injury can result from direct strikes or side flashes. Current can travel on the surface of the body rather than through it, producing a "splashed-on" pattern of skin burn.

  2. **Complications** include **cardiopulmonary arrest** (more common with alternating current) (*Br Heart J.* 1987;57:279), **thrombosis, associated fractures** related to fall or severe muscle contraction (*Am J Surg.* 1977;134:95), **spinal cord injury** (*Neurology.* 2003;60:182), and **cataracts** (*J Burn Care Rehabil.* 1991;12:458). **Rhabdomyolysis** may occur and result in myoglobin release from injured cells of deep tissues. Precipitation of protein in the renal tubules can cause acute renal failure (*Burns.* 2004;30:680). Dark urine is the first clinical indication of myoglobinuria, and intravenous lactated Ringer's solution should be administered to maintain a urine output greater than 2 mL/kg/hr. Although somewhat controversial, concomitant administration of intravenous sodium bicarbonate and mannitol to solubilize hemochromogens can potentially minimize nephrotoxicity from myoglobinuria.

C. **Chemical injury** may result from contact with alkali, acid, or petroleum compounds. Removal of the offending agent is the cornerstone of treatment. Dry chemicals should be brushed off or aspirated into a closed suction container before irrigating with **copious** amounts of water for at least 20 to 30 minutes. Alkali burns penetrate more deeply than acid burns and require longer periods of irrigation. Irrigation has a threefold effect: it dilutes the chemicals already in contact with the skin, washes unreacted agent from the skin, and helps to correct the hygroscopic effects that some agents have on tissues (*ANZ J Surg.* 2003;73:45). Neutralizing the chemicals is not recommended because the resulting reaction generates heat, which can exacerbate the injury. All chemical injuries to the eye are potentially blinding and require copious irrigation with several liters of water and prompt referral to an ophthalmologist (*BMJ.* 2004;328:36). Tar can cause ongoing burns which can be quite deep if not removed promptly.

Treat them by cooling the tar with cold water followed by removing any remaining tar with adhesive remover.

D. **Cold injury**

1. **Hypothermia** is defined as a core body temperature less than 35°C. Mild hypothermia is classified as a core body temperature of 32°C to 35°C; moderate hypothermia is 30°C to 32°C; and severe hypothermia is less than 30°C (*CMAJ.* 2003;168:305). The elderly and children are particularly susceptible. Signs of hypothermia include reduced levels of consciousness, dysrhythmias, and skin that appears cold, gray, or cyanotic. Moderate to severe hypothermia is a medical emergency and necessitates maintenance of airway, breathing, and circulation. Core body temperature should be monitored by means of an esophageal or rectal probe. The heart becomes increasingly irritable at core temperatures below 34°C, and cardiac monitoring should be routine in all hypothermic patients (*Ann Emerg Med.* 1989;18:72). Asystole may occur below 28°C, and cardiopulmonary resuscitation should be started and maintained until the patient is rewarmed to at least 36°C. Rewarming can be passive or active. Passive rewarming involves using blankets to cover the body and head. The warming rate ranges between 0.5°C and 2°C per hour. Active external warming includes the use of heating blankets or a heated forced-air system, which can increase rewarming rates by 1°C per hour as compared with simple cotton blankets (*Ann Emerg Med.* 1996;27:479). Active internal rewarming can be started immediately in the case of severe hypothermia and includes the use of warmed intravenous fluids and oxygen, together warming at a rate of 1°C to 2°C per hour (*Resuscitation.* 1998;36:101). Although used rarely, active invasive rewarming methods can warm faster, at a rate 1°C to 4°C per hour. Examples of this approach include warmed peritoneal lavage, thoracostomy lavage, and bladder lavage. Extracorporeal rewarming of blood via a continuous venovenous bypass circuit or heated hemodialysis can rewarm at a rate of 1°C to 2°C every 5 minutes (*N Engl J Med.* 1997;337:1500).

2. **Frostbite** results from the formation of intracellular ice crystals and microvascular occlusion. Factors affecting severity are temperature, duration of exposure, and environmental conditions promoting rapid heat loss such as wind velocity, moisture, immobilization, and open wounds. The fingers, toes, and ears are most commonly injured, particularly when reduced tissue perfusion has resulted from other causes such as shock.

   a. **Classification**

      (1) **First-degree:** hyperemia and edema, without skin necrosis.

      (2) **Second-degree:** superficial vesicle formation containing clear or milky fluid surrounded by hyperemia, edema, and partial-thickness necrosis.

      (3) **Third-degree:** hemorrhagic bullae and full-thickness necrosis.

      (4) **Fourth-degree:** gangrene with full-thickness involvement of skin, muscle, and bone.

b. Treatment consists of rapid rewarming in a warm water bath between 40°C and 42°C until the tissue perfusion returns, which also may help to minimize tissue loss (*Surg Clin North Am.* 1991;71:345). Splinting and elevation of the frostbitten extremity may reduce edema and promote tissue perfusion. Because mechanical pressure or friction can injure the tissue further, massage and weightbearing are discouraged. Rewarming can be painful, and therefore intravenous analgesia should be provided. Any ruptured blisters should be debrided and covered with a topical antimicrobial and gauze. Tetanus prophylaxis is administered, and follow-up over several weeks is recommended to allow for demarcation of full-thickness injury. Escharotomy may be required for severe injury. Early amputation is not recommended because improvement in tissue viability can occur weeks after injury.

25 Skin and Soft-Tissue Tumors

Amber L. Traugott and Bruce L. Hall

DIAGNOSIS OF SKIN LESIONS AND SOFT-TISSUE MASSES

The surgical management of cutaneous oncology has dramatically changed over the last 100 years. As our understanding of tumor cell biology and immunology has improved through dedicated research, so has our ability to apply surgical efforts in a more directed fashion. When a patient presents to a surgeon with a lesion, a focused history and physical examination are crucial to derive the correct diagnosis. Biopsy to obtain a tissue sample followed by histologic examination remains the gold standard for the accurate diagnosis of cutaneous lesions. For large or deep soft-tissue tumors, radiologic evaluation often precedes biopsy.

I. **SKIN LESIONS**

A. **History.** Pigmented lesions with a change in size, borders, and coloration are of concern for malignancy. In addition, the itching, bleeding, or ulceration should be assessed.

B. **Physical examination.** The color, size, shape, borders, elevation, location, firmness, and surface characteristics should be noted for each skin lesion. If possible, photographs should also be taken. Uniformly colored, small, round, circumscribed lesions are more likely benign. Irregularly colored, larger, asymmetric lesions with indistinct borders and ulceration are worrisome for malignancy.

C. **Biopsy.** A tissue diagnosis is needed for lesions that have worrisome features or *change* after a period of observation. Optimally, a full-thickness tissue is obtained via punch or excisional biopsy. Punch biopsy uses a cylindrical blade to remove a small core of skin: The sample should be obtained from the thickest portion of the lesion, avoiding areas of crusting, ulceration, or necrosis that may underestimate the thickness of the tumor. Excisional biopsy is the same as for soft-tissue masses, discussed in Section II.D. Use of non–full-thickness shave biopsy is generally discouraged because it may lead to inaccurate tumor thickness measurements; nevertheless, it does not appear to affect overall patient outcome (*Am J Surg.* 2005;190:913). A second consideration is that a shave biopsy site heals by secondary intention, giving an inferior cosmetic outcome.

II. **SOFT-TISSUE MASSES**

A. **History.** Focused history includes location, duration, change in size, and presence of associated symptoms. An enlarging, painless mass is the most common presentation. There is frequently a perceived antecedent trauma. Pain is usually a late symptom. Lesions may be misdiagnosed as hematomas or strained muscle. Any symptom or perception of enlargement is concerning for malignancy.

B. **Physical examination.** Key features are size, anatomic relationships with surrounding structures, borders, and mobility. A neurovascular examination of the affected area should be performed.

C. Radiologic evaluation

1. **Magnetic resonance (MR) scan** is the best choice for imaging soft-tissue masses. It can be difficult to distinguish edematous normal tissue from tumor; T2-weighted images and gadolinium enhancement aid in this distinction.

2. **Computed tomography (CT)** is used to assess character and extent of larger, deeper tumors. Involvement of adjacent structures and surgical access to the tumor can be determined. CT-guided core-needle biopsy can be attempted for tumors with difficult surgical access. A CT scan of the chest is useful in patients with soft-tissue sarcomas (STSs) due to its specific pattern of metastasis. CT can also be helpful in evaluating the pelvis and retroperitoneum.

D. **Biopsy.** Ideally, the surgical oncologist who performs the definitive resection should perform the biopsy.

1. **Incisional biopsy** is the gold standard. A small incision should be made that can be excised at subsequent operation: It should be oriented parallel to the long axis of the extremity. Incisional biopsy rather than excisional biopsy should be performed for a mass greater than 3 cm (or >5 cm if it is consistent with a lipoma) in diameter. Drains should be avoided; meticulous hemostasis to prevent hemorrhage from spreading tumor is critical. If drains are needed, drain sites should be in line with the incision, to be excised at subsequent operation.

2. **Core-needle biopsy** provides a section of intact tissue for histologic analysis; it can provide the same information as an incisional biopsy if a good core of tissue is obtained. A very small incision allows easy entrance of the needle into the skin. Most indeterminate or negative results should be confirmed by incisional or excisional biopsy.

3. **Excisional biopsy** is performed for tumors that are probably benign or less than 3 cm in diameter. The usual approach is an elliptical incision around the tumor oriented parallel to the long axis of the limb and, when possible, along the skin lines of minimal tension. The tumor should be excised completely with a thin margin of normal tissue. Primary closure should be employed whenever possible.

4. **Fine-needle aspiration** (FNA) is the least invasive, but can be the least informative, method of tissue diagnosis. Multiple passes are made through a mass in various directions; the plunger is released before removing the needle from the mass. The specimen is then fixed and sent for cytopathologic evaluation. FNA usually cannot give the grade, but often it can determine the presence of malignancy and the

histologic type. Indeterminate results should be followed by further evaluation. FNA is the biopsy method of first choice in the head and neck.

BENIGN LESIONS

I. **SEBORRHEIC KERATOSES** are benign skin growths that originate in the epidermis. These lesions characteristically appear in older people as multiple, raised, irregularly rounded lesions with a verrucous, friable, waxy surface and variable pigmentation from yellowish to brownish black. Common locations include the face, neck, and trunk. If removal is desired, treatment may consist of excision or curettage followed by electrodesiccation, as well as topical agents, such as trichloroacetic acid, or cryotherapy with liquid nitrogen.

II. **ACTINIC KERATOSES** are caused by sun exposure and are found predominantly in elderly, fair-skinned patients. These lesions are small, usually multiple, flat-to-slightly elevated with a rough or scaly surface ranging from red to yellowish brown to black and are found in areas of chronic sun exposure. Unlike seborrheic keratoses, these lesions have malignant potential. Indeed, 15% to 20% of lesions become squamous cell carcinoma, although metastases are rare. Benign-appearing actinic keratoses may be observed. When indicated, treatment consists of topical application of 5-fluorouracil twice a day for 2 to 6 weeks.

III. **NEVI** Junctional nevus cells actually are located in the epidermis and at the dermal–epidermal junction. These nevi are small (<6 mm), well-circumscribed, light brown or black macules found on any area of the body. Nevi rarely develop in people older than 40 years, and any new lesion in someone older than 40 years should be considered a possible early melanoma.

IV. **EPIDERMAL INCLUSION CYSTS** are lined by epidermal cells containing lipid and keratinous material. Asymptomatic cysts may be removed for diagnosis, prevention of infection, or cosmesis. Excision of the cyst should include the entire cyst lining, preferably without interruption of the lining to prevent recurrence, and should include any skin tract or drainage site.

V. **NEUROFIBROMAS** are benign tumors that arise from Schwann cells and are seen most frequently in the setting of neurofibromatosis (von Recklinghausen disease). Neurofibromas are soft, pendulous, sometimes lobulated subcutaneous masses that vary widely in size. The overwhelming majority of these tumors do not require excision. These tumors are removed for symptoms of pain, an observed increase in size, or cosmetic reasons.

VI. **GANGLION CYSTS** are subcutaneous cysts attached to the joint capsule or tendon sheath of the hands and wrists; they are most commonly seen in young and middle-aged women. These lesions present as firm, round masses often seen on the dorsum of the wrist, but can also be found on the radial volar wrist, along the flexor tendon sheaths of the hand, or in the dorsum of the distal interphalangeal joint. After surgical excision, there is an extremely low recurrence rate. To prevent recurrence, the capsular attachment and a small portion of the joint capsule should be removed.

VII. **LIPOMAS** are benign tumors consisting of fat and are perhaps the most common human neoplasms. There is very little potential for malignancy; sarcomatous elements occur in less than 1% of cases. They are soft, fatty, subcutaneous masses and vary widely in size. Asymptomatic small tumors can be followed clinically, but symptomatic or rapidly growing tumors are of concern and should be removed. Large tumors (>5 cm) should be evaluated by core or incisional biopsy. Every effort should be made to excise lipomas cleanly at the first operation to prevent recurrence.

MALIGNANT LESIONS

I. **DERMATOFIBROSARCOMA PROTUBERANS (DFSP)** is a locally aggressive tumor that does not metastasize. Margins of 2 to 5 cm should be achieved if possible. Alternatively, Mohs micrographic surgery involves serial excisions of the tumor, with microscopic examination for areas of positive margins that have been mapped and are then re-excised, one section at a time, until a negative margin is reached. Although time consuming and expensive, this surgery has been advocated in the management of DFSP for improved tissue conservation, cosmetic advantages, and low recurrence rates (*Curr Opin Oncol.* 2006;18:341). DuBay et al. reviewed 62 patients treated for DFSP with wide local excision, Mohs surgery, or a combination approach. At a median follow-up of 4.4 years, there were no local or distant recurrences. Eighty-five percent of the lesions treated initially with Mohs surgery had histologically negative margins. This suggests that Mohs surgery can be effective and that negative margin resection should be achieved (*Cancer.* 2004;100:1008).

II. **DESMOID TUMORS** are nonmetastasizing but locally aggressive tumors that arise from connective tissue. Wide excision with a margin of normal tissue should be performed if possible, but limb function should be spared. Local recurrences are common, and re-excision is often required. Tamoxifen, nonsteroidal anti-inflammatory drugs (e.g., sulindac), or a combination have been used with only anecdotal success and may be attempted as an alternative to surgery. These drugs have been advocated in recurrent or unresectable cases as well. Recommendations regarding future pregnancies are conflicting and unclear. Patients with a desmoid tumor should undergo colonoscopy to exclude the diagnosis of familial adenomatous polyposis (*Fam Cancer.* 2006;5:275).

III. **MELANOMA.** The incidence of melanoma continues to rise at an epidemic rate (101.5% increase from 1970s to 1990s). Melanoma represents the fifth-most-common type of cancer (*CA Cancer J Clin*. 2006;56:106). The estimated direct costs of treatment of melanoma by Medicare alone were $249 million in 1996, with 51% of the costs for patients with stage III or IV melanoma. (*Arch Dermatol*. 2010;146:250).

A. **Lesions.** Most pigmented lesions are benign, but approximately one-third of all melanomas arise from pigmented nevi. It is essential to differentiate among benign, premalignant, and malignant lesions.

1. **Premalignant lesions**
   a. **Dysplastic nevi** have variegated color (tan to brown on a pink base); are large (5 to 12 mm); appear indistinct, with irregular edges; and have macular and papular components. There exists a familial association between dysplastic nevi and a high incidence of melanoma. Melanomas may develop *de novo* or from preexisting dysplastic nevi (*N Engl J Med*. 2003;349:2233).
   b. **Congenital nevi** are notable by their presence since birth and are commonly referred to as "birthmarks." They can be premalignant: There is an increased risk of melanoma developing from these lesions, particularly for nevi greater than 20 cm in diameter.

2. **Malignant lesions**
   a. **Superficial spreading melanoma** (SSM) is the most common form of melanoma (80%), with approximately one-half arising from a preexisting mole. The lesions usually are slow growing and brown, with small discrete nodules of differing colors. SSM tends to spread laterally but can be slightly elevated. SSM is found most commonly on the back in men and women and on the lower extremities of women.
   b. **Nodular melanoma** is the most aggressive form, rapidly becoming a palpable, elevated, firm nodule that may be dense black or reddish blue-black. A distinct convex nodular development indicates deep dermal invasion. Nodular melanomas arise from the epidermal–dermal junction and invade deeply into the dermis and subcutaneous tissue. Approximately 5% are amelanotic.
   c. **Lentigo maligna melanoma** usually is found on older patients as a large melanotic freckle on the temple or malar region known as **Hutchinson freckle.** It usually is slow growing but becomes large, often reaching 5 to 6 cm in diameter. Initially, it is flat, but it becomes raised and thicker, with discrete brown to black nodules and irregular edges.
   d. **Acral lentiginous melanoma** occurs on the palms, soles, and nail beds, occurs primarily in dark-skinned people, and metastasizes more frequently than do other melanomas, possibly related to later stage at presentation.
   e. **In-transit metastases** and **satellites** both signify a poor prognosis with a high risk of local recurrence and distant metastasis. In-transit metastases are lesions in the skin more than 2 cm from the primary lesion; they arise from tumor cells in intradermal lymphatics. Satellites are metastatic lesions in the skin within 2 cm of the primary tumor.

B. **History and risk factors.** A history for melanoma should include an assessment of risk factors and family history.

1. **Risk factors.** Each of the risk factors listed is considered to carry a more-than-threefold increase in risk for melanoma; the presence of three or more risk factors carries approximately 20 times the risk (*Curr Probl Surg.* 2006;43:781).

    a. Family or personal history of melanoma.
    b. Blond or red hair.
    c. Freckling of the upper back.
    d. Three or more blistering sunburns before age of 20 years.
    e. Presence of actinic keratosis.
    f. Blue, green, or gray eyes.

C. **Clinical features.** Early melanoma and dysplastic lesions can be recognized by the features highlighted in the mnemonic **ABCD: *A*symmetry, *b*order** irregularity, *c*olor variegation, and *d*iameter greater than 6 mm. Advanced lesions are more readily apparent and may be nodular or ulcerated.

D. **Staging and prognosis.** Tumor thickness is the most important factor in staging the tumor. Tumors less than 1 mm thick have 10-year survival of 92%, whereas 10-year survival for lesions more than 4 mm thick is 50% (*J Clin Oncol.* 2009;27:6199). Thickness is also correlated with the risk of regional node and distant metastasis (*J Clin Oncol.* 2001;19:3622). The Breslow thickness is a physical depth measurement of the primary tumor and is used to classify the tumor (see "T Classification" in Table 25-1). In contrast, the *Clark level* describes the *anatomic* level of invasion (Table 25-2). The Clark level was historically used as a staging criterion for melanoma; however, it is no longer used for this purpose as recent studies have shown it is not an independent prognostic factor. Mitotic rate of the primary melanoma has emerged as a better predictor of clinical outcomes in recent studies and has been incorporated into recent staging systems. The revised American Joint Committee on Cancer (AJCC) system of TNM (tumor, node, metastasis) classification for melanoma (Tables 25-1 and 25-3) is the standard classification system. This system was revised in 2009 to provide more accurate and precise information regarding patient prognosis (*J Clin Oncol* 2009;27:6199). Older age, male gender, satellitosis, ulceration, and location on the *b*ack, posterolateral *a*rm, *n*eck, or *s*calp (the BANS region) all carry a worse prognosis. The presence of regional node metastasis severely worsens prognosis (10-year survival, 20% to 60%). Distant metastases have a dismal prognosis (median survival, 2 to 11 months).

E. **Treatment**

1. **Surgery**

    a. **Wide local excision** is the primary treatment for most melanomas and premalignant lesions. Melanoma in situ (MIS) should be excised to clean margins. For all other malignant melanomas, the width of the surgical margin depends on the Breslow tumor thickness: Thin melanomas (Breslow thickness <1 mm) should have a margin of 1 cm; lesions thicker than 1 mm and all scalp lesions should have a margin of at least 2 cm. Several prospective, randomized trials

TABLE 25-1	American Joint Committee on Cancer TNM (Tumor, Node, Metastasis) Definitions of Melanoma	
T classification	—	—
Tis	Melanoma in situ	—
T1	≤1.0 mm	a. Without ulceration and mitosis <1/mm^2
	—	b. With ulceration or mitoses ≥1/mm^2
T2	1.01–2.0 mm	a. Without ulceration
	—	b. With ulceration
T3	2.01–4.0 mm	a. Without ulceration
	—	b. With ulceration
T4	>4.0 mm	a. Without ulceration
	—	b. With ulceration
Regional lymph nodes (N)	—	—
N1	One lymph node	a. Micrometastasis[a]
	—	b. Macrometastasis[b]
N2	2–3 lymph nodes	a. Micrometastasis[a]
	—	b. Macrometastasis[b]
	—	c. In-transit met(s)/ satellite(s) without metastatic lymph node(s)
N3	≥4 metastatic lymph nodes, matted lymph nodes, or in-transit met(s)/satellite(s) with metastatic lymph node(s)	
Distant metastasis (M)	—	—
M1a	Distant skin, subcutaneous, or lymph node mets	Normal LDH
M1b	Lung mets	Normal LDH
M1c	All other visceral mets	Normal LDH
	Any distant mets	Elevated LDH

[a]Micrometastases are diagnosed after sentinel or completion lymphadenectomy (if performed).
[b]Macrometastases are defined as clinically detectable lymph node metastases confirmed by therapeutic lymphadenectomy or when any lymph node metastasis exhibits gross extracapsular extension.
LDH, lactic dehydrogenase; mets, metastases.
Modified from Balch CM, Gershenwald JE, Soong SJ, et al. Melanoma of the skin. In: Edge SE, Byrd DR, Carducci MA, et al., eds. *AJCC Cancer Staging Manual.* 7th ed. New York, NY: Springer; 2010: 325–44.

TABLE 25-2	Clark's Classification (Level of Invasion) of Melanoma
Level I	Lesions involving only the epidermis (in situ melanoma); not an invasive lesion
Level II	Invasion of the papillary dermis but does not reach the papillary–reticular dermal interface
Level III	Invasion fills and expands the papillary dermis but does not penetrate the reticular dermis
Level IV	Invasion into the reticular dermis but not into the subcutaneous tissue
Level V	Invasion through the reticular dermis into the subcutaneous tissue

have investigated margin requirements. A seminal trial addressed the efficacy of 2-cm versus 4-cm margins for Breslow thickness 1 to 4 mm (*Ann Surg.* 1993;218:262). There was no significant difference in the local recurrence rate, disease-free survival, or overall survival between the two groups at 10 years of follow-up (*Ann Surg Oncol.* 2001;8:101). These data suggest that a 2-cm margin is both safe and effective for primary melanomas between 1 and 4 mm, with a significant decrease in the need for skin grafting. In general, excisions should be closed primarily, with flaps or skin grafts reserved for large defects. Mohs micrographic surgery has been advocated for areas where wide and deep excisions are difficult, such as the face, or for MIS. Several single-institution series using Mohs techniques for facial lentigo maligna melanoma have shown highly variable recurrence rates ranging from 0% to 33% (*Int J Dermatol.* 2010;49:482).

b. **Elective lymph node dissection (ELND).** The term "elective" refers here to lymph node dissection done in the absence of clinically evident, palpable nodes (for palpable nodes, see Section 1.d of this part on therapeutic lymph node dissection). In the past, ELND was at times performed for the staging of patients presenting with localized melanoma. ELND provided an element of local control and reasonably accurate staging for patients with occult lymph node metastases (*Ann Surg.* 1991;214:491). Several large trials, such as the World Health Organization trial number 1, World Health Organization trial number 14, the Mayo Clinical Surgical Trial, and the Intergroup Melanoma Surgical Trial, investigated whether ELND provides benefit to patients, particularly regarding survival. The Intergroup Trial showed that ELND in patients with intermediate-thickness tumors (Breslow thickness 1 to 4 mm) improved survival, especially for patients under the age of 60 years.

Stage	Clinical Staging[a]			Pathologic Staging[b]		
0	Tis	N0	M0	Tis	N0	M0
IA	T1a	N0	M0	T1a	N0	M0
IB	T1b	N0	M0	T1b	N0	M0
	T2a	N0	M0	T2a	N0	M0
IIA	T2b	N0	M0	T2b	N0	M0
	T3a	N0	M0	T3a	N0	M0
IIB	T3b	N0	M0	T3b	N0	M0
	T4a	N0	M0	T4a	N0	M0
IIC	T4b	N0	M0	T4b	N0	M0
III[c]	Any T	≥N1	M0	—	—	—
IIIA	—	—	—	T1–4a	N1a	M0
—	—	—	—	T1–4a	N2a	M0
IIIB	—	—	—	T1–4b	N1a	M0
—	—	—	—	T1–4b	N2a	M0
—	—	—	—	T1–4a	N1b	M0
—	—	—	—	T1–4a	N2b	M0
—	—	—	—	T1–4a	N2c	M0
IIIC	—	—	—	T1–4b	N1b	M0
—	—	—	—	T1–4b	N2b	M0
—	—	—	—	T1–4b	N2c	M0
—	—	—	—	Any T	N3	M0
IV	Any T	Any N	M1	Any T	Any N	M1

TABLE 25-3 American Joint Committee on Cancer Stage Groupings for Cutaneous Melanoma

[a]Clinical staging includes microstaging of the primary melanoma and clinical/radiologic evaluation for metastases. By convention, it should be used after complete excision of the primary melanoma with clinical assessment for regional and distant metastases.

[b]Pathologic staging includes microstaging of the primary melanoma and pathologic information about the regional lymph nodes after partial or complete lymphadenectomy, except for pathologic stage 0 or stage Ia patients, who do not need pathologic evaluation of their lymph nodes.

[c]There are no stage III subgroups for clinical staging.

Modified from Balch CM, Gershenwald JE, Soong SJ, et al. Melanoma of the skin. In: Edge SE, Byrd DR, Carducci MA, et al., eds. *AJCC Cancer Staging Manual*. 7th ed. New York, NY: Springer; 2010: 325–344.

ELND has not been conclusively shown to benefit other subgroups (*Ann Surg.* 1996;224:255). This remains a controversial issue.

c. **Sentinel lymph node biopsy (SLNB).** SLNB has greatly enhanced accurate staging of patients with melanoma. This technique is based on the documented pattern of lymphatic drainage of melanomas to a specific, initial lymph node, termed the *sentinel lymph node*, before further spread. The histology of the SLN is highly (although not perfectly) reflective of the rest of the nodal basin. If the SLN is negative for metastases, a more radical and morbid lymph node dissection can be avoided. This procedure requires expertise and a multidisciplinary approach involving radiology/nuclear medicine and pathology. The SLN can be accurately identified 96% of the time using radiolymphoscintigraphy and intraoperative dye injection and radioprobe guidance. SLNB appears to be most beneficial for intermediate-thickness melanomas (Breslow thickness 1 to 4 mm) (*Ann Surg.* 2001;233:250). Data from the Multicenter Sentinel Lymphadenectomy Trial (MSLT)-I, a prospective, randomized, multinational trial, support the role of SLN and immediate (vs. delayed) complete lymphadenectomy if the SLN is positive. In MSLT-I, 1,269 patients with intermediate-thickness melanomas (1.2 to 3.5 mm) were randomized to either wide excision only followed by observation (no SLNB) or to wide excision and SLNB. In the observation-only group, complete lymphadenectomy was performed only when there was clinical evidence of nodal recurrence (delayed), whereas the SLNB group underwent a complete (immediate) lymphadenectomy if nodal micrometastases were detected in any of the SLNs. The results from this landmark trial showed that the mean estimated 5-year disease-free survival rate was significantly higher in the SLNB group than in the observation-only group (78.3% vs. 73.1%, respectively; $p = 0.009$) (*N Engl J Med.* 2006;355:1307). Although 5-year melanoma-specific survival rates were similar in the two groups, the presence of metastatic disease within the SLN was found to be the most important prognostic factor predictive of overall survival. The 5-year survival rate was 72.3% in those patients with tumor-positive SLNs and 90.2% in those with tumor-negative SLNs. For thin melanomas (≤ 1 mm thickness), the incidence of positive SLN is 2 to 5% in retrospective series (*Surg Oncol Clin N Am.* 2007;16:35). Factors which were predictive of a positive SLN in patients with thin melanomas included Breslow thickness, Clark level, mitotic rate, and younger age (*Arch Surg.* 2008;143:892). Current practice guidelines issued by the National Comprehensive Cancer Network (NCCN) recommend that SLNB be considered for patients with high-risk stage IA melanoma and discussed and offered to patients with stage IB-IIC melanomas (*NCCN Clinical Practice Guidelines in Oncology—Melanoma.* 2010, v. 2).

d. **Therapeutic lymph node dissection** should be performed for involved axillary and superficial inguinal lymph nodes unless unresectable distant metastases are present. Ideally, therapeutic LND provides optimal locoregional control of disease and a chance of cure, with 5-year survival rates of 20% to 40% (*Ann Surg Oncol.* 1998;5:473). Surgical therapy of the inguinal region includes a superficial inguinal lymphadenectomy with inclusion of the deep pelvic region for either clinical evidence of disease (palpable pelvic nodes) or radiographic or intraoperative evidence of obvious lymph node involvement. Intraoperative pathologic analysis of clinically suspicious lymph nodes may be necessary to determine the presence of metastases and possibly the need for more extensive nodal dissection. The highest superficial inguinal node (Cloquet node) can also be analyzed by frozen section to help determine the need for deep dissection. Deep inguinal node dissection should be reserved for patients whose survival is thought to justify the potential morbidity of the procedure. Hughes et al. noted that patients who underwent a superficial and deep nodal dissection (*n* = 72) had a lower regional recurrence rate than those who underwent a superficial dissection only (*n* = 60), although there was no statistical difference in overall survival (*Br J Surg.* 2000;87:892). In some cases, nodal dissection does not benefit patients with advanced disease and should therefore be carefully considered.

e. **Resection of metastases.** The surgical options for patients with metastatic melanoma can be divided into two categories: Curative or palliative. Curative interventions for metastatic melanoma should carefully weigh the risks of the surgery against the potential benefits. Recent data on the surgical management of metastatic melanoma note that certain factors are associated with an improved overall survival: (1) ability to achieve a complete resection with negative margins, (2) the initial site of metastasis, (3) extent of metastatic disease (single or multiple sites), (4) disease-free interval after surgical removal of the primary melanoma, and (5) stage of initial disease (*Curr Opin Oncol.* 2004;16:155). Favorable sites for resection include the skin, subcutaneous tissue, lymph nodes, lung, and gastrointestinal (GI) tract. Skin and subcutaneous metastases demonstrated the best long-term results after resection, with a 20% to 30% 5-year survival and a median survival of 48 months. Unfavorable sites include metastases to the brain, adrenal, and liver (*Arch Surg.* 2004;139:961).

2. **Isolated limb perfusion (ILP)** is used for recurrent limb melanoma that is locally advanced and cannot be resected by simple surgical means. ILP delivers high-dose regional chemotherapy and establishes a hyperthermic environment to an extremity though its circulation has been isolated from the rest of the body. Melphalan is commonly used. A large, retrospective meta-analysis reported complete response rates for melphalan with mild hyperthermic ILP range from 40% to 82% (median 54%) (*Eur J Surg Oncol.* 2006;32:371). Adding tumor necrosis factor (TNF)-α to melphalan has been suggested to increase the complete response rate to 60% to 85%. Randomized, multicenter data collected through the American College of Surgeons Oncology Group (ACOSOG) comparing hyperthermic ILP with melphalan alone to

melphalan plus TNF suggested that addition of TNF did not significantly enhance short-term response rates in locally advanced extremity melanoma; however, addition of TNF was found significantly to increase the overall complication rate (*J Clin Oncol.* 2006;24:4196). Patients who are elderly or who have medical comorbidities or systemic metastases are generally not suitable for this therapy.

3. **Immunotherapy.** Endeavors in both animals and humans have established that the immune system can damage or destroy even very large established tumors (*N Engl J Med.* 1984;313:1485, *J Exp Med.* 2005;202:907). Complete and durable regression of stage IV melanoma has been reported using interleukin-2 (IL-2)–based immunotherapy alone (*J Clin Oncol.* 1999;17:2105). However, treatment using IL-2 in conjunction with vaccine therapy may be more effective. Patients with metastatic melanoma who received IL-2 therapy in conjunction with gp209–2M peptide vaccine had a response rate of 22.3%, compared with 12.8% in those treated with only IL-2 ($p = 0.01$) and 13.8% in those treated with IL-2 plus other vaccines ($p = 0.009$) (*Clin Cancer Res* 2008;14:5612). High-dose interferon also has been studied in several randomized clinical trials. A pooled analysis of these trials, in patients with resected stage IIb or stage III melanoma treated with high-dose interferon versus observation, showed a significant benefit for relapse-free survival [hazard ratio (HR) = 1.3 for observation, $p = 0.006$], but no benefit in overall survival (*Clin Cancer Res.* 2004;10:1670). A recent trial of pegylated interferon versus observation in patients with resected stage III melanoma similarly showed a significant improvement in 4-year relapse-free survival (45.6% vs. 38.9%, $p = 0.01$), but no benefit for overall survival. The choice to initiate interferon therapy should be made only after a discussion with the patient about the considerable adverse effects of the drug in the context of these limited benefits.

F. **Hereditary tumor syndromes.** Melanoma is familial in approximately 10% of cases, and in these cases, it is often associated with multiple atypical moles. **Familial atypical multiple-mole melanoma syndrome (FAMMM)** has also been called *dysplastic nevus syndrome, B-K syndrome,* and *large atypical nevus syndrome.* A National Institutes of Health Consensus Conference defined FAMMM using the following criteria: (1) the occurrence of malignant melanoma in one or more first- or second-degree relatives, (2) a large number of melanocytic nevi, usually more than 50, some of which are atypical and variable in size, and (3) melanocytic nevi that have certain histopathologic features, including architectural disorder with asymmetry, subepidermal fibroplasia, and lentiginous melanocytic hyperplasia with spindle or epithelial melanocyte nests. These lesions predominantly occur on the trunk but are also found on the buttocks, scalp, and lower extremities. The relative risk for developing melanoma when multiple atypical moles are present ranges from 5 to 11 based on multiple studies. The median age for melanoma diagnosis is 34. *CDKN2,* a cell cycle protein gene, has been found to contain germline mutations in some kindreds with familial melanoma (*Nat Genet.* 1994;8:15). Other malignancies have been related to mutations in the *CDKN2* gene, especially pancreatic cancer. There may be other genes contributing to FAMMM. **Screening** for FAMMM begins at around puberty and consists of yearly physical examinations, including a total-body skin examination. For patients who have a large number of moles, baseline photographs or computerized scanning are helpful. Patients should examine their skin regularly. Suspicious lesions should undergo biopsy. Sun exposure should be avoided. Regular ophthalmologic examinations should be performed due to the increased risk of ocular nevi and ocular melanoma.

OTHER MALIGNANT SKIN TUMORS

I. **BASAL CELL CARCINOMA** is the most common malignant neoplasm of the skin; it derives from the basal cells of the epidermis and adnexal structures. They are slow growing and rarely metastasize (<0.1%) but can be locally aggressive. Sun exposure is the most significant epidemiologic factor; consequently, this neoplasm is found most commonly on the skin of the head and neck (85%) in fair-skinned patients older than 40 years.

A. **Lesions.** It is particularly important to identify the morpheaform carcinoma because it is more aggressive, with a tendency toward deep infiltration and local recurrence. These carcinomas are flat, indurated lesions with a smooth, whitish, waxy surface and indistinct borders. The noduloulcerative form is the most common and is characterized by shiny, translucent nodules with a central umbilication that often becomes ulcerated, with pearly, rolled, telangiectatic edges.

B. **Treatment**

1. **Excisional biopsy** is adequate treatment for small tumors, with intraoperative frozen-section analysis (to confirm negative margins) and primary closure. Larger tumors may be diagnosed by incisional or punch biopsy followed by complete removal. A margin of 2 to 4 mm on all sides of visible tumor should be obtained, and positive margins on frozen-section analysis should be re-excised. Margins of dysplasia or actinic changes need not be re-excised because local recurrence generally does not occur in these cases. The patient should be warned about possible pigmentation persistence.

2. **Mohs micrographic surgery** may be useful for recurrent tumors or in situations in which tissue conservation is important.

3. **Curettage with electrodesiccation** can be performed for small superficial tumors, with little risk of recurrence.

4. **Liquid nitrogen** can be used for tumors less than 1 cm in diameter.

5. **Radiation therapy** can be used in certain situations for areas difficult to reconstruct, such as the eyelids. It also can be used for palliation in patients who have large tumors and who might refuse an extensive operation, especially the elderly. Although re-excision is indicated for recurrences or positive margins, radiation therapy can be used in individual circumstances.

II. **SQUAMOUS CELL CARCINOMA** is the second-most-common skin cancer in fair-skinned people and is the most common cancer in darkly pigmented people. As with the other skin malignancies, sunlight is the major etiology, with the greatest risk in elderly men who have a history of chronic sun exposure. The mean age of presentation is 68 years, and men predominate two to one. Squamous cell carcinoma can be found on any sun-exposed area, including mucous membranes. It also is known to develop from draining sinuses, radiation, chronic ulcers, and scars (particularly burn scars, in which case it is called a ***Marjolin ulcer***).

A. **Lesions.** Squamous cell carcinoma presents as small, firm, erythematous plaques with a smooth or verrucous surface and indistinct margins with progression to raised, fixed, and ulcerated lesions. Ulceration tends to occur earlier in aggressive lesions. Most lesions are preceded by actinic keratosis, which results in a slow-growing, locally invasive lesion without metastases. If not preceded by actinic keratosis, the cancer tends to be more aggressive, with more rapid growth, invasion, and metastatic spread. Perineural invasion has a poorer prognosis and higher recurrence rate.

B. **Treatment** is similar to that for basal cell carcinoma. Tumor-free margins of 5 mm for tumors of less than 1 cm and tumor-free margins of 1 to 2 cm for tumors of more than 2 cm in diameter should be obtained. Curettage with electrodesiccation and laser vaporization has been used for small, superficial squamous carcinomas, but there is no way to assess margins of treatment. Solitary metastases should be resected if possible because there is a relatively high cure rate compared to other cancers.

SOFT-TISSUE SARCOMAS

Soft-tissue sarcomas represent a heterogeneous group of malignant tumors derived from mesodermal tissues. STS are rare, constituting approximately 1% of adult malignant neoplasms and causing 3,100 deaths annually; many general surgeons will see few of these tumors during their careers. Most of these tumors arise *de novo,* rarely from premalignant tumors. In a minority of cases, STSs are associated with cancer predisposition syndromes such as von Recklinghausen disease, Werner syndrome, or Li–Fraumeni syndrome. Lymphedema and radiation have been shown to be etiologic factors in certain rare sarcomas (*Am Surg.* 2006;72:665).

I. **LESIONS.** Sarcomas are classified by histologic cell type of origin and grade. The most common subtype is malignant fibrous histiocytoma (40%), followed by liposarcoma (25%). Patients typically present with an asymptomatic lump or mass that has grown to be visible or palpable. Retroperitoneal tumor can reach massive proportions before increased abdominal girth and vague symptoms bring it to the physician's attention. Tumors also may grow unnoticed to large sizes in the thigh or trunk.

II. **DIAGNOSIS.** Biopsy (usually core or incisional) is necessary for diagnosis. Care is needed to orient incisions to aid in the definitive operation. Even small, apparently benign lesions should be biopsied or excised. Adequate tissue must be provided to pathology for histologic assessment.

TABLE 25-4	American Joint Committee on Cancer Staging System for Soft-Tissue Sarcoma

Tumor grade (G)	**Stage IA**
GX: Grade cannot be assessed	G1/GX, T1a, N0, M0
G1: Well differentiated	G1/GX, T1b, N0, M0
G2: Moderately differentiated	**Stage IB**
G3: Poorly differentiated	G1/GX, T2a, N0, M0
G4: Undifferentiated	G1/GX, T2b, N0, M0
Primary tumor (T)	**Stage IIA**
TX: Primary tumor cannot be assessed	G2–3, T1a, N0, M0
T0: No evidence of primary tumor	G2–3, T1b, N0, M0
T1: Tumor ≤ 5 cm in greatest dimension	**Stage IIB**
T1a: Superficial tumor[a]	G2, T2a, N0, M0
T1b: Deep tumor[a]	G2, T2b, N0, M0
T2: Tumor >5 cm in greatest dimension	**Stage III**
T2a: Superficial tumor[a]	G3, T2a, N0, M0
T2b: Deep tumor[a]	G3, T2b, N0, M0
Regional lymph nodes (N)	Any G, any T, N1, M0
NX: Regional lymph nodes cannot be assessed	**Stage IV**
N0: No regional lymph node metastasis	Any G, any T, any N, M1
N1: Regional lymph node metastasis	—
Distant metastasis (M)	—
MX: Distant metastasis cannot be assessed	—
M0: No distant metastasis	—
M1: Distant metastasis	—

[a]Superficial tumor is located exclusively above the superficial fascia without invasion of the fascia; deep tumor either is located exclusively beneath the superficial fascia or superficial to the fascia with invasion of or through the fascia or is located superficial and beneath the fascia. Retroperitoneal, mediastinal, and pelvic sarcomas are classified as deep tumors.

Modified from Soft tissue sarcoma. In: Edge SE, Byrd DR, Carducci MA, et al., eds. *AJCC Cancer Staging Manual.* 7th ed. New York, NY: Springer: 2010; 291–298.

III. **STAGING AND PROGNOSIS (TABLE 25-4).** The AJCC staging system is based on tumor size, nodal status, histologic grade, and metastasis. Of these, size and grade are the most important.

   A. **Grade.** The grade of the tumor is the major prognostic factor. Grade is obtained from histopathologic analysis of biopsy tissue and is generally based on the mitotic index, nuclear morphology, and degree of anaplasia. However, interobserver variability is high, with some centers having different criteria: Rates of discordance even among expert pathologists of up to 40% have been observed.

   B. **Staging** for STS includes physical examination and CT or MR scan to assess the size and extent of tumor. Metastases most commonly are found in the lungs; CT scan of the lungs is a required study for grade II and III lesions. Abdominal CT scan is required for evaluation of retroperitoneal sarcomas. This study can assess for hepatic metastases, which are more common for this primary. Retroperitoneal and truncal STS have worse prognoses than extremity STS.

C. **Prognosis.** Almost 80% of metastases are to the lungs and occur within 2 to 3 years of diagnosis. If the pulmonary disease is resectable, 30% survival at 3 years can be expected. In addition, tumor size, grade, tumor rupture during surgery, margins after resection, and anatomic location all have an impact on various outcome measures such as local recurrence, overall survival, and tumor-free survival. Local recurrence should be resected aggressively, and long-term follow-up is required because late recurrences may occur.

IV. SURGICAL TREATMENT

A. **Resection.** Smaller, grade I tumors can be excised with a minimum 1-cm margin, usually without adjuvant radiation. Larger tumors may benefit from a larger margin or radiation to prevent recurrence. Grade II and III tumors, in general, require radiation therapy in addition to excision to avoid more radical surgery. Depending on the size and grade of tumor, compartment resection may be indicated.

B. **Limb-sparing resection** combined with radiation therapy offers survival equivalent to that achieved with amputation (*Ann Surg*. 1982;196:305). Limb-sparing procedures have a distinct psychological as well as functional advantage and are the procedures of choice for most tumors. The tumor should be removed with an envelope of normal tissue surrounding it, if possible. The resection should include the area of previous incision and biopsy and any drain sites. The resection field should be marked with clips to guide radiation therapy.

C. **Gastrointestinal stromal tumors (GISTs)** are sarcomatous tumors of the GI tract. These tumors are rare and most commonly arise from the stomach. GIST can present with acute or subacute GI bleeding, vague abdominal pain, a palpable abdominal mass, or as an incidental mass found on CT scan of the abdomen. These tumors are distinguished from other tumors of the GI tract by expression of c-*kit* (CD117). Surgical resection with microscopically negative margins is standard treatment. Imatinib mesylate (Gleevec), a tyrosine kinase inhibitor, has been approved to treat patients with unresectable or metastatic GIST. Patients with GIST that is resistant to imatinib may have a response to sunitinib, which has been approved as second-line treatment for these tumors.

D. **Retroperitoneal sarcomas** are considerably more difficult to treat because the tumors often involve vital structures. Operative intervention employs resection of as much tumor as possible with a wide margin. Organs associated with the tumor should be resected *en bloc* to completely remove the tumor. A recent large retrospective study demonstrated a 5-year recurrence rate of 48% for simple removal of involved tissues versus 28% for *en bloc* resection, with a non-significant trend towards improved overall survival with more aggressive surgery (*J Clin Oncol*. 2009;27:24). An initial tissue diagnosis is often obtained by core biopsy. Postoperative irradiation may be used in some cases but is associated with relatively high morbidity, often due to irradiation of normal intestines and other organs. Wide margins are often not achievable in the retroperitoneum and limit the effectiveness of surgery. For these reasons, preoperative irradiation therapy, with the tumor in place displacing normal organs, is increasingly favored. Studies are beginning to reveal recurrence and survival benefits. Some surgeons, however, remain concerned about irradiation making surgical dissection more difficult. For tumor recurrences, surgical resection is the therapy of choice. Gronchi et al. studied 167 consecutive patients who underwent operation for retroperitoneal STS; complete resection of all gross disease was achieved in 88% of patients. Overall survival at 10 years was 27%, and disease-free survival was 16%. The 10-year disease-free survival rate was 27% for patients who underwent resection for primary sarcomas compared with 5% for patients who underwent resection for recurrent retroperitoneal sarcoma (*Cancer.* 2004;100:2448). The data suggest that novel treatment approaches are needed for prevention of local, regional, and distant recurrences.

V. OTHER ADJUVANT THERAPY

A. **Interstitial perioperative radiation therapy (brachytherapy)** involves the use of catheters or implants placed at the time of surgery to provide radiation directly to the tumor bed. Afterloading involves loading of the radiation source through catheters postoperatively to deliver localized high-dose radiation to the tumor bed. Brachytherapy has at least two advantages: It requires a short course of in-hospital treatment rather than 5 to 6 weeks of outpatient external-beam radiation therapy, and it can provide dose control near sensitive areas, such as joints and blood vessels. There is evidence that it is effective at decreasing local recurrence for high-grade tumors when combined with surgery.

B. **Chemotherapy.** Several randomized, prospective trials have failed to show any improvement in survival with adjuvant chemotherapy for adult grade II or III sarcomas. The two drugs with the greatest efficacy are doxorubicin and ifosfamide; however, even these have, at best, a 40% to 60% response rate. Recent data from two institutional prospective sarcoma databases identified patients who underwent resection for high-grade extremity liposarcoma greater than 5 cm in size. Using contemporary cohort analysis, the authors concluded that doxorubicin is not associated with improved disease-specific survival, but that ifosfamide is associated with improved disease-specific survival (*Ann Surg.* 2004;240:697). Doxorubicin, ifosfamide, and dacarbazine are all used as single agents or in combination therapy. Gemcitabine–docetaxel combination therapy has also demonstrated improved progression-free survival and overall survival for metastatic STS (*J Clin Oncol.* 2007;25:2755).

C. **ILP** provides increased delivery of therapy (e.g., hyperthermic therapy and chemotherapy) to an extremity sarcoma while reducing systemic toxicity. There is some suggestion of decreased local recurrence with definite downstaging of the tumor, but there is no improvement in survival (*Ann Surg Oncol.* 2007;14:230).

VI. **HEREDITARY TUMOR SYNDROMES: SARCOMAS.** Soft-tissue sarcomas have been identified in several familial cancer syndromes, including Li–Fraumeni syndrome, hereditary retinoblastoma, and neurofibromatosis types 1 and 2. The prognosis is highly dependent on the tumor grade.

26 Hernia

Lora Melman and Brent D. Matthews

I. INGUINAL HERNIA

A. **Incidence. The true incidence and prevalence of inguinal hernia worldwide is unknown.** The etiology of inguinal hernia formation is a by-product of genetic, environmental, and metabolic factors, combined with individual patient factors that can vary over time such as activity level, immune status, infection(s), medications, personal habits (e.g., smoking), and change in body mass index (*Surg Clin North Am.* 2008;88:179–201). Laparoscopic studies have reported rates of contralateral defects as high as 22%, with 28% of these going on to become symptomatic during short-term follow-up. The male-to-female ratio is greater than 10:1. Lifetime prevalence is 25% in men and 2% in women. Two-thirds of inguinal hernias are indirect. Nearly two-thirds of recurrent hernias are direct. Approximately 10% of inguinal hernias will become incarcerated, and a portion of these may become strangulated. Recurrence rates after surgical repair are less than 1% in children and vary in adults according to the method of hernia repair.

B. **Terminology and anatomy**

1. **The inguinal canal** (Fig. 26-1) is a tunnel that traverses the layers of the abdominal wall musculature, bounded on the lateral deep aspect by an opening in the transversalis fascia/transversus abdominis muscle (internal inguinal ring), and travels along the fused edges of the transversus abdominis/internal oblique/inguinal ligament (iliopubic tract) posteriorly and layers of the external oblique musculature anteriorly, ending on the medial superficial aspect at an opening in the external oblique aponeurosis (external inguinal ring). The inguinal canal houses the spermatic cord (males) or the round ligament (females) and is subject to hernia formation due primarily to decreased mechanical integrity of the internal ring and/or transversalis fascia, allowing intra-abdominal contents to encroach into this space, forming a characteristic bulge.

2. **Direct hernias** occur as a result of weakness in the posterior wall of the inguinal canal, which is usually a result of attenuation of the transversalis fascia. The hernia sac protrudes through Hesselbach's triangle, which is the space bounded by the inferior epigastric artery, the lateral edge of the rectus sheath, and the inguinal ligament.

3. **Indirect hernias** pass through the internal inguinal ring lateral to Hesselbach's triangle and follow the spermatic cord in males and the round ligament in females. During dissection, an indirect hernia sac is typically found on the anteromedial aspect of the spermatic cord. Indirect hernias may become incarcerated at either the internal or external ring.

4. **In combined (pantaloon) hernias,** direct and indirect hernias coexist.

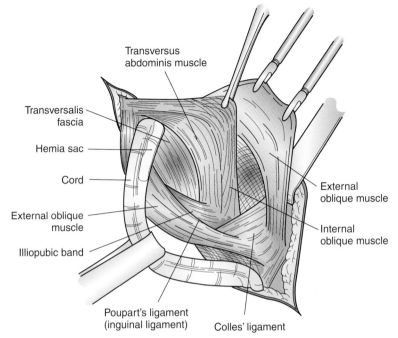

Figure 26-1. Anatomy of the right inguinal region.

Labels in figure:
- Transversus abdominis muscle
- Transversalis fascia
- Hernia sac
- Cord
- External oblique muscle
- Illiopubic band
- External oblique muscle
- Internal oblique muscle
- Poupart's ligament (inguinal ligament)
- Colles' ligament

5. A **sliding hernia** (usually indirect inguinal) denotes that a part of the wall of the hernia sac is formed by an intra-abdominal viscus (usually colon, sometimes bladder). In a **Richter hernia,** part (rather than the entire circumference) of the bowel wall is trapped. A **Littré hernia** is one that contains a Meckel's diverticulum. An **Amyand hernia** is one that contains the appendix.

6. **Incarcerated hernias** cannot be reduced into the abdominal cavity, whereas strangulated hernias have incarcerated contents with vascular compromise. Frequently, intense pain is caused by ischemia of the incarcerated segment.

C. Diagnosis

1. **Clinical presentation**

   a. **Most inguinal hernias** present as an intermittent bulge that appears in the groin. In males, it may extend into the scrotal sac. Symptoms are usually related to exertion or long periods of standing. The patient may complain of unilateral discomfort without noting a mass. Often, a purposeful Valsalva maneuver can reproduce the symptoms and/or the presence of a bulge. In infants and children, a groin bulge is often noticed by caregivers during episodes of crying or defecation. Only in rare cases do patients present with bowel obstruction without the presence of a groin abnormality. All patients presenting with small bowel obstruction must be questioned carefully and examined for all types of hernia (i.e., inguinal, umbilical, incisional, etc.) as a possible etiology of obstruction.

   b. Physical examination. The main diagnostic maneuver for inguinal hernias is palpation of the inguinal region. The patient is best examined while standing and straining (cough or Valsalva). Hernias manifest as bulges with smooth, rounded surfaces that become more evident with straining. The hernia sac can also be examined more clearly by invaginating the hemiscrotum to introduce an index finger through the external inguinal ring. This may become uncomfortable for the patient and is unnecessary if an obvious bulge is present. It is often difficult, if not impossible, to determine whether the hernia is direct or indirect based solely on physical examination. Incarcerated inguinal hernias present with pain, abdominal distention, nausea, and vomiting due to intestinal obstruction.

   2. Radiographic evaluation. X-ray studies are rarely indicated. Ultrasonography or computed tomographic (CT) scan may occasionally be used to diagnose an occult groin hernia, particularly in the obese patient. Plain abdominal radiographs may verify intestinal obstruction in cases of incarceration.

D. Differential diagnosis. Inguinal hernias should be distinguished from femoral hernias, which protrude below the inguinal ligament. Inguinal adenopathy, lipomas, dilation of the saphenous vein, epididymitis, testicular torsion, groin abscess, and vascular aneurysms/pseudoaneurysms all should be considered.

E. Treatment

   1. Preoperative evaluation and preparation. Most patients with hernias should be treated surgically, although "watchful waiting" may be appropriate for individuals with asymptomatic hernias or for elderly patients with minimally symptomatic hernias (*JACS*. 2006;203:458–468). Associated conditions that lead to increased intra-abdominal pressure such as chronic cough, constipation, or bladder outlet obstruction should be evaluated and remedied to the extent possible before elective herniorrhaphy. In patients with symptoms of altered bowel habits (i.e., frequent straining/constipation), one may wish to assess the risk of underlying colorectal malignancy, depending on the age and family history of the patient. In cases of intestinal obstruction and possible strangulation, broad-spectrum antibiotics and nasogastric suction may be indicated. Correction of volume status and electrolyte abnormalities is important when there is associated small bowel obstruction.

   2. Reduction. Temporary management includes manual reduction. In uncomplicated cases, the hernia reduces with palpation over the inguinal canal with the patient supine. If this does not occur, the physician applies gentle pressure over the hernia with the concavity of the palm of his or her hand and fingers. The palm of the physician's hand exerts a steady but gentle pressure and also maintains the direction to be followed: craniad and lateral for direct hernias, craniad and posterior for femoral hernias. If the herniated viscera do not reduce, gentle traction over the mass with compression may allow bowel gas to leave the herniated segment, making the mass reducible. Sedation and Trendelenburg position may be required for reduction of an incarcerated hernia, but the difficulty of distinguishing between acute incarceration and strangulation should be noted, as the inguinal canal can become quite tender with or without ischemic contents. When an incarcerated hernia is reduced nonsurgically, the patient should be observed for the potential development of peritonitis caused by perforation or ischemic necrosis of a loop of strangulated bowel. Strong suspicion of strangulation (i.e., erythema over hernia site, pain out of proportion to examination, patient appears toxic, or persistent pain after reduction) is a surgical emergency; the patient should be expeditiously taken to the operating room to reduce the risk of death from intra-abdominal sepsis.

3. **Surgical treatment**
   a. **Choice of anesthetic.** Local anesthesia, which has several advantages over general or regional (spinal or epidural) anesthesia, is the preferred anesthetic for elective open repair for small- to moderate-sized hernias. Local anesthesia results in better postoperative analgesia, a shorter recovery room stay, and a negligible rate of postoperative urinary retention; it is the lowest-risk anesthetic for patients with underlying cardiopulmonary disorders. Commonly, a mixture of a short-acting agent (lidocaine 1%) and longer-acting agent (bupivacaine 0.25% to 0.50%) is used. The dose limits for local anesthesia are 4.5 mg/kg plain lidocaine or 7 mg/kg lidocaine with epinephrine and 2 mg/kg plain bupivacaine or 3 mg/kg bupivacaine with epinephrine. Use of local anesthesia for herniorrhaphy in our hospital is routinely supplemented by monitored anesthesia care and administration of intravenous midazolam and propofol. Virtually all patients who undergo hernia repair under local anesthesia can be managed as outpatients unless associated medical conditions or extenuating social circumstances necessitate overnight observation in the hospital. Laparoscopic hernia repair is almost always performed under general anesthesia to facilitate tolerance of pneumoperitoneum.
   b. **Treatment of the hernia sac.** For indirect hernias, the sac (peritonealized abdominal contents) is dissected from the spermatic cord and cremasteric fibers [Figure 26-1]. The sac can be ligated deep into the internal ring with an absorbable suture after reduction of herniated contents, or just invaginated back into the abdomen without ligation. Large, indirect sacs that extend into the scrotum should not be dissected beyond the pubic tubercle because of an increased risk of ischemic orchitis. Similarly, one should avoid translocating the testicle into the inguinal canal during hernia repair owing to the risk of ischemia or torsion. Cord lipomas are frequently encountered during repair and should be excised or reduced into the preperitoneal space to avoid future confusion with a recurrent hernia. Sliding hernia sacs can usually be managed by reducing the sac and attached viscera. Direct sacs are usually too broadly based for ligation and should not be opened. The redundant attenuated

tissue may be inverted and the inguinal floor reconstructed with a few interrupted sutures before placement of mesh.

c. **Primary tissue repairs** without mesh were the mainstay of hernia surgery for decades, prior to the development of synthetic meshes. While primary repair avoids placement of foreign prosthetic material, disadvantages of this approach include higher recurrence rates (5% to 10% for primary repairs and 15% to 30% for repair of recurrent hernias) due to tension on the repair and a slower return to unrestricted physical activity. Although the vast majority of hernias are now treated with a tension-free mesh repair, a primary tissue repair can be considered in contaminated wounds, in which placement of synthetic material is contraindicated. The principal features of the more commonly performed tissue repairs are the following:

(1) **Bassini repair.** The inferior arch of the transversalis fascia or conjoint tendon is approximated to the shelving portion of the inguinal ligament (iliopubic tract) with interrupted, nonabsorbable sutures. The Bassini repair has been used for simple, indirect hernias, including inguinal hernias in women.

(2) **McVay repair.** The transversalis fascia is sutured to the Cooper ligament medial to the femoral vein and the inguinal ligament at the level of, and lateral to, the femoral vein. This operation usually requires placement of a relaxing incision medially on the aponeuroses of the internal oblique muscle to avoid undue tension on the repair. The McVay repair closes the femoral space and therefore, unlike the Bassini repair, is effective for femoral hernias.

(3) **Shouldice repair.** In this repair, the transversalis fascia is incised (and partially excised if weakened) and reapproximated. The overlying tissues (the conjoint tendon, iliopubic tract, and inguinal ligament) are approximated in multiple, imbricated layers of running nonabsorbable suture. The experience of the Shouldice Clinic with this repair has been excellent, with recurrence rates of less than 1%, but higher recurrence rates have been reported in nonspecialized centers.

(a) **Open tension-free repairs.** The most common mesh inguinal hernia repairs performed today are the tension-free mesh hernioplasty (Lichtenstein repair) and the patch-and-plug technique. In the Lichtenstein repair, a piece of polypropylene mesh approximately 5 × 3 in. is used to reconstruct the inguinal floor (Fig. 26-2). The mesh is sutured to the fascia overlying the pubic tubercle inferiorly, the transversalis fascia and conjoint tendon medially, and the inguinal ligament laterally. The mesh is slit at the level of the internal ring, and the two limbs are crossed around the spermatic cord and then tacked to the inguinal ligament, effectively re-creating a new internal ring. This repair avoids the approximation of attenuated tissues under tension, and recurrence rates with this technique have been consistently 1% or less. Moreover, because the repair is

Figure 26-2. Lichtenstein tension-free hernia repair.

without tension, patients are allowed to return to unrestricted physical activity in 2 weeks or less. The mesh plug technique entails placement of a preformed plug of mesh in the hernia defect (e.g., internal ring) that is sutured to the rings of the fascial opening. An onlay piece of mesh is then placed over the inguinal floor, which may or may not be sutured to the fascia. Mesh plugs may be ideally suited for the repair of small, tight defects such as femoral hernias. Another technique involves the use of a bilayer mesh in which the posterior leaflet is placed in the preperitoneal space and the anterior leaflet is sutured to the same layers as that in the Lichtenstein repair.

(b) **Laparoscopic inguinal hernia repair.** The laparoscopic hernia repair is based on the technique of Stoppa, who used an open preperitoneal approach to reduce the hernia and placed a large piece of mesh to cover the entire inguinal floor and myopectineal orifice. Laparoscopic hernia repair is typically advocated in the elective setting; it is nonoptimal for patients presenting with signs and symptoms of incarceration or strangulation. Other contraindications to the laparoscopic approach include inability to tolerate general anesthesia and/or pneumoperitoneum, or the presence of a hernia with a significant scrotal component, which is more difficult to reduce laparoscopically. There are two approaches to laparoscopic repair of inguinal hernias:

(i) **Transabdominal preperitoneal (TAPP) repair.** In the TAPP technique, the peritoneal space is entered by conventional means at the umbilicus, the peritoneum overlying the inguinal floor is dissected away as a flap, the hernia is reduced, mesh is fixed over the internal ring opening in the preperitoneal space, and the peritoneum is reapproximated. The advantages of the TAPP approach are that a large working space is retained, familiar anatomic landmarks are visible, and the contralateral groin can be examined for an occult hernia.

(ii) **Totally extraperitoneal repair (TEP).** In the TEP technique, the preperitoneal space is developed with a dissecting balloon inserted between the posterior rectus sheath and the rectus abodominis and directed toward the pelvis inferior to the arcuate ligament (Fig. 26-3). The other ports are inserted into this preperitoneal space without ever entering the peritoneal cavity. The advantages of the TEP repair are that the peritoneum is not opened, which minimizes exposure of the mesh to the intra-abdominal viscera, thereby minimizing the risk of intestinal adhesions.

In either the TAPP or TEP technique, a large piece of mesh (6 × 4 in.) is placed over the inguinal floor and fixed superiorly to the posterior abdominal wall fascia on either side of the inferior epigastric vessels, medially to the Cooper ligament and the midline, and superolateral to the fascia above the internal ring. Staples/tacks must not be placed inferomedial to the internal ring or inferior to the iliopubic tract because of the risk of injury to the external iliac vessels (triangle of doom) and ilioinguinal, genitofemoral, lateral femoral cutaneous, and femoral nerves (triangle of pain). Studies comparing laparoscopic and open approaches to inguinal hernia repair have shown that laparoscopic repair is associated with less postoperative pain and faster recovery than open repair but that hospital costs have been higher for the laparoscopic technique. Operative times, complications, and recurrence rates (<3% for both laparoscopic and open repairs) have been similar. Recent randomized controlled trials, including the LEVEL trial of 660 patients randomized to Lichtenstein or TEP repair, concluded that laparoscopic repair was associated with earlier discharge from hospital, quicker return to normal activity and work, and significantly fewer postoperative complications than open

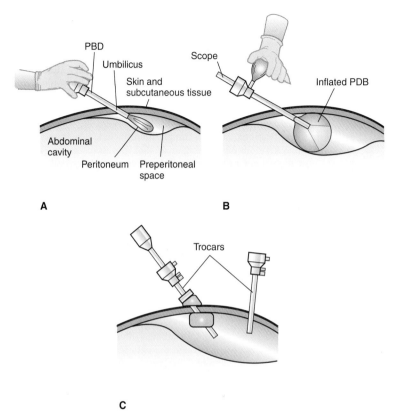

Figure 26-3. Laparoscopic total extraperitoneal approach with preperitoneal balloon dilation (PBD).

inguinal hernia repair. Operating times were significantly longer for laparoscopic repairs (p <0.001), but recurrence rate at mean follow-up of 49 months was similar (p = 0.64) (*Ann Surg.* 2010;251:819–824; *Int J Surg.* 2010;8:25–28). Another randomized trial comparing open and laparoscopic mesh inguinal hernia repairs at 14 Veterans Affairs (VA) institutions concluded that the open technique is superior to the laparoscopic technique for mesh repair of primary hernias due to decreased recurrence (4% vs. 10.1%) and complication rates (33.4% vs. 39%) (*N Engl J Med.* 2004;350:1819).

Special circumstances in which laparoscopic repair may also be favored include (1) recurrent hernias to avoid the scar tissue in the inguinal canal, (2) bilateral hernias, because both sides of the groin can be repaired with the same three small incisions used for the unilateral repair, (3) individuals with a unilateral hernia for whom a rapid recovery is critical (e.g., athletes and laborers), and (4) obese patients. Laparoscopic hernia repair is contraindicated in patients who have large scrotal hernias or who have undergone prior extensive lower abdominal or pelvic surgery.

d. **Complications.** Surgical complications include hematoma, infection, nerve injury (ilioinguinal, iliohypogastric, genital branch of the genitofemoral, lateral femoral cutaneous, femoral), vascular injury (femoral vessels, testicular artery, pampiniform venous plexus), vas deferens injury, ischemic orchitis, and testicular atrophy. Recurrence rates after tension-free mesh repairs for primary hernias are 1% to 2% or less.

e. **Recurrent inguinal hernias** are more difficult to repair because the scar makes dissection difficult and the disease process has continued. Recurrence within 1 year of initial repair suggests an inadequate initial attempt, such as overlooking an indirect hernia sac. Recurrence after 2 or more years suggests progression of the disease process that caused the initial hernia (e.g., increased intra-abdominal pressure, degeneration of tissues). Recurrences should be repaired because the defect usually is small with fixed edges that are prone to complications such as incarceration or strangulation. Repair can be done by an anterior approach through the old operative field or by a posterior (open preperitoneal or laparoscopic) approach. Prosthetic mesh is almost always used to reinforce attenuated tissues unless the operative field is contaminated.

F. **Prosthetic mesh in inguinal hernia repairs.** The choice of mesh for inguinal hernia repair is expanding rapidly as industries compete to produce the ideal prosthetic material that provides the right combination of strength to prevent recurrence and flexibility to minimize chronic postoperative pain and/or the sensation of feeling a foreign body. Examples of the three basic classes of synthetic meshes available to surgeons for use in inguinal hernia repair are summarized in Table 26-1. Recent randomized clinical trials demonstrate that lightweight polypropylene meshes for Lichtenstein hernia repair does not affect recurrence rates and offer improved aspects of postoperative pain and discomfort (*Hernia*. 2010;14:253–258). These results support the use of newer, lighter-weight mesh materials in inguinal hernia repair.

II. FEMORAL HERNIAS

A. **Incidence.** Femoral hernias constitute up to 2% to 4% of all groin hernias; 70% occur in women. Approximately 25% of femoral hernias become incarcerated or strangulated, and a similar number are missed or diagnosed late.

TABLE 26-1 Weight Classes of Mesh Used in Inguinal Hernia Repair

	Marlex[a] (Heavyweight)	Prolene Soft[b] (Midweight)	Ultrapro[b] (Lightweight)
Material	Polypropylene	Polypropylene	Polypropylene, poliglecaprone
Weight (g/m^2)	95	45	28
Pore size (mm)	0.6	2.4	4
Burst strength (newtons)	1,218	590	576
Stiffness (newtons/cm)	59.1	49.1	43.2

[a]Davol, Inc., Cranston, RI.
[b]Ethicon, Inc., Somerville, NJ.
Adapted from Cobb WS, Burns JM, Peindl RD, et al. Textile analysis of heavy weight, midweight, and light weight polypropylene mesh in a porcine ventral hernia model. *J Surg Res.* 2006;136(1):1–7.

B. **Anatomy.** The abdominal viscera and peritoneum protrude through the femoral canal into the upper thigh. The boundaries of the femoral canal are the lacunar ligament medially, the femoral vein laterally, the iliopubic tract anteriorly, and the Cooper ligament posteriorly.

C. **Diagnosis**

1. **Clinical presentation**

    a. **Symptoms.** Patients may complain of an intermittent groin bulge or a groin mass that may be tender. Because femoral hernias have a high incidence of incarceration, small bowel obstruction may be the presenting feature in some patients. Elderly patients, in whom femoral hernias occur most commonly, may not complain of groin pain, even in the setting of incarceration. Therefore, an occult femoral hernia should be considered in the differential diagnosis of any patient with small-bowel obstruction, especially if there is no history of previous abdominal surgery.

    b. **Physical examination.** The characteristic finding is a small, rounded bulge that appears in the upper thigh just below the inguinal ligament. An incarcerated femoral hernia usually presents as a firm, tender mass. The differential diagnosis is the same as that for inguinal hernia.

    c. **Radiographic evaluation.** Radiographic studies are rarely indicated. Occasionally, a femoral hernia is found on a CT scan or gastrointestinal contrast study performed to evaluate a small bowel obstruction.

D. **Treatment.** The surgical approach can be inguinal, preperitoneal, or femoral.

1. **Inguinal approach.** A Cooper ligament repair (McVay) using the inguinal canal approach allows reduction of the hernia sac with visualization from above the inguinal ligament and closure of the femoral space. Occasionally, it may be necessary to divide the inguinal ligament to reduce the hernia. The repair can be performed with or without mesh.

2. **Preperitoneal approach.** A transverse suprainguinal incision permits access to the extraperitoneal spaces of Bogros and Retzius. The hernia is reduced from inside the femoral space, and the hernia defect is repaired preperitoneally, usually with mesh, but can be repaired primarily. This approach is especially useful for incarcerated or strangulated femoral hernias. Uncomplicated femoral hernias can also be repaired laparoscopically.

3. **Femoral approach.** A horizontal incision is made over the hernia, inferior and parallel to the inguinal ligament. After the hernia sac is dissected free, it can be resected or invaginated. The femoral canal is closed by placing interrupted stitches to approximate the Cooper ligament to the inguinal ligament or by using a plug of prosthetic material.

4. **Complications.** Complications are similar to those for inguinal hernia repair. The femoral vein may be especially susceptible to injury because it forms the lateral border of the femoral canal.

III. INTERNAL HERNIA

A. **Incidence.** Of patients who present with acute intestinal obstruction, less than 5% have an internal hernia. When internal hernias are complicated by intestinal volvulus, there is an 80% incidence of strangulation or gangrene.

B. **Etiology.** Internal hernias occur within the abdominal cavity owing to congenital or acquired causes. Congenital causes include abnormal intestinal rotation (paraduodenal hernias) and openings in the ileocecal mesentery (transmesenteric hernias). Other, less frequent types are pericecal hernias, hernias through the sigmoid mesocolon, and hernias through defects in the transverse mesocolon, gastrocolic ligament, gastrohepatic ligament, or greater omentum. Acquired causes include hernias through mesenteric defects created by bowel resections or ostomy formation. Internal hernia is also a common cause of small bowel obstruction after laparoscopic gastric bypass surgery, as the small bowel can herniate through a residual mesenteric defect. Adhesive bands from prior operations may also cause or contribute to mechanical obstruction.

C. **Diagnosis**

1. **Clinical presentation.** These hernias usually are diagnosed because an intestinal segment becomes incarcerated within the internal defect, resulting in small-bowel obstruction. Patients with congenital causes usually have not had prior abdominal surgery. The reported mortality in acute intestinal obstruction secondary to internal hernias is 10% to 16%. **Symptoms** usually are of intestinal obstruction without evidence of an external hernia. When there is intestinal obstruction or intestinal

strangulation, the diagnosis is based on clinical rather than on laboratory findings.

   2. **Radiographic studies.** Plain abdominal films may show small-bowel obstruction. An abdominal CT scan can sometimes establish the diagnosis of an internal hernia preoperatively. Contrast studies may also sometimes be useful.

   D. **Differential diagnosis** includes other causes of intestinal obstruction, such as adhesions, external hernia, malignancy, gallstone ileus, and intussusception.

   E. **Surgical treatment.** The diagnosis of internal hernia is often made at laparotomy for small-bowel obstruction. Intestinal loops proximal to the obstruction are dilated, friable, and edematous above the obstruction and collapsed distal to it. Once the hernia is reduced, intestinal viability is assessed and nonviable intestine is removed. If a large percentage of bowel is of questionable viability, a limited bowel resection followed by a second-look laparotomy in 24 to 48 hours may preserve small-bowel length. The hernia defect should be closed primarily with nonabsorbable suture.

IV. ABDOMINAL WALL HERNIA

   A. Incidence and etiology

   1. **Incisional hernias** occur at sites of previous incisions at which there has been a division of abdominal wall fascia. Contributing factors include obesity, wound infection, malnutrition, smoking, and technical errors in wound closure. Hernias occur in up to 20% of patients undergoing abdominal operations and are most commonly seen with midline incisions. Most incisional hernias are now repaired with a mesh prosthetic via open or laparoscopic approach.

   2. **Umbilical hernias** are congenital defects. They are more frequent in African Americans than in whites. Most newborn umbilical hernias close spontaneously by the second year of life. However, umbilical hernias are also common in adults. Patients with ascites have a high incidence of umbilical hernias. Small umbilical hernias can be present for years without causing symptoms and may even go unnoticed. Over time, however, these hernias can enlarge and become incarcerated, usually with preperitoneal fat or omentum. Umbilical hernias greater than 3 cm should be repaired with a prosthetic mesh.

   3. **Epigastric hernias** are hernias of the linea alba above the umbilicus. They occur more frequently in athletically active young men. When small or in obese individuals, epigastric hernias may be hard to palpate, making the diagnosis difficult as well. Usually, they produce epigastric pain that may be falsely attributed to other abdominal diagnoses. The diagnosis is made by palpation of a subcutaneous epigastric mass; most such hernias occur within a few centimeters of the umbilicus and are associated with a small (1 to 2 cm) fascial defect.

   4. **Spigelian hernias** protrude through the spigelian fascia, near the termination of the transversus abdominis muscle along the lateral edge

of the rectus abdominis near the junction of the linea semilunaris and linea semicircularis. Because the herniated visceral contents are intraparietal (between the abdominal wall muscles), these hernias can be difficult to diagnose and therefore are included in the differential diagnosis of obscure abdominal pain. Ultrasonography, CT scan, or laparoscopy can be useful confirmatory tools in patients with focal symptoms in the appropriate region.

5. The most **common type of lumbar hernia** is an incisional hernia from a previous retroperitoneal or flank incision. Lumbar hernias may also occur in two different triangles: the Petit triangle and the Grynfeltt triangle. Lower lumbar hernias of the Petit triangle are located in a weak area limited posteriorly by the latissimus dorsi, anteriorly by the external oblique muscle, and inferiorly by the iliac crest. Grynfeltt hernias are upper lumbar in location, below the lowest rib.

6. **Obturator hernias** are very rare hernias that occur predominantly in thin, older women and are difficult to diagnose. Patients classically present with bowel obstruction and focal tenderness on rectal examination. Pain along the medial aspect of the thigh with medial thigh rotation, known as the *Howship–Romberg sign,* results from obturator nerve compression and, when present, may aid in the clinical diagnosis of an obturator hernia.

B. **Treatment and operative management.** Small epigastric, umbilical, obturator, and spigelian hernias may be repaired primarily. Most incisional hernias as well as lumbar and obturator hernias require the use of a prosthetic mesh because of their size and high recurrence rates after primary repair.

1. **Open repairs.** The principles for ventral hernia repair include dissection and identification of all defects and repair with nonabsorbable sutures placed in healthy tissue. Most sizable incisional hernias are now repaired with some types of mesh prosthesis that should be anchored by nonabsorbable sutures placed in healthy fascial tissue several centimeters beyond the margins of the defect. The mesh should be durable and well tolerated by the patient, with a low risk for infection. A variety of mesh products are available for repair, including polypropylene, polytetrafluoroethylene ([PTFE], Gore-Tex), and a composite mesh of polypropylene and PTFE. Several newer composite mesh products (Table 26-2) with absorbable barriers coating polypropylene or polyester mesh are available to minimize tissue attachment to intraabdominal structures. One should try to avoid placing polypropylene mesh in direct contact with the intestine because of the risk of adhesion formation and fistulization.

2. **Laparoscopic repairs.** The laparoscopic approach is an increasingly used alternative method for repair of incisional hernias. The repair generally involves placement of a mesh prosthesis to cover the hernia defect. The contents of the hernia are reduced and the mesh is anchored in place with sutures and tacks with a minimum of 4 cm overlap past the edge of the hernia defect on all sides. A recent meta-analysis of 45 published series comparing open and laparoscopic ventral hernia repairs

TABLE 26-2	Commonly Used Biomaterials for Incisional Hernia Repair		
	Product Trade Name	Manufacturer	Components
Absorbable barrier composite meshes	Sepramesh	Genzyme Corp., Cambridge, MA	Polypropylene mesh on one side, absorbable sodium hyaluronate/ carboxymethylcellulose on the other side
	C-Qur	Atrium Medical, Hudson, NH	Lightweight polypropylene mesh (Prolite) coated with omega-3 fatty acid
	Paritex, Parientene	Sofradim Corp., Trevoux, France	Polyester mesh with bovine type I collagen coating covered with absorbable PEG/ glycerol layer
	Proceed	Ethicon, Inc., Somerville, NJ	Polypropylene mesh encapsulated in polydioxanone coated on one side with oxidized regenerated cellulose
Nonabsorbable, barrier composite mesh	Bard Composix	C.R. Bard, Inc., Murray Hill, NJ	Macroporous bilayer mesh; polypropylene and microporous PTFE
	Gore-Tex Dual Mesh	W.L. Gore & Associates, Flagstaff, AZ	PTFE with different architecture on the peritoneal (intra- abdominal) and parietal (abdominal wall) surfaces of the mesh
Bioremodelable materials (aka biologic meshes)	Surgisis	Cook Biotech, Inc., West Lafayette, IN	Acellular, extracellular matrix material derived from porcine small intestinal submucosa
	Alloderm	LifeCell Corp., Branchburg, NJ	Acellular dermal matrix harvested from cadaveric human dermis

(continued)

TABLE 26-2	Commonly Used Biomaterials for Incisional Hernia Repair *(Continued)*		
Product Trade Name	**Manufacturer**	**Components**	
Flex HD	Musculoskeletal Transplant Foundation, Edison, NJ	Acellular dermal matrix harvested from cadaveric human dermis	
Strattice	LifeCell Corp., Branchburg, NJ	Acellular porcine dermal matrix	
Permacol	Tissue Science Laboratories, Covington, NJ	Acellular, cross-linked porcine dermal matrix	

PEG, polyethylene glycol; PTFE, polytetrafluoroethylene.

concluded that laparoscopic repair is associated with fewer wound-related (3.8% vs. 16.8%) and overall complications (22.7% vs. 41.7%) and has a lower rate of recurrence (4.3% vs. 12.1%) than open repairs (*Surg Endosc.* 2007;21:378–386). Contraindications to laparoscopic ventral hernia repair include inability to establish pneumoperitoneum safely, an acute abdomen with strangulated or infarcted bowel, loss of abdominal domain, or the presence of peritonitis.

C. **Prosthetic mesh in abdominal wall hernia repairs.** The recurrence rate for ventral incisional hernia repair is 31% to 54% when primarily repaired. The placement of prosthetic biomaterials in the retrorectus, preperitoneal space to repair ventral, incisional hernias as popularized by Rives, Stoppa, and Wantz has reduced the recurrence rate to between 4% and 24%. Long-term follow-up of a randomized controlled trial showed that the use of mesh results in a lower recurrence rate and less abdominal pain and does not result in more complications than primary repair (*Hernia.* 2006;10:236–242). Microporous PTFE remains a popular choice of mesh due to its adhesion-resistant properties for intra-abdominal placement. The microporous architecture and hydrophobicity of ePTFE prevent cellular penetration of intestine or abdominal viscera. There are also several absorbable barrier-coated meshes. Each product has its own characteristics, making it useful in various circumstances. This is summarized in Table 26-2. Currently, there is little outcomes data to support the use of one product over another. However, the use of mesh is superior to primary repair for incisional hernias.

27 | Breast Diseases

Lauren Steward and Julie A. Margenthaler

ANATOMY

I. **THE BREAST.** Breast tissue is located between the subcutaneous fat and the fascia of the **pectoralis major** and **serratus anterior** muscles. It extends from the second/third rib to the inframammary fold. The lateral border is the anterior or midaxillary line and the medial border is the lateral edge of the sternum. Posterior to the breast and anterior to the pectoralis fascia is the *retromammary space*, which contains small lymphatics and vessels. Breast tissue can extend to the clavicle, into the axilla (axillary tail of Spence), to the latissimus dorsi, and to the top of the rectus muscle. Running through the breasts from the deep fascia to the skin are *suspensory ligaments* (**Cooper's ligaments);** involvement of these ligaments by cancer may cause skin dimpling.

A. **Vasculature.** The arterial supply is from the **internal thoracic artery (or internal mammary artery),** via perforating branches, and the **axillary artery,** via the long thoracic and thoracoacromial branches. Additional blood supply to the breast comes from branches of the second to fifth intercostals, subscapular, and thoracodorsal arteries. Venous drainage is mainly to the **axillary vein,** as well as the internal thoracic, lateral thoracic, and intercostals veins.

B. **Lymphatic drainage.** A superficial subareolar plexus (Sappey's plexus, which primarily drains the skin and some central portions of the breast) converges with a deep lymphatic plexus (which receives lymphatic drainage from the breast parenchyma) to form the perilobular and deep subcutaneous plexuses, which ultimately drain into the axillary and internal mammary lymph nodes.

C. **Innervation.** Lateral and anterior cutaneous branches of the second to sixth intercostals nerves innervate the breasts.

II. **THE AXILLA.** The borders of the axilla are defined as the **axillary vein** superiorly, **latissimus dorsi** laterally, and the **serratus anterior** muscle medially.

A. **Axillary lymph nodes** are classified according to their anatomic location relative to the **pectoralis minor** muscle.
 1. **Level I** nodes. *Lateral* to the pectoralis minor muscle.
 2. **Level II** nodes. *Posterior* to the pectoralis minor muscle.
 3. **Level III** nodes. *Medial* to the pectoralis minor muscle and most accessible with division of the muscle.
 4. **Rotter's** nodes. *Between* the pectoralis major and the minor muscles.

B. **Axillary nerves.** Three motor and several sensory nerves are located in the axilla. Preservation of all is preferred during an axillary lymph node dissection

(ALND); however, direct tumor invasion may require resection along with the specimen.

1. **Long thoracic nerve** travels from superiorly to inferiorly along the chest wall at the medial aspect of the axilla and innervates the serratus anterior muscle. Injury to this nerve causes a "winged" scapula in which the medial and inferior angle of the scapula abduct away from the chest wall with arm extension.

2. **Thoracodorsal nerve** courses along the posterior border of the axilla from superiorly to inferiorly on the subscapularis muscle and innervates the latissimus dorsi. Injury to this nerve causes weakness in arm abduction and external rotation.

3. **Medial pectoral nerve** travels from the posterior aspect of the pectoralis minor muscle around the lateral border of the pectoralis minor to the posterior aspect of the pectoralis major muscle. It innervates the lateral third of the pectoralis major; injury to this nerve results in atrophy of the lateral pectoralis major muscle.

4. **Intercostal brachial** sensory nerves: travel laterally in the axilla from the second intercostal space to the medial upper arm. Transection causes numbness in the posterior and medial surfaces of the upper arm.

CLINICAL ASSESSMENT

I. **HISTORY.** **Patients seek medical attention** most commonly for an abnormal mammogram, a breast mass, breast pain, nipple discharge, or skin changes. History should include the following:

- Duration of symptoms, change over time, associated pain or skin changes, relationship to pregnancy or the menstrual cycle, previous trauma.
- Date of last menstrual period and regularity of the menstrual cycle.
- Age of menarche.
- Number of pregnancies and age at first full-term pregnancy.
- Lactational history.
- Age at menopause or surgical menopause (i.e., oophorectomy).
- Previous history of breast biopsies or breast cancer.
- Mammogram history.
- Oral contraceptive and hormonal replacement therapy.
- Family history of breast and gynecologic cancer, including the age at diagnosis. This should include at least two generations as well as any associated cancers, such as ovary, colon, prostate, gastric, or pancreatic.

A. **Assessment of cancer risks**

1. Hormonal, environmental exposure and genetics are correlated to an increased risk for breast cancer. A family history of breast cancer in a first-degree relative is associated with a doubling of risk. If two first-degree relatives (e.g., a mother and a sister) have breast cancer, the risk is further elevated. *These familial effects are enhanced if the relative had either early-onset cancer or bilateral disease.* Breast-feeding may exert a protective effect against the development of breast cancer.

Overall, factors that increase a patient's risk by 1.5- to 4-fold include the following:

    a. Increased estrogen or progesterone exposure due to early menarche (before 12 years of age) or late menopause (age >55 years).

    b. Late age at first full-term pregnancy: women with a first birth after the age of 30 years have twice the risk of those with a first birth before the age of 18 years.

    c. High body mass index after menopause.

    d. Exposure to ionizing radiation.

2. BRCA1 and BRCA2 are breast cancer susceptibility genes associated with 80% of hereditary breast cancers but account for only 5% of all breast cancers. Women with BRCA1 mutations have an estimated risk of 85% for breast cancer by the age of 70 years, a 50% chance of developing a second primary breast cancer, and a 20% to 40% chance of developing ovarian cancer. BRCA2 mutations carry a slightly lower risk for breast and ovarian cancer and account for 4% to 6% of all male breast cancers. Screening for BRCA gene mutations should be reserved for women who have a strong family history of breast or ovarian cancer. The criteria for referral for genetic counseling, adopted from the National Comprehensive Cancer Network guidelines, are as follows:

    a. Personal history of breast cancer diagnosed at age less than 40, less than 50 if of Ashkenazi Jewish ancestry, less than 50 with at least one first- or second-degree relative with breast cancer at age less than 50, and/or epithelial ovarian cancer at any age.

    b. Personal history of epithelial ovarian cancer, diagnosed at any age, particularly if of Ashkenazi Jewish ancestry.

    c. Personal history of male breast cancer, particularly if one first or second degree relative with breast cancer and/or epithelial ovarian cancer.

    d. Relatives of individuals with a deleterious BRCA1 or BRCA2 mutation.

3. Previous breast biopsies. Some pathologic features are associated with increased cancer risk.

    a. *No* increased risk is associated with adenosis, cysts, duct ectasia, or apocrine metaplasia.

    b. There is a slightly increased risk with moderate or florid hyperplasia, papillomatosis, and complex fibroadenomas.

    c. Atypical ductal hyperplasia (ADH) or atypical lobular hyperplasia (ALH) carries a four- to five-fold increased risk of developing cancer; the risk increases to 10-fold if there is a positive family history. Patients with increased risk should be counseled appropriately and should be followed with semiannual physical examinations and yearly mammograms.

4. Models for breast cancer risk. The original Gail model estimates the absolute risk (probability) that a woman in a program of annual screening will develop breast cancer over a defined age interval. The risk factors in this model include current age, age at menarche, age at first full-term pregnancy, previous breast biopsies, presence of ADH on earlier biopsy, and number of affected first-degree relatives. This model has been validated in white women, but may underestimate the risk of breast cancer in black women. It has not been validated in other populations. The National Surgical Adjuvant Breast and Bowel Project (NSABP) modified this model to project the absolute risk of developing only invasive breast cancer. This modified Gail model has been used to define eligibility criteria for entry into chemoprevention trials. The NSABP and the National Cancer Institute offer an interactive online risk assessment tool, which is available at http://www.cancer.gov/bcrisktool.

II. PHYSICAL EXAMINATION

A. **Inspect the breasts** with the patient both in the upright and supine positions. With the patient in the upright position, examine with the patient's arms relaxed and then raised, looking for shape asymmetry, deformity, and skin changes (erythema, edema, dimpling). With the patient in the supine position, examine the entire breast systematically with the patient's ipsilateral arm raised above and behind the head.

1. If a mass is found, determine its size, shape, texture, tenderness, location, fixation to skin or deep tissues, and relationship to the areola. Evaluate the nipples for retraction, discoloration, inversion, ulceration, and eczematous changes.

2. For nipple discharge, note its color and quality, where pressure elicits discharge, and whether it is from a single duct or associated with a mass.

B. **The axillary, supraclavicular, and infraclavicular lymph nodes** should be palpated with the patient in the upright position, with arms relaxed. The size, number, and fixation of nodes should be noted.

III. BREAST IMAGING

A. Screening for breast cancer. **Screening mammogram** lowers mortality from breast cancer. It is performed in the **asymptomatic** patient and consists of two standard views, mediolateral oblique (MLO) and craniocaudal (CC). The current recommendation from the National Cancer Institute and American College of Surgeons is **annual screening mammography for women aged 40 years and older.** Breast lesions on mammograms are classified according to the American College of Radiology by **BI-RADS (Breast Imaging Reporting and Database System)** scores:
- **0** = Needs further imaging; assessment incomplete.
- **1** = Normal; continue annual follow-up (risk of malignancy: 1/2,000).
- **2** = Benign lesion; no risk of malignancy; continue annual follow-up (risk of malignancy: 1/2,000).
- **3** = Probably benign lesion; needs 4 to 6 months follow-up (risk of malignancy: 1% to 2%).

- **4** = Suspicious for breast cancer; biopsy recommended (risk of malignancy: 25% to 50%).
- **5** = Highly suspicious for breast cancer; biopsy required (75% to 99% are malignant).
- **6** = Known biopsy-proven malignancy.

1. Malignant mammographic findings
   a. New or spiculated masses.
   b. Clustered microcalcifications in linear or branching array.
   c. Architectural distortion.

2. Benign mammographic findings
   a. **Radial scar.** Generally due to fibrocystic breast condition (FBC); associated with proliferative epithelium in the center of the fibrotic area in approximately one third of cases. Appearance often mimics malignancy; a biopsy is needed to rule out malignancy.
   b. **Fat necrosis.** Results from local trauma to the breast. It may resemble carcinoma on palpation and on mammography. The fat may liquefy instead of scarring, which results in a characteristic oil cyst. A biopsy may be needed to rule out malignancy.
   c. **Milk of calcium.** Associated with FBC; caused by calcified debris in the base of the acini. Characteristic microcalcifications appear discoid on CC view and sickle shaped on MLO view. These are benign and do not require biopsy.
   d. **Cysts** cannot be distinguished from solid masses by mammography; ultrasound is needed to make this distinction.

3. **Screening in high-risk patients:** For patients with *known BRCA mutations,* annual mammograms and semiannual physical examinations should **begin at the age of 25 to 30 years.** In patients with a *strong family history of breast cancer but undocumented genetic mutation,* annual mammograms and semiannual physical examinations should begin **10 years earlier than the age of the youngest affected relative and no later than the age of 40 years.**

4. **Magnetic resonance imaging (MRI)** is recommended for screening in *selected* **high-risk patients** with:
   a. A **lifetime risk of breast cancer greater than 20%** as defined by available risk assessment tools (e.g., BRCAPRO, Gail, Claus, and Tyrer-Cuskick models).
   b. BRCA mutations.
   c. A first-degree relative (parent, sibling, child) with a BRCA1 or BRCA2 mutation.
   d. History of radiation to the chest wall between the ages of 10 to 30 years (e.g., Hodgkin lymphoma patients).
   e. Li-Fraumeni, Cowden, or Bannayan–Riley–Ruvalcaba syndromes.

B. **Diagnostic imaging**

1. **Diagnostic mammograms** are performed in the symptomatic patient or to follow up on an abnormality noted on a screening mammogram. Additional views (spot-compression views or magnification views) may be used to further characterize any lesion. The false-negative and

false-positive rates are both approximately 10%. A normal mammogram in the presence of a palpable mass does **not** exclude malignancy and further workup should be performed with an ultrasound, MRI, and/or biopsy.

2. **Ultrasonography** is used to further characterize a lesion identified by physical examination or mammography. It can determine whether a lesion is solid or cystic and can define the size, contour, or internal texture of the lesion. Although not a useful screening modality by itself due to significant false-positive rates, when used as an adjunct with mammography, ultrasonography may improve diagnostic sensitivity of benign findings to greater than 90%, especially among younger patients for whom mammographic sensitivity is lower due to denser breast tissue. In the patients with a known cancer, ultrasound is sometimes used to detect additional suspicious lesions and/or to map the extent of disease.

3. **MRI** is useful as an adjunct to mammography to determine extent of disease, to detect multicentric disease in the dense breast, to assess the contralateral breast, to evaluate patients with axillary metastases and an unknown primary, and in patients in whom mammogram, ultrasound, and clinical findings are inconclusive. It is also useful for assessing chest wall involvement.

IV. BREAST BIOPSY

A. **Palpable masses**

1. Fine-needle aspiration biopsy (FNAB) is reliable and accurate, with sensitivity greater than 90%. FNAB can determine the presence of malignant cells and estrogen receptor (ER) and progesterone receptor (PR) status but does not give information on tumor grade or the presence of invasion. Nondiagnostic aspirates require an additional biopsy, either surgical or core needle biopsy (*Am J Surg.* 1997;174:372).

2. Core biopsy is preferred over FNAB. It can distinguish between invasive and noninvasive cancer and provides information on tumor grade as well as receptor status. For indeterminate specimens, a surgical biopsy is necessary.

3. Excisional biopsy should primarily be used when a core biopsy cannot be done. In general, this should be an infrequent diagnostic method. It is performed in the operating room; incisions should be planned so that they can be incorporated into a mastectomy incision should that subsequently be necessary. Masses should be excised as a single specimen and labeled to preserve three-dimensional orientations.

4. Incisional biopsy is indicated for the evaluation of a large breast mass suspicious for malignancy but for which a definitive diagnosis cannot be made by FNAB or core biopsy. For inflammatory breast cancer with skin involvement, an incisional biopsy can consist of a skin punch biopsy.

B. **Nonpalpable lesions.** Minimally invasive breast biopsy is the optimal initial tissue acquisition method and procedure of choice for obtaining a pathologic diagnosis of image-detected abnormalities. Correlation between pathology results and imaging findings is mandatory. Patients with histologically benign findings on percutaneous biopsy do not require open biopsy if imaging and pathological findings are concordant. Patients with high-risk lesions on image-guided biopsy (ADH, ALH, lobular carcinoma *in situ* (LCIS), radial scar) may have malignancy at the same site and should undergo a surgical biopsy.

1. **Stereotactic core biopsy** is used for nonpalpable mammographically detected lesions, such as microcalcifications, which cannot be seen with ultrasonography. Tissue can be collected from several foci in disparate quadrants of the breast. Using a computer-driven stereotactic unit, two mammographic images are taken to triangulate the lesion in three-dimensional space. A computer determines the depth of the lesion and the alignment of the needle, which can be positioned within 1 mm of the intended target. Biopsies are taken, and postfire images are obtained of the breast and specimen. Contraindications include lesions close to the chest wall or in the axillary tail and thin breasts that may allow needle strikethrough. Superficial lesions and lesions directly beneath the nipple-areolar complex are also often not approachable with stereotactic techniques. Nondiagnostic and insufficient specimens should undergo needle-localized excisional biopsy (NLB, see later discussion), as should discordant pathologic findings on core needle stereotactic biopsy.

   a. **Vacuum-assisted biopsy** is generally used during stereotactic core biopsies and ultrasound-guided core biopsies. These devices employ large needles (9 to 14 gauge) to contiguously acquire tissue, which is pulled into the bore of the needle by vacuum suction. Multiple contiguous samples of tissue are collected while the probe remains in the breast. Volumes up to 1 mL can be collected during a single insertion. A metallic marking clip is usually placed through the probe after sampling is complete to allow for identification of the biopsy site if excisional biopsy or partial mastectomy were necessary. This is the preferred approach for lesions presenting with microcalcifications without a visible or palpable mass.

2. **Ultrasound-guided biopsy** is the preferred method if a lesion can be visualized with ultrasound because it is generally easier to perform than a stereotactic core biopsy. Lesions with a cystic component are better visualized with ultrasound, and ultrasound-guided biopsy can be used to aspirate the cyst as well as to provide core biopsy specimens.

3. **NLB.** A needle and hookwire are placed into the breast adjacent to the concerning lesion under mammographic guidance. The patient is then brought to the operating room for an excisional biopsy. Using localization mammograms as a map, the whole hookwire, breast lesion, and a rim of normal breast tissue are removed *en bloc.* The specimen is oriented, and a radiograph is performed to confirm the presence of the lesion within the specimen.

BENIGN BREAST CONDITIONS

I. **FIBROCYSTIC BREAST CHANGE (FBC)** encompasses several of the following pathologic features: stromal fibrosis, macro- and microcysts, apocrine metaplasia, hyperplasia, and adenosis (which may be sclerosing, blunt-duct, or florid).

   A. FBC is common and may present as breast pain, a breast mass, nipple discharge, or abnormalities on mammography.

   B. The patient presenting with a breast mass or thickening and suspected FBC should be reexamined in a short interval, preferably on day 10 of the menstrual cycle, when hormonal influence is lowest. Often, the mass will have diminished in size.

   C. A persistent dominant mass must undergo further radiographic evaluation, biopsy, or both to exclude cancer.

II. **BREAST CYSTS** frequently present as tender masses or as smooth, mobile, well-defined masses on palpation. If tense with fluid, its texture may be firm, resembling a solid mass. Aspiration can determine the nature of the mass (solid vs. cystic) but is not routinely necessary. Cyst fluid color varies and can be clear, straw-colored, or even dark green.

   A. Cysts discovered by mammography and confirmed as simple cysts by ultrasound are usually observed *if asymptomatic.*

   B. *Symptomatic* simple cysts should be aspirated. If no palpable mass is present after drainage, the patient should be evaluated in 3 to 4 weeks. If the cyst recurs, does not resolve completely with aspiration, or yields bloody fluid with aspiration, then mammography or ultrasonography should be performed to exclude intracystic tumor. Nonbloody clear fluid does not need to be sent for cytology.

III. **FIBROADENOMA** is the most common discrete mass in women younger than 30 years of age. They typically present as smooth, firm, mobile masses. In approximately 20% of cases, multiple fibroadenomas may be present in the ipsilateral or contralateral breast.

   A. They may enlarge during pregnancy and involute after menopause.

   B. They have well-circumscribed borders on mammography and ultrasound.

   C. They may be managed conservatively if clinical and radiographic appearance is consistent with a fibroadenoma and is less than 2 cm. If the mass is symptomatic, greater than 2 cm, or enlarges, it should be excised.

IV. **MASTALGIA.** Most women (70%) experience some form of breast pain or discomfort during their lifetime. The pain may be cyclic (worse before a menstrual cycle) or noncyclical, focal or diffuse. Benign disease is the etiology in the majority of cases. However, pain may be associated with cancer in up to 10% of patients. **Features that raise the suspicion of cancer are *noncyclic* pain in a focal area and pain associated with a mass or bloody nipple discharge.** *Once cancer has been excluded*, most patients can be managed successfully with symptomatic therapy and reassurance; a well-fitting supportive bra is an important first step in pain relief. In 15% of patients, the pain may be so disabling that it interferes with activities of daily living.

A. **Cyclic breast pain.** Often described as a heaviness or tenderness and is usually worse before a menstrual cycle. It may be maximal in the upper outer quadrant and radiate to the inner surface of the upper arm. It resolves spontaneously in 20% to 30% of women but tends to recur in 60%. Many patients experience symptomatic relief by reducing caffeine intake or by taking vitamin E, although there is no scientific evidence supporting this.

B. **Noncyclic breast pain.** Described as burning or stabbing and frequently occurs in the subareolar area or medial aspect of the breast. It responds poorly to treatment but tends to resolve spontaneously in 50% of women.

C. **Treatment of mastalgia**

1. **Topical nonsteroidal anti-inflammatory drugs (NSAIDs)** (diclofenac gel) have been proven in a randomized, blinded, placebo-controlled study to have significant efficacy with minimal side effects and should be considered **first-line treatment** (*J Am Coll Surg.* 2003;196:525).

2. **Tamoxifen** (an estrogen antagonist) has been shown to provide good pain relief in placebo-controlled trials with tolerable side effects (*Lancet.* 1986;1:287), although concerns over increased risks of endometrial cancer limit long-term use.

3. **Danazol** (a derivative of testosterone) has been shown to be efficacious and has been used historically for severe breast pain (*Gynecol Endocrinol.* 1997;11:393), but significant side effects (hirsutism, voice changes, acne, amenorrhea, and abnormal liver enzymes levels) limit its use.

4. **Bromocriptine** and **gonadorelin analogs** should be reserved for severe refractory mastalgia due to significant side effects.

5. **Evening primrose oil** is often used but has been shown to have no benefit over placebo in clinical trials (*Am J Obstet Gynecol.* 2002;187:1389).

D. **Superficial thrombophlebitis** of the veins overlying the breast (**Mondor disease)** may present as breast pain. The thrombosed vein or "cord" may be palpated. NSAIDs and hot compresses can provide symptomatic relief. Antibiotics are not generally indicated.

E. **Breast pain in pregnancy and lactation** can occur from engorgement, clogged ducts, trauma to the areola and nipple from pumping or nursing, or any of the aforementioned sources. Clogged ducts are usually treated with warm compresses, soaks, and massage.

F. **Tietze syndrome or costochondritis** may be confused with breast pain. Patients are locally tender in the parasternal area. Treatment is with NSAIDs.

G. **Cervical radiculopathy** can also cause referred pain to the breast.

V. NIPPLE DISCHARGE

A. **Lactation** is the most common physiologic cause of nipple discharge and may continue for up to 2 years after cessation of breast-feeding. In parous nonlactating women, a small amount of milk may be expressed from multiple ducts. This requires no treatment.

B. **Galactorrhea** is milky discharge unrelated to breast-feeding. Physiologic galactorrhea is the continued production of milk after lactation has ceased and menses resumed and is often caused by continued mechanical stimulation of the nipples.

1. **Drug-related galactorrhea** is caused by medications that affect the hypothalamic–pituitary axis by depleting dopamine (tricyclic antidepressants, reserpine, methyldopa, cimetidine, and benzodiazepines), blocking the dopamine receptor (phenothiazine, metoclopramide, and haloperidol), or having an estrogenic effect (digitalis). Discharge is generally bilateral and nonbloody.

2. **Spontaneous galactorrhea** in a **nonlactating** patient may be due to a pituitary **prolactinoma.** Amenorrhea may be associated. The diagnosis is established by measuring the serum prolactin level and performing a computed tomography (CT) or MRI scan of the pituitary gland. Treatment is bromocriptine or resection of the prolactinoma.

C. **Pathologic nipple discharge** is either (1) bloody or (2) spontaneous, unilateral, and originates from a single duct. *Normal physiologic discharge* is usually nonbloody, from multiple ducts, can be a variety of colors (clear to yellow to green), and requires breast manipulation to produce.

1. **Pathologic discharge** is serous, serosanguineous, bloody, or watery. The presence of blood can be confirmed with a guaiac test.

2. Cytologic evaluation of the discharge is not generally useful.

3. **Malignancy is the underlying cause in 10% of patients.**

4. If physical examination and mammography are negative for an associated mass, the most likely etiologies are **benign intraductal papilloma, duct ectasia,** or **fibrocystic changes.** In lactating women, serosanguineous or bloody discharge can be associated with duct trauma, infection, or epithelial proliferation associated with breast enlargement.

5. A solitary **papilloma** with a fibrovascular core places the patient at marginally increased risk for the development of breast cancer. Patients with persistent spontaneous discharge from a single duct require a surgical microdochectomy, ductoscopy, or major duct excision.

   a. **Microdochectomy:** Excision of the involved duct and associated lobule. Immediately before surgery, the involved duct is cannulated, and radiopaque contrast is injected to obtain a **ductogram,** which identifies lesions as filling defects. The patient is then taken to the operating room, and the pathologic duct is identified and excised, along with the associated lobule.

   b. **Ductoscopy** utilizes a 1-mm rigid videoscope to perform an internal exploration of the major ducts of the breast. Once a ductal lesion is identified, this single associated duct with the lesion is excised.

   c. **Major duct excision** may be used for women with bloody nipple discharge from multiple ducts or in postmenopausal women with bloody nipple discharge. It is performed through a circumareolar incision, and all of the retroareolar ducts are transected and excised, along with a cone of tissue extending up to several centimeters posterior to the nipple.

VI. BREAST INFECTIONS

A. **Lactational mastitis** may occur either sporadically or in epidemics.

1. The most common causative organism is ***Staphylococcus aureus.***

2. It presents as a swollen, erythematous, and tender breast; purulent discharge from the nipple is *uncommon.*

3. In the early cellulitic phase, the treatment is antibiotics. The frequency of nursing or pumping should be *increased.* Approximately 25% progress to abscess formation.

4. **Breast abscesses** occur in the later stages and are often *not* fluctuant. The diagnosis is made by failure to improve on antibiotics, abscess cavity seen on ultrasound, or aspiration of pus. Treatment is cessation of nursing and surgical drainage.

B. **Nonpuerperal abscesses** result from duct ectasia with periductal mastitis, infected cysts, infected hematoma, or hematogenous spread from another source.

1. They usually are located in the peri/retroareolar area.

2. **Anaerobes** are the most common causative agent, although antibiotics should cover both **anaerobic and aerobic** organisms.

3. Treatment is surgical drainage.

4. **Unresolved or recurring infection requires biopsy to exclude cancer.** These patients often have a chronic relapsing course with multiple infections requiring surgical drainage.

5. Repeated infections can result in a chronically draining periareolar lesion or a mammary fistula lined with squamous epithelium. Treatment is excision of the central duct along with the fistula once the acute infection resolves. The fistula can recur even after surgery.

VII. GYNECOMASTIA is hypertrophy of breast tissue in men. It usually occurs secondary to an imbalance between the breast stimulatory effects of estrogen and the inhibitory effects of androgens. Possible etiologies include overproduction of estrogens, enhanced extraglandular conversion of estrogen precursors to estrogen, or decreased secretion of androgens from the testes.

A. **Pubertal** hypertrophy occurs in adolescent boys, is usually bilateral, and resolves spontaneously in 6 to 12 months.

B. **Senescent** gynecomastia is commonly seen after the age of 70 years, as testosterone levels decrease.

C. **Drugs** associated with this are similar to those that cause galactorrhea in women, for example, digoxin, spironolactone, methyldopa, cimetidine, tricyclic antidepressants, phenothiazine, reserpine, and marijuana. Drugs used for androgen blockade, such as luteinizing hormone releasing hormone analogues for the treatment of prostate cancer and 5-alpha reductase inhibitors for the management of benign prostatic hypertrophy, may also result in gynecomastia.

D. **Tumors** can cause gynecomastia secondary to excess secretion of estrogens: testicular teratomas and seminomas, bronchogenic carcinomas, adrenal tumors, and tumors of the pituitary and hypothalamus.

E. Gynecomastia may be a manifestation of **systemic diseases** such as hepatic cirrhosis, renal failure, hyperthyroidism, and malnutrition.

F. During the workup of gynecomastia, cancer should be excluded by mammography and subsequently by biopsy if a mass is found. The cause of gynecomastia should be identified and corrected if possible. If workup fails to reveal a medically treatable cause or if the enlargement fails to regress, excision of breast tissue via a periareolar incision can be performed.

MALIGNANCY OF THE BREAST

I. **EPIDEMIOLOGY.** Breast cancer is the **most common cancer in women,** with a lifetime risk of **one in eight women.** In 2010, approximately 209,000 new cases of invasive breast cancer and 54,000 new cases of noninvasive *in situ* carcinoma of the breast will be diagnosed (*Cancer Facts & Figures, American Cancer Society, 2010*). Approximately 40,000 women will die in 2010 due to breast cancer, making it the second-leading cause of cancer death in women (led by lung cancer).

II. **STAGING.** The management of breast cancer is guided by the extent of disease and the biologic features of the tumor. Treatment is multidisciplinary, involving surgeons, radiation oncologists, and medical oncologists. The disease is staged by the TNM (tumor, node, and metastasis) system (Tables 27-1 and 27-2). Workup should include the following (in addition to breast-specific imaging):
- Complete blood cell count, complete metabolic panel, and chest x-ray.
- A bone scan, if the alkaline phosphatase or calcium level is elevated.
- CT scan of the liver if liver function panel is abnormal.
- **Patients with clinical stage III** disease should undergo bone scan and CT scan of the chest/abdomen/pelvis due to a high probability of distant metastases.

III. **TUMOR BIOMARKERS AND PROGNOSTIC FACTORS** should be evaluated on all tumor specimens.

Tumor size and **grade** are the most reliable pathologic predictors of outcome for patients **without axillary nodal involvement.** The **Nottingham score** combines histologic grade based on *glandular differentiation, mitotic count,* and *nuclear grade.* A higher grade is a *poor* prognostic factor.

A. **Hormone receptors.** Expression of **ERs** and **PRs** should be evaluated by immunohistochemistry. Intense ER and PR staining is a *good* prognostic factor.

B. *Her2/neu (ERB2): Her2/neu* is a member of the epidermal growth factor family and is involved in cell growth regulation. Overexpression due to gene amplification is seen in approximately 30% of patients with breast cancer. *Her2/neu* expression is measured by immunohistochemistry; and if

TABLE 27-1	American Joint Committee on Cancer TNM (Tumor, Node, Metastasis) Staging for Breast Cancer

Stage	Description
Tumor	
TX	Primary tumor not assessable
T0	No evidence of primary tumor
Tis	Carcinoma *in situ*
T1	Tumor ≤2 cm in greatest dimension
T1 mic	Microinvasion ≤0.1 cm in greatest dimension
T1a	Tumor >0.1 cm but not >0.5 cm
T1b	Tumor >0.5 cm but not >1 cm
T1c	Tumor >1 cm but not >2 cm
T2	Tumor >2 cm but <5 cm in greatest dimension
T3	Tumor >5 cm in greatest dimension
T4	Tumor of any size with direct extension into the chest wall or skin
T4a	Extension to chest wall (ribs, intercostals, or serratus anterior)
T4b	*Peau d'orange,* ulceration, or satellite skin nodules
T4c	T4a + T4b
T4d	Inflammatory breast cancer
Regional Lymph Nodes	
NX	Regional lymph nodes not assessable
N0	No regional lymph node involvement
N1	Metastasis to movable ipsilateral axillary lymph nodes
N2	Metastases to ipsilateral axillary lymph nodes fixed to one another or to other structures
N3	Metastases to ipsilateral internal mammary lymph node with or without axillary lymph node involvement, or in clinically apparent clavicular lymph node.
Distant Metastases	
MX	Presence of distant metastases not assessable
M0	No distant metastases
M1	Existent distant metastases (including ipsilateral supraclavicular nodes)

With permission from Fleming ID, Cooper JS, Henson DE, et al., eds. *AJCC Cancer Staging Manual,* 5th ed. Philadelphia, PA: Lippincott Williams & Wilkins; 1998.

equivocal by fluorescence *in situ* hybridization. Overexpression of *Her2/neu* is a *poor* prognostic factor, as it results in an increased rate of metastasis, decreased time to recurrence, and decreased overall survival. Patients with Her2/neu amplified tumors are treated with targeted monoclonal antibody therapies, such as trastuzumab (Herceptin) or lapatinib (Tykerb).

TABLE 27-2	American Joint Committee on Cancer Classification for Breast Cancer Based on TNM (Tumor, Node, Metastasis) Criteria		
Stage	Tumor	Nodes	Metastases
0	Tis	N0	M0
I	T1	N0	M0
IIA	T0, 1 T2	N1 N0	M0 M0
IIB	T2 T3	N1 N0	M0 M0
IIIA	T0, 1, 2 T3	N2 N1, 2	M0 M0
IIIB	T4 Any T	Any N N3	M0 M0
IV	Any T	Any N	M1

With permission from Fleming ID, Cooper JS, Henson DE, et al., eds. *AJCC Cancer Staging Manual*, 5th ed. Philadelphia, PA: Lippincott Williams & Wilkins; 1998.

C. Other **negative markers** include those tumors that do not express any tumor biomarkers (**"triple negative"**), the presence of **lymphovascular invasion,** and other indicators of a high proliferative rate (>5% of cells in the **S phase;** >20% **Ki-67**).

IV. **NONINVASIVE (*in situ*) Breast Cancer.** Ductal carcinoma *in situ* (**DCIS**) or LCIS are lesions with malignant cells that have not penetrated the basement membrane of the mammary ducts or lobules, respectively.

A. **DCIS,** or intraductal carcinoma, is treated as a **malignancy** because DCIS has the potential to develop into invasive cancer.
   - It is usually detected by mammography as clustered pleomorphic calcifications.
   - Physical examination is normal in the majority of patients.
   - It may advance in a segmental manner, with gaps between disease areas.
   - It can be **multifocal** (two or more lesions >5 mm apart within the same index quadrant) or **multicentric** (in different quadrants).
   1. Histology
      a. There are **five architectural subtypes:** papillary, micropapillary, solid, cribriform, and comedo. Specimens are also grouped as *comedo* versus *noncomedo.*

    b. The **high-grade subtype** is often associated with microinvasion, a higher proliferation rate, aneuploidy, gene amplification, and a higher local recurrence rate.

    c. ER and PR expression levels should be obtained if hormone therapy is being considered.

2. Treatment

    a. **Surgical excision** alone (via partial mastectomy) with **margins greater than 10 mm** is associated with a local recurrence rate of 14% at 12 years (*Am J Surg.* 2006;192:420). The addition of adjuvant radiation reduces the local recurrence rate to 2.5%. Approximately half of the recurrences present as invasive ductal carcinomas. **Surgical options** depend on the extent of disease, grade, margin status, multicentricity of disease, and patient age.

        (1) **Partial mastectomy:** For unicentric lesions. Needle localization is required to identify the area to be excised in most cases. Bracket needle localization (two or more wires to map out the extent of disease to be resected) for more extensive lesions is occasionally used.

        (2) **Mastectomy:** Total (simple) mastectomy with or without immediate reconstruction is recommended for patients with multicentric lesions, extensive involvement of the breast (disease extent relative to breast size), or persistently positive margins with partial mastectomy.

    b. Assessment of axillary lymph nodes: axillary dissection is not performed for pure DCIS.

        (1) **Sentinel lymph node biopsy (SLNB,** see later discussion) may be considered when there is a reasonable probability of finding invasive cancer on final pathologic examination (e.g., >4 cm, palpable, or high grade).

        (2) Some surgeons perform SLNB in all patients with DCIS undergoing mastectomy because SLNB cannot be performed postmastectomy if an occult invasive cancer is found. This is an area of ongoing controversy and research.

        (3) **A positive sentinel node indicates invasive breast cancer** and changes the stage of the disease; a **completion axillary dissection** is then indicated.

    c. Adjuvant therapy

        (1) For pure DCIS, there is no added benefit from systemic chemotherapy because the disease is confined to the ducts of the breast. However, in those patients with **ER-positive DCIS,** adjuvant **tamoxifen** can reduce the risk of breast cancer recurrence by 37% over 5 years and the risk of developing a new contralateral breast cancer (NSABP B-24 trial). However, there is no survival benefit. **Aromatase inhibitors** (e.g., **anastrozole, exemestane, letrozole**), which block the peripheral conversion of androgens into estrogens by inhibiting the enzyme aromatase but does not affect estrogen produced by the ovaries, are sometimes used as an alternative in postmenopausal patients.

TABLE 27-3	Van Nuys Scoring System[a]		
	Score		
	1	**2**	**3**
Size (mm)	d15	>15–40	>40
Margins (mm)	S10	<10 but >1	<1
Histology	Non–high grade without necrosis	Non–high grade with necrosis	High grade with or without necrosis

[a]A score of 13 points is given for each of the prognostic factors described, resulting in a total index score ranging from 3 to 9. Scores of 3 and 4 are considered low index values; scores of 5, 6, or 7 are considered intermediate; and scores of 8 or 9 are considered high.
Modified from Silverstein MJ, Lagios MD, Craig PH, et al. A prognostic index for ductal carcinoma *in situ* of the breast. *Cancer.* 1996;77:226–227.

       (2) **Adjuvant radiation** should be given to patients with DCIS treated with partial mastectomy to **decrease the local recurrence rate** (NSABP B-17 trial). This is especially true for younger women with close margins or large tumors. However, there is no survival benefit. For older patients with smaller, widely excised DCIS of low or intermediate grade, the benefit of radiation therapy is less clear and adjuvant radiation may not be necessary.

      d. **The Van Nuys Prognostic Index** (Table 27-3) is a numerical algorithm (based on lesion size, margin, tumor grade, presence of necrosis, and age) used to stratify patients with DCIS into three groups to determine which patient is at greatest risk of recurrence and would therefore benefit the most from a more aggressive treatment approach. The low-scoring group may be treated with partial mastectomy alone. The intermediate-scoring group has been shown to benefit from adjuvant radiation therapy, and the high-scoring group should undergo mastectomy because the risk of recurrence with partial mastectomy with or without radiation is high (*Adv Surg.* 2000;34:29).

  B. LCIS is not considered a preinvasive lesion but rather an indicator for increased breast cancer risk of approximately 1% per year (~20% to 30% at 15 years) (*JNCCN* 2006;4:511) and is not treated as a breast cancer.

    1. It may be multifocal and/or bilateral.

    2. The cancer that develops may be invasive ductal or lobular and may occur in either breast.

    3. LCIS has loss of **E-cadherin** (involved in cell–cell adhesion), which can be stained for on pathology slides to clarify cases that are borderline DCIS versus LCIS.

4. **Pleomorphic LCIS** is a particularly aggressive subtype of LCIS that is treated more like DCIS; it tends to have less favorable biological markers.

5. **Treatment options** are (1) lifelong close **surveillance,** (2) **bilateral total mastectomies** with immediate reconstruction for selected women with a strong family history after appropriate counseling, or (3) prophylaxis with **tamoxifen or raloxifene** (raloxifene has only been validated in the postmenopausal setting).

V. INVASIVE BREAST CANCER

A. **Histology** consists of five different subtypes: *infiltrating ductal* (75% to 80%), *infiltrating lobular* (5% to 10%), *medullary* (5% to 7%), *mucinous* (3%), and *tubular* (1% to 2%).

B. Surgical options for stage I and II breast cancer:

1. **Mastectomy** with or without reconstruction.

   a. **Radical mastectomy** involves total mastectomy, complete ALND (levels I, II, and III), removal of the pectoralis major and minor muscles, and removal of all overlying skin. This surgical approach is largely historical and is rarely, if ever, performed in modern practice.

   b. **Modified radical mastectomy** (MRM) involves total mastectomy and ALND. It is indicated for patients with clinically positive lymph nodes or a positive axillary node based on previous SLNB or FNAB.

   c. **Total (simple) mastectomy with SLNB** is for patients with a clinically negative axilla. A skin-sparing mastectomy (preserves skin envelope and inframammary ridge) may be performed with immediate reconstruction, resulting in improved cosmesis: the nipple-areolar complex, a rim of periareolar breast skin, and any previous excisional biopsy or partial mastectomy scars are excised.

   d. **Immediate reconstruction** at the time of mastectomy should be offered to eligible patients. Options include latissimus dorsi myocutaneous flaps, transverse rectus abdominis myocutaneous flaps, and inflatable tissue expanders followed by exchange for saline or silicone implants. Immediate reconstruction has been shown not to affect patient outcome adversely. The detection of recurrence is not delayed, and the onset of chemotherapy is not changed.

   e. **Follow-up after mastectomy:** physical examination every 3 to 6 months for 3 years, then every 6 to 12 months for the next 2 years, and then annually (*J Clin Oncol.* 2006;24:5091). Mammography of the contralateral breast should continue yearly. Regular gynecologic follow-up is recommended for all women (tamoxifen increases risk of endometrial cancer).

2. **Breast conservation therapy (BCT): partial mastectomy** and SLNB (or ALND; see later discussion) followed by breast irradiation.

   a. Several trials have demonstrated that BCT with adjuvant radiation therapy has similar survival and recurrence rates to those for MRM (*J Clin Oncol.* 1992;10:976).

b. **Contraindications for BCT:** not every patient is a candidate for BCT. Contraindications include patients who may be unreliable with follow-up or radiation therapy (may involve radiation treatment 5 days a week for 5 to 6 weeks); when the extent of disease prevents adequate negative margins; a high tumor-to-breast size ratio, which prevents adequate resection without major deformity; persistently positive margins on re-excision partial mastectomy; and inability to receive adjuvant radiation (e.g., prior radiation to the chest wall; first- and second-trimester pregnancy in which the delay of radiation to the postpartum state is inappropriate; collagen vascular diseases such as scleroderma).

c. For patients with large tumors who desire BCT, **neoadjuvant chemotherapy** or **neoadjuvant hormonal therapy** may be offered to attempt to reduce the size of the tumor to make BCT attempt possible.

d. **Partial mastectomy** incisions should be planned so that they can be incorporated into a mastectomy incision should that prove necessary. Incisions for partial mastectomy and either SLNB or ALND should be separate.

e. **Adjuvant radiotherapy** decreases the breast cancer recurrence rate from 30% to less than 7% at 5 years and is a required component of BCT.

f. **Follow-up after BCT.** Physical examinations are the same as those for mastectomy (see earlier discussion). A posttreatment mammogram of the treated breast is performed to establish a new baseline, no earlier than 6 months after completion of radiation therapy. Mammograms are then performed every 6 to 12 months after the new baseline mammogram until the surgical changes stabilize and then annually. Contralateral breast mammography remains on an annual basis. Regular gynecologic follow-up is recommended.

3. **Management of the axilla.** Approximately 30% of patients with clinically negative exams will have positive lymph nodes in an **ALND** specimen. The presence and number of lymph nodes involved affect staging and thus prognosis. However, complications are not infrequent (see later discussion). Thus, **SLNB** was developed to provide sampling of the lymph nodes without needing an ALND.

a. **SLNB** has been established as a standard of care for predicting axillary involvement in most patients with breast cancer. The procedure requires a multidisciplinary approach, including nuclear medicine, pathology, and radiology.

(1) It involves injection of blue dye (either **Lymphazurin or methylene blue**) in the operating room and/or **technetium-labeled sulfur colloid** (in the nuclear medicine department, radiology suite, or sometimes by the surgeon). The combination of blue dye and radioisotope provides higher node identification rates and increases the sensitivity of the procedure. The goal is to identify the primary draining lymph node(s) in the axillary nodal basin.

(2) A variety of injection techniques are used: **intraparenchymal** versus **intradermal** (intradermal methylene blue will cause skin necrosis at the injection site); **peritumoral** versus **periareolar.**

(3) The SLN is identified by its blue color, and/or by high activity detected by a handheld gamma probe, or by a blue lymphatic seen to enter a non-blue node. Palpable nodes are also sentinel nodes, even if not blue or radioactive.

(4) Twenty percent to 30% of the time more than one SLN is identified.

(5) Experienced surgeons (those who have performed at least 30 SLNBs, with ALND for confirmation) can identify the SLN in greater than 90% of patients, accurately predicting the patients' remaining axillary lymph node status in greater than 97% of cases.

(6) **If the SLN is positive for metastasis** (micrometastasis 0.2 mm or larger, *not isolated tumor cells*), **a standard completion ALND is the current recommendation.** A recent randomized trial compared the overall survival and axillary recurrence rates for patients with limited SLN metastatic disease who received breast conservation and systemic therapy and either had ALND versus no further axillary procedures (*JAMA.* 2011;305(6):569). There was no difference in the two groups, leading many to defer completion ALND for this subgroup of patients. All patients underwent lumpectomy, whole breast radiation, and systemic therapy; thus, the results cannot be generalized to all patients with a positive SLN.

(7) Serial sectioning and immunohistochemical staining of SLNB specimens may improve accuracy in detecting micrometastatic disease.

(8) Currently, **isolated tumor cells are considered N0** disease, and therapeutic decisions should *not* be based on finding these.

b. **ALND.** Patients with clinically positive lymph nodes should undergo ALND for local control. ALND involves the following:

(1) Removal of **level I** and **level II nodes** and, *if grossly involved,* possibly level III nodes. Motor and sensory nerves are preserved unless there is direct tumor involvement.

(2) An ALND should remove **10 or more nodes.** The number of nodes identified is often pathologist dependent.

(3) Patients with **4 or more positive lymph nodes** should undergo **adjuvant radiation to the axilla.** Selective patients with 1 to 3 positive nodes may also benefit from radiation therapy to the axilla.

(4) **Intraoperative complications:** potential injury to the axillary vessels and neuropathy secondary to injury to the motor nerves of the axilla (the long thoracic, thoracodorsal, and medial pectoral nerves).

(5) Most frequent **postoperative complications:** wound infections and seromas. Persistent seroma may be treated with repeated aspirations or reinsertion of a drain. Other complications include pain and numbness in the axilla and upper arm, impaired shoulder mobility, and **lymphedema.**

Lymphedema occurs in approximately 10% to 40% of women undergoing axillary dissection; radiation to the axilla increases the risk of this complication. The most effective therapy is early intervention with intense physiomassage; graded pneumatic compression devices and a professionally fitted compression sleeve can also provide relief and prevent worsening of lymphedema. Blood draws, blood pressure cuffs, and intravenous lines should be avoided in the affected arm, mainly to avoid infection in it. Infections of the hand or arm should be treated promptly and aggressively with antibiotics and arm elevation because infection can damage lymphatics further and cause irreversible lymphedema. Lymphedema itself increases the risk of developing **angiosarcoma.**

C. **Adjuvant systemic therapy** is given in appropriate patients after completion of surgery.

1. All node-positive patients should receive adjuvant chemotherapy.

   a. Regimens are guided by the tumor biomarkers. Typical regimens comprise four to eight cycles of a combination of cyclophosphamide and an anthracycline, followed by a taxane administered every 2 to 3 weeks.

   b. Patients with **ER-positive tumors** receive **adjuvant hormonal therapy** for 5 years. **Tamoxifen** is given to premenopausal women, and **aromatase inhibitors** are given to postmenopausal women (aromatase inhibitors are not used in premenopausal women because decreased feedback to the hypothalamus and pituitary increases gonadotropin secretion, stimulating the ovary to secrete more substrate).

   c. In postmenopausal women older than 70 years, chemotherapy is performed less frequently. In postmenopausal women with tumors with ER or PR positivity, tamoxifen or an aromatase inhibitor is frequently the sole adjuvant medical therapy.

   d. In patients with *Her2/neu*-**positive tumors,** polychemotherapy is combined with biological therapy targeting the *Her2/neu* protein: **trastuzumab** is a recombinant monoclonal antibody that binds to *Her2/neu* receptor to prevent cell proliferation. The NSABP trial B-31 and the North Central Cancer Treatment Group trial N9831 showed that adding trastuzumab to a chemotherapy regiment of doxorubicin, cyclophosphamide, and paclitaxel was associated with an increase in the disease-free survival by 12% and a 33% reduction in the risk of death at 3 years. It is usually administered intravenously monthly for 12 months. The most serious toxicity with the regiment was cardiac failure (*N Engl J Med.* 2005;353:1673).

2. **Node-negative patients** may have increased disease-free survival from adjuvant chemotherapy and/or hormonal therapy. An individualized approach is crucial and requires thorough discussion with the patient regarding the risks of recurrence without adjuvant therapy, the cost and toxicities treatment, and the expected benefit in risk reduction and survival.

   a. Up to 30% of node-negative women die of breast cancer within 10 years if treated with surgery alone.

b. Node-negative patients who are at **high risk** and benefit the most from adjuvant chemotherapy include those with tumors greater than 1 cm, higher tumor grade, *Her2/neu* expression, aneuploidy, Ki-67 expression, increased percentage in S phase, lymphovascular invasion, and ER/PR-negative tumors.

c. The NSABP B-20 trial and the International Breast Cancer Study Group trial IX showed that **polychemotherapy in combination with tamoxifen was superior to tamoxifen alone** in increasing disease-free and overall survival, especially in ER-negative patients, regardless of tumor size.

d. The St. Gallen Consensus Panel in 1998 suggested that patients who have node-negative disease and whose tumors are 1 cm or less and ER-positive may be spared adjuvant chemotherapy but still may benefit from adjuvant endocrine therapy.

e. The Web site http://www.adjuvantonline.com provides an online tool for physicians to use to calculate the added benefit of hormonal and chemotherapeutic therapies.

D. Adjuvant radiation

1. **Indications** for adjuvant radiation to the chest wall and axilla **after mastectomy** include T3 and T4 tumors, attachment to the pectoral fascia, positive surgical margins, skin involvement, involved internal mammary nodes, inadequate or no axillary dissection, four or more positive lymph nodes, and residual tumor on the axillary vein. Presence of one to three positive axillary nodes is a relative indication.

2. Randomized, prospective trials have shown a significantly decreased recurrence and improved survival in premenopausal women with these indications treated with chemotherapy and radiation therapy (*N Engl J Med.* 1997;337:949).

3. Adjuvant whole-breast radiation **after BCT** decreases the breast cancer recurrence rate from 30% to less than 7% at 5 years.

4. **Complications.** Radiation to the chest wall can cause skin changes. Infrequent complications include interstitial pneumonitis, spontaneous rib fracture, breast fibrosis, pericarditis, pleural effusion, and chest wall myositis. Radiation to the axilla can increase the incidence of lymphedema and axillary fibrosis. **Angiosarcoma** can occur as a late complication.

E. Locally advance breast cancer (LABC) comprises T3 or T4, N1 or greater, and M0 cancers **(stages IIIA and IIIB).**

1. **Staging in LABC.** Because of the frequency of distant metastasis at the time of presentation, all patients should receive complete blood cell count, complete metabolic panel, bone scan, and CT scan of chest and abdomen before treatment.

2. **Noninflammatory LABC** (chest wall or skin involvement, skin satellites, ulceration, fixed axillary nodes)

   a. Patients should receive **neoadjuvant chemotherapy** (often cyclophosphamide combined with an anthracycline and taxane), followed by surgery and radiation. The high response rates seen with this regimen for **stage IIIB** allow **MRM** to be carried out, with primary skin closure. Neoadjuvant chemotherapy also provides information regarding tumor response to treatment that may aid to guide further adjuvant therapy. Adjuvant radiation to the chest wall and regional nodes chemotherapy follow surgery; additional adjuvant chemotherapy is also necessary in select cases. SLNB may be used in selected patients with a clinically negative axilla.

- **b.** Patients with **stage IIIA** disease receiving neoadjuvant chemotherapy who can be converted to **BCT** candidates have no difference in overall survival outcome.
- **c.** Approximately 20% of patients with stage III disease present with distant metastases after appropriate staging has been performed.

3. Inflammatory LABC (T4d)
- **a.** This is characterized by erythema, warmth, tenderness, and edema (*peau d'orange*).
- **b.** It represents 1% to 6% of all breast cancers.
- **c.** An underlying mass is present in 70% of cases. Associated axillary adenopathy occurs in 50% of cases.
- **d.** It is often misdiagnosed initially as mastitis.
- **e.** **Skin punch biopsy** confirms the diagnosis: in two third of cases, tumor emboli are seen in dermal lymphatics.
- **f.** Approximately 30% of patients have distant metastasis at the time of diagnosis.
- **g.** Inflammatory breast cancer requires **aggressive multimodal therapy** because median survival is approximately 2 years, with a 5-year survival of only 5%.

4. Follow-up. Because of higher risk for local and distant recurrence, patients should be examined every 3 months by all specialists involved in their care.

F. **Locoregional recurrence.** Patients with locoregional recurrence should have a **metastatic workup** to exclude visceral or bony disease and should be considered for systemic chemotherapy or hormonal therapy.

1. Recurrence in the breast after BCT requires total (simple) mastectomy. Provided margins are negative, survival is similar to that for patients who received mastectomy initially.

2. Recurrence in the axilla requires surgical resection followed by radiation to the axilla and systemic therapy.

3. Recurrence in the chest wall after mastectomy occurs in 4% to 5% of patients. One third of these patients have distant metastases at the time of recurrence, and greater than 50% will have distant disease within 2 years. Multimodal therapy is essential. For an isolated local recurrence, excision followed by radiotherapy results in excellent local control. Rarely, patients require radical chest resection with myocutaneous flap closure.

VI. CHEMOPREVENTION

A. The NSABP P-1 trial was the first large prospective, randomized chemopreventive trial to evaluate the efficacy of the estrogen antagonist **tamoxifen** to reduce breast cancer incidence in women at risk.

1. Women taking tamoxifen achieved an overall reduction in the risk of developing invasive breast carcinoma of 49% and a reduction in the risk of developing noninvasive breast cancer of 50%.

2. In subgroups of women with a history of **LCIS** and with a history of **ADH,** tamoxifen reduced the risk of developing invasive breast cancer by 65% and 86%, respectively.

B. The NSABP B-24 trial showed that tamoxifen provided a 37% overall risk reduction for all breast cancers (invasive and noninvasive) in women with **DCIS treated with lumpectomy and radiation.**

1. The **toxicities** of the drug include an increased risk of endometrial cancer, thrombotic vascular events, and cataract development. Women on tamoxifen also reported increased vasomotor symptoms (hot flashes) and vaginal discharge.

2. Tamoxifen also provided a significant reduction in hip fractures in women older than 50 years of age. There was no difference noted in the incidence of ischemic heart disease for women taking tamoxifen.

3. Tamoxifen has been approved by the Food and Drug Administration (FDA) for (1) the treatment of metastatic breast cancer, (2) adjuvant **treatment of breast cancer,** and (3) **chemoprevention of invasive or contralateral breast cancer in high-risk women.**

4. The **dosage** for chemoprevention is 20 mg/day for 5 years. It is estimated that chemoprevention could prevent as many as 500,000 invasive and 200,000 noninvasive breast cancers over 5 years in the United States alone.

5. The Study of Tamoxifen and Raloxifene (STAR) trial compared tamoxifen to **raloxifene** (a selective ER modulator). Raloxifene has not been approved by the FDA for chemoprevention, but was shown to provide equal risk reduction for the development of invasive breast cancers as tamoxifen. It was not as effective at reducing the risk of developing noninvasive breast cancer. Its side effect profile is somewhat different than that of tamoxifen, so it can be considered in patients with relative contraindications to tamoxifen.

SPECIAL CONSIDERATIONS

I. BREAST CONDITIONS DURING PREGNANCY

A. **Bloody nipple discharge** may occur in the second or third trimester. It results from epithelial proliferation under hormonal influences and usually resolves by 2 months postpartum. If it does not resolve by then, standard evaluation of pathologic nipple discharge should be performed.

B. **Breast masses** occurring during pregnancy include **galactoceles, lactating adenoma, simple cysts, breast infarcts, fibroadenomas,** *and* **carcinoma.** Fibroadenomas may grow during pregnancy due to hormonal stimulation.

1. Masses should be evaluated by ultrasound, and a core needle biopsy should be performed for any suspicious lesion.

2. Mammography can be performed with uterine shielding but is rarely helpful due to increased breast density.

3. If a breast lesion is diagnosed as malignant, the patient should be given the **same surgical treatment** options, stage for stage, as a nonpregnant woman, and the **treatment should not be delayed** because of the pregnancy.

C. **Breast cancer during pregnancy** may be difficult to diagnose due to the low level of suspicion and breast nodularity and density.

1. It occurs in approximately 1 in 5,000 gestations and accounts for almost 3% of all breast cancers.

2. **Workup is the same as in a nonpregnant woman.** The standard preoperative staging workup is performed. Laboratory values such as alkaline phosphatase may be elevated during pregnancy. For advanced-stage disease, MRI scan or ultrasound may be used in lieu of CT scan for staging. Excisional biopsy can be safely performed under local anesthesia if there is some contraindication to the preferred core needle biopsy.

3. **Therapeutic decisions** are influenced by the clinical cancer stage and the trimester of pregnancy and must be **individualized.** MRM has been the standard surgical modality for pregnant patients with breast cancer, but BCT can be offered to selected patients. The radiation component of BCT cannot be applied during pregnancy, and delaying radiation therapy is not ideal. For these reasons, BCT is usually not recommended to patients in their first or second trimester. For patients in the third trimester, radiation can begin after delivery. SLNB is starting to be used more frequently; the commonly used radioisotope is approved for use during pregnancy.

4. **Chemotherapy** may be given by the mid-second trimester.

II. **PAGET DISEASE OF THE NIPPLE** is characterized by eczematoid changes of the nipple, which may involve the surrounding areola.

A. Burning, pruritus, and hypersensitivity may be prominent symptoms.

B. Paget disease is almost always accompanied by an underlying malignancy, either invasive ductal carcinoma or DCIS.

C. Palpable masses are present in approximately 60% of patients.

D. Mammography should be performed to identify other areas of involvement. If clinical suspicion is high, a pathologic diagnosis should be obtained by wedge biopsy of the nipple and underlying breast tissue.

E. Treatment is mastectomy or BCT with excision of the nipple-areolar complex (sometimes called a central lumpectomy), followed by radiation therapy. The prognosis is related to tumor stage.

III. BREAST CANCER IN MEN accounts for less than 1% of male cancers and less than 1% of all breast cancers. BRCA2 mutations are associated with approximately 4% to 6% of these cancers.

   A. Patients generally present with a nontender hard mass. This contrasts with unilateral gynecomastia, which is usually firm, central, and tender.

   B. Mammography can be helpful in distinguishing gynecomastia from malignancy. Malignant lesions are more likely to be eccentric, with irregular margins, and are often associated with nipple retraction and microcalcifications. Biopsy of suspicious lesions is essential, and core needle biopsy is preferred.

   C. MRM was traditionally the surgical procedure of choice; however, SLNB has been shown to be effective in men. Thus, total (simple) mastectomy with SLNB is a valid option in men.

   D. Eighty-five percent of malignancies are infiltrating ductal carcinoma and are positive for ER.

   E. Adjuvant hormonal, chemotherapy, and radiation treatment criteria are the same as in women. Overall survival *per stage* is comparable to that observed in women, although men tend to present in later stages.

IV. PHYLLODES TUMORS account for 1% of breast neoplasms.

   A. They present as a large, smooth, lobulated mass and may be difficult to distinguish from fibroadenoma on physical exam.

   B. They can occur in women of any age, but most frequently between the ages of 35 and 55 years.

   C. Skin ulcerations may occur secondary to pressure of the underlying mass.

   D. FNAB cannot reliably diagnose these tumors; at least a core needle biopsy is needed. Histologically, stromal overgrowth is the essential characteristic for differentiating phyllodes tumors from fibroadenomas.

   E. Ninety percent are benign; 10% are malignant. The biologic behavior of malignant tumors is similar to that of **sarcomas.**

   F. Treatment is **wide local excision to tumor-free margins or total mastectomy.** Axillary assessment with either SLNB or ALND is **not** indicated unless nodes are clinically positive (which is rare).

   G. Currently, there is no role for adjuvant radiation; however, tumors greater than 5 cm in diameter and with evidence of stromal overgrowth may benefit from adjuvant chemotherapy with doxorubicin and ifosfamide (*Cancer.* 2000;89:1510).

   H. Patients should be followed with semiannual physical examinations and annual mammograms and chest radiographs.

28

Otolaryngology: Head and Neck Surgery

Sunitha M. Sequeira and Bruce H. Haughey

I. THE EAR

A. Anatomy and physiology

1. **External ear.** The auricle (pinna) is composed of elastic cartilage and channels sound waves to the external auditory canal, which is bone medially and cartilage laterally.

2. **Middle ear.** The middle ear is a mucosa-lined sinus in the temporal bone containing the ossicular chain. The tympanic membrane (TM) vibrates in response to sound waves, and transmits this mechanical energy via the ossicles (malleus, incus, and stapes) to the oval window of the cochlea. The difference in surface area between the TM and oval window, along with the lever action of the ossicles, results in a 22-fold amplification of sound energy. The eustachian tube (ET) connects the middle ear with the nasopharynx, allowing aeration of the middle ear, drainage of fluid, and protection from pharyngeal pathogens. It is opened by contraction of the tensor veli palatini muscle, during swallowing or yawning.

3. **Inner ear.** The end-organs of hearing and balance are surrounded by thick bone, the otic capsule. The cochlea is a snail-shaped structure containing the organ of Corti. The vestibular system consists of three semicircular canals, which sense angular acceleration, and the saccule and utricle, which sense linear acceleration, yielding a sense of spatial orientation and movement. The cochlea and vestibular system convert mechanical energy into neuroelectric inputs, which are transmitted to the pons via cranial nerve (CN) VIII, the **vestibulocochlear nerve.**

4. The **facial nerve** (CN VII) travels a complex path through the temporal bone, where it is vulnerable to trauma, and the middle ear. It innervates the facial musculature, stapedius muscle, and taste sensation for the anterior 2/3 of the tongue via the chorda tympani.

B. Infectious/Inflammatory disorders

1. **Otitis externa** ("swimmer's ear") is inflammation of the external auditory canal. Moisture and local trauma (e.g., q-tips) allow bacterial infection, causing severe ear pain, drainage, pruritus, canal swelling, and conductive hearing loss (CHL). It may progress to auricular swelling and facial cellulitis. Common pathogens include *pseudomonas aeruginosa* and fungus. Treatment includes topical antibiotic drops, antiseptic drying drops, and aural toilet.

   a. Persistent otitis externa in a diabetic or immunocompromised patient should raise concern for **necrotizing otitis externa** (malignant otitis externa), a potentially fatal skull base osteomyelitis that can spread intracranially. Patients have long-standing otalgia, otorrhea, and granulation tissue in the external auditory canal. Work-up includes computed tomography (CT) or magnetic resonance imaging (MRI) and radionuclide bone scans. Treatment is intravenous (IV) antibiotics and surgical debridement.

   b. A nonhealing, weepy erythematous ear canal lesion in an adult should undergo biopsy, for concern of squamous cell carcinoma (SCC).

2. **Acute otitis media** (AOM) is acute inflammation of the middle ear, usually of infectious etiology. Common in children, it presents with fevers, otalgia, irritability, decreased appetite, hearing loss, and a thickened, red, bulging TM. Typical pathogens are *Streptococcus pneumoniae, haemophilus influenzae,* and *Moraxella catarrhalis.* Risk factors include day-care attendance, cigarette smoke exposure, young age (immature immune system), male sex, winter months, and genetics. **ET dysfunction** significantly contributes to AOM—young children have immature, weak, and more horizontal ET cartilage, contributing to poor aeration of the middle ear and poor protection from pharyngeal pathogens. Breastfeeding is protective. Because spontaneous resolution often occurs, watchful waiting is preferred for children older than 2 years or nontoxic children older than 6 months (without severe otalgia or high fevers), to reduce antibiotic usage and resistance. Treatment (first line is amoxicillin) is indicated for symptoms longer than 48 to 72 hours or children younger than 6 months. For recurrent OM more frequent than three to four episodes in 6 months or four to six episodes in a year (recommendations vary), tympanostomy tube placement reduces the frequency of ear infections, facilitates diagnosis (as OM then manifests as ear drainage), and reduces the necessity for systemic antibiotics (by allowing topical treatment via ear drops). Adenoidectomy also reduces number of infections, and is performed if repeat ear tubes are needed.

3. **Otitis media with effusion** (OME), or **serous OM,** is fluid present in the middle ear without acute infection. It may result from resolving AOM or ET dysfunction. Patients present with hearing loss, aural fullness/pressure, and a dull, gray, or yellow TM with reduced mobility. OME usually resolves spontaneously. Tympanostomy tube placement is indicated for bilateral OME for greater than 3 months, unilateral OME for more than 6 months, and in children with hearing loss and concerns for speech/language delay. Adults with persistent unilateral OME should undergo evaluation of the nasopharynx for masses causing ET obstruction.

4. Complications from OM are uncommon and include TM perforation, tympanosclerosis, mastoiditis, facial nerve palsy, labyrinthitis, meningitis, intracranial abscess, sigmoid sinus thrombosis, and otitic hydrocephalus.

   a. Tympanosclerosis is hyalinization and calcium deposition onto the middle ear and TM, resulting in white plaques, in response to inflammation or trauma (e.g., tympanostomy tubes). It is usually asymptomatic but can cause ossicular fixation and hearing loss.

b. Mastoiditis is a clinical diagnosis, based on history of fevers, otalgia, postauricular tender swelling and a proptotic pinna. CT shows severity of infection, including subperiosteal abscess and intracranial complications. Mastoid fluid on CT without clinical correlation is not diagnostic of mastoiditis. Treatment is IV antibiotics; tympanostomy and/or mastoidectomy are indicated for no response or complications.

C. **Hearing loss** is classified as conductive, sensorineural, or mixed.

1. CHL is caused by pathology of the external auditory canal, TM, and middle ear, resulting in attenuation of sound energy delivered to the inner ear. In adults, the most common cause is impacted cerumen (wax). In kids, it is OM. Other causes include TM perforation, ossicular discontinuity or fixation, otosclerosis, and cholesteatoma.

2. **Sensorineural hearing loss** (SNHL) involves the cochlea or auditory neural pathway. The most common causes are presbycusis (age-related hearing loss), noise exposure, and hereditary. Other etiologies include viral or bacterial infections, ototoxicity (due to aminoglycosides, platinum-based chemotherapy, loop diuretics), vestibular schwannomas, temporal bone trauma, and autoimmune disease. Congenital SNHL occurs in 1 to 2 in 1,000 newborns, with approximately 50% from genetic etiology.

3. **Evaluation of hearing**

    a. **Tuning fork testing.** Bedside assessment of hearing is performed with a 512 Hz tuning fork. In the **Weber** test, the tuning fork is placed on patient's midline forehead or maxillary incisor teeth. Those with normal hearing perceive the sound as equal intensity in both ears. In CHL, sound is louder in the affected ear. In SNHL, sound is heard louder in the contralateral ear. In the **Rinne** test, the tuning fork is held lateral to the auricle (air conduction), and placed on the mastoid tip (bone conduction). In normal hearing, air conduction is perceived as louder; in CHL, bone conduction is louder.

    b. **Audiometry.** An audiogram tests air and bone conduction hearing to pure-tone sounds and speech sounds. Tympanometry measures ear canal volume, TM integrity and compliance, as well as the stapedial reflex (seventh/eighth CN reflex arc). SNHL is diagnosed as equal losses of bone and air conduction; CHL is loss of air conduction with normal bone conduction, resulting in an air-bone gap. In mixed hearing loss, there is an air-bone gap and a loss of bone conduction. Decreased word-discrimination scores out of proportion to pure-tone hearing loss suggest retrocochlear pathology (e.g., vestibular schwannoma). Reduced TM peak compliance on tympanometry is consistent with middle ear pathology (e.g., middle ear effusion).

    c. **Newborn screening.** Universal hearing screening leads to early detection of congenital hearing loss and early intervention to facilitate language development. Newborn hearing screens are performed with **otoacoustic emission** (OAE) testing, which detects sound waves generated by cochlear outer hair cells in response to sound. **Auditory brainstem response** (ABR) measures neural activity from the cochlea along the cochlear nerve (CN VIII) to the midbrain. Behavioral audiometry can be done when a child is approximately 9 months. In adults, ABR is useful for detection of vestibular schwannoma.

4. **Treatment of hearing loss**
   a. Most of hearing loss is treated with behavioral modification and hearing aids. Idiopathic sudden SNHL can be treated with high-dose systemic or intratympanic steroids.
   b. Profoundly deaf individuals who do not benefit from hearing aids are candidates for cochlear implant (CI), in which an electrode array is placed into the cochlea. A microphone worn near the ear receives and transmits acoustic signals to the implanted electrode, which then stimulates the cochlear nerve. Preimplant evaluation and postimplant rehabilitation are crucial factors in the effectiveness of the implant.
   c. CHL can often be treated successfully by restoring the sound conduction pathway. This may be done through repair of the TM (tympanoplasty), ossicular chain reconstruction, stapedectomy (for otosclerosis), or removal of cholesteatoma. Bone anchored hearing aids (BAHA) are implantable hearing aids that bypass the sound conduction pathway.

D. **A cholesteatoma** is a nonneoplastic epithelial-lined cyst containing keratinous debris that expands and causes bony erosion. Patients may present with hearing loss, otorrhea, otalgia, and a pearly-white mass in their middle ear or on their TM. It may also cause vertigo from perilymphatic fistula, facial paresis, and similar complications to OM. Treatment is surgical resection, with tympanoplasty and mastoidectomy. Cholesteatomas often recur.

1. *Primary-acquired* cholesteatoma results from ET dysfunction and negative pressure in the middle ear. A retraction pocket develops in the pars flaccida (the superior segment of the TM), collects squamous debris, and expands into the middle ear and mastoid.

2. *Secondary-acquired* cholesteatoma arises from a TM perforation with medial migration of squamous epithelium bordering the perforation.

3. *Congenital* cholesteatoma presents as a white mass in the anterosuperior quadrant with no prior history of otologic surgery, and an intact TM.

E. **Vestibular schwannoma** (acoustic neuroma) is a benign neoplasm of CN VIII arising in the internal auditory canal (IAC). They can be nonhereditary or associated with neurofibromatosis type 2. Symptoms include unilateral hearing loss, vertigo, imbalance, or facial paralysis due to facial nerve compression in the IAC. As they grow into the cerebropontine angle, they may cause additional CN deficits and headaches from elevated intracranial pressure. Work-up includes audiogram and MRI. ABR may be used to screen. Treatment is surgical excision via craniotomy. Many are slow growing and may be closely monitored, particularly in patients not suitable for surgery.

F. **Dizziness.** True **vertigo** originates from the inner ear, and is described as a sensation of spinning or moving. This must be distinguished from *nonotologic dizziness,* characterized by unsteadiness, lightheadedness, or syncope. Causes of this may be cardiovascular (orthostatic hypotension, vertebrobasilar insufficiency, cerebellar/brainstem infarction), metabolic (hypoglycemia, hypothyroidism, drug-induced), neurogenic (migraines, multiple sclerosis, neoplasm), or psychogenic. Diagnosis is primarily from history and physical exam (particularly provocation of nystagmus). Vestibular testing is complementary, and includes electronystagmography, caloric testing, rotational chair analysis, and dynamic posturography. Causes of vertigo are best organized by the chronology of symptoms:

1. **Seconds to minutes. Benign paroxysmal positional vertigo** (BPPV) is the most common cause of transient vertigo. It is precipitated by changes in head position and is caused by stimulation of the vestibular system by free-floating calcium carbonate crystals within the semicircular canals, usually in the posterior semicircular canal. It is diagnosed by the Dix–Hallpike maneuver. Canalith repositioning maneuvers (Epley technique) are immediately effective in 80% of patients with BPPV (*Otolaryngol Head Neck Surg.* 2006;135:529). Refractory cases may undergo semicircular canal plugging.

2. **Hours. Ménière disease** (endolymphatic hydrops) is characterized by episodic vertigo, hearing loss, tinnitus, and aural fullness. Treatment is salt restriction, diuretics, and vestibular suppressants. Intratympanic dexamethasone or gentamicin injection may be effective. Refractory cases can undergo endolymphatic sac surgery, labyrinthectomy, or vestibular nerve sectioning.

3. **Days. Viral labyrinthitis/viral neuronitis** (inflammation of the inner ear labyrinth or nerve, respectively) can cause days to even weeks of vertigo. Disequilibrium may persist for months. Treatment is supportive; vestibular rehabilitation can be helpful. Other causes include temporal bone trauma and vestibular schwannoma.

G. **Trauma**

1. An **auricular hematoma** presents as a tender, fluctuant subperichondrial swelling effacing the normal anatomy of the pinna. It can result in cartilage necrosis and a "cauliflower" ear deformity. Treatment is incision and drainage (I&D), with bolster placement to prevent reaccumulation.

2. **Foreign bodies** should be removed under binocular microscopy. If organic material is present, irrigation or topical drops should not be used, as this causes painful expansion of the material and difficult removal. Batteries (in the ear canal or upper aerodigestive tract) must be removed urgently, as leakage of contents can cause burns and later stenosis.

3. Traumatic **TM perforation** usually resolves spontaneously. Antibiotic drops may be prescribed prophylactically, and the patient should avoid

water entry into the ear canal. Chronic perforations may undergo surgical repair.

4. **Temporal bone fracture** results from high-velocity blunt trauma,
often due to motor-vehicle accidents. Physical exam findings include
Battle's sign (postauricular ecchymosis) and hemotympanum. Most
fractures can be diagnosed by head CT, which is usually sufficient in
an asymptomatic patient. High-resolution temporal bone CT is useful
in the presence of facial weakness, cerebrospinal fluid (CSF) fistula,
vascular injury, and for operative planning. Fractures are categorized
as longitudinal (80%) or transverse (20%) with respect to the petrous
apex. Transverse fractures are more likely to cause SNHL or facial
nerve injury. Acute facial paralysis warrants surgical exploration and
nerve decompression. Delayed facial weakness is likely secondary to
nerve edema, and usually recovers spontaneously. CSF fistula/leak is
a serious sequela of temporal bone fracture, and may present with
middle ear effusion, clear rhinorrhea (drainage via ET), or clear otorrhea via a TM perforation. Most CSF leaks resolve spontaneously
with conservative measures such as bed-rest and lumbar drain. Surgical repair is typically indicated for CSF leaks persistent for more than
1 week, as these are less likely to spontaneously close and are associated with risk of meningitis. In any case, patients should undergo formal audiometry 4 to 6 weeks after injury (allowing hemotympanum
to clear) to assess hearing.

II. THE NOSE AND PARANASAL SINUSES

A. Anatomy and Physiology

1. The **nose** and **septum** are composed of bone superiorly and posteriorly, and cartilage anteriorly. The turbinates (superior, middle, inferior,
and supreme) are mucosa-covered bony prominences from the lateral
nasal cavity that humidify, warm, and filter inhaled air. The choanae
open the nasal cavity into the nasopharynx. The nasopharynx contains
the ET orifices bilaterally, and the adenoid pad centrally, which involute in late childhood. Superiorly, the olfactory nerve (CN I) penetrates
the cribriform plate with receptors that sense smell. The nasal cavity is
lined by ciliated mucosa rich in mucus glands, nerves, blood vessels,
and inflammatory cells.

2. The **paranasal sinuses** are pneumatized cavities in the skull named for
the bone in which they lie (frontal, sphenoid, ethmoid, maxillary). They
reduce the weight of the skull, contribute to the resonance of voice, and
cushion the cranial contents against trauma. They are lined with ciliated respiratory epithelium that directs clearance of mucus and inhaled
particles into the nose, and then into the pharynx. Obstruction of the
outlets of drainage, or ostia, can occur from anatomic abnormalities,
inflammation, or masses, causing fluid accumulation and symptoms.

B. Congenital disorders

1. Congenital nasal masses include encephaloceles, dermoid cysts, and
gliomas. They may present intranasally or extranasally as a midline

nose or lower forehead mass. MRI evaluates for intracranial extension. Treatment is surgical excision.

2. **Choanal atresia** is the persistence of the embryologic nasobuccal membrane, preventing communication between the nose and the nasopharynx. Bilateral choanal atresia presents with respiratory distress soon after birth, typically requiring intubation, as neonates are obligate nasal breathers. Diagnosis is confirmed by failure to pass a nasogastric tube. Unilateral choanal atresia often presents later in life. Choanal atresia is more commonly unilateral, associated with other anomalies, and in females. Choanal atresia is repaired surgically.

C. **Infectious/inflammatory disorders**

1. **Acute rhinosinusitis** arises from infectious, allergic, and drug-induced etiologies. Although most acute rhinosinusitis is viral, bacterial superinfection may occur, typically with *S. pneumoniae, H. influenzae, M. catarrhalis,* or *S. aureus.* Criteria for diagnosis include **two** of the following **major features:** facial pain/pressure, nasal discharge, nasal obstruction, anosmia or hyposmia, fevers (for acute sinusitis), and purulence in nasal cavity on exam; and **two minor criteria:** dental pain, halitosis, cough, ear discomfort, fatigue, and fevers (for chronic sinusitis). Treatment consists of saline nasal irrigations to improve mucociliary clearance, mucolytics to thin secretions, hydration, and antibiotics for bacterial sinusitis (first-line amoxicillin). Nasal topical steroids reduce symptom duration. Topical decongestion (e.g., oxymetalozone) aids in symptomatic relief; however, use *should not exceed three days,* as may result in rebound congestion, or *rhinitis medicamentosa.* Antihistamines dry mucous secretions, and therefore are not recommended unless allergy symptoms are present. Intraorbital or intracranial infectious complications may rarely occur.

2. **Chronic rhinosinusitis** is symptoms for more than 12 weeks with signs of inflammation on exam (nasal polyps, polypoid mucosal changes, or purulent drainage). Sinus CT may show mucosal thickening, sinus opacification, obstruction of the osteomeatal complex, and anatomic/bony abnormalities. Treatment typically includes combination of antibiotics, nasal saline irrigation, and topical nasal and/or oral steroids. Patients refractory to medical therapy benefit from **functional endoscopic sinus surgery (FESS)** (*Curr Opin Otolaryngol Head Neck Surg.* 2007;15:6). The objectives of FESS are to reestablish the patency of the sinus ostia, ventilate the sinuses, and selectively remove diseased mucosa or polyps.

3. **Fungal sinusitis**

   a. *Noninvasive fungal sinusitis,* caused by *Aspergillus* infection, includes mycetoma (fungus ball) and allergic fungal sinusitis. It is treated with steroids, saline irrigations, and FESS.

   b. *Acute invasive fungal sinusitis* is an aggressive, potentially fatal mucormycosis. Immunocompromised patients, particularly those with hematologic malignancies or diabetic ketoacidosis, are at risk. Management is IV antifungal therapy and surgical debridement of necrotic tissue.

D. **Nasal airway obstruction** has many causes, from rhinosinusitis to anatomic obstructions.

   1. **Adenoid hypertrophy.** The adenoids are lymphoid tissue present in the posterior nasopharynx that hypertrophy during childhood and then atrophy with age. Adenoid hypertrophy can cause nasal obstruction, snoring, sleep-disordered breathing, and recurrent OM. Adenoidectomy is often performed in conjunction with tonsillectomy.

   2. **Nasal polyposis.** Nasal polyps are inflammatory, edematous, hyperplastic regions of nasal mucosa that often obstruct sinus drainage. The etiology of nasal polyps is unknown, but they are commonly associated with systemic diseases (cystic fibrosis, allergies, chronic rhinosinusitis, or Samter's triad: aspirin sensitivity, asthma, and nasal polyposis). Nasal polyps are usually treated with nasal or systemic steroids and surgical debulking.

   3. **Nasal septal deviation** results from nasal trauma or differential growth. The role of septal deviation in sinus disease is controversial (*Otolaryngol Head Neck Surg.* 2005;133:190). Septal deviation can be corrected (septoplasty) in conjunction with FESS if nasal obstruction and sinus disease are present.

E. **Epistaxis** has many causes, including trauma, neoplasm, environmental irritants, rhinitis, coagulopathies, and granulomatous diseases (e.g., Wegener's disease and sarcoidosis). Unilateral recurrent epistaxis with nasal airway obstruction should prompt evaluation for a mass. Most epistaxis is minor. However, due to the significant vascularity of the nose, hemorrhage can be life threatening. Address ABCs first (airway, breathing, circulation) and treat underlying causes. The patient should pinch the cartilaginous nose and lean forward to avoid swallowing blood; a vasoconstrictor such as oxymetalozone spray should be applied. Much of epistaxis resolves with these measures. The most common site of bleeding is Kisselbach's plexus, on the anterior caudal septum. Bleeding can be cauterized with silver nitrate or electrocautery. The nose can also be packed using epistaxis balloons, gauze, or absorbable hemostatic agents. Arterial embolization is reserved for refractory cases. Preventative measures involve moisturization via nasal saline spray, Vaseline application, and humidification of air.

F. Neoplasms

   1. **Benign**
      a. The most common benign lesion is the **inverted papilloma,** a wart-like growth usually arising from the lateral nasal wall. It has a 10% incidence of malignant transformation into SCC. Wide local excision is necessary to prevent recurrence.
      b. **Juvenile nasopharyngeal angiofibromas** are vascular tumors usually presenting in adolescent boys with nasal obstruction and recurrent epistaxis. Treatment is surgical excision, with preoperative embolization to reduce blood loss.

   2. **Malignant**
      a. **Nasopharyngeal SCC** is most common in Asia and Africa, where it is often associated with the Epstein–Barr virus (EBV). Treatment

is chemotherapy and radiation, with surgical resection reserved for residual disease. Cervical metastasis is very common, in up to 80% at presentation.

b. Other sinonasal cancers include adenocarcinoma, adenoid cystic carcinoma, olfactory esthesioneuroblastoma, mucosal melanoma, and sinonasal undifferentiated carcinoma; other nasopharyngeal tumors include lymphoepithelioma and lymphoma.

G. **Trauma.** Maxillofacial fractures are usually due to blunt trauma. Operative repair is indicated for functional restoration and cosmesis.

1. **Nasal bone fractures** may result in cosmetic deformity and nasal airway obstruction. Epistaxis and airway management are the first priority. Closed reduction should be done 3 to 14 days after injury to allow improvement in swelling and avoidance of bony healing.

2. **Nasal septal hematoma** may occur with any nasal trauma. Blood collects between the septal mucoperichondrium and cartilage, which can cause cartilage ischemia, necrosis, and septal perforation. Large septal perforations can cause a "saddle nose" deformity. Treatment is I&D.

3. **Orbital blowout fractures** usually involve the medial and inferior orbit walls. Patients may have diplopia and hypesthesia of the cheek due to fracture along the infraorbital canal. Surgery is indicated for entrapment of the inferior rectus muscle causing restricted ocular movement, defects greater than 50%, or enophthalmos/hypophthalmos. Ophthalmologic evaluation for intraocular injury is also recommended.

4. **Le Fort fractures** involve the pterygoid plates (and other bones according to classification), mobilizing the maxilla from the skull base. Le Fort I fracture separates the maxillary alveolus from the upper maxilla via transverse fractures across the maxillary sinus and nasal septum. Le Fort II fracture creates a mobile pyramidal nasomaxillary segment by extending superiorly through the maxilla, across the orbital floor and nasal bones. Le Fort III fracture, or craniofacial disjunction, separates the entire midface from the cranium, extending through the zygoma and transversely through the orbits and nasal bones. The midface withstands the forces of mastication via the vertical and horizontal buttresses. Operative goals are to stabilize the buttresses, restore occlusion (dental relationship), and cosmesis.

III. ORAL CAVITY AND PHARYNX

A. **Anatomy and physiology**

1. **The oral cavity plays a crucial role in articulation and deglutition.** The oral cavity extends from the vermillion border of the lips anteriorly to the circumvallate papillae and junction of the hard and soft palate posteriorly. The pharynx is divided into the nasopharynx, oropharynx (which includes the lingual and palatine tonsils, and soft palate), and hypopharynx. Swallowing is a complex sensorimotor task involving soft palate elevation, elevation and retrusion of the tongue, laryngeal elevation, glottic closure, epiglottic retroflexion, and pharyngeal/esophageal peristalsis.

B. **Congenital disorders**

1. **Pierre–Robin sequence** is micrognathia, glossoptosis, and cleft palate, often resulting in significant airway obstruction and feeding difficulties. Airway obstruction can be treated with prone positioning, glossopexy, mandibular advancement, or tracheostomy.

2. **Cleft lip and palate.** Failure of the midface processes to fuse during embryogenesis results in clefts. Ideal management is by a multidisciplinary team, to address feeding, respiratory, hearing, cosmetic, speech, and psychosocial issues. Cleft palate causes abnormal insertion of the tensor veli palatini muscle, resulting in ET dysfunction, recurrent AOM, and OME. The otolaryngologist typically manages airway concerns, ear disease, velopharyngeal insufficiency, and sometimes cleft repair. Timing of repair is variable; cleft lips are often repaired after 10 weeks of age, and cleft palates by 1 year (to improve speech development).

C. **Infectious/inflammatory disorders**

1. **Ulcers** in the oral cavity are common and are usually related to viral infections, nutritional deficiencies, or glandular changes. Treatment is generally supportive. A variety of oral rinses are available that contain antifungal, antihistamine, antibiotic, steroid, and coating agents. Non-healing ulcers should be biopsied for malignancy.

2. **Tonsillopharyngitis** is usually viral; bacterial infection (typically group A β-hemolytic streptococci) is seen in approximately 40% of children and 10% adults. Antibiotic treatment is reserved for rapid test (or culture) positive cases. Treatment is penicillin (β-hemolytic streptococci are generally not resistant) or clindamycin for penicillin-allergic patients. Current guidelines recommend tonsillectomy (+/– adenoidectomy), in children with seven to eight or more episodes per year, or five episodes per year for 2 years, or three episodes per year for 3 years. Tonsillectomy reduces frequency of episodes but may not eliminate tonsillopharyngitis.

3. **Peritonsillar abscess** (PTA) refers to purulence between the tonsil bed and capsule. It is characterized by fevers, severe throat pain, trismus, drooling, and a muffled "hot potato voice." Physical exam reveals a bulging, erythematous soft palate with uvular, and tonsillar deviation. Treatment is needle aspiration or I&D, and antibiotics.

4. **Retropharyngeal abscess** occurs primarily in children younger than 2 due to suppuration of retropharyngeal lymph nodes. Children present with irritability, fever, stiff neck, muffled speech, cervical lymphadenopathy, and posterior pharyngeal swelling. Contrast-enhanced CT delineates the extent of infection. Some patients may respond to IV antibiotics, otherwise oral intubation and transoral drainage is performed.

D. **Neoplasms**

1. **Benign**

    a. **Ameloblastoma** is a locally invasive tumor arising from odontogenic epithelium, most frequently occurring in the mandible. It often requires segmental mandibulectomy with reconstruction.

    b. Other neoplasms include papillomas and hemangiomas.

    c. Premalignant lesions include leukoplakia (white hyperkeratotic patches) and erythroplakia (velvet-red patches).

2. Malignant

    a. SCC is the most common neoplasm of the head and neck. Tobacco and alcohol abuse synergistically increase risk for SCC. Human papilloma virus (HPV; genotypes 16 and 18) infection is also a causative agent in a subset of SCC, particularly of the lingual and palatine tonsils, and is seen in younger patients, often without significant tobacco or alcohol use. SCC is also associated with chronic inflammation, chronic trauma (e.g., poorly-fitting dentures), betel-nut chewing, Plummer–Vinson syndrome, and sun exposure (for lip cancer). Work-up includes a thorough head-and-neck history and physical examination, contrast-enhanced CT, biopsy, and possibly positron emission tomography (PET) and MRI. Operative endoscopic biopsies are done to assess extent of the tumor, detect synchronous primaries, and provide tissue for pathologic analysis. Staging follows the TNM (primary Tumor, regional Nodal metastases, distant Metastasis) site-specific guidelines from the American Joint Committee on Cancer (AJCC). Treatment involves a multidisciplinary team consisting of head and neck surgeons, radiation oncologists, medical oncologists, pathologists, and speech/swallowing therapists. Treatment of SCC is complex and based on location, nodal involvement, local invasion, and metastasis. Early stage (I–II) cancers are usually treated with single modality therapy (surgery or radiation), and advanced stage (III–IV) with combined modalities (surgery and chemoradiation).

    b. Oral cavity and oropharyngeal SCC may present with a metastatic neck mass, nonhealing painful oral ulcers, otalgia, odynophagia, dysphagia, trismus, and/or dysphonia. Typical treatment is surgical resection of primary, and neck dissection for clinically palpable nodes or in cases where risk of metastasis exceeds 20%. Postoperative radiation is indicated for high-risk tumors: advanced T-stage, perineural invasion, close/positive margins, multiple malignant lymph nodes, and/or lymph node extracapsular extension. Chemotherapy may be added to radiation for extracapsular spread and positive margins. Lingual and palatine tonsil SCC associated with HPV infection is more responsive to therapy, with improved survival (*Laryngoscope.* 2010;120(9):1756–1772). Emerging approaches such as transoral laser microsurgery provide good oncologic and functional outcome. Primary chemoradiation may be used for large oropharyngeal cancers (in which resection would cause significant morbidity), with goal of protecting speech and swallowing function; however, chemoradiotherapy itself usually causes significant swallowing dysfunction.

    c. Other oral cavity and oropharyngeal cancers include minor salivary gland carcinomas, verrucous carcinoma, lymphoma, mucosal melanoma, and Kaposi's sarcoma.

E. **Obstructive sleep apnea (OSA)** is dysfunctional respiration during sleep due to upper airway obstruction. Symptoms of OSA in children often include behavioral, learning, and growth problems, whereas OSA in adults is usually manifest by excessive daytime sleepiness. Untreated OSA can lead to pulmonary hypertension and cor pulmonale. The most common cause of OSA in children is adenotonsillar hypertrophy, whereas in adults it is obesity. Overnight polysomnography is the gold standard for diagnosing OSA. Adenotonsillectomy is first-line treatment in children, improving polysomnography parameters and quality of life (*Laryngoscope.* 2007;117(10):1844–1854). In adults, OSA is usually successfully treated with continuous positive airway pressure (CPAP). Surgery (uvulopalatopharyngoplasty, tongue base reduction, maxillomandibular advancement, or tracheostomy) is reserved for refractory cases.

F. Trauma

1. **Mandible fractures** (MFs) occur most commonly at the angle and parasymphysis, as well as at the condylar neck. Fractures present with dental malocclusion, halitosis, and pain with crepitus while chewing or on manipulation. Panorex radiographs are usually sufficient to diagnose MF and visualize postreduction; however, high-resolution maxillofacial CT may be more sensitive. Imaging modality is usually influenced by surgeon preference. Minimally displaced fractures can be treated by closed reduction and external fixation (mandibulomaxillary fixation, or "wiring the jaw shut"), for 4 weeks. Open reduction and internal fixation with lag screws and/or plates are used for treating displaced or comminuted fractures. Fixation within 3 days has been shown to result in more favorable outcomes (*Laryngoscope.* 2005;115:769). Complications of MF include wound infection, malocclusion, nonunion, tooth loss, temporomandibular joint ankylosis, and paresthesias.

IV. THE SALIVARY GLANDS

A. Anatomy and physiology

1. There are three pairs of major salivary glands (parotid, submandibular, and sublingual) and many minor salivary glands in the mucosa of the oral cavity, oropharynx, and nasopharynx. These produce 1 to 1.5 L of saliva per day, which provides lubrication during mastication, inhibits bacterial growth, and contains digestive enzymes.

2. The largest salivary gland, the **parotid gland,** lies over the masseter muscle, and is the predominant producer of saliva during mastication, secreting serous saliva. The parotid duct (Stensen's duct) exits the buccal mucosa opposite the second maxillary molar. The facial nerve (CN VII) travels through the parotid gland, artificially dividing the gland into superficial and deep lobes. The **submandibular gland** is inferomedial to the mandible, and produces a mixture of mucinous and serous saliva. The submandibular duct (Wharton's duct) empties into the floor of the mouth just lateral to the lingual frenulum. The **sublingual gland** lies beneath the floor of the mouth mucosa, and secretes mucinous saliva.

B. **Inflammatory diseases**

1. **Acute sialadenitis** usually involves the parotid gland, presenting as a tender, indurated preauricular swelling, often with purulence expressible from Stensen's duct. It occurs from retrograde bacterial contamination from the oral cavity (usually *S. aureus* and oral anaerobes) due to stasis of inspissated saliva or stones. Postoperative, dehydrated, diabetic, and/or immunocompromised patients are particularly susceptible. Contrast-enhanced CT may be performed to evaluate for abscess or mass. Treatment is hydration, warm compresses, massage, antibiotics, and sialogogues (stimulants of saliva flow, such as lemon wedges).

2. **Sialolithiasis** (ductal calculi) most frequently affects the submandibular glands, causing transient swelling and pain when eating, and is diagnosed by palpation or radiography. Ductal stones are removed transorally using probing instruments, via open excision, or minimally invasively via sialoendoscopy. Symptomatic parenchymal calculi are treated with surgical removal of the gland.

3. **Chronic sialadenitis** is caused by stones or duct stenosis, and can result in gland hypertrophy and fibrosis. Those with significant pain can undergo resection of the gland.

4. **Viral infections** that can cause salivary gland inflammation include HIV (lymphoepithelial hyperplasia) and paramyxovirus (mumps, causing acute parotitis).

5. Noninfectious inflammatory systemic diseases such as Sjogren's disease and autoimmune disorders may cause bilateral parotid swelling due to lymphoid infiltration.

C. **Neoplasms.** Up to 80% of salivary gland neoplasms occur in the parotid gland, and of these 75% are benign. Half of submandibular neoplasms are malignant; the proportion of sublingual and minor salivary gland malignancies is even higher. The treatment of benign and malignant neoplasm is excision; however FNAB (US-guided if necessary) during the work-up is useful for surgical planning and patient counseling—to determine extent of resection, management of the facial nerve, and treatment of neck nodes. Other work-up includes CT and/or MRI. A history of skin cancer should be elicited, as scalp and facial skin cancer (e.g., SCC and melanoma) can metastasize to the parotid gland.

1. **Benign.** The most common neoplasm is **pleomorphic adenoma,** followed by **Warthin's tumor.** These tumors grow slowly, are painless, and usually occur in the parotid gland. Facial weakness is rare. Warthin's tumors may be bilateral and are associated with cigarette smoking. Treatment is excision with a cuff of normal parotid tissue, sometimes necessitating superficial parotidectomy, with facial nerve preservation. Both tumor types have a propensity for local recurrence.

2. **Malignancy** is suspected when pain, facial nerve paresis, fixation, and cervical lymphadenopathy are present. The most common malignancy is **mucoepidermoid carcinoma,** followed by **adenoid cystic carcinoma.** Other types include acinic cell carcinoma, adenocarcinoma, carcinoma ex-pleomorphic adenoma, and primary SCC. Treatment is

parotidectomy, with facial nerve sacrifice if involved in tumor, possible neck dissection, and possible adjuvant radiation therapy.

D. Trauma. Cheek lacerations can involve the parotid parenchyma, Stensen's duct, and branches of the facial nerve. Loss of facial function mandates exploration and epineural repair of the nerve if proximal (posterior) to a vertical line drawn at the lateral canthus. Injury to the parotid duct requires repair of the duct over a stent.

V. THE LARYNX

A. Anatomy and physiology

1. The larynx is divided into the **supraglottis** (which includes the epi-glottis, arytenoid cartilages, false vocal cords/folds, and ventricles), the **glottis** (true vocal cords/folds), and **subglottis** (from the true vocal cords inferiorly to the cricoid cartilage). The thyroid and cricoid carti-lages and the hyoid bone provide rigid support for the larynx.

2. The **superior laryngeal nerve** supplies sensory innervation to the sup-raglottic mucosa and motor innervation to the cricothyroid muscle. The **recurrent laryngeal nerve** provides sensory innervation to the remain-ing laryngeal mucosa and motor innervation to the intrinsic laryngeal muscles. Both are derived from the vagus nerve (CN X).

3. The larynx is a critical part of the aerodigestive tract for airway protec-tion, deglutition, and phonation. Laryngeal elevation, glottic closure, and retroflexion of the epiglottis help to prevent aspiration during swallowing. Coughing occurs when the expiratory muscles contract to increase subglottic pressure against a closed glottis; the glottis then sud-denly opens, resulting in a rapid outflow of air and expulsion of mucus from the airway.

4. Laryngeal or tracheobronchial obstruction results in **stridor.** Inspira-tory stridor is usually from supraglottic obstruction. Biphasic stridor is caused by glottic or proximal tracheal obstruction. Expiratory stridor results from obstruction of the distal trachea or bronchi.

B. Congenital disorders

1. **Laryngomalacia** is the most common congenital disorder. Infants present with inspiratory stridor, typically exacerbated by feeding or cry-ing. The etiology is likely neuromuscular hypotonia causing inspiratory supraglottic collapse. Awake flexible fiberoptic laryngoscopy demon-strates prolapse of the arytenoid mucosa into the airway on inspiration, shortened aryepiglottic folds, and often an omega-shaped epiglottis. Symptoms often worsen for the first 9 months of life and then improve, with 75% of patients asymptomatic by 18 months of age. Endoscopic supraglottoplasty is indicated for difficulty feeding and failure to thrive, apnea, cyanosis, or cardiopulmonary sequelae.

2. **Vocal cord paralysis** is the second most common laryngeal abnor-mality in the newborn, causing inspiratory or biphasic stridor (bilat-eral cord paralysis), aspiration, and weak cry. Etiologies include birth

trauma, neurologic disease (e.g., Arnold–Chiari malformation), and iatrogenic (e.g., patent ductus arteriosus ligation); it is often idiopathic. Diagnosis is made by awake flexible laryngoscopy. Work-up includes brain MRI and modified barium swallow (to evaluate for aspiration). Most noniatrogenic unilateral paralysis resolves spontaneously within the first year of life. Alternative feeding routes (nasogastric or gastrostomy tube) and speech therapy is utilized until then. Bilateral cord paralysis often requires tracheotomy.

3. **Subglottic stenosis** can cause inspiratory or biphasic stridor. Congenital stenosis is due to abnormally formed cricoid cartilage. Acquired stenosis is usually the sequelae of intubation. Mild stenosis often presents during upper respiratory infection (URI), resulting in croup-like symptoms. In less than 50% stenosis, patients often improve as they grow. Otherwise, surgical laryngotracheal reconstruction or cricotracheal resection may be necessary.

4. Other congenital laryngeal abnormalities include laryngeal atresia, webs, cysts, laryngeal clefts, and hemangiomas.

C. **Infectious/inflammatory disorders**

1. **Viral croup,** or viral laryngotracheitis, is glottic and subglottic inflammation usually from parainfluenza virus. It most frequently occurs in children younger than three, in the winter. Diagnosis is clinical— patients have a prodromal URI, followed by a barking cough, hoarseness, and inspiratory stridor. Lateral airway X-ray may show the "steeple sign" from subglottic edema. Treatment includes humidified air, glucocorticoids for moderate to severe croup, racemic epinephrine, and heliox. Recurrent croup should undergo rigid laryngoscopy and bronchoscopy after resolution to evaluate for underlying anatomic anomalies.

2. **Epiglottitis** is rare (due to *H. influenzae* type B vaccination), but a medical emergency. The presentation is acute (hours) with high fever, muffled voice, drooling, dyspnea, inspiratory stridor, and sitting upright. Treatment is urgent airway management and IV antibiotics.

3. **Acute laryngitis** is inflammation of the laryngeal mucosa and vocal cords resulting in hoarseness. Most cases occur in adults and are of viral origin. It is usually self-limited and treated by hydration and voice rest. Adult smokers with persistent hoarseness should undergo fiberoptic laryngoscopy to evaluate for lesions concerning for malignancy.

4. **Laryngopharyngeal reflux (LPR)** is characterized by hoarseness, cervical dysphagia, globus sensation, sore throat, cough, and chronic throat clearing, caused by retrograde movement of gastric contents. It is the most common cause of chronic laryngitis. In infants, it exacerbates laryngomalacia. Patients often do not have the heartburn/esophagitis associated with gastroesophageal reflux disease (GERD), and ancillary studies diagnostic of GERD may be inconclusive in LPR. Fiberoptic laryngoscopy primarily demonstrates laryngeal edema, but also can show erythema and thickening of the posterior glottic mucosa. Treatment is diet and behavioral modifications, as well as high-dose

proton-pump inhibitors (PPI). Treatment with twice-daily PPI for at least 3 months significantly improves symptoms and laryngeal appearance (*Otolaryngol Head Neck Surg.* 2008;139(3):414–420).

5. Other inflammatory lesions that affect the larynx include sulcus vocalis, contact ulcers, vocal cord nodules, granulomas, and smoker's laryngitis.

D. **Neuromuscular disorders**

1. **Vocal cord paralysis** occurs from recurrent laryngeal nerve injury, often due to surgery, neoplasm, or trauma to the neck or thorax. Recognized iatrogenic injuries should be repaired by primary epineural anastomosis or cable grafting. Patient with no history of surgery should undergo CT scan and/or MRI of the neck and chest. Unilateral paralysis may cause dysphonia and aspiration, depending on vocal cord position. Treatment consists of speech therapy and observation, as recovery often occurs over several months. Temporary vocal cord medialization via injection helps prevent aspiration and improve voice during nerve recovery, lasting up to 6 months. If significant problems persist, thyroplasty and laryngeal reinnervation are other surgical options. Bilateral paralysis can cause stridor from airway obstruction and is treated with arytenoidectomy, cordectomy, or tracheostomy.

2. **Chronic aspiration** is caused by loss of the protective functions of the larynx due to impaired motor activity or sensory loss. Aspiration can result in bronchopulmonary infection and airway obstruction. Patients may have coughing or choking during swallowing, or silent aspiration, which may present with sequelae such as fever and productive cough. Etiology includes cerebral compromise (stroke, brainstem neoplasm, traumatic brain injury), degenerative neurologic diseases (Parkinson disease, amyotrophic lateral sclerosis, multiple sclerosis), neuromuscular disorders (myasthenia gravis, muscular dystrophies), vagal or recurrent laryngeal nerve palsy, anatomic abnormalities (Zenker's diverticulum), and alteration of the larynx (cancer resection or radiation). Work-up includes chest X-ray and modified barium swallow study or functional endoscopic evaluation of swallowing (FEES) by speech therapy. Physical therapy with a speech therapist corrects many cases. Refractory cases may be treated with nasogastric or gastrostomy tube feedings or parenteral nutrition. Surgical treatments include tracheostomy, vocal cord medialization, and laryngectomy.

3. **Spasmodic dysphonia (laryngeal dystonia)** is laryngeal motion disorder with unclear pathophysiology. It is treated with botulinum toxin injections into the laryngeal musculature.

E. **Neoplasm**

1. **Benign**

a. **Recurrent respiratory papillomatosis (RRP)** is the most common laryngeal neoplasm in children. Bulky papillomas, caused by HPV 6 and 11, arise on the larynx and tracheobronchial tree, causing hoarseness and airway obstruction. The mode of transmission is unclear, but thought to be vertical transmission during delivery from genital HPV infection. Treatment is repeated excision (with laser or microdebrider). Lesions usually recur. Malignant transformation to SCC can occur, but is rare.

2. **Malignant.** More than 90% of laryngeal malignancies are SCC (see Section III.D.2 for discussion of SCC). In the United States, glottic cancer is the most prevalent, followed by supraglottic cancer; subglottic cancer is rare. Presenting symptoms include dysphonia, odynophagia, dysphagia, otalgia, dyspnea, stridor, hemoptysis, and neck mass. Early stage (I or II) tumors are treated with surgery or primary radiotherapy. Advanced stage (III or IV) are treated with combination of surgery, radiotherapy, or chemoradiation. The oncologic gold standard is total laryngectomy. Organ-preservation treatments such as partial laryngectomy or primary chemoradiation offer good oncologic and functional outcomes, although the latter results in severe late toxicities in about 40%. Transoral laser microsurgery further reduces morbidity of partial laryngectomy compared with open partial procedures. Neck dissection is performed for supraglottic malignancies as rate of metastasis exceeds 20%. Glottic cancer has a low metastatic rate due to paucity of glottic lymphatics.

F. **Trauma**

1. Blunt or penetrating laryngeal trauma requires rapid airway assessment and management, often requiring intubation or awake tracheostomy. Work-up involves fiberoptic laryngoscopy, CT, and operative endoscopy. Laryngeal hematomas and small lacerations are managed conservatively with airway observation and humidified air. Displaced fractures and laryngeal instability require urgent tracheostomy followed by open reduction and internal fixation.

VI. THE NECK

A. **Anatomy and physiology**

1. The **anterior triangle** is defined by the body of the mandible superiorly, the anterior border of the sternocleidomastoid muscle laterally, and the midline anteriorly. It further divides into the submental, submandibular, carotid, and muscular spaces. The anterior triangle contains the carotid artery, internal jugular vein, nerves (CNs IX–XII and ansa cervicalis), larynx, trachea, pharynx, esophagus, submandibular, thyroid, and parathyroid glands, and strap muscles. The posterior triangle is bounded by the sternocleidomastoid muscle, the clavicle, and the trapezius muscle. It contains the spinal accessory nerve (CN XI), cervical and brachial plexuses, and thyrocervical trunk arising from the subclavian vessels.

2. The **cervical fascia** provides planes for passage of infection, hemorrhage, and surgical dissection. The superficial cervical fascia lies just beneath the skin. The deep cervical fascia has three layers: the superficial (or investing) layer, which is just deep to the platysma muscle and invests the sternocleidomastoid and trapezius muscles; the middle

(or visceral) layer, which envelops the thyroid gland, trachea, and esophagus; and the internal (or prevertebral) layer, which surrounds the deep neck musculature and cervical vertebrae.

3. The neck has an extensive **lymphatic system,** which is divided into six levels. Level I contains the submental and submandibular lymph nodes, level II through IV parallel the jugular vein, level V is the nodes of the posterior triangle, and level VI is the central compartment medial to the carotid artery. The retropharyngeal, suboccipital, and postauricular nodes are also distinct groups.

B. A **neck mass** is a common presenting complaint in which methodical work-up is important. History must focus on duration, progression, location, and associated symptoms (pain, URI symptoms, fevers, weight loss, dysphagia, voice changes, otalgia), past medical history, and social history (tobacco and alcohol use, travel history, animal exposures, sick contacts). Differential diagnosis is most strongly influenced by age. Neck masses in adults (particularly >40 years) are *presumed malignant until proven otherwise.* In contrast, neck masses in children are usually inflammatory; congenital etiology is less common and neoplasm is rare.

1. **Adult neck masses.** A neck mass that has not resolved after several weeks needs further evaluation. Eighty percent of adult neck masses are neoplastic, most commonly metastatic SCC from an aerodigestive primary. A complete head and neck exam, with inspection of all mucosal and cutaneous sites, including indirect or fiberoptic laryngoscopy reveals a primary source in most cases. Work-up includes contrast-enhanced CT or MRI and, of paramount importance, fine needle aspiration biopsy (FNAB). PET is also important; however, because of low specificity, it should be ordered only once the patient is thoroughly evaluated by an experienced head and neck surgeon. If FNAB is negative, it should be repeated; ultrasound (US) guidance markedly improves yield. Unless lymphoma is suspected, core and excisional biopsies are avoided. Open/excisional biopsy of cervical metastatic SCC is not recommended since it is associated with increased risk of distant metastases and late locoregional recurrence. If excisional biopsy is deemed necessary, for example, when lymphoma or other unusual diagnosis is found on FNA, intraoperative frozen histologic analysis should be done and, if diagnostic of SCC, followed immediately by comprehensive neck dissection. Lymphoma requires fresh tissue processing.

2. **Pediatric neck masses.** Children often have palpable hyperplastic lymph nodes; however, persistent masses larger than 2 cm should be investigated. Initial work-up is US, as this spares children radiation exposure, IV contrast, and sedation involved in CT and MRI. CT should be reserved for deep neck space infections, such as retropharyngeal abscesses. Additional studies include WBC with differential and specific serologic tests for infectious etiologies.

C. **Congenital neck masses** are often cystic and may swell during a URI. The acute infection should be treated with antibiotics. I&D should be avoided, as it increases the difficulty of future excision (done when the inflammation has subsided). If necessary, needle aspiration may be performed for decompression. A cystic mass in adults should undergo FNAB as tonsillar SCC and papillary thyroid carcinoma can manifest as a cystic neck masses.

1. **Branchial cleft anomalies** comprise up to a third of congenital masses. The persistence of embryologic pharyngobranchial ducts can result in cysts, sinuses, or fistulae. The most common anomaly is of the second branchial cleft, which presents as a nontender, fluctuant mass anterior to the sternocleidomastoid muscle, with a deep tract that travels between the internal and external carotid arteries to the tonsillar fossa. Much less common are first branchial cleft anomalies, which present near the angle of the mandible or around the ear and may be associated with the facial nerve and ear canal. Third branchial cleft anomalies are rare; they present as a lower neck mass with tracts that end in the thyrohyoid membrane or pyriform sinus.

2. **Thyroglossal duct cysts** also make up a third of congenital neck masses. They arise from the failure of the thyroglossal duct to obliterate after the embryologic descent of the thyroid from the foramen cecum at the base of tongue to the low anterior neck. Patients present with a midline neck mass that moves vertically with swallowing and tongue protrusion, as the cyst tract is closely involved with the hyoid bone. Definitive treatment is the Sistrunk procedure, involving resection of the cyst, its tract, and the central portion of the hyoid bone, which reduces recurrence. Preoperative thyroid US ensures the cyst is not the sole functioning thyroid tissue. Transformation into papillary thyroid carcinoma may rarely occur.

3. A **hemangioma** presents as a reddish-bluish compressible mass in infancy that may have a bruit on auscultation, and increases in size with crying or straining. Cervical hemangiomas may be associated with subglottic, gastrointestinal, and spine vascular malformations. Hemangiomas typically grow rapidly during the first year of life, followed by slow involution at 18 to 24 months. Ninety percent resolve without need for treatment. Treatment is indicated for airway compromise, ulceration, dysphagia, thrombocytopenia, and cardiac failure. Recently, propranolol has been found to be an effective treatment (*N Engl J Med.* 2008;358(24):2649–2651; *Laryngoscope.* 2010;120(4):676–681). Steroids, laser therapy, and surgical resection are also other options.

4. **Lymphatic malformations** are soft, doughy, compressible lesions that may swell with URI. CT or MRI is done to evaluate extent. Treatment is indicated for cosmesis or symptomatic relief. Complete excision is difficult because of its infiltrative nature; debulking may be effective. Alternative treatments involve sclerotherapy.

5. Other congenital masses include laryngocele, dermoid cyst, teratoma, plunging ranula, and thymic cyst.

D. **Infectious/inflammatory disorders**

1. **Reactive lymphadenopathy** is commonly associated with viral URI, and is self-limited.

2. **Suppurative bacterial lymphadenitis** is common in children, usually from *S. aureus* or group A streptococcal infections. Treatment is IV antibiotics, with I&D for poor response.

3. **Acute mononucleosis,** caused by EBV infection, is a frequent etiology of cervical lymphadenopathy in young adults. It is associated with fevers, tonsillitis, and hepatosplenomegaly. Diagnosis is via monospot and/or EBV titers. Treatment is supportive.

4. **Deep neck space infections. Infections** can spread easily into potential spaces along the fascial planes of the neck. Etiology is most frequently dental infection, and also tonsillitis, trauma, or suppurative lymph nodes. Pathogens include streptococcal, staphylococcal, and oral anaerobic bacteria. Neck abscesses present with fevers, acute neck swelling, induration, redness, and tenderness. Dysphagia, odynophagia, and stridor/stertor may result from compression. Treatment is I&D and IV antibiotics. Ludwig's angina is cellulitis of the submandibular and submental spaces, causing retrusion of the tongue, a woody, firm floor of mouth, and potential for airway compromise. Treatment is airway control (intubation or tracheotomy) and IV antibiotics.

5. **Sialadenitis/sialolithiasis** (see Section IV.B).

6. Other infectious causes of lymphadenopathy include cat-scratch disease, atypical mycobacterial infection (subacute mass with violaceous overlying skin), and HIV (diffuse hyperplastic adenopathy).

7. Causes of noninfectious inflammatory lymphadenopathy include sarcoidosis, Kawasaki's disease, and Castleman syndrome. A low anterior midline mass may be thyroiditis.

E. **Neoplasm**

1. **Benign**

   a. **Paragangliomas** are vascular tumors arising from paraganglionic cells of the autonomic nervous system. These are classified as jugulotympanic, vagal, sinonasal, laryngeal, and carotid body (most common) tumors. Catecholamine production, more commonly associated with multiple or familial presentation, is rare (3%). Treatment is surgical excision with preoperative embolization.

   b. Other benign tumors include lipomas, schwannomas, infiltrative fibromatosis, neurofibromas (associated with neurofibromatosis type I), and salivary gland neoplasms (see Section IV.C).

2. **Malignant.** The most common malignant neck mass in adults is metastatic SCC, and in children, lymphoma. Location of the mass is suggestive of primary site, based on patterns of lymphatic drainage. Oral cavity cancers usually metastasize to the submandibular triangle. Lateral metastatic SCC at levels II and III typically arises from base of tongue, tonsil, or supraglottic larynx. Nasopharyngeal, scalp, and cutaneous tumors can metastasize to the posterior triangle. Central neck masses may be primary thyroid neoplasms. Papillary thyroid cancer can metastasize to any level of the neck. Masses in the supraclavicular fossa should elicit evaluation of the skin, trunk, lungs, and abdomen.

a. **SCC** of aerodigestive mucosa metastasizes to the neck at significant rates in oral cavity, nasopharynx, oropharynx, and supraglottic larynx primaries. (SCC is also discussed in Sections III and IV.) The neck is treated with lymphadenectomy, with possible adjuvant radiation and chemotherapy, often with combined modalities. Neck dissections are termed *therapeutic* for clinically palpable metastases or *elective* in the absence of clinical lymphadenopathy. *Radical* neck dissection includes resection of all lymph nodes, the sternocleidomastoid muscle, internal jugular vein, and spinal accessory nerve. *Modified radical* neck dissection reduces morbidity by sparing one or more of these structures. *Selective* neck dissection removes only nodal groups at greatest probability for containing metastases for a particular primary site.

   (1) A special diagnostic dilemma is cervical SCC with unknown primary. In addition to the above work-up and treatment, patients should undergo operative panendoscopy with biopsies of the nasopharynx, and palatine and/or lingual tonsillectomy, as these are the usual sites of origin. Up to 40% of ipsilateral tonsil tissue harbors malignancy. PET/CT may also detect a primary source.

b. **Thyroid carcinoma.** Palpable thyroid nodules occur in 5% of women and 1% of men. Incidental diagnosis on imaging can approach 30%. Most patients are asymptomatic, but some may have dysphagia, difficulty breathing, and hoarseness. Up to 20% of nodules are carcinoma. Ninety percent of thyroid carcinomas are differentiated; 85% of these are papillary carcinoma, 10% follicular, and 3% Hurthle cell. Rare pathologies include lymphoma, metastatic lesions (e.g., melanoma), and anaplastic carcinoma. Initial work-up is TSH and US. Nodules larger than 1 cm, with suspicious US findings, or in high-risk patients, should undergo US-guided FNAB. Risk of malignancy is associated with older age, male sex, history of radiation exposure, and family history. Total thyroidectomy is indicated for FNAB diagnostic of malignancy, or in cases of suspected malignancy (suggestive FNAB or possibly high-risk patients). Lobectomy may be performed for indeterminate specimens (as incidence of malignancy is 20%), and low risk, small tumors. Tumor extent, completeness of resection, age, and metastases are important variables affecting prognosis. Up to 50% of patients with differentiated thyroid carcinoma have clinical cervical metastasis, particularly to the central compartment, although papillary carcinoma can metastasize to any level of the neck. For biopsy-positive lateral neck nodes, initial comprehensive *en-bloc* neck dissection is preferred to node-plucking. Postoperative radioactive iodine (in tumors able to take it up) is indicated for gross extrathyroidal extension, metastases, and large (>4 cm) tumors. Subsequent TSH suppression with levothyroxine reduces recurrence. Unresectable or anaplastic disease may undergo external beam radiation therapy. Chemotherapy is not routinely indicated.

   c. **Lymphoma.** The majority of head-and-neck lymphomas present in cervical lymph nodes, but also manifest in the tonsils, nasopharynx, paranasal sinuses, thyroid, and salivary glands. Up to 85% of Hodgkin's lymphoma presents as painless cervical lymphadenopathy, often with bulky, matted nodes. Patients are commonly pruritic, and may have "B symptoms" (fevers, night sweats, weight loss). Non-Hodgkin's lymphoma presents with similar symptoms, varying with subtype. Surgery aids in diagnosis and is not curative. FNAB provides cytologic material; tissue samples (obtained from core or excisional biopsy) are often required for architectural detail, flow cytometry, and immunophenotyping. Treatment is chemotherapy and radiation.

   d. **Adenocarcinoma** may be a primary salivary gland neoplasm or metastasis from the sinonasal airway, nasopharynx, salivary glands, and lungs.

F. **Trauma.** The neck is divided into three zones: zone I is the area inferior to the cricoid to 1 cm below the claviculomanubrial junction, zone II is between the cricoid and angle of mandible, and zone III is above the angle of mandible to the skull base.

   1. **Penetrating neck injuries** are wounds that violate the platysma. Zone II is most commonly involved. ABC's should be initially assessed, and ATLS protocol followed. Emergent surgical exploration is indicated for imminently life-threatening signs such as expanding hematoma, airway compromise, hemorrhage, and hemodynamic instability. In stable patients, mandatory versus selective neck exploration is controversial, as many explorations are negative. Management may be therefore directed by physical exam and adjunctive studies, with close observation for asymptomatic, hemodynamically stable patients (*J Oral Maxillofac Surg.* 2007;65(4):691–705). Signs such as bruits, crepitus, stridor, CN deficits, and hemoptysis support neck exploration. Vascular, laryngotracheal, and pharyngoesophageal injuries are evaluated by angiography (usually CT-angiography), water-soluble contrast esophagoscopy, and endoscopy. Hypopharyngeal injuries may be managed conservatively, with gastric decompression by nasogastric tube and IV antibiotics. Esophageal injuries close to the thorax can have considerable morbidity and mortality if gastric spillage occurs, and repair is recommended.

29 Plastic and Hand Surgery

Noopur Gangopadhyay and Thomas H. Tung

Plastic surgery has no defined anatomic territory and thus is a specialty built on principles and techniques rather than specific procedures. Plastic surgeons must optimize form and function in the setting of trauma, burns, congenital defects, postoncologic wounds, general reconstruction, and elective cosmetic improvements. Subspecialties include pediatrics, hand surgery, craniofacial surgery, peripheral nerve surgery, microsurgery, and aesthetic surgery. As the scope of plastic surgery is too broad to cover in one chapter, we discuss topics pertinent to the general surgeon that may be applied to a number of surgical situations.

BASIC TECHNIQUES AND PRINCIPLES

I. **THE RECONSTRUCTIVE LADDER.** When planning reconstruction, the simplest approach is often the best. The reconstructive ladder of soft-tissue coverage begins with consideration of the simplest approach (healing by secondary intention) and ends with the most complex (free tissue transfer), maximizing opportunities for success.

   A. Healing by **secondary intention** is the simplest approach but is not always feasible. Absolute contraindications include exposed vessels, nerves, tendons, viscera, or bone. Relative contraindications include a large or poorly vascularized wound with a prolonged (>3 weeks) anticipated period of healing and undesirable aesthetic consequences.

   B. **Primary closure** may provide the most aesthetically pleasing result, but excessive tension on the skin may cause displacement of neighboring structures (e.g., lower eyelid) or necrosis of the skin flaps.

   C. **Skin grafting** is the most common method of large-wound closure. Skin grafts require a healthy, uninfected bed and protection from shear forces to survive. Wound surfaces such as bare tendon, desiccated bone or cartilage, radiation-damaged tissue, or infected wounds will not support skin graft survival. Exposed vessels, nerves, or viscera are relative contraindications for skin grafting.

   D. **Local tissue transfers** of skin, fascia, and muscle may be used in regions with healthy tissue nearby. If the adjacent tissue cannot be adequately mobilized or the wound requires more bulk than is locally available, local flaps alone may not be adequate.

   E. **Distant tissue transfers** were the mainstay of difficult wound closure until the advent of free tissue transfer in the 1970s. This involves transferring healthy tissue into the wound bed while leaving it attached to its native blood supply. The vascular pedicle is divided in a subsequent procedure.

Disadvantages of this technique include multiple operations, prolonged wound healing, immobilization for at least 3 weeks, and a limited choice of donor sites.

F. **Free tissue transfer** is the most technically demanding approach to wound closure but has several advantages, including single-stage wound closure, a relatively wide variety of flaps tailored to specific wound closure needs, and, in many cases, an acceptable aesthetic outcome.

G. **Negative-pressure wound therapy** has altered wound management by decreasing bacterial load and accelerating granulation. Wounds that previously would not have healed by secondary intention may now be treated adequately with vacuum-assisted closure. Furthermore, it may convert a wound that would otherwise need adjacent or free tissue transfer into a wound that needs only split-thickness skin grafting. Contraindications include the presence of malignancy, ischemic wounds, or inadequately débrided tissue beds.

II. TYPES OF GRAFTS

A. Skin grafts

1. **Split-thickness grafts** consist of epidermis and a variable thickness of dermis. Thinner grafts (<0.016 in.) have a higher rate of engraftment, whereas thicker grafts, with a greater amount of dermis, are more durable and aesthetically acceptable. Common donor sites are the thigh, buttock, and scalp.

2. **Full-thickness grafts** include epidermis and a full layer of dermis. Common donor sites include groin and postauricular and supraclavicular sites, but the hypothenar eminence and instep of the foot can also be used. The donor site is usually closed primarily. These grafts are generally used in areas for which a high priority is placed on the aesthetic result (e.g., face and hand). Thinner grafts have greater secondary contraction and do not grow commensurate with the individual. They have fewer adnexal cells and therefore have variable pigment, less hair, and less sebum, with a proclivity toward dryness and contractures. Full-thickness grafts, with more dermis and the requisite adnexal structures, exhibit less contraction and better cosmesis.

3. Grafts can be meshed in **expansion ratios** from 1.5:1 to 6:1. Meshing a graft allows coverage of a wider area using the same-size donor site and decreases the risk of seroma accumulating under the graft without a method of drainage. The interstices are covered within 1 week by advancing keratinocytes. However, because the entire area is not covered by dermis, meshed grafts are less durable, and the meshing pattern remains after healing, making them inappropriate for aesthetically important areas, such as the face.

4. **Graft healing.** Initial metabolism is supported by **imbibition** or diffusion of nutrients from the wound bed. Revascularization occurs between days 3 and 5 by ingrowth of recipient vessels into the graft (inosculation). Therefore, for a graft to take, the bed must be well vascularized and free of infection, and the site must be immobilized for a

minimum of 3 to 5 days. Prevention of shear forces is important during this period of inosculation. Although bare bone and tendon do not engraft, periosteum and peritenon can support skin grafts, especially if they are first left to form a layer of granulation tissue. Graft failures are most often the result of hematoma, seroma, or shear force prohibiting diffusion and vascular ingrowth.

B. **Tendon grafts** are used to replace or augment tendons. Preferred donor sites are palmaris longus and plantaris tendons.

C. **Bone grafts** are used for repair of bony defects. Iliac bone is used for donor cancellous bone, and ribs or outer table of cranium are used for donor cortical bone.

D. **Cartilage grafts** are used to restore the contour of the ear, nose, and eyelid. Preferred donor sites include costal cartilage, concha of ear, and nasal septum.

E. **Nerve grafts** are used to repair damaged nerves when primary repair is not feasible. Preferred donor sites include the sural nerve and lateral or medial antebrachial cutaneous nerves. Allogeneic nerve grafting has been described using a short course of immunosuppression (*Exp Neurol.* 2010;223(1):77–85).

F. **Dermal or dermal-fat grafts** are used for contour restoration. Preferred donor sites include back, buttock, and groin. The long-term survival of grafted fat is variable but is generally unreliable.

III. **TYPES OF FLAPS.** A flap is any tissue that is transferred to another site with an intact blood supply.

A. **Classification based on blood supply**

1. **Random cutaneous flaps** have a blood supply from the dermal and subdermal plexus without a single dominant artery. They generally have a limited length-to-width ratio (usually 3:1, although this varies by anatomic region (e.g., the face has a ratio of up to 5:1). These flaps are usually used locally to cover adjacent tissue defects but can be transferred to a distant site by use of a staged procedure. Depending on the size of the defect to be covered, moving a local tissue flap can create a donor defect, which may require skin grafting. All local flaps are comparatively easier to use with the loose skin of the elderly.

   a. **Flaps that rotate** around a pivot point include rotation flaps (Fig. 29-1) and transposition flaps (Fig. 29-2). Planning for shortening of the effective length through the arc of rotation is important when designing these flaps. More complex rotation flaps include bilobed flaps (Fig. 29-3) and rhomboid flaps (Fig. 29-4).

   b. **Advancement of skin** directly into a defect without rotation can be accomplished with a simple advancement, a V-Y advancement (Fig. 29-5), or a bipedicle advancement flap.

2. **Axial cutaneous flaps** contain a single dominant arteriovenous system. This results in a potentially greater length-to-width ratio.

   a. **Peninsular flaps** are those in which the skin and vessels are moved together as a unit.

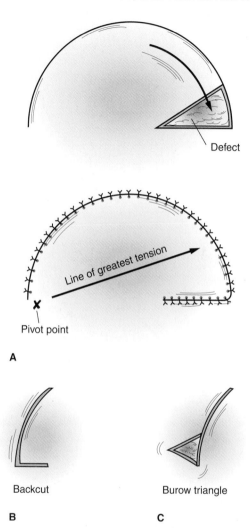

Figure 29-1. Rotation flap. **A:** The edge of the flap is four to five times the length of the base of the defect triangle. **B, C:** A backcut or Burow triangle can be useful if the flap is under tension.

    b. Island flaps are those in which the skin is divided from all surrounding tissue but maintained on an isolated, intact vascular pedicle.

    c. Free flaps are those in which the vascular pedicle is isolated and divided. The flap and its pedicle are then moved to a new location and microsurgically anastomosed to vessels at the recipient site, allowing for long-distance transfer of tissue.

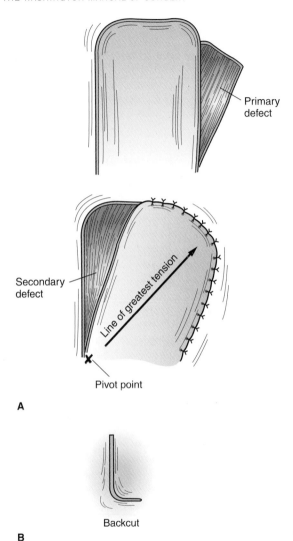

Figure 29-2. **A:** Transposition flap. The secondary defect is typically covered with a skin graft. **B:** A backcut may be added to reduce tension at the pivot point.

B. Classification based on tissue type

1. Cutaneous flaps include the skin and subcutaneous fat. These are generally random flaps because the axial blood supply is deep to the fat.

2. Fasciocutaneous flaps are axial flaps with a single dominant blood supply contained in the deep fascia along with the overlying fat and

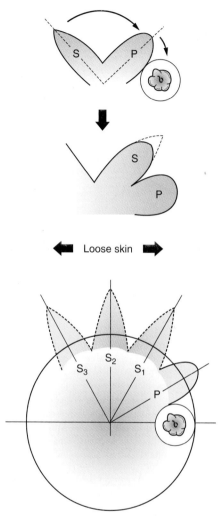

Loose skin

Figure 29-3. Bilobed flap. After the lesion is excised, the primary flap (P) is transposed into the initial defect, and the secondary flap (S) is moved to the site vacated by the primary flap. The bed of the secondary flap is then closed primarily. The primary flap is slightly narrower than the initial defect, whereas the secondary flap is half the width of the primary flap. To be effective, this must be planned in an area where loose skin surrounds the secondary flap site. Three choices for the secondary flap are shown (S_1, S_2, S_3).

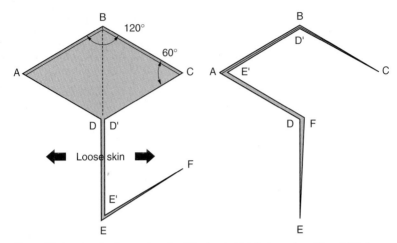

Figure 29-4. Rhomboid or Limberg flap. The rhomboid defect must have 60- and 120-degree angles so that the length of the short diagonal is the same as the length of the sides. The short diagonal is extended by its own length to point *E*. The line *EF* is parallel to *CD,* and they are equal in length. There are four possible Limberg flaps for any rhomboid defect; the flap should be planned in an area where loose skin is available to close the donor defect primarily.

skin. A wide variety of fasciocutaneous flaps have been described, but those commonly used include radial forearm, anterolateral thigh, lateral arm, and groin flaps. These flaps are often utilized for coverage of mobile structures such as tendons.

3. **Muscle flaps** use the specific axial blood supply of a muscle to provide well-vascularized soft-tissue bulk. These flaps can often be transferred with the overlying skin as a myocutaneous flap. Alternatively, they may be transferred without the overlying skin to fill a cavity or may be covered with a skin graft. Considerations include the pattern of circulation,

Figure 29-5. V-Y advancement. The skin to the sides of the V is advanced.

arc of rotation, donor-site contour, and donor-site functional defects. Commonly used muscle flaps include the latissimus dorsi, pectoralis major, rectus abdominis, gastrocnemius, soleus, gracilis, tensor fascia lata, trapezius, and gluteus maximus, but any muscle can potentially be transferred as a flap.

4. **A musculocutaneous flap** involves transfer of a muscle with the overlying skin and subcutaneous tissue. The skin is vascularized via myocutaneous or septocutaneous perforating vessels.

C. Specialized flaps

1. **Fascial flaps** are used when thin, well-vascularized coverage is needed (e.g., for coverage of ear cartilage or the dorsum of the hand or foot). The temporoparietal fascia flap is a classic example, but other fasciocutaneous flaps can be transferred without the overlying skin.

2. **Vascularized bone flaps** are designed to meet specific reconstructive needs, as dictated by loss of bony structure. Because they must be transferred to a specific location, they are generally transferred as free flaps. They may or may not include muscle and/or overlying skin. Commonly used bone flaps include free fibula, scapular spine, iliac (with overlying internal oblique muscle), and rib (with pectoralis major or intercostal muscle).

3. **Functional muscle** may be transferred with its accompanying dominant nerve. Common functional muscle transfers include transfer of gracilis for restoration of facial movement or latissimus for replacement of biceps function.

4. **Segmental muscle flaps** can be used when multiple sources provide blood supply to the muscle. A portion of the muscle is used as a flap, leaving behind a vascularized, innervated, functional muscle. This technique minimizes donor-site functional loss. Portions of the serratus anterior and gluteus maximus can be transferred as segmental flaps.

IV. **TISSUE EXPANSION** is a reconstructive technique that uses an inflatable silicone balloon to serially expand surrounding skin. This expansion adjacent to the wound provides donor tissue of similar color, texture, thickness, and sensation, with minimal scar formation and donor-site morbidity. The technique takes advantage of the skin's ability to accommodate a slowly enlarging mass beneath it by increasing its surface area. The idea is to create and develop donor tissue, harvest it, and leave the original donor site preserved.

A. **The advantages** include lower donor-site morbidity and the provision of donor tissue of similar quality to the recipient tissue. Tissue expansion is a simple and versatile technique that provides robust tissue.

B. **The disadvantages** are that it is a staged technique, there is a visible deformity during the period of expansion, it requires frequent visits for expansion, and there is a relatively high rate of complications, including infection and extrusion of the implant.

C. Technique

1. **Preoperative planning** involves assessing the defect size, locating matching tissue to be expanded, and deciding where final scars will be.

2. **Expander placement** is usually performed through an incision at the junction of the lesion and the area of proposed expansion. The length of the incision is controversial. Some authors propose one-third the length of the expander (it should be big enough to ensure full pocket creation). The filling port can be incorporated into the expander or placed in a separate pocket. In addition, the port may be externalized to minimize anxiety and pain during filling, especially in the pediatric population. Partially filling the expander on initial placement may reduce the duration of the expansion phase and reduce mechanical implant failure due to folding.

3. **The expansion phase** begins 2 to 3 weeks after expander placement. The expander is inflated weekly with saline, using sterile technique. The amount infused with each fill depends on patient comfort, skin tension, and blanching of overlying skin. A rough guide is 10% of expander volume per injection. The duration of the expansion phase can vary from 6 weeks to 3 months. Waiting 2 to 3 weeks after the desired volume is achieved allows the expanded skin to soften, decreasing the contraction at the time of flap transposition.

4. **Removal of expander** is straightforward. However, infection, exposure, or rupture may necessitate premature removal.

5. **The expanded tissue** is usually in the form of a random flap (rotation, advancement, or transposition). If more than one flap is necessary using expanded tissue, one must ensure that all flaps have adequate blood supply.

D. The **origin of the new tissue** is not completely understood. One potential source is new tissue created in response to the expansion process. Alternatively, tissue may derive from recruitment of adjacent tissues by stretching or creep and by stress relaxation. These possibilities are not mutually exclusive. Studies have shown that expansion gives rise to an increase in the thickness of the epidermis, a decrease in the thickness of the dermis, and atrophy of the underlying muscle and fat (*Plast Reconstr Surg.* 1994;93:1428–1432).

E. **Tissue expanders are indicated** for patients who cannot, or choose not to, tolerate the longer operative procedures or rehabilitation associated with more distant flaps. In areas where little suitable tissue is available (e.g., scalp), tissue expansion can be the aesthetically superior option. The patient must be motivated and understand the process. Common indications include burn alopecia, congenital nevi, male pattern baldness, and postmastectomy breast reconstruction.

F. **Relative contraindications** include malignancy or an open wound, active infection, and unwillingness to comply with multiple procedures. Similarly, tissue expanders cannot be placed under burned tissue, scar, skin graft, or a prior incision. In addition, tissue expanders are less effective in areas that will be irradiated because the skin in those areas thickens, scars, and contracts, minimizing the degree of expansion possible.

G. **Complications** include pain, seroma, hematoma (rates widely variable), infection (1% to 5%), exposure or extrusion (5% to 10%), and skin necrosis. Less common complications include striae, resorption of underlying bone, and neurapraxia.

ACUTE INJURIES

I. FACIAL TRAUMA

A. **Examination.** A facial trauma exam should assess soft tissue, nerve, and underlying bony injuries, with special attention to periorbital injuries. Note the location of lacerations, abrasions, and missing tissue that may indicate underlying facial nerve injuries or fractures. Gingival lacerations, malocclusion, and step-offs between the teeth may be a sign of a mandibular fractures. The examiner should query the five branches of the facial nerve (temporal, zygomatic, buccal, marginal mandibular, cervical) by having the patient raise the eyebrows, squeeze the eyelids shut, smile, and frown, noting any paresis or asymmetry. The facial skeleton should be palpated for bony step-offs indicating fractures. A brief ocular exam should include an assessment of gross vision, pupil reactivity, and intact extraocular movements. Examine the ears for lacerations as well as intact tympanic membranes. One should note gross deviations in the nose externally, and examine the nasal septum with an otoscope to assess for septal hematoma. Inspect the mouth for tongue or intraoral lacerations and avulsed teeth.

B. **Imaging.** A computed tomography (CT) scan with fine axial and coronal cuts through the facial bones is a fast, sensitive, and specific means of determining the location and orientation of facial fractures. A Panorex may be useful in the setting of isolated mandible fractures; however, many facial reconstructive surgeons want a more complete picture of the anatomy with a CT scan as a guide for the reconstructive plan, regardless of the diagnosis of a fracture on plain film.

C. **Other work-up.** Any patient with a mandible fracture should be examined for C-spine injuries. Mandible fractures are associated with a 10% incidence of C-spine fractures. Patients with bony orbital fractures should have an ophthalmology evaluation to rule out associated ocular injuries.

D. **Soft-tissue repair.** Facial lacerations should be copiously irrigated, and obviously devitalized tissue should be débrided. Local anesthesia may be used to block facial nerve branches prior to wound repair. The wound edges may be reapproximated using a few interrupted deep dermal 4-0 Vicryl or Monocryl sutures. A running superficial layer of 6-0 fast gut suture may be used to close the epidermis. If nonabsorbable sutures are used on the face, they should be removed within 5 days to prevent permanent suture marks.

   1. Eyelid lacerations should be referred to a facial reconstructive surgeon or ophthalmologist. Full-thickness lacerations of the ear and nose should be copiously irrigated, cartilage reapproximated with an absorbable monofilament suture [polydioxanone (PDS)], and skin closed in the usual manner. Full-thickness lip lacerations may be repaired using a three-layer closure. The orbicularis oris muscle should be reapproximated with 5-0 PDS, the mucosa repaired with 5-0 chromic, and the vermillion carefully aligned with 6-0 fast gut suture. Lacerations overlying fractures should be copiously irrigated and closed until definitive fracture fixation can be achieved.

E. **Fractures.** In the absence of airway compromise or ocular muscle entrapment, most facial and mandible fractures may be fixed electively within 1 to 2 weeks with good results and low incidence of infection. Patients with mandible fractures may be temporized until definitive fixation with a liquid diet, pain control, antibiotics covering intraoral flora (clindamycin), and good oral hygiene including Peridex (chlorhexidine) swish and spit three times per day. Indications for fracture reduction and fixation include alteration in dental occlusion with mandible and midface fractures, ocular muscle entrapment and inadequate eye support associated with orbital fractures, midface instability, and displaced fractures with obvious cosmetic implications. In light of these indications, not all facial fractures require operative intervention.

F. **Special situations**

1. Facial nerve injuries may be managed expectantly if they are medial to the lateral canthus because facial nerve branches, such as the buccal branch, are extensively arborized in these locations. Function will usually return without operative intervention, and it is exceedingly difficult to localize and repair nerve branches in this area. Facial nerve injuries should be referred to a facial plastic surgeon as soon as possible.

2. Eyelid lacerations situated in the medial aspect of the lid may be associated with injury to the lacrimal drainage system. These injuries should be evaluated by a facial plastic surgeon or ophthalmologist.

II. HAND TRAUMA

A. **Assessment** must be done using a systematic, efficient, and reproducible approach. Underestimating the extent of a hand injury or infection can lead to extended recovery or permanent loss of function.

1. **History.** The mechanism and timing of the injury, hand position at the time of injury, hand dominance, and patient occupation are all important to diagnosis and treatment.

2. **Examination**

   a. **Inspect the position of the patient's hand,** paying attention to the resting position of the digits and any swelling or asymmetry as compared with the contralateral hand.

   b. **Vascular assessment** requires observation of color, temperature, capillary refill, and the presence of pulses (palpable or Doppler) and an Allen test to verify the integrity of the palmar arches. Bleeding is controlled by application of direct pressure, not by blindly clamping tissue, because this often results in serious injury to surrounding structures. The use of tourniquets should be reserved for life-threatening exsanguinations only.

   c. **Motor examination,** both active and passive, involves testing for integrity of the tendons.

      (1) **Flexor digitorum profundus (FDP)** is tested by stabilizing the proximal interphalangeal (PIP) joint in extension and having the patient flex the distal interphalangeal (DIP) joint.

TABLE 29-1	Unambiguous Tests of Hand Nerve Function		
Test	**Radial Nerve**	**Median Nerve**	**Ulnar Nerve**
Sensory	Dorsum first web	Index fingertip	Little fingertip
Extrinsic motor	Extend wrist	FDP index	FDP small
Intrinsic motor	None	Abduct thumb perpendicular to palm	Cross long finger over index (interossei)

FDP, flexor digitorum profundus.

     (2) Flexor digitorum superficialis (FDS) is tested by stabilizing all other fingers in full extension and asking the patient to flex at the PIP joint.

     (3) Extensor tendons are tested by having the patient extend each finger individually. It should be noted that connections between neighboring tendons (juncturae tendinum) can mask a proximal laceration.

  d. Sensory testing includes gross examination of the ulnar, radial, and median nerves, which innervate the muscles in the hand and forearm (Table 29-1). It also involves careful examination of two-point discrimination on the palmar aspect of both the radial and ulnar sides of the digits and comparison with the uninjured hand. Normal two-point discrimination is 3 to 6 mm at the distal tip of the digit. The Strauch 10–10 test is also extremely useful in determining degrees of sensory loss. For this test, the patient rates his or her level of light touch sensation in an injured area on a scale of 1 to 10 as compared to the contralateral normal region, which is by definition a 10. This test should be used over multiple visits to chart the patient's subjective improvement with operative intervention or spontaneous reinnervation.

  e. Skeletal examination involves palpating for any tenderness, soft-tissue swelling, or deformity of the bones. Joint integrity is assessed by gently stressing the ligaments and noting any instability, crepitus, or pain. Any suspicion of fracture or dislocation requires radiographic examination.

3. Diagnostic radiology. Plain radiographs of the injured area, including the joint above and below if the physical examination warrants it, are indicated for almost all hand trauma and should be considered in cases of hand infections, particularly in penetrating trauma. Images should include true posteroanterior, lateral, and oblique views. If the injury involves the digits, separate laterals of the involved digits are indicated. The description of the fracture pattern should include the following: the bone(s) involved, open versus closed injury, simple versus comminuted, displaced versus nondisplaced, transverse versus oblique versus spiral, angulation or rotation of the distal fragment, and intra-articular versus extra-articular. Fractures in children involving the growth plate use the Salter–Harris classification.

B. **Fractures**

1. **Principles of management**

   a. **Reduction in displaced fractures** can be attempted in the emergency room using local or regional anesthesia. However, early referral to a hand surgeon is essential for all hand fractures.

   b. **Postreduction radiographs** should be done for all fractures after splinting or casting.

   c. **Splinting the fracture** in a position that does not impair function during the healing phase is imperative. A splint made of plaster or fiberglass, appropriately padded and with the hand in the "intrinsic-plus" position, may be used for almost all hand injuries. The intrinsic-plus position places ligamentous structures in their longest position and minimizes stiffness should immobilization be required to treat the fracture. The interphalangeal (IP) joints are in full extension, the metacarpophalangeal (MCP) joints are at 60 to 90 degrees of flexion, and the wrist is at 20 to 30 degrees of extension. Individual digits can be splinted without involving the remainder of the patient's hand and wrist. A thumb spica splint is used for fractures that involve the thumb proximal to the IP joint. The MCP joint is placed in extension, the thumb abducted, and the wrist placed in 20 to 30 degrees of extension. Even if operative management of the fracture is planned, a reduction with splinting in the emergency room is still appropriate for patient comfort and to prevent stiffness.

   d. **Early motion** is used whenever possible to minimize joint stiffness.

   e. **Operative intervention** is considered if closed treatment does not obtain or maintain reduction in the fracture. Contaminated open fractures, associated soft-tissue injuries, malalignment (uncorrected rotated, angulated, or shortened deformities of the digit), and articular incongruity of greater than 1 mm are also indications for operative management.

2. **Specific fractures**

   a. **Phalangeal fractures** require closed reduction and protective splinting for 4 to 6 weeks. Fractures of the distal phalanx may involve the nail bed apparatus or insertion of either the flexor or extensor mechanisms. Disruption of the extensor mechanism at the distal phalanx results in a mallet finger deformity and can be treated by splinting the DIP joint in extension. Other fractures of the distal phalanx can generally be treated with a protective splint. Stable middle and proximal phalanx fractures can be adequately treated by buddy-taping the injured finger to its neighbor. Certain fracture patterns are considered unstable and require operative fixation. As always, the goal of early motion is desirable.

   b. **Boxer's fracture** is a common transverse fracture at the distal portion of the ring or small finger metacarpal, with volar angulation of the distal fragment. Volar angulation of the distal fragment of up to 45 degrees is acceptable in the fifth metacarpal because of its mobility, although this may cause prominence of the metacarpal head in the palm. Less angulation is accepted in the fourth metacarpal, and angulation greater than 15 degrees is unacceptable in the second and third metacarpals. Any rotation or scissoring of the finger must be corrected by reduction as well. It is unnecessary to immobilize the MCP joint, and protection with a volar splint brought to the middle palmar crease is used until the patient sees a hand surgeon. Buddy taping of the ring and small fingers may also be helpful.

c. **Transverse metacarpal shaft fractures** are caused by axial loading and follow the same guidelines as neck fractures in terms of angulation. Oblique and spiral fractures result from torsional forces and are often best treated with operative fixation, protective splinting, and early range-of-motion exercises.

d. **Bennett's fracture** is an intra-articular fracture at the base of the first metacarpal resulting from an axial load to the thumb. The distal fragment subluxes radially through the pull of the abductor pollicis longus and angulates volarly through the force of the adductor pollicis. The ulnar fragment of the base is held fixed by the volar beak ligament. Closed reduction and splinting often yield a reduction that is anatomic; however, the deforming forces usually move the fragments out of reduction, and these fractures are best treated with open reduction and fixation. Less common is the "baby Bennett's," or "reverse Bennett's," fracture of the fifth metacarpal base; it is similar to the Bennett's fracture, with the extensor carpi ulnaris representing the deforming force on the distal fragment.

e. **Epiphyseal fractures in children** can lead to alterations in the growth of the involved bone. Treatment is similar to that for adults, although healing is often faster and immobilization is more acceptable because joint stiffness is less of a problem in children. Although reduction in the fracture is important, bone remodeling allows for angulation deformities of up to 20 or 30 degrees in the phalanges and metacarpals, provided it is in the anteroposterior plane. Rotatory deformity or radial or ulnar deviation should not be accepted because remodeling does not correct these deformities (*Emerg Med Clin North Am.* 2010;28:85–102).

f. **Open fractures** require adequate irrigation, reduction, and fixation as necessary, with prophylactic antibiotic coverage.

C. **Dislocations and ligament injuries**

1. **Principles of management**

   a. **Pre- and postreduction films** to confirm joint alignment and look for associated fractures.

   b. **Joint stability assessment** by stressing the periarticular structures and putting the joint through its range of motion. If instability is demonstrated, operative management should be considered. A stable joint is managed with protective splinting and early range-of-motion exercise.

   c. **Distal neurovascular assessment** before and after manipulation.

2. **Specific dislocations**
   a. **DIP joint and thumb IP joint dislocations** are uncommon injuries treated with closed reduction followed by splinting for 3 weeks, along with early protective range-of-motion exercise, provided tendon function is normal.
   b. **PIP joint injuries** are commonly known as "jammed fingers" and require careful assessment and follow-up to prevent long-term stiffness.
      (1) **Dislocations may be dorsal or volar.** Volar dislocations may be difficult to reduce owing to interposition of the extensor apparatus. Volar dislocations may also result in disruption of the extensor tendon central slip and need close observation to watch for boutonnière deformity. Postreduction care consists of early hand therapy, or operative management if unstable or irreducible.
      (2) **Volar plate injuries** are common and result from hyperextension of the PIP joint. The ligament can be strained, ruptured, or avulsed from the base of the middle phalanx with or without a bone fragment. If the injury is to soft tissue only or the avulsion represents less than 20% of the articular surface with a stable joint, treatment involves buddy-taping or extension block splinting with the joint in 30 degrees of extension and immediate range of motion. If the bone fragment represents 20% or more of the articular surface and there is associated instability, open reduction and internal fixation or volar plate arthroplasty are required.
   c. **Finger MCP joint dislocations** are usually caused by forced hyperextension and are most often seen in the index and small fingers. The dislocation is usually dorsal and is usually reducible in the emergency room. If the volar plate is interposed in the joint, however, open reduction may be required. If the joint is stable after reduction, it should be splinted for protection and early motion started. Occasionally, the metacarpal head can be held volarly by the flexor tendons on one side and the intrinsic muscles on the other side such that longitudinal traction tightens the "noose" around the head and prevents reduction. Open reduction is required in these situations.
   d. **Thumb MCP joint dislocations** are uncommon. The dislocation is usually dorsal and results from forced abduction. Closed reduction with a thumb spica splint and early range of motion is the usual treatment. The ulnar collateral ligament can be partially or completely torn and may avulse with a bone fragment from the proximal phalanx. If there is joint stability and congruity, the MCP joint is splinted for 4 weeks, leaving the IP joint free. If the joint is unstable or the proximal portion of the torn ulnar collateral ligament is displaced superficial to the adductor pollicis (Stener lesion), open reduction and internal fixation are required. **Of note, a stable lesion may be converted into an unstable (Stener) lesion by inexperienced examiners aggressively stressing the joint.**

e. **Carpometacarpal injuries** are usually dislocations with or without fractures. Ligamentous injuries are less common because the carpometacarpal articulation has less movement than do other joints. Dorsal dislocations with and without fractures result from a direct blow and are more common on the ulnar part of the hand. Closed reduction is frequently possible, but maintaining the reduction often requires percutaneous pinning of the joint.

D. Tendon injuries

1. **Flexor tendons** are frequently lacerated during everyday activities. Assessment and management of these injuries by a hand surgeon are critical to a satisfactory outcome.

   a. **The assessment** involves a careful history and examination; the examiner should look for a change in the resting tone of the digits (cascade) and assess the profundus and superficialis tendons independently. If flexion against resistance elicits pain, a partial laceration must be suspected. A careful neurovascular examination, including two-point discrimination, should be performed to evaluate for concomitant nerve or vessel injury.

   b. **Emergency room management** involves a thorough examination, then irrigation and closure of the wound, dorsal splinting with the patient's wrist in 20 to 30 degrees of flexion, the MCP joint at 90 degrees of flexion, and the IP joints in extension. Operative exploration and repair are appropriate for all lacerations through the tendon sheath because wrist and digit position at the time of injury can result in significant retraction with respect to skin laceration.

   c. **Anatomy: flexor tendon zones**
      (1) **Zone I:** at the DIP level, distal to the FDS insertion.
      (2) **Zone II:** from proximal A1 pulley (MCP joint) to FDS insertion.
      (3) **Zone III:** from distal transverse carpal ligament (carpal tunnel) to A1 pulley.
      (4) **Zone IV:** within the carpal tunnel.
      (5) **Zone V:** proximal to the carpal tunnel.

   d. **Technique of repair** involves a core, locking suture and an epitendinous repair. For tendon ruptures and lacerations within 1 cm of the FDP insertion, advancement and reinsertion of the tendon are used. A dorsal splint is applied, and a strict protected motion protocol directed by a hand therapist is started within 24 to 72 hours after repair and continues for 6 to 8 weeks.

2. **Extensor tendon injuries** result from lacerations and closed axial loading of the digits.

   a. **Zone I: over the DIP joint.** Mallet finger is a very common injury that results from forced flexion of the tip of the finger, with rupture of the terminal tendon from the distal phalanx. This leads to inability to extend the DIP. Mallet finger may be associated with an avulsion fracture or joint subluxation. These injuries are treated with splinting of the DIP joint in extension for 6 weeks. Operative management with reduction in the fracture and joint is only occasionally indicated. For open injuries, the tendon should be repaired and the joint pinned or splinted in extension for 6 weeks.

b. Zone II: over the middle phalanx. Lacerations in this zone should be repaired using a figure-of-eight or mattress technique. The DIP joint may be transfixed with a pin or splinted for 4 to 6 weeks.

c. Zone III: over the PIP joint. A complicated injury, since injury can occur to the central slip or lateral bands. A clue to central slip injury is the inability of the patient to initiate PIP extension from 90 degrees. If the patient is able to fully extend the PIP and DIP, at least one lateral band is intact. If untreated, these injuries can result in a boutonnière deformity (PIP flexion and DIP hyperextension). For open injuries, the tendon should be repaired and the joint transfixed with an oblique pin for 3 to 5 weeks. For tendon injuries associated with a fracture that is displaced, reduction and fixation of the fracture are advised. Protective splinting of the joint should be maintained for 6 weeks.

d. Zone IV: over the proximal phalanx. The lacerations are often partial because of the width of the tendon at this level. Splinting of the PIP joint in extension for 3 to 4 weeks is often sufficient for these injuries. Repair of the tendon is required if there is any extension lag of the IP joints.

e. Zone V: over the MCP joint. These injuries often occur as a result of a punching incident, particularly with a blow to the mouth. Contamination of the wound with oral flora can produce serious infection. Aggressive wound exploration must be undertaken to rule out joint space involvement because intra-articular infection can rapidly destroy cartilaginous surfaces. This often requires elongation of the laceration for adequate visualization and irrigation of the full extent of the wound. Only after the full extent of the wound has been evaluated and the wound aggressively cleansed can the tendon or tendons be repaired and the joint splinted in 20 to 30 degrees of flexion. The wrist is splinted in 30 degrees of extension. Dynamic splinting is useful to avoid adhesions and improve early motion.

f. Zone VI: over the dorsum of the metacarpals and carpus. Repair and splint as for zone V injuries.

g. Zone VII: at the level of the extensor retinaculum. Repair and splint as for zone V.

h. Zone VIII: proximal to the extensor retinaculum. Injury is often at the musculotendinous junction. Repair and splinting for 4 to 6 weeks are required.

E. Amputation

1. Replantation or revascularization

a. Indications for replantation include amputation of the thumb, amputation of multiple digits, amputation at the metacarpal, wrist, or forearm level, and amputation at any level in a child. More controversial indications include amputation of the proximal arm and amputation of a single digit distal to the FDS insertion.

  b. Contraindications for replantation include coexisting serious injuries or diseases that preclude a prolonged operative time, multiple levels of amputation, severe crush or degloving injury to the part, and prolonged ischemia time (12 hours for fingers and 6 hours for proximal limb amputations). Avulsion injury is a relative contraindication to replantation because of the extensive vascular and soft-tissue trauma.

  c. Preparation for transfer involves a moist dressing on the stump and splinting for comfort. The amputated part should be wrapped in saline-moistened gauze and placed in a clear plastic bag on a mixture of ice and water. The part should never be placed directly on ice or immersed in saline. Radiographs of the stump and the amputated part are essential and can be done at the transferring facility, provided that this does not significantly delay transfer to the microsurgery center. Intravenous fluids, prophylactic antibiotics, and tetanus toxoid, when indicated, should be begun immediately to facilitate prompt transfer to the appropriate facility for replantation. The sequence of repair involves identification of neurovascular structures and tendons and preparation of the bone for fixation. After providing bony stability, the arteries are repaired, followed by repair of the tendons and then veins, nerves, and skin. The postoperative care involves careful monitoring of the splinted part (temperature, color, and turgor) and adequate intravenous hydration in a warm environment.

2. **Revision amputation (nonreplantable amputation) management**
   a. Principles
      (1) **Complete assessment,** including radiographs.
      (2) **Antibiotics** when bone is involved or soft tissues are crushed or contaminated.
      (3) **Preservation of length.**
      (4) **Maintenance of sensation and motion.**
      (5) **Aesthetics.**
      (6) **Early motion.**
   b. Fingertip injuries are optimally managed using primary closure without shortening. If this is not possible, lateral V-Y advancement or volar advancement flaps or skin grafts can be used to obtain closure. An alternative for small wounds (with no vital structures exposed) is closure by secondary intention.
   c. More proximal amputations involve shortening and contouring the bone, shortening the tendons, and identifying digital nerves and allowing them to be transposed away from the skin closure.
   d. A protective dressing that allows joint motion is recommended, with early referral to a hand therapist for range-of-motion exercises and later desensitization of the tip of the stump.

F. **Infections**
   1. **Management.** Infections in the hand can progress rapidly via potential spaces and may risk the viability of tendons, bones, joints, and

neurovascular structures by creating increased pressure from pus and edema in closed spaces.

- **a. Surgical drainage** is required in most hand infections.
- **b. Antibiotic coverage** should be directed against common skin flora such as *Staphylococcus aureus, Staphylococcus epidermidis,* and *Streptococcus* species.
- **c. Gram stain and culture of wound.**
- **d. Splinting and elevation of the hand.**
- **e. Tetanus prophylaxis when appropriate.**

2. **Local infections**
   - **a. Paronychia** is a soft-tissue infection of the skin and soft tissue of the lateral nail fold; an **eponychial infection** may extend from this and involves the proximal nail fold. These localized infections often arise from self-inflicted trauma by nail biting or foreign-body penetration, such as a needle-stick. Treatment requires incision and drainage, with removal of the nail when the infection extends deep to the nail plate. Oral antibiotics are used if a cellulitis is present. **Chronic paronychia** is sometimes associated with underlying osteomyelitis or fungal organisms. Treatment may require marsupialization.
   - **b. Felon** is a localized infection involving the volar pulp of the digit and usually originates with a puncture wound, although a paronychial infection may spread volarly. Purulent fluid is usually under pressure in the fibrous septa of the tip of the digit. Management involves incision and drainage of the abscess (which can be between septa) and systemic antibiotics if there is an associated cellulitis. In general, the incision is located where the felon is "pointing"; however, it should be carefully planned to avoid sensitive scars and destabilization of the pulp of the finger. As with a paronychia, aggressive cleansing with soap and water after incision and drainage promotes drainage and avoids premature closing of the wound.
   - **c. Cellulitis** in the hand usually occurs secondary to a laceration, abrasion, or other soft-tissue injury. Management involves draining an abscess if present. The fluid should be sent for culture and sensitivity, and oral or intravenous antibiotics should be administered, depending on the severity. When associated with swelling of the digits and hand, splinting in the intrinsic-plus position and elevation prevent stiffness.
   - **d. After an animal bite,** the wound must be thoroughly irrigated to decrease the bacterial load and to remove any foreign body, such as a tooth. Bite wounds should be treated with oral antibiotics prophylactically and with intravenous antibiotics when an established infection is present. Although a greater percentage of cat bites become infected than do dog bites, the jaws of a dog are significantly more powerful and can inflict other injuries. The organisms most often involved from dog or cat bites include *Pasteurella multocida, S. aureus, Bacteroides* species, and *Streptococcus viridans.* Recommended oral antibiotics are amoxicillin–clavulanate or clindamycin with either ciprofloxacin or trimethoprim–sulfamethoxazole.

e. **Human bites** can involve particularly virulent organisms and frequently present in association with extensor tendon injuries or fractures sustained during physical altercations. An open wound, particularly if it overlies the dorsum of the hand with signs of infection or underlying soft-tissue or bony injuries, should prompt patient questioning about the source of the laceration. Typical organisms cultured from human bite wounds are *S. viridans, S. epidermidis,* and *S. aureus,* as well as anaerobic bacteria, such as *Eikenella corrodens* and *Bacteroides* species. Amoxicillin–clavulanate should be used prophylactically, and when signs of infection are present, treatment with ampicillin–sulbactam, cefoxitin, or clindamycin plus either ciprofloxacin or trimethoprim–sulfamethoxazole is recommended. Wound exploration should be carried out.

G. **Surgical emergencies**

1. **Compartment syndrome** is seen in the hand and forearm and results from increased pressure within an osseofascial space, leading to decreased perfusion pressure. If it is left untreated, muscle and nerve ischemia may progress to necrosis and fibrosis, causing Volkmann ischemic contracture.

   a. **Etiology.** Fractures that cause bleeding, crush and vascular injuries, circumferential burns, bleeding dyscrasias, reperfusion after ischemia, or tight dressings can lead to the syndrome.

   b. **Diagnosis** is based on a high index of suspicion, clinical examination, and symptoms of pain that are exacerbated with passive stretch of the compartment musculature, paresthesias, paralysis, or paresis of ischemic muscles. Pulselessness may occur and indicates a late finding (and is usually also a sign of irreversible damage) or the presence of major arterial occlusion rather than compartment syndrome. Measurement with a pressure monitor of a compartment pressure of greater than 30 mm Hg confirms diagnosis.

   c. **Treatment** of incipient compartment syndrome involves close observation and frequent examinations and should include removal of tight casts and dressings. Elevation of the extremity to, or slightly above, the level of the heart is recommended. Acute or suspected compartment syndrome requires urgent fasciotomies of the involved areas. Decompression within 6 hours of established compartment pressures is necessary to prevent irreversible muscle ischemia. Forearm fasciotomies involve volar, carpal tunnel, and dorsal compartments. Hand fasciotomies include dorsal incisions for interossei and adductor pollicis, thenar, and hypothenar compartments, as well as midaxial incisions of the digits (ulnar for the index, long, and ring fingers and radial for the thumb and small finger).

2. **Suppurative tenosynovitis** involves infection of the flexor tendon sheath, which is usually caused by a puncture wound to the volar aspect of the digit or palm.

   a. **Diagnosis: cardinal signs of Kanavel**
      (1) **Finger held in flexion.**
      (2) **Fusiform swelling of the finger.**

        (3) **Tenderness along the tendon sheath.**

        (4) **Pain on passive extension.**

    b. **Management** involves urgent incision and drainage in the operating room, with placement of an irrigating catheter in the sheath for continuous irrigation with saline. Irrigation is maintained for 24 to 48 hours. Intravenous antibiotics are administered. Frequent reassessment to verify resolution is critical to avoiding ischemic injury to the tendon secondary to the contained infection.

3. **Palmar abscess** is usually associated with a puncture wound. The fascia divides the palm into thenar, midpalmar, and hypothenar spaces; each involved space must be incised and drained. As with other infections, splinting, elevation, and intravenous antibiotics are required.

4. **Necrotizing infections** threaten both limb and life. The incidence of invasive group A streptococcal infection is on the rise (*N Engl J Med.* 1996;335:547) and can occur after surgery or trauma. Aggressive surgical débridement, high-dose penicillin, and supportive management are the mainstays of treatment. Additional therapy with gentamicin or clindamycin provides antibacterial synergy and blocks production of bacterial toxins. Immune globulin and hyperbaric oxygen are adjuvant therapies.

5. **High-pressure injection injuries** result from grease or paint injected at up to 10,000 lb/in^2. Although the external wounds are often small and unassuming, deep-tissue injury can be severe. Injury to the tissue is the result of both direct physical damage and chemical toxicity, and it leads to edema, thrombosis, and subsequent infection. Management involves urgent, thorough débridement, irrigation, decompression, systemic antibiotics, and splinting, with frequent reassessments and repeat débridement in 24 hours as required. When a digit has sustained significant injection, amputation may be required.

SPECIFIC PROBLEMS IN RECONSTRUCTIVE PLASTIC SURGERY

I. PERIPHERAL NERVE

A. **Clinical assessment** of neuropathy requires evaluation of both motor and sensory function as well as electrodiagnostic evaluation of nerve conduction and muscle innervation.

1. **Standard classification schemes** are available for classification of motor nerve function (Table 29-2). In addition, specific testing of moving or static two-point discrimination, vibration and pressure thresholds, or grip strength may be appropriate.

2. **Diagnostic studies** for quantification of nerve dysfunction include nerve conduction studies (NCSs) and electromyography (EMG). An NCS characterizes the conduction of large-diameter, myelinated nerves, and normal values may be present despite partial nerve injury. NCSs are useful in determining the degree of nerve dysfunction, the presence of segmental demyelination or axonal degeneration, the site

TABLE 29-2	Classification of Motor Function
Grade	Motor Function
M0	No contraction
M1	Perceptible contraction in proximal muscles
M2	Perceptible contraction in proximal and distal muscles
M3	All important muscles powerful enough to act against gravity
M4	Muscles act against strong resistance; some independent movement possible
M5	Normal strength and function

Adapted from SE Mackinnon, AL Dellon. *Surgery of the Peripheral Nerve.* New York: Thieme; 1988:118.

of injury, and whether the injury is unifocal, multifocal, or diffuse. EMG samples the action potentials from muscle fibers and can detect individual motor unit potentials, which may indicate early reinnervation and fibrillations, which represent denervation owing to axonal degeneration.

B. **Acute nerve injury** results from transection, crush, or compression and represents the loss of nerve function distal to the area of injury. Axons are myelinated by Schwann cells and organized into fascicles surrounded by the perineurium. The fascicles are bundled into nerves by the epineurium. The prognosis of injury to a peripheral nerve is dictated by which structures are disrupted. It is important to recognize in the acute setting that an injured nerve may be responsive to stimuli distally for 48 to 72 hours after transection. The severity of nerve injury has been organized into a grading scheme (Table 29-3). Operative repair is indicated for fourth-through sixth-degree injury.

1. **The technique of nerve repair** affects the eventual degree of recovery. Several basic concepts are used to optimize outcome.
   a. **Microsurgical technique** should be used, including magnification and microsurgical instruments and sutures. When conditions allow, a **primary repair** should be performed. The repair should be tension free.
   b. Positioning a limb or digit in extreme flexion or extension to facilitate an end-to-end repair is discouraged because of the joint and ligamentous problems that result. If a tension-free repair cannot be achieved in **neutral position,** transposing the nerve or placing an interposition nerve graft should be used.

TABLE 29-3	Classification of Nerve Injuries		
Sunderland[a]	Seddon[b]	Structure Injured	Prognosis
First degree	Neurapraxia	Schwann cell (demyelination)	Complete recovery within 12 wk
Second degree	Axonotmesis	Axon (Wallerian degeneration)	Complete recovery regeneration 1 mm/d
Third degree		Endoneurium	Incomplete recovery
Fourth degree		Perineurium	No recovery
Fifth degree	Neurotmesis	Epineurium	No recovery
Sixth degree		Mixed injury, neuroma incontinuity[c]	Unpredictable recovery

[a]Sunderland S. A classification of peripheral nerve injuries producing loss of function. *Brain.* 1951;74:491.
[b]Seddon HJ. Three types of nerve injury. *Brain.* 1943;66:237.
[c]Mackinnon SE. New direction in peripheral nerve surgery. *Ann Plast Surg.* 1989;22(3):257–273.

    c. An **epineural repair** is typically performed, but a grouped fascicular repair should be performed whenever the internal topography of the nerve is segregated into motor, sensory, or regional components.

    d. **Postoperative motor and sensory reeducation** will help to optimize outcome.

2. **Indications** for peripheral nerve repair include partial or complete transection or in-continuity conduction block. These represent fourth- to sixth-degree nerve injuries and can be difficult to distinguish from lesser grades of injury based on clinical examination alone. This is true because all grades of injury can lead to complete loss of function. Some guidelines for surgical intervention are listed in the following sections.

    a. **Nerves inadvertently divided** during operation are fifth-degree injuries and should be repaired immediately.

    b. **Closed-nerve injuries that localize near an anatomically restrictive site** (e.g., the ulnar nerve at the elbow or the common peroneal nerve at the knee) can result in neurologic deficit secondary to conduction block from edema and compression. If no recovery occurs within 3 weeks, management includes surgical decompression at that site. Iatrogenic nerve deficit from positioning during long operative procedures is managed similarly.

c. **Closed-nerve injury from blunt trauma or traction** is usually a first-, second-, or third-degree injury, and full recovery can be expected in most cases. Patients are closely followed for signs of recovery, including an advancing Tinel sign, indicating regenerating axons. Baseline NCS and EMG are obtained at 6 weeks. If there is no evidence of return of function at 3 months, repeat studies are obtained. If there is no improvement, the nerve is explored and repaired.

d. **Nerve deficit after sharp trauma** (e.g., a stab wound) usually is the result of partial or complete transection, and the nerve should be explored and repaired urgently.

e. **Loss of nerve function after gunshot or open blunt trauma** is usually the result of first- or second-degree injury, and recovery can be expected in most cases. These cases are usually treated as for closed injuries. If the nerve is visible or the wound is explored for other reasons (e.g., vascular repair), the nerve is explored. If the nerve is in continuity, it is managed as for a closed injury. If the nerve is not in continuity, it is usually best to tag the ends of the nerve for ease of identification and delay definitive repair until the zone of injury to the nerve is clearer (generally by 3 weeks).

f. **Nerve deficit from compartment syndrome** is treated by emergent fasciotomy. If decompressed early (within 6 hours), there is usually a rapid return of function.

g. **Decompression of injured nerves** (e.g., ulnar nerve transposition or carpal tunnel release) at sites distal to trauma can be useful to avoid retardation of nerve regeneration across these areas. Multiple sites of injury or compression can have additive effects, and for first- through third-degree injuries, decompression can improve outcome.

h. **Division of a sensory nerve** can lead to a painful neuroma as the regenerating axons grow into the surrounding soft tissue. If the resulting neural deficit results in loss of function or protective sensation, these nerves can be repaired. If not, the neuroma is excised and the cut end of the nerve is transposed proximally well away from the wound, preferably into a nearby muscular environment.

C. **Compression neuropathy** due to compression or repetitive trauma is a common clinical problem. Typically involved nerves include the median nerve at the wrist (carpal tunnel syndrome), the ulnar nerve at the elbow or wrist (cubital tunnel syndrome), the anterior or posterior interosseous nerves in the forearm, the brachial plexus at the thoracic outlet, the common peroneal nerve at the knee, and the posterior tibial nerve at the ankle (tarsal tunnel syndrome).

1. **Clinical assessment** of these conditions involves assessment of motor and sensory function, as well as provocative testing (reproducibility of symptoms with extrinsic nerve compression) and determination of whether the Tinel sign is present. EMG and NCS are appropriate if the clinical picture is unclear.

2. **Initial management** is usually physical therapy, behavior modification, and splinting to avoid repetitive compression. A period of at least 6 weeks of nonsurgical management without improvement is usually recommended before operation, although nerve compression at the cubital tunnel or thoracic outlet typically requires prolonged nonsurgical management. Operations generally involve **decompression** of the affected nerve or transposition to an unrestricted site.

II. SCALP, CALVARIAL, AND FOREHEAD RECONSTRUCTION

A. **Anatomy**

1. The **scalp** consists of five layers: skin, subcutaneous tissue, galea aponeurotica, loose areolar tissue, and pericranium.

2. **Five major paired vessels** provide the scalp with an ample collateral blood supply: the supraorbital, supratrochlear, superficial temporal, posterior auricular, and occipital arteries.

3. The **scalp receives sensory innervation** from the supraorbital and supratrochlear, branches of cranial nerve V1, the lesser occipital branch of C2 or C3, the greater auricular nerve, and the auriculotemporal branch of cranial nerve V3. The motor innervation to the frontalis derives from the frontal branch of the facial nerve.

B. **Scalp lacerations** are common concomitant sequelae of blunt trauma to the head. As such, there may be associated skull, cervical spine, or intracranial injuries. The rich blood supply to the scalp can produce significant blood loss, and hemostasis is important to prevent subgaleal hematoma. Radical débridement is seldom indicated, and primary repair is usually feasible. Repair of the galea generally helps to prevent hematoma formation.

C. **Partial-thickness scalp loss** from avulsion usually occurs at the subaponeurotic layer. Large avulsions may be skin grafted. One can expect 20% to 40% contraction of the skin graft over the first 6 to 8 months. After this has leveled off, the grafted area can be removed by serial excisions.

D. **Full-thickness scalp loss** can occur from trauma or tumor extirpation. The optimal treatment varies depending on the size of the defect.

1. **Small defects** (<3 cm) can often be closed primarily after undermining of flaps. Local flaps, either random or based on blood supply, can be raised. Scoring the galea in a grid pattern of perpendicular lines spaced 1 cm apart can allow for expansion of the flap. Rotation flaps should involve a margin of at least five times the length of the defect. Bipedicled flaps are well suited for coverage of the poles of the head (forehead, temporal areas, and nape of neck).

2. **Medium-sized defects** (3 to 10 cm) are usually covered with a scalp flap combined with skin grafting of the donor pericranium. Several specific flaps have been described for medium-sized defects, including the pinwheel flap, three-flap, and four-flap techniques described by Orticochea. All have been used with variable success.

3. **Large defects** (>10 cm) often require free tissue transfer. If the deficit is due to trauma, replant may be attempted. Because most of these

injuries are from industrial accidents involving avulsion, however, the injury to the arterial intima can extend far into the scalp. Latissimus dorsi or omental free flaps with split-thickness skin grafts are described for complete scalp loss.

E. Calvarial defects in the parietal or occipital regions require cranioplasty for protection. Temporal defects are somewhat protected by the temporalis muscle.

 1. **Alloplastic material** can be used to cover these defects, including titanium mesh, calcium hydroxyapatite, and methylmethacrylate. Polymethylmethacrylate (PMMA) is the most commonly employed because it is both durable and easy to use. However, it is exothermic on initial application and has reported infection rates of approximately 5% to 30%. Newer alloplastic materials are being developed to promote bony ingrowth and decrease the risk of infection. Some can be custom-made, based on three-dimensional reconstructions of computed tomographic scans.

 2. **Autogenous tissue** for cranioplasty includes split-rib grafts, split-table calvarial bone grafts, and bone paste. These are somewhat more difficult to use but have the advantage of a lower complication rate.

III. TRUNK

 A. **Breast**

 1. **Postmastectomy breast reconstruction** offers restoration of an important symbol of femininity and sexual intimacy. Reconstruction of breast symmetry can lead to a significant improvement in body image and is an important part of cancer rehabilitation for many women (*J Natl Cancer Inst.* 2000;92:1422–1429).

 a. **The aims of reconstruction** are to create symmetric breast mounds and, if desired, a new nipple-areola complex. The aesthetic goal is defined by the patient and includes a symmetric appearance both clothed and unclothed. Extensive preoperative consultation is required to allow women to explore their options. It should be emphasized that each approach to breast reconstruction usually requires at least two procedures and that the reconstructed breast will never completely replicate the original. Reconstruction can be accomplished with or without the use of an implant, and most procedures can be performed either immediately at the time of the mastectomy or in a delayed fashion.

 b. **Reconstruction of the breast mound** is accomplished with an implant in approximately two thirds of cases (*Probl Gen Surg.* 1996;13:75). In most cases, enough skin is removed with the mastectomy that the desired size of the breast precludes closure of the wound without tension. When this is the case, a tissue expander is placed and serial expansions performed until the desired size is reached (usually after 6 weeks of expansion). At this time, the expander is replaced with a permanent implant filled with silicone gel or saline. The advantages of this approach to reconstruction are minimal additional operative time, fewer additional scars, and a shorter recovery period. The disadvantages include the risks of permanent implants (rupture, infection) and the inability to reproduce certain natural contours.

c. **Autologous tissue** can be used to recreate a breast mound in the form of pedicled (rectus abdominis, latissimus dorsi) or free (rectus abdominis, gluteus maximus) myocutaneous flaps. The advantages include a more natural appearance for some patients, permanent reconstruction without the potential for future procedures to replace a ruptured implant, and fewer complications with subsequent radiation therapy. Disadvantages include a relatively long procedure, additional scars, and potential donor-site morbidity.

d. **Reconstruction of the nipple-areola complex** is chosen by approximately 50% of patients undergoing breast reconstruction. Methods include local flaps or nipple-sharing grafts to reconstruct a nipple-like prominence. Split-thickness skin grafting or tattooing can be used to recreate an areola.

e. **Procedures on the contralateral breast to improve symmetry** may be performed concomitantly or subsequently and include modification of an inframammary fold, removal of dog ears, liposuction of flaps, or reduction mammoplasty or mastopexy of the contralateral side. Symmetry procedures are almost always covered by insurance.

2. **Reduction mammoplasty** is performed for women with a variety of physical complaints and aberrations in body image.
   a. **Common symptoms** are listed as follows and are considered indications for reduction mammoplasty:
      (1) **Personal embarrassment and psychosocial problems.**
      (2) **Shoulder and back pain.**
      (3) **Grooving of the soft tissue of the shoulders by bra straps.**
      (4) **Chronic inframammary skin breakdown, rash, or infection (intertrigo).**
      (5) **Inability to engage in vigorous exercise.**
      (6) **Symptoms of brachial plexus compression (rare).**
   b. A variety of procedures are designed to **reduce breast size.** All of them move the nipple-areola complex superiorly on the chest wall. The nipple-areola complex is maintained on a pedicled blood supply when possible, but in certain instances (e.g., pedicle length >15 cm or a patient who smokes), tenuous blood supply to the nipple-areola complex may require a full-thickness graft. There are always scars resulting from the movement of the nipple and resection of excess skin, and the configuration of these scars varies by the procedure chosen.

B. **Chest wall reconstruction**
   1. **Before beginning chest wall reconstruction,** one must ensure complete resection of tumor and radiation-damaged or infected tissue.
   2. **Dead space** in the chest allows for potential empyema and may be obliterated. This space is best filled with pedicled muscle (latissimus dorsi, pectoralis major, serratus anterior, or rectus abdominis) or omental flaps.

3. **Skeletal stabilization** is required if more than four rib segments or 5 cm of chest wall are missing. This can be achieved using autologous (rib, dermis, or fascial grafts or bulky muscle flaps) or prosthetic (Prolene mesh, Gore-Tex, Marlex-methylmethacrylate sandwich) material.

4. **Optimal soft-tissue coverage** usually requires pedicled myocutaneous flaps but can be achieved with pedicled muscle or omentum covered with split-thickness skin graft. Rarely, free tissue transfer is required.

5. **Median sternotomy dehiscence** owing to infection occurs in 1% to 2% of cardiac procedures. Predisposing factors include bilateral internal mammary artery harvest, diabetes mellitus, obesity, and multiple operations. Closure requires removal of wires and débridement of all infected tissue, including bone and cartilage. Closure of the resultant dead space is usually accomplished by advancing or rotating the pectoralis major and/or rectus abdominis muscles. The rectus abdominis muscle cannot be used as a rotational flap if the ipsilateral internal mammary artery has been harvested. Pedicled omental flaps are reserved as alternatives in case of initial failure.

C. Abdominal wall reconstruction

1. **Reconstruction of full-thickness abdominal wall defects** includes recreation of a fascial barrier and skin coverage. Restoration of a functional muscle layer is also helpful in maintaining abdominal wall functionality.

2. **Complete absence of all layers of the anterior abdominal wall** is usually the result of direct trauma or infection, with or without intra-abdominal catastrophe. The open abdomen can be temporized by skin grafts placed directly on bowel serosa, omentum, or absorbable mesh through which granulation tissue has formed. This allows for resolution of intra-abdominal edema and maturation of adhesions but usually results in a large ventral hernia.

3. **Primary closure of fascial defects** represents the best approach and can be assisted by sliding myofascial advancement flaps. Lateral release of the external oblique fascia, or "component separation," is ideal for midline musculofascial defects greater than 3 cm in size. Using bilateral relaxing incisions and release, a total of 10, 18, and 6 to 10 cm of advancement may be obtained in the upper, middle, and lower thirds of the abdomen, respectively (*Plast Recon Surg.* 1990;86:519). The anterior sheath of one or both rectus muscles can be divided and turned over to provide additional fascia for closure. Synthetic mesh may be used when fascial defects cannot be primarily closed. Allo-Derm, freeze-dried cadaveric dermis devoid of antigenic cells, also may be utilized for large fascial defects. AlloDerm may also be preferred when infection is a concern because it is revascularized and more resistant to infection. However, it stretches with time and therefore synthetic mesh is preferred especially for extensive defects. Myofascial flaps are required when the existing fascia is insufficient for closure after advancement and there is insufficient skin for primary closure. The most frequently used flaps are the tensor fascia lata, rectus femoris,

and vastus lateralis with overlying fascia. These flaps are usually not useful for closing more distant defects of the upper abdomen.

4. **Skin coverage** is accomplished with split-thickness skin grafts, the cutaneous portion of a myocutaneous flap, or local tissue rearrangement (e.g., bipedicled flap and V-Y advancement flap). Because skin grafts cannot survive directly on synthetic mesh, a muscle flap may be required to provide an adequate bed for skin grafting.

D. **Pressure sores**
   1. The **etiology and staging criteria** are described in prior chapters.
   2. **Principles of nonoperative management** of pressure sores include (1) relief of pressure by positioning changes and appropriate cushioning; (2) bedside débridement of devitalized tissue; (3) optimization of the wound environment with aggressive wound care; (4) avoidance of maceration, trauma, friction, or shearing forces; and (5) reversal of underlying conditions that may predispose to ulcer development as well as optimizing nutritional status. This type of aggressive nonoperative management is often optimally coordinated by specially trained wound care nurses.
   3. **Operative management** with soft-tissue flap closure is only indicated for large, deep, or complicated ulcers and then only in patients who are able to care for their wounds. A high degree of cooperation from the patient and caregivers is essential because the recurrence of pressure sores at the same site or new sores at other sites after operation is high. This is especially true for individuals who have spinal cord injuries, whose rate of recurrence is 13% to 61% (*Am J Surg.* 2004;188:42–51). This is most likely the result of breakdown in the postoperative support and care systems in this population. Most surgeons, therefore, require demonstration of the patient's ability to care for wounds before embarking on operative closure. Flaps commonly used for closure of pressure ulcers around the pelvic girdle include gluteus maximus, tensor fascia lata, hamstring, or gracilis-based rotation or advancement flaps.

IV. **LOWER EXTREMITY.** Soft-tissue defects from trauma to the lower extremity are common. A multidisciplinary approach involving orthopedic, vascular, and plastic surgeons provides optimal care.

   A. Lower-extremity injuries are first assessed according to **advanced trauma life support guidelines.** The general sequence of priorities is as follows:
      1. The first priority is assessment for **concomitant life-threatening injuries and control of active bleeding.** Blood loss from open wounds is often underestimated, and patients must be adequately resuscitated.
      2. The **neurovascular status** is determined. If a nerve deficit is progressive during observation in the emergency room, it is likely the result of ischemia from arterial injury or compartment syndrome.
      3. **Bony continuity** is assessed by radiographs of all areas of suspected injury.

4. **Operative management** addresses bone stabilization followed by venous and arterial repair. Fasciotomies are indicated for compartment pressures greater than 30 mm Hg and by clinical suspicion from preoperative neurovascular examination. Fasciotomy must be performed within 6 hours to avoid ischemic contracture. Nonviable tissue is débrided, and an assessment is made about delayed or immediate soft-tissue coverage.

B. **Soft-tissue defects of the thigh** are usually closed by primary closure, skin grafts, or local flaps. The thick muscular layers ensure adequate local tissue for coverage of bone and vessels and adequate vascular supply to any fracture sites.

C. **Open tibial fractures** frequently involve degloving of the thin layer of soft tissue covering the anterior tibial surface. The distal tibia is a watershed zone, and fracture with loss of periosteum or soft tissue leads to increased rates of infection and nonunion.

1. Open tibial fractures are classified according to the scheme of **Gustilo** (Table 29-4).

2. **Gustilo types IIIb and IIIc** frequently require flap coverage of exposed bone.

   a. The **proximal third** of the tibia or knee can often be covered by a pedicled hemigastrocnemius flap.

TABLE 29-4	Gustilo Open Fracture Classification
Classification	**Characteristics**
I	Clean wound <1 cm long
II	Laceration >1 cm long with extensive soft-tissue damage
III	Extensive soft-tissue laceration, damage, or loss; open segmental fracture; or traumatic amputation
IIIa	Adequate periosteal cover of the bone despite extensive soft-tissue damage; high-energy trauma with small wound or crushing component
IIIb	Extensive soft-tissue loss with periosteal stripping and bone exposure requiring soft tissue flap closure; usually associated with massive contamination
IIIc	Vascular injury requiring repair

Adapted from RB Gustilo, JT Anderson. Prevention of infection in the treatment of one thousand and twenty-five open fractures of long bones: retrospective and prospective analysis. *J Bone Joint Surg Am.* 1976;58A:453.

    b. The **middle third** of the tibia is often covered by a pedicled hemi-soleus flap.

    c. **Large defects of the distal third** of the tibia generally require coverage by free muscle transfer.

D. Limb salvage reconstruction for neoplasm differs from that for trauma in that large segments of bone, nerve, or vessels may require replacement. **Skeletal replacement** can be accomplished using an endoprosthesis, allogeneic bone transplant, or vascularized free bone (fibula) transfer.

E. The foot is divided into regions for purposes of soft-tissue defects caused by trauma or ischemic, diabetic, or infectious ulceration. Optimal coverage of the plantar surface provides a durable, sensate platform.

    1. Small defects of the heel can be covered using the non–weight-bearing skin of the midsole. Larger defects require free muscle transfer and split-thickness skin grafting.

    2. The metatarsal heads are often successfully covered using plantar V-Y advancement and fillet of toe flaps. Multiple fillet of toe flaps or free muscle transfer may be required for large defects.

    3. For fitting of proper footwear, coverage of the dorsum of the foot must be thin. If peritenon is present, the dorsum can usually be covered with a skin graft. Small areas of exposed tendon may granulate, but larger areas require thin fascial free flaps (temporoparietal, parascapular, or radial forearm) covered by skin grafts.

30 Cardiac Surgery

Anson M. Lee and Ralph J. Damiano Jr.

This chapter focuses on providing background and practical information regarding the treatment of adult patients undergoing common cardiac operations, particularly coronary artery bypass grafting (CABG) and valve repair or replacement. It also discusses the surgical treatment of heart failure and arrhythmia.

I. ANATOMY

A. **Coronary arteries.** The left and right coronary arteries arise from within the sinuses of Valsalva just distal to the right and left coronary cusps of the aortic valve.

1. The **left main coronary artery** travels posterior toward the pulmonary artery, then divides into its main branches, the **left anterior descending artery (LAD)** and the **left circumflex artery (LCx).** The LAD runs in the interventricular groove and arborizes into **septal** and **diagonal** branches. The LCx runs in the posterior atrioventricular (AV) groove and gives off **obtuse marginal** branches. In 10% to 15% of patients, the LCx gives off the **posterior descending artery (PDA),** termed a **left dominant coronary circulation.**

2. The **right coronary artery (RCA)** descends in the anterior AV groove, where, in **right dominant coronary circulation** (80% to 85% of cases), it gives off the PDA. In addition, the RCA gives off **acute marginal** branches.

B. **Coronary veins.** There are three principal venous channels for coronary venous drainage.

1. The **coronary sinus** is located in the posterior AV groove and receives venous drainage mainly from the left ventricular system. Its main tributaries are the great, middle, and small cardiac veins.

2. **Thebesian veins** are small venous channels that drain directly into the cardiac chambers.

3. The **anterior cardiac veins** drain the right coronary system, ultimately into the right atrium.

C. **Valves.** The valves of the heart are critical to its pump function. Their proper functioning is essential for the maintenance of pressure gradients and antegrade flow through the heart chambers.

1. **AV valves.** The function of the AV valves is to prevent atrial regurgitation during ventricular contraction. These valves are fibrous and continuous with the **annuli fibrosi** at the base of the heart. Furthermore, the leaflets are joined at their commissures and are further secured by **chordae tendineae,** which attach the free leaflets to the intraventricular papillary muscles.

a. The **tricuspid valve** separates the right chambers and consists of a large anterior leaflet, a posterior leaflet, and a septal leaflet attached to the interventricular septum.

b. The **mitral (bicuspid) valve** separates the left chambers and consists of a large anterior (aortic) leaflet and a posterior (mural) leaflet.

2. **Semilunar valves.** The **pulmonary** and **aortic** valves are essentially identical, except that the coronary arteries arise just distal to the aortic valve. The valves consist of three cusps, and each cusp comprises two lunulae. The lunulae extend from the commissure and meet at the midpoint, a thickening known as the **nodulus of Arantius.** During diastole, the three nodules coapt, forming a seal. Just distal to the valves are gentle dilations of the ascending aorta, known as **sinuses of Valsalva.** These structures play an important role in the maintenance of sustained laminar blood flow.

II. PHYSIOLOGY

A. **Electrophysiology.** Like all neuromuscular tissue, the myocardium depends on efficient and predictable electrical activation. The myocardium has specialized tissue responsible for the rapid and orderly dispersal of myocardial electrical activation. The myocardial cells communicate through **gap junctions.**

1. The **sinoatrial (SA) node** is located at the junction of the anteromedial aspect of the superior vena cava and the right atrium. The **cardiac pacemaker** is determined by the cells that have the most frequent rate of spontaneous depolarization. In most instances, the pacemaker is at the SA node **(sinus rhythm),** which represents an area in the right atrium with the fastest **automaticity,** that is, spontaneous depolarization. In general, all myocardium demonstrates automaticity.

2. The **AV node** is located in the interatrial septum, on the ventricular side of the orifice of the coronary sinus. It is designed to protect the ventricle from high atrial rates. In the event of SA node dysfunction, the AV node can assume a pacemaker role because this specialized tissue often has the next highest rate of spontaneous depolarization.

3. The **bundle of His** originates in the AV node and descends through the membranous interventricular septum, just inferior to the septal cusp of the tricuspid valve. Also referred to as **Purkinje fibers,** it separates into the right and left branches at the junction of the membranous and muscular portions of the interventricular septum. In normal anatomy, this is the only electrical connection between the atria and the ventricles. The bundle of His functions to rapidly distribute the depolarization to the ventricular myocardium, starting with the ventricular septum; to the apex; then throughout the ventricle via the Purkinje fiber network.

B. **Mechanics.** The heart functions to convert electrical stimuli to chemical energy and eventually to mechanical energy. The mechanical forces are governed by the pressure, volume, and contractile state of the cardiac chambers. The determination of **rate, rhythm, preload, afterload,** and

contractility are critical to understanding effective cardiac mechanical function.

1. The **cardiac cycle** describes the relationship between the electrical status of myocardial membranes and the mechanical condition of the cardiac chambers. As the mitral valve opens, diastolic filling commences. Following atrial depolarization and contraction, the ventricle depolarizes and isovolumetric contraction begins [at **end-diastolic volume** (EDV)]. Once intraventricular pressure exceeds aortic pressure, the aortic valve opens and **ventricular ejection** occurs. As the aortic pressure overcomes ventricular pressure, the aortic valve closes. Isovolumetric relaxation commences until intraventricular pressure is lower than left atrial pressure, and the mitral valve opens.

2. **Preload** is defined as the EDV of the ventricle. It is practically measured by central venous pressure (CVP) or more accurately by **pulmonary capillary wedge pressure.**

3. **Afterload** is most widely defined as "resistance to ejection." It is more practically described as the **aortic pressure gradient** across the aortic valve.

4. **Starling's law** describes the relationship between EDV and contractility. As EDV is increased, ventricular contraction increases as the optimal sarcomere length is reached. However, once the optimal length is exceeded, contractility can decrease, as can be seen in pathologic states. This relationship is particularly important to optimize in right heart failure.

III. **PREOPERATIVE EVALUATION.** The preoperative evaluation of patients undergoing cardiac surgery is similar to the evaluation of patients undergoing any major operation. All patients should have a complete history and physical examination. Laboratory studies usually include a complete blood cell count; serum electrolytes, creatinine, and glucose levels; prothrombin (PT) and partial thromboplastin times (PTT); and urinalysis. An arterial blood gas measurement is indicated in patients with a history of chronic obstructive pulmonary disease, heavy tobacco abuse, or other pulmonary pathology. In general, 2 to 4 units of packed red blood cells should be available for use during the operation. For elective operations, this may be predonated autologous blood. A chest radiograph (posteroanterior and lateral) should be obtained to evaluate for calcification of the aorta and to examine for the presence of other intrathoracic pathology. In redo patients, a chest computed tomography (CT) scan is recommended to evaluate the proximity of the heart and aorta to the underside of the sternum. CT angiography also is helpful in determining the relationship of the previous bypass grafts to the sternum. The height and weight of the patient should be measured, and the body-surface area (in square meters) should be calculated.

A. Organ-specific evaluation

1. **Neurologic complications** after cardiac surgery can be devastating. Perioperative cerebrovascular accidents (CVA) occur in 4% of CABGs and up to 10% of triple valve cases (*Ann Thorac Surg.* 2003;75:472). CVA may result from aortic atherosclerotic or air emboli that are

loosened by cannulation, cross-clamping, or construction of proximal anastomoses. Postoperative arrhythmias such as atrial fibrillation (AF) are also a common cause of CVA following cardiac surgery. Underlying cerebrovascular disease in conjunction with alterations in cerebral blood flow patterns during cardiopulmonary bypass (CPB) may play a role in some patients. Patients with carotid bruits, known peripheral vascular disease, a history of transient ischemic attack, amaurosis fugax, or CVA should undergo noninvasive evaluation of the carotid arteries with Doppler ultrasonography before operation. Because of the strong association between carotid artery and left main coronary stenoses, patients with left main disease should undergo carotid Doppler examination preoperatively. In general, carotid stenoses greater than or equal to 80% are addressed by carotid endarterectomy or stenting before or in combination with the planned cardiac surgical procedure.

2. **Pulmonary disease,** particularly the obstructive form, occurs commonly in patients with cardiac pathology because cigarette smoking is a risk factor for both disease processes. A preoperative chest X-ray may demonstrate suspicious pulmonary pathology and can be used in combination with a preoperative arterial blood gas evaluation to identify patients who are at high risk for difficulty in being weaned from the ventilator postoperatively. Pulmonary function tests are indicated in high-risk patients. Smoking should be discontinued before operation, when possible.

3. **Peripheral vascular examination.** The presence and quality of arterial pulses in the radial, brachial, femoral, popliteal, dorsalis pedis, and posterior tibial arteries should be documented preoperatively as a baseline for comparison if postoperative arterial complications arise. Blood pressure (BP) should be measured in both arms to evaluate for subclavian artery stenosis. Significant subclavian artery stenosis may preclude the use of an internal thoracic (mammary) artery (ITA) as a conduit. A preoperative Allen test should also be performed to assess the palmar arch and the feasibility of using the radial artery for bypass conduit. For patients with varicosities of the saphenous veins or a history of vein stripping, preoperative vein mapping with ultrasonography can be done to assess the availability and quality of the saphenous vein conduit.

4. **Infection.** Operation should be delayed, if possible, in patients with systemic infection or sepsis and in those with cellulitis or soft-tissue infection at the site of planned incisions. Specific infections should be identified preoperatively and treated with appropriate antibiotic therapy. In patients who have fever or leukocytosis but require an immediate operation, cultures should be obtained from all potential sources (including central venous catheters), and broad-spectrum intravenous (IV) antibiotics should be administered preoperatively.

5. **Medications.** The cardiac surgery patient usually is taking a variety of preoperative medications. In general, nitrates and β-adrenergic blocking agents should be continued throughout the entire perioperative period (*Circulation.* 1991;84(5, Suppl):III236). Unless a specific contraindication exists, statins should be given to all patients because of their ability to reduce recurrent coronary artery disease (CAD) and

postoperative stroke rates (*Eur J Cardiothorac Surg.* 2006;30:300). If possible, antiplatelet agents (e.g., Plavix) are stopped before surgery to prevent hemorrhagic complications. Aspirin is continued in patients with acute coronary syndromes where the benefit of aspirin outweighs the risk of bleeding (*Eur J Cardiothorac Surg.* 2008;34:73). Digoxin and calcium channel blockers generally are discontinued at the time of operation and restarted only as needed in the postoperative period. For patients receiving heparin preoperatively for unstable angina, the heparin should not be discontinued before the operation because this may precipitate an acute coronary syndrome. For patients receiving warfarin preoperatively (including patients with mechanical valves), the warfarin should be discontinued several days before operation. Once the PT time [International Normalized Ratio (INR)] has normalized, anticoagulation can be accomplished using IV heparin.

B. **Cardiac testing**

1. The **electrocardiogram** (ECG) is an important tool diagnostic tool. It demonstrates the electrical activity of the cardiac cycle. Stress testing is used to detect CAD or to assess the functional significance of coronary lesions. The exercise ECG is used to evaluate patients who have symptoms suggestive of angina but no symptoms at rest. A positive test is the development of typical signs or symptoms of angina pectoris and/ or ECG changes (ST-segment changes or T-wave inversion).

2. A **pulmonary artery catheter (Swan–Ganz)** is often used in the perioperative setting; it is placed prior to the start of a cardiac procedure. The PA catheter allows for measurement of intravascular and intracardiac pressures, cardiac output, and mixed-venous oxygen saturation (see Table 30-1).

3. The use of **echocardiography** is essential in modern practice. The real-time assessment of chamber size, wall thickness, ventricular function, and valve appearance and motion are possible. It also is an invaluable aid in assessing the presence of intracardiac air prior to weaning from CPB. With the addition of Doppler imaging, blood flow characteristics can be determined. Both transthoracic and transesophageal echocardiography are widely available. Transesophageal imaging is particularly helpful intraoperatively.

4. **Thallium imaging** is used to identify ischemic myocardium. The thallium in the blood is taken up by cardiac myocytes in proportion to the regional blood flow. Decreased perfusion to a region of the myocardium during exertion with subsequent reperfusion suggests reversible myocardial ischemia, whereas the lack of reperfusion suggests irreversibly scarred, infarcted myocardium. In patients who cannot exercise, thallium imaging can be performed after administration of the coronary vasodilator dipyridamole or adenosine.

5. **Coronary arteriography** is used to document the presence and location of coronary artery stenoses. Separate injections are made of the right and left main coronary arteries. In general, the atherosclerotic process involves the proximal portions of the major coronary arteries,

TABLE 30-1	Normal Hemodynamic Parameters	
Parameter	Normal Value	Unit
Central venous pressure	2–8	mm Hg
Right ventricular pressure (syst/diast)	15–30/2–8	mm Hg
Pulmonary artery pressure (syst/diast)	15–30/4–12	mm Hg
Pulmonary capillary wedge pressure	2–15	mm Hg
Left ventricular pressure (syst/diast)	100–140/3–12	mm Hg
Cardiac output	3.5–5.5	L/min
Cardiac index	2–4	L/min/m^2 BSA
Stroke volume index	1	mL/kg
Pulmonary vascular resistance	20–130	dynes · sec/cm^5
Systemic vascular resistance	700–1,600	dynes · sec/cm^5
Mixed-venous oxygen saturation	65–75	Percent

BSA, body-surface area; diast, diastolic; syst, systolic.

particularly at or just beyond branch points. A 75% decrease in cross-sectional area (50% decrease in luminal diameter) is considered a significant stenosis. Indications for coronary arteriography include suspected CAD (e.g., positive stress test), preparation for coronary revascularization, typical or atypical clinical presentations with normal or borderline stress testing when a definitive diagnosis of CAD is needed, and planned cardiac surgery (e.g., valve surgery) in patients with risk factors for CAD. Concomitant ventriculography can be used for assessing left ventricular function.

6. **CT angiography** is a relatively new technique for the detection of CAD. Its main application is for evaluating chest pain in patients with typical symptoms of angina pectoris but with low-to-intermediate risk factors for CAD, as it has a very high negative predictive value (99%) but a low positive predictive value (48%) for detecting CAD in these patients (*J Am Coll Cardiol.* 2005;52:1724).

IV. MECHANICAL CARDIOPULMONARY SUPPORT AND OFF-PUMP CABG

A. **CPB,** first introduced in 1954 by Gibbon, allowed for the development of modern cardiac surgery. It is intended as a support system during surgery and requires systemic anticoagulation.

1. A **venous reservoir** stores blood volume and allows for the escape of bubbles prior to infusion. A **membrane oxygenator** is used to perform the gas exchange function. A **heat exchanger** is necessary to maintain hypothermia when needed and to assist with patient rewarming. The **arterial pump** is usually a roller pump and requires frequent calibration to ensure accurate flows. The **cannulae** and pump tubing are constructed of Silastic or latex, which remain supple when cold. A **left atrial vent** can be used to remove any blood that enters the left-side circulation.

2. **Myocardial protection** strategies are critical to a good outcome. Hyperkalemic perfusate (warm or cold) based on blood or crystalloid may be infused into the aortic root and coronary ostia (antegrade) or via the coronary sinus (retrograde).

3. During CPB, the perfusionist, working with the surgeon, can effectively control perfusion rate, temperature, hematocrit, pulmonary venous pressure, and glucose and arterial oxygen levels.

4. CPB is generally considered safe, but side effects do exist. Most notably, **postperfusion syndrome** is characterized by a diffuse, whole-body inflammatory reaction that can lead to multisystem organ dysfunction. It is believed that most patients experience some form of inflammatory reaction following CPB, but only a fraction develop this syndrome. Other factors contributing to poor CPB tolerance are length of support (e.g., >4 hours) and patient age.

B. **Extracorporeal membrane oxygenation (ECMO)** is primarily used in infants with severe cardiopulmonary failure but can be used in adults. It is not a practical long-term therapeutic modality but rather an intermediate-term (days to weeks) artificial heart and lung support system. Most commonly, it is used to allow patients to recover from reversible myocardial dysfunction, adult respiratory distress syndrome, or pulmonary insufficiency of various etiologies.

C. **Off-pump coronary bypass** is an alternative method of doing CABG. In recent years, this method has been promoted by some as a way to decrease morbidity associated with the use of CPB. This technique of doing bypass grafting on the beating heart while supporting the myocardium with stabilizers has shown a decrease in morbidity by some groups (*J Thorac Cardiovasc Surg.* 2003;125:797; *BMJ.* 2006;332:1365). However, it is more technically challenging than on-pump techniques, and long-term outcomes were similar in a multicenter, randomized trial comparing on- and off-pump CABG in low-risk patients (*JAMA.* 2007;297:701). Long-term patency rates were also similar in a recent long-term follow-up study of two randomized control trials (*J Thorac Cardiovasc Surg.* 2009;137:295). A large VA-based, multicenter trial demonstrated worse patency and mortality at 1-year follow-up for patients undergoing off-pump CABG (*NEJM.*

2009;361:1827). Patients at high risk (e.g., those with severe atheromatous aortic plaque or renal failure or the elderly) may benefit, especially when done by surgeons experienced with this technique.

V. DISEASE STATES AND THEIR TREATMENT

A. **CAD** is the leading cause of death in adults in North America. Risk factors for CAD include cigarette smoking, hypertension, diabetes mellitus, hyperlipidemia, male gender, obesity, advanced age, rheumatoid arthritis, and a family history of CAD. The clinical presentation of CAD is determined by the distribution of the atherosclerotic lesions, the severity of stenosis, the level of myocardial oxygen demand, and the relative acuity or chronicity of the oxygen supply–demand mismatch. The three most common presentations for patients with CAD are angina pectoris, myocardial infarction (MI), and chronic ischemic cardiomyopathy.

1. **Angina pectoris** is a symptom complex resulting from reversible myocardial ischemia without cellular necrosis. Patients typically complain of retrosternal chest pain or pressure that often radiates to the left shoulder and down the left arm or into the neck. Angina occurs during times of increased myocardial oxygen demand (e.g., exercise) and resolves with rest or the administration of nitrates. Unstable angina refers to chest pain that occurs at rest or episodes of pain that are increasing in frequency, duration, or severity. Silent myocardial ischemia occurs when there is ECG evidence of myocardial ischemia in the absence of any angina or angina-equivalent symptoms.

2. **Acute MI** results when there is a critical decrease or interruption of myocardial oxygen supply with irreversible muscle injury and cell death. The patient typically presents with protracted and severe chest pain, at times associated with nausea, diaphoresis, or shortness of breath. There are accompanying increases in the troponin isozyme, creatine kinase-MB isozyme, or serum lactate dehydrogenase. ECG changes include ST-segment elevation, T-wave inversions, and the development of new Q waves. Early and late sequelae of acute MI can include atrial or ventricular arrhythmias, heart failure, rupture of the interventricular septum or ventricular free wall, dysfunction or rupture of the papillary muscle(s) and new mitral regurgitation (MR), and the development of a ventricular aneurysm.

   a. **Arrhythmias** are common during the first 24 hours after acute MI. In addition to potentially fatal ventricular arrhythmias, patients can develop supraventricular tachycardia, AF, atrial flutter, heart block of any degree, or junctional rhythms.

   b. **Congestive heart failure (CHF)** may result when a large portion (usually >25%) of the left ventricular myocardium is infarcted. Cardiogenic shock and death often occur with loss of more than 40% of the left ventricular myocardium. The extent to which the patient's activity is limited can be graded according to the **New York Heart Association (NYHA) classification:** class I, no symptoms; class II, symptoms with heavy exertion; class III, symptoms with mild exertion; class IV, symptoms at rest. There is additional discussion of CHF in Section D.

c. **Rupture of the interventricular septum** occurs in approximately 2% of patients after MI (anterior wall in 60%, inferior wall in 40%) and leads to a **ventricular septal defect (VSD).** Septal perforation typically occurs when the myocardium is at its weakest, approximately 3 to 5 days after an acute MI, but it may develop 2 or more weeks later. An acute VSD is suggested by a new holosystolic murmur and an oxygen step-up from the right atrium to the pulmonary artery, as evaluated with a pulmonary artery catheter. This is determined by comparing the oxygen saturation of samples drawn simultaneously from the central venous port and the distal pulmonary artery port. A step-up of greater than 9% is generally held to be diagnostic of a left-to-right shunt. The diagnosis can be confirmed with echocardiography. More than 75% of patients survive the initial event and are candidates for urgent surgical repair of the VSD before they develop the sequelae of low-output syndrome (i.e., multiorgan system failure), which greatly increases the operative risk. An intra-aortic balloon pump (IABP) is indicated to support the failing circulation until surgical correction is possible. Ventricular free-wall rupture results in hemopericardium and cardiac tamponade, which often is fatal. For those patients who survive, emergent surgical repair is indicated.

d. **Acute MR** is caused by papillary muscle dysfunction or rupture after an infarction that has extended into the region of the papillary muscles (usually the posteroinferior wall). The failing circulation should be supported with an IABP or temporary mechanical support, if necessary, until emergent operation can be performed.

e. **Ventricular aneurysm,** a well-defined fibrous scar that replaces the normal myocardium, develops in 5% to 10% of individuals after acute MI. The majority of aneurysms develop at the anteroseptal aspect of the left ventricle after infarction in the distribution of the LAD coronary artery. Large dyskinetic left ventricular aneurysms can reduce the left ventricular ejection fraction (EF) substantially, resulting in signs and symptoms of CHF. These scars can also serve as the substrate for ischemic reentrant ventricular arrhythmias. In addition, the pooled blood that collects in the aneurysm can clot and shower emboli into the peripheral circulation.

3. **Chronic ischemic cardiomyopathy** can develop after several MIs. Diffuse myocardial injury results in diminishing ventricular function and, eventually, signs and symptoms of heart failure. This presentation is most common in patients with diffuse small-vessel disease (e.g., in patients with diabetes mellitus).

4. **Coronary revascularization** may be accomplished via percutaneous transluminal coronary angioplasty (PTCA) or CABG. Indications depend on the patient but generally include intractable symptoms and proximal coronary stenoses that place a significant portion of myocardium at risk.

a. **PTCA** is often used for focal symmetric stenoses in proximal coronary vessels. It is generally contraindicated if there is significant left main coronary disease, three-vessel disease, or complex obstructive lesions (*N Engl J Med.* 2005;352:2174). PTCA is associated with restenosis, which may be reduced with the concomitant placement of **drug-eluting stents (DESs),** which inhibit neointimal hyperplasia. DESs have been associated with improved outcomes but have not eliminated the problem of restenosis or the need for reintervention (*J Am Coll Cardiol.* 2007;49:616).

b. **CABG** is indicated for patients with documented atherosclerotic CAD in several settings: (1) patients with unstable angina for whom maximal medical therapy has failed; (2) patients with severe chronic stable angina who have multivessel disease or left main or proximal LAD stenoses; (3) patients with severe, reversible left ventricular dysfunction (documented by stress thallium scan or dobutamine echocardiography); (4) patients who develop coronary occlusive complications during PTCA or other endovascular interventions; (5) patients who develop life-threatening complications after acute MI, including VSD, ventricular free-wall rupture, and acute MR; and (6) patients with diabetes mellitus and multivessel disease (*J Am Coll Cardiol.* 2004;44:1146).

c. Compared with balloon angioplasty alone, the need for repeat revascularization has dramatically decreased for patients in whom a stent was placed, from 50% of angioplasty patients to approximately 20% of stented patients at 1 year (*Lancet.* 2002;360:965). More recent studies have shown the reintervention rate to be lower, from 5% to 7% depending on the type of stent used (*J Am Coll Cardiol.* 2007;49:616). This decrease has been due to improved delivery systems and the development of DES. For patients with hemodynamic instability or refractory angina after failed angioplasty, IABP support or percutaneous CPB may be helpful before an emergent operation can be performed.

d. **CABG** results in initial elimination of angina in more than 90% of patients. Perioperative mortality ranges from 1% to 2% in low-risk patients to more than 10% to 15% in high-risk patients. Graft patency after CABG is related to the bypass conduit used and the outflow vessel. In one study, the left internal thoracic artery patency at 5 years was 98%, at 10 years it was 95%, and at 15 years it was 88%. The right ITA patency at 5 years was 96%, at 10 years it was 81%, and at 15 years it was 65%. The radial artery patency at 1 year was 96%, and at 4 years it was 89% (*Ann Thor Surg.* 2004;77:93). At 10 years, it was 83% (*J Thorac Cardiovasc Surg.* 2010;140:73). Reverse saphenous vein grafts have 10-year patency rates of approximately 80% to the LAD and 50% to the circumflex or RCA. Antiplatelet therapy using aspirin (81 to 325 mg/day) and Plavix beginning immediately after operation is recommended to increase the graft patency rate.

B. Valvular heart disease

1. **Aortic valve**
   a. **Aortic stenosis (AS).** Left ventricular outflow obstruction can occur at the subvalvular, the supravalvular, or (most commonly)

the valvular level. Aortic valvular stenosis is usually the result of senile degeneration and calcification of a normal or a congenitally bicuspid aortic valve. Less frequently, AS develops many years after an episode of acute rheumatic fever. AS places a pressure overload on the left ventricle. Adequate cardiac output is usually maintained until late in the course of AS, but at the expense of **left ventricular hypertrophy.** Physical signs include a systolic ejection murmur, diminished carotid pulses, and a sustained, forceful, nondisplaced apical impulse. Symptoms often develop when the valve area decreases to 1 cm^2 or less. **Angina pectoris** develops in approximately 35% of patients with severe AS and results from ventricular hypertrophy (e.g., increased myocardial oxygen demand and reduced coronary perfusion) and the high incidence of concomitant CAD. **Syncope** (15% incidence) probably results from fixed cardiac output and decreased cerebral perfusion during systemic vasodilatation. **CHF** is the presenting symptom in approximately one half of patients and usually manifests as dyspnea on exertion. The effect of aortic valve replacement (AVR) on patients with aortic valve stenosis is dramatic and well documented by several studies. For example, survival was 87% at 3 years in operated and 21% in unoperated patients in one study (*Circulation.* 1982;66:1105).

b. **Aortic insufficiency (AI)** is usually the result of valve leaflet pathology from rheumatic heart disease (often associated with mitral valve disease) or myxomatous degeneration. AI also may result from other causes of leaflet dysfunction or aortic root dilation, including endocarditis, syphilis, connective tissue diseases (e.g., Marfan syndrome), inflammatory disease (e.g., ankylosing spondylitis), hypertension, and aortic dissection. Chronic AI results in volume overload of the left ventricle, causing chamber enlargement and wall thickening (although a relatively normal ratio of wall thickness to volume is usually maintained). Gradual myocardial decompensation often progresses either without symptoms or with subtle symptoms (e.g., weakness, fatigue, or dyspnea on exertion). Physical signs include a hyperdynamic circulation with markedly increased systemic arterial pulse pressure, known as **Corrigan's water-hammer pulse;** forceful and laterally displaced apical impulse; and a decrescendo diastolic murmur. Acute AI is not well tolerated because of the lack of compensatory chamber enlargement and thus often results in fulminant pulmonary edema, myocardial ischemia, and cardiovascular collapse.

c. **AVR** is indicated for symptomatic patients with severe AS (defined as valve area <1 cm^2, or mean gradient >40 mm Hg or jet velocity >4 m/second). Surgery is also indicated in asymptomatic patients with severe AS undergoing CABG or other cardiac surgery and in patients with severe AS and left ventricular systolic dysfunction (i.e., EF <0.50). AVR may also be considered for (1) asymptomatic patients with severe AS and hypotension or symptoms with exercise, (2) patients who have a high likelihood of rapid progression (age, calcification, and CAD), (3) patients undergoing CABG who have mild-to-moderate AS with moderate-to-severe calcification of the valve, and (4) low-risk patients with extremely severe AS (valve area <0.6 cm^2 or gradient >60 mm Hg or jet velocity >5 m/second). Elderly patients (>80 years old) have had acceptable morbidity and mortality rates undergoing AVR, with greater than 50% 5-year survival (*Ann Thorac Surg.* 2007;83(5):1651).

For symptomatic patients with AI, indications for surgery include (1) severe AI, (2) chronic moderate to severe AI and left ventricular dysfunction (EF <0.5), and (3) patients with chronic severe AI who are undergoing other cardiac surgery. Patients without symptoms and normal left ventricular function but who have severe left ventricular dilatation (end diastolic dimension >75 mm) are also reasonable candidates (*J Am Coll Cardiol.* 2006;48:e1).

d. Transcatheter aortic valve interventions have received commercial approval for use in Europe and are undergoing multicentered randomized trials for approval in the United States. The Edwards Sapien valve is the closest to being approved in the United States. These valves can be implanted through a transfemoral or transapical approach without the use of CPB. Early results with both approaches have been reported in patients with high operative risk based on EuroSCORE calculations. In patients with risk of operative mortality averaging 27.6%, transapical implantation achieved 94% procedural success with 92%, 74%, and 71% 1-month, 6-month, and 1-year survival, respectively (*Eur J Cardiothorac Surg.* 2007;31:9). In the recently reported PARTNERS trial, there was a 20% absolute reduction in mortality at 1 year for transcatheter AVR in patients considered to be inoperable compared to maximal medical therapy (*NEJM.* 2010;363:1597).

2. Mitral valve

a. Mitral stenosis (MS) is caused by rheumatic fever in most cases. Other, less common causes include collagen vascular diseases, amyloidosis, and congenital stenosis. MS places a pressure overload on the left atrium, with relative sparing of ventricular function. Left atrial dilation to more than 45 mm is associated with a high incidence of AF and subsequent thromboembolism. A transvalvular pressure gradient is present when the valve area is less than 2 cm^2, and critical MS occurs when the valve area is 1 cm^2 or less. Physical signs include an apical diastolic murmur, an opening snap, and a loud S_1. Symptoms usually develop late and reflect pulmonary congestion (e.g., dyspnea), reduced left ventricular preload (e.g., low–cardiac-output syndrome), or AF (e.g., thromboembolism).

b. MR results from abnormalities of the leaflets (e.g., rheumatic disease, myxomatous degeneration, endocarditis), annulus (e.g., calcification, dilation usually due to a cardiomyopathy, or destruction), chordae tendineae (e.g., rupture from endocarditis or MI, fusion, or elongation), or ischemic papillary muscle dysfunction or rupture. The most common cause of MR in the United States is myxomatous degeneration. MR places a volume overload on the left ventricle and atrium, causing chamber enlargement and wall thickening, although a relatively normal ratio of wall thickness to volume is usually maintained. Systolic unloading into the compliant left atrium allows enhanced emptying of the left ventricle during systole, with only slight increases in oxygen consumption. AF often develops due to left atrial dilation. Physical signs include a hyperdynamic circulation and a brisk, laterally displaced apical impulse; a holosystolic murmur; and a widely split S_2. Gradual myocardial decompensation often progresses in the absence of symptoms (e.g., dyspnea on exertion, fatigue). In acute MR, adaptation is not possible, and fulminant cardiac decompensation often ensues.

  c. **Repair of the mitral valve** is preferred over replacement whenever possible. Surgery is indicated in patients with moderate-to-severe MS, and symptoms or asymptomatic patients with severe pulmonary hypertension. Moderate MS is defined by a pressure gradient of 25 to 40 mm Hg across the valve or a valve area 1.0 to 1.5 cm², and severe MS is defined by a pressure gradient of >40 mm Hg or a valve area less than 1.0 cm² on echocardiography. Percutaneous mitral balloon valvuloplasty can be performed in selected patients. Surgery is indicated in symptomatic patients with acute or chronic severe MR with NYHA class II, III, or IV symptoms. Asymptomatic patients with chronic severe MR and mild-to-moderate left ventricular dysfunction (EF <0.6) are also candidates for surgery. MV repair is also indicated for asymptomatic patients with chronic severe MR when (1) there is evidence of LV dysfunction (EF <0.6 or end systolic diameter > 40 mm) or (2) the likelihood of successful repair is greater than 90% or (3) there is new onset of AF or (4) pulmonary hypertension (*J Am Coll Cardiol.* 2006;48:e1). Patients with AF and indications for MR repair/replacement should be considered for a Cox-Maze procedure at the time of surgery.

3. **Tricuspid valve**
  a. **Tricuspid insufficiency (TI)** most often results from a functional dilation of the valve annulus caused by pulmonary hypertension, which, in turn, may be caused by intrinsic mitral or aortic valve disease. Causes of primary TI include rheumatic heart disease, bacterial endocarditis (often in IV drug users), carcinoid tumors, Ebstein anomaly, and blunt trauma. Patients have a systolic murmur, a prominent jugular venous pulse, and a pulsatile liver. Mild-to-moderate TI usually is well tolerated.

  b. Significant **tricuspid regurgitation** may be repaired at the time of surgery for other cardiac anomalies. Intervention for isolated TI is uncommon. The majority of tricuspid valves can be repaired with annuloplasty techniques rather than replacement.

4. **Selection of a prosthetic valve** must be individualized for each patient. Despite many years of research, there still is no ideal prosthetic valve. The general considerations for selecting an appropriate prosthetic valve are summarized in Table 30-2.

  a. **Bioprostheses** are made from animal tissues, usually the porcine aortic valve or bovine pericardium. Examples include the Carpentier-Edwards, Hancock, St. Jude Biocor, and Edwards Perimount

TABLE 30-2	Selection of a Prosthetic Valve
Bioprosthetic valve	
Reoperation unlikely	
Age >60 y	
Previous thrombosed mechanical valve	
Limited life expectancy	
Anticoagulant-related complication or intolerance	
Unreliable anticoagulant risk	
Young women who wish to become pregnant	
Mechanical valve	
Reoperation likely	
Age <60 y	
Long life expectancy	
Small aortic annulus in a large patient	
Patient fear of reoperation	

stented valves and the St. Jude Toronto SPV, Sorin, and Medtronic Freestyle stentless valves. These prostheses are associated with a low rate of thromboembolism, even without long-term anticoagulation. However, they are less durable than mechanical valves. Their rate of deterioration depends on the patient's age and is relatively faster in younger patients and slower in the elderly. Overall, the mean time to failure is approximately 10 to 15 years. However, the bioprosthetic material life may be prolonged in newer valves due to modern preservation methods. In general, bioprostheses are the preferred valves for older patients (>60 years) or patients with a contraindication to anticoagulation (e.g., young women who desire future pregnancies).

b. **Mechanical valves** have excellent long-term durability, but the high rate of thromboembolic complications (0.5% to 3% per year) necessitates lifelong anticoagulation. All of these valves are manufactured from **pyrolytic carbon,** which was first discovered in 1966 and has the unique quality of thromboresistance. Examples include the St. Jude, Medtronic-Hall, Sorin, and MRCI (Medical Carbon Research Institute) valves. These valves typically are used in young patients who have a long life expectancy and can tolerate lifelong anticoagulation.

c. **Allograft and autograft valves** are useful for replacement of the aortic valve, particularly in the setting of endocarditis (*J Heart Valve Dis.* 1994;3:377). These prostheses have reasonable durability and a low incidence of thromboembolism, but experience with them is limited by the supply of allografts and the relative difficulty of the autograft (Ross) procedure, in which a patient's pulmonic valve is used to replace the diseased aortic valve.

5. **Endocarditis.** The main indications for operation include hemodynamic instability, CHF, recurrent septic emboli, and persistent evidence of infection despite appropriate antibiotic therapy. Relative indications include severe acute mitral or aortic valvular insufficiency, heart block, intracardiac fistulas, fungal endocarditis, or infections with especially virulent organisms like oxacillin-resistant *Staphylococcus aureus*. The risk for reoperation for recurrent infective endocarditis is about 17% for IV drug users and 5% for non-IV drug users (*Ann Thorac Surg.* 2007;83:30). Antibiotic therapy alone may be sufficient for the first, uncomplicated episode of prosthetic valve endocarditis, but valve replacement is often required for the treatment of prosthetic valve endocarditis.

6. **Perivalvular leak** occurs when the implanted valve separates from the valve annulus. This may lead to clinically significant valvular regurgitation, which can be defined by echocardiography. Hemolytic anemia may be documented by an increased reticulocyte count, increased serum lactate dehydrogenase level, and increased urinary iron excretion. Replacement of the valve is indicated for perivalvular leak associated with symptoms, severe valvular regurgitation, or severe hemolysis.

7. **Thrombosis and thromboembolism.** Thrombus formation may occur on the surface of the artificial valve and lead to valve thrombosis or embolism. Embolic complications may include transient ischemic attack, stroke, or embolism other vital organs or the extremities. The use of appropriate anticoagulation with mechanical valves may reduce the risk of thromboembolism to the level (approximately 0.5% per year) associated with bioprosthetic valves (*Chest.* 2004;126:457S). The target INR for aortic valves is 2 to 3 and for mitral valves is 3 to 4.

8. **Hypertrophic obstructive cardiomyopathy (HOCM)** is characterized by asymmetric hypertrophy and fibrosis of the myocardium, causing obstruction of the outflow tract. The overall annual death rate of patients with HOCM is about 2% per year. In hypertrophic cardiomyopathy without obstruction of the outflow tract, the annual death rate is about 1% per year. Hypertrophic cardiomyopathy (with or without obstruction) is the most common cause of sudden cardiac death in young people. Medical therapy with β-blockade or calcium channel blockade is the preferred first-line treatment. Nifedipine, nitroglycerin,

angiotensin-converting enzyme inhibitors, and angiotensin II blockers are all generally contraindicated due to their vasodilatory properties, which can exacerbate the outflow tract obstruction. Surgical treatment of HOCM is myectomy, with a postoperative mortality of 1% or less (*Ann Thorac Surg.* 2000;69:1732). By convention, surgery is recommended for symptomatic patients who have failed medical therapy with a documented at-rest outflow tract gradient of at least 30 mm Hg. Long-term results have been excellent with symptomatic relief in over 80% of patients (*J Thor Cardiovasc Surg.* 1996;111:586). An alternate therapy is catheter-based septal alcohol ablation. Short-term results with success rates greater than 90% have been reported for catheter-based septal alcohol ablation (*Circulation.* 2005;112:293), but some long-term data have shown myectomy to be superior to septal ablation (*Circ Heart Failure.* 2010;3:162). There is a much higher rate of pacemaker implantation with alcohol ablation. Generally, alcohol ablation is reserved for the elderly or patients considered high risk for surgery.

C. **AF** affects more than 2 million people in the United States, with approximately 160,000 new cases per year. It affects nearly 10% of individuals older than the age of 80 years. Morbidity includes patient discomfort, hemodynamic compromise, and thromboembolism.

   1. Nonsurgical management of AF includes antiarrhythmic drugs, cardioversion, and catheter ablation. Although drugs can induce **chemical cardioversion,** the failure rate is high (50% at 2 years in some series) (*JAMA.* 2008;300:1784). In patients in AF, the use of chronic anticoagulation for stroke prevention has significant associated morbidity. Because the pulmonary veins have been shown to be the source of ectopic foci in many patients with paroxysmal AF (*Circulation.* 1999;100:1879), the use of catheter-based ablation and isolation of the pulmonary veins has gained popularity. Success rates have been improving, with the best centers achieving success rates of greater than 70% in patients with paroxysmal AF (*Heart Rhythm.* 2007;4:816). In patients with persistent or long-standing persistent AF, results have been worse.

   2. The indications for the surgical ablation AF are (1) symptomatic AF in patients undergoing other cardiac procedures, (2) selected asymptomatic AF patients undergoing cardiac surgery in whom the ablation can be performed with minimal risk, and (3) standalone AF surgery should be considered for symptomatic AF patients who prefer a surgical approach, have failed one or more attempts at catheter ablation, or are not candidates for catheter ablation (*Heart Rhythm.* 2007;4:816). The **Cox-Maze procedure,** first performed in the late 1980s, was designed to eliminate multiple macroreentrant circuits in the atria that were felt to be responsible for fibrillation. Through a median sternotomy or right thoracotomy, a series of incisions on both atria, excision of the atrial appendages, and isolation of the pulmonary veins was performed. Long-term results have been outstanding, with a freedom from symptomatic AF of 97% at a median of 5.4 years and an operative mortality of less than 2% (*J Thorac Cardiovasc Surg.* 2003;126:1822). This

"cut and sew" procedure was difficult to perform, and consequently only a few groups adopted the operation. Recently, less invasive surgical procedures have been developed that have replaced the surgical incisions with linear lines of ablation. These ablation techniques have included cryosurgery, radiofrequency or microwave energy, and ultrasound. These new approaches have broadened procedural adoption and have had promising success rates (*Ann Surg.* 2006;244:583). If the entire Cox-Maze lesion set is performed, ablation-assisted procedures with appropriate ablation technology have had identical success rates to the original cut-and-sew procedure (*J Thorac Cardiovasc Surg.* 2007;133:389). Freedom from AF, off antiarrhythmic drugs approaches 80% at 1 year (*J Thorac Cardiovasc Surg.* 2008;135:870).

Other surgical approaches have included pulmonary vein isolation, with or without extended left atrial ablation lines, and with or without ganglionated plexi ablation. The advantage of these procedures has been that they can be performed with small incisions or thoracoscopically without the use of CPB (*J Thorac Cardiovasc Surg.* 2005;130:797). Results have been variable from center to center, but generally have been better with paroxysmal as opposed to long-standing persistent AF (*J Interv Card Electrophysiol.* 2007;20:89).

D. Heart failure. It is estimated that approximately 250,000 people suffer from advanced heart failure in the United States (*Curr Heart Fail Rep.* 2010;7:140). The management of heart failure involves medical and surgical care and both acute and chronic interventions. The surgical management of heart failure is discussed here.

1. The **IABP** is used as the first-line device to provide circulatory support in acute heart failure (*Ann Thorac Surg.* 1992;54:11).

   a. **Physiology.** The principal effect of the IABP is a reduction in left ventricular afterload. This occurs due to deflation of the balloon at the time of the opening of the aortic valve. The resulting effects include improved ventricular ejection and reduction in myocardial oxygen consumption. The IABP inflates during early diastole, increasing diastolic BP and thus also diastolic coronary artery blood flow.

   b. **Indications for the IABP** vary in relation to the timing of operation. In the preoperative period, the IABP is indicated for low-cardiac-output states and for unstable angina refractory to medical therapy (e.g., nitrates, heparin, and β-adrenergic blocking agents). Intraoperatively, the IABP is used to permit weaning from CPB when inotropic agents alone are not sufficient. In the postoperative period, the IABP is used primarily for low-cardiac-output states. The IABP can be used to support the circulation during periods of refractory arrhythmias and can also be used to provide support to the patient awaiting cardiac transplantation.

   c. **Insertion of the IABP** generally is accomplished percutaneously via the common femoral artery. Sheathless devices, because of their narrower diameter, may have decreased the incidence of lower-extremity ischemic complications. Correct placement should be confirmed by chest X-ray. The radiopaque tip of the balloon is positioned just below the aortic knob and just distal to the left subclavian artery. At operation, the IABP may be placed directly into the transverse aortic arch, with the balloon positioned down into the descending aorta. Before **removal of the IABP,** the platelet count, PT, and PTT should be normal. Manual pressure should be applied for 20 to 30 minutes after removal to achieve hemostasis and avoid the formation of a femoral artery pseudoaneurysm or arteriovenous fistula.

d. **Management** of the device after placement focuses on ensuring proper diastolic inflation and deflation. The ECG and the femoral (or aortic) pressure waveform are monitored continuously on a bedside console. The device may be triggered using either the ECG or the pressure tracing for every heartbeat (1:1) or less frequently (1:2, 1:3). Anticoagulation during IABP support is optional. If the balloon must be repositioned or removed, the device should be turned off first. IABP support is withdrawn gradually by decreasing the augmentation frequency from 1:1 to 1:3 in steps of several hours each.

e. **Complications of IABP** therapy include incorrect placement of the device, resulting in perforation of the aorta; injury to the femoral artery; and reduction in blood flow to the visceral or renal arteries. Ischemia of the lower extremity, evidenced by diminished peripheral pulses or other sequelae, may necessitate removal of the IABP or performance of an inflow arterial bypass procedure (e.g., femoral-to-femoral artery). Rupture of the balloon is an indication for immediate removal because blood may clot within the ruptured balloon, necessitating operative removal.

f. **Percutaneous Assist Devices** are devices that can be deployed via catheter-based approach and function as ventricular assist devices (VADs) without the need for open surgery. They are typically used only for short-term support, such as temporary support during high-risk percutaneous coronary interventions. Two examples of these are the TandemHeart and the Impella devices (*Expert Rev Cardiovasc Ther.* 2010;8:1247).

2. **Ventricular remodeling.** The progression of heart failure leads to dilation and structural changes in the ventricle by a process known as remodeling. Initially, these changes are compensatory, but eventually they result in pathologic states—including high wall stress, increased neurohormonal levels, and increased inflammatory mediators—that lead to CHF.

a. **Partial left ventriculectomy.** There are several techniques described to reduce the diameter of the left ventricle. In most series, after an initial improvement, heart failure parameters returned to their preoperative state. For the most part, these procedures have been abandoned in favor of assist devices and transplantation. A randomized control trial recently reported no difference between CABG alone and CABG with surgical ventricular remodeling in mortality and cardiac hospitalizations at 4 years (*N Engl J Med.* 2009;360:1705).

3. **Mitral valve surgery** has gained recent popularity for the therapy of CHF. MR secondary to heart failure and ventricular dilatation results from mitral annular dilatation and leaflet lengthening, leading to poor leaflet coaptation. The use of a mitral ring annuloplasty has been shown to be safe and effective for improving NYHA class, left ventricular EF, cardiac output, and left ventricular EDV (*J Thorac Cardiovasc Surg.* 2006;136:568). In fact, it has been estimated that up to 10% of patients undergoing heart transplant evaluation may benefit from mitral valve repair (*J Heart Valve Dis.* 2002;11:S26). However, the long-term results of mitral valve repair remain controversial (*J Heart Valve Dis.* 2000;9:364; *Circulation.* 2006;114:167). In cases in which papillary muscle dysfunction due to ischemia has changed valvular geometry dramatically, mitral valve replacement rather than repair may be more appropriate.

4. **Biventricular pacing** for cardiac resynchronization has emerged as a valid treatment modality for patients with heart failure and concomitant intraventricular conduction delay manifested by QRS complex greater than 120 ms. Absolute risk reduction in all cause mortality in two trials was about 10% at 1 year (*Cardiol Clin.* 2008;26:419). Cardiac resynchronization therapy is an important adjunct in this subset of patients with NYHA class III and IV heart failure.

5. **VADs** may be used to support the left side of the circulation (LVAD) or the right side of the circulation (RVAD). When both an LVAD and an RVAD are used, the combination is termed a **biventricular assist device (BiVAD).**

   a. The **physiologic effect** of a VAD is decompression of the left or right ventricle (or both) and restoration of cardiac output, resulting in decreased myocardial oxygen consumption. The goal of VAD therapy is either to permit recovery of myocardium that is not irreversibly injured (e.g., "stunned" myocardium) or to support the circulation in patients with a failing heart until a heart transplantation is possible. More recently, VAD therapy has been used in patients with end-stage CHF who are not candidates for transplantation.

   b. There are no formal **indications** for VAD implantation. Instead, VADS have been used in three separate broad categories. They are used for patients in which there is (1) an inability to separate from CPB despite inotropic and IABP support ("bridge to recovery"), (2) for intermediate-term cardiac support ("bridge to transplant"), and (3) for permanent replacement therapy ("destination therapy").

   c. **VAD subtypes.** Historically, there have been many different subtypes of VADs and a comprehensive review is beyond the scope of this text. Broadly, there are nonpulsatile devices, which include **centrifugal pumps** and **axial flow pumps,** and pulsatile devices, which include **external devices** and **long-term implantable devices.** No single type has been shown to be superior to the others, and device selection depends on surgeon familiarity and on practical advantages and disadvantages with each particular device.

      (1) **Centrifugal pumps** (BioMedicus Biopump and 3M Sarns Delphin) have been used most frequently as bridges to recovery in patients with postcardiotomy cardiogenic shock.

(2) **Axial flow pumps** (Jarvik 2000 Flowmaker, MicroMed DeBakey VAD, Thoratec HeartMate II) are small pumps, consume less power, and are completely implantable. These devices are designed for longer-term support (months to years). The devices have an impeller suspended by bearings and provide continuous flow. The speed of the pump and the adequacy of left ventricular preload determine output. All of these pumps have a cable that is externalized from the right lower quadrant of the abdomen that connects to the controller system. Many examples of these devices are undergoing clinical trials in the United States and some have Food and Drug Administration (FDA)-approved indications as bridge to transplant or destination therapy. Newer devices in development use magnetically suspended impellers to reduce friction and provide device longevity.

(3) **External pulsatile devices** (Abiomed BVS 5000, Abiomed AB5000, and Thoratec Intracorporeal Ventricular Assist Device) generally have the same indications as centrifugal pumps, although the duration of support may be somewhat longer. They consist of pneumatically driven compression sacs or chambers and mimic the native function of the heart. These devices can be used as a bridge to recovery in patients with acute fulminant myocarditis or MI. Typically these devices are implanted in a preperitoneal pocket.

(4) **Long-term implantable pulsatile devices** (WorldHeart Novacor and Thoratec HeartMate) are used primarily as bridges to transplantation in patients with chronic heart failure. They also are typically pneumatically driven devices with a compression chamber (see destination therapy in Section V.D.4.g below).

d. **Insertion** of VADs. In general, RVADs receive inflow from the right atrium and return outflow to the pulmonary artery using flexible cannulae or grafts. LVADs receive inflow from the left atrium or ventricle and return outflow to the ascending aorta.

e. **Management** of the VAD after placement focuses on maintaining proper function and adequate anticoagulation. The activated clotting time should be monitored frequently and maintained at approximately 200 seconds. Factors that affect **a low-flow-state status post-LVAD** include right ventricular dysfunction, pulmonary hypertension, hypovolemia, and tamponade. It is therefore critical that adequate ventilatory support be provided to correct hypoxemia and acidosis. Pulmonary vasodilators such as NO or inhaled prostacyclin are frequently used to lower pulmonary vascular resistance.

f. **Complications** of VAD therapy include excessive bleeding, thrombus formation, embolization, and hemolysis, which are most common with temporary support devices. Associated complications not related to the device specifically include respiratory failure (due to infection or fluid overload) and renal failure. For chronic devices, long-term complications include infections at the drive-line site, thromboembolism, and device failure.

g. **Destination therapy.** The recent Randomized Evaluation of Mechanical Assistance for the Treatment of Congestive Heart Failure (REMATCH) trial compared assist devices with best medical therapy and demonstrated an increased survival at 2 years (23% vs. 8%). In addition, there was a significant quality-of-life improvement (*N Engl J Med.* 2001;345:1435). The Thoratec HeartMate XVE Left Ventricular Assist System (LVAS) has been approved for destination therapy by the FDA for patients with chronic heart failure.

6. **Cardiac transplantation** can provide relief from symptoms in patients with end-stage cardiomyopathy who are functionally incapacitated despite optimal medical therapy and who are not candidates for any other cardiac corrective procedures. The first successful heart transplant occurred in 1967 in South Africa. There were 2,163 heart transplants performed in the United States in 2008, making this intervention an infrequently used but important modality in the management of heart failure. The 1-year survival following heart transplant is 88% for males and 77% females (American Heart Association Heart Disease and Stroke Statistics 2010 update).

   a. **Accepted indications for heart transplant** include cardiomyopathy that is ischemic, idiopathic, postpartum, or chemotherapy induced. Patients are generally in class III or IV NYHA CHF, have a Heart Failure Survival Score of high risk (score derived from a predictive model based on clinical factors and peak oxygen consumption), and have a peak oxygen consumption of less than 14 mL/kg/minute after reaching an anaerobic threshold. Relative indications include instability in fluid balance or renal function despite best medical therapy, recurrent unstable angina not amenable to revascularization, and intractable ventricular arrhythmias.

   b. **Relative contraindications to transplantation** include age older than 65 years, irreversible pulmonary hypertension (>4 Wood units), active infection, recent pulmonary embolus, renal dysfunction (serum creatinine >2.5 mg/dL or creatinine clearance <25 mL/minute), hepatic dysfunction (bilirubin >2.5 or alanine aminotransferase/aspartate aminotransferase >2× normal), active or recent malignancy, systemic disease such as amyloidosis, significant carotid or peripheral vascular disease, active or recent peptic ulcer disease, brittle diabetes mellitus, morbid obesity, mental illness, substance abuse, or psychosocial instability.

   c. **Donor pool expansion.** Because of the shortage of acceptable donors, the use of an expanded donor pool has been advocated. Some centers have tolerated size mismatch, increased age (>55 years), malignancy, infection, or even donor bypass grafting for carefully selected high-risk recipients.

   d. **Immunosuppressive therapy** generally includes a calcineurin inhibitor (cyclosporine or tacrolimus), steroids, and an antimetabolite (mycophenolate or mofetil). Recently, tacrolimus has replaced cyclosporine as the calcineurin inhibitor of choice. When rejection episodes occur, the majority can be reversed with bolus doses of IV steroids. When rejection episodes are resistant to increased steroid doses, the monoclonal antibody OKT3 or rabbit antithymocyte serum can be added to the treatment regimen. Immunosuppression is covered in more detail in Chapter 23.

e. **Acute allograft rejection** is diagnosed by **endomyocardial biopsy.** Biopsy forceps are passed into the right ventricle percutaneously, using fluoroscopic or echocardiographic guidance, usually via the right internal jugular or femoral vein, and several biopsies are taken to document the presence and degree of rejection histologically. During the early postoperative period, biopsies are performed several times each month. After the first 6 months, the frequency of biopsies is decreased to one or two times per year. Whenever a patient develops evidence of a rejection episode, a biopsy is performed. Complications of endomyocardial biopsy are rare but include ventricular perforation, pneumothorax, injury to the tricuspid valve, transient ventricular or supraventricular arrhythmias, hematoma, and infection. **Coronary artery vasculopathy (CAV),** thought to represent **chronic vascular rejection,** occurs in a significant percentage of cardiac transplant recipients and is a major limitation on the long-term success of cardiac transplantation, being responsible for 30% of deaths in transplanted patients after 5 years (*J Heart Lung Transplant.* 2007;26:769). CAV is usually not amenable to conventional revascularization owing to small-vessel, nonfocal disease and often requires retransplantation. Routine echocardiography is also performed frequently to evaluate allograft function.

7. **Future therapy for heart failure**
   a. **Device therapy.** There has been a substantial improvement in devices over the last two decades. They have become smaller, more durable, and less prone to thrombotic complications. Continued advances in this area will likely expand the indications for these devices for long-term support (destination therapy).
   b. **Myocyte regeneration.** Several approaches, including those using embryonic stem cells, cardiomyocytes, cryopreserved fetal cardiomyocytes, skeletal myoblasts, bone marrow-derived mesenchymal cells, and dermal fibroblasts, are under investigation.
   c. **Xenotransplantation.** The primary difficulty in xenotransplantation is the management of rejection and cross-species infection. To date, such management has been unsuccessful, and the data do not yet justify clinical trials.

VI. **POSTOPERATIVE MANAGEMENT.** Postoperative care of the cardiac surgery patient is provided in three phases: in the intensive care unit (ICU), on the ward, and after discharge from the hospital.

A. Intensive care. ICU care resources generally are required for 1 to 3 days after an operation requiring CPB.

1. **Initial assessment.** Information on the patient's history, indications for operation, and technical details of the operation (e.g., coronary

arteries bypassed, conduits used, CPB time, and aortic cross-clamp time) should be related to the ICU staff by the surgeon. The anesthesiologist should relate information about the intraoperative course, including preoperative and intraoperative hemodynamic parameters (especially cardiac filling pressures) and current medications. A thorough physical examination should be performed, with attention to the cardiovascular system. A chest X-ray, ECG, complete blood count, basic metabolic panel, arterial blood gas, prothrombin and PTT, and magnesium level are usually obtained.

2. **Monitoring in the immediate postoperative period.** Continuous recordings are made of arterial, central venous, and occasionally pulmonary artery pressures (PAPs); the ECG; and arterial oxygen saturation using pulse oximetry. The pulmonary artery wedge pressure is measured from the Swan–Ganz catheter as indicated by the patient's status, and calculations are made of the cardiac output, cardiac index (cardiac output per unit of body-surface area), stroke volume, pulmonary vascular resistance, and systemic vascular resistance (by thermodilution technique). Normal values for these parameters are listed in Table 30-1. Immediate attention is necessary to determine the etiology and to correct deviations from normal values of any of these parameters. **Body temperature** is monitored continuously using a pulmonary artery thermistor or rectal thermometer. Because early postoperative hypothermia may increase afterload (systemic vascular resistance) and adversely affect blood clotting, hypothermia is treated aggressively (e.g., air-warming blankets). Warming is discontinued when the core temperature reaches 36°C. For patients with persistent fever, a search should be made for active infection and efforts made to decrease the patient's body temperature.

3. **Cardiovascular. Cardiac pump function** is assessed as described earlier. A cardiac index of 2 L/minute/m^2 is generally a minimum acceptable value. A mixed-venous oxygen saturation of less than 60% suggests inadequate peripheral tissue perfusion and increased peripheral oxygen extraction. Etiologies include reduced oxygen-carrying capacity (e.g., low hematocrit), reduced cardiac output, and increased oxygen consumption (e.g., shivering). Common causes of low cardiac output in the early postoperative period are hypovolemia, increased systemic vascular resistance due to persistent hypothermia or increased circulating catecholamines, and decreased contractility secondary to myocardial stunning or intrinsic myocardial dysfunction.

   a. **Preload** is increased by administering crystalloid solution (e.g., lactated Ringer's solution) or colloid solution (e.g., 6% hetastarch, 5% albumin) as needed to maintain the pulmonary arterial wedge pressure in the target range, as determined by the patient's diastolic compliance and systolic performance. Using blood products in a judicious manner is mandatory. At our institution, blood transfusion is indicated in patients with a hemoglobin below 8 g/dL.

   b. **Afterload reduction** in the volume-restored patient increases EF and cardiac output and decreases myocardial oxygen consumption.

The body temperature should be returned to the normal range, and hypertension should be controlled. In general, the mean arterial BP should be maintained near the preoperative level. For patients with valve replacement or aortic replacement, the systolic BP should be carefully controlled to prevent postoperative bleeding. Afterload is often initially titrated with parenteral infusions of sodium nitroprusside, nitroglycerin, or nicardipine, followed by a change to longer-acting parenteral or enteral agents once the patient's hemodynamic status has been stabilized.

c. **Contractility. Inotropic agents** are used only after ensuring an adequate preload and an appropriate afterload. Selection of a particular inotropic agent must be individualized based on the agent's specific effects on the heart rate, BP, cardiac output, systemic vascular resistance, and renal blood flow. All of these agents increase the work of the heart and increase myocardial oxygen consumption and thus should be used judiciously. Typically used agents include dobutamine (a beta-1 adrenergic agonist), milrinone (a phosphodiesterase inhibitor), and epinephrine (a nonspecific adrenergic agonist) at doses of 1 to 5 μg/kg/minute, 0.375 to 0.750 μg/kg/minute, and 0.01 to 0.1 μg/kg/minute, respectively. **Mechanical support** in the form of an IABP or a VAD can be considered if other measures are ineffective in restoring adequate ventricular ejection.

d. **Rate control.** The heart can be paced using temporary epicardial pacing electrodes (placed at the time of operation) at 80 to 100 beats/minute to increase the cardiac output. Pacing can be performed using only the atrial leads (atrial pacing, or AAI mode), only the ventricular leads (ventricular pacing, or VVI mode), or with both sets of leads (AV sequential pacing or atrial tracking with ventricular pacing). Optimal pacing always involves maintaining AV synchrony. VVI pacing should only be used in patients with atrial tachyarrhythmias. If epicardial pacing is not necessary, the epicardial pacemaker generator is set in a backup mode to provide ventricular pacing only in the event of marked bradycardia. The pacemaker output threshold (in milliamperes) should be set to approximately twice the minimum threshold required to capture.

e. **Arrhythmias,** including bradycardia from resolving hypothermia, heart block secondary to persistent cardioplegia effect, and supraventricular and ventricular tachyarrhythmias can be associated with reduced cardiac output and should be corrected. **Arrhythmias** occur in 40% to 60% of patients after cardiac surgical procedures and are more common in patients who receive inotropic support. Advanced cardiovascular life support guidelines should be followed.

(1) **Supraventricular arrhythmias** (AF, atrial flutter, atrial tachycardia) are most common and are associated with an increased risk of transient or permanent neurologic deficits (*J Card Surg.* 2005;20:425). Postoperative AF occurs in approximately 30% of patients and has a peak incidence on postoperative day 2 (*J Thorac Cardiovasc Surg.* 2011;141:559). To reduce the incidence of postoperative

arrhythmias, patients receiving β-adrenergic blocking agents and/or statins preoperatively should continue to be given these medications postoperatively. Patients with supraventricular arrhythmias and hemodynamic compromise should undergo immediate electrical cardioversion (with 50 to 100 joules). Because a frequent etiology is hypoxia or hypokalemia, the new onset of a supraventricular arrhythmia should be evaluated by measurement of the arterial oxygen saturation and the serum potassium. In many patients with hemodynamically stable arrhythmias, prompt correction of the partial pressure of oxygen (to >70 mm Hg) and the serum potassium level (to >4.5 mg/dL) may terminate the arrhythmia. For patients with **atrial flutter,** overdrive pacing may be used to terminate the arrhythmia. The patient's atrial temporary epicardial pacing wires are connected to a pacemaker generator, and either burst pacing (700 to 800 beats/minute for 3 to 4 seconds) or decremental pacing (stepwise decrease from 10% above the flutter rate to 180 beats/minute) is used. For patients who persist in AF for greater than an hour despite adequate rate control, consideration should be given for the initiation of rhythm control with amiodarone. A loading dose is given, orally if possible, and the patient is reassessed for a maintenance dose. For patients who persist in AF for greater than 8 hours despite amiodarone, anticoagulation should be considered to avoid the complication of stroke. IV heparin as a bridge to oral Coumadin with a goal INR of 2.0 to 3.0 should be started.

    (2) Ventricular arrhythmias in the postoperative period are treated as they are in other patients. Ventricular arrhythmias other than premature ventricular contractions suggest underlying ischemic pathology. The drugs of choice for treatment have been lidocaine and amiodarone.

f. Cardiac tamponade is a potentially lethal cause of low cardiac output early after operation. Clinical features include narrowed pulse pressure, increased jugular venous distention, rising cardiac filling pressures, muffled heart sounds, pulsus paradoxus, widened mediastinal silhouette on chest radiograph, and decreased urine output. Definitive diagnosis is usually made by the equalization of diastolic heart pressures on Swan–Ganz catheter pressure recordings or transthoracic or transesophageal echocardiography.

g. Perioperative MI occurs in approximately 1% to 2% of patients and can be diagnosed by ECG changes, biochemical criteria (e.g., elevated troponin-I or creatine kinase-MB), or echocardiography. Long-term and acute survival may be adversely affected, especially if complications such as cardiogenic shock or ventricular arrhythmias develop.

h. Postoperative hemorrhage is relatively common after cardiac surgery and necessitates reexploration in up to 5% of patients. Hematologic parameters (complete blood count, PT, PTT) are measured on admission to the ICU and as needed. CPB requires heparinization, causes platelet dysfunction and destruction, and activates the fibri-nolytic system. Initial focus is on adequate BP control, metabolic stability, maintenance of normothermia, and adequate reversal of heparin with protamine. For patients with significant postopera-tive bleeding (>200 mL/hour), consideration should be given to platelet transfusion to maintain the platelet count at greater than 100,000/μL and transfusion of fresh-frozen plasma if the INR is abnormal. Although definitive randomized studies have not been conducted, the use of recombinant factor VIIa in patients expe-riencing life-threatening, unresponsive bleeding has been effective in rare cases and should be considered in this situation (*Ann Thorac Surg.* 2007;83:707). Some surgeons advocate stripping the chest tubes every hour to prevent clotting. If clotting becomes appar-ent, sterile suction tubing can be used to evacuate blood clot. The formation of undrained clot in the mediastinum may result in cardiac tamponade. Indications for operative reexploration for bleeding include (1) prolonged bleeding (>200 mL/hour for 4 to 6 hours), (2) excessive bleeding (>1,000 mL), (3) a sudden increase in bleeding, and (4) cardiac tamponade. Pleural and mediastinal chest tubes generally are removed when the drainage is less than 200 mL in 8 hours.

4. **Pulmonary. Mechanical ventilation** is used in the initial postopera-tive period with typical settings: intermittent mandatory ventilation, 10 to 16 breaths/minute; inspired oxygen concentration, 100%; tidal volume, 10 to 15 mL/kg; and positive end-expiratory pressure, 5 cm H_2O. The patient can be extubated when (1) he or she is fully awake and has had a normal neurologic examination; (2) weaning parameters are satisfactory (e.g., respiratory rate <20 breaths/minute; minute ven-tilation <12 L/minute; negative inspiratory pressure >20 mm H_2O); (3) the arterial blood gas, with only continuous positive airway pres-sure, is satisfactory (pH approximately 7.40; CO_2 tension <45 mm Hg; oxygen tension >70 mm Hg); (4) there is little mediastinal bleed-ing (<100 mL/8 hours); and (5) there is hemodynamic stability. Most patients can be extubated shortly after operation. After extubation, oxygen is administered by high-humidity facemask with an initial inspired oxygen concentration of 0.4. The oxygen can be weaned, as tolerated, to keep the arterial oxygen saturation above 94%.

5. **Renal. Renal dysfunction** in the postoperative period can be due to decreased perfusion pressure during CPB or to inadequate perfusion of the kidneys in the postoperative period. Treatment of acute renal insufficiency in the postoperative period includes ensuring adequate hydration and avoiding nephrotoxic medications. Fluid and electro-lyte balance is evaluated immediately after operation and then hourly as needed. Early after operation, IV fluids are administered slowly (<30 mL/hour). A useful acute measure of a patient's intravascular volume status is the CVP, PAP, or pulmonary capillary wedge pres-sure. If these are not available and the patient is on the ward, the body weight, which is measured daily and compared to the preoperative

weight, can be used. Serum potassium levels are maintained at greater than 4.5 mg/dL to prevent atrial and ventricular arrhythmias, and concomitant repletion of magnesium is warranted (to >2 mg/dL). Metabolic acidosis can reflect a low-cardiac-output state.

6. **Neurologic. Neurologic examination** of the patient is performed on admission to the ICU and periodically as needed. Changes in the neurologic examination warrant immediate investigation. Shivering increases oxygen consumption and should be treated in the early postoperative period by warming the patient or by the administration of meperidine (50 to 100 mg intramuscularly or intravenously every 3 hours) or, for the ventilated patient, pancuronium (0.04 to 0.10 mg/kg intravenously) or vecuronium (0.08 to 0.10 mg/kg slow IV bolus, then 1 to 5 mg/hour IV continuous infusion). **Pain control** is accomplished using parenteral narcotics or nonsteroidal anti-inflammatory agents, or both, during the early postoperative period.

7. **Nutrition.** The patient is given nothing by mouth until after extubation. A clear liquid diet then is begun and is advanced to a regular diet as tolerated. Patients with prolonged ventilation should receive enteral feedings or if this is not possible, parenteral nutrition.

8. **Infection.** Infectious complications are uncommon after cardiac surgical procedures but may lead to substantial morbidity and mortality. Perioperative antibiotics should be started prior to surgery and administered for 24 hours. Prophylaxis with a second-generation cephalosporin has been associated with a fivefold decrease in wound infection rates compared to placebo in a meta-analysis (*J Thorac Cardiovasc Surg.* 1992;104:590). **Wound infection** occurs in 1% to 2% of sternotomy incisions and a higher proportion of saphenous vein harvest sites. Risk factors for deep sternal wound infection include diabetes mellitus, male gender, obesity, and, possibly, the use of bilateral ITAs during CABG procedures in patients older than 74 years (*Ann Thorac Surg.* 1998;65:1050). Serous drainage from the skin incision is worrisome and should be treated by application of a sterile dressing twice daily and the administration of IV or oral antibiotics. Purulent wound drainage, a sternal click, gross movement of the sternal edges, or substernal air on the chest X-ray may indicate a deep sternal infection. A CT scan of the chest can confirm this diagnosis. In general, deep sternal infections require operative débridement of devitalized sternal and substernal tissues, with cultures of the tissue; administration of broad-spectrum IV antibiotics; and vascularized muscle flap closure of the soft-tissue defect.

9. **Gastrointestinal. Gastrointestinal (GI) complications** are uncommon after cardiac surgical procedures. Stress gastritis can occur after CPB and is thought to be secondary to subclinical ischemia of the gut mucosa. Although overt GI hemorrhage is uncommon, when it does occur, it is associated with a high mortality. Patients should receive proton-pump inhibitor or H_2-receptor–antagonist therapy until a regular diet is begun. GI bleeding may arise from throughout the GI tract. Acute cholecystitis, usually acalculous, is associated with a high mortality.

B. **Ward.** Ward care focuses on convalescence, management of fluid balance, activity level, and diet.

1. **Fluid status.** The patient is weighed daily. Patients who were receiving diuretics preoperatively resume their regimen postoperatively. For patients who were not receiving diuretics preoperatively, oral diuretics are administered until the patient's weight falls to the preoperative value. For most patients, no restrictions are placed on the daily oral fluid intake.

2. **Activity.** The patient is encouraged to be out of bed to a chair and to ambulate as soon as possible after operation. Patients are instructed not to perform any heavy lifting (>10 lb) for a period of 4 weeks postoperatively.

3. **Diet.** A mild postoperative ileus may be present for several days after operation. A regular diet is begun as early as possible after operation. Some patients require a stool softener. Attention should be paid to maintaining a prudent diet that is low in salt and cholesterol.

C. **Postdischarge care.** Care after hospital discharge focuses on continued risk factor modification and surveillance for late complications. Common difficulties during the first 6 to 8 weeks after operation include decreased motivation, decreased appetite, depression, and insomnia. In general, these conditions are temporary, and the physician can provide reassurance.

1. **Physical rehabilitation** with a daily exercise program begins early after operation and continues after discharge from the hospital. Vigorous walking, with increasing distances and longer periods of activity, is the most useful form of exercise for most patients. Bicycling and swimming are acceptable alternatives after 6 to 8 weeks. Patients who were working before operation should return to work within 4 to 6 weeks after operation.

2. **Risk factor modification** may slow or possibly reverse the progression of atherosclerosis in bypass grafts after CABG.

   a. **Smoking** should be discontinued. Referral to organizations with smoking cessation programs should be made before operation, if possible.

   b. **Obesity.** Patients should reach an ideal body weight through planned exercise and dieting.

   c. **Hyperlipidemia** is a major risk factor for the development of graft atherosclerosis and should be treated aggressively, with diet modification and treatment with statins.

   d. **Hypertension** must be controlled.

   e. **Antiplatelet therapy** with aspirin and/or Plavix in patients who underwent coronary artery bypass should be initiated.

   f. **Postpericardiotomy (Dressler) syndrome** is a delayed pericardial inflammatory reaction characterized by fever, anterior chest pain, and pericardial friction rub, and it may lead to mediastinal fibrosis and premature graft occlusion. Treatment includes nonsteroidal anti-inflammatory drugs for 2 to 4 weeks or corticosteroids for refractory cases.

31 General Thoracic Surgery

Ankit Bharat and Bryan F. Meyers

Thoracic surgery encompasses the management of benign and malignant conditions of the esophagus, lung, pleura, and mediastinum. In this chapter, we focus on the systematic evaluation and treatment of the most common thoracic conditions. Disease processes of the esophagus, clearly within the realm of thoracic surgery, are discussed in a separate chapter.

I. **LUNG CANCER.** Lung cancer was a rare disease in the early 20th century. The incidence of lung cancer began to accelerate in the 1930s that mirrored the increased prevalence of cigarette smoking. Dr Alton Oschner was among the first to suggest the association between smoking and lung cancer. Cigarette smoking is the leading risk factor and smoking history influences risk stratification in the evaluation of a suspicious lesion. Currently, lung cancer is the second most common nonskin malignancy, following prostate in men and breast in women. Because of the high case fatality rate, lung cancer is responsible for a larger fraction of cancer deaths in both men and women (29% and 26%, respectively, *www.cancer.org*). An estimated 222,520 cases of lung cancer were diagnosed in 2010 and 157,300 patients died of the disease. Unfortunately, most newly diagnosed cases are not amenable to surgical resection and have poor prognosis. Lung cancer carries an overall 15% 5-year survival. In addition to smoking history, increasing age also increases the probability of lung cancer. Although trials conducted more than two decades ago to screen for lung cancer by either sputum cytology or chest X-ray imaging failed to show benefit, annual spiral computed tomography (CT) scanning can detect lung cancers that are curable (*N Engl J Med.* 2006;355:1822–1824). However, questions remain as to whether the test is sufficiently effective to justify screening people at high risk for lung cancer.

A. **Radiographic presentation**

1. **Solitary pulmonary nodule (SPN).** Because of the widespread application of CT technology, an estimated 200,000 SPNs are diagnosed each year. By conventional definition, these are circumscribed lung lesions in an asymptomatic individual. Lesions greater than 3 cm are called "masses."

2. **Radiographic imaging by CT** is used to both follow these lesions and predict outcome. The first step in the evaluation of an SPN is to evaluate any prior films. Factors favoring a benign lesion include absence of growth over a 2-year period, size of the lesion, and pattern of calcification. Calcifications that are diffuse, centrally located, "onion skinned"

(laminar), or popcornlike are generally benign. Eccentric or stippled calcifications may indicate malignancy. Lesion size greater than 2 cm, intravenous contrast enhancement, and irregular borders all predict malignancy.

3. **Positron emission tomography (PET) scanning** has demonstrated 95% sensitivity and 80% specificity in characterizing SPNs. PET imaging has a high negative predictive value for most lung cancers; however, bronchoalveolar carcinoma and carcinoid tumor can be negative by PET scan, and inflammatory and infectious processes can be falsely positive. The patient's overall risk factor profile must be considered. In the setting of low risk (e.g., young age, nonsmoker, and favorable features on CT), a negative PET scan has a high negative predictive value, but the same result in an elderly smoker is less reassuring, and further evaluation is warranted.

4. **Tissue biopsy** remains the gold standard for diagnosis. Tissue may be obtained by bronchoscopy in patients with central lung lesions or by CT-guided biopsy. This latter technique has 80% sensitivity for a malignant process and requires technical expertise. Surgical biopsy of SPN by either percutaneous radiographic needle biopsy or minimally invasive surgical techniques like video thoracoscopy and radial endobronchial ultrasound (EBUS) can provide a definitive diagnosis and definitive treatment.

B. **Pathology.** The two main classes of lung tumors are small-cell (oat cell) carcinoma and non-small-cell carcinoma.

1. **Small-cell carcinoma** accounts for approximately 20% of all lung cancers. It is highly malignant, usually occurs centrally near the hilum, occurs almost exclusively in smokers, and rarely is amenable to surgery because of wide dissemination by the time of diagnosis. These cancers initially respond to chemotherapy, but overall 5-year survival remains less than 10%.

2. **Non-small-cell carcinomas** account for 80% of all lung cancers and make up the vast majority of those treated by surgery. The three main subtypes are **adenocarcinoma** (30% to 50% of cases), **squamous cell** (20% to 35%), and **large cell** (4% to 15%). Most tumors are histologically heterogeneous, possibly indicating common origin. **Bronchioloalveolar carcinoma** is a variant of adenocarcinoma and is known for its ability to produce mucin and its multifocal nature. Over the last decade, it has been appreciated that carcinoid tumors (grade I), atypical carcinoid tumors (grade II), large-cell carcinoma, and small-cell tumors represent important subgroups of bronchogenic neuroendocrine carcinoma. This may explain the more aggressive behavior of large-cell carcinoma relative to other non-small-cell cancers.

C. **Symptomatic presentation** of lung cancer implies a worsening stage and is associated with an overall lower rate of survival.

1. **Bronchopulmonary features** include cough or a change in a previously stable smoker's cough, increased sputum production, dyspnea, and new wheezing. Minor hemoptysis causing blood-tinged sputum,

even as an isolated episode, should be investigated with flexible bronchoscopy, especially in patients with a history of smoking who are 40 years of age or older. Lung cancer may also present with postobstructive pneumonia.

2. **Extrapulmonary thoracic symptoms** include chest wall pain secondary to local tumor invasion, hoarseness from invasion of the left recurrent laryngeal nerve near the aorta and left main pulmonary artery, shortness of breath secondary to malignant pleural effusion or phrenic nerve invasion, and superior vena cava syndrome causing facial, neck, and upper-extremity swelling. A Pancoast tumor (superior sulcus tumor) can lead to brachial plexus invasion, as well as invasion of the cervical sympathetic ganglia, which causes an ipsilateral Horner syndrome (ptosis, miosis, and anhidrosis). Rarely, lung cancer can present as dysphagia secondary to compression or invasion of the esophagus by mediastinal nodes or by the primary tumor.

   The most frequent **sites of distant metastases** include the liver, bone, brain, adrenal glands, and the contralateral lung. Symptoms may include pathologic fractures and arthritis from bony involvement. Brain metastasis may cause headache, vision changes, or changes in mental status. Adrenal involvement infrequently presents with Addison disease. Lung cancer is the most common tumor causing adrenal dysfunction.

3. **Paraneoplastic syndromes** are frequent and occur secondary to the release of endocrine substances by tumor cells. They include Cushing syndrome (adrenocorticotropic hormone secretion in small-cell carcinoma), syndrome of inappropriate antidiuretic hormone (SIADH), hypercalcemia (parathyroid hormone-related protein secreted by squamous cell carcinomas), hypertrophic pulmonary osteoarthropathy (clubbing of the fingers, stiffness of joints, and periosteal thickening on X-ray), and various myopathies.

D. **Accurate clinical and pathologic staging is critical** in the management of patients with non-small-cell carcinoma because surgery is the primary mode of therapy for many stage I and II patients and selected stage III patients who have enough physiologic reserve to tolerate resection. It is critical to exclude metastatic disease prior to resection. The essential elements of staging include evaluation for lymph node involvement and evaluation for adrenal, brain, and bone metastasis. An anatomic staging system using the classification for tumor, nodal, and metastatic status was most recently modified in 2009 (AJCC 7th edition; Table 31-1).

1. **Chest CT to include the upper abdomen** provides useful information on location, size, and local involvement of tumor and also allows evaluation for liver and adrenal metastasis. CT scanning alone does not accurately determine the resectability of tumor adherent to vital structures. Patients with localized disease may require intraoperative staging to determine resectability. CT also can identify mediastinal lymphadenopathy. However, the sensitivity for identifying metastatic lymph nodes by CT is only 65% to 80% and the specificity is only 65%. With nodes larger than 1 cm, the sensitivity decreases but the specificity increases.

| TABLE 31-1 | American Joint Committee on Cancer Staging System of Lung Cancer |

Tumor Status (T)

T1a	≤2 cm
T1b	>2–3 cm
	No invasion of visceral pleura or more proximal than lobar bronchus
T2a	>3–5 cm
T2b	>5–7 cm
	Involvement of bronchus ≥2 cm distal to the carina
	Invasion of visceral pleura
	Associated atelectasis or obstructive pneumonitis not involving entire lung
T3	>7 cm or tumor with any of the following characteristics:
	Invasion of chest wall, diaphragm, phrenic nerve
	Invasion of mediastinal pleura or parietal pericardium
	Associated atelectasis or obstructive pneumonitis of entire lung
	Tumor within main bronchus <2 cm from carina but does not involve carina
	Satellite nodules in the same lobe
T4	Tumor with any of the following characteristics:
	Mediastinal invasion
	Invasion of heart of great vessels
	Invasion of carina, trachea, esophagus, or recurrent laryngeal nerve
	Invasion of vertebral body
	Separate tumor nodules in a different but ipsilateral lobe

Nodal Involvement (N)

N0	None
N1	Hilar, interlobar, or peripheral lymph node zones
N2	Ipsilateral mediastinal lymph nodes, subcarinal, or aortopulmonary lymph nodes
N3	Contralateral mediastinal, hilar, or aortopulmonary lymph nodes; ipsilateral or contralateral scalene or supraclavicular lymph nodes

Distant Metastases (M)

M0	None
M1	Distant metastases present

TABLE 31-1	American Joint Committee on Cancer Staging System of Lung Cancer *(Continued)*

Stage		5-y Survival
Ia	T1a/T1b N0 M0	50%–80%
Ib	T2a N0 M0	47%
IIa	T1a/T1b, N1 M0	36%
	T2a N1 M0	
	T2b N0 M0	
IIb	T2b N1 M0	26%
	T3 N0 M0	
IIIa	T1/ T2 N2M0	19%
	T3 N1/N2 M0	
	T4 N0/N1 M0	
IIIb	T4 N2 M0	7%
	Any T with N3 M0	
IV	Any T, any N, M1	2%

2. **PET imaging** is often used to stage patients with non-small-cell carcinoma, but its accuracy for detecting primary tumors and metastatic disease may be limited by the presence of inflammation and ongoing infection. In regions endemic for inflammatory processes such as tuberculosis and histoplasmosis, the usefulness of PET imaging for investigating mediastinal lymph nodes is limited. However, it can be useful for identifying occult distant metastatic disease to the liver, adrenals, and bone.

3. **Lymph node staging** of the mediastinum is done using either **EBUS**-guided fine needle aspiration or **mediastinoscopy.** The pretracheal, paratracheal, and subcarinal lymph nodes can be easily accessed by these techniques. With experience, the sensitivity and specificity of EBUS can approach that of mediastinoscopy. For sampling aortopulmonary nodes, either **Video-assisted thoracoscopic surgery (VATS)** or, less commonly, **anterior mediastinoscopy (chamberlain procedure)** is performed. Mediastinoscopy still remains the gold standard. Although invasive, it is safe, with less than a 1% complication rate. Routine use of these technique in the staging of patients with non–small-cell carcinoma should be favored, with the exception of select patients with clinical stage I lung cancer staged by CT and PET with no abnormal lymphadenopathy. These patients benefit little from lymph node staging (*J Thorac Cardiovasc Surg.* 2006;131:822–829). The timing of mediastinoscopy, whether at the time of thoracotomy or before a planned resection, is controversial and depends on the surgeon's preference and the availability of accurate pathologic evaluation of mediastinal lymph node frozen sections.

4. **CT or magnetic resonance (MR) imaging of the brain** to identify brain metastases is mandatory in the patient with neurologic symptoms but is controversial as a routine part of the work-up of symptomatic patients. Given the reported, albeit low, incidence of CNS metastasis in the setting of even small primary tumors, we advocate the routine use of brain imaging.

5. **Bone scan** is sometimes obtained in patients with specific symptoms of skeletal pain and selectively as part of the general preoperative metastatic work-up. The routine use of PET imaging in many centers has eliminated the routine use of this modality.

6. **Fiberoptic bronchoscopy** is important in diagnosing and assessing the extent of the endobronchial lesion. Although peripheral cancers rarely can be seen with bronchoscopy, preoperative bronchoscopy is important for excluding synchronous lung cancers (found in approximately 1% of patients) prior to resection. Bronchial washings with culture can be taken at the time of bronchoscopy in patients with significant secretions.

E. **Preoperative assessment of pulmonary** function and estimation of postoperative pulmonary assessment is the most critical factor in planning lung resection for cancer.

1. **Pulmonary function tests** and **arterial blood gas analysis** are the standard by which the risk of developing postoperative pulmonary failure is determined. In general, pulmonary resection is associated with a 1% to 2% mortality risk if preoperative FEV_1 (forced expiratory volume in 1 second) is greater than 1.5 L for lobectomy, greater than 2 L for pneumonectomy and is greater than 80% predicted. Predicted postoperative FEV_1 is less than 0.8L or less than 40% is associated with high mortality. **Diffusion capacity, quantitative ventilation–perfusion scan, and exercise testing** are indicated in patients with marginal function for accurate assessment of postoperative function. These tests allow the surgeon to estimate how much the planned target for resection contributes to the overall pulmonary function. Postoperative predicted FEV_1 postpneumonectomy = Preoperative FEV_1 × (1-fraction of total perfusion of the resected lung). Postoperative predicted FEV_1 postlobectomy = preoperative FEV_1 × (1-y/z), where y = functional or unobstructed segments to be resected and z = total number of functional segments. Preoperative diffusion capacity (DLCO) less than 80% is associated with two- or threefold increased risk of pulmonary complication and less than 60% with increased mortality. In general, an estimated postresection FEV_1 of 800 cc or greater suggests that the patient will tolerate a pneumonectomy. Preoperative hypercapnia (arterial carbon dioxide tension >45 mm Hg) may preclude resection.

2. **Evaluation of cardiac disease** is critical for minimizing perioperative complications. Patients with lung cancer are often at high risk for coronary disease because of extensive smoking histories. A detailed history and physical examination to elicit signs and symptoms of ischemia and a baseline electrocardiogram (ECG) are the initial steps. Any abnormal

findings should be aggressively pursued with stress tests or coronary catheterization.

3. **Smoking cessation** preoperatively for as little as 2 weeks can aid in the regeneration of the mucociliary function and pulmonary toilet and has been associated with fewer postoperative respiratory complications.

F. In summary, all patients should have a chest CT scan to evaluate the primary tumor and the mediastinum and to check for metastatic disease to the brain and adrenals. PET imaging or bone scan is useful to exclude bone metastasis. Lymph node staging with either EBUS or mediastinoscopy should be performed to exclude mediastinal lymph node metastasis prior to resection, except possibly in patients with clinical stage Ia disease. All patients should undergo a fiberoptic bronchoscopy by the surgeon before thoracotomy; this is usually done at the same setting as lymph node staging.

G. Operative principles. In the patient able to tolerate any resection, the minimal extent of resection is usually an anatomic lobectomy. Even in stage I disease, a limited resection, such as a wedge resection, results in a threefold higher incidence of local recurrence and a decreased overall and disease-free survival. Patients with limited pulmonary reserve may be treated by segmental or wedge resection. Most centers report operative mortality of less than 2% with lobectomy and 6% with pneumonectomy. Minimally invasive techniques for anatomic resection are becoming common and it is speculated that most resections will soon be performed via VATS.

H. **Five-year survival rates range** from 70% to 80% for stage Ia (T1N0) disease and 40% to 60% for stage Ib (T2aN0) disease. Stage I disease is generally treated with surgical resection alone. The presence of ipsilateral intrapulmonary lymph nodes decreases the overall survival to 36% for stage IIa (T1N1, T2aN1) disease and 26% for stage IIb (T2bN1) disease. Stage II cancers are also treated with surgical resection. However, adjuvant chemotherapy has been associated with improved 5-year survival and is now routinely recommended in patients with stage II or stage III disease. Adjuvant radiation therapy is considered in patients with close surgical margins or central N1 lymph node metastasis.

Certain patients with stage IIIa disease appear to benefit form surgical resection alone (T3N1M0). However, selected patients with mediastinal lymph node metastasis (N2 disease) may be candidates for surgical resection after neoadjuvant chemoradiation therapy. Patients with bulky, diffuse mediastinal lymphadenopathy are typically treated using definitive chemoradiation. The optimal regimen of chemotherapy, radiation, or a combination of both is being investigated in clinical trials. Stage IIIb tumors involve the contralateral mediastinal or hilar lymph nodes, the ipsilateral scalene or supraclavicular lymph nodes, extensive mediastinal invasion, intrapulmonary metastasis, or malignant pleural effusions. These tumors are considered unresectable. Stage IV tumors have distant metastases and are also considered unresectable. However, selected patients with node-negative lung cancer and a solitary brain metastasis have achieved long-term survival with combined resection.

II. **TUMORS OF THE PLEURA.** The most common tumor of the pleura is the rare but aggressive **mesothelioma.** Less common tumors include lipomas, angiomas, soft-tissue sarcomas, and fibrous histiocytomas.

A. Malignant mesothelioma

1. *Incidence:* Selikoff et al. first reported the link between asbestos and mesothelioma in 1968. It is estimated that asbestos exposure is associated with mesothelioma in 80% of the cases. Incidence of mesothelioma has been increasing since 1980 and about 2,500 to 3,000 cases occur each year in United States. Taking the latency period of 20 to 50 years from asbestos exposure, the peak incidence of mesotheliomas will be encountered by 2020.

2. *Epidemiology:* Mesothelioma is primarily a disease of men in the fifth through seventh decades of life. Patient presentation may be variable. Although benign mesothelioma variants are not associated with asbestos exposure and are asymptomatic, patients with the more common malignant form often report chest pain, malaise, cough, weakness, weight loss, and shortness of breath with pleural effusion. One-third of patients report paraneoplastic symptoms of osteoarthropathy, hypoglycemia, and fever.

3. *Diagnosis:* Tissue is necessary for definitive diagnosis. Cytology of pleural fluid has a 30% to 62% diagnostic yield. Needle biopsy of pleural is used in some centers and has a reported yield of 68%. However, thoracoscopy is the best modality with greater than 90% diagnostic yield. Further, it allows evaluation of pleural, pericardial, and diaphragmatic surfaces for staging. CT scan is useful in differentiating pleural from parenchymal disease. Malignant mesothelioma usually appears as markedly thickened, irregular, pleural-based mass, or thickened pleura with pleural effusion. Occasionally, only a pleural effusion is seen. Routine use of MRI is not recommended but it is superior to CT for identifying transdiaphragmatic extension of tumor into the abdomen or mediastinal invasion. PET scan is being increasingly used as it can identify distant metastatic disease that is missed by CT scan (*J Thorac Cardiovasc Surg.* 2003;126:11–15).

4. *Classification:* The most common and favorable subtype is epithelioid (50%), followed by sarcomatoid (15% to 20%), mixed, and desmoplastic. Careful distinction using histology and immunostaining is required between malignant mesothelioma, especially epithelioid type, and adenocarcinoma.

5. *Staging and treatment:* Three staging systems have been described: American Joint Commission against Cancer (AJCC), Brigham and Women's Hospital (BWH), and the Butchart. Median survival of patients with untreated malignant mesothelioma is 8 to 10 months. Smoking, male gender, advanced stage, and asbestos exposure are prognostic of worse survival. Epithelioid histotype has the most favorable survival. The treatment consists of a multimodal therapy comprising surgery, combination chemotherapy, and radiation. Surgical options include extrapleural pneumonectomy or pleurectomy/decortication.

Consensus is lacking on the choice of surgical procedure. However, for early stage cases, extrapleural pneumonectomy may offer the best chance of cure. The best reported 5-year survival following completion of the multimodal therapy in patients without nodal metastasis is 53% (*J Clin Oncol.* 2009;27:1413–1418).

III. **TUMORS OF THE MEDIASTINUM.** The location of a mass in relation to the heart helps the surgeon to form a differential diagnosis (Table 31-2). On the lateral chest X-ray, the mediastinum is divided into thirds, with the heart comprising the middle segment.

A. **Epidemiology.** In all age groups, lymphoma is the most common mediastinal tumor. Neurogenic tumors are more likely in children. The likelihood of malignancy is greatest in the second to fourth decades of life. The presence of symptoms is more suggestive of a malignant lesion. Symptoms are often nonspecific and include dyspnea, cough, hoarseness, vague chest pain, and fever.

TABLE 31-2	Differential Diagnosis of Tumors Located in the Mediastinum	
Anterior	**Middle**	**Posterior**
Thymoma	Congenital cyst	Neurogenic
Germ cell	Lymphoma	Lymphoma
Teratoma	Primary cardiac	Mesenchymal
Seminoma	Neural crest	
Nonseminoma		
Lymphoma		
Parathyroid		
Lipoma		
Fibroma		
Lymphangioma		
Aberrant thyroid		

Modified from Young RM, Kernstine KH, Corson JD. Miscellaneous cardiopulmonary conditions. In: Corson JD, Williamson RCN, eds. *Surgery.* Philadelphia: Mosby; 2001.

B. **Evaluation.** Chest X-ray is often used as a screening tool and can lead to the diagnosis of a mass. This should be followed by a CT scan to further delineate the anatomy.

C. **Tumors.** Because of the prevalence of germ cell tumors, all anterior mediastinal masses should be evaluated with biochemical markers β-human chorionic gonadotropin (β-HCG) and α-fetoprotein (AFP).

1. **Teratomas** are usually benign and often contain ectodermal components such as hair, teeth, and bone. Elevation of both β-HCG and AFP is very rare, and it suggests a malignant teratoma. Treatment is surgical resection.

2. **Seminomas** do not present with an elevation in AFP, and fewer than 10% present with an elevation in β-HCG. Their treatment is primarily nonsurgical (radiation and chemotherapy), except in the case of localized disease.

3. **Nonseminomatous germ cell** tumors present with an elevation of both tumor markers. Again, the treatment is primarily nonsurgical, with the exception of obtaining tissue for diagnosis and resecting residual masses after definitive chemotherapy.

4. Tissue diagnosis is often crucial for the diagnosis and treatment of **lymphoma.** Treatment is primarily nonsurgical. Cervical lymph node biopsy, CT-guided biopsy, or mediastinoscopy with biopsy may be required. These lesions often present as irregular masses on CT scan.

5. Patients with paravertebral or posterior mediastinal masses should have their catecholamine levels measured to rule out **pheochromocytomas.**

IV. THYMUS GLAND

A. The physiologic role of thymus is still poorly understood. Tumors of thymus (thymomas) are composed of cytologically bland epithelial cells with a variable admixture of lymphocytes. Because these tumors are relatively rare, consensus on the classification and management of these tumors is lacking. Most behave as if benign, but the presence of invasion of its fibrous capsule defines malignancy. Whereas 15% of myasthenia gravis patients have a thymoma, approximately 50% of patients with a thymoma have some version of paraneoplastic syndromes, including myasthenia gravis, hypogammaglobulinemia, and red cell aplasia.

Although the role of the thymus gland in myasthenia gravis is poorly understood, it appears to be important in the generation of autoreactive antibodies directed against the acetylcholine receptor. Greater than 80% of cases demonstrate complete or partial response to thymectomy. Chances of improvement are increased if thymectomy is performed early in the course of disease (first signs of muscle weakness) or if the myasthenia is not associated with a thymoma.

B. **Preoperative preparation** of the patient with myasthenia gravis involves reduction in corticosteroid dose, if appropriate, and the weaning of anticholinesterases. Plasmapheresis can be performed preoperatively to aid in discontinuation of anticholinesterase agents. Muscle relaxants and atropine should be avoided during the anesthetic.

C. **Operative approach** for thymectomy for myasthenia in cases in the absence of a thymoma or a mass lesion is controversial. The options range from median sternotomy to a transcervical thymectomy. The transcervical approach involves a low-collar incision and is facilitated by using a table-mounted retractor to elevate the manubrium and expose the thymic tissue for resection. The transcervical approach has lower morbidity, but there are questions as to whether it is as efficacious as the transsternal approach. In bulky thymic disease, and for any tumors of the thymus, a median sternotomy approach is preferred to provide maximal exposure for complete resection.

V. PNEUMOTHORAX

A. Pneumothorax is the presence of air in the pleural cavity, leading to separation of the visceral and parietal pleura. This disruption of the potential space disrupts pulmonary mechanics, and, if left untreated, it may progress to tension physiology. In tension pneumothorax, cardiac compromise occurs and presents a true emergency. The etiology may be spontaneous, iatrogenic, or due to trauma. The etiology will determine the most appropriate short- and long-term management strategies.

B. **Physical examination** may demonstrate decreased breath sounds on the involved side if the lung is more than 25% collapsed. Hyperresonance on the affected side is possible. Common symptoms include dyspnea and chest pain. Careful examination for signs of tension pneumothorax (including deviation of the trachea to the opposite side, respiratory distress, and hypotension) must be performed. If there is no clinical evidence of tension pneumothorax, an upright chest X-ray will be required to establish the diagnosis. Smaller pneumothoraces may only be evident on expiration chest X-rays or CT scan. The clinical setting will influence their management.

C. **Management options** include observation, aspiration, chest tube placement with or without pleurodesis, and surgery. The etiology of the pneumothorax influences management strategy.

1. **Observation** is an option in a healthy, asymptomatic patient. This should only be reserved for small pneumothoraces. Generally speaking, if there is a lateral extension of pneumothorax on a plain radiograph, an intervention should be considered. Supplemental oxygen may help to reabsorb the pneumothorax by affecting the gradient of nitrogen in the body and in the pneumothorax.

2. **Aspiration** of the pneumothorax may be done using a small catheter attached to a three-way stopcock. This should be reserved for situations with low suspicion of an ongoing air leak.

3. **Percutaneous catheters** may be placed using Seldinger technique. Multiple commercial kits (like Cook's Thal-Quick) exist and allow for the catheter to be placed to a Heimlich valve or to suction. The catheters in

these kits are generally of small caliber, and their use is limited to situations of simple pneumothorax. Also, if there is any concern for lung adhesions, bedside percutaneous catheters should be avoided.

4. **Tube thoracostomy** remains the gold standard, especially for larger pneumothoraces, for persistent air leaks, when there is an expected need for pleurodesis, or for associated effusion.

    a. Chest tubes may be connected either to a Heimlich flutter valve, to a simple underwater-seal system, or to vacuum suction. The two most commonly used systems are the Pleurovac and Emerson systems. Both systems may be placed to a water seal (providing -3-cm to -5-cm H_2O suction) or to vacuum suction (typically -20 cm). Digital chest tube monitoring systems are also available now and can track the pleural pressure and air leak continuously.

    b. If the water-seal chamber bubbles with expiration or with coughing, this is evident that an air leak persists. In most cases, the tube stays in until the air leak stops.

5. **Bedside pleurodesis.** Sclerosing agents may be administered through the chest tube to induce fusion of the parietal and visceral pleural surfaces. Doxycycline, bleomycin, and talc have all been described.

    a. Bedside pleurodesis can be associated with an inflammatory pneumonitis in the lung on the treated side. In patients with limited pulmonary reserve, this may present as clinically significant hypoxia. Pleurodesis can be quite uncomfortable for the patient, and adequate analgesia is mandatory. Patient-controlled analgesic pump and bolus administration of ketorolac (if tolerated) are effective.

    b. Doxycycline is often used as the sclerosing agent for benign processes.

        (1) It is administered as 500 mg in 100 mL of normal saline. Doxycycline is extremely irritating to the pleural surfaces; therefore, 30 mL of 1% lidocaine can be administered via the chest tube before the doxycycline is given and used to flush the drug again. The total dose of lidocaine should not exceed the toxic dose, which is usually 5 mg/kg.

        (2) In patients with large air leaks, the chest tube should not be clamped, to prevent the development of a tension pneumothorax. Instead, the drainage kit should be elevated to maintain the effective water-seal pressure at -20 cm H_2O while keeping the sclerosant in the pleural space.

        (3) The patient (with assistance) is instructed to roll from supine to right lateral decubitus to left lateral decubitus every 15 minutes for 2 hours. Prone, Trendelenburg, and reverse Trendelenburg positions should also be part of the sequence if the patient is able to tolerate it.

        (4) The chest tube is unclamped and returned to suction after the procedure.

    c. Talc is a less painful sclerosing agent. Because of largely unfounded concern about introducing a potentially carcinogenic agent and permanent foreign body, it is generally limited to older patients with underlying malignant conditions (see Effusions, Section VII.A.4.a).

   (1) Talc, 5 g in 180 mL of sterile saline split into 360-mL catheter syringes, is administered via the chest tube and then flushed with an additional 60 mL of saline. A handy aerosol is available for use in the operating room.

   (2) The patient is instructed to change positions as described previously.

6. Surgery is performed using a video-assisted approach or by thoracotomy. Patients who have a persistent air leak secondary to a ruptured bleb but are otherwise well should be considered for surgery. By this point, patients have already undergone stabilization by chest tube placement (see Section V.D.3 for specific indications for surgery).

   a. Etiology

   (1) Iatrogenic pneumothoraces usually are the result of pleural injury during central venous access attempts, pacemaker placement, or transthoracic or transbronchial lung biopsy. Hence, a postprocedure chest X-ray is mandatory. Often the injury to the lung is small and self-limited. The extent of pneumothorax and associated injury should determine the need for invasive procedures. Observation or percutaneous placement of a chest tube may be appropriate in a patient who is not mechanically ventilated.

   (2) Spontaneous pneumothorax is typically caused by rupture of an apical bleb. Up to 80% of patients are tall, young adults, and men outnumber women by 6 to 1; it is more common in smokers than in nonsmokers. The typical patient presents with acute onset of shortness of breath and chest pain on the side of the collapsed lung. Patients older than 40 years usually have significant parenchymal disease, such as emphysema. These patients present with a ruptured bulla and often have a more dramatic presentation, including tachypnea, cyanosis, and hypoxia. There is a significant risk of recurrence, and pleurodesis or surgical intervention is considered after the first or second occurrence. Other etiologies of spontaneous pneumothorax include cystic fibrosis and, rarely, lung cancer.

   (3) Indications for operation for spontaneous pneumothorax include (1) recurrent ipsilateral pneumothoraces, (2) bilateral pneumothoraces, (3) persistent air leaks on chest tube suction (usually >5 days), and (4) first episodes occurring in patients with high-risk occupations (e.g., pilots and divers) or those who live at a great distance from medical care facilities. The risk of ipsilateral recurrence of a spontaneous pneumothorax is 50%, 62%, and 80% after the first, second, and third episodes, respectively.

Operative management consists of stapled wedge resection of blebs or bullae, usually found in the apex of the upper lobe or superior segment of the lower lobe. Pleural abrasion (pleurodesis) should be done to promote formation of adhesions between visceral and parietal pleurae. Video-assisted thoracoscopic techniques have allowed procedures to be less invasive in most cases. Using two or three small port incisions on the affected side, thoracoscopic stapling of the involved apical bulla and pleurodesis can be done. Alternatively, a transaxillary thoracotomy incision gives excellent exposure of the upper lung through a limited incision.

7. **Traumatic** pneumothoraces may be caused by either blunt or penetrating thoracic trauma and often result in lung contusion and multiple rib injury.

   a. **Evaluation and treatment** begin with the initial stabilization of airway and circulation. A chest X-ray should be obtained.

   b. **Prompt chest tube insertion** is performed to evacuate air and blood. In 80% of patients with penetrating trauma to the hemithorax, exploratory thoracotomy is unnecessary, and chest tube decompression with observation is sufficient. Indications for operation include immediate drainage of greater than 1,500 mL of blood after tube insertion or persistent bleeding of greater than 200 mL/hour. Patients with multiple injuries and proven pneumothoraces or significant chest injuries should have prophylactic chest tubes placed before general anesthesia because of the risk of tension pneumothorax with positive-pressure ventilation.

   c. **Pulmonary contusion** is associated with traumatic pneumothorax. The contusion usually is evident on the initial chest X-ray (as opposed to aspiration, in which several hours may elapse before an infiltrative pattern appears on serial radiographs), and it appears as a fluffy infiltrate that progresses in extent and density over 24 to 48 hours.

   d. The contusion may be associated with multiple rib fractures, leading to a **flail chest.** This occurs when several ribs are broken segmentally, allowing for a portion of the chest wall to be "floating" and to move paradoxically with breathing (inward on inspiration). The paradoxical movement and splinting secondary to pain and the associated pain lead to a reduction in vital capacity and to ineffective ventilation.

   e. All patients with suspected contusions and rib fractures should have aggressive pain control measures, including patient-controlled analgesia pumps, epidural catheters, and/or intercostal nerve blocks.

   f. **Intravenous fluid should be minimized** to the extent allowed by the patient's clinical status because of associated increased capillary endothelial permeability. Serial arterial blood gas measurements are important for close monitoring of respiratory status. Close monitoring and a high index of suspicion for respiratory decompensation are necessary. Intubation, positive-pressure ventilation, and even tracheostomy are sometimes necessary.

g. A traumatic bronchopleural fistula can occur after penetrating or blunt chest trauma. If mechanical ventilation is ineffective secondary to the large air leak, emergent thoracotomy and repair are usually necessary. On occasion, selective intubation of the uninvolved bronchus can provide short-term stability in the minutes before definitive operative treatment.

h. The unusual circumstance known as a **sucking chest wound** consists of a full-thickness hole in the chest wall greater than two thirds the diameter of the trachea. With inspiration, air flows through the wound because of the low resistance to flow and the lung collapses. This requires immediate coverage of the hole with an occlusive dressing and chest tube insertion to reexpand the lung. If tube thoracostomy cannot be immediately performed, coverage with an occlusive dressing taped on three sides functions as a one-way valve to prevent the accumulation of air within the chest, although tube thoracostomy should be performed as soon as possible.

VI. HEMOPTYSIS can originate from a number of causes, including infectious, malignant, and cardiac disorders (e.g., bronchitis or tuberculosis, bronchogenic carcinoma, and mitral stenosis, respectively).

A. Massive hemoptysis requires emergent thoracic surgical intervention, often with little time for formal studies before entering the operating room. The surgeon is called primarily for significant hemoptysis, which is defined by some as more than 600 mL of blood expelled over 48 hours or, more often, a volume of blood that is impairing gas exchange. Because the volume of the main airways is approximately 200 mL, even smaller amounts of blood can cause severe respiratory compromise. Prompt treatment is required to avoid life-threatening airway obstruction. As baseline lung function decreases, a lower volume and rate of hemoptysis is capable of severely compromising gas exchange.

1. A **brief focused history** can often elucidate the etiology of the bleed, such as a history of tuberculosis or aspergillosis. A recent chest X-ray may reveal the diagnosis in up to half of cases. Chest CT is rarely helpful in the acute setting and is thus unsafe and contraindicated in patients who are unstable. Smaller amounts of hemoptysis can be evaluated by radiologic examinations in conjunction with bronchoscopy.

2. **Bronchoscopy** is the mainstay of diagnosis and initial treatment of major episodes of hemoptysis. Although it may not eliminate later episodes of bleeding, it can allow for temporizing measures, such as placement of balloon-tipped catheters and topical or injected vasoconstrictors. In a setting of massive hemoptysis, the patient should be prepared for a rigid bronchoscopy, which is best performed in the operating room under general anesthesia. Asphyxiation is the primary cause of death in patients with massive hemoptysis. Rigid bronchoscopy allows for rapid and effective clearance of blood and clot from the airway, rapid identification of the bleeding side, and prompt protection of the remaining lung parenchyma (with cautery, by packing with epinephrine-soaked gauze, or by placement of a balloon-tipped catheter in the lobar orifice).

3. In cases in which the **etiology** and the precise bleeding source are not identified by bronchoscopy, ongoing bleeding requires protection of the contralateral lung. Selective ventilation, either with a double-lumen tube or by direct intubation of the contralateral mainstem bronchus, may be critical to avoid asphyxiation.

4. **After isolation of the bleeding site, angiographic embolization** of a bronchial arterial source may allow for lung salvage without the need for resection. The bronchial circulation is almost always the source of hemoptysis. Bleeding from the pulmonary circulation is seen only in patients with pulmonary hypertension.

5. **Definitive therapy** may require thoracotomy with lobar resection or, rarely, pneumonectomy. Infrequently, emergent surgical resection is necessary to control the hemoptysis. The etiology of the bleeding and the pulmonary reserve of the patient are important because many patients are not candidates for surgical resection.

VII. PLEURAL EFFUSION

A. Pleural effusion may result from a wide spectrum of benign, malignant, and inflammatory conditions. By history, it is often possible to deduce the etiology, but diagnosis often depends on the analysis of the pleural fluid. The presentation of symptoms depends on the underlying etiology, and treatment is based on the underlying disease process.

1. **Chest X-ray** is often the first diagnostic test. Depending on radiographic technique, an effusion may remain hidden. Although decubitus films are the most sensitive for detecting small, free-flowing effusions, the same volume may remain hidden in a standard antero-posterior film. A concave meniscus in the costophrenic angle on an upright chest X-ray suggests at least 250 mL of pleural fluid. CT scan and ultrasound can be particularly helpful if the fluid is not free flowing or if history suggests a more chronic organizing process such as empyema.

2. **Thoracentesis**

   a. The technique of thoracentesis is described in Chapter 37.

   b. The fluid should be sent for culture and Gram stain, biochemical analyses [pH, glucose, amylase, lactate dehydrogenase (LDH), and protein levels], and a differential cell count and cytology to rule out malignancy.

   c. In general, thin, yellowish, clear fluid is common with transudative effusions; cloudy and foul-smelling fluid usually signals infection or early empyema; bloody effusions often denote malignancy; milky white fluid suggests chylothorax; and pH less than 7.2 suggests bacterial infection or connective tissue disease.

   d. Larger volumes (several hundred milliliters) can often aid the cytopathologists in making a diagnosis. White blood cell count greater than $10,000/mm^3$ suggests pyogenic etiology. A predominance of lymphocytes is noted with tuberculosis. Glucose is decreased in infectious processes as well as in malignancy.

    e. Pleural effusions are broadly categorized as either **transudative** (protein-poor fluid not involving primary pulmonary pathology) or **exudative** (resulting from increased vascular permeability as a result of diseased pleura or pleural lymphatics). Protein and LDH levels measured simultaneously in the pleural fluid and serum provide the diagnosis in nearly all settings.

    f. Exudative pleural effusions satisfy at least one of the following criteria: (1) ratio of pleural fluid protein to serum protein greater than 0.5, (2) ratio of pleural fluid LDH to serum LDH greater than 0.6, or (3) pleural fluid LDH greater than two thirds the upper normal limit for serum.

3. **Transudative pleural effusion** can usually be considered a secondary diagnosis; therefore, therapy should be directed at the underlying problem (e.g., congestive heart failure, cirrhosis, or nephrotic syndrome). Therapeutic drainage is rarely indicated because fluid rapidly reaccumulates unless the underlying cause improves.

4. **Exudative pleural effusion** may be broadly classified based on whether its cause is benign or malignant.

    a. **Malignant** effusions are most often associated with cancers of the breast, lung, and ovary and with lymphoma. Diagnosis is often made by cytology, but in the event that this process is not diagnostic, pleural biopsy may be indicated. Given the overall poor prognosis in these patients, **therapy offered by the thoracic surgeon is generally palliative.**

        (1) **Drainage** of effusion to alleviate dyspnea and improve pulmonary mechanics by reexpanding the lung may be done with chest tube placement or indwelling pleurX catheters.

        (2) **Pleurodesis** with talc or doxycycline may prevent reaccumulation of the effusion.

    b. **Benign exudative effusions** are most often a result of pneumonia (parapneumonic). The process begins with a sterile parapneumonic exudative effusion and leads to a suppurative infection of the pleural space, empyema, if the effusion becomes infected. The initially free-flowing fluid becomes infected and begins to deposit fibrin and cellular debris (5 to 7 days). Eventually, this fluid becomes organized, and a thick, fibrous peel entraps the lung (10 to 14 days).

        (1) **Empyema.** Fifty percent of empyemas are complications of pneumonia; 25% are complications of esophageal, pulmonary, or mediastinal surgery; and 10% are extensions from subphrenic abscesses. Thoracentesis is diagnostic but is sufficient treatment in only the earliest cases.

        (2) The **clinical presentation** of empyema ranges from systemic sepsis requiring emergent care to chronic loculated effusion in a patient who complains of fatigue. Other symptoms include pleuritic chest pain, fever, cough, and dyspnea.

        (3) The **most common offending organisms** are Gram-positive cocci (*Staphylococcus aureus* and streptococci) and Gram-negative organisms (*Escherichia coli* and *Pseudomonas* and *Klebsiella* species). *Bacteroides* species are also common.

(4) Management includes control of the infection by appropriate antibiotics, drainage of the pleural space, and obliteration of the empyema space. Once the diagnosis is made, treatment should not be delayed. Specific management depends on the phase of the empyema, which depends on the character of the fluid. If the fluid does not layer on posteroanterior and lateral and decubitus chest X-ray, a CT scan should be done.

(a) Early or **exudative empyema** is usually adequately treated with simple tube drainage.

(b) Fibropurulent empyema may be amenable to tube drainage alone, but the fluid may be loculated. The loculations of empyema cavities are composed of fibrin.

(c) In advanced or **organizing empyema,** the fluid is thicker and a fibrous peel encases the lung. Thoracotomy may be necessary to free the entrapped lung.

(d) If a patient has a **persistent fluid collection with an adequately placed tube** as evidenced by chest CT, intrapleural fibrinolytic therapy may be indicated. Intrapleural streptokinase, 250,000 units, is divided into three doses, each in 60 mL of normal saline. A dose is administered and flushed with 30 mL of normal saline. The tube is clamped and the patient rolled as described for pleurodesis; then the tube is returned to suction. The procedure is repeated every 8 hours. Alternatively, 250,000 units can be administered daily for 3 days. The adequacy of treatment is determined by resolution of the fluid collection and complete reexpansion of the lung.

(e) A **postpneumonectomy empyema** is one of the most difficult complications to manage in thoracic surgery. Typically, there is a dehiscence of the bronchial stump and contamination of the pneumonectomy space with bronchial flora. The finding of air in the pneumonectomy space on chest X-ray is often diagnostic. The incidence of major bronchopleural fistula after pulmonary resection varies from 2% to 10% and has a high mortality (16% to 70%). Initial management includes thorough drainage (either open or closed) of the infected pleural space, antibiotics, and pulmonary toilet.

(f) Definitive surgical repair of the fistula may include primary closure of a long bronchial stump or closure of the fistula using vascularized muscle or omental flaps. The residual pleural cavity can be obliterated by a muscle transposition, thoracoplasty, or delayed Clagett procedure.

(i) Initially, a chest tube is inserted to evacuate the empyema. Great caution should be taken in inserting chest tubes into postpneumonectomy empyemas. A communicating bronchial stump–pleural fistula can contaminate the contralateral lung rapidly when decompression of the empyema is attempted. The patient should be positioned with the affected side down so that the remaining lung is not contaminated with empyema fluid. This procedure might best be handled in the operating room.

(ii) **After the patient is stabilized,** the next step usually is the creation of a **Clagett window thoracostomy** to provide a venue for daily packing and to maintain external drainage of the infected pleural space. This typically involves reopening the thoracotomy incision at its anterolateral end and resecting a short segment of two or three ribs to create generous access to the pleural space. The pleura is then treated with irrigation and débridement. After a suitable interval (weeks to months), the wound edges can be excised, and the pneumonectomy space is closed either primarily or with a muscle flap after it has been filled with 0.25% neomycin solution. Alternatively, the space can be filled with vascularized muscle flap.

VIII. CHRONIC OBSTRUCTIVE PULMONARY DISEASE (COPD), LUNG VOLUME REDUCTION, AND TRANSPLANTATION

A. The long-term consequences of smoking lead not only to lung cancer but also to **COPD.**

1. **Destruction of lung parenchyma** occurs in a nonuniform manner. As lung tissue loses its elastic recoil, the areas of destruction expand. This expansion of diseased areas, in combination with inflammation, leads to poor ventilation of relatively normal lung.

2. This leads to the **typical findings of hyperexpanded lungs** on chest X-ray: flattened diaphragms, widened intercostal spaces, and horizontal ribs. On pulmonary function testing, patients present with increased residual volumes and decreased FEV_1.

3. Despite maximal medical and surgical treatment, the **disease is progressive.** Surgical treatment is generally reserved for the symptomatic (dyspnea) patient who has failed maximal medical treatment, with the goal of improving symptoms.

4. The **goals of surgery** are to remove diseased areas of lung and allow improved function of the remaining lung tissue.

B. The mainstays of surgical treatment have been bullectomy, lung volume reduction, and transplantation. Prior to any surgical intervention, patients must be carefully selected. Smoking cessation for at least 6 months is mandatory, as is enrollment in a supervised pulmonary rehabilitation program.

1. **Bullectomy.** Patients with emphysema may have large bullous disease. Emphysematous bullae are giant air sacs and may become secondarily infected.

2. **Lung volume reduction** may be indicated in symptomatic patients who have predominantly apical disease, with FEV_1 greater than 20%

of predicted, and patients who may be too old for transplantation. However, several patients have undergone lung volume reduction prior to getting a lung transplant. Through a bilateral VATS approach or a sternotomy incision, one or both lungs have areas of heavily diseased lung resected. Patients with diffuse homogeneous emphysema are not candidates for this procedure.

3. Emphysema and α_1-antitrypsin deficiency have become the leading indications for lung transplantation. Other common indications include cystic fibrosis, pulmonary fibrosis, and pulmonary hypertension.

   a. Patients selected for lung transplantation generally are younger, have diffuse involvement of emphysema, and have FEV_1 less than 20%.

   b. Both single-lung and bilateral-lung transplantation have been performed for emphysema, although bilateral transplant patients have improved long-term survival.

   c. The only absolute indication for bilateral lung transplantation is cystic fibrosis because single-lung transplantation would leave a chronically infected native lung in an immunocompromised patient.

   d. Long-term, chronic allograft dysfunction in the form of bronchiolitis obliterans occurs in 50% of patients.

IX. ISSUES IN THE CARE OF THE THORACIC PATIENT

A. Postoperative care of the thoracic surgery patient focuses on three factors: control of incisional pain, maintenance of pulmonary function, and monitoring of cardiovascular status.

   1. The **thoracotomy incision is one of the most painful and debilitating** in surgery. Inadequate pain control contributes heavily to nearly all postoperative complications. Chest wall splinting contributes to atelectasis and poor pulmonary toilet. Pain increases sympathetic tone and myocardial oxygen demand, provoking arrhythmias and cardiac ischemic episodes. The routine use of epidural catheter anesthesia perioperatively and during the early recovery period has improved pain management significantly. Other effective analgesic maneuvers include intercostal blocks with long-acting local anesthetic before closure of the chest and intrapleural administration or local anesthetic via catheters placed at the time of thoracotomy.

   2. **Maintenance of good bronchial hygiene** is often the most difficult challenge facing the postthoracotomy patient. A lengthy smoking history, decreased ciliary function, chronic bronchitis, and significant postoperative pain all contribute to the ineffective clearance of pulmonary secretions. Even aggressive pulmonary toilet with incentive spirometry and chest physiotherapy delivered by the respiratory therapist, along with adequate analgesia, are insufficient on occasion. Diligent attention must be paid, including frequent physical examination and daily chest X-ray and arterial blood gas evaluation to detect any

changes in gas exchange. Atelectasis and mucus plugging can lead to ventilation–perfusion mismatch and ensuing respiratory failure. The clinician should make liberal use of nasotracheal suctioning, bedside flexible bronchoscopy, and mechanical ventilatory support if needed.

3. All physicians caring for the postthoracotomy patient should be familiar with chest tube placement, maintenance, and removal. The purpose of chest tube placement after thoracotomy and lung resection is to allow drainage of air and fluid from the pleural space and to ensure reexpansion of the remaining lung parenchyma.

   a. **Chest-tube drainage** is not used routinely with pneumonectomy unless bleeding or infection is present. Some surgeons place a chest tube on the operative side and remove it on postoperative day 1. Balanced pneumonectomy drainage systems have been advocated to balance the mediastinum during the first 24 to 48 hours. A chest tube in the patient with a pneumonectomy space should never be placed to conventional suction because of the risk of cardiac herniation and mediastinal shift.

   b. **Chest tubes are removed after the air leak has resolved and fluid drainage decreased** (usually <100 mL over 8 hours). Chest tubes usually are removed one at a time. The tube is removed swiftly and the site is simultaneously covered with an occlusive dressing. The technique of swift chest tube removal is critical to preventing air entry through the removal site.

4. **Cardiovascular complications** in the postoperative period are second in frequency only to pulmonary complications because the population that develops lung cancer is at high risk for heart disease. The three most common sources of cardiac morbidity are arrhythmias, myocardial infarctions, and congestive heart failure. A negative preoperative cardiac evaluation does not preclude the development of postoperative complications.

   a. **Cardiac arrhythmias** occur in up to 30% of patients undergoing pulmonary surgery. The most common arrhythmia is atrial fibrillation. The highest incidence occurs in elderly patients undergoing pneumonectomy or intrapericardial pulmonary artery ligation. All patients should have cardiac rhythm monitoring after thoracotomy for at least 72 hours.

   b. A number of trials have failed to reach consensus on optimal regimen for prophylaxis.

   c. **Treatment** of any rhythm disturbance begins with an assessment of the patient's hemodynamic status. Manifestations of these arrhythmias vary in acuity from hemodynamic collapse to palpitations. If the patient is hemodynamically unstable, the advanced cardiac life support protocol should be followed. After the patient has been examined and hemodynamic stability confirmed, an ECG, arterial blood gas sample, and serum electrolyte panel should be obtained. Frequently, supplementary oxygen and aggressive potassium and magnesium replenishment are the only treatment necessary. Premature ventricular contractions often are signs of myocardial ischemia.

They should be treated expediently with electrolyte correction, optimization of oxygenation, and evaluation for ischemia.

d. Chest pain associated with myocardial infarction often goes unnoticed by caretakers and patients due to thoracotomy incisional pain and narcotic administration.

e. Perioperative fluid management of thoracic surgery patients differs from that of patients after abdominal surgery. Pulmonary surgery does not induce large fluid shifts. In addition, collapse and reexpansion of lungs during surgery can lead to pulmonary edema. Pulmonary edema should be treated with aggressive diuresis. This is largely due to the limited pulmonary reserve, most graphically demonstrated in the pneumonectomy patient in whom 100% of the cardiac output perfuses the remaining lung. Judicious fluid management, including avoiding fluid overload and pulmonary edema, is critical in patients with limited pulmonary reserve. Discussions regarding intraoperative fluid management should be held with the anesthesiologist before surgery. Physicians may need to accept transiently decreased urine output and increased serum creatinine. Mild hypotension may be treated with intravenous α-agonists such as phenylephrine. Cardiac dysfunction may also be the source of postoperative oliguria, pulmonary edema, and hypotension and should always be considered in patients who are not responding normally. Echocardiography or placement of a Swan–Ganz catheter may guide treatment.

X. THORACOSCOPY

A. **Diagnostic thoracoscopy**

1. **VATS pleuroscopy** is performed in patients after thoracentesis and percutaneous pleural biopsy have failed to provide a diagnosis of suspected pleural disease. VATS frequently is used to diagnose malignancy in a solitary peripheral nodule. It is contraindicated in patients with extensive intrapleural adhesions or those who are unable to tolerate single-lung ventilation.

2. **VATS is approximately 95% accurate** for diagnosis of pleural disease.

B. **Therapeutic thoracoscopy**

1. **VATS is routinely performed** for a wide variety of thoracic procedures including lung biopsy/wedge resections, closure of leaking blebs, pleurodesis, sympathectomies, pericardiectomy, excision of mediastinal cysts, thymectomy, lobectomies, and bilobectomies. In fact, many centers are even performing VATS for pneumonectomies and esophagectomies. As this field continues to develop, there will be increasing trend toward the use of minimally invasive techniques in thoracic surgery. Robotics has also impacted thoracic surgery and lung resections are being performed at several centers with the robot.

   a. **Absolute contraindications** include extensive intrapleural adhesions or the inability to tolerate single-lung anesthesia.

  b. Relative contraindications include previous thoracotomy, tumor involvement of the hilar vessels, and previous chemotherapy or radiotherapy for lung or esophageal tumors.

2. The **patient is placed** in the lateral decubitus or semioblique position. Thoracoscopy requires selective intubation to allow collapse of the ipsilateral lung and to create a working space within the thorax (thus, insufflation gases are not needed). For most procedures, two to three incisions are required. The thoracoscope is placed through a port in the seventh or eighth intercostal space in the midaxillary line. Working ports for instruments generally are at the fourth or fifth intercostal space in the anterior axillary line and posteriorly near the border of the scapula. The endoscopic stapler, electrocautery, or laser can be used for resection. A chest tube is generally placed through one of the port sites.

3. **Complications** include hemorrhage, perforation of the diaphragm, air emboli, prolonged air leak, and tension pneumothorax.

4. **Postoperative thoracoscopy management**
   a. **A chest X**-ray is taken and checked for residual air or fluid.
   b. **Chest tubes,** if any, are removed when there is no air leak and the drainage decreases to satisfactory levels.
   c. **Analgesia** is provided by patient-controlled anesthesia or orally administered medication as needed.
   d. **Diet** is usually advanced by postoperative day 1.
   e. **Physical activity** is as tolerated with a chest tube. Depending on the procedure and diagnosis, patients can return to work in approximately 1 week.

32

Pediatric Surgery

Amy C. Fox and Patrick A. Dillon

Pediatric surgery is predicated on the fundamental fact that children differ from adults in anatomy, physiology, and their reaction to operative trauma, thereby making adjustments in care not merely matters of scale. Although some disease processes are managed similar to those in adults, this chapter addresses the more pediatric-specific surgical issues.

I. SPECIAL CONSIDERATIONS IN PRE- AND POSTOPERATIVE CARE

A. Fluid, electrolytes, and nutrition

1. **Fluid requirements.** Normal daily fluid requirements for children (Table 32-1) are higher than those of adults due to greater insensible losses. Infants have a high ratio of body surface area to volume and a limited ability to concentrate urine due to immature kidneys. Total body water is a higher percentage of body weight (75% in children vs. 60% in adults). Total blood volume in a full-term newborn measures approximately 85 mL/kg and decreases with age. Postoperative fluid replacement should be adjusted to support urine output between 1 and 2 mL/kg/hour.

2. **Electrolytes.** Maintenance fluids for children younger than 6 months old should include 10% dextrose in 0.25% saline with 20 mEq/L of potassium chloride. However, children older than 6 months old can be given 5% dextrose in 0.45% saline with 20 mEq/L of potassium chloride. Daily sodium requirements are 2 to 3 mEq/kg. Daily potassium requirements are 1 to 2 mEq/kg.

3. **Nutrition.** Normal daily caloric requirements per kilogram decrease as children age (Table 32-2). These estimated requirements must be increased to take into account altered metabolic states such as fevers, traumas, and burns.

   a. A newborn is expected to gain weight at about 15 to 30 g/day.

   b. Most infant formulas contain 20 kcal/oz. Caloric needs can be calculated by the following formula:
   Weight (kg) × 6 oz = Volume of formula needed to deliver 120 kcal/kg

   c. Carbohydrates should supply 50%, lipids 40%, and protein 10% of total calories in the diet.

B. Preoperative preparation

1. **Nothing-by-mouth status** (Table 32-3). Studies indicate that clear liquids ingested 2 hours before induction of anesthesia do not increase the risk of aspiration in children at normal risk of aspiration during anesthesia. In addition, children permitted fluids in a less restrictive fashion have a more comfortable preoperative experience in terms of thirst and hunger (*Cochrane Database Syst Rev.* 2009;(4):CD005285).

TABLE 32-1	Normal Fluid Requirements in Children

Weight (kg)	24-hr Fluid Requirements
<2 (premature)	150 mL/kg
1–10	100 mL/kg
11–20	1,000 mL + 50 mL/kg for each kg >10
>20	1,500 mL + 20 mL/kg for each kg >20

Weight (kg)	Hourly Fluid Requirements
0–10	4 mL/kg
10–20	2 mL/kg
>20	1 mL/kg

TABLE 32-2	Normal Daily Caloric Needs in Children

Age (y)	REE (kcal/kg/d)	Average (kcal/kg/d)
<36 wk	63	120
0–0.5	53	108
0.5–1	56	98
1–3	57	102
4–6	48	90
7–10	40	70
11–14	32	55
15–18	27	45

REE, resting energy expenditure.

TABLE 32-3	Nothing-by-Mouth Requirements in Children

Age	Clear Liquids	Solids/Formula/Breast Milk
<6 mo	2 hr	4 hr
>6 mo	2 hr	6 hr

2. Indications for preoperative antibiotic prophylaxis include patients with cardiac anomalies, ventriculoperitoneal shunts, and those with implanted prosthetic material.

C. Vascular access

1. Peripheral venous access can be obtained from the dorsal veins of the hand or foot, antecubital vein, saphenous vein, external jugular vein, or scalp veins.

2. Central venous access may be needed if peripheral access is exhausted or if drugs or nutrition need to be given centrally. Central veins can be accessed directly or via peripheral veins (i.e., peripherally inserted central catheter). Common sites for direct access are the subclavian, internal jugular, external jugular, and femoral veins.

3. Intraosseous (IO) access can be used in an emergency setting when attempts at obtaining vascular access have failed. A location 1 to 3 cm distal to the tibial tuberosity is recommended. The needle should be directed inferiorly during insertion. Alternatively, the femur may be reached by inserting the needle in a cephalad direction 3 cm proximal to the condyles. A bone marrow aspiration needle or a 16G to 19G butterfly needle is adequate. Contraindications to IO access include a fracture of the bone or previous IO catheter.

4. Arterial catheters are needed in some children. The potential sites for an arterial catheter include the umbilical, radial, femoral, posterior tibial, and temporal arteries. For the neonate, the umbilical artery can often be cannulated through the umbilical stump within the first 2 to 4 days of life.

II. ABDOMINAL PAIN IN CHILDREN

A. Abdominal pain is a common complaint in the pediatric age group with various etiologies (Table 32-4).

B. The differential diagnosis of abdominal pain must take the following into consideration: age, gender, duration of symptoms, circumstances at onset, and modifying factors.

C. The **history of present illness** is often difficult to obtain from a child; therefore, parents should be present to corroborate accurate information. While characteristics of the pain should be elicited, associated symptoms such as emesis (bilious, nonbilious, bloody), diarrhea, constipation, melena, hematochezia, or fever may be more likely to suggest surgical etiologies.

D. The **physical examination** is critical in determining how toxic a patient may be. A patient's ease and comfort are integral to a thorough and accurate physical exam.

1. Peritonitis may be elicited by various maneuvers such as palpation, percussion, manipulation of the hip, deep respiratory movements, or rectal examination.

2. Bimanual pelvic exam may be necessary in age-appropriate patients.

TABLE 32-4	Etiologies of Pediatric Abdominal Pain	
Very Common Causes	**Less Common Causes**	**Rare Causes**
Acute appendicitis	Intussusception	Henoch–Schönlein purpura
Viral infection	Lower lobe pneumonia	Nephrotic syndromes
Gastroenteritis	Intestinal obstruction	Pancreatitis
Constipation	Urinary tract obstruction	Hepatitis
Genitourinary tract infection	Inguinal hernia	Diabetic ketoacidosis
Trauma	Meckel diverticulum Cholecystitis Intra-abdominal mass	Lead poisoning Acute porphyria Herpes zoster Sickle cell anemia

III. NEONATAL SURGICAL PROBLEMS

A. **Congenital diaphragmatic hernia (CDH).** Incomplete diaphragm development at 8 weeks of gestation can result in herniation of abdominal organs into the chest which can prevent normal lung development. Posterolateral (Bochdalek) defects occur 85% of the time with over 90% of these occurring on the left side. CDH occurs in a 1:1 male-to-female ratio. CDH can be a lethal condition with mortality rates dependent on associated anomalies, the severity of pulmonary hypertension, and the degree of pulmonary hypoplasia. The less common Morgagni defect occurs in a parasternal anterior location and is usually associated with fewer pulmonary and systemic complications.

1. Diagnosis
   a. Signs and symptoms
      (1) Cardiorespiratory distress such as tachypnea, retractions, and cyanosis
      (2) Asymmetric chest
      (3) Reduced breath sounds on the affected side
      (4) Scaphoid abdomen
   b. Imaging
      (1) **Antenatal ultrasound and maternal–fetal magnetic resonance imaging (MRI)** are used to determine polyhydramnios and location of the fetal liver and give an estimation of fetal lung volumes.
      (2) Chest x-rays may demonstrate bowel in the thorax, a loss of the normal diaphragm contour, or mediastinal shift.

2. Management

 a. Immediate postnatal care includes supplemental oxygen or endotracheal intubation if the patient is in significant respiratory distress. Excessive bag-mask ventilation should be avoided as it can exacerbate gastrointestinal (GI) distension which further impedes lung ventilation. Decompression by orogastric or nasogastric intubation reduces distension of the stomach in the thoracic cavity.

  (1) Conventional ventilation

 b. Initial peak inspiratory pressures (PIP) less than 25 cm H_2O to minimize barotrauma.

 c. Maintain preductal oxygen saturation greater than 85% with minimal PIP.

 d. When stable, wean fraction of inspired oxygen (FIO_2) for preductal oxygen saturation greater than 85%.

 e. In order to minimize PIP, arterial carbon dioxide tension of 45 to 60 mm Hg is acceptable.

 f. Maintain pH>7.2.

 g. Ventilator rates of 40 to 60 breaths per minute and 3 to 5 positive end-expiratory pressure (PEEP) are often required for adequate oxygenation and ventilation.

  (1) High-frequency oscillating ventilation is associated with decreased barotrauma and may be used if conventional ventilation fails.

  (2) Inhaled agents—nitric oxide or epoprostenol and sildenafil— may decrease the severity of pulmonary hypertension.

  (3) Extracorporeal membrane oxygenation (ECMO) is considered for patients with severe preductal hypoxemia or right-to-left shunting due to severe pulmonary hypertension. Patients with severe pulmonary hypoplasia may not be candidates for ECMO.

 h. Operative intervention is deferred until the patient has been stabilized.

  (1) A subcostal incision on the affected side allows the herniated abdominal contents to be reduced into the peritoneal cavity.

  (2) The diaphragmatic defect is repaired primarily or with a synthetic patch if the defect is large.

  (3) A laparoscopic or thoracoscopic approach may be utilized for repair in carefully selected patients.

B. Tracheoesophageal malformations are a spectrum of anomalies including esophageal atresia and tracheoesophageal fistula (TEF) separately or in combination (Fig. 32-1). There is a 1:1 male-to-female ratio. Over 50% of patients will have associated anomaly and 25% will have a VACTERL association (e.g., *v*ertebral defects, imperforate *a*nus, *c*ardiac defects, *t*racheo*e*sophageal malformations, *r*enal dysplasia, and *l*imb anomalies).

1. Diagnosis

 a. Signs and symptoms

  (1) Excessive drooling

  (2) Regurgitation of feedings

  (3) Choking, coughing, or cyanosis during feeding

  (4) Resistance when passing a nasogastric tube

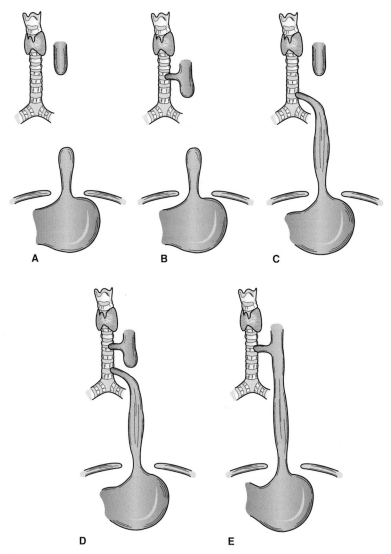

Figure 32-1. Variants of TEF. **A:** Atresia without fistula (5% to 7% of cases). **B:** Proximal fistula and distal pouch (<1% occurrence). **C:** Proximal pouch with distal fistula (85% to 90% of cases). **D:** Atresia with proximal and distal fistulas (<1% of cases). **E:** Fistula without atresia (H type) (2% to 6% occurrence).

- **b.** Chest radiograph
    - **(1)** Coiled orogastric tube in the esophageal pouch
    - **(2)** Gas in the GI tract implies a distal TEF
    - **(3)** Infiltrates suggestive of aspiration pneumonia
- **2.** Management
    - **a. Preoperative management** includes prevention of aspiration through elevation of the head of the bed 30 degrees and placing an orogastric or nasogastric tube into the proximal esophageal pouch for decompression. An ECHO should be obtained to evaluate the location of the aortic arch which helps determine the operative approach.
    - **b. Operative intervention** is typically through a right extrapleural posterolateral thoracotomy. The fistula is ligated and the atresia is repaired in a one-stage procedure when possible. H type fistulas are often approached through a right transverse cervical incision.

- **C. Necrotizing enterocolitis (NEC)** is an acute, fulminating inflammatory disease of the intestine associated with focal or diffuse ulceration and necrosis of the small bowel, colon, and rarely the stomach. While the cause is unknown, the pathogenesis is thought to be multifactorial involving an immature gut barrier defense and virulent bacteria. The incidence of NEC is 1 to 3 per 1,000 live births and is the most common GI emergency of neonates. It primarily affects premature infants and occurs in 10% of all babies born weighing less than 1,500 g.
    - **1. Diagnosis.** A high index of suspicion is needed in making a diagnosis of NEC.
        - **a.** Signs and symptoms
            - **(1)** Patients may be lethargic, apneic, or have temperature instability.
            - **(2)** Patients may have emesis, bilious nasogastric tube drainage, or high gastric residuals. The abdomen is often distended.
            - **(3)** Bowel movements may be bloody.
            - **(4)** Edema or erythema of the abdominal wall may indicate peritonitis, a localized response to inflamed bowel, or perforation of bowel. The skin may show pallor or mottling.
        - **b.** Other adjunct studies
            - **(1) Laboratory studies** may reveal a metabolic acidosis, thrombocytopenia, leukocytosis, or leukopenia.
            - **(2) Plain radiographs** of the abdomen may reveal dilated loops of bowel, pneumatosis intestinalis, portal vein gas, or pneumoperitoneum. Contrast imaging is often avoided due to the risk of perforation.
    - **2.** Management
        - **a.** Nonoperative management
            - **(1)** Patients are placed on bowel rest with nasogastric decompression and parenteral nutrition. Broad-spectrum antibiotics are initiated.
            - **(2)** Serial abdominal examinations, plain radiographs, and laboratory studies help determine the progress of nonoperative management.

b. Operative management

   (1) Indications for operative treatment include pneumoperitoneum, bowel obstruction, intra-abdominal abscess, or sepsis unresponsive to treatment.

   (2) The two main surgical options are laparotomy or primary peritoneal drainage. A randomized controlled trial (RCT) suggests that the operation performed for perforated NEC does not alter mortality rates, dependence on parenteral nutrition 90 days after operation, or hospitalization duration (*N Engl J Med.* 2006;354(21):2225–2234).

c. Laparotomy includes resection of necrotic bowel and creation of stomas. If intestinal viability is questionable, re-exploration within 24 hours is essential.

d. Primary peritoneal drainage may be used as a temporizing measure in critically ill infants until they can tolerate a laparotomy or as a primary therapy.

D. Gastroschisis and omphalocele are congenital abdominal wall defects that differ in etiology and severity.

   1. Gastroschisis is an abdominal wall defect (usually <4 cm) that is believed to arise from an isolated vascular insult in the developing mesenchyme. It typically occurs to the right of the normal umbilical cord with abdominal organs herniating through the defect. In contrast to omphalocele, there is no membranous sac covering the eviscerated abdominal organs. The incidence of associated anomalies in gastroschisis is low, but approximately 10% may have an intestinal atresia.

   2. Omphalocele is an abdominal wall defect (usually >4 cm) of the umbilical ring in which the intestines protrude through the base of the umbilical cord and herniate into a sac. The high incidence (50%) of associated congenital anomalies (cardiac, chromosomal) often dictates the prognosis for infants with omphalocele.

   3. Diagnosis

   a. A **gastroschisis** defect is to the **right** of the umbilical cord with abdominal organs herniating through the defect. There is **no encompassing sac,** and the exposed bowel may develop a serositis.

   b. An **omphalocele** defect is at the **base** of the umbilical cord and can vary from a few centimeters to absence of most of the abdominal wall. A **sac** covers the herniated viscera. While rupture of the sac is infrequent, it can be distinguished from gastroschisis by the presence of residual sac in continuity with the umbilical cord and normal appearing bowel.

   c. Radiologic exams

   (1) Prenatal ultrasound may demonstrate either defect after 13 weeks of gestation.

   (2) A finding of omphalocele mandates a thorough search for other birth defects given the high incidence of related anomalies.

   4. Management

   a. Prenatal management. Serial ultrasounds may be necessary. If bowel dilation and mural thickening of the eviscerated bowel are detected, delivery at the time of lung maturity may be indicated. However, a systematic review found insufficient evidence to support induction of labor (*Br J Obstet Gynaecol.* 2009;116(5):626–636). Delivery should be planned at a tertiary care center with high-risk obstetrics and pediatric surgical expertise.

b. Postnatal management

(1) **Heat and fluid losses** can be decreased by covering the exposed bowel in gastroschisis defects with moistened gauze and then wrapping the bowel with plastic wrap or placing the infant in a plastic bag to cover the lower body and defect. Fluids should be given as a bolus (20 mL/kg) to start resuscitation and then titrated to achieve a urine output of 1.5 to 2 mL/kg/hour.

(2) The neonate can be positioned in a lateral position to prevent kinking of the mesentery and vascular compromise of the bowel.

c. Operative intervention

(1) Viscera may be reduced primarily. If this is not possible, viscera are placed in a spring-loaded or self-made silo which is secured beneath the fascial edge. The silo and viscera can be reduced gradually over time (*J Pediatr Surg.* 2009;44(11):2126–2129).

(2) The abdominal wall defect is then repaired in a primary fashion on an elective basis. Fewer complications may arise with this method of management compared to immediate reduction of viscera and primary closure (*J Pediatr Surg.* 2006;41(11):1830–1835).

(3) The fascial defect can be extended in the midline for 1 to 2 cm if the bowel mesentery appears to be compressed by a narrow opening.

IV. ALIMENTARY TRACT OBSTRUCTION

A. Congenital causes of alimentary tract obstruction

1. Intestinal malrotation results when the intestine fails to undergo its normal rotation and fixation during embryologic development. Symptoms most often present in the neonatal period but may present in adulthood. Malrotation places the intestine at greater risk for volvulus which is a surgical emergency.

   a. Diagnosis

   (1) Signs and symptoms

   (a) Bilious emesis in the newborn mandates evaluation for intestinal malrotation with volvulus.

   (b) The abdomen may be distended or tender. Patients may have hematemesis or hematochezia.

   (2) Radiologic studies

   (a) Plain radiographs commonly show a normal bowel gas pattern but may also show a "double-bubble" which is indicative of duodenal obstruction but is not diagnostic of volvulus.

   (b) An upper GI series is necessary to establish the diagnosis. Failure of the duodenum to cross to the right of the midline with a right-sided jejunum characterizes intestinal malrotation. Hallmark signs for volvulus include the "bird's beak" sign and a corkscrew appearance of the proximal small intestine.

   b. Management. The operative intervention is a Ladd procedure. The bowel is eviscerated and rotated counterclockwise to correct the volvulus. Peritoneal (Ladd) bands are divided. The colon is positioned to the left and the small bowel to the right side of the abdomen. An appendectomy completes the procedure.

2. Intestinal atresia or stenosis usually results from an intrauterine vascular accident; however, duodenal atresia results from failure of recanalization of the duodenum.

   a. Location. Distal ileum > proximal jejunum > duodenum > colon.

   b. Diagnosis

   (1) Prenatal ultrasound may show polyhydramnios or dilated bowel loops.

   (2) Signs and symptoms

   (a) Symptoms appear shortly after birth for atresia but may take weeks to months for stenosis or intestinal web.

   (b) Patients may have bilious emesis or abdominal distension.

   (c) Other symptoms include failure to pass meconium, failure to thrive, or poor feeding.

   (3) Radiology

   (a) A "double-bubble" sign is diagnostic of duodenal obstruction.

   (b) Contrast enema may identify a distal intestinal atresia and can also identify obstruction secondary to meconium ileus or meconium plug syndrome.

   c. Management

   (1) Preoperative management includes nasogastric decompression and resuscitation with intravenous (IV) fluids. Antibiotics should be given preoperatively.

   (2) Operative intervention

   (a) Dependent on the site of atresia but a primary anastomosis is usually attempted for small bowel atresia and may require resection and/or tapering of the dilated proximal segment.

   (b) Atresia involving the colon usually requires initial colostomy with delayed anastomosis.

   (c) A duodenoduodenostomy or duodenojejunostomy is created to bypass the obstruction in duodenal atresia.

   (d) Saline should be infused into the distal bowel to rule out synchronous intestinal atresias.

3. Hirschsprung disease is intestinal aganglionosis of the hindgut. The segment of aganglionosis can vary but over 80% of patients have a transition point in the rectosigmoid area. It can be familial or sporadic, and up to 7.8% of cases occur in patients for whom more than one family member is affected. Mutations in the *RET* protooncogene have been found in both familial and sporadic cases.

   a. Diagnosis

     (1) Signs and symptoms

       (a) Neonates may present with abdominal distention, failure to pass meconium within the first 48 hours of life, infrequent defecation, or enterocolitis with sepsis.

       (b) Older infants and children present with chronic constipation or failure to thrive.

     (2) Radiology

       (a) Plain radiographs show a pattern of distal bowel obstruction.

       (b) Contrast enema usually demonstrates a transition zone between distal nondilated bowel and proximal dilated bowel; however, total colonic aganglionosis does not have a transition zone.

     (3) Pathology is essential for making the diagnosis and requires a rectal biopsy. Full-thickness specimens are the ideal tissue samples to demonstrate the absence of ganglion cells. In neonates, rectal suction biopsy is often sufficient for diagnosis.

   b. Management

     (1) Preoperative management includes colonic decompression to prevent enterocolitis. Saline enemas may be used to evacuate impacted stool. A nasogastric tube should be placed if the child is vomiting.

     (2) Operative goals are removal of aganglionic bowel and reconstruction of the intestinal tract by bringing innervated bowel down to the anus while maintaining normal sphincter function. There are multiple "primary pull-through" variations which achieve this goal such as the Swenson, Duhamel, Soave, laparoscopic endorectal pull-through (Georgeson), and transanal endorectal pull-through (Langer).

       (a) Each of these operations has been modified to improve functional results and may be performed in the newborn period; however, surgery may be delayed to allow for increased weight gain or resolution of enterocolitis.

       (b) Transanal endorectal pull-through is associated with fewer complications and fewer episodes of enterocolitis compared to transabdominal approaches without higher rates of incontinence (*J Pediatr Surg.* 2010;45(6):1213–1220).

       (c) A diverting colostomy may be performed proximal to the aganglionic segment in patients who are unstable or who have massively dilated bowel.

 4. Anorectal anomalies refer to various congenital defects (noted below) which can produce neonatal intestinal obstruction. The lesions may be classified as low, intermediate, or high depending on whether the atresia is below, at the level of, or above the puborectalis sling, respectively. These anomalies are associated with other congenital defects such as the VACTERL syndromes or cardiovascular defects.

    • Males: Perineal fistula, rectourethral bulbar fistula, rectourethral prostatic fistula, rectovesical (bladder neck) fistula, imperforate anus without fistula, rectal atresia and stenosis.

- Females: Perineal fistula, vestibular fistula, imperforate anus with no fistula, rectal atresia and stenosis, persistent cloaca.
  a. Diagnosis
     (1) Physical examination may demonstrate various findings from no anus to perineal fistulas. Meconium on the perineum within 24 hours of birth may signify a perineal fistula (low defect).
     (2) Plain radiographs such as an obstructive series or an invertogram may be obtained. Sacral abnormalities may be identified. A contrast study may demonstrate a fistulous tract.
  b. Management
     (1) A perineal fistula (low defect) may be safely repaired without a colostomy. A high defect with probable rectourethral or rectovaginal fistula requires a colostomy and mucous fistula for initial management.
     (2) For the more complex anorectal anomalies, a three-step procedure is advocated with a diverting colostomy after birth, posterior sagittal anorectoplasty, and colostomy closure.

5. Meconium ileus is a neonatal intestinal obstruction caused by inspissated meconium that may occur in the setting of cystic fibrosis.
  a. Diagnosis
    (1) Prenatal ultrasound may demonstrate polyhydramnios.
    (2) Signs and symptoms may include abdominal distention, bilious emesis, failure to pass meconium within 24 to 48 hours of life, pneumoperitoneum, peritonitis, abdominal wall inflammation, hypovolemia, or sepsis.
    (3) Plain abdominal radiographs can show dilated loops of small bowel and a ground-glass appearance of air and meconium mixture. Given the thick meconium, air–fluid levels are often absent. Intra-abdominal calcifications suggest prenatal perforation and subsequent meconium peritonitis. Ascites or pneumoperitoneum also suggest perforation. However, up to 35% of infants with complicated meconium ileus show no radiographic abnormalities.
    (4) Water-soluble contrast enema can confirm the diagnosis by demonstrating a microcolon and inspissated meconium in the ileum.
  b. Management
    (1) Nonoperative management includes hydration with IV fluids and broad-spectrum antibiotics. A water-soluble contrast enema can be both diagnostic and therapeutic. This solution draws fluid into the bowel lumen and causes an osmotic diarrhea.
    (2) Operative intervention is indicated for complicated meconium ileus or when enema therapy fails.
      (a) An enterotomy is made followed by irrigation with 1% to 2% acetylcysteine solution. If gentle irrigation does not flush out the meconium, a 14-French ileostomy tube may be placed and routine irrigations are done beginning on postoperative day one.

(b) If intestinal volvulus, atresia, perforation, or gangrene complicates the illness, the nonviable bowel is resected and an end ileostomy with mucus fistula is created. Routine irrigations are started. A primary anastomosis is delayed for 2 to 3 weeks later.

6. Meconium plug syndrome refers to altered colonic motility or viscous meconium believed to cause impaired stool transit and obstruction of the colonic lumen. Unlike meconium ileus, patients do not have cystic fibrosis. While diagnosis is similar to meconium ileus, operative intervention is rarely needed to relieve the obstruction. Suction biopsy is needed to rule out Hirschsprung disease. A sweat chloride test is needed to rule out cystic fibrosis.

7. Intestinal duplications are cystic or tubular structures lined by various types of normal GI mucosa. They are located dorsal to the true alimentary tract. They frequently share a common muscular wall and blood supply with the normal GI tract. In 20% of cases, enteric duplications communicate with the true GI tract. They are most commonly located in the ileum but may occur anywhere from the mouth to the anus.

   a. Diagnosis
      (1) Signs and symptoms are nonspecific and can include emesis, abdominal pain, abdominal distension, or an abdominal mass.
      (2) Abdominal ultrasound or GI contrast studies may show external compression or displacement of the normal alimentary tract. Technetium radioisotope scans may aid in diagnosis if the cyst contains gastric mucosa.

   b. Management involves resection of the duplication or internal drainage. Internal drainage may be indicated if the resection would require an extensive amount of bowel being removed. Internal drainage minimizes the risk of damage to the biliary system in the case of a duodenal duplication. When gastric mucosa is found in a cyst, it is stripped, and the cyst lumen is joined to the adjacent intestine.

B. **Acquired causes of alimentary tract obstruction**

   1. Pyloric stenosis is the most common surgical cause of nonbilious vomiting in infants. It occurs in 1 of 400 live births. The male-to-female ratio is 4:1. It occurs generally in neonates who are 2 to 5 weeks of age. Patients often present with a hypochloremic hypokalemic metabolic alkalosis.

      a. Diagnosis
         (1) Signs and symptoms
            (a) Nonbilious, projective vomiting occurring 30 to 60 minutes after feeding is typical. Patients can also have formula intolerance which does not resolve with change of feeds.
            (b) Signs of dehydration include lethargy, the absence of tears, a sunken anterior fontanelle, dry mucous membranes, or decreased urine output.
            (c) The "olive" mass refers to a thickened pylorus which can be palpated to the right and superior to the umbilicus. It is approximately 2 cm in diameter, firm, and mobile.

  (2) Radiologic studies
   (a) Abdominal ultrasonography notes a pyloric diameter greater than 14 mm, muscular thickness greater than 4 mm, and pyloric length greater than 16 mm. This is diagnostic of pyloric stenosis with approximately 99.5% sensitivity and 100% specificity (*Semin Pediatr Surg.* 2007;16(1):27–33).
   (b) An upper GI contrast study shows an enlarged stomach, poor gastric emptying, and an elongated, narrow pyloric channel or "string sign."
 b. Management
  (1) Preoperative management involves aggressive fluid resuscitation which often requires a bolus (20 mL/kg) and then 5% dextrose in normal saline to achieve a urine output of 2 mL/kg/hour. Addition of potassium and changing to 5% dextrose in 0.45% normal saline occurs when urine output is adequate.
  (2) Operative intervention is indicated only after adequate resuscitation and correction of the metabolic alkalosis. A pyloromyotomy is division of the hypertrophied pyloric muscle, leaving the mucosa intact. This can be done through an open incision or laparoscopically. A double-blind RCT suggests that while both procedures are safe, laparoscopy results in decreased time to achieve full enteral feeds and a decreased postoperative length of stay over open pyloromyotomy without any additional complications (*Lancet.* 2009;373(9661):390–398).
  (3) Postoperative management. An electrolyte solution can typically be started by mouth 6 hours after pyloromyotomy. Over the next 12 hours, formula or pumped breast milk can be started and should reach goal within 24 hours. Parents should be advised that vomiting may occur postoperatively as a result of swelling at the pyloromyotomy, but this problem is self-limited. If the pyloric mucosa is perforated and repaired during surgery, nasogastric drainage is recommended for 24 hours.

2. Intussusception refers to an invagination of proximal intestine into adjacent distal bowel with resultant obstruction of the lumen (most common: ileocolic intussusception). A lead point of the intussusception is identified in only 5% of patients and is most commonly a Meckel diverticulum. This obstruction may compromise the arterial inflow and venous return. The highest incidence is at 5 to 10 months of age.
 a. Diagnosis
  (1) A typical history is a previously healthy infant who presents with periods of abrupt crying and retraction of the legs up to the abdomen. Attacks usually subside over a few minutes but recur every 10 to 15 minutes. In 30% of cases, a recent viral gastroenteritis or upper respiratory infection may precede onset of symptoms.
  (2) Physical findings include a dark-red mucoid stool ("currant jelly" stool). Hyperperistaltic rushes may be heard during an episode. A sausage-shaped abdominal mass may be palpated or the tip of the intussusception may be felt on rectal examination.

       (3) Ultrasound can be used for screening in suspected cases of intussusception.

       (4) Barium or air-contrast enema confirms the diagnosis by demonstrating a "coiled spring" sign.

  b. Management

       (1) Nonoperative management includes nasogastric drainage, IV fluid resuscitation, broad-spectrum antibiotics, and an early surgical consultation.

          (a) Pneumatic or hydrostatic reduction is attempted under radiographic guidance if no evidence of peritonitis exists and the patient is stable. This technique has a 90% success rate. The maximum safe intraluminal air pressure is 80 mm Hg for young infants and 110 to 120 mm Hg for older children. Recurrent intussusception in children less than 1 year old can be treated with repeated enema therapy.

          (b) Postreduction a patient should be observed for 24 hours. A liquid diet with advancement can be started once the child is alert. Recurrent intussusception occurs in 8% to 12% of patients.

       (2) Operative indications include failure of nonoperative reduction, peritonitis, sepsis, or shock. Recurrence after enema reduction in an older child is also an indication to operate as small bowel tumors which can serve as the lead point are more frequent in this age group.

          (a) During laparotomy, a transverse incision is made to deliver the bowel. Gentle retrograde pressure is applied to the telescoped portion of the intestine in an attempt at manual reduction. Proximal and distal segments should not be pulled apart because of the risk of bowel injury.

          (b) If manual reduction is not possible, resection of the involved segment and primary anastomosis should be done.

          (c) An incidental appendectomy should also be performed.

          (d) Recurrence of intussusception after operative treatment is approximately 1%.

3. Distal intestinal obstruction syndrome (DIOS), formerly known as *meconium ileus equivalent,* is caused by impaction of inspissated intestinal contents in older patients with cystic fibrosis. This problem occurs in 10% to 40% of patients with cystic fibrosis who are followed long term.

  a. Diagnosis requires a high index of suspicion in a child with cystic fibrosis who presents with chronic or recurrent abdominal pain and distention, vomiting, and constipation. An inciting cause such as abrupt cessation of pancreatic enzyme supplementation, dehydration, a dietary change, or exacerbation of respiratory symptoms is present.

       (1) Plain abdominal radiographs may show a ground-glass appearance of the intestine. Dilated small bowel with air–fluid levels is present.

       (2) Water-soluble contrast enemas demonstrate the inspissated intestinal contents.

  b. Management

  (1) Nonoperative management includes a water-soluble contrast enema to induce an osmotic diarrhea to flush the intestine and relieve the obstruction. GoLYTELY solution may be used in selective cases to relieve the obstruction from above.

  (2) Operative management is indicated when enemas or conservative therapy are unsuccessful. It is also indicated when intussusception or volvulus complicates DIOS.

V. JAUNDICE IN CHILDREN

- This is a yellowing of the skin that reflects hyperbilirubinemia.
- In jaundiced infants, the total serum bilirubin usually exceeds 7 mg/dL.
- This elevated bilirubin may reflect a rise in either the **conjugated (direct)** or **unconjugated (indirect)** bilirubin, or both. This distinction is integral for establishing a differential diagnosis for jaundice.

A. Unconjugated hyperbilirubinemia occurs when bilirubin that has not been metabolized in the liver rises above normal serum values. Common causes include hemolytic disorders, breast-feeding, and physiologic jaundice of the newborn. More rare causes of unconjugated hyperbilirubinemia include indirect causes of increased enterohepatic circulation of bilirubin such as meconium ileus, Hirschsprung disease, and pyloric stenosis. Treatment typically involves phototherapy and correction of primary diseases.

B. Conjugated hyperbilirubinemia occurs when excess monoglucuronides and diglucuronides in the liver result in elevated levels of bilirubin in the serum. The most common causes include biliary obstruction, hepatitis (infectious, toxic, or metabolic etiology), or TORCH (*to*xoplasmosis, *r*ubella, *c*ytomegalovirus, and *h*erpes simplex virus) infections. Two surgical causes of conjugated hyperbilirubinemia include biliary atresia and choledochal cysts.

  1. Biliary atresia is the most common cause of infantile jaundice that requires surgical correction. The etiology is unknown. The disease is characterized by progressive obliteration and sclerosis of the biliary tree. With age, obliteration of the extrahepatic bile ducts, proliferation of the intrahepatic bile ducts, and liver fibrosis progress at an unpredictable rate.

  a. Diagnosis

  (1) Signs and symptoms are often nonspecific such as jaundice, acholic stools, dark urine, and hepatomegaly.

  (2) Percutaneous liver biopsy results range from classic biliary tree fibrosis to those unable to be differentiated from $\alpha 1$-antitrypsin deficiency or neonatal hepatitis.

  (3) Technetium-99m iminodiacetic acid hepatobiliary imaging aids in differentiation between liver parenchymal disease and biliary obstructive disease. In biliary atresia, the liver readily takes up the tracer molecule, but no excretion into the extrahepatic biliary system or duodenum is seen.

  (4) Ultrasonography notes shrunken extrahepatic ducts and a noncontractile or absent gallbladder.

b. **Management**
   (1) Open liver biopsy and cholangiogram
      (a) The common bile duct is visualized by cholangiography in only 25% of patients with biliary atresia.
      (b) Cholangiography in the remaining 75% of patients demonstrates an atretic biliary tree.
   (2) **Operative intervention**
      (a) The obliterated extrahepatic ducts are excised with subsequent hepaticojejunostomy in a **Kasai procedure.** When the distal common bile duct is patent, a choledochojejunostomy is constructed.
      (b) **Jaundice improves in two-thirds of patients after a Kasai procedure, but only one third will retain their liver after the first decade of life (*Eur J Pediatr.* 2010;169(4):395–402).**
      (c) **Liver transplantation** is the recommended option when liver failure occurs or the Kasai procedure fails.

2. **Choledochal cysts** are a spectrum of diseases characterized by cystic dilation of the extrahepatic and intrahepatic biliary tree. They are believed to be an embryologic malformation of the pancreaticobiliary system. Approximately 50% of children present within the first 10 years of life. There are five types:
   • **Type I:** Fusiform cystic dilation of common bile duct (most common)
   • **Type II: Diverticulum of the extrahepatic bile duct**
   • **Type III: Choledochocele**
   • **Type IV:** Cystic disease of the intra- or extrahepatic bile ducts
   • **Type V:** Single or multiple intrahepatic ducts
   a. Diagnosis
      (1) **Signs and symptoms** include nonspecific findings such as jaundice, abdominal pain, abdominal mass, cholangitis, pancreatitis, portal hypertension, hepatic abscess, or cyst rupture.
      (2) These cysts can be demonstrated on various radiologic tests such as ultrasonography, hepatobiliary scintigraphy, transhepatic cholangiography, magnetic resonance cholangiopancreatography, or endoscopic retrograde cholangiopancreatography.
   b. **Management**
      (1) The entire cyst is excised when possible. It is important to identify the pancreatic duct entrance into the biliary tree before excision.
      (2) **Choledochojejunostomy**
      (3) **Hepatic resection** if disease is intrahepatic and limited to a lobe or segment of the liver.
      (4) **Liver transplantation** for diffuse intrahepatic disease.

VI. GROIN MASSES

A. **Indirect inguinal hernias** affect approximately 1% to 5% of children. Boys are affected more than girls, with an 8:1 ratio. Prematurity increases the incidence of inguinal hernia to between 7% and 30%. The incidence of bilateral hernias ranges from 10% to 40%. Bilateral hernias occur more frequently in premature infants and girls.

1. **Diagnosis** is made by a history and physical examination. A groin bulge is noted which extends toward the scrotum or vulva either by history or observation. This is sometimes reproduced only when the child laughs, cries, or stands. Boys may have a thickened spermatic cord.

2. **Management**
   a. Reducible hernias are repaired with high ligation of the sac through a low abdominal incision. The hernia sac is anterior and medial to the spermatic cord in boys and more difficult to locate among the muscle fibers running through the external ring in girls. The sac can contain small bowel, omentum, or ovary.
   b. Incarcerated hernias can often be reduced with gentle direct pressure on the hernia. Simultaneously applying caudal traction on the testicle in addition to direct pressure on the hernia may be necessary in some cases.
   c. Strangulated hernias require emergent operative repair. Even if a severely incarcerated/strangulated hernia is reduced, the child should be admitted and scheduled for urgent herniorrhaphy. If viability of sac contents is in question, the bowel must be examined before abdominal closure.

B. **Hydroceles** are fluid collections within the processus vaginalis that envelop the testicles. They occur in approximately 6% of full-term male newborns.

1. **Communicating hydroceles** allow the free flow of peritoneal fluid down to the scrotum. The processus vaginalis is patent. This must be regarded as a hernia, with elective repair encouraged to prevent subsequent incarceration.

2. **Noncommunicating hydroceles** confine the fluid to the scrotum. A portion of the processus vaginalis obliterates normally. This is usually a self-limiting process and resolves in 6 to 12 months.

VII. TUMORS AND NEOPLASMS

A. **Neuroblastoma** is a neoplasm of the sympathochromaffin system with an incidence of approximately 8 million cases per year. It is the most common extracranial tumor of childhood and accounts for 10% of all pediatric malignancies. The median age at diagnosis is 2 years, with 85% of the tumors being diagnosed before age 5 years.

1. **Diagnosis.** Neuroblastoma is often an incidental finding on radiographic studies performed for other reasons. Patients may have an abdominal mass on exam. Rarely, children present with symptoms of fever, malaise, or abdominal pain. At the time of discovery, up to 75% of neuroblastomas are metastatic.

2. **International Neuroblastoma Staging System**
   a. This system places patients in low-, intermediate-, or high-risk groups on the basis of age, surgical staging, and status of the **N-*myc* oncogene** as these factors significantly predict outcome.
   b. Children younger than 12 months at the time of diagnosis have a better prognosis for cure, whereas older patients are more likely to have disseminated disease and a poorer prognosis.

TABLE 32-5	International Neuroblastoma Staging System

Stage	Characteristics
1	Localized tumor confined to the area of origin; complete gross excision with or without microscopic residual disease; identifiable ipsilateral and contralateral lymph nodes negative microscopically
2A	Unilateral tumor with incomplete gross excision; identifiable ipsilateral and contralateral lymph nodes negative microscopically
2B	Unilateral tumor with complete or incomplete gross excision; with positive ipsilateral regional lymph nodes; identifiable contralateral lymph nodes negative microscopically
3	Tumor infiltrating across the midline with or without regional lymph node involvement; or unilateral tumor with contralateral regional lymph node involvement; or midline tumor with bilateral tumor involvement
4	Dissemination of tumor to distant lymph nodes, bone, bone marrow, liver, or other organs (except as defined in stage 4S)
4S	Localized primary tumor as defined for stage 1 or 2 with dissemination limited to liver, skin, or bone marrow

      c. The staging system incorporates **clinical, radiographic,** and **surgical** information to define the tumor stage (Table 32-5). While operative evaluation may be necessary for accurate staging, various tests are also used to stage patients: Plain radiographs of the chest and skull, bone scan, computed tomography (CT) scan, bone marrow aspirate, ^{131}I-meta-iodobenzylguanidine scan.

   3. **Surgical treatment**

      a. **Local disease** is treated through complete excision of the tumor with lymph node sampling.

      b. **Bulky** or **metastatic** disease is treated with chemotherapy and radiotherapy after undergoing tumor biopsy. If tumor shrinkage occurs with chemotherapy and radiation, delayed resection can take place.

  B. **Wilms tumor** accounts for 6% of all malignancies in children and is the most common renal malignancy in children. Most children are diagnosed between 1 and 3 years of age with an annual incidence of approximately 5 to 7.8 per 1 million children younger than 15 years. The gender distribution is equal. Five percent of cases are bilateral.

   1. Diagnosis

      a. **History.** Patients typically present with vague symptoms of abdominal pain or fever; however, they may also have hematuria or a urinary tract infection.

| TABLE 32-6 | Wilms Tumor Staging System |

Stage	Characteristics
1	Tumor confined to the kidney and completely removed by surgery
2	Tumor grew beyond the kidney (e.g., nearby fatty tissue or into blood vessels) but the kidney and affected tissue were completely removed surgically
3	Tumor is not completely removed. Tumor remaining after surgery is limited to the abdomen (e.g., abdominal lymph nodes, positive margin, peritoneal implants)
4	Tumor has spread through the bloodstream to other organs far away from the kidneys (e.g., lungs, liver, bone or distant lymph nodes)
5	Tumors are in both kidneys at the time of diagnosis

     b. Physical examination. A palpable flank mass is present in 85% of children. Wilms tumors are associated with other anomalies such as Beckwith–Wiedemann syndrome, hemihypertrophy, aniridia, and genitourinary anomalies.

     c. Diagnostic studies. Ultrasound can be helpful in determining tumor extension into the renal vein or vena cava. **Chest and abdominal CT** scans are necessary for staging (Table 32-6) to evaluate the contralateral kidney and to screen for pulmonary metastases. **Histologic examination** confirms the diagnosis.

  2. Management

     a. Surgery and **chemotherapy** together result in a better than 90% chance of cure.

     b. Surgical intervention includes a radical nephrectomy with sampling of para-aortic lymph nodes. The hilar vessels are isolated and the contralateral kidney is also examined. If the Wilms tumor is found initially to be unresectable because of size or bilaterality, a second-look operation can be done after chemotherapy.

     c. Chemotherapy. Vincristine, doxorubicin, and dactinomycin are used, depending on the stage of the Wilms tumor.

     d. Radiotherapy is used for advanced stages of Wilms tumor.

C. Hepatic tumors make up fewer than 5% of all intra-abdominal malignancies. They are malignant in 70% of cases.

- Hepatoblastoma
- 39% of liver tumors
- 90% occur before 3 years of age
- 60% are diagnosed by 1 year of age
- Hepatocellular carcinoma

- Presents in older children
- Approximately one-third of these patients have cirrhosis secondary to an inherited metabolic abnormality
    1. **Diagnosis.** Patients may present with abdominal pain or an enlarging abdominal mass. Serum alpha fetoprotein (AFP) may be elevated. CT or MR scan may demonstrate the lesion.
    2. **Management.** Surgical intervention typically includes primary tumor resection and lymph node sampling. Intraoperative histologic analysis of the liver margins is necessary to confirm complete removal of the tumor. Hepatoblastoma that is not initially resectable undergoes chemotherapy and re-exploration for curative resection.

D. **Teratomas** are composed of tissues from all germ layers (endoderm, ectoderm, and mesoderm). In neonates, sacrococcygeal teratomas are the most common. They are more common in girls (4:1). Complications of teratomas include hemorrhage and a high rate of recurrence if the coccyx is incompletely resected.

1. **Diagnosis** can be made with prenatal ultrasound. CT scan can also be useful. A rectal exam must be completed.

2. **Management**
    a. Antenatal diagnosis may necessitate delivery by cesarean section.
    b. Surgical intervention is typically during the first week of life.
        (1) A chevron-shaped buttock incision is made.
        (2) Resection of the tumor includes preservation of the rectal sphincter muscles, resection of the coccyx with the tumor, and early control of the mid-sacral vessels that supply the tumor.
        (3) Resection may require combined abdominal and perineal approaches for large intra-abdominal teratomas.
    c. Chemotherapy for malignant teratomas may shrink the tumor and allow for resection.

E. **Soft-tissue sarcomas** account for 6% of childhood malignancies. Greater than one half are rhabdomyosarcomas.

1. **Diagnosis** is made with a CT or MR scan. However, **incisional biopsy** is usually required to determine the histologic type preoperatively.

2. **Management**
    a. A multidisciplinary approach involving medical and radiation oncology is advised prior to starting therapy.
    b. Non-rhabdomyosarcomas require wide surgical excision.
    c. Rhabdomyosarcoma
        (1) Treatment is determined by the location of the tumor.
        (2) Complete resection of **head and neck tumors** is rarely possible, and they are usually managed with biopsy followed by chemotherapy.
        (3) **Trunk and retroperitoneal tumors** are treated with wide excision.
        (4) **Extremity tumors** are treated with wide excision, but resection of muscle groups and the use of radiotherapy or brachytherapy should also be considered.
        (5) A biopsy of the regional lymph nodes should be included in all procedures.

33 Neurosurgical Emergencies

Matthew R. Reynolds and Michael R. Chicoine

Neurosurgical emergencies involve a broad spectrum of illness, including traumatic injury to the brain and spine. Several nontraumatic settings also require emergent intervention. Among these are intracranial hemorrhage, elevated intracranial pressure (ICP), spinal cord compression, and infections.

NEUROSURGICAL TRAUMA

I. INTRACRANIAL TRAUMA

A. **Evaluation.** Initial management of head injury focuses on hemodynamic stabilization through establishment of an adequate airway, ventilation, and support of circulation, followed by the rapid diagnosis and treatment of intracranial injuries. The initial evaluation of patients with trauma has been discussed in detail previously (see Chapter 22) and will only briefly be discussed here with emphasis on the neurosurgical patient.

1. **Airway and ventilation.** Severe head injury frequently leads to failure of oxygenation, ventilation, and airway protection. Intubation in these cases is essential, and a low threshold for intubation in agitated patients requiring sedation must also be present. A rapid neurologic assessment performed before sedation and paralysis are induced is critical. When possible, cervical spine imaging and neurologic examination should be performed before intubation. Associated cervical spine injuries should always be assumed in the patient with a head injury until they are ruled out. Two-person in-line intubation is performed, with the second person securing the patient's neck with axial traction to avoid neck extension. Short-acting neuromuscular blocking agents are preferred in the acute setting. Nasal intubation can be performed in the absence of craniofacial injuries.

2. **Circulatory support** requires aggressive fluid resuscitation for treatment of arterial hypotension. In the absence of profuse scalp bleeding, however, intracranial hemorrhage is almost never the sole cause of systemic hypotension. Mental status examination should be performed after the mean arterial pressure (MAP) and cerebral perfusion pressure (CPP) (CPP = MAP − ICP) have normalized (e.g., CPP ≥60 mm Hg). In addition, the use of hypotonic fluids should be avoided in patients with head injuries because this could exacerbate cerebral edema.

B. Neurologic evaluation

1. **A rapid but systematic** neurologic examination is performed on the scene and is repeated frequently during transport and on initial presentation to the emergency room. Examination focuses on the three components of the **Glasgow Coma Scale** (GCS) (Table 33-1): Eye

TABLE 33-1	Glasgow Coma Scale[a]
Component	Points
Eye opening	—
Spontaneous	4
To voice	3
To stimulation	2
None	1
Motor response	—
To command	6
Localizes	5
Withdraws	4
Abnormal flexion	3
Extension	2
None	1
Verbal response	—
Oriented	5
Confused but comprehensible	4
Inappropriate or incoherent	3
Incomprehensible (no words)	2
None	1

[a]Glasgow Coma Score = Best eye opening + best motor response + best verbal response. If patient is intubated, the verbal score is omitted and an addendum of "T" is given to the best eye opening + best motor response score.

opening, verbal response, and motor response (*Lancet.* 1974;2:81). This score indicates injury severity and measures changes in the impairment of consciousness. Overall level of consciousness may be graded as normal (awake, alert, oriented, and conversant), somnolent (arousable to voice), lethargic (arousable to deep stimulation), or comatose (nonarousable to any stimulation). The cranial nerves (e.g., pupillary response, extraocular movements, facial symmetry, and tongue protrusion) should be examined. Unilateral pupillary dilatation may herald the onset of early brain herniation (see Section V.A.2). For this reason, the pupils of a head-injured patient should never be pharmacologically dilated in the acute setting. Strength and symmetry of the extremities should be noted, and sensory examination should be performed as thoroughly as the level of consciousness permits. Reflexes and sphincter tone should also be assessed. In the critically ill patient, examination is performed while the patient is off sedation and paralytic medications. Finally, the head-injured patient has a high incidence of associated injuries. Cervical spine evaluation is obligatory (see Sections IV.A.2 and IV.A.3) given the high incidence of injury to this region (~4% to 8%) in patients with traumatic brain injury (*J Neurosurg.* 2002;96 (3, Suppl):285).

2. **Systemic causes** of mental status impairment must be ruled out including metabolic (electrolyte or acid–base abnormalities, hypo- and hyperglycemia), toxic (drugs, uremia), hypothermic, or respiratory (hypoxia, hypercapnia) derangements. Seizures or cardiac arrest can also impair neurologic function.

C. **Radiographic evaluation** may begin with cervical spine plain radiographs, including anteroposterior, lateral, open-mouth (odontoid) views, and a lateral swimmer's view if needed (see Section IV.A.3.a). In many trauma centers, however, the rapidity and diagnostic accuracy of computed tomographic (CT) technology has supplanted X-ray imaging. A growing body of evidence demonstrates increased sensitivity of CT in detecting spine fractures in patients with blunt trauma compared to plain radiography (*J Trauma.* 2006;61:382). The initial emergency room evaluation should proceed rapidly to noncontrast head CT, and delay caused by evaluation of non–life-threatening injuries should be avoided until the patient's head is imaged. Centers without this capability should transfer the patient expeditiously to a facility with CT scanning and neurosurgical facilities. A normal CT scan without altered level of consciousness, neurologic deficit, or open injuries may allow the patient to be discharged to home with reliable supervision. Any exceptions may indicate a more severe injury with a higher risk of associated or delayed lesions and may require the patient to be admitted for observation.

D. **Seizures** should be controlled rapidly in patients with head injury. Intravenous lorazepam (Ativan) can be administered in 1 to 2 mg boluses and repeated until seizures are controlled. Airway protection must be available if significant doses of benzodiazepines are to be given. Phenytoin (Dilantin) should also be administered for seizures and is indicated for seizure prophylaxis in patients at high risk for early post-traumatic seizures

(GCS = 10 or less, intracranial hematoma, depressed skull fracture, cortical contusion visible on CT, penetrating or open injuries) for a duration of no more than 7 days if the patient remains seizure free (*N Engl J Med.* 1990;323:497). A loading dose of phenytoin or fosphenytoin (Cerebyx) in patients with poor intravenous (IV) access or status epilepticus may be given (15 to 20 mg/kg). Maintenance doses of phenytoin should then be started and drug levels followed to guide dosing. Alternatively, levetiracetam (Keppra) may be loaded orally, or intravenously, at 1,000 mg and then continued at 500 to 1,000 mg orally twice daily. The latter agent does not require serum drug level monitoring, has an acceptable side-effect profile, and is preferable in patients with hepatic disease. Levetiracetam appears to be as effective as phenytoin in the prevention of early post-traumatic seizures and may provide improved long-term outcomes in patients with severe traumatic brain injury (*Neurocrit Care.* 2010;12:165).

II. TYPES OF HEAD INJURY

A. **Focal (mass) lesions** are best diagnosed by CT scan of the head without contrast. Hemiparesis, unilateral pupillary dysfunction (the fixed and dilated pupil), or both can herald brainstem herniation from mass lesions, but these are imperfect localizing signs (*Neurosurgery.* 1994;34:840). Relative indications for surgical evacuation include neurologic symptoms referable to the mass lesion, midline shift greater than 5 to 10 mm, and elevated ICP that is refractory to medical management. Posterior fossa mass lesions can be particularly dangerous because brainstem herniation may have very few specific warning signs before death occurs (see Section V.A.2.b).

1. **Epidural hematomas (EDHs)** can cause rapid neurologic deterioration and usually require surgical evacuation if they cause significant mass effect (e.g., are greater than 1 cm in width) or clinical symptoms. Classically, EDH presents with a "lucid interval" after injury, which precedes rapid deterioration. This sign is inconsistent and nonspecific, however, and may also be seen with other forms of severe brain injury. EDH typically results from laceration of the middle meningeal artery due to fracture of the squamosal portion of the temporal bone. They appear on head CT scan as biconvex hyperdensities that typically respect the suture lines (Fig. 33-1, panels A and B). Location in the low-to-mid temporal lobe is particularly dangerous, given their propensity for midbrain compression and uncal herniation.

2. **Acute subdural hematomas (aSDH)** typically appear on head CT scan as hyperdense crescents as the blood spreads around the surface of the brain (Fig. 33-1, panel C). Often, aSDH results from high-speed acceleration or deceleration trauma and portend severe underlying intracranial injury. These injuries typically result from shearing/tearing forces applied to small bridging (emissary) veins that drain the underlying neural tissue into the dural sinuses. If surgical evacuation is indicated and delayed for more than 4 hours, these lesions have a high mortality (*J Neurosurg.* 1991;74:212, *N Engl J Med.* 1981;304:1511).

Figure 33-1. Noncontrast head CTs showing **(A)** large right-sided epidural hematoma with mass effect and midline shift, **(B)** bone windows from panel "A" demonstrating associated linear temporal bone fracture (*asterisk,* see inset), **(C)** left-sided acute subdural hematoma with significant midline shift, **(D)** bilateral mixed-density subdural hematomas with both acute (hyperdense) and chronic (hypodense) components, **(E)** bilateral frontal and right-sided temporal hemorrhagic contusions with surrounding edema (hypodense), and **(F)** large left-sided basal ganglia intraparenchymal hemorrhage (nontraumatic, likely related to hypertension) with intraventricular extension resulting in acute hydrocephalus.

3. **Chronic SDHs (cSDH)** can present, especially in the elderly and alcoholic population, days to weeks after the initial head injury. cSDH may cause focal neurologic deficits, mental status changes, metabolic abnormalities, and/or seizures. If necessary, a symptomatic cSDH can be treated with burr-hole drainage and subdural drain placement (*J Neurosurg.* 1986;65:183). Prophylactic anticonvulsants should be considered and steroids may be beneficial, though this remains unclear. Diagnosis is best made with a noncontrast head CT that typically shows a hypodense crescentic collection tracking between the dura and the brain (Fig. 33-1, panel D).

4. **Cerebral contusions** manifest on noncontrast head CT scan as small, punctuate hyperdensities that are commonly located in the basal frontal and temporal lobes (Fig. 33-1, panel E). These injuries may occur during blunt trauma to the head or with acceleration/deceleration injury. In many cases, damage occurs when the brain comes into contact with the sharp bony ridges on the interior skull base. Contusions may be observed in a "coup" pattern, whereby injury to the cerebral cortex occurs in the region immediately underlying the site of impact as the brain collides with the inert table of the skull. Alternatively, a "contrecoup" pattern occurs when the brain comes into contact with the opposite pole of the skull following the initial impact. Cerebral contusions may be appreciated in a significant proportion of patients with severe traumatic brain injury and have a tendency to progress in size and mass effect (*J Neurosurg.* 2010;112:1139).

5. **Intraparenchymal hemorrhage (IPH).** While also caused by hypertension, coagulopathy, hemorrhagic transformation of ischemic stroke or tumor, venous outflow obstruction, or a ruptured aneurysm or vascular malformation, IPH may be precipitated by trauma. These injuries manifest on noncontrast head CT as focal areas of hyperdensity, typically with hypodense surrounding areas of edema (Fig. 33-1, panel F). IPH can occur with high-energy traumatic mechanisms or in the setting of a low-to-moderate energy mechanism in a coagulopathic patient. Typically, laceration of larger cerebral vessels is the inciting event. Mechanical complications of mass effect may quickly progress to brain herniation in severe cases. Extension of bleeding into the ventricular system may result in **intraventricular hemorrhage** with increased risk of communicating or noncommunicating hydrocephalus due to impaired cerebrospinal fluid (CSF) reabsorption by the arachnoid granulations or a focal blockade of CSF flow, respectively.

B. **Nonfocal** sequelae of head injury include **cerebral edema** and **diffuse axonal injury (DAI).** Hallmarks of cerebral edema on head CT scan include obliteration of the basal cisterns and coronal sulci with loss of differentiation of the gray and white matter. In DAI, severe head injury and neurologic dysfunction can be associated with minimal changes on head CT scan (*J Neurosurg.* 1982;56:26). DAI represents the pathologic result of shearing forces on the brain. Often, small hemorrhages are seen in the corpus callosum, midbrain, or deep white matter.

C. **Open skull fractures** require operative irrigation, débridement of non-viable tissues, and dural closure. Evaluation of scalp lacerations should include attention to the integrity of the galeal layer and the underlying skull fractures. Prophylactic antibiotics may reduce the risk of infection. Surgical treatment of **depressed skull fractures** usually is required for depressions greater than the thickness of the skull table. Open, depressed skull fractures require elevation and débridement of depressed bony fragments as well as devitalized tissue, followed by a course of antibiotics. Fractures through the paranasal air **sinuses,** especially with associated pneumocephalus and dural tears, may require repair. The prophylactic use of broad-spectrum antibiotics to prevent meningitis in these cases is controversial.

D. **Basilar skull fractures** can be complicated by **CSF** leaks and are mostly managed nonoperatively. The use of prophylactic antibiotics is controversial in these cases. If drainage continues or recurs, a lumbar drain or surgical repair may be required because persistent leakage can lead to meningitis. Temporal bone fractures can be associated with damage to the seventh and eighth cranial nerves, the middle ear apparatus, or both.

E. **Missile injuries** require débridement, closure, and prophylactic antibiotics similar to those used for other open-head injuries. However, injuries from gunshot wounds present several associated problems. Shock waves can result in widespread destruction of brain tissue and vasculature. Operative management must address removal of accessible foreign bodies and bone fragments, evacuation of intracranial hematomas, débridement of entrance and exit wounds, and closure of dura and scalp. Overaggressive débridement near large vessels should be avoided to prevent further damage to vascular structures.

III. MANAGEMENT OF ELEVATED INTRACRANIAL PRESSURE

A. Monitoring

1. **Indications.** ICP monitoring is recommended if serial neurologic examinations cannot be used as a reliable indicator of progressive intracranial pathology. The current standard for ICP monitoring is in patients with an abnormal head CT scan and a GCS score less than 8. Alternatively, ICP monitoring should be performed in patients with a normal head CT scan and GCS score greater than 8 if two of the following three criteria are met: (i) Age greater than 40 years, (ii) unilateral or bilateral motor posturing, and (iii) systemic blood pressure less than 90 mm Hg on admission (*J Neurosurg.* 1982;56:650).

2. **ICP pressure monitors** are of several types. The **parenchymal bolt** consists of a fiberoptic or strain gauge catheter tip that measures ICP at the brain surface. **Intraventricular catheters** (ventriculostomy) are placed in the lateral ventricle with the tip at the foramen of Monro. These devices allow for drainage of CSF in the treatment of elevated ICP in addition to ICP monitoring. Newer monitors include those that measure ICP, cerebral temperature, and brain tissue oxygenation, and the utility of such devices is under investigation.

B. Treatment

1. **If elevated ICP** is suspected, such as with signs of herniation or acute neurologic deterioration, therapy should be empirically initiated until the ICP can be measured. If the patient is hemodynamically stable with adequate renal function, high-dose **mannitol** (0.5 to 1.0 g/kg IV bolus) is effective in acutely controlling elevated ICP. Fluid balance, serum electrolytes, and serum osmolarity should be carefully monitored, and a Foley catheter is placed to closely follow the osmotic diuresis. Mannitol is generally held if the serum osmolarity exceeds 320 mOsm/L. Hypotension should be avoided in these patients as data suggests that better outcomes occur with maintenance of CPP (MAP – ICP) of 60 mm Hg or greater (see Section III.C.1). A euvolemic, hyperosmolar situation is desirable; fluid replacement is usually necessary to avoid hypotension which may precipitate an ischemic episode that could worsen the underlying brain injury. Treatment is aimed at keeping ICP less than 20 mm Hg (*J Neurosurg.* 1991;75:S59). If elevated ICP is refractory to a single mannitol bolus, then standing high-dose mannitol therapy may be instituted at 0.5 to 1.0 g/kg IV every 6 hours.

2. **Hypertonic saline** is a useful adjunct to mannitol in the control of elevated ICP (*Crit Care Med.* 2003;31:1683). Hypertonic saline (23.4%), or "super salt," is effective for acutely reducing ICP in patients with severe traumatic brain injury (*J Trauma.* 2009;67:277). This agent may be preferable in hypovolemic patients, but requires central venous access for administration and frequent plasma sodium monitoring. Plasma sodium levels should not exceed 160 mmol/L. Hypertonic saline (23.4%, 30 to 60 mL IV every 6 hours) can be alternated with mannitol therapy in cases of refractory ICP.

3. Ventilatory support to maintain a mildly hypocapnic partial pressure of carbon dioxide (Pco_2) (~35 mm Hg) should be instituted, and **hyperventilation** (Pco_2 ~30 mm Hg) may be used in the acute setting for brief periods. Prolonged use of hyperventilation may worsen ischemia by compromising cerebral blood flow.

4. In addition to the initial treatment of elevated ICP (e.g., hyperosmolar therapy, mechanical ventilation), **simple measures** are taken, such as head elevation to 30 degrees (a neutral head position to enhance venous drainage), avoidance of circumferential taping around the patient's neck when securing the endotracheal tube, appropriate fitting of cervical spine collars if indicated, and adequate sedation before any stimulation. Elevated intrathoracic pressures (as with coughing, straining, or high positive end-expiratory pressure) can elevate ICP. Fever can also exacerbate ICP; aggressive treatment with antipyretics, cooling blankets, and intravascular cooling devices should be instituted to prevent hyperthermia.

5. **Sedation** can also be used to control ICP. Benzodiazepine or narcotic (e.g., fentanyl) infusions can be given and titrated to effect, with a goal of 3 on the Ramsay sedation scale (*Br Med J.* 1974;11:659). Intubation and mechanical ventilation usually are needed. Refractory elevation of ICP may require neuromuscular paralysis or even barbiturate coma with invasive hemodynamic monitoring.

6. **Surgical interventions** are directed primarily at removal of **mass lesions,** if present. In the absence of a mass lesion, uncontrollable ICP and a deteriorating neurologic examination may require **craniectomy,** with removal of a large bone flap to relieve pressure on the intracranial contents. Retrospective studies suggest that decompressive hemicraniectomy for uncontrolled intracranial hypertension may decrease mortality and improve outcomes in certain patients (*J Neurosurg.* 2006;104:469). Multicenter, prospective studies are underway to better evaluate the indications for surgical intervention in this difficult patient population (*Acta Neurochir Suppl.* 2006;96:17). Removal of CSF by **ventriculostomy** can reduce ICP; however, the small intracranial volume occupied by the CSF limits this effect.

C. **Considerations when managing elevated ICP**

1. **Cardiac considerations.** Adequate blood pressure should be maintained in the setting of elevated ICP, with care taken to avoid hypotension (systolic blood pressure <90 mm Hg), which has been associated with inferior outcome in severely head-injured patients (*Br J Neurosurg.* 1993;7:267). Maintenance of CPP greater than 60 mm Hg (or MAP >80 to 90 mm Hg) can be used as a treatment guideline (*Crit Care.* 2000;9(6):R670).

2. **Fluid and electrolytes.** Head-injured patients are at risk for development of either diabetes insipidus or the syndrome of inappropriate antidiuretic hormone (SIADH). Initially, the use of isotonic saline (with glucose and, if necessary, potassium) avoids exacerbating cerebral edema. Close monitoring of electrolytes is essential because alterations in sodium and water balance are common. **Diabetes insipidus** can develop rapidly and must be treated aggressively. Fluid hydration should match output. Often, the process is self-limiting, but persistent output of large amounts (>300 mL/hour) of urine with a low specific gravity (<1.005) may necessitate vasopressin treatment [desmopressin (DDAVP), 1 μg IV every 12 hours]. If SIADH with hyponatremia develops, treatment with restriction of free water intake usually is sufficient, although infusion of hypertonic (1.5% NaCl) saline may be necessary.

3. **Coagulopathy,** if present, should be corrected as expeditiously and safely as possible. For patients with an intracranial hemorrhage being treated with systemic anticoagulation for other medical morbidities (e.g., atrial fibrillation, deep venous thrombosis, pulmonary emboli), all anticoagulant agents should be discontinued. Blood products and other agents should be administered for a goal of international normalized ratio (INR) ≤1.4, prothrombin time (PTT) ≤40 seconds, and platelets ≥100,000. For patients on systemic antiplatelet agents (e.g., full-dose aspirin, clopidogrel [Plavix]), consideration should be given to platelet transfusion even in the setting of a normal platelet count. Recombinant factor VII may be given under circumstances of life-threatening intracranial hemorrhage with coagulopathy and the need for immediate normalization of coagulation parameters. Disseminated intravascular coagulopathy can also occur with severe head injury, such

as missile injuries, often developing several hours after the disruption of brain tissue. Coagulopathies should be aggressively treated with fresh-frozen plasma and vitamin K, especially if intracranial hemorrhage is present.

4. **Nutrition.** Nutritional demands are increased in head injury (*Neurosurg Clin North Am.* 1991;2:301). High-osmolarity tube feedings can reduce the risk of cerebral edema and provide adequate caloric intake. If tube feedings are not tolerated, parenteral nutrition may be necessary.

5. **Deep venous thrombosis prophylaxis.** Patients with severe head injury are at high risk for deep venous thrombosis and subsequent pulmonary embolism. Early use of intermittent pneumatic compression devices is highly recommended. Although efficacy remains controversial, recent studies suggest no increased risk of intracranial hemorrhage in head-injured patients who receive subcutaneous heparin (*J Trauma.* 2002;53:38) or enoxaparin (*Arch Surg.* 2002;137:701) within 72 hours of admission.

IV. **SPINAL TRAUMA. Evaluation** for spinal injury is indicated if focal pain, neurologic examination, or mechanism of injury warrants. Neurologic deficit involving the lower extremities after trauma may require evaluation of the entire spine to find an injury.

A. **Initial support**

1. As with all patients with trauma, attention should first focus on airway, breathing, and circulation (see Chapter 22 for initial evaluation of the patient with trauma). In the setting of known or suspected spinal cord injury, several additional points are worthy of mention. First, intubation should be performed early in patients demonstrating respiratory fatigue or otherwise requiring airway protection or ventilatory support. With cervical spine injury, fiberoptic intubation should be performed as this procedure requires less manipulation and reduces the risk of further neurologic injury. Second, in the paraplegic or quadriplegic patient who becomes hypotensive without an obvious source of internal or external hemorrhage, **neurogenic (or spinal) shock** should be considered. Hypotension associated with the loss of sympathetic tone seen in some high thoracic and cervical spine injuries does not respond to fluid challenge alone. Vasopressors (e.g., dopamine) reduce peripheral vasodilatation and improve cardiac output. Excessive fluid administration can worsen respiratory difficulty and spinal cord edema.

2. **Neurologic examination** includes a careful assessment of motor function, sensory function, and deep tendon reflexes. Multiple sensory modalities (light touch, pinprick, temperature sensation, and joint position sense) should be assessed, especially in the patient with an incomplete lesion. Useful landmarks for sensory dermatomes include the nipple (T4 level) and the umbilicus (T10 level). Sphincter tone as well as cremasteric and bulbocavernosus reflexes should be documented. Incomplete lesions are common and, as with sacral sparing of sensory function, carry prognostic significance (*Neurosurgery.* 1987;20:742).

3. Radiographic evaluation

a. Standard radiographic evaluation of the cervical spine includes **anteroposterior, lateral, and open-mouth (odontoid)** views. A **swimmer's** view may be necessary to visualize C7 and the C7–T1 interspace, which is essential in the complete evaluation of the cervical spine. CT scanning with coronal and sagittal reconstructions is necessary if adequate plain films cannot be obtained and is replacing radiography as the standard of care in patients with blunt trauma (*J Trauma.* 2006;61:382). Of note, flexion/extension films remain the best means of surveying for fractures or subluxations that may suggest occult ligamentous instability that may not be visualized on CT. Anteroposterior and lateral views of the thoracic and lumbar spine are obtained as indicated or may be reconstructed from chest, abdominal, and pelvic CT if available. If a spinal fracture is found, the entire spine should be imaged because of the high rate of coincident injuries (*J Spinal Disord.* 1992;5:320).

b. Other imaging modalities include **CT scans** to further evaluate known or suspected fractures. **Magnetic resonance imaging (MRI)** is sensitive for ligamentous injuries, intraspinal hemorrhage, and protruded intervertebral discs (*J Neurosurg.* 1993;79:341), which can cause deficit with or without bony abnormalities seen on plain films. Damage to the vertebral artery can occur with cervical injuries, especially if fracture through the foramen transversarium occurs. CT angiography, conventional digital subtraction angiography, or magnetic resonance angiography are pursued if neurologic damage is referable to vertebral artery injury.

B. Instability. Spinal instability must be suspected until ruled out. Ligamentous injury can occur in the absence of fracture, and instability can occur with normal plain films. Point tenderness, severe midline pain, or apprehension of neck movement also warrants careful assessment. In the minimally symptomatic, alert patient, cervical flexion/extension films can aid in the assessment of spinal stability. Flexion and extension must be done under the patient's own power, and motion should be stopped if pain or other symptoms arise. Limited flexion and extension motion on physical exam may significantly decrease the utility of flexion/extension radiography in detecting ligamentous instability (*J Trauma.* 2002;53:426). These patients should be left in a cervical collar and may require additional cross-sectional imaging to exclude occult injury.

C. Treatment

1. Methylprednisolone is recommended only as an option in the treatment of spinal cord injury, given the increased risk of medical complications associated with its use (*Neurosurgery.* 2002;50:S63). Patients seen between 3 and 8 hours after injury may be treated with methylprednisolone, **30 mg/kg IV bolus** over 15 minutes, followed 45 minutes later by a **5.4 mg/kg/hour IV infusion** continued over the next 48 hours (*J Am Med Assoc.* 1997;277:1597). If steroids are administered within 3 hours of injury, IV infusion is given for only 24 hours. If patients are seen more than 8 hours after injury, this protocol is not of proven benefit and is contraindicated. Steroids are also contraindicated in cases of penetrating spinal injury (*Neurosurgery.* 1997;41:576) and have been associated with increased postoperative complications after thoracolumbar spine stabilization (*J Trauma.* 2010;69:1479).

2. **Immobilization and reduction.** Suspected or known spine injuries require immobilization, initially with a rigid cervical collar and long backboard. Cervical spine subluxations and dislocations must be reduced under neurosurgical supervision. Fractures may be treated by external immobilization (e.g., halo external fixation) or by operative fusion, depending on the nature of the fracture and degree of instability. Thoracic and lumbar spine fractures are managed with operative stabilization or immobilization with an orthosis. Injuries with associated neurologic deficit, excessive displacement or angulation of the spinal column, or loss of vertebral body height are more likely to require operative stabilization. Before stabilization, patients are managed with bed rest and frequent log rolling. Although early surgical decompression and stabilization promote mobilization of the patient, the timing of surgery and the role of emergency surgery in the patient with acute neurologic deficit remain somewhat controversial (*Neurosurgery.* 1994;35:240).

3. **Cervical collar management.** If a patient with trauma has a normal level of alertness, no evidence of intoxication, no focal neurological deficit, no painful distracting injuries, no posterior midline cervical spine tenderness, and normal cervical spine range of motion, then no cervical spine imaging is required and cervical immobilization may be discontinued (*J Orthop Trauma.* 2010;24:100). If posterior cervical tenderness is present in the setting of negative cervical spine imaging, the collar may be cleared radiographically following adequate flexion/extension radiographs or a normal cervical spine MRI within 48 hours of the injury. If flexion/extension films are inadequate (e.g., due to pain and/or effort), the films may be repeated in 10 to 14 days while maintaining cervical spine precautions. In the obtunded patient with normal cervical spine imaging, the cervical collar may be cleared by normal flexion/extension radiographs taken under fluoroscopy, a normal cervical spine MRI taken within 48 hours of injury, or at the discretion of the treating physician (*Neurosurgery.* 2002;50 (3 Suppl):S36).

4. **Cervical spine injuries** are associated with the development of acute respiratory distress syndrome, hyponatremia, hypotension, bradyarrhythmias, ileus, and urinary retention. Patients with cervical spine injuries may require cardiorespiratory monitoring, isotonic fluid support, nasogastric decompression, urinary catheter placement, laxatives, and stool softeners to address these issues. Bladder and bowel dysfunction also are seen with lower spine injuries, although autonomic problems are rare in injuries below the upper thoracic spine.

5. **Penetrating injuries** to the neck and torso may result in fractures of the spine or penetration of the spinal canal.

6. **Venous thromboembolism risk** is significantly elevated in patients with spinal cord injury. Intermittent pneumatic compression devices with subcutaneous heparin or enoxaparin have been demonstrated to be equally safe in the acute management of spinal cord injury (*J Trauma.* 2003;54:1116).

V. OTHER EMERGENCIES

A. Nontraumatic intracranial hypertension and herniation syndromes

1. **Etiology.** Elevation of ICP may lead to compression of neurologic structures and irreversible neurologic damage. Nontraumatic causes include hemorrhagic and nonhemorrhagic mass lesions.

   a. Spontaneous **IPHs** may occur owing to hypertension, vascular malformations (arteriovenous malformations or aneurysms), tumor, angiopathy, vasculitis, or secondary hemorrhage into a large infarction.

   b. **Nonhemorrhagic lesions** include tumor, infection, and mass effect from edema after cerebral infarction.

2. Clinical **herniation syndromes** represent shift of the normal brain through or across regions within the skull secondary to increased ICP and/or mass effect. These syndromes are typically caused by a mass lesion and exist with presentations referable to the location of the lesion (Fig. 33-2).

   a. **Supratentorial** sites of herniation include uncal, central (transtentorial), and cingulate (subfalcine) herniation. **Uncal** herniation often results from temporal lobe mass lesions given the proximity of the temporal lobe to the midbrain. In this circumstance, the medial temporal lobe (uncus) is pushed over the tentorial incisura and exerts pressure on the midbrain. Unilateral pupillary dilatation may occur in the absence of a complete third cranial nerve palsy due to the compression of the parasympathetic fibers which travel on the exterior surface of the nerve (e.g., superficial to the motor fibers). Progressive lethargy (due to increased ICP), contralateral hemiparesis (due to compression of the cerebral peduncle/corticospinal tract), and contralateral visual deficits (due to compression of the posterior cerebral artery) also suggest uncal herniation. **Central (transtentorial)** herniation results from downward compression of brainstem structures through the tentorial incisura. Unresponsiveness, deep coma, and cranial nerve dysfunction are observed. Central herniation suggests a bilateral process or an interhemispheric lesion. **Cingulate (subfalcine)** herniation results from lesions causing a shift across the inferior aspect of the falx cerebri and can present with only lethargy or lower-extremity weakness (the latter from injury to the anterior cerebral arteries). Both falcine and uncal herniation can progress to a central transtentorial picture as further structures are compressed.

   b. **Infratentorial** herniation results from posterior fossa masses compressing the brainstem or from herniation of the cerebellar tonsils

Figure 33-2. Brain herniation syndromes may be classified as supratentorial (above the tentorial notch) or infratentorial (below the tentorial notch). **(A)** Represents normal anatomy. **(B)** Shows herniation due to a mass lesion. Uncal *(1)*, transtentorial *(2)*, and subfalcine *(3)* are examples of supratentorial herniation. Tonsillar *(4)*, or downward cerebellar, herniation may be observed in the infratentorial compartment.

through the foramen magnum. Signs of infratentorial herniation include lower cranial nerve dysfunction and the rapid onset of respiratory or cardiac arrest with little warning.

3. **Treatment** of herniation requires control of ICP. The obtunded patient must have their airway controlled. Mannitol can be used, often with ICP monitoring (see Section III.A and III.B) to guide medical treatment. Mass lesions may need to be evacuated.

B. **Nonhemorrhagic lesions.** Diffuse cerebral edema also can produce ICP elevations that require treatment. **Metabolic derangements,** such as those seen in hepatic encephalopathy, can elevate the ICP. Edema can also develop secondary to large **infarctions** in the cerebral hemispheres, leading to delayed deterioration. Management of elevated ICP may be indicated in large cerebral infarctions, whether hemorrhagic or nonhemorrhagic.

1. **Brain tumors** rarely are surgical emergencies. Presenting symptoms include progressive headache, seizures, and localizing neurologic deficits. Uncommonly, acute neurologic deterioration is seen, usually suggestive of hemorrhage into the tumor. Evaluation and treatment are similar to those for any other acute intracranial mass lesion. High-dose **steroids** may have a potent effect on the brain edema associated with tumors. Urgent **surgical resection** of the mass lesion occasionally is required.

2. **Hydrocephalus** may result from various causes and can lead to rapid neurologic deterioration.

   a. **Cerebellar tumors** or other mass lesions may cause fourth ventricle obstruction without preceding symptoms. Tuberculosis and bacterial meningitis also can cause hydrocephalus. Patients classically present with lethargy, headache, papilledema, sixth nerve palsy, or abnormalities of upward gaze ("setting-sun" sign). **Treatment** involves urgent placement of a catheter for external **ventricular drainage** (see Section III.A.2) to relieve the buildup of CSF.

   b. **Shunt malfunction.** Internal ventricular drainage systems (shunts) require special attention. Malfunction can present with warning symptoms, such as headache or nausea, or with rapid deterioration of mental status, such as somnolence. Imaging, such as a head CT scan, can help in the diagnosis, but emergent operative revision may be indicated if mental status deterioration is present and shunt malfunction is suspected. A shunt series (plain films of the head, neck, chest, and abdomen) can visualize the entire course of the shunt and its connections, possibly leading to identification of a shunt tube fracture or stricture. Importantly, evaluation of shunt patency should always be performed under the guidance of a neurosurgeon given that as many as 33% of all shunt malfunctions will not have radiographic evidence of failure (e.g., large ventricles, grossly disconnected catheter) (*Pediatrics.* 1998;101:1031).

C. **Intracranial hemorrhage.** Spontaneous intracranial hemorrhage requires emergent intervention, and the sequelae of the associated mass effect also need to be addressed.

Figure 33-3. Noncontrast head CT depicting acute subarachnoid blood within the basal cisterns, bilateral sylvian fissures, and interhemispheric fissure. The anterior tips of the temporal horns may be visualized bilaterally (*asterisks*), representing early signs of hydrocephalus.

1. **Subarachnoid hemorrhage (SAH)** secondary to aneurysmal hemorrhage is a common neurosurgical emergency. The clinical **presentation** usually includes a history of severe sudden headache, nuchal rigidity, photophobia, lethargy, agitation, or a comatose state. Acute blood from a SAH appears hyperdense on a noncontrast head CT and is typically seen in the basal cisterns or sylvian fissure (Fig. 33-3). Lumbar puncture can make the diagnosis if the history is suggestive, even with a normal CT scan, but is not required when the scan is diagnostic. Treatments including surgical clipping and endovascular techniques aim to prevent rebleeding. Without intervention, rebleeding occurs in 50% of patients with a ruptured aneurysm in the first 6 months (*J Neurosurg.* 1985;62:321).

2. **Spontaneous intracranial hemorrhage** most commonly results from chronic hypertension, but other causes may include vascular malformations (e.g., aneurysm, arteriovenous malformation), arteriopathy (e.g., cerebral amyloid angiopathy, moyamoya disease), altered hemostasis, and hemorrhagic transformation of a tumor or infarct. While the optimal management of spontaneous supratentorial intracranial hemorrhage remains unclear, one large randomized trial suggests that early hematoma evacuation has no impact on outcome and mortality at 6 months as compared to initial conservative therapy (*Lancet.* 2005;356:387).

3. **Spontaneous intraventricular hemorrhage** may be an isolated event or result from extension of an IPH into the ventricular system. Patients are observed for the development of hydrocephalus, which may require external CSF drainage (ventriculostomy). In cases of unclear etiology, cerebral angiography may be helpful to delineate the cause.

4. Pituitary apoplexy occurs after hemorrhage into the pituitary gland, usually related to an underlying pituitary adenoma. Patients typically present with acute headache and visual symptoms, such as decreased acuity, visual field cut, ptosis, or diplopia, which result from compression of nearby cranial nerves. Life-threatening panhypopituitarism can occur. Treatment involves hormonal replacement, correction of any electrolyte abnormalities, and emergent CT or MRI scan to evaluate for hemorrhagic pituitary lesions. Emergent evacuation of hematoma may preserve vision.

D. Infections

1. Cerebral abscesses can result from hematogenous or local traumatic spread of a septic process. Infections may also involve the epidural or subdural spaces. Underlying abnormalities are common, such as an immunocompromised state or systemic arteriovenous shunting. Presenting symptoms include those of increased ICP, focal deficits, and seizures. An MRI or head CT scan with IV contrast shows an enhancing lesion. Early-stage cerebral abscess may respond to medical management alone. Abscesses larger than 3 cm, failure of medical management, and the need for tissue diagnosis are common indications for surgical drainage by open craniotomy or stereotactic drainage. Prolonged IV antibiotics are indicated.

2. Spinal epidural abscesses can become a surgical emergency. Severe neck or back pain in the setting of fever should raise concern. Although neurologic deficit may not occur initially, often progressive evidence of cord compression exists. MRI scan or myelography demonstrates the lesion. Surgical evacuation is most often necessary, although antibiotics alone can be attempted if neither neurologic compromise nor a large collection is present. Even with surgical drainage, an extended course of antibiotics is required. Disc space infection and spinal osteomyelitis can occur in association with, or separately from, spinal epidural abscesses. Antibiotic therapy usually is effective. An elevated erythrocyte sedimentation rate generally is present and falls with effective treatment.

E. Spinal cord compression

1. Diagnosis. Nontraumatic spinal cord compression can result from metastatic tumor or another adjacent mass lesion. Patients present initially with pain, followed by progressive or sudden neurologic symptoms. Lung, breast, and prostate are the most common sources of metastases (*Neurosurgery.* 1987;21:676). Examination usually reveals weakness, long-tract signs (spasticity, hyperactive reflexes, upgoing toes), or sphincter dysfunction. It is important to distinguish **myelopathy** from **radiculopathy.** The latter presents with pain, sensory changes, and weakness in a dermatomal pattern. Emergent MRI scan or myelography to demonstrate the presence and level of the lesion confirms diagnosis of cord compression. Imaging should extend to higher spinal levels if no lesion is found because, for example, a cervical lesion can present with only lower-extremity symptoms; alternatively, multilevel involvement can be present.

2. **Treatment** begins with **steroids** (dexamethasone, 10 mg intravenously, followed by 4 to 10 mg orally or intravenously every 6 hours; higher doses frequently are given for severe deficits). These are administered immediately if spinal cord compression is suspected. The neurosurgical priorities include **decompression** if a deficit is present and spinal **stabilization and fusion** if bony destruction is prominent (*Neurosurgery.* 1985;17:424). Vertebral corpectomy and reconstruction with internal fixation is often required because a simple laminectomy may not be helpful (*Lancet.* 2005;366(9486):643). Emergent **radiation therapy** to the area of compression may be preferable to surgical intervention in some cases.

34 Orthopedic Injuries

Kathleen E. McKeon and Michael J. Gardner

TREATMENT OF ORTHOPEDIC INJURIES

I. INITIAL ASSESSMENT

A. **Priorities of management. Assessment and management of ABCs** (*a*irway, *b*reathing, and *c*irculation) take precedence over extremity injuries. Multisystem-injured patients benefit from early aggressive treatment of extremity and pelvic trauma.

B. **History.** In addition to standard medical history, the mechanism of injury, especially the relative energy associated with the injury (e.g., low-energy fall vs. high-energy motor vehicle crash), is important to elucidate. An orthopedic history should also include preinjury functional level, especially previous occupation and ambulatory status.

C. **Examination**

1. An orthopedic examination includes inspection, palpation, range of motion, strength, stability, and body region–specific tests. Severe or multiple injuries can mask other injuries. Especially important in this setting is a complete primary evaluation where each joint and bone is inspected, and then a repeat secondary survey. **Inspect** the extremities for bruising, swelling, lacerations, abrasions, deformity, and asymmetry. Systematically **palpate** all extremities, noting tenderness, crepitus, and deformity of the underlying bone. In suspected cervical spine (C-spine) injury, maintain immobilization in a cervical collar until C-spine injury is ruled out radiographically and/or clinically. Logroll the patient to examine and palpate the spine.

2. **Assess extremity vascular status** by checking pulses, capillary refill, temperature, and color and comparing to the opposite side.

3. **Sensorimotor evaluation** (see Table 34-1). Muscle strength evaluation in the setting of acute spinal cord injury or peripheral nerve injury is critical, and serial exams are often required. A sensory examination includes light touch in dermatomal and peripheral nerve distributions. In upper-extremity or C-spine trauma, two-point discrimination of the fingers should be assessed. A normal peripheral nerve exam is often documented as "SILT (sensation intact to light touch) A/R/M/U and + EPL/APB/FDP2,5/IO" in the upper extremity and "SILT DP/SP/T and + TA/GS/EHL/FHL" in the lower extremity.

II. RADIOLOGIC EXAMINATION.
All trauma and unconscious patients should have screening chest x-ray, anteroposterior (AP) pelvis x-ray, and C-spine

TABLE 34-1	Peripheral Nerve Exam		
Nerve	**Sensory**	**Motor**	**Muscle**
Deep peroneal (DP)	Web space between great and second toe	Ankle and great toe dorsiflexion	Tibialis anterior (TA), Extensor hallucis longus (EHL)
Superficial peroneal (SP)	Lateral dorsum of foot	—	—
Tibial (T)	Plantar surface of foot	Ankle and great toe plantarflexion	Gastrocnemius and soleus (GS), flexor hallucis longus (FHL)
Axillary (A)	Lateral deltoid	Shoulder abduction	Deltoid
Radial (R)	Dorsal web space between thumb and index	Extension of thumb IP joint	Extensor pollicis longus (EPL)
Median (M)	Two-point discrimination of thumb, index, long	Abduct thumb perpendicular to palm, flex index DIP joint	Abductor pollicis brevis (APB), flexor digitorum profundus to index (FDP2)
Ulnar (U)	Two-point discrimination of ring, small	Spread fingers apart, flex small finger DIP joint	Interossei (IO), flexor digitorum profundus to small (FDP5)

IP, interphalangeal; DIP, distal interphalangeal.

radiographs or computed tomography (CT) scan. Although C-spine CT scans have replaced radiographs as an initial screening tool at many institutions, radiographs can be a useful adjunct. The overall alignment of the C-spine can be better appreciated on plain radiographs than on CT scan, so plain radiographs are mandatory if any injury is identified on the CT scan. Plain radiographs, especially flexion and extension views, are also mandatory if there is concern for any ligamentous injury. Lateral C-spine radiographs must visualize all cervical vertebrae to the C7–T1 junction.

Assessment of extremity fractures and dislocations should include a minimum of two views 90 degrees to each other (usually AP and lateral views) of the affected area and should include both the joint above and the joint below the injury. **Dislocations should be reduced as soon as possible,** without the benefit of radiographs if necessary, because they are often associated with neurovascular and soft-tissue compromise.

III. FRACTURES AND DISLOCATIONS

A. How to describe a fracture

1. Accurate descriptions of fractures and dislocations begin with the bone or joint involved. For fractures, the **anatomic region** refers usually to the proximal, middle, or distal portion of the bone. *Epiphyseal, metaphyseal,* and *diaphyseal* are commonly used descriptive terms of the fracture location. The **quality** of the fracture is described on the basis of its **orientation** and the **number of fracture fragments.** A fracture is **transverse** if it runs relatively perpendicular to the long axis of the bone and **oblique** if it is angled. **Spiral** fractures propagate around and along a long bone and are caused by a twisting injury. **Comminuted** fractures have, by definition, more than two fragments. **Intra-articular** fractures involve the joint surface.

2. **Alignment** always references the distal fragment relative to the proximal fragment. Key components are **angulation, translation, rotation,** and **shortening. Angulation** is angular deformity in the coronal or sagittal plane, **rotation** is deformity about the long axis of the bone, **translation** is nonangular coronal or sagittal displacement with decreased bony **apposition,** and **shortening** is loss of bone length though the fracture.

3. **Stable** fractures and dislocations are not likely to displace after reduction (the "setting" of a fracture or dislocation) and appropriate immobilization, whereas **unstable** fractures are either unable to be reduced or are likely to lose reduction despite adequate immobilization.

4. **Soft-tissue injury. Open** fractures are those with a disruption of the overlying skin and tissue such that the fracture communicates with the external environment. **Closed** fractures are those that do not communicate with the external environment. Abrasions or lacerations that do not communicate with the fracture site are considered closed, but should be carefully probed and examined before that determination is made. Fractures complicated by associated neurovascular, ligamentous, or muscular injury require prompt recognition and injury-specific treatment.

5. Joint **subluxation** refers to joint disruption and instability with decreased contact between joint surfaces. **Dislocation** refers to complete loss of contact between joint surfaces. Both are described by the position of the distal bone in relation to its proximal articulation.

B. **General management principles**
1. **Dislocation.** All dislocated joints, especially in the setting of **neu-rovascular compromise,** should be reduced **emergently,** even before initial radiographs are taken if possible. This can generally be accomplished via gentle longitudinal traction. Successful reduction reduces the risk and degree of soft-tissue injury (e.g., pressure necrosis) and neurovascular compromise. Postreduction radiographs are essential to confirm adequate reduction and to re-evaluate for associated fractures previously not visualized because of deformity associated with the dislocation. Persistently diminished or absent pulses may require arteriography and further evaluation.
2. **Fractures: Pediatric versus adult**
   a. **Management of pediatric fractures can be significantly different from the management of adult fractures. Children, especially those with open growth plates, have a greater potential for bony remodeling than adults,** and therefore a greater amount of malalignment is acceptable. In children, at least limited reduction of deformity is often necessary to decrease the risk of permanent deformity. Whereas in the adult, inability to achieve and obtain an acceptable reduction is a relative indication for surgical treatment. Fracture evaluation principles of history, physical exam, and radiographs are the same as in the adult. **Throughout this chapter, we will focus primarily on management of injuries in adult patients unless otherwise specified.**
   b. **Physeal plate injuries** ("growth plate") are common because this is the weakest part of the bone. The Salter–Harris classification categorizes these fractures into five types of increasing severity and likelihood of future growth disturbance (see Table 34-2 and Fig. 34-1).

TABLE 34-2	Salter–Harris Classification of Growth Plate Injuries
Type 1	Fracture through the growth plate without any metaphyseal or epiphyseal involvement
Type 2	Fracture through the growth plate is associated with a metaphyseal fracture
Type 3	Fracture through the growth plate is associated with an epiphyseal fracture
Type 4	Fracture through the metaphysis, across the growth plate, and exiting the epiphysis
Type 5	Severe crush injury to the growth plate

The Salter-Harris Classification of Growth Plate Injuries

Figure 34-1. The five types of Salter–Harris growth plate injuries.

IV. SOFT-TISSUE INJURY

A. **Principles of management.** In general, isolated soft-tissue injuries, such as ligament sprains and muscle strains, are treated with *r*est, *i*ce, *c*ompression bandage, and *e*levation **(RICE therapy)** with or without immobilization.

1. **Skin lacerations/defects.** All devitalized tissue should be débrided. If the wound cannot be closed due to excessive tension, it should be covered with a moist saline dressing, and a delayed primary closure or skin grafting should be planned.

2. **Muscle**
   a. **Mechanism. Strains** of the **musculotendinous unit** are usually secondary to violent contraction or excessive stretch. Injury spans the range from stretch of the fibers to a complete tear with loss of function.
   b. **Physical examination. Swelling, tenderness, and pain with movement occur.** A defect may be palpable. RICE-type treatment of the muscle involved is adequate for most such injuries.

3. **Tendon.** Lacerated, ruptured, or avulsed tendons, especially those of the upper extremity, should be surgically repaired because such injuries result in loss of function. Examination reveals loss of motion or weakness. Open wounds with a tendon laceration are irrigated thoroughly, débrided, and closed primarily with early planned repair of the tendon in the operating room (OR). In grossly contaminated wounds, incision and débridement in the OR are needed. Splints are applied with the extremity in a functional position.

4. **Ligament.** Ligament **sprains** range from mild stretch to complete tear and are commonly sports related. Pain, localized tenderness, and joint instability may be present on examination. Radiographs may reveal joint incongruence. If the joint is clinically or radiographically unstable, treatment involves immobilization in a reduced position. If no evidence of instability is present, treatment based on the RICE principle is used, and early range of motion is encouraged.

V. SPECIFIC INJURIES BY ANATOMIC LOCATION

A. Shoulder

1. Fractures: Clavicle, proximal humerus, and scapula

   a. Clavicle fractures

   (1) **Typical mechanism.** A fall onto an outstretched hand or onto a shoulder.

   (2) **Typical physical signs.** A visible or palpable **deformity** is often present at the fracture site.

   (3) **Radiographic evaluation.** Two views of the clavicle and a chest x-ray to allow a comparison of clavicle length with the contralateral side.

   (4) **Typical management.** Most clavicle fractures heal with non-operative treatment and can be managed with a sling. Figure-of-eight splints offer no benefit over a sling, are usually poorly tolerated by patients, and therefore are usually not indicated. A severe deformity with tenting of the overlying skin is an indication for surgical intervention.

   b. Proximal humerus fractures

   (1) **Typical mechanism.** Commonly caused by a low-energy fall in the elderly.

   (2) **Typical physical signs.** Decreased range of motion, swelling, ecchymosis, and pain. The neurovascular exam is critical to rule out any associated injury to the brachial plexus.

   (3) **Radiographic evaluation.** Radiographic evaluation of the shoulder and proximal humerus should include three orthogonal views: An AP of the glenohumeral joint, scapular Y, and axillary. A dislocation can be missed if one relies solely on an AP and scapular Y-view, and an axillary view is mandatory.

   (4) **Typical management.** If nondisplaced and stable, can be treated with a sling and early, controlled mobilization. Significant comminution, especially of the greater and lesser tuberosities, and displacement place the humeral head at risk of avascular necrosis and are indications for surgical reduction and fixation, especially in the young. For such a fracture in the elderly, a primary shoulder arthroplasty (replacement) may be considered if stable internal fixation cannot be achieved.

   (5) **When associated with dislocation.** Fracture dislocations of the shoulder are difficult to reduce closed. If there is an associated neurovascular compromise, these should be taken emergently to the OR for open reduction. Closed reduction, if performed, should be done cautiously to avoid neurovascular injury and to avoid displacement of an otherwise nondisplaced fracture.

   c. Scapula fractures

   (1) **Typical mechanism.** Scapula fractures are a marker of very high-energy chest trauma, usually involving a motor vehicle.

   (2) **Typical physical signs.** Tenderness to palpation over the scapula. Observe for signs of pneumothorax or other chest trauma with scapula fractures.

(3) **Usual radiographic evaluation.** Often first noted on chest CT in the evaluation of coexisting chest injuries. CT is the best way to evaluate for joint involvement.

(4) **Typical management.** Treatment in a sling unless intra-articular glenoid displacement necessitates surgical fixation.

2. Dislocations
   a. **Shoulder dislocations (glenohumeral dislocation)**
      (1) **Typical mechanism.** Anterior shoulder dislocations (most common, ~85%) occur with forced shoulder abduction or external rotation (or both). Less common posterior shoulder dislocations are associated with seizure and electrical shock.
      (2) **Typical physical signs.** Shoulder dislocation presents with decreased and painful range of motion and the humeral head may be palpable anteriorly or posteriorly. A "sulcus sign," or indentation between the acromion and humeral head, is suggestive of dislocation. Whereas with fractures, a thorough neurovascular examination is critical and should be documented prior to and following any reductions.
      (3) **Radiographic evaluation (see radiographic evaluation of proximal humerus fractures).** Posterior shoulder dislocations can be missed with traditional films if there is not an adequate axillary view. Evidence of glenoid rim fractures (Bankart lesion) or humeral head impaction fractures (Hill-Sachs lesion) associated with shoulder dislocations should be sought.
      (4) **Typical management.** Reduction is performed under sedation with axial traction and bringing the arm up into full abduction above the head. Care should be taken with the elderly with any reduction because it is possible to fracture osteoporotic bone with minimal force. The arm is then immobilized in the position of greatest stability: Internal rotation for anterior dislocations and external rotation for posterior dislocations. Radiographs should be repeated to demonstrate reduction, and a postreduction neurovascular exam should be done. The redislocation rate is inversely proportional to patient's age and correlated with activity level and demand.
   b. **Acromioclavicular (AC) dislocations ("a separated shoulder")**
      (1) **Typical mechanism.** Fall directly onto the shoulder or a direct blow to the shoulder.
      (2) **Typical physical signs.** Variable deformity and instability can be seen. Assess side-to-side asymmetry. Pain with shoulder motion and tenderness to palpation can be seen with sprains or dislocations of the AC joint.
      (3) **Radiographic evaluation** (see proximal humerus and clavicle fracture sections). Stress views of the AC joint are taken holding 5- to 10-lb weights, comparing side to side for displacement; however, this can be quite uncomfortable and is not generally necessary.

(4) **Typical management.** AC joint dislocations can be treated with a sling and early motion in most cases. Significant displacement and deformity may require reduction and fixation, especially if the skin or soft tissue is tented or otherwise at risk.

c. **Sternoclavicular dislocations**

(1) **Typical mechanism.** Anterior dislocations can occur after a force is applied to the anterolateral shoulder. Posterior dislocations are usually secondary to a direct blow to the distal clavicle.

(2) **Typical physical signs.** Localized pain, swelling, and tenderness are seen. **Hoarseness, dyspnea, dysphagia, or engorged neck veins are red flags** for posterior sternoclavicular joint dislocations with neurovascular compromise and should prompt emergent evaluation and treatment.

(3) **Radiographic evaluation. Although often subtle, asymmetry can be seen on chest x-ray.** A CT scan may be indicated to evaluate the sternoclavicular joint to determine anterior or posterior displacement and to visualize adjacent neurovascular structures.

(4) **Typical management. Anterior sternoclavicular dislocation** can be treated with a sling or shoulder immobilizer, whereas **posterior dislocations** commonly require reduction because of potential neurovascular and airway compromise. This should be done in the OR under general anesthesia with general or thoracic surgery backup in case of injury to the lung or great vessels.

3. **Soft-tissue injury**

a. **Rotator cuff tears.** In the young, rotator cuff tears are caused by repetitive overuse (throwing in athletes) or by acute trauma. In the elderly, tears are commonly degenerative and chronic, but they can be acute. History reveals shoulder pain and weakness, especially with overhead activities, and decreased range of motion. In the young, treatment consists of open or arthroscopic tendon repair. In the elderly, function may not be as severely affected, and physical therapy for improved strength and motion may suffice.

b. **Pectoralis major rupture.** This is most often caused by heavy lifting. In addition to weakness and pain, there is often significant bruising, a palpable defect, and a visibly changed muscle contour. Initial treatment in the emergency room (ER) consists of sling immobilization. An open repair gives best results when performed early.

B. **Arm and elbow**

1. **Fractures**

a. **Humeral shaft fractures**

(1) **Typical mechanism.** Commonly caused by a fall onto an outstretched arm, especially in the elderly.

(2) **Typical physical signs.** Deformity of the upper arm, pain, ecchymosis. Evaluate closely for small lacerations that may represent open fractures. A careful neurovascular exam should

be performed. In mid-diaphyseal fractures, the radial nerve is especially vulnerable to injury because it is directly adjacent to the posterior humeral shaft in this region.

(3) **Radiographic evaluation.** Two orthogonal views of the humerus, including the shoulder and elbow joints.

(4) **Typical management.** Closed fractures are placed in a coaptation splint or Sarmiento brace. Secondary (following closed reduction) radial nerve palsy is considered an indication for surgical management to rule out incarceration of the nerve within the fracture. However, primary radial nerve dysfunction usually resolves spontaneously (over a period of months) and can be treated nonoperatively. Other indications for surgical fixation include open fractures, injuries to multiple extremities, concurrent injury below the elbow ("floating elbow"), or a body habitus that is not amenable to bracing.

b. Distal humerus fractures

(1) **Typical mechanism.** Fall onto an outstretched hand or directly onto the elbow. Supracondylar humerus fractures are the most common fracture seen in children, especially between the ages of 4 and 7 years.

(2) **Typical physical signs.** Swelling, pain, ecchymosis, and decreased elbow range of motion. In children, displaced supracondylar fractures are frequently associated with peripheral nerve injuries. Patients should undergo serial exams to rule out the development of compartment syndrome.

(3) **Radiographic evaluation.** Orthogonal views of the elbow should be taken. For supracondylar fractures in adults, stress views taken with gentle longitudinal traction can help to delineate the fracture pattern, especially in cases with significant comminution or deformity. A CT scan may be indicated for additional fracture characterization to aid in surgical planning. Nondisplaced elbow fractures in children may present only with a "sail sign" caused by the superior displacement of the anterior and posterior elbow fat pads by a joint effusion.

(4) **Typical management. Supracondylar fractures in children** can be treated in a splint acutely if they are nondisplaced but require percutaneous pinning and casting if they are displaced. Significant swelling and neurovascular embarrassment are indications for urgent reduction followed by close observation. In adults, displaced fracture, especially with intra-articular displacement, is an indication for open reduction with internal fixation.

c. Radial head fractures

(1) **Typical mechanism.** Fall onto an outstretched arm.

(2) **Typical physical signs.** These present with tenderness to palpation and pain with forearm rotation. An elbow effusion is present. Range of motion of the elbow is typically limited.

(3) **Radiographic evaluation.** Three views of the elbow joint, an AP, oblique, and a lateral, are obtained. These can present with

only subtle x-rays findings, and occasionally only an elbow effusion can be seen on plain x-ray. CT scans can be helpful in determining the size, location, and nature of a radial head fracture.

(4) **Typical management.** Radial head fractures with minimal involvement of the articular surface (<30%) can be treated nonoperatively with early range-of-motion exercises. Increasing head involvement is an indication for surgical management. Open reduction and internal fixation are performed when stable fixation is achievable (usually three or fewer fragments). In adults, radial head excision or replacement is performed if comminution precludes adequate repair.

d. Olecranon fractures

(1) **Typical mechanism.** Fall directly onto the elbow or a direct blow to the posterior elbow.

(2) **Typical physical signs.** A palpable defect may be present. If the entire triceps insertion is involved, the patient may not be able to actively extend the elbow.

(3) **Radiographic evaluation.** Three views of the elbow are obtained. The lateral view is typically the most useful in evaluating these fractures.

(4) **Typical management.** Nondisplaced **olecranon fractures** are treated with a posterior splint followed by early range of motion, but when they are displaced, surgical fixation is indicated.

2. Elbow dislocations (ulnohumeral)

a. Typical mechanism. Fall onto an outstretched hand.

b. Typical physical signs. Examination reveals pain, swelling, bruising, and deformity with loss of elbow flexion and extension and forearm supination and pronation. Posterior dislocations are most common but can also occur anteriorly, medially, or laterally. The dislocated segment can often be palpated. Whereas with other elbow injuries, a careful neurovascular exam should be performed.

c. Radiographic evaluation. AP and lateral radiographs of the elbow confirm the diagnosis and reveal the direction of dislocation and major associated fractures. Postreduction radiographs are essential to demonstrate concentric joint reduction and more reliably identify any associated fractures. Coronoid process and radial head fractures are frequently seen with elbow dislocations. A CT scan may aid in complex fracture dislocations.

d. Typical management. Initial treatment consists of prompt reduction (typically accomplished with axial traction and flexion) and assessment of stability by carefully extending the elbow after the reduction has been done. The joint should be splinted in a stable position, with arm flexed less than 90 degrees. Postreduction radiographs are taken, and postreduction neurovascular status is documented. Stable dislocations benefit from early, controlled motion, whereas unstable elbows may require surgical stabilization of fractures and/or ligament reconstruction.

3. **Soft-tissue injury**
   a. **Biceps tendon rupture/avulsion** is usually secondary to violent contracture or excessive stretch. Loss of power, pain with resisted elbow flexion, local swelling, and ecchymosis are seen, along with an abnormal muscle contour ("Popeye sign"), proximal retraction. Examine for side-to-side differences. Initial treatment is sling immobilization followed by early surgical repair or nonoperative management, depending on the patient's activity level.

C. **Forearm, wrist, and hand**
   1. **Fractures**
      a. **Radius and ulna fractures (aka "both bone forearm fractures")**
         (1) **Typical mechanism.** These are commonly caused by falls onto the elbow or outstretched arm and are common in both children and the elderly. A direct blow can cause a "night-stick fracture," a typically mid-shaft fracture of the ulna caused by a forceful blow to the arm positioned to protect the face, often with a bat or club during an assault.
         (2) **Typical physical signs.** Examination reveals deformity, pain, and focal tenderness. Variable amounts of swelling can be seen, and diaphyseal fractures can cause a compartment syndrome, so careful, serial examination may be needed (see Section VI.B). A Galeazzi fracture is a fracture of the distal half of the radius associated with disruption of the distal radioulnar joint; this joint must be tested for stability in all radius fractures. A distal fracture with spread of the hematoma into the carpal tunnel may present as an acute carpal tunnel syndrome with associated median nerve sensory and motor dysfunction. Note wrist swelling and ecchymosis, and test two-point discrimination of the fingers (normally <5 to 7 mm) and test motor strength of the thumb abductors.
         (3) **Radiographic evaluation.** AP and lateral radiographs that include the entire forearm including the elbow and wrist are the minimum required. Splinted postreduction films are obtained to confirm reduction.
         (4) **Typical management.** In children, most diaphyseal and wrist fractures can be managed with closed reduction and sugar-tong splinting. If an adequate reduction cannot be achieved in the ER, these are treated with closed reduction and pinning or with insertion of intramedullary thin flexible rods. In adults, shaft fractures that involve both bones are almost always treated with open reduction internal fixation (ORIF) after initial closed reduction and splinting is done in the ER to limit the stress on the surrounding soft tissues. Isolated radius and ulna fractures can be treated nonoperatively if they are minimally displaced. **Associated acute carpal tunnel syndrome is a surgical emergency.**
      b. **Distal radius fractures**
         (1) **Typical mechanism.** Fall on an outstretched hand.

(2) **Typical physical signs.** Pain, deformity, swelling, ecchymosis, focal tenderness. Similarly to diaphyseal fractures, there can be an associated compartment syndrome or acute carpal tunnel syndrome, both of which are surgical emergencies.

(3) **Radiographic evaluation.** Three views of the wrist with an AP, lateral, and oblique view. CT scans can be helpful in comminuted intra-articular fractures.

c. **Scaphoid fractures**

(1) **Typical presentation.** A fall onto an outstretched hand with the wrist in radial deviation.

(2) **Typical physical signs.** Local swelling, pain with wrist motion, and focal tenderness in the "anatomic snuffbox."

(3) **Radiographic evaluation.** Three views of the wrist, an AP, lateral, and oblique as well as a scaphoid view taken with wrist in ulnar deviation. These fractures may not be visualized on plain x-rays at the time of injury.

(4) **Typical management.** Nondisplaced scaphoid fractures are treated in a thumb spica splint. Suspected scaphoid fractures, with pain in the anatomic snuffbox but no fracture seen on x-ray, should be treated as nondisplaced fractures and immobilized in the ER. Fractures with greater than 1 mm of displacement are at risk of nonunion and avascular necrosis and benefit from internal fixation.

d. **Metacarpal fractures**

(1) **Typical mechanism.** Crush injury or axial load onto a closed fist.

(2) **Typical physical signs.** Swelling and bruising, often with flexion of the distal fragment causing the knuckle to be less prominent; the most common is the distal fifth metacarpal or so-called "boxer's fracture." Check for rotational deformity by observing for finger divergence with flexion of the metacarpal phalangeal joints and comparing with the contralateral side.

(3) **Typical management.** Reduction and splinting in an ulnar gutter or volar slab splint with fingers in intrinsic plus position (see Section VII.A.2.c), re-examining for rotational malalignment. If unstable, significantly angulated, or rotationally malaligned, these may require closed reduction and pinning or ORIF.

e. **Distal phalanx fractures**

(1) **Typical mechanism.** Crush injury.

(2) **Typical physical signs.** These are typically associated with lacerations of the fingertip or nail-bed injuries.

(3) **Radiographic evaluation.** Any patients with a laceration to the fingertip should have an AP and lateral of the finger to rule out any underlying fracture.

(4) **Typical management.** While these are technically open fractures, they can be adequately irrigated and débrided in the ER

and do not require a formal I&D in the OR. If there is any question of a nail-bed injury, the nail should be removed. After irrigation and débridement, nail-bed lacerations should be repaired with 5-0 or 6-0 chromic gut. Lacerations in the skin can be repaired with 4-0 nylon. Preformed Alumafoam finger splints are used to immobilize the fracture.

2. **Dislocations**
   a. **Perilunate dislocations**
      (1) **Typical mechanism.** Lunate and perilunate dislocations usually occur after forced wrist hyperextension.
      (2) **Typical physical signs. Perilunate dislocations** present with pain, limited wrist motion, tenderness, and possibly signs of median neuropathy caused by compression of the median nerve in the carpal tunnel by the displaced lunate. Observe closely for signs of acute carpal tunnel syndrome.
      (3) **Radiographic evaluation.** AP and lateral views of involved joints are the minimum required. Perilunate dislocations can be subtle on plain x-ray, and a high index of suspicion is necessary. Oblique views aid in evaluating the position of displaced carpal bones. Scaphoid, capitate, and radial styloid fractures should be ruled out as associated injuries with lunate dislocations.
      (4) **Typical management.** Perilunate dislocations are reduced using axial traction and hyperextension of the wrist while pressure is applied to the lunate. Avoid splinting the wrist in a flexed position because this increases risk of median nerve compression. After closed reduction in the ER, these usually require surgical treatment with stabilization of associated fractures and disrupted intercarpal ligaments.
3. **Soft-tissue injury**
   a. **Subungual hematomas** are decompressed by burning a hole in the nail with electrocautery or with a large-bore needle after a digital block.
   b. **Nail-bed injuries** require removal of the overlying nail with repair of the nail bed using absorbable suture and splinting open of the nail fold with sterile Vaseline-impregnated gauze or with the Betadine-soaked nail.
   c. **Tip amputations** involving only soft tissue can often be allowed to heal by secondary intent or, if the area is greater than 1 cm², treated with local flaps. Exposed bone is resected back to a level that allows soft-tissue coverage.

D. **Pelvic fractures**
   1. **Disruptions of the pelvic ring**
      a. **Typical mechanism.** Pelvic ring injuries are typically of very high energy, as from a motor vehicle collision or a fall from tall heights.
      b. **Typical physical signs.** Crepitus, pelvic instability, or pain with iliac wing compression or distraction should alert the examiner to

possible pelvic ring injury. Inspect for soft-tissue injury including a degloving injury. Rectal and vaginal examinations are performed to check for blood, open communication with a fracture, or a high-riding prostate. Blood at the urethral meatus at time of catheterization is a sign of lower urogenital injury. Pelvic bleeding may result in a loss of 2 to 3 L of blood or more, and signs of hypovolemic shock must be monitored along with aggressive fluid replacement. High-energy pelvic fractures rarely occur in isolation, and significant associated injuries are likely. Palpate for spinal tenderness or step-offs, and treat all patients initially with spinal precautions. A thorough primary and secondary survey must be undertaken and documented.

c. **Radiographic evaluation.** An AP pelvis view is part of the standard trauma panel. The use of an abdominal–pelvic CT scan is becoming standard part of the trauma workup and is extremely useful in evaluating pelvic, sacral, and lumbar spine fractures. An L5 transverse process fracture suggests posterior pelvic ligamentous disruption. Once stabilized, pelvic ring fractures are further evaluated with pelvic inlet and outlet views. If genitourinary injury is suspected, a retrograde urethrogram and cystogram should be obtained. Other standard radiographs such as chest and C-spine films should be reviewed.

d. **Typical management.** The initial treatment consists of adherence to standard trauma ABCs. Maintenance of adequate intravascular volume and systolic blood pressure is essential in the hemodynamically unstable patient. In the persistently unstable patient, sources of bleeding other than the pelvis should be ruled out followed by emergent fixation of the pelvic ring in the emergency department, usually with a linen sheet tied around the pelvis or with a specialized pelvic binder to reduce pelvic volume until an anterior pelvic external fixation can be applied. Pelvic binders that remain in place for more than several hours must be often re-evaluated to rule out associated pressure necrosis of the skin. Because binders can cause increased patient discomfort and skin breakdown, they should be removed if patients remain hemodynamically stable or the fracture pattern does not allow decreased pelvic volume with lateral compression. Angiogram and embolization of bleeding pelvic vessels may precede or follow placement of provisional external fixation. If the patient is hemodynamically and otherwise stable, surgical intervention can be delayed to allow complete assessment of associated injuries and resuscitation of the patient. An open pelvic fracture has a very high morbidity, and a diverting colostomy should be considered. Patients are at high risk of developing a deep venous thrombosis (DVT) in association with these injuries, and appropriate prophylaxis should be initiated. Sacral fractures and sacroiliac joint disruptions can often be treated with percutaneous screws.

2. **Pubic rami fractures**
   a. **Typical mechanism.** Same level falls in an elderly patient.
   b. **Typical physical signs.** Groin pain, pain with weight bearing.

    c. **Usual radiographic evaluation.** An AP pelvis and inlet and outlet views are all used to evaluate the pubic rami. A CT is usually not required.

    d. **Typical management.** These patients are allowed to bear weight as tolerated, but frequently have significant pain with weight bearing initially. Intensive physical therapy is important to prevent these patients from becoming bedridden.

3. Acetabular fractures

    a. **Typical mechanism.** Usually the result of high-energy trauma such as an motor vehicle collision (MVC) or fall from height.

    b. **Typical physical signs.** Hip pain, pain with logroll. In cases with an associated hip dislocation, the limb may be shortened and externally rotated. A sciatic palsy is also possible with a posterior hip dislocation. Since these patients have usually been in a high-energy trauma, they may have several associated injuries and should have a carefully secondary exam.

    c. **Radiographic evaluation.** These fractures are usually identified on an AP pelvis taken as part of the initial trauma work-up. Judet (oblique) views of the pelvis and a CT scan with fine cuts through the acetabulum are also needed.

    d. **Typical management.** Skeletal traction may be indicated for fractures of the acetabulum, depending on the size and location of the fracture and an associated dislocation (see also Section V.F.2). Fractures involving the weight-bearing portion of the acetabulum are usually treated with surgical reduction and fixation.

E. Hip and femur

1. Fractures of the hip and femur

    a. **Hip fractures (femoral neck and intertrochanteric fractures)**

        (1) **Typical mechanism.** Commonly the result of low-energy falls or direct blows in the elderly, but in the young they are generally a result of more significant trauma. A stress fracture of the femoral neck typically presents as groin or medial thigh pain associated temporally with a recent increase in activity level or training.

        (2) **Typical physical signs.** Shortening of the limb may be seen in addition to pain with motion and the inability to bear weight. Rotational stability is typically lost with displaced hip fractures, with the leg falling into a shortened, externally rotated posture. A high index of suspicion must be maintained in the elderly after a low-energy fall presenting with complaints of groin or medial thigh pain (site of referred pain from the hip joint) because these may be the only signs of a nondisplaced hip fracture.

        (3) **Radiographic evaluation.** An AP pelvis view and hip films (AP and lateral views) are usually diagnostic. The femoral neck can easily be evaluated on a trauma pelvic CT if available. If history suggests a hip fracture in the elderly or a stress fracture in the young but no fracture is seen, magnetic resonance

imaging (MRI) or bone scan is indicated to rule out the occult fracture.

(4) **Typical management.** Displaced femoral neck fractures in the young require urgent anatomic reduction and internal fixation to reduce the **risk of avascular necrosis,** whereas stress fractures are treated with protected weight bearing. In the elderly, surgical treatment is generally the rule for hip fractures. Stable femoral neck fractures are usually treated with internal fixation (most commonly, percutaneous screws) and unstable femoral neck fractures with hip arthroplasty (hemi- or total hip arthroplasty). Peritrochanteric fractures are treated with various internal fixation methods, including the use of compression screw and plate or intramedullary nail. The utility of skin traction to increase patient comfort prior to surgery is controversial.

b. **Femoral shaft fractures**

(1) **Typical mechanism.** Usually high-energy injuries or gun shot wounds.

(2) **Typical physical signs.** Patients usually have gross deformity and instability. Even small lacerations that seem to be far away from the level of the fracture should be carefully evaluated to rule out open fractures.

(3) **Radiographic evaluation.** An AP and lateral of the femur, which include the high and knee joints, are usually the only x-rays required. Ipsilateral femoral neck fractures should be excluded.

(4) **Typical management.** Initial long-leg splinting and occasionally skeletal traction to increase comfort and stability while maintaining length and protecting the soft tissues (traction splints placed by emergency personnel should be promptly removed at the time of initial evaluation). Even closed femur fractures can be a source of significant blood loss, and appropriate blood replacement, especially in the multiply injured patient, is important. Most shaft fractures are treated with intramedullary nailing soon after the injury to allow early mobilization and decrease the risk of additional complications. In the unstable, multiply injured patient, external fixation may be the initial treatment of choice to minimize adverse systemic effects caused by the additional trauma of surgery. DVTs are common after pelvic and leg bone fractures, so prophylaxis (mechanical with or without chemical) is essential.

2. **Hip dislocations**

a. **Typical mechanism.** High-energy motor vehicle crash, often associated with acetabular fracture. In patients with previous hip replacement, dislocation is typically atraumatic, caused primarily by noncompliance with positioning precautions given after hip replacement.

b. **Typical physical signs.** Anterior dislocations typically leave the extremity abducted and externally rotated. Posterior dislocations cause greater shortening with an adducted and internally rotated posture. Sciatic nerve function should be assessed for palsy with posterior dislocations (the peroneal division is most commonly affected).

c. **Radiographic evaluation.** Obtain appropriate pelvic films to evaluate for acetabular, femoral head, or hip fracture (see previous section) and to determine the direction of dislocation (requires adequate lateral view). In hip replacement, check for component positioning, loosening, or periprosthetic fractures.

d. **Typical management.** In a native hip, once a hip dislocation is identified, **immediate closed reduction,** prior to an additional imaging, to reduce **risk of avascular necrosis** should be done. Most failed attempts at closed reduction are due to inadequate sedation and muscle relaxation, which are essential. Assessment of stability and postreduction neurologic exam are necessary. If stable once reduction is achieved, the leg is kept abducted with an abduction pillow. Skeletal traction is indicated when the hip remains unstable after a reduction is performed. Postreduction radiographs, including AP, lateral, and Judet views, are needed to confirm reduction and assess for associated fractures. Associated fractures are stabilized surgically. Patients with dislocated hip arthroplasties can usually be reduced closed, placed in an abduction brace, and discharged home.

F. **Knee and tibia**

1. **Fractures**

a. **Supracondylar femur fractures**

(1) **Typical mechanism.** Can be low energy in the elderly, generally higher energy in younger patients.

(2) **Typical physical signs.** Deformity and swelling about the knee. Evaluate carefully for any open wounds.

(3) **Radiographic evaluation.** Four views of the knee (AP, lateral, and two obliques) help to identify fractures involving the knee. Traction views taken with gentle longitudinal traction for comminuted and displaced periarticular fractures may be necessary to understand the fracture pattern. A CT scan may be helpful for preoperative planning for complex intra-articular fractures.

(4) **Typical management.** These fractures are initially reduced and splinted in the ER. Almost all these will require ORIF to restore anatomic alignment to the joint surface.

b. **Patellar fractures**

(1) **Typical mechanism.** Patella fractures are commonly caused by falling directly onto the knee or striking a dashboard.

(2) **Typical physical signs.** Patella fractures often have a palpable defect and have an associated inability to perform a straight-leg raise.

(3) **Radiographic evaluation.** Four views of the knee (AP, lateral, and two obliques) help to identify fractures involving the knee. A sunrise view can also be helpful in evaluating the patella.

(4) **Typical management.** Patella fractures with displacement, joint incongruity, or loss of active knee extension require reduction and surgical fixation. Nondisplaced fractures can be treated with a knee immobilizer and weight bearing as tolerated.

c. **Tibial plateau fractures**

(1) **Typical mechanism.** Motor vehicle collision, fall from a height, direct blow, and pedestrian versus car are all common.

(2) **Typical physical signs.** Large knee effusion, significant swelling in the lower leg, ecchymosis, and deformity. Tibial plateau fractures should be carefully monitored for compartment syndrome.

(3) **Radiographic evaluation.** Tibial shaft fractures require an AP and lateral of the tibia and views of the knee and ankle. A CT scan is usually required for preoperative planning.

(4) **Typical management.** Tibial plateau fractures are treated with splinting and early motion if they are nondisplaced and stable but require reduction and internal fixation for articular incongruity, significant displacement, deformity, or instability. Most plateau fractures associated with significant soft-tissue swelling or compartment syndrome are treated with a temporary, spanning external fixator across the knee followed by ORIF.

d. **Tibial shaft fractures**

(1) **Typical mechanism.** Motor vehicle collision, motorcycle collision, fall from height, and gun shot wound are all common mechanisms. Spiral fractures of the tibia are caused by twisting injury.

(2) **Typical physical signs.** Gross deformity and instability is usually present. The subcutaneous location of the tibia predisposes to open fractures. Observation and probing lacerations and skin defects for communication to underlying bone or fracture are necessary. Check nerve function and pulses and foot perfusion compared with the contralateral side. The patients should be carefully monitored to rule out compartment syndrome.

(3) **Radiographic evaluation.** AP and lateral x-rays of the tibia, including both the ankle and knee joints, are usually the only imaging required.

(4) **Typical management.** Stable tibial shaft fractures can be treated with casting; however, most are treated with intramedullary nailing to allow early weight bearing and motion. Open tibial shaft fractures often require multiple surgical débridements and soft-tissue coverage.

2. **Knee dislocations**

a. **Typical mechanism.** Knee dislocations are very high-energy injuries and require multiple ligamentous disruption to occur. In extremely obese persons, these can occur with a same level fall or even walking on uneven surfaces. These are very different from patella dislocations, which usually occur with a twisting force while in extension, often during sports, and usually reduce spontaneously.

b. **Typical physical exam.** Knee dislocations present with deformity, shortening, ligamentous instability, and often signs of significant neurovascular compromise. Check side-to-side differences in pulse examination serially. Knee dislocations that have reduced spontaneously are easy to miss in the acute setting, and the knees should be examined for ligamentous instability in the setting of high-energy trauma.

c. **Usual radiographic evaluation.** Look for associated fractures with knee dislocations with four views of the knee *after* reduction. Angiography or CT angiography is often performed with knee dislocations (see later comments). Obtain an MRI of the knee in the subacute setting to evaluate the associated ligamentous injuries.

d. **Typical management.** Knee dislocations require immediate, emergent reduction. These should be reduced even before radiographs are taken if possible. The incidence of concomitant vascular injury is approximately 30%, and pedal pulse examination has a low sensitivity (79%) for detecting significant vascular injury. One should have a very low threshold for arteriography; and a vascular surgery consultation is mandatory in the presence of questionable pulses. If vascular repair is necessary, a spanning external fixator can be placed to stabilize the knee. After any vascular repair, prophylactic fasciotomy should be considered. Often, delayed ligamentous reconstruction is necessary to restore knee stability.

3. **Soft-tissue injuries**
   a. **Quadriceps and patellar tendon ruptures** are caused by violent contraction or excessive stretch. Palpable defects and a high-riding (with patella tendon rupture) or low-riding (with quadriceps rupture) patella on physical exam or lateral radiographs are hallmarks. Partial tears that do not affect the integrity of the extensor mechanism can be managed without surgery with protected motion. Injuries affecting the extensor mechanism require surgical repair.

   b. **Knee ligament disruption** is commonly seen with sports injuries involving a pivoting injury or a bending moment. A hemarthrosis is common. Physical exam demonstrates joint instability with testing. Common ligamentous injuries include anterior cruciate and medial collateral ligaments.

   c. **Meniscal tears** are more common than ligamentous injury and often occur in association with them. They present with a joint effusion, pain with deep flexion, and joint line tenderness. Rarely, a displaced segment can cause locking of the knee joint. Meniscal tears can be treated nonoperatively or, if symptoms persist, with arthroscopic débridement or repair.

G. **Distal tibia and ankle**
   1. **Fractures**
      a. **Pilon fractures**
         (1) **Typical mechanism.** Distal tibial intra-articular fractures (pilon fractures) are associated with an axial loading mechanism such as falls from a height or floor board injury from a motor vehicle accident.

    (2) Typical physical signs. Deformity, instability, swelling, and ecchymosis about the ankle. Note soft-tissue injury, which is often significant with pilon injuries, including location of fracture blisters and whether the blisters are blood filled (marker of deeper injury).

    (3) Radiographic evaluation. Obtain three views of the ankle (AP, lateral, and mortise). Foot films are used to evaluate for concomitant talus, calcaneus, or other foot fractures associated with high-energy pilon fractures. Traction views and a postreduction CT of pilon fractures help with fracture characterization and surgical planning.

    (4) Typical management. Pilon fractures with significant shortening, comminution, or soft-tissue injury are best managed initially with closed reduction and placement of a spanning external fixator. External fixation is then maintained until the soft tissues can tolerate a formal open procedure. Soft-tissue management is critical in the presence of these injuries, especially pilon fractures.

b. Ankle fractures

    (1) Typical mechanism. Ankle fractures are commonly caused by a twisting mechanism.

    (2) Typical physical signs. Note deformity and instability of the lower leg and ankle joint. Perform and document a neurovascular exam. With ankle fractures, note the precise location of tenderness and swelling.

    (3) Radiographic evaluation. Obtain three views of the ankle (AP, lateral, and mortise). With ankle fractures of questionable joint stability, obtain a stress mortise view by stabilizing the distal tibia and externally rotating the patient's foot and look for widening of greater than 2 mm of the medial joint space. Comparison views to the uninjured ankle can be helpful.

    (4) Typical management. Stable, nondisplaced fractures of the ankle can be treated with immobilization and protected weight bearing. Unstable fractures (one with both medial and lateral injuries) and fractures with joint subluxation benefit from delayed open reduction and internal fixation once the swelling has decreased. All fractures should be reduced in the ER with postreduction radiographs demonstrating adequate joint and fracture reduction. If adequate joint reduction cannot be achieved or maintained, early surgical treatment (usually a spanning external fixator) is indicated to prevent further joint damage.

2. Ankle dislocations

  a. Typical mechanism. Simple (not associated with fracture) ankle dislocations are uncommon. Fracture dislocations are caused by similar, but higher energy, mechanisms as those in other ankle fractures.

  b. Typical physical exam. Look for deformity and pain with inability to bear weight. Dislocations are often associated with open fractures about the ankle. Document a neurovascular exam because significant soft-tissue injury and deformity place neurovascular structures at risk.

    c. Usual radiographic examination. Same as for ankle fractures.

    d. Typical management. These should be reduced emergently, even before radiographs are taken. Open injuries should be treated appropriately (see Section VI.C). Dislocations represent unstable injuries, and associated fractures are treated surgically. Whereas with pilon fractures, spanning external fixation may be an appropriate initial treatment.

  3. Soft-tissue injuries

    a. Ankle sprains are commonly caused by inversion or eversion of the foot. Patients present with swelling, ecchymosis, and maximal tenderness along the injured ligaments medially or laterally. Radiographs are normal or reveal insignificant cortical avulsions. Initial treatment with rest, ice, and elevation is usually adequate, followed by physical therapy for proprioceptive training to reduce the risk of reinjury. Immobilization is generally not indicated.

    b. A ruptured Achilles tendon usually occurs during running, jumping, or vigorous activity, with sudden pain and difficulty in walking. Examination can reveal a palpable defect, weak plantar flexion, and (if a complete rupture) no passive ankle plantar flexion on squeezing the patient's calf (positive Thompson sign). Nonoperative treatment in a splint with the ankle plantar flexed is one treatment option, but is associated with higher rerupture rates than surgical repair.

H. Foot

  1. Fractures

    a. Calcaneus fractures

      (1) Typical mechanism. Calcaneus fractures are the most common tarsal fracture and are usually the result of an axillary load such as a fall from height, often in a young laborer.

      (2) Typical physical signs. Calcaneal fractures are associated with considerable swelling and blister formation, heel widening, and significant tenderness and ecchymosis extending to the arch. Associated fractures are common and include those seen with an axial loading mechanism.

      (3) Radiographic evaluation. Obtain three views each of the ankle and the foot. A Harris view evaluates the calcaneal width and profiles the subtalar joint. A CT scan is usually obtained with displaced calcaneal fractures. Obtain lumbar spine films to evaluate for associated fracture.

      (4) Typical management. Calcaneal fractures should be placed in a well-padded splint and observed for compartment syndrome. Significant subtalar joint depression and comminution may require open reduction with internal fixation once soft-tissue swelling allows. Regardless of treatment, outcomes are often disappointing and result in significant disability.

b. Talus fractures

(1) **Typical mechanism.** Talus fractures (the second most common) are also generally higher energy (motor vehicle collision or falls) and are usually caused by forced dorsiflexion (e.g., slamming on the brake at the time of impact).

(2) **Typical physical signs.** Talus fractures can also present with significant swelling, and when they are associated with a dislocation of the tibiotalar joint and/or the subtalar joint, a significant deformity can be present. A careful neurologic exam should be performed and followed.

(3) **Radiographic evaluation.** Obtain three views each of the ankle and the foot. CT scans are often helpful with talus fractures as well to evaluate the myriad of articular surfaces of the tibiotalar and subtalar joints, which are difficult to evaluate properly with plain radiographs.

(4) **Typical management.** Talus fractures can be treated with cast immobilization if they are absolutely nondisplaced, but most talar neck fractures are treated with ORIF to decrease the risk of nonunion and avascular necrosis.

c. Metatarsal fractures

(1) **Typical mechanism.** Metatarsal fractures can be seen with lower energy trauma. Stress fractures can occur in runners or others who have recently increased their distance or activity.

(2) **Typical physical signs.** Stress fractures may present only with tenderness to palpation at the level of the injury.

(3) **Radiographic evaluation.** Three views (AP, lateral, and oblique) of the foot. Metatarsal stress fractures, if suspected and not apparent on initial radiographs, may be seen on MRI or bone scan.

(4) **Typical management.** Metatarsal fractures can generally be treated nonoperatively with splinting. First metatarsal fractures may be treated operatively if displaced. Transverse fractures of the proximal fifth metatarsal diaphysis (Jones fracture), due to being in a vascular watershed region, are prone to healing complications and require more aggressive treatment than other metatarsal fractures, including either strict non-weight bearing with cast immobilization or surgery. An avulsion of the base of the fifth metatarsal, the so-called "pseudo-Jones fracture," can be treated with early weight bearing.

d. Toe fractures. Toe injuries are best treated by "buddy taping" to the adjacent digit and giving the patient a hard-soled shoe for more comfortable ambulation. Distal phalanx fractures with nail-bed injuries or soft-tissue lacerations are treated the same as similar injuries in the fingers (see Section V.C.1.e).

e. Fractures in diabetic feet. Diabetics with peripheral neuropathy and injuries to the foot or ankle require special attention and care. Because of neuropathic changes, casts and splints must be well padded and adapted to any deformity of the foot. Typically, foot and ankle fractures in the diabetic require twice the normal period of immobilization. A hot, swollen foot in a diabetic patient should be examined radiographically for neuropathic fractures (the Charcot foot) and immobilized. This should be differentiated from cellulitis and infection with laboratory tests, although they can occur simultaneously.

2. Dislocations
   a. Talar dislocations
      (1) Typical mechanism. The level of energy is similar to that for calcaneal and talar fractures. Talar dislocation occurs with forced foot inversion.
      (2) Typical physical signs. With talar dislocations, there is often significant deformity. Dislocation of the talar body can commonly impinge on adjacent neurovascular structures and can be entrapped by tendons. Neurovascular compromise is possible and must be identified and treated emergently.
      (3) Radiographic evaluation. With a talus dislocation, obtain views of both the ankle and the foot. If it is associated with a fracture, perform imaging as noted previously.
      (4) Typical management. Talar dislocations are treated with emergent reduction to decrease the risk of avascular necrosis, neurovascular injury, and skin compromise. Soft-tissue interposition can prevent closed reduction, in which case open reduction is required. Associated fractures must be anatomically reduced and stabilized as described previously.

   b. Lisfranc dislocations
      (1) Typical mechanism. Lisfranc injuries are disruptions of the tarsal–metatarsal joints by either dislocation or fracture dislocation and are caused by a bending or twisting force through the mid-foot.
      (2) Typical physical signs. Lisfranc injuries are associated with significant swelling and mid-foot tenderness. Compartment syndrome of the foot may be present.
      (3) Radiographic evaluation. Lisfranc fractures are diagnosed radiographically by incongruity of the tarsometatarsal joints, most commonly between the medial base of the second metatarsal and the medial edge of the middle cuneiform, which are normally collinear. A CT scan may be useful if a significant fracture component is present.
      (4) Typical management. Lisfranc injuries are splinted, iced, and elevated in preparation for eventual operative reduction and fixation. An attempt at closed reduction should be made to help decrease soft-tissue swelling.

VI. OTHER ORTHOPEDIC CONDITIONS

A. Orthopedic infections
   1. Septic arthritis. Can occur in otherwise healthy persons, especially in children, but usually occurs in association with immunosuppression,

systemic infection, preexisting joint disease, previous joint surgery, or intravenous (IV) drug abuse. It is of special concern in patients with joint replacements.

a. **Examination** reveals tenderness, effusion, increased warmth, and **pain with passive motion.** Laboratory tests may demonstrate an elevated erythrocyte sedimentation rate (ESR), C-reactive protein (CRP), and/or white blood cell (WBC) count. Diagnosis is confirmed by needle aspiration and laboratory analysis of synovial fluid for cell count and differential, Gram stain, routine aerobic and anaerobic cultures, and crystal analysis. **Baseline radiographs** are obtained at the time of presentation (note that significant changes occur late, after 7 to 10 days).

b. **Treatment** with broad-spectrum IV antibiotics should be initiated **after** adequate joint fluid specimens are obtained. If septic arthritis is diagnosed, some means of joint lavage should be performed (serial aspirations, arthroscopic or open débridement) to prevent progressive cartilage degradation and further systemic illness.

2. **Osteomyelitis.** Childhood osteomyelitis most commonly results from hematogenous spread of bacteria to the metaphysis. Adult osteomyelitis typically occurs from direct inoculation via surgery, an open fracture, or chronic soft-tissue ulceration. Hematogenous spread may occur in cases of IV drug abuse, sickle cell disease, and immunosuppression.

a. **Physical examination** findings are similar to those in septic arthritis, if located about a joint, but may also reveal bony tenderness and drainage. Assess the soft tissues about the region. Examine for infective sources.

b. Appropriate **imaging studies** should always start with plain radiographs of the area. If typical changes are seen on plain x-ray, advanced imaging is usually not required. Of the advanced imaging modalities, MRI is the most useful in detecting occult osteomyelitis. Bone scans and tagged WBC scans are rarely useful unless the patient cannot undergo an MRI (*Semin Ultrasound CT MR.* 2010;31:100–106; *Int J Low Extrem Wounds.* 2010;9:24–30). Laboratory examination includes ESR, CRP, peripheral WBC count, and blood cultures.

c. **Treatment** typically involves 6-week-long course of empiric IV antibiotics (guided by cultures if available). Response to treatment is gauged clinically and with trends in the ESR and CRP. If response is inadequate, bone biopsy can be done to obtain further cultures for sensitivities. Débridement of the infected bone is sometimes required, especially in the presence of intramedullary or subperiosteal abscess. Associated septic arthritis is treated as outlined previously.

3. **Suppurative flexor tenosynovitis.** Patients present with tenderness along the flexor sheath, the finger held in a semiflexed position, and fusiform swelling of the entire finger (**Kanavel signs**). The patient will also have pain with palpation of the tendon in the palm and with wrist extension. Look for associated skin wounds (may appear quite innocuous). Immediate surgical decompression, irrigation, and débridement are indicated.

4. **Abscess**
   a. **Hand.** There are numerous potential spaces in the hand that can become infected. Surgical drainage is required, either in the ER or OR, depending on the extent of the abscess.
   b. **Olecranon and prepatellar bursa** can become infected and present with pain, redness, heat and fluctuance, often with a zone of cellulitis. Treatment is decompression and packing in the ER in addition to a course of oral antibiotics. A significant cellulitis may necessitate a brief course of IV antibiotics.

B. **Compartment syndrome** is characterized by an increase in tissue pressure within a closed osteofascial space sufficient to compromise microcirculation, leading to irreversible damage to tissues within that compartment, including death of muscle and nerves. The end result can be devastating, with a chronically wasted, contracted, paralytic extremity.

1. **Location.** Although it occurs most frequently in the anterior, lateral, or posterior compartments of the leg or the volar or dorsal compartments of the forearm, it can also occur about the elbow or in the thigh, hand, or foot.

2. **Causes.** Long-bone fracture, crush, or vascular injuries are common risk factors. Increased capillary permeability secondary to postischemic swelling, trauma, or burns may also contribute to compartment syndrome. Muscle hypertrophy, tight dressings, and pneumatic antishock garments (e.g., military antishock trousers) are less common causes.

3. **Examination**
   a. On the basis of injury and physical findings, patients at risk for compartment syndrome should be identified early and examined frequently. The **five "P's"** are classically used to aide in diagnosis: The earliest and most important sign is pain out of proportion to the injury, particularly an increasing and disproportionate narcotic demand and unexpectedly poor response to appropriate pain medication, and **pain with passive motion** of involved muscles or tendons traversing the involved compartment. This sign alone is enough to diagnose compartment syndrome, and the patient should not be further observed for the development of any other signs. **Paresthesias** in the distribution of the peripheral nerves traversing the involved compartment occurs at an intermediate time. **Paralysis, pallor, and pulselessness** are late signs and likely indicate irreversible soft-tissue injury. If pulses are altered or absent, major arterial occlusion rather than compartment syndrome should be considered in the diagnosis.
   b. In the awake patient, compartment syndrome **is a clinical diagnosis.** However, when the clinical picture and physical examination are sufficiently uncertain or in the unresponsive patient, **compartment pressures** should be measured. Multiple measurements should be taken in different locations. Comparison to uninvolved compartments may be helpful. For pressures within 30 mm Hg of the diastolic blood pressure with equivocal clinical examination, fasciotomy is in order.

4. **Treatment.** Circumferential bandages, splints, or casts should be removed. Extremities should be elevated to above the level of the heart. Excessive elevation can be counterproductive. If the clinical picture deteriorates or physical examination worsens, then fasciotomy should be performed emergently.

C. **Open fractures and joints.** Lacerations or wounds near fractures or joints can communicate and should be carefully evaluated. If exposed bone is not evident, wounds should be probed to determine whether communication to fracture is present. Joints may be distended with sterile saline to check for extravasation from adjacent wounds, but this method is associated with poor sensitivity, and is not routinely used. Air in the joint on x-ray and fat droplets in blood from the wound also confirm communication with a joint or fracture, respectively.

1. **Treatment.** Assess wounds, remove any obvious gross contamination, apply moist saline or Betadine-soaked dressing, reduce the fracture or joint, and splint the extremity. Administer tetanus prophylaxis and IV antibiotics based on fracture severity. Type I and type II open fractures, defined as having a skin opening less than 1 cm for type I or less than 10 cm without gross contamination or significant bone stripping for type II, require a first-generation cephalosporin, usually cefazolin (Ancef). Vancomycin is used in patients with a penicillin allergy. With type III injuries (skin opening >10 cm, gross contamination, and/or significant soft-tissue stripping from bone), an aminoglycoside, usually gentamicin, should be added.

2. **Gunshot injuries**
   a. It is helpful to identify the **weapon caliber and type.** High-energy injuries (shotgun, rifle, or high-caliber (.357 or .44) handguns) with large associated soft-tissue wounds are treated like open fractures and require antibiotic prophylaxis and operative débridement. With lower energy injuries (most handguns, .22 rifles), antibiotic prophylaxis and débridement are generally not needed because less damage and contamination occur.
   b. **Physical exam.** Neurovascular status should be checked closely and followed. Deficits are usually due to concussive injury and not laceration, but developing deficits are a sign of compartment syndrome. Obtain radiographs to assess for bony involvement. If the wound is near a joint with concern for intra-articular involvement, aspirate to check for hemarthrosis.
   c. **Treatment.** Clean the skin, débride the wound edges, and irrigate thoroughly. Isolated soft-tissue injury is typically treated with local wound care with or without oral antibiotics. If a fracture is found, management of the bony injury is usually the same despite the mechanism.

3. **Traumatic amputation. A team approach is needed** to evaluate for possible reimplantation, and all necessary consultants should be contacted early.
   a. **Management. The proximal stump is cleaned,** and a compressive dressing is applied. Tourniquets are not used. Amputated parts are wrapped in moist gauze, placed in a bag, and cooled by placing on

ice (must avoid freezing damage). The amputated part can be sent to the OR before the patient for preparation. Reimplantation is most likely to be successful with a sharp amputation and not likely possible with crush injuries or other injuries with a wide zone of injury. Timing is of the essence, and a rapid and efficient evaluation is critical. Indication for reimplantation of fingers includes injury in a child, involvement of the thumb, multiple involved digits, and injury distal to the middle phalanx.

VII. PRACTICAL PROCEDURES

A. **Common splints and casts.** Splints and casts stabilize bones and joints and limit further soft-tissue injury and swelling and help to minimize pain. Splints are not circumferential and allow for more swelling than traditional casts but are less durable. Air splints are used only in the emergency setting because they increase pressure in the extremity and can compromise blood flow.

1. **Preparation and application.** Prefabricated splints and immobilizers can be used if available. Plaster splints consist of plaster and cast padding. The required length to include a joint above and below the injury is measured from the uninjured side. Any required reduction maneuvers are performed prior to splint application. Three to four layers of soft roll are applied against the skin, and extra padding is placed over bony prominences. A 10-layer-thick stack of plaster splint material is wetted in cold to lukewarm water and squeezed until damp. Hot water should be avoided because increased water temperature can lead to burns. The splint is applied over the soft-roll padding and wrapped lightly with an elastic bandage. The extremity is held in the appropriate position (any required molding to hold the reduction in place is done without making sharp indentations that can lead to skin breakdown) until the plaster is firm.

2. **Upper-extremity splints.** Removal of all of the patient's jewelry on the affected extremity is mandatory.

    a. **Commercial shoulder immobilizers, Velpeau dressing, and sling and swathe** are used for shoulder dislocations, humerus fractures, and some elbow fractures. A pad is placed in the axilla to prevent skin maceration.

    b. **Posterior and sugar-tong splints** are used in elbow, forearm, and wrist injuries. They are applied with the patient's elbow flexed to less than 90 degrees, the wrist in neutral to slight extension, and forearm in neutral rotation. Posterior splints consist of plaster along the posterior aspect of the arm, with a shorter "A-frame" piece on the lateral aspect across the elbow for added stability. Sugar-tong splints consist of one long strip of plaster that extends from the volar surface of the palm, down the volar forearm, around the posterior elbow, and along the dorsal surface of the forearm to the dorsal surface of the palm.

    c. **Thumb spica, ulnar/radial gutter, and volar/dorsal forearm splints** are used for forearm, hand, and wrist injuries. Finger injuries may be treated with prefabricated aluminum splint material.

For hand injuries, immobilization is performed with the patient's hand and wrist in a so-called **safe position or "intrinsic plus" position:** The wrist in 20 to 30 degrees of extension, the metacarpophalangeal joints in 70 to 80 degrees of flexion, and the interphalangeal joints extended.

3. **Lower extremity splints**
    a. **Thomas/Hare traction splints** are used by primary responders for femur fractures. Traction is applied by an ankle hitch, with counter traction across the ischial tuberosity. These should be replaced with an alternate form of immobilization as quickly as possible, because sloughing of the skin can occur around the ankle and groin.
    b. A **Jones dressing, consisting of bulky cotton padding underneath the plaster layers,** is used in acute knee, ankle, calcaneus, and tibial pilon fractures or any other foot or lower leg injury where a reduction is not needed in the ER and considerable swelling is expected. The injured extremity is wrapped with bulky Jones cotton, and then plaster splints can be applied to the posterior, medial, and lateral aspects as usual.
    c. **Short leg splints** are used in acute leg or foot trauma. They extend from below the knee to the toes and include posterior, medial, and lateral plaster slabs. Posterior slabs alone are inadequate. The ankle should be immobilized in the neutral position, with the foot as dorsiflexed as possible.

B. **Local anesthesia for fracture and joint reduction**
    1. **Digital nerve block.** The digital nerves of the fingers or toes can be blocked by infiltrating 2 to 5 mL of local anesthetic **without epinephrine** into the web spaces adjacent to the injured digit ensuring infiltration to the palmar or plantar skin. Ring blocks are needed for the thumb and great toes and involve circumferential subcutaneous infiltration about the digit.
    2. **Hematoma block** involves direct injection of lidocaine into a fracture site and is especially effective with fractures of the distal radius. Using sterile technique, a 21-gauge needle is inserted into the fracture site through the dorsal forearm. Aspiration of blood confirms the appropriate position of the needle in the fracture site. Approximately 8 to 10 mL of 1% of lidocaine without epinephrine is then infiltrated.
    3. **Intra-articular injection** is used to provide analgesia for reduction of intra-articular fractures and dislocations. Similar needle placement is used for joint aspirations. Under **sterile conditions,** the joint is entered with a needle with verification of placement by aspiration of blood (in the case of fracture) and the easy flow of the anesthetic from the syringe. The **ankle** may be entered anteriorly adjacent to either malleolus, and the **elbow** laterally in the triangle formed by the lateral epicondyle, radial head, and olecranon. Finally, the shoulder is entered either anteriorly 1 cm lateral to the coracoid process or posteriorly 2 cm distal and 2 cm medial to the posterolateral edge of the acromion aiming toward the coracoid.

Urologic Surgery

Samay Jain and Arnold Bullock

The discipline of **urologic surgery** encompasses the diagnosis and treatment of benign and malignant conditions of the genitourinary system including the kidneys, ureters, bladder, urethra, and the male external genitalia.

I. **HEMATURIA,** or blood in the urine, warrants a complete urologic work-up. Gross hematuria is visibly bloody urine, whereas microscopic hematuria is defined as *three or more red blood cells per high-power field* on microscopic evaluation of urinary sediment from two of three properly collected urinalysis (UA) specimens (*Am Fam Physician.* 2001;63:1145–1154).

A. **Evaluation** consists of laboratory, radiologic, and urine studies.

1. Urinalysis (macro- and microscopic), urine culture, and urine cytology should be obtained from a *freshly voided* specimen.

2. A complete blood count, coagulation panel, and serum creatinine should be obtained.

3. Radiographic imaging should be obtained to evaluate *both the renal parenchyma and the renal collecting system.* Cross-sectional imaging provides the most information with respect to total abdominal and pelvic anatomy. *Computed tomography* (CT) *urogram* is the preferred imaging modality; however, *magnetic resonance (MR) urogram* and *renal ultrasound with retrograde pyelograms* are adequate in appropriately selected patients (i.e., intravenous (IV) dye allergy, pregnancy).

4. Cystoscopy is the *gold standard* for evaluating the lower urinary tract.

5. If the etiology of the hematuria remains unclear, the patient should have a repeat UA, urine cytology, and blood pressure measurement at 6, 12, 24, and 36 months (*Urology.* 2001;57:604).

B. Treatment of symptomatic gross hematuria

1. Patients in **clot retention** require urologic consultation and bladder drainage with a large-caliber (larger than 22 French) three-way Foley catheter. The catheter should be manually irrigated and aspirated with normal saline or sterile water irrigant until the bladder is clot free. Continuous bladder irrigation (CBI) *should not be initiated* until the bladder is clot free.

2. **Persistent gross hematuria from a lower urinary tract source (bladder, prostate, urethra)** requires operative management via *cystoscopy and fulguration* of the bleeding source. A *cystogram* is usually performed at the same time to rule out bladder perforation and/or vesicoureteral reflux (VUR).

3. **Pharmaceutical options for lower tract bleeding**
   a. *Alum 1% and silver nitrate 1%* are astringents that act by protein precipitation over bleeding surfaces. They can be added to the CBI

fluid and used to irrigate the bladder, given there is no bladder perforation or VUR.

b. ε-*Aminocaproic acid (Amicar)* is an inhibitor of plasmin that can be administered intravenously, orally, or intravesically with CBI. It is absolutely contraindicated in patients with upper tract bleeding or DIC and can be associated with thromboembolic complications.

4. Persistent hematuria from an upper urinary tract source (kidney, ureter) is usually from a hemorrhagic renal mass, angiomyolipoma, arterial–venous fistula or renal trauma. These patients require intervention by either urology or interventional radiology. Upper tract bleeding may need to be managed by angioembolization of the source of bleeding.

II. DISEASES OF THE KIDNEY

A. Renal masses can be categorized as cystic or solid masses.

1. Renal cysts occur in approximately 50% of persons older than 50 years and the vast majority are benign. Renal cysts can be diagnosed and evaluated with CT, MRI, or ultrasound. Cysts are graded according the *Bosniak* grading system which attempts to predict their malignant potential based on various radiographic criteria (*Urology.* 2005;66(3):484–488).

a. Bosniak I describes a benign simple cyst with a hairline thin wall that does not contain septa, calcifications, or solid components. Category I cysts have no risk of malignancy and do not require further imaging or follow-up.

b. Bosniak II includes cysts that contain a few hairline septa or minor wall calcification. Uniformly high attenuation lesions (high-density cysts) that do not enhance on contrast imaging are included in this group. Category II cysts have no risk of malignancy and do not require further imaging or follow-up.

c. Bosniak IIF is a subgroup of cysts that contain multiple *nonenhancing* hairline septa sometimes with nodular or thick calcifications. Approximately 5% to 20% of these lesions may be malignant, which can be determined by serial imaging.

d. Bosniak III describes indeterminate lesions with numerous, thick or irregular septa, in which measurable enhancement is present. Category III cysts have more than a 50% malignant potential and require surgical management.

e. Bosniak IV type cysts are clearly malignant and have all the features of Category III cysts in addition to soft-tissue components. Category IV cysts have more than a 90% malignancy potential and mandate surgical management.

2. Solid renal masses should be considered malignant until proven otherwise. The majority of renal masses are discovered incidentally. Approximately 13% to 27% of abdominal imaging will reveal a renal mass (*N Engl J Med.* 2010;362:624–634). The historical triad of flank pain, hematuria, and flank mass occurs less than 10% of the time. Most solid masses are **renal cell carcinoma** (85% to 90%); transitional cell cancer, oncocytoma (benign in most cases), sarcoma, lymphoma, and various metastatic tumors (lung, breast, gastrointestinal, prostate, pancreas, and melanoma) can also present as a renal mass.

   a. Evaluation of a renal mass requires radiographic characterization and assessment for metastatic disease.

   (1) CT scan and MRI are ideal studies to assess renal masses. All patients with a solid renal mass must have a noncontrast study followed by a contrast study to **assess for enhancement.** In patients with contraindications to IV contrast or gadolinium, ultrasonography can determine whether a mass is cystic or solid; Doppler ultrasonography is useful for evaluating the renal vein and vena cava.

   (2) Chest radiography is required to rule out metastasis. Bone scan is indicated in patients with an abnormal alkaline phosphates or bone-related complaints with known renal mass.

   b. The role of percutaneous **renal mass biopsy** has expanded in recent times with diagnostic accuracy approaching greater than 90% while maintaining a low complication rate (<5%) (*J Urol.* 2008;179(1):20–27).

   c. Staging of renal masses is described in **Table 35-1**.

3. Paraneoplastic syndromes occur in 10% to 40% of renal cell carcinomas.

   a. Renin overproduction can present as hypertension.

   b. *Stauffer syndrome* is nonmetastatic hepatic dysfunction which resolves after tumor removal.

   c. Hypercalcemia is frequently caused by the production of parathyroid hormone–like protein (PTHrP) produced by the tumor.

   d. Erythrocytosis can result secondary to production of erythropoietin by the tumor.

B. Management of renal masses

1. Benign cystic renal lesions require no intervention (see Section II.A.1).

2. The management of solid renal masses depends on the tumor stage (*Eur Urol.* 2010;58:398–406).

   a. **T1 lesions.** Nephron-sparing surgery via partial nephrectomy.

   b. **T2 lesions.** Nephron-sparing surgery is preferred whenever possible; otherwise, radical nephrectomy is considered the standard of care.

   c. T3 and T4 lesions mandate radical nephrectomy.

3. Metastatic renal cell carcinoma is resistant to radiation and chemotherapy. Targeted therapy with agents such as bevacizumab, sorafenib, and sunitinib as well as immunotherapy with interleukin-2 and IFN-α has shown survival benefit in select patients (*BMC Cancer.* 2009;9:34).

III. DISEASES OF THE URETER

A. Ureteropelvic junction obstruction (UPJO)

1. UPJO is often a **congenital anomaly** that results from a stenotic segment of ureter. Acquired lesions may include tortuous or kinked ureters as a result of VUR, benign tumors such as fibroepithelial polyps,

TABLE 35-1	AJCC 2010 TNM Staging for Renal Cell Carcinoma

Primary Tumor (T)

Tx	Primary tumor cannot be assessed
T0	No evidence of primary tumor
T1	Tumor 7 cm or less in greatest dimension, limited to kidney
T1a	Tumor 4 cm or less in greatest dimension, limited to kidney
T1b	Tumor greater than 4 cm but not larger than 7 cm and limited to kidney
T2	Tumor greater than 7 cm in greatest dimension and limited to kidney
T2a	Tumor greater than 7 cm but less than 10 cm and limited to kidney
T2b	Tumor greater than 10 cm and limited to kidney
T3	Tumor extends into the major veins or perinephric tissues but not into the ipsilateral adrenal or beyond Gerota fascia
T3a	Tumor grossly extends into the renal vein or its segmental branches or tumor invades perirenal and/or renal sinus fat but not beyond Gerota fascia
T3b	Tumor grossly extends into the vena cava below the diaphragm
T3c	Tumor grossly extends into the vena cava above the diaphragm or invades the wall of the IVC
T4	Tumor invades beyond Gerota fascia

Regional Lymph Nodes—Clinical Stage (N)

Nx	Regional lymph nodes cannot be assessed
N0	No regional lymph node metastasis
N1	Metastasis in regional node(s)

Distant Metastasis (M)

M0	No distant metastasis
M1	Distant metastasis

or scarring as a result of stone disease, ischemia, or previous surgical manipulation of the urinary system. The role of crossing vessels (present in one third of cases) has not been firmly established, although their presence may be associated with treatment failures.

2. **Presentation.** Although UPJO can be a congenital problem, patients may present at any age. Common symptoms are flank pain (which may be intermittent), hematuria, infection, and, rarely, hypertension.

3. **Radiographic studies** help to determine the **site** and **functional significance** of the obstruction. Diuretic renal scintigraphy is both a functional and anatomic study that can diagnose obstruction and give the relative functions of both kidneys. Ultrasound and retrograde pyelography may demonstrate hydronephrosis, but neither is diagnostic of functional obstruction.

4. **Treatment** (*Curr Urol Rep.* 2010;11:74–79)
   a. Observation is recommended for poor surgical candidates or patients who are completely asymptomatic with a known nonfunctioning kidney.

b. Endopyelotomy is a minimally invasive procedure where the obstructed ureter is incised via a ureteral catheter through a cystoscope; however, success rates are lower than pyeloplasty (53% to 94%).

c. Pyeloplasty is the gold standard for treatment which allows for concurrent removal of ureteral stones, if present. Although more invasive than endopyelotomy, success rates for pyeloplasty are consistently higher, with most series reporting success rates more than 90%. The trend for repair has shifted from open to laparoscopic and robotic-assisted with success rates being similar, but with less morbidity with respect to pain control and days of hospitalization.

B. Urolithiasis

1. Urolithiasis frequently presents as the acute onset of severe, intermittent flank pain often associated with nausea and vomiting. Although patients may present with microscopic or gross hematuria, 15% of patients may have no hematuria. Stone formation commonly occurs between the third and fifth decade and tend to have a male predominance.

2. Risk factors for stone formation are both environmental and patient-related. Relative hydration and diets that contain high animal protein or oxalate promote stone formation. Various medications including high doses of vitamins C and D, acetazolamide, triamterene, and indinavir (*Lancet.* 1997;349:1294) favor stone formation. Disease states including inflammatory bowel disease, type I renal tubular acidosis (RTA) or cystinuria, and hyperparathyroidism can increase patient risk for stones.

3. Types of calculi

a. Calcium stones are radiopaque, make up the majority of all stones, and form in a wide range of pH. Risk factors for forming calcium-based stones include increased intestinal absorption, increased renal excretion, hyperparathyroidism, sarcoidosis, immobilization (causing calcium resorption from bone), and type I RTA.

b. Uric acid stones (10% of stones) are radiolucent and form in acidic pH (<6.0); they can be associated with gout or Lesch–Nyhan disease.

c. Cysteine stones (4% of stones) are radiopaque and form in acidic pH (<6.0). Risk factors include defective tubular resorption of cysteine that is inherited in an autosomal recessive manner.

d. Magnesium ammonium phosphate or **struvite stones** (15% of stones) are radiopaque, form in alkaline urine, and are associated with urea-splitting organisms.

4. Evaluation of urolithiasis

a. UA and urine culture should be performed.

b. Serum electrolytes (including calcium and creatinine levels), uric acid, and parathyroid hormone levels are part of the standard work-up.

c. Noncontrast CT scan has replaced IVP as the diagnostic study of choice in the acute setting to evaluate for stones (*Eur Radiol.* 2002;12(1):256–257).

d. **KUB (kidneys, ureters, bladder)** is useful to monitor for stone passage of radiopaque stones and to assess whether the stone is amenable for extracorporeal shock

5. The clinician should determine if the patient's urolithiasis is most appropriately managed as an outpatient, inpatient, or with surgery. Patients with intractable pain, nausea, or emesis not adequately controlled by oral medication require **hospital admission** for hydration and analgesia. **Surgical intervention** is indicated in patients with as above findings but also including infection or signs of sepsis, obstructed solitary kidney, bilateral obstruction, large stone size, or azotemia.

   a. **Medical expulsive therapy.** Approximately 70% of stones smaller than 5 mm will pass spontaneously. Spontaneous stone passage can be aided with prescription of narcotic pain medication as well as daily alpha blocker therapy (tamsulosin) which has been shown to improve stone passage rates by up to 20%. Urine should be strained with each void and radio opaque stones can be tracked with KUB (*J Urol.* 1997;178:2418–2434).

   b. **Surgical treatment.** In the acute setting, patients meeting surgical criteria can be managed by ureteral stenting or percutaneous nephrostomy tube placement. With a negative urine culture and lack of stone progression, surgical options include extracorporeal shockwave lithotripsy, ureteroscopic stone extraction, and percutaneous nephrolithotomy.

IV. DISEASES OF THE URINARY BLADDER

A. **Acute bacterial cystitis** is a common urologic problem which can present with suprapubic pain, dysuria, hesitancy, and frequency. Risk factors included recent bladder instrumentation, postmenopausal state, urinary retention, fistulae from GI tract, and female gender. Evaluation of patients requires **urine culture** with sensitivities. Males with a recurrent urinary tract infection (UTI) should have upper tract imaging (renal US), measurement of posturinary residual, and cystoscopy. Uncomplicated UTI (young women with no previous history of instrumentation and normal anatomy) should receive 3 days of empiric/culture-specific antibiotic treatment. Complicated UTI (male, previous manipulation, or abnormal anatomy) should receive 7 days of culture specific antibiotics and management of any underlying problem.

B. Bladder cancer. Bladder cancer is found in up to 10% of patients with microscopic hematuria.

1. **Urothelial cell carcinoma** (UCC) accounts for more than 90% of bladder tumors in the United States; squamous cell carcinoma and adenocarcinoma are less common. UCC has been linked to smoking, aniline dye, aromatic amine exposure, chronic phenacetin use, chronic indwelling Foley, chronic parasitic infection (*Schistosoma haematobium*), cyclophosphamide, radiation exposure.

2. **UCC is categorized as superficial or invasive.** Staging is outlined in Table 35-2. Evaluation for UCC requires cystoscopy, voided urine

TABLE 35-2 AJCC 2010 TNM Staging for Urothelial Cell Carcinoma

Primary Tumor (T)

Tx	Primary tumor cannot be assessed
T0	No evidence of primary tumor
Ta	Noninvasive papillary carcinoma
Tis	Carcinoma *in situ;* "Flat Tumor"
T1	Tumor invades the subepithelial connective tissue
T2	Tumor invades the muscularis propria
pT2a	Tumor invades superficial muscularis propria
pT2b	Tumor invades deep muscularis propria
T3	Tumor invades perivesical tissue
pT3a	Microscopic invasion
pT3b	Macroscopic invasion
T4	Tumor invades any of the following: prostatic stroma, seminal vesicles, uterus, vagina, pelvic/abdominal wall

Regional Lymph Nodes—Clinical Stage (N)

Nx	Regional lymph nodes cannot be assessed
N0	No regional lymph node metastasis
N1	Single regional lymph node in the true pelvis
N2	Multiple regional lymph nodes in the true pelvis
N3	Lymph node metastasis to the common iliac lymph nodes

Distant Metastasis (M)

M0	No distant metastasis
M1	Distant metastasis

cytology, upper tract imaging via CT/MR urogram, or ultrasound with retrograde pyelography to rule out concurrent upper tract disease, although this is rare (1.8%; *Eur Urol.* 2008;54:303–331).

a. **Superficial tumors** (stages Tis, Ta, T1) are exophytic papillary lesions that do not invade the muscular bladder wall. These tumors can be treated and staged with transurethral resection (TUR). Instillation of mitomycin C within 24 hours of TUR has been shown to decrease recurrence by 12% (*Eur Urol.* 2008;54:303–314). Between 65% and 85% of superficial tumors recur; therefore, diligent follow-up is necessary. Recurrent tumors are treated with TUR and intravesical therapy (bacillus Calmette–Guérin or mitomycin C).

b. **Muscle-invasive UCC** (stage ≥T2) is treated with radical cystectomy and urinary diversion. Radical cystectomy involves radical cystoprostatectomy (removal of bladder, prostate, and possibly urethra) in the male and anterior exenteration (removal of bladder, urethra, uterus, cervix, and anterior wall of vagina) in the female. Appropriate metastatic evaluation for patients with invasive bladder cancer includes chest radiograph, CT urogram, bone scan, and liver function tests. Despite this aggressive management, only 50% of patients with invasive bladder cancer are rendered completely free of tumor because many have occult metastases at the time of surgery.

c. **Chemotherapy** is the treatment of choice for locally advanced or metastatic bladder cancer. Both neoadjuvant and adjuvant chemotherapy have been shown to benefit patients with advanced UCC (≥T2) who also undergo surgery (*New Engl J Med.* 2003;349,9: 859–866; *Eur Urol.* 2009;55,2:348–358).

V. DISEASES OF THE PROSTATE

A. **Prostate cancer** is the most common noncutaneous malignancy in American men and the second leading cause of cancer death. Twenty percent of men with prostate cancer die of the disease. Prostate cancer rarely causes symptoms until it becomes locally advanced or metastatic. Risk factors for prostate cancer include being African American, advanced age, and family history (Table 35-3).

TABLE 35-3	AJCC 2010 TNM Staging for Prostate Carcinoma
Primary Tumor (T)	
Tx	Primary tumor cannot be assessed
T0	No evidence of primary tumor
T1	Clinically inapparent tumor neither palpable nor visible by imaging
T1a	Tumor incidental histologic finding in 5% or less of tissue resected
T1b	Tumor incidental histologic finding in more than 5% of tissue resected
T1c	Tumor identified by needle biopsy via screening (PSA, DRE)
T2	Tumor confined to the prostate
T2a	Tumor involves one-half of one lobe or less
T2b	Tumor involves more than one-half of one lobe, but not both lobes
T2c	Tumor involves both lobes
T3	Tumor extends through the prostatic capsule
T3a	Extracapsular extension
T3b	Seminal vesicle invasion
T4	Tumor is fixed or invades adjacent structures other than the SVs, such as external sphincter, rectum, bladder, levator muscles, and/or pelvic wall
Regional Lymph Nodes—Clinical Stage (N)	
Nx	Regional lymph nodes cannot be assessed
N0	No regional lymph node metastasis
N1	Metastasis in regional node(s)
Distant Metastasis (M)	
M0	No distant metastasis
M1	Distant metastasis
M1a	Nonregional lymph node(s)
M1b	Bone(s)
M1c	Other site(s) with or without bone disease

Modified from Prostate. In: Edge SE, Byrd DR, Carducci MA, et al., eds. *AJCC Cancer Staging Manual.* 7th ed. New York, NY: Springer; 2010:525–538.

1. Screening for prostate cancer includes digital rectal examination (DRE) and measurement of serum prostate-specific antigen (PSA).
   a. **Digital rectal exam.** DRE and PSA provide a better sensitivity for screening than either alone; therefore, DRE is an essential aspect of screening for prostate cancer (*J Urol.* 1994;151(5):1308–1309; *Nat Clin Pract Urol.* 2009;6(2):68–69). The normal prostate measures 3.5 cm wide at the base, 2.5 cm long, and 2.5 cm deep; it weighs approximately 20 g. The prostate should feel smooth and have the consistency of the contracted thenar eminence of the thumb.
   b. **PSA screening** remains controversial based on contradictory conclusions from two large, prospective randomized trials (*N Engl J Med.* 2009;360:1310–1319, 1320–1328). Current AUA guidelines recommend initial PSA screening at 40 years of age and then yearly screening at 50 years of age. Abnormal PSA results require detailed discussion with a urologist to determine the next best step in patient care (American Urological Association Clinical Guidelines 2008).
   c. Abnormalities in either the DRE (manifest as indurated nodules) or the PSA greater than 2.5 ng/mL should be evaluated by **trans-rectal ultrasound and needle biopsy of the prostate** (*National Comprehensive Cancer Network Clinical Practice Guidelines in Oncology* 2006, http://www.nccn.org).
2. Prostate cancer is diagnosed and graded by the **Gleason scoring system** (*J Urol.* 2010;183(2):433–440) This grading system relies on the overall architecture of the biopsy core and assigns a grade from 2 to 5 of the two most prominent architectural patterns to give a sum of 5 to 6 (low-grade disease), 7 (intermediate grade), or 8 to 10 (high grade).
3. Staging of prostate cancer is selectively completed.
   a. **Bone scan** should be obtained for patients with a life expectancy greater than 5 years and a PSA ≥20 ng/mL or Gleason 8 disease or T3-T4 disease or having symptomatic bone complaints.
   b. **CT/MRI of the abdomen and pelvis** should be obtained in patients with T3-T4 disease or if patients have a ≥20% probability of lymph node involvement based on current prostate cancer nomograms.
4. **Treatment options** for men with organ-confined prostate cancer include active surveillance (AS), radical prostatectomy (RP), and radiation therapy (RT, either external-beam or interstitial). These are stratified based on the aggressiveness of the cancer and the patient's life expectancy (NCCN Clinical Proactive Guidelines in Oncology, V.3.2010, www.nccn.org).
   a. **Very low risk** is classified as t1c, Gleason ≤6, PSA less than 6, fewer than three biopsy cores positive, ≤50% cancer in each core, PSA density less than 0.15 ng/mL/g.
   b. **Low risk** is classified as T1-T2, Gleason ≤6, PSA less than 10.
   c. **Intermediate risk** is classified t2b-T2c or Gleason 7 or PSA 10 to 20.
   d. **High risk** is classified as T3a or Gleason 8 to 10 or PSA more than 20.

e. Treatment of **locally advanced disease** (t3b-T4) is tailored to the patient based on various factors and may consist of RT, RP, or androgen deprivation therapy.

f. **Metastatic disease** is treated with androgen deprivation therapy.

Life Expectancy	Risk			
	Very Low	**Low**	**Intermediate**	**High**
<10 years	AS	AS	AS, RT, RP	RT, RP
≥10 years		AS, RT, RP	RT, RP	

5. **Prostatitis** is a diagnosis that spans a spectrum of disease entities. The classification and diagnostic criteria for the different forms of prostatitis recently have been changed in an effort to standardize diagnosis to improve research and clinical treatment. Prostatitis encompasses four clinical entities (*Am Fam Physician.* 2010;82(4):397–406).

a. **Acute bacterial prostatitis (ABP)** presents with **signs and symptoms of urinary tract infection;** many patients have significant voiding complaints, fevers, and malaise. ABP requires prompt treatment with antibiotics. Urine should be cultured prior to initiating treatment. Most common organisms are *Escherichia coli, Klebsiella, Proteus* and *Pseudomonas*, and occasionally *Enterococcus.* Prostate exam will reveal tender, boggy enlarged prostate. Prostatic massage should not be performed as this could be potentially harmful. Empiric treatment should be started at the time of diagnosis and tailored to culture specific therapy when appropriate. Mildly to moderately ill-appearing patients are treated with a 6-week course of sulfamethoxazole (Bactrim) or ciprofloxacin. Severely ill-appearing or septic patients require hospital admission for IV antibiotics (ampicillin and gentamicin) until afebrile, before transitioning to oral medications listed above. If a patient does not improve on the prescribed antibiotic regimen, imaging of the prostate should be obtained by either a CT scan or transrectal ultrasound to rule out abscess.

b. **Chronic bacterial prostatitis** is differentiated from other categories by the documented recurrent bacterial infection of expressed prostatic secretions, postprostatic massage urine, or semen. Treatment is with 4 to 6 weeks of antibiotics; fluoroquinolones have excellent prostatic penetration.

c. **Chronic pelvic pain syndrome** is diagnosed in patients with continued pelvic pain but with no bacteria infection isolated from expressed prostatic secretions.

d. **Asymptomatic prostatitis** is an incidental finding and usually does not require treatment.

B. **Benign prostatic hyperplasia (BPH)** is a histologic diagnosis and represents an increase in several epithelial and stromal elements of the prostate.

Men with BPH and benign prostatic enlargement on examination do not necessarily have lower urinary tract symptoms (LUTS).

1. **Evaluation.** Common signs and symptoms of BPH include hesitancy, decreased force of stream, frequency, urgency, postvoid dribbling, double voiding, incomplete bladder emptying, and nocturia. LUTS is a symptom complex of obstructive and irritative voiding problems. Bladder outlet obstruction is objective evidence of obstructive voiding problems and can include a demonstrated decrease in maximum urinary flow rate, increase postvoid residual urine, and cystoscopic findings of obstruction (American Urological Association Clinical Guidelines 2003).

2. Treatment
   a. **Watchful waiting** is best suited for patients without bothersome symptoms.
   b. **Medical therapy.** Men with **LUTS without BPH** are best treated by long-acting selective alpha blocker (tamsulosin, terazosin, doxazosin, alfuzosin). In patients with **LUTS and BPH,** the standard of care is combination therapy with an alpha blocker (i.e., tamsulosin) and a 5α reductase inhibitor (i.e., dutasteride or finasteride) based on the results of two large, prospective, randomized trials in which the risk of overall clinical progression of LUTS was lower with combination therapy than treatment with either drug alone (*N Engl J Med.* 2003;349:2387, *Eur Urol.* 2010;571):123–131).
   c. **Surgical therapy** is indicated in patients who have failed medical therapy or have severe symptoms of LUTS (complete urinary retention, bladder stones, persistent UTI, gross hematuria, renal failure). The gold standard is transurethral resection of the prostate, but transurethral laser ablation/vaporization offers similar functional results with less morbidity (*Eur Urol.* 2010;58(3):349–355).

VI. **URINARY RETENTION** may result from BPH, prostate cancer, or urethral stricture disease. Retention also can be associated with pelvic trauma, neurologic conditions, or various medications or the postoperative setting.

A. **Evaluation.** A history usually elicits the cause of retention. Patients with BPH who are treated with decongestants containing an α-agonist may develop urinary retention from increased smooth-muscle tone at the bladder neck and the prostate.

B. **Physical examination** reveals a distended lower abdomen. Prostatic enlargement is common on DRE. Serum electrolytes including creatinine level, UA, and urine culture should be obtained. Serum PSA concentration obtained during acute urinary retention often is spuriously elevated and is best measured at least 4 to 6 weeks after the acute event.

C. **Treatment**

1. **Bladder decompression with a Foley catheter is the mainstay of treatment.** The proper technique of urethral catheter placement involves passing the catheter to the hub and inflating the balloon *only* after the return of urine.

2. **When a standard Foley catheter cannot be passed easily,** sterile 2% viscous lidocaine can be injected through the urethra. This anesthetizes and relaxes the sphincter, allowing gentle passage of a 16- to 22-French Coudé tip catheter. The catheter is passed gently with the tip directed upward. If the Coudé tip catheter does not pass easily, a urology consultation is required.

3. **Catheterization should not be attempted when a urethral injury is suspected.** Urethral stricture requires calibration and dilation or placement of a suprapubic tube by a urologist. Urinary clot retention usually requires bladder irrigation.

4. **Patients should be monitored for postobstructive diuresis, especially if the patient is azotemic.** This is a self-limited, physiologic response to a hypervolemic state. Occasionally, it can become a pathologic diuresis and may warrant hospital observation, with fluid and electrolyte replacement. Five-percent dextrose in 0.45% saline should be used for hydration. Urine output greater than 200 mL/hour for more than 2 hours should be replaced with 0.5 mL of IV 0.45% saline for each 1 mL of urine. Electrolytes should be checked every 6 hours initially and replaced as needed.

VII. DISEASES OF THE PENIS

A. **Priapism** is a persistent penile erection that continues hours beyond, or is unrelated to, sexual stimulation and typically only affects the corpora cavernosa. Priapism can be classified as nonischemic or ischemic.

1. **Non ischemic priapism** is a nonsexual erection caused by unregulated cavernous arterial flow usually brought about by perineal or genital trauma. A traumatic pudendal arterial fistula or cavernosal artery laceration may give rise to a high-flow state. Diagnosis is confirmed ultrasound demonstrating increased flow or by aspiration of bright-red, well-oxygenated blood. Blood gas analysis can be helpful in differentiating low-flow priapism from high-flow priapism. Treatment of nonischemic priapism *is not an emergency* as 60% of cases will resolve with observation. Selective arterial embolization of the ipsilateral branch of the pudendal artery embolization can be attempted after outpatient discussion of risks of the procedure [i.e., erectile dysfunction (ED)]. Surgical ligation of abnormal vessel(s) is reserved as a last resort as complications, such as ED, are higher with this approach.

2. **Ischemic priapism** is a nonsexual, persistent erection characterized by little or no cavernous blood flow. This is a **urologic emergency.** Symptoms include pain and tenderness. History should elicit various etiologies of priapism including: (i) Hematologic abnormalities, such as **sickle cell disease;** (ii) **drugs,** including antihypertensives (hydralazine, guanethidine, prazosin), anticoagulants, antidepressants, and psychotropic agents (especially trazodone), alcohol, marijuana, cocaine, and intracavernous injection of vasoactive substances (prostaglandin E_1, phentolamine, papaverine) used to treat ED; and (iii) **neoplasm (especially leukemia),** with venous occlusion, stasis, and emboli.

Physical examination reveals firm corpora and a flaccid glans. Stasis, thrombosis, fibrosis, and scarring of the corpora cavernosa eventually can result in ED if priapism is not treated promptly. Of note, phosphodiesterase type 5 (PDE5) inhibitors, which are used for the treatment of ED (see Section VII.B.4), are rarely associated with ischemic priapism.

  a. Treatment (American Urological Association Clinical Guidelines 2008)

    (1) First-line treatment involves corporal irrigation and aspiration of old blood from the corpora via a large bore needle (larger than 21 G).

    (2) Intracorporal injection of an α-**adrenergic agent** (phenylephrine, 250 to 500 μg/mL) is a useful adjunct to corporal irrigation. Doses should be administered every 2 to 5 minutes until detumescence is achieved. Patients should be monitored for hypertension and reflex bradycardia.

    (3) For patients with sickle cell disease, treatment involves aggressive hydration, supplemental oxygen, and blood transfusion if the hematocrit is low.

    (4) Surgical shunting should be considered only if multiple attempts at aspiration/irrigation and injection of a-adrenergic agents fail. Distal corpus cavernosum-to-glans penis (corpus spongiosum) shunting (**Winter or Al-Ghorab shunt**) is the initial surgical treatment. If distal shunting fails, then a more proximal **side-to-side cavernosospongiosal shunt (Quackel shunt) or cavernosaphenous shunt** may be necessary. Insertion of a malleable, temporary penile prosthesis can be used in cases where shunting has failed. The aim is to prevent corporal fibrosis to allow for elective revision of the prosthesis at a later date.

B. Erectile dysfunction is the inability to achieve or maintain an erection sufficient for satisfactory sexual performance. ED affects 52% of men aged 40 to 70 years according to the Massachusetts Male Aging Study; incidence increases with age, but the degree of mild ED remains fairly constant from age 40 to 70 years. Unfortunately, only 20% of men with ED discuss this condition with a health care provider. The overwhelming majority of men have an organic etiology of their ED.

  1. Initial evaluation entails a frank discussion of the complaint to define the true sexual disorder; one must differentiate ED from premature ejaculation, inability to climax, infertility, and loss of libido. Unlike men with organic ED, those with psychogenic ED have sudden onset and continue to have nocturnal erections. Loss of libido may signal hormonal disturbances. A complete history and physical examination is done to elicit possible underlying causes of ED, including heart disease, hypertension, diabetes, dyslipidemia, renal insufficiency, and endocrine disease (hypogonadism). Smokers have a twofold higher incidence of ED. Previous pelvic or penile surgery may be associated with ED.

2. **Attention should be paid to medications,** such as antihypertensives [central-acting agents (clonidine), α-adrenergic blocking agents (prazosin), β-blocking agents], antipsychotics, tricyclic antidepressants, and histamine (H_2) blockers, which may be associated with ED. Heavy use of alcohol and social drugs can also lead to ED.

3. **Physical examination** should focus on genital development and signs of endocrinologic or neurologic abnormalities.

    Appropriate laboratory testing includes serum chemistries, creatinine, CBC, UA, and a morning testosterone level. If the testosterone is abnormal, prolactin, FSH, and LH are obtained.

4. **Treatment.** The initial recommendation should be for lifestyle modification and management of the underlying disease. Smoking cessation, diet modification, and exercise have all been shown to improve erectile function and overall health. It is appropriate to counsel patients about available nonsurgical and surgical options for treatment and to encourage treatment until a satisfactory solution is found (AUA Clinical Guidelines 2009).

    a. **PDE-5 inhibitors (i.e., sildenafil)** are considered first-line therapy. PDE5 inhibitors inhibit the breakdown of cyclic guanosine monophosphate, allowing smooth-muscle relaxation in the corpus cavernosum. Side effects include headache, facial flushing, and dyspepsia. PDE5 inhibitors are contraindicated in patients who are taking nitrates because of a synergistic effect that results in hypotension. All are metabolized by the liver, so doses should be adjusted accordingly in liver failure patients.

    b. **Intracavernosal therapy.** Injection of vasoactive medications, such as alprostadil (prostaglandin E_1), directly into the corpus cavernosum is effective in 70% to 80% of patients. Side effects are pain with injection, hematoma or ecchymosis, and priapism. An **intraurethral alprostadil (MUSE)** suppository is also available and is effective in some men.

    c. **Vacuum erection device (VED).** For men who fail or are not candidates for medical therapy, a vacuum pump is efficacious, but many couples find it cumbersome and uncomfortable. Patients with difficulty in maintaining an erection due to cavernosal venous insufficiency may benefit from a constriction band.

    d. **Surgical options.** For patients who are refractory to noninvasive therapy, consideration may be given to a surgically placed penile implant. These devices have a high degree of success, and they are placed via small genital incisions. There are potential complications, such as infection (2%) and mechanical malfunction (2%).

VIII. DISEASES OF THE SCROTUM AND TESTICLES

Acute scrotal pathology can result in significant morbidity, testicular loss, and infertility. The diagnosis can be difficult to make and may require scrotal exploration.

A. **Testicular torsion** is the rotation of the testicle on its vascular pedicle that results in ischemia. This is a true urologic emergency which develops most often in the peripubertal (12 to 18 years old) age group, although it can occur at any age.

1. The **clinical picture** is one of acute onset of testicular pain and swelling, commonly associated with nausea and vomiting. Some patients give a history of a prior episode that spontaneously resolved (intermittent torsion). There usually is no history of voiding complaints, dysuria, fever, or exposure to sexually transmitted diseases. Risk factors include cryptorchidism (undescended testis) and "bell clapper" anatomy of the testicle, although this cannot be determined outside of scrotal exploration.

2. **Physical examination** reveals an extremely tender, swollen testicle high riding in the scrotum with a transverse lie. The cremasteric reflex (elicited by stroking the inner thigh) is absent on the affected side. In contrast to epididymitis, elevation of the scrotum does not provide relief of pain (Prehn sign) in torsion. Normal UA and the absence of leukocytosis help to rule out epididymitis. Testicular torsion is a clinical diagnosis, and, if enough suspicions exist, the patient needs to be explored without delay.

   a. **History.** Acute onset of testicular pain and swelling often associated with visceral complaints of abdominal pain and nausea and vomiting. LUTS and trauma are typically absent.

3. Testicular torsion is a **clinical diagnosis** and treatment should not be delayed to obtain imaging. However, if clinical diagnosis is equivocal or suspicion is low, color Doppler ultrasound can help to confirm or exclude the diagnosis with reported sensitivity and specificity greater than 95% (*Urology.* 2010;75(5):1170–1174).

4. **Treatment.** If testicular torsion is suspected based on history and physical exam, the patient should be taken for immediate scrotal exploration and bilateral orchiopexy. Manual detorsion of the testicle may be attempted in the emergency room, but bilateral orchiopexy is still indicated.

B. **Torsion of testicular appendage (appendix testis)** presents with symptoms similar to those of torsion of the testicle, usually in a prepubertal boy. The onset commonly is over 12 to 24 hours. Extreme tenderness over a palpable, nodular appendage, usually on the superior aspect of the testicle is frequently present. The "blue dot" sign may be present when the ischemic appendage can be seen through the scrotal skin (*Urology.* 1973;1(1):63–66). The testicle has a normal position, lies, and is freely mobile. The spermatic cord is nontender and there is usually a cremasteric reflex present. Similar to testicular torsion, torsion of an appendix testis is a clinical diagnosis. Imaging can be obtained if the clinical picture is unclear or for documentation. Unlike true testicular torsion, this is not an emergency. Treatment is **expectant** with anti-inflammatory agents; light physical activity and scrotal support can manage the symptoms until resolution over 7 to 14 days.

C. **Epididymitis** usually presents with a 1- to 2-day onset of unilateral testicular pain and swelling sometimes associated with dysuria, urethral discharge, or LUTS.

1. Typically, the **findings** include a painful, indurated epididymis, and pyuria. Urinalysis, urine culture, and CBC count are obtained. When clinically indicated, urethral swabs for gonococci and chlamydiae are sent for culture.

2. With **appropriate antibiotic coverage,** these patients can be managed as outpatients. Treatment is empiric with an oral fluoroquinolone for 3 to 4 weeks; antibiotics should be tailored based on culture results. Appropriate antibiotic therapy should be instituted for any diagnosed sexually transmitted disease. Nonsteroidal analgesics and scrotal elevation can reduce inflammation and provide symptomatic relief.

3. Moderate-to-severe cases of epididymitis may require hospital admission. Symptoms usually have been present for several days. Fever and leukocytosis are present. Broad-spectrum antibiotics and supportive measures of bed rest with scrotal elevation should be instituted. Ultrasonography can be useful to rule out abscess formation and assess testicular perfusion.

D. **Fournier gangrene** is a severe polymicrobial soft-tissue infection involving the genitals and perineum. Although the term *Fournier gangrene* usually is applied to men, necrotizing fasciitis of this area can occur in women. Prompt diagnosis and institution of treatment may be lifesaving. Roughly 19% of the patients have a genitourinary source (urethral stone, urethral stricture, and urethral fistulae), 21% have an colorectal source (ruptured appendicitis, colonic carcinoma, diverticulitis, perirectal abscesses, and/or fistulae), 24% have a dermatologic source, and nearly 36% have an unidentified source (*Br J Surg.* 2000;87:718). Diabetic, alcoholic, and other immunocompromised patients appear to be more susceptible. The clinical course is one of abrupt onset with pruritus, rapidly progressing to edema, erythema, and necrosis, often within a few hours. Fever, chills, and malaise are accompanying signs.

1. **Physical examination** reveals edema and erythema of the skin of the scrotum, phallus, and perineal area. This may progress rapidly to frank necrosis of the skin and subcutaneous tissues, with extension to the skin of the abdomen and back, reaching as high as the clavicles and down the thighs. Crepitus in the tissues suggests the presence of gas-forming organisms.

2. **Laboratory evaluation** should include a CBC, serum electrolytes, creatinine, arterial blood gas, coagulation parameters, UA, urine, and blood cultures. A KUB plain film may reveal subcutaneous gas. Cross-sectional imaging (CT scan) can be obtained to determine the source of infection, any undrained abscesses, and the subcutaneous gas, but should never delay definitive, operative treatment.

3. **The patient should be stabilized and prepared emergently for the operating room.** Broad-spectrum antibiotics that are active against both aerobic and anaerobic organisms should be started immediately. Aerobic and anaerobic wound cultures are usually polymicrobial.

4. **Wide débridement** is required, with aggressive postoperative support. The testicles are often spared because they have a blood supply discrete from the scrotum; orchiectomy is rarely indicated. Wound closure and

dermal coverage often is an extensive process, and recovery requires intense physical therapy and wound care. Despite improvements in critical care, antibiotics, and surgical technology, **mortality** ranges from 3% to 45% (*Br J Surg.* 2000;87:718).

E. **Nonacute scrotal masses**

1. **Hydroceles** generally are asymptomatic fluid collections around the testicle that **transilluminate.** Ultrasound evaluation is recommended to rule out serious underlying causes such as testicular malignancies. If hydroceles do enlarge and become symptomatic, they can be repaired by various transscrotal techniques. Hydroceles in infants may be associated with a patent processus vaginalis; parents give a history of intermittent scrotal swelling. These hydroceles usually resolve by 1 year of age. Those that persist or cause symptoms can be repaired by an inguinal approach.

2. **Spermatoceles** are benign cystic dilations involving the tail of the epididymis or proximal vas deferens.

3. **Varicoceles** are abnormal tortuosities and dilations of the testicular veins within the spermatic cord. On physical examination, they feel like a "bag of worms." A varicocele may diminish in size when the patient is supine. Because the left gonadal vein drains directly into the renal vein, varicoceles are much more common on the left side. Right-sided varicoceles may be associated with obstruction of the inferior vena cava. Varicoceles are the most common surgically correctable cause of male infertility; nevertheless, most men with varicoceles remain fertile. Varicocele repair results in improved semen quality in approximately 70% of patients. Surgical treatment of varicoceles is indicated for diminished testicular growth in adolescents, infertility, or significant symptoms. Any patient who presents with a **new-onset varicocele later in life warrants retroperitoneal imaging** to rule out a malignancy causing venous obstruction.

F. **Testicular tumors** are the most common solid tumors in 15- to 35-year-old men. The estimated lifetime risk for testicular malignancy is 1 in 500. Owing to improved multimodality therapy, overall 5-year survival for testis cancer is now 95%. Risk factors associated with testicular tumors include cryptorchidism, HIV infection, and gonadal dysgenesis with Y chromosome (Table 35-4).

1. **The typical clinical finding is a painless testicular mass,** although one third of patients may present with pain. Pulmonary or gastrointestinal complaints or an abdominal mass may reflect advanced disease. Scrotal sonography is mandatory; seminomas appear as a hypoechoic lesion, and nonseminomatous tumors appear inhomogeneous. α-Fetoprotein, β-human chorionic gonadotropin, and lactic acid dehydrogenase are serum tumor markers that help to identify the tumor type and completely stage the tumor. The markers are used to monitor the effectiveness of therapy and to screen for recurrence.

2. **Staging of testicular tumors** is outlined in Table 35-5. All patients with testicular carcinoma should have cross-sectional imaging of the retroperitoneum and pelvis as well as a chest X-ray to assess for distant disease.

| **TABLE 35-4** | AJCC 2010 TNM Staging for Testes Carcinoma |

Primary Tumor (T)

pTx	Primary tumor cannot be assessed
pT0	No evidence of primary tumor
pTis	Intratubular germ cell neoplasia
pT1	Tumor limited to testis and epididymis without vascular/lymphatic invasion; tumor may invade the tunica albuginea but not the tunica vaginalis
pT2	Tumor limited to testis and epididymis with vascular/lymphatic invasion, or tumor extending through into the tunica vaginalis
pT3	Tumor invades the spermatic cord with or without vascular/ lymphatic invasion
pT4	Tumor invades the scrotum with or without vascular/lymphatic invasion

Regional Lymph Nodes—Clinical Stage (N)

Nx	Regional lymph nodes cannot be assessed
N0	No regional lymph node metastasis
N1	Metastasis with a lymph node mass 2 cm or less in greatest dimension, or multiple nodes, none greater than 2 cm in greatest dimension
N2	Lymph node mass >2 cm but <5 cm or multiple nodes with one mass >2 cm, but none >5 cm
N3	Lymph node mass >5 cm in greatest dimension

Distant Metastasis (M)

M0	No distant metastasis
M1	Distant metastasis
M1a	Nonregional nodal or pulmonary metastasis
M1b	Distant metastasis other than to nonregional nodes and lung

Serum Tumor Markers (S)

S0	Marker study levels within normal limits
S1	LDH <1.5× normal and hCG <5,000 and AFP <1,000
S2	LDH 1.5 to 10× normal or hCG 5–50,000 or AFP 1,000–10,000
S3	LDH > 10× normal or hCG >50,000, or AFP >10,000
Sx	Marker studies not available or not performed

Modified from Testis. In: Edge SE, Byrd DR, Carducci MA, et al., eds. *AJCC Cancer Staging Manual.* 7th ed. New York, NY:Springer; 2010:539–543.

3. **Initial therapy** for all testicular tumors is radical inguinal orchiectomy. The type of tumor and the stage of the disease determine further therapy.

a. **Seminomas** constitute 60% to 65% of germ-cell tumors. Low-stage seminomas are treated with adjuvant RT to the retroperitoneum. Advanced disease is usually treated with a platinum-based chemotherapy regimen.

b. **Nonseminomatous tumors** include the histologic types of embryonal carcinoma, teratoma, choriocarcinoma, and yolk sac elements, alone or in combination. Nonseminomatous tumors are more likely

TABLE 35-5	AAST Organ Injury Severity Scale	

Grade	Type	Description
I	Contusion	Microscopic or gross hematuria, urological studies normal
	Hematoma	Subcapsular, not expanding with no parenchymal laceration
II	Hematoma	Not expanding perirenal hematoma confined to renal retroperitoneum
	Laceration	<1.0 cm parenchymal depth of renal cortex with no urinary extravasation
III	Laceration	>1.0 cm parenchymal depth of renal cortex with no collecting system rupture or urinary extravasation
IV	Laceration	Parenchymal laceration extending through renal cortex, medulla, and collecting system
	Vascular	Main renal artery or vein injury with contained hemorrhage
V	Laceration	Completely shattered kidney
	Vascular	Avulsion of renal hilum

to present with advanced disease. Patients with clinically negative retroperitoneal nodes with normal tumor markers are treated with retroperitoneal lymph node dissection, prophylactic chemotherapy, or close observation. Patients with high-stage disease with elevated markers receive platinum-based chemotherapy followed by retroperitoneal node dissection if there is residual disease.

IX. **GENITOURINARY TRAUMA** is relatively uncommon and associated with only 10% of all traumas. Injuries should be identified during the secondary survey after life-threatening injuries have been addressed and initial resuscitation has been undertaken.

A. **Renal trauma**

1. The kidneys are the most commonly injured urologic organ occurring in 1.2% to 3.3% of all traumatic injuries. Over 80% are blunt in nature and anywhere from 4% to 10% are penetrating (*Br J Urol.* 2004;93(7):937–954). The grading system for renal injuries is shown in Table 35-5.

2. **Microscopic hematuria** (>three RBCs per high-power field) or gross hematuria is present in more than 95% of patients with a renal injury. A voided specimen is best for UA, but if the patient cannot void or is unconscious and no blood is at the meatus, a well-lubricated urethral catheter should gently be passed.

3. All patients with **gross hematuria and blunt trauma** should be evaluated with a CT scan using IV contrast. If the patient is stable, 10-minute-delayed imaging is helpful to evaluate for collecting system injuries. Patients with microscopic hematuria and shock (systolic blood pressure <90 mm Hg) should be imaged with a CT scan after they are stabilized. Patients with microscopic hematuria, no shock, and no evidence of significant deceleration or renal injury do not need radiographic evaluation of their urinary system (*J Urol.* 1989;141:1095).

4. The **degree of hematuria** does not correlate with the severity of the injury (*Br J Urol.* 2004;93(7):937–954), and any patient with a suspected renal injury due to rapid deceleration requires radiographic evaluation. Disruption of the ureteropelvic junction should be considered in children with deceleration or hyperextension injuries.

5. Most **blunt renal injuries** can be managed conservatively; fewer than 10% of blunt renal injuries require surgery or procedural intervention. Ongoing hemorrhage can be managed with selective renal artery angioembolization.

6. **Penetrating renal trauma** with microscopic hematuria (>three RBCs per high-power field) or gross hematuria requires radiographic assessment with CT scan. Preferably, this is done before exploration to evaluate the injured kidney and to confirm function of the contralateral kidney. A normal contralateral kidney may influence the surgeon's decision (repair vs. nephrectomy) on management of the injured kidney. Intraoperative palpation of a contralateral kidney may be misleading.

7. **Absolute indications for intraoperative renal exploration** include hemodynamic instability, persistent and life-threatening hemorrhage from renal injury, expanding or pulsatile perirenal mass, or renal pedicle avulsion. Selective exploration can be advocated in patients with a perirenal hematoma secondary to penetrating trauma and instability precluding evaluation with cross-sectional imaging.

B. **Ureteral injuries** account for approximately 3% of all urologic traumas and are most often associated with **penetrating trauma and multiple associated injuries** (*Br J Urol.* 2004;94(3):277–289). A high index of suspicion often is necessary to make the diagnosis, and many ureteral injuries have a delayed presentation. The absence of gross or microscopic hematuria has been documented in 30% of patients.

1. **Radiographic findings** include extravasation and, more commonly, delayed function; proximal dilation; and deviation of the ureter. A CT may demonstrate medial extravasation; delayed images are necessary to assess ureteral patency.

2. **Adequately visualizing the ureter during laparotomy** is important for diagnosing ureteral injury; IV or intraureteral injection of indigo carmine or methylene blue may help to assess the integrity of the urothelium.

3. For purposes of determining the **type of repair,** the ureter is divided into thirds:

   a. Injuries to the distal one third of the ureter are best managed by **ureteral reimplantation.** Additional length to provide a tension-free anastomosis may be gained by using a Psoas hitch and, if necessary, a Boari bladder flap.

   b. Injuries of the middle or upper third of the ureter are best managed by **ureteroureterostomy.** An omental wrap may be used to protect the repair. Stents and drains are recommended for all ureteral repairs.

C. Bladder injuries present in 2% of all blunt trauma and 6% of all pelvic fractures (*Br J Urol.* 2004;94(1):27–32).

   1. Ninety-five percent of bladder injuries present with **gross hematuria** (*Urol Clin North Am.* 2006;33:676). CT cystogram should be obtained in any patient with gross hematuria and pelvic fracture. Relative indications for a cystogram include gross hematuria without a pelvic fracture, microscopic hematuria with pelvic fracture, or isolated microscopic hematuria.

   2. CT cystogram is the most sensitive imaging modality for bladder injury. The bladder should be filled retrograde by gravity via an indwelling Foley catheter with 350 mL of dilute (3% to 5%) contrast. Postdrainage films are not necessary; merely clamping the Foley to allow bladder filling with excreted contrast does not constitute an adequate study.

   3. Treatment

   a. All patients with penetrating trauma to the bladder and **intraperitoneal extravasation** of contrast require **surgical exploration and repair** of the bladder (*Urol Clin North Am.* 2006;33:67).

   b. Patients with blunt trauma and **extraperitoneal extravasation** of contrast can be managed nonoperatively with **catheter drainage** for 10 days. A cystogram should be performed prior to catheter removal. Greater than 85% will have healed by the 10th day from injury. Surgical repair is indicated if the bladder does not heal over the catheter after 3 weeks, or if concomitant vaginal or rectal injury, or bladder neck injury/avulsion, or in patients undergoing pelvic fracture plating.

D. Urethral injuries occur in 5% of patients with pelvic fractures and should be suspected when blood is at the meatus or the mechanism of injury is such that urethral injury might have occurred. Physical examination in patients with urethral injury may reveal penile and scrotal edema and ecchymosis. Rectal examination can reveal a high-riding prostate or boggy hematoma in the expected position of the prostate. If a urethral injury is suspected, a **retrograde urethrogram** must be performed prior to Foley catheter placement.

   1. Posterior urethral injuries involve the prostatic and membranous urethra to the level of the urogenital diaphragm. These injuries are caused mainly by blunt trauma, and management is dependent on the degree of injury. Partial disruption of the urethra is best managed with urethral catheterization when possible. Complete disruption requires suprapubic catheter placement in the acute setting with attempt at endoscopic primary realignment within 72 hours. After realignment, primary repair is performed in the delayed setting (3 to 6 months from injury). Unstable patients require suprapubic tube placement and realignment when stable. Primary surgical repair of a posterior urethral injury is not recommended in the acute setting as it is complicated by higher rates of impotence, incontinence, and stricture (*Urol Clin North Am.* 2006;33:87).

2. Anterior urethral injuries include injuries to the bulbous and penile urethra distal to the urogenital diaphragm. Straddle injuries and penetrating trauma are the most common causes of these types of injuries. Injuries contained by Buck fascia often have a characteristic "sleeve of penis" pattern, whereas urethral or penile injuries in which Buck fascia is disrupted are contained by the Colles fascia and have a "butterfly" appearance on the perineum. These injuries are best managed with urethral catheterization and delayed surgical repair (3 months after injury).

E. Penile trauma

1. Penile fracture occurs when excessive bending force is applied to the erect penis resulting in a tear of the tunica albuginea. Patients describe an auditory "pop" heard during intercourse followed by rapid detumescence and swelling of the penis/scrotum. Inability to void or blood at the meatus indicates concomitant urethral injury, seen in 15% to 20% of penile fractures. Physical exam demonstrated edema and ecchymosis/hematoma confined to penis if Buck fascia is intact or in butterfly pattern in perineum if hematoma is contained within Colle fascia. Imaging is generally **not indicated,** unless urethral injury is suspected. Hematuria, inability to void, or blood at the meatus are all indications for **urethrography/urethroscopy.** Immediate/early surgical exploration with repair is the standard of care and is associated with better outcomes than delayed repair (>36 hours).

2. Minor penile lacerations and contusions can be managed in the emergency room.

3. Serious blunt or penetrating trauma with injury to the corpus cavernosum requires surgical exploration, débridement, and repair of the corporal injury. A retrograde urethrogram or flexible cystoscopy is necessary to rule out urethral injury. Broad-spectrum antibiotics should be given, particularly in human bite injuries.

F. Testicular injury may occur as a result of blunt or penetrating trauma. History and physical examination are the keys to diagnosis of testicular rupture. The presentation is marked by acute and severe pain, often with associated nausea and vomiting. Physical examination may reveal a hematoma or ecchymosis of overlying skin. All penetrating scrotal gunshot wounds deep to the dartos fascia require surgical exploration. **Ultrasonography** can help to diagnose testicular injury associated with blunt trauma with a 100% sensitivity and a specificity of 93.5% (*J Urol.* 2006;175:175). The orchiectomy rate is less than 10% for ruptured testicles explored within 72 hours after injury. Repair consists of hematoma evacuation, débridement of the necrotic tubules, and closure of the tunica albuginea (*Br J Urol.* 2004;94(4):507–515).

G. Scrotal avulsion and skin loss are most often a result of motor vehicle accidents. Because of the redundancy and vascularity of scrotal skin, various options are available for local flaps and coverage of the testicles. Wounds should be copiously irrigated and débrided; clean wounds may be closed in layers, whereas grossly contaminated wounds should be cleaned and packed with sterile gauze dressings.

36 Obstetric and Gynecologic Surgery

Lindsay M. Kuroki and Premal H. Thaker

OBSTETRIC AND GYNECOLOGIC DISORDERS

I. **VAGINAL BLEEDING.** A thorough history including pattern and intensity of bleeding, date of last menstrual period, and physical examination is sufficient to determine the etiology. A pregnancy test must be performed in all women of reproductive age. Hemoglobin (Hgb) and hematocrit (Hct) should be drawn to determine whether the abnormal bleeding is chronic or heavy. An endometrial biopsy should be performed in all postmenopausal women with bleeding to rule out endometrial carcinoma.

A. **Obstetric etiologies.** Bleeding during pregnancy has different etiologies depending on the trimester. Differential diagnosis of first trimester bleeding includes spontaneous abortions (SABs), postcoital bleeding, ectopic pregnancy (see Section IIA), lower genital tract lesions/lacerations, and expulsion of a molar pregnancy. Third trimester bleeding occurs in 4% to 5% of pregnancy and most commonly is caused by placenta previa, abruption, vasa previa, preterm labor, and lower genital tract lesions/lacerations. Overall, 30% to 40% of all pregnancies are associated with vaginal bleeding and approximately half of these result in SABs.

1. **Terminology**
   a. **Threatened abortion:** any vaginal bleeding during the first half of pregnancy without cervical dilation or expulsion of products of contraception (POCs); cervix closed.
   b. **Missed abortion:** fetal death before 20 weeks' gestation with retention of POCs; cervix closed.
   c. **Inevitable abortion:** cervical dilation with or without ruptured membranes.
   d. **Incomplete abortion:** partial passage of POCs; cervix open.
   e. **Complete abortion:** expulsion of all POCs from the uterine cavity; cervix closed.

2. **Presentation and clinical features.** Classically, patients present with vaginal bleeding and crampy, midline, lower abdominal pain. Bleeding from the urethra or rectum, and cervical/vaginal lacerations, should be excluded. Passage of tissue may represent a complete or incomplete abortion.

3. **Physical examination.** Vital signs are within normal ranges unless extensive vaginal bleeding or septic abortion occurs with resultant

tachycardia and hypotension. Septic abortions can cause elevated temperatures, marked suprapubic tenderness, or purulent discharge through the cervical os.

4. **Laboratory investigation**
   a. **Hgb and Hct.** Plasma volume expansion in pregnancy may result in a lower mean Hgb during the second trimester. With acute blood loss, the Hgb/Hct can be normal until compensatory mechanisms restore normal plasma volume.
   b. **White blood cell (WBC) count with differential** is useful to evaluate febrile morbidity. Septic abortion is associated with a left shift and an elevated WBC count.
   c. **Blood type and screen** are essential to identify Rh-negative patients at risk for isoimmunization. Any woman with pregnancy-related vaginal bleeding who is Rh negative should be given Rho immunoglobulin (RhoGAM) if she has not received it within the last 12 weeks (see Section I.A.6.g).
   d. **Quantitative β subunit of human chorionic gonadotropin (hCG).** The sensitivity of a pregnancy test (urine or serum) can vary depending on the type of test performed (i.e., latex agglutination, enzyme-linked immunosorbent assays, radioimmunoassay). A urine pregnancy test gives a rapid qualitative result, although the sensitivity is variable. Serum pregnancy tests are more sensitive and yield a quantitative level of hCG that assists in evaluating the status of a pregnancy. Serial serum hCG values along with ultrasonography can help to distinguish an early, viable intrauterine pregnancy (IUP) from an abnormal pregnancy. In most normal IUPs near 6 weeks' gestation, hCG increases by at least 66% every 48 hours (ACOG Practice Bulletin 94. *Obstet Gynecol.* 2008;111:1479). Patients with stable clinical examinations can be followed with serial hCG values until they reach the sonographic threshold values at which an IUP can be visualized (see Section I.A.5).
   e. **Progesterone levels** are prognostic, independent of hCG levels. Values less than 5 ng/mL have 100% specificity in confirming an abnormal pregnancy. Levels more than 20 ng/mL are usually associated with a normal IUP.

5. **Imaging studies.** Ultrasonography may be useful in demonstrating a viable pregnancy. Vaginal probe ultrasonography should demonstrate an intrauterine gestational sac (if it exists) at hCG levels more than 1,500 to 2,000 mIU/mL versus an abdominal ultrasonography, where the threshold is more than 6,000 mIU/mL. Cardiac activity can be seen at 10,000 mIU/mL.

6. **Treatment**
   a. **Threatened abortion.** Patients with a pregnancy that is viable or of indeterminate viability who present with vaginal bleeding and a closed internal cervical os are followed expectantly with a repeat ultrasound in 7 days, repeat hCG in 48 hours, or both.

b. **Missed abortion.** Patients may be followed expectantly or undergo surgical or medical therapy. Expectant management should include weekly coagulation studies [i.e., complete blood cell (CBC) count, prothrombin time, partial thromboplastin time, fibrinogen, and fibrin degradation products] because of the risk of disseminated intravascular coagulopathy (DIC). Patients should bring any tissue passed to the hospital for pathologic verification. If POCs have not passed within 3 weeks, evacuation should be scheduled.

c. **Inevitable abortion.** Patients occasionally are followed expectantly with monitoring for infection but typically undergo uterine evacuation (see Section I.6.f). If fever develops, intravenous (IV) antibiotics with polymicrobial coverage are administered, followed by evacuation. These patients require admission and careful monitoring of coagulation factors because they are at risk of DIC.

d. **Incomplete abortion.** Uterine evacuation is indicated. If POCs are not recovered, an ectopic pregnancy should be ruled out.

e. **Complete abortion.** Only short-term observation is necessary, given that all POCs are expelled, the cervix is closed, and bleeding and cramping are minimal.

f. **Evacuation of the uterus.** Suction curettage is done safely in the first trimester and can be performed in the emergency department if significant cervical dilation exists. A stable patient with a first trimester missed abortion can undergo dilation and curettage (D&C) as an outpatient. In the second trimester, a dilation and evacuation or medical induction of labor under gynecologic consultation is performed. After curettage, prophylactic antibiotics [doxycycline 100 mg orally (PO) two times a day for 7 days], ergot alkaloids (methylergonovine maleate 0.2 mg PO three times a day for 2 to 3 days) for uterine contraction, and antiprostaglandins (ibuprofen 600 mg PO every 6 hours as needed for pain) commonly are prescribed. If heavy vaginal bleeding, abdominal pain, or fever occurs after evacuation, investigation for retained POCs, uterine perforation, and endometritis is warranted.

g. RhoGAM is given to any pregnant patient with vaginal bleeding who is Rh negative with a negative antibody screen. The recommended dose of RhoGAM for first trimester events is 50 μg intramuscularly (IM); anytime thereafter, 300 μg IM is sufficient [ACOG Practice Bulletin 4. *Obstet Gynecol.* 1999;93(5):771–774].

h. **Pathology.** Any tissue passed or obtained from uterine evacuation must be evaluated for chorionic villi. If villi are not identified, further investigation is necessary to exclude ectopic pregnancy or incomplete abortion. Hydatidiform mole should also be excluded on final pathology.

B. **Nonobstetric etiologies of vaginal bleeding (Table 36-1).**

TABLE 36-1 Nonobstetric Causes of Vaginal Bleeding

Differential Diagnosis	Laboratory Data	Signs and Symptoms	Treatment
Menses	CBC count, urine hCG	Cyclic bleeding every 21–35 days	Iron therapy if indicated
Dysfunctional uterine bleeding	CBC count, urine hCG, endometrial biopsy if >35 y, duration >6 mo	Non-cyclic bleeding; may have associated dysmenorrhea, fatigue, or dizziness	Hormonal therapy if patient is hemodynamically stable; if unstable, transfuse as needed, IV estrogen or high-dose OCPs
Infection: gonorrhea/*Chlamydia* cervicitis	Cervical culture, wet prep	Purulent vaginal discharge, possible spotting	Ceftriaxone, 125 mg IM × 1; azithromycin, 1 g PO × 1
Trichomonas vaginitis	Wet prep	Yellow-green frothy vaginal discharge, possible spotting	Metronidazole, 500 mg PO bid × 7 days or 2 g PO × 1 (if pregnant, defer until second trimester)
Sexual trauma	Rape kit	Vaginal bleeding and/or discharge	Emergency contraception, prophylactic treatment for STDs; if laceration, pack vagina, possible surgical repair
Malignancy	Endometrial biopsy, Papanicolaou test smear, cervical biopsy	Postmenopausal, postcoital, or intermenstrual bleeding	Refer to gynecologic oncologist

bid, twice daily; CBC, complete blood cell; hCG, human chorionic gonadotropin; OCPs, oral contraceptive pills; STDs, sexually transmitted diseases; IM, intramuscular; IV, intravenous; PO, oral.

II. **ABDOMINAL PAIN.** The differential diagnosis for nongynecologic etiologies includes appendicitis, gastroenteritis, irritable bowel, ischemic bowel, cholecystitis, ureteral colic, and urinary tract infection. Pregnancy should be excluded in all reproductive age women.

A. **Ectopic pregnancy** occurs when the blastocyst implants outside the uterine cavity; 97% of pregnancies occur in a fallopian tube (tubal pregnancy).

1. **Presentation and clinical features.** More than 90% of patients with tubal pregnancies have abdominal or pelvic pain, although some may be asymptomatic. Early unruptured ectopic pregnancies often present with amenorrhea, vaginal spotting, and colicky, vague lower abdominal pain, whereas, patients with a ruptured ectopic pregnancy may report severe pain, syncope, and dizziness. Pleuritic chest pain and shoulder pain from diaphragmatic irritation by blood can also occur. A ruptured ectopic pregnancy is a true surgical emergency, as it can quickly result in rapid hemorrhage, shock, and even death.

2. **Physical examination.** Vital signs vary greatly, from normal blood pressure and pulse to hypotension and tachycardia due to cardiovascular collapse secondary to hemorrhage. Although patients with unruptured ectopic pregnancy may demonstrate only mild tenderness, peritoneal signs (e.g., tenderness, rigidity, guarding, rebound) can also be present. Pelvic masses sometimes are palpable, but lack of one does not exclude ectopic pregnancy. The uterus may appear small for presumed gestational date.

3. **Laboratory investigation**
   a. **CBC count**. Hgb/Hct may indicate the degree of hemorrhage, except in acute blood loss. The WBC typically is normal/slightly elevated and does not demonstrate increased percentage of immature neutrophils.
   b. **Blood type and screen** should be obtained to identify Rh-negative patients and, if appropriate, order cross-match blood on hold for possible transfusion (see Section I.A.6.g).
   c. **hCG.** Although ectopic pregnancy can occur with any quantitative serum hCG value, these data can be useful for ultrasound interpretation. Serial hCG values that do not increase appropriately are suspicious for an ectopic pregnancy (see Section I.A.4.d).
   d. **Progesterone** values rarely aid in the diagnosis of ectopic pregnancy (see Section I.A.4.e).

4. **Imaging studies.** Ultrasonography is most useful in excluding an ectopic pregnancy by demonstrating an intrauterine gestational sac or fetus. Stable patients with an hCG less than 1,500 mIU/mL should be followed with serial hCG titers. An hCG more than 2,500 mIU/mL and absence of a gestational sac in the uterus indicate either a nonviable intrauterine or an ectopic pregnancy. Ultrasound findings consistent with ectopic pregnancy include a uterus without a well-formed gestational sac—although a pseudosac (intrauterine fluid collection) may be present—free intraperitoneal fluid, and sometimes an adnexal mass representing a tubal pregnancy.

5. **Diagnostic studies**
   a. **Culdocentesis** is useful for detecting hemoperitoneum, although it is used infrequently because sonographic evaluation for free intraperitoneal fluid often is sufficient. A culdocentesis is performed by passing a needle aseptically into the posterior vaginal fornix. Aspiration of clear yellow fluid is normal; no fluid is nondiagnostic. Aspiration of clotting blood is likely from an intravascular source and nondiagnostic, whereas nonclotting blood with an Hct above 15% is consistent with hemoperitoneum.
   b. **D&C** can be performed to differentiate between an ectopic pregnancy and incomplete abortion after excluding a normal early IUP. Curettage products that float in saline are suggestive of chorionic villi. If villi are not identified, laparoscopy to exclude ectopic pregnancy is indicated.

6. **Treatment**
   a. **Surgical therapy.** Comparing systemic methotrexate with tube-sparing laparoscopic surgery in hemodynamically stable patients, randomized trials have consistently shown no difference in overall tubal preservation, tubal patencies, repeat ectopic pregnancies, or future pregnancies. The mainstay of surgical management for ectopic pregnancy is a conservative approach that preserves the tubes.
      (1) **Laparoscopy** is preferred for diagnosis and treatment of tubal pregnancy; however, laparotomy is indicated if the patient is hemodynamically unstable.
      (2) **Conservative surgical therapy** is recommended in patients who wish to preserve reproductive potential. **Linear salpingostomy** in the antimesosalpinx portion of the tube performed with fine-tip electrocautery is preferable when the ectopic pregnancy is unruptured and located in the ampulla of the tube. After removal of the pregnancy from the tube, the base is irrigated and hemostasis is achieved with cautery. The tube is left to heal by secondary intention. **Segmental resection** often is performed when the tube is ruptured and the ectopic pregnancy is in the isthmic portion of the tube.
      (3) **Nonconservative surgical therapy** includes **salpingectomy** (removal of tube) for tubal rupture or severe hemorrhage and **cornual resection** for interstitial pregnancies. Pregnancy rates after salpingectomy have been shown to be equivalent to those following linear salpingostomy, although the incidence of recurrent ectopic pregnancy may be slightly higher with salpingostomy.
      (4) **Follow-up.** Patients treated with conservative surgical management or after rupture or spillage of trophoblastic tissue have a 5% incidence of persistent, viable trophoblastic tissue. Weekly quantitative hCG values should be followed until negative. If the levels plateau or increase, reevaluation is indicated.

b. **Medical therapy** with methotrexate, a folic acid antagonist, can be used in compliant outpatients who are hemodynamically stable. Success depends on treatment regimen, gestational age, and hCG levels. Candidates for treatment with methotrexate include gestational sac less than 3.5 cm in diameter, an intact tube, no fetal heart motion, no evidence of hemoperitoneum, and no history of hepatic, renal or hematologic dysfunction. Baseline laboratory tests, which include hCG, Rh factor, CBC count, hepatic enzymes, and serum creatinine, should be obtained. The most common adverse effects of therapy are bloating and flatulence, followed by stomatitis, hair loss, and anemia. A transient rise in hepatic enzymes may be observed. Repeat quantitative hCG levels should be drawn on days 4 and 7. If hCG levels fail to decline less than 15% between days 4 and 7, a second dose of methotrexate should be administered and a new day 1 assigned. Quantitative hCG values are followed until negative. Approximately 20% of patients have an inappropriate fall in hCG levels and require surgical intervention. *Separation pain* refers to the increase in abdominopelvic discomfort that is commonly experienced by patients undergoing treatment and is thought to be caused by tubal stretching during resolution of the pregnancy. Patients are counseled to rest and take oral analgesics but cautioned to seek immediate reevaluation to rule out rupture if pain does not resolve within 1 hour. While undergoing treatment, patients should avoid alcohol and folic acid because these may interfere with methotrexate; refrain from intercourse, as this may increase the risk of rupture (ACOG Practice Bulletin 94. *Obstet Gynecol.* 2008;111:1479).

B. **Pelvic inflammatory disease (PID)** is a polymicrobial infection of the upper genital tract. The majority of cases occur in sexually active 15- to 30-year-old women. It rarely occurs in nonmenstruating women and during pregnancy. Factors promoting progression of infection from the lower to upper genital tract include events that cause breakdown of the cervical mucus barrier, such as douching, intrauterine device insertion, hysteroscopy, D&C, endometrial biopsy, and hysterosalpingography. Risk factors include a history of sexually transmitted diseases (STDs) or PID, multiple sexual partners, and age younger than 25 years. Causative pathogens are primarily *Neisseria gonorrhoeae* and *Chlamydia trachomatis*, although other vaginal flora microorganisms (e.g., anaerobes, *Gardnerella vaginalis*, *Haemophilus influenzae*, enteric gram-negative rods, *Streptococcus agalactiae*), as well as cytomegalovirus (CMV), *Mycoplasma hominis*, *Ureaplasma urealyticum*, and *Mycoplasma genitalium*, have been associated with PID.

1. **Presentation and clinical features.** Patients with PID typically have lower abdominal and pelvic pain, which may be constant, dull, sharp, or crampy. PID is aggravated by movement and often occurs around or during menses. Other signs/symptoms include purulent vaginal discharge (75%), abnormal vaginal bleeding (<50%), fever (<33%), dyspareunia, and dysuria. Nausea and vomiting with associated ileus may occur but are usually late symptoms.

2. **Physical examination** reveals lower abdominal tenderness, including peritoneal signs of rebound and guarding, adnexal tenderness with or without fullness or palpable mass, mucopurulent vaginal discharge, and cervical motion tenderness. Cervical motion tenderness is not pathognomonic of PID, because it is a nonspecific sign of peritoneal irritation that can be elicited in any patient with peritonitis from any cause.

3. **Laboratory investigation.** Pregnancy must be excluded. Leukocytosis and an elevated erythrocyte sedimentation rate (ESR) suggest a severe infection. Evaluation of a saline mount of vaginal secretions under high magnification usually reveals numerous WBCs. If none are present and the discharge appears normal, PID is unlikely. A cervical swab for DNA probe analysis of *N. gonorrhoeae* and *C. trachomatis* should be obtained, although bloody samples may give false-negative results. Alternatively, a voided urine assay (URI probe) may be used. Women with PID should also be screened for other STDs including HIV and hepatitis B and for rapid plasma reagin (RPR).

4. **Imaging studies.** Ultrasonography is used to detect tubo-ovarian abscess (TOA) if a mass is palpable on examination or if no improvement is noted after 48 hours of antibiotics. Abdominal plain films, magnetic resonance imaging (MRI), or computed tomography (CT) scan may also be used to investigate other etiologies of a patient's pain if the diagnosis is uncertain.

5. **Diagnostic studies**
   a. The Centers for Disease Control and Prevention (CDC) issued guidelines for the diagnosis of acute PID that are intended to serve as clinical criteria for initiating treatment. **Minimum criteria** include lower abdominal tenderness, adnexal tenderness, and cervical motion tenderness. **Additional criteria** include abnormal cervical/vaginal discharge, temperature more than 101°F (38.3°C), elevated ESR, elevated C-reactive protein level, and documented infection with *N. gonorrhoeae* or *C. trachomatis.* **Definitive criteria** include histopathologic evidence of endometritis on endometrial biopsy, transvaginal ultrasonography showing fluid-filled tubes or TOA, and laparoscopic abnormalities consistent with PID.
   b. **Culdocentesis** seldom is necessary to make the diagnosis of PID. However, aspiration of purulent material confirms an infectious process (see Section II.A.5.a).
   c. **Laparoscopy** revealing erythema and edema of the fallopian tubes and purulent material confirms the diagnosis and provides the opportunity to collect direct cultures of infected organs. However, laparoscopy should not be considered a routine means of establishing a diagnosis.

6. **Treatment** of PID depends on the severity of the infection.
   a. **Inpatient therapy** is indicated for patients with nausea and vomiting, possible surgical emergencies, pregnancy, suspicion for TOA, immunodeficiency, failed outpatient therapy, or for patients in whom preservation of reproductive potential is important. According to 2007 CDC guidelines, inpatient parenteral treatment

regimens include cefotetan 2 g IV every 12 hours or cefoxitin 2 g IV every 6 hours and doxycycline 100 mg PO/IV every 12 hours. Oral doxycycline is preferred because of pain with IV administration. Alternative regimens include (1) clindamycin 900 mg IV every 8 hours and gentamicin 2 mg/kg IV load followed by 1.5 mg/kg IV every 8 hours and (2) ampicillin/sulbactam 3 g IV every 6 hours and doxycycline 100 mg PO/IV every 12 hours. Inpatient treatment is continued until the patient is afebrile for 48 hours and has decreased pain on pelvic examination. Patients then are transitioned to PO doxycycline ± metronidazole for a total of 14 days. Those with discrete pelvic fluid collections and TOAs may be candidates for ultrasound-guided vaginal aspiration and pelvic drain placement by interventional radiologists; concurrent antibiotics should be administered.

b. Outpatient therapy. Clinical outcomes among women treated with PO therapy are similar to those treated with IV therapy. Oral regimens include (1) one dose of ceftriaxone 250 mg IM, plus doxycycline 100 mg PO twice daily ± metronidazole 500 mg PO twice daily for 14 days; (2) cefoxitin 2 g IM and probenacid 1 g PO administered concurrently in a single dose plus doxycycline ± metronidazole; or (3) third-generation cephalosporin (e.g., cefotaxime) plus doxycycline ± metronidazole. Patients should follow-up within 48 to 72 hours to ensure improvement.

c. Surgery should be considered for patients with symptomatic pelvic masses, or ruptured TOAs, who do not clinically improve after 48 hours of IV antibiotics.

C. Corpus luteal cysts develop from mature follicles in the ovary. Intrafollicular bleeding can occur 2 to 4 days after ovulation creating a hemorrhagic cyst. Corpus luteal cysts usually are 4 cm or more in diameter but can be more than 12 cm. Diagnosis can be difficult in pregnancy because a cyst may be confused with an ectopic pregnancy.

1. **Presentation and clinical features.** Patients can be asymptomatic or may present with unilateral, dull lower abdominal/pelvic pain. If the cyst has ruptured, the patient may complain of sudden onset of severe pain.

2. **Physical examination** reveals adnexal enlargement, tenderness, or both with or without peritoneal irritation if the cyst has ruptured. It is important to ensure hemodynamic stability because some patients can bleed significantly from a hemorrhagic cyst.

3. **Laboratory investigation.** A CBC count and hCG should always be obtained. Ultrasonography can aid in visualizing a cyst or free fluid in the pelvis, indicative of recent cyst rupture. Culdocentesis may be performed to search for blood in the cul-de-sac in cases of suspected cyst rupture.

4. **Treatment** usually is conservative, allowing for spontaneous resolution. Oral contraceptive pills (OCPs) can be used to suppress ovulation and future cyst formation. Nonsteroidal anti-inflammatory drugs

(NSAIDs) or short courses of narcotics are commonly prescribed for pain control. Surgical treatment with laparoscopic cystectomy is rarely indicated unless significant ongoing intraperitoneal hemorrhage is present.

D. **Adnexal torsion** accounts for an estimated 3% of gynecologic surgical emergencies. Torsion occurs when the ovary, tube, or both structures twist on the infundibulopelvic ligament. Incomplete torsion results in occlusion of the venous and lymphatic channels, causing cyanotic and edematous adnexa. Complete torsion interrupts the arterial supply with subsequent ischemia and necrosis of the adnexa. Torsion occurs most commonly in the reproductive age group, more frequently on the right side, and typically with large ovaries or benign ovarian masses (50% to 60%). Concurrent pregnancy is present in 15% of cases.

1. **Presentation and clinical features.** History and physical examination are critical, as adnexal torsion is primarily a clinical diagnosis. Patients with torsion present with acute, severe, sharp, intermittent, unilateral lower abdominal or pelvic pain and nausea. Intermittent torsion may present with periodic pain for days to weeks from twisting and untwisting of the adnexa. The pain often is related to a sudden change in position.

2. **Physical examination** can reveal tachycardia or bradycardia (from vagal stimulation) and fever if there is necrosis. Unilateral abdominal tenderness or a tender adnexal mass often is found on pelvic examination. Peritoneal signs may be present as the ovary undergoes necrosis.

3. **Diagnostic studies.** Ultrasonography may visualize an adnexal mass. Doppler ultrasonography has moderate sensitivity and specificity in diagnosing torsion. Blood flow around the adnexa is reassuring but does not exclude torsion, which is mainly a clinical diagnosis. Visualization by laparoscopy confirms the diagnosis.

4. **Treatment** involves immediate surgical intervention. If only partial torsion or no evidence of tissue necrosis exists and the patient desires future fertility, preservation of adnexa with untwisting and transfixation of the ovarian pedicle is possible. Cyst resection and exclusion of underlying malignancy (rare) should be performed. If necrosis of the adnexa is present or the ovary is felt to be nonviable, a salpingo-oophorectomy should be performed.

E. **Fibroids or leiomyomas** are benign tumors of uterine smooth muscle that vary in size from less than 1 cm to more than 20 cm.

1. **Presentation and clinical features.** Although most fibroids are asymptomatic, one-third of patients have dysmenorrhea or abnormal menstrual bleeding, including menorrhagia (heavy menses) or metrorrhagia (intermenstrual bleeding). Symptoms can also result from pressure on the bladder or rectum. Fibroid degeneration may cause fever and acute pain that is self-limited and usually responsive to NSAIDs.

2. **Physical examination** may reveal an enlarged, irregular uterus.

3. **Diagnostic studies.** Ultrasonography confirms uterine size and the presence of myomas. In patients older than 35 years with abnormal bleeding, an endometrial biopsy should be performed to rule out endometrial pathology, including hyperplasia and carcinoma.

4. **Treatment** is determined by symptoms and the patient's desire for future fertility. Prostaglandin synthetase inhibitors (e.g., ibuprofen or naproxen sodium) are useful for pain control; hormonal therapy (e.g., OCPs and medroxyprogesterone acetate) can be used to regulate bleeding; and gonadotropin-releasing hormone agonists (e.g., Lupron) can also be used to shrink fibroids. Uterine artery embolization by interventional radiology (IR) is another alternative in which the uterine arteries are embolized using polyvinyl alcohol particles of trisacryl gelatin microspheres with or without metal coils causing uterine leiomyoma devascularization and involution. Surgery (myomectomy or hysterectomy) is reserved for patients who have failed medical management and no longer desire future fertility (ACOG Practice Bulletin 96. *Obstet Gynecol.* 2008;112:387).

F. **Dysmenorrhea** is painful lower abdominal cramping that occurs just before and during menses. It affects 40% of women of reproductive age and is often accompanied by other symptoms including diaphoresis, tachycardia, headache, nausea, vomiting, and diarrhea.

1. The **etiology** of dysmenorrhea is thought to be related to increased prostaglandin levels.

2. **Treatment** includes prostaglandin synthetase inhibitors (e.g., ibuprofen or naproxen sodium) beginning before the onset of menses or OCPs to suppress ovulation.

G. **Adnexal masses** are often found incidentally either on pelvic examination or in the operating room. In the United States, women have a 5% to 10% lifetime risk of undergoing surgery for a suspected ovarian neoplasm, with 13% to 21% of these cases resulting in a diagnosis of malignancy. To guide surgeons in their management, criteria have been developed that aid in assessing the malignant potential of adnexal masses (ACOG Practice Bulletin 83. *Obstet Gynecol.* 2007;110:201).

1. **Presentation and clinical features.** Most adnexal masses are asymptomatic unless they are associated with torsion or are large enough to compress surrounding structures. Less than 2% of adnexal masses are malignant, although up to 34% may be malignant in postmenopausal women.

2. **Physical examination** may reveal adnexal fullness or a discrete mass. Attention should be paid to the size, number (unilateral vs. bilateral), mobility, texture (solid, cystic, nodular), and presence of ascites.

3. **Diagnostic studies.** Ultrasonography can reveal the size and characteristics of adnexal masses (i.e., complex, simple, nodular, septations, papillary excrescences, etc.) as well as the assessing free fluid in the pelvis. A CT scan is less useful for visualizing the pelvis.

4. **Treatment.** A large (>10 cm) adnexal mass warrants surgical exploration. Smaller masses in premenopausal women may be observed for 6 to 8 weeks unless certain factors make it likely to be malignant. Patients undergoing expectant management should be counseled on the warning signs of torsion. If the mass grows or persists on repeat ultrasonography, surgery is indicated. Controversy exists regarding the management of small, asymptomatic adnexal masses in postmenopausal women. Small, unilocular cysts may be observed for some time, although most physicians have a lower threshold for surgery in these patients because the risk of malignancy increases with increasing age. Laparoscopy has been shown to be as effective and safe as laparotomy for the removal of masses of size less than 10 cm, with decreased morbidity and shorter hospital stay. Fixed and solid masses or those associated with ascites require laparotomy and a gynecologic oncologist on standby. Benign adnexal masses frequently encountered include cystic teratomas (dermoid cysts), endometriomas, and serous and mucinous cystadenomas. Dermoids and serous cystadenomas are frequently bilateral and necessitate a close inspection of the contralateral ovary. Mucinous cystadenomas can be associated with pseudomyxoma peritonei and therefore warrant evaluation of the appendix because appendiceal mucoceles and carcinomas can also result in pseudomyxoma. Other benign, solid ovarian tumors include Brenner tumors, fibromas, and thecomas.

III. **NONOBSTETRIC SURGERY IN THE PREGNANT PATIENT.** Common indications for surgery in the pregnant patient are appendicitis, adnexal mass, and cholecystitis. It is preferable to treat pregnant patients conservatively and, if safely possible, defer surgery to the postpartum period. However, delay of an indicated surgical procedure can be devastating. If nonemergent surgery is required, it is safest to proceed in the second trimester. Surgery in the first trimester carries a risk of fetal loss and malformation because organogenesis occurs, whereas surgery in the third trimester carries a risk of inducing preterm labor.

A. **Preoperative considerations.** Pregnant patients are at increased risk for aspiration because of upward displacement of the stomach and the inhibitory effects of progesterone on gastrointestinal motility. A nonparticulate antacid should be given shortly before induction of anesthesia. In the second half of pregnancy, patients should be placed in the left lateral position to decrease vena caval and aortic compression. If the fetus is of viable gestational age, continuous fetal monitoring should be employed; otherwise, heart tones should be documented pre and postoperatively. Patients between 24 and 34 weeks' gestation should be given a course of antenatal glucocorticoids (betamethasone or dexamethasone) more than 48 hours prior to surgery to promote fetal lung maturity should preterm delivery occur.

B. **Laparoscopy in pregnancy.** The second trimester is the optimal time to safely perform laparoscopy in pregnancy because the uterus is not large enough to obstruct visualization, allowing for minimal uterine manipulation. Current practice techniques are based on the Society of American Gastrointestinal Endoscopic Surgeons (SAGES) Guidelines of Laparoscopic Surgery During Pregnancy (*Surg Endosc.* 1998;12:189). To highlight, trocar placement is best accomplished by an open Hasson technique, with the additional trocars inserted under direct visualization. Carbon dioxide pneumoperitoneum at 12 to 15 mm Hg appears safe and is unlikely to result in fetal hypoxia or acidosis. Any cervical or uterine manipulator should be avoided in pregnant patients, as it can cause artificial rupture of membranes, preterm labor, or injury to fetus. Overall, laparoscopic surgical procedures may result in decreased morbidity and mortality, a reduced cost with shorter hospitalizations, and a decreased risk of thromboembolic disease compared with laparotomy.

C. **Anesthetic** selection is based on the maternal condition and the planned surgical procedure. For general anesthesia, all patients should be intubated using cricoid pressure to minimize the risk of aspiration. Anesthetic inhalation agents and narcotic analgesia are commonly used. Regional anesthesia may be complicated by hypotension, which is potentially poorly tolerated by patient and fetus.

D. **Postoperatively,** fetal-uterine monitoring and tocolytic agents are used depending on gestational age and degree of maternal symptoms. Document fetal well-being.

IV. TRAUMA IN PREGNANCY

A. **Presentation and clinical features.** Trauma is the leading cause of morbidity and mortality in the United States in women younger than 40 years and complicates approximately 1 in 12 pregnancies. After initial interventions are aimed at stabilizing the mother according to advanced cardiac trauma life support protocols and assessing the extent of injury, fetal well-being should be established by calculating gestational age, monitoring fetal heart tones, determining viability, and administering antenatal glucocorticoids if appropriate for fetal lung maturity.

B. **Types of abdominal trauma**

1. **Penetrating trauma** places the uterus and fetus at great risk during the later stages of pregnancy. Evaluation and treatment are similar to those in the nonpregnant patient; surgical exploration is usually necessary. Amniocentesis to establish fetal lung maturity or to detect bacteria or blood may be helpful if time permits.

2. **Blunt trauma** in pregnancy is associated most often with motor vehicle accidents. Despite the concern for abdominal seat-belt injuries, restrained pregnant patients fare better than those who are unrestrained. Intrauterine or retroplacental hemorrhage must be considered because 20% of the cardiac output in pregnancy is delivered to the uteroplacental unit.

3. **Abruptio placentae** occurs in 1% to 5% of minor and 40% to 50% of major blunt traumas. Focal uterine tenderness, vaginal bleeding, hypertonic contractions, and fetal compromise frequently occur. DIC may

occur in almost one-third of abruptions. Work-up includes a DIC panel including coagulation factors, fibrinogen, as well as a Kleihauer–Betke screen to assess for fetal-maternal hemorrhage in Rh-negative patients.

a. **Management of abruptio placentae** depends on fetal age, degree of placental separation, and estimated blood loss determined by ultrasonography. At viability, continuous fetal heart monitoring is performed and the mode of delivery is dictated by both fetal and maternal cardiovascular stability. The immediate maternal and fetal threat must be weighed against the morbidity associated with pre-maturity, with the threshold for delivery decreasing with increasing gestational age.

C. **Special considerations of trauma in pregnancy**

1. **Fetal-uterine monitoring** is effective in determining fetal distress, abruptio placentae, and preterm labor caused by trauma for pregnancies of more than 20 weeks. Doppler auscultation of fetal heart tones is sufficient for previable pregnancies (>12 weeks' gestation).

2. **Ultrasonography** is an effective tool for establishing gestational age, fetal viability, placental characteristics, and placental location.

3. In **positioning** the pregnant patient, avoid placing her supine to optimize venous return. During cardiopulmonary resuscitation, a 15-degree wedge into the left lateral decubitus position should be used if possible.

4. **Tetanus prophylaxis** in a pregnant patient should be administered in the same manner and for the same indications as in the nonpregnant patient.

5. **Peritoneal lavage,** usually by the open, above-the-fundus technique, can be used to detect intraperitoneal hemorrhage while avoiding the uterus, which is localized by examination and ultrasonography [ACOG Practice Bulletin 251. *Obstet Gynecol.* 1999;92(3):394–397].

6. **Radiation** in the form of diagnostic studies places the fetus at potential risk for SAB (first several weeks of pregnancy), teratogenesis (weeks 3 to 12), and growth retardation (>12 weeks' gestational age). These effects and secondary childhood cancers are unlikely at doses of more than 10 rads (chest x-ray film, <1 rad; CT scan of abdomen and pelvis, 5 to 8 rads). Uterine shielding should be used when possible. Studies should be ordered judiciously, but imaging deemed important for evaluation should not be omitted (ACOG Committee Opinion 299. *Obstet Gynecol.* 2004;104:647).

7. **Perimortem or postmortem cesarean delivery** should be accomplished within 10 minutes of maternal cardiopulmonary arrest to optimize neonatal prognosis and maternal response to resuscitation.

8. **Isoimmunization** must be considered in the Rh-negative patient, and RhoGAM should be administered when fetal maternal hemorrhage is suspected (see Section I.A.6.g).

9. All **blood products** should be screened and negative for CMV.

10. **Prophylactic cephalosporins** are safe in all trimesters of pregnancy.

V. GYNECOLOGIC MALIGNANCIES. The female genital tract accounts for more than 83,750 new cases of invasive carcinoma annually in the United States, resulting in approximately 27,710 deaths in 2010 (*CA Cancer J Clin.* 2010;60:260–267). Mortality can be reduced by earlier detection. Five-year survival rates after proper treatment of cancers diagnosed at stage I (confined to primary organ) approach 90%, but fall to 30% to 50% when diagnosed at advanced stages. A brief overview of vulvar, cervical, endometrial, and ovarian cancers is presented with emphasis on diagnosis and initial management. A complete discussion of gynecologic malignancies including less common cancers (vaginal, fallopian tube, and gestational trophoblastic disease) is beyond the scope of this manual. Patients should be referred to a gynecologic oncologist for comprehensive management.

A. **Vulvar carcinoma** is primarily a disease of postmenopausal women, and the average age at diagnosis is 68 years. The etiology has been linked to human papillomavirus (HPV) infection in younger patients and is associated with chronic vulvar conditions including dystrophies, lichen sclerosis, and condylomata. Squamous cell histology predominates (90%), followed by melanoma and adenocarcinoma.

 1. **Presentation and clinical features.** Vulvar cancer often presents as a hyper- or hypopigmented lesion. It may be ulcerated, pruritic, painful, or asymptomatic and may have been treated with a variety of antibiotics and ointments before diagnosis.

 2. **Diagnosis.** Accurate diagnosis requires biopsy and histopathologic evaluation of suspicious areas.

 3. **Treatment** of vulvar cancer depends on the stage. Surgery ranging from local excision to radical vulvectomy with bilateral inguinal lymph node dissection generally is the primary treatment. Local, groin, and pelvic adjuvant radiation is administered depending on the pathologic findings. Basal cell carcinoma requires only a wide local excision.

 4. **Prognosis** depends on stage (Table 36-2). A landmark paper by Homesley et al. showed that the extent of nodal disease and tumor diameter are independent predictors of survival. Patients with stage I tumors have a 5-year survival of 90% or better, whereas those with positive lymph nodes have a 5-year survival of approximately 50% to 60%, depending on the number and location of positive lymph nodes (*Am J Obstet Gynecol.* 1991;164:997). Improved 5-year survival rates for intermediate- and high-risk patients may be attributed to advancements in adjuvant chemoradiation therapy as well as diagnosing younger patients with less advanced disease (*Gynecol Oncol.* 2007;106:521).

B. **Cervical carcinoma.** Although detection of preinvasive disease has increased, the incidence of invasive cervical cancer has dramatically decreased in the United States because of widespread screening by cervical cytology (Papanicolaou smears). However, cervical cancer remains the leading cause of cancer-related deaths among women in developing countries (National Cervical Cancer Coalition Web site, http://www.ncccconline.org/). In the United States, approximately 12,200 new cases and

TABLE 36-2		Vulvar Cancer Staging
TNM	**FIGO**	**Definition**
T1	I	Tumor confined to the vulva
T1a	IA	Lesions ≤2 cm in size with stromal invasion ≤1 mm
T1b	IB	Lesions >2 cm in size or with stromal invasion >1 mm
T2	II	Tumor of any size, extending to adjacent perineal structures (lower one-third urethra, lower one-third vagina, anus) with negative nodes
T3	III	Tumor of any size with or without extension to adjacent perineal structures (lower one-third urethra, lower one-third vagina, anus) with positive inguinofemoral lymph nodes
T3a	IIIA(i) IIIA(ii)	With 1 lymph node metastasis (≥5 mm) 1–2 lymph node metastasis(es) (<5 mm)
T3b	IIIB(i) IIIB(ii)	With ≥2 lymph node metastasis (≥5 mm) ≥3 lymph node metastasis(es) (<5 mm)
T3c	IIIC	With positive lymph nodes with extracapsular spread
T4	IVA(i) IVA(ii)	Invades two-third upper urethral, two-third upper vagina, bladder/rectal mucosa, or fixed to pelvic bone, or Fixed or ulcerated inguinofemoral lymph nodes
M1	IVB	Distant metastasis including pelvic nodes

FIGO, International Federation of Gynecology and Obstetrics; TNM, tumor, node, metastasis.

4,210 deaths occur annually. The goal of evaluating abnormal Papanicolaou smears with colposcopy-guided biopsies for appropriate patients is to diagnose and treat preinvasive disease (*JAMA.* 2001;285:1500). Risk factors for cervical cancer include a history of STDs, HIV infection, multiple sexual partners, early age of first intercourse, lower socioeconomic status, smoking, and HPV infection. Because the majority of squamous cell cancers of the cervix contain high-risk HPV DNA, especially from HPV 16 and 18, HPV vaccines (Gardasil and Cervarix) have been developed and are recommended for females aged 9 to 26 and 10 to 25 years, respectively, although the impact in eradicating cancer will take several decades.

1. **Presentation and clinical features.** Patients may be asymptomatic or present with irregular or postcoital vaginal bleeding or a foul-smelling/watery discharge. Advanced stages may present with leg pain (sciatic nerve involvement), flank pain (ureteral obstruction), renal failure, or rectal bleeding.

2. **Diagnosis** is by biopsy via speculum examination of a visible or palpable lesion. Staging remains clinical and is based on a thorough bimanual and rectovaginal examination, cystoscopy, and proctoscopy. Appropriate adjuvant radiographs include chest radiogram, IV pyelogram, and barium enema. Positron emission tomographic scan is a useful diagnostic modality for assessing distant disease activity. Stage, which is never changed by intraoperative findings, remains the most important prognostic factor, with 5-year survival rates of 88% for stage I disease and 38% for stage III disease, respectively (Table 36-3).

3. **Treatment** depends on stage and lymph node status.

   a. **Microinvasive disease** [stage IA1, depth of invasion less than 3 mm, diameter less than 7 mm, negative lymph vascular space invasion (LVSI)] can be treated with cervical conization alone or with extrafascial hysterectomy. Reproductive age patients desiring fertility with stages IA1 with LVSI, IA2, or IB1 (preferably with a cervical lesion <2 cm and no extracervical disease) may be offered a radical vaginal or abdominal trachelectomy with a lymph node dissection and cerclage placement (*Gynecol Oncol.* 2010;117:350). Lesions with greater depth of invasion, multifocal disease, or upper-vaginal involvement (stages IA2 to IB1) require a radical hysterectomy (removing the parametria and upper vagina) and a complete pelvic and sometimes para-aortic lymphadenectomy. Although radical hysterectomy is only appropriate for a subset of patients, radiotherapy is applicable to any patient with early-stage cervical cancer. The most common complication after radical hysterectomy is bladder dysfunction. Ureteral fistulas, infection, hemorrhage, and lymphocyst formation are less common.

   b. **Radiotherapy** is the appropriate treatment for advanced-stage disease. Combined surgery and radiotherapy for advanced stages does not improve survival but dramatically increases the rate of treatment-related complications such as ureteral and bowel obstruction, strictures, and fistula formation. The nature of radiation is based on stage, lesion size, and lymph node status. Both external beam (teletherapy) and intracavitary (brachytherapy) radiation are used in various combinations. Complications from radiotherapy depend on dose, volume, and tissue tolerance. Acute complications include transient nausea and diarrhea. Early complications including skin ulceration, cystitis, and proctitis occur within the first 6 months after treatment. Late complications (>6 months after treatment) may include bowel obstruction secondary to strictures, fistulas, hemorrhagic cystitis, and chronic proctosigmoiditis. Recent studies indicate that adding cisplatin to radiation decreases the risk of dying from cervical cancer by 30% to 50% over radiation alone (*Lancet.* 2001;358:781).

TABLE 36-3		Cervical Cancer Staging
TNM	**FIGO**	**Definition**
T1	I	Cervical carcinoma confined to the cervix (disregard extension to the corpus).
T1a	IA	Preclinical invasive carcinoma, diagnosed by microscopy only. Deepest invasions ≤5 mm and largest extension ≥7 mm
T1a1	IA1	Microscopic stromal invasion ≤3 mm in depth and extension ≤7 mm
T1a2	IA2	Tumor with stromal invasion between 3 and 5 mm in depth and extension <7 mm
T1b	IB	Clinically visible tumor confined to the cervix but larger than IA2
T1b1	IB1	Clinical lesions ≤4 cm in size
T1b2	IB2	Clinical lesions >4 cm in size
T2	II	Invades beyond the cervix but not to the pelvic side wall or the lower one-third of the vagina
T2a	IIA	Tumor without parametrial involvement
T2a1	IIA1	Tumor ≤4 cm
T2a2	IIA2	Tumor >4 cm
T2b	IIB	Tumor with parametrial involvement
T3	III	Extends to the pelvic side wall and/or involves the lower one-third of the vagina and/or causes hydronephrosis or nonfunctioning kidney
T3a	IIIA	Invades lower one-third of the vagina with no extension to the pelvic side wall
T3b	IIIB	Extends to the pelvic side wall and/or causes hydronephrosis or a nonfunctioning kidney
T4	IVA	Invades mucosa of the bladder/rectum and/or extends beyond the true pelvis
M1	IVB	Distant metastasis

FIGO, International Federation of Gynecology and Obstetrics; TNM, tumor, node, metastasis.

    c. Patients with **pelvic recurrence** after radical hysterectomy are often treated with radiation. Those with isolated central recurrence may be candidates for pelvic exenteration. Five-year survival ranges from 20% to 62% after exenteration, with an operative mortality of 10%. Response to chemotherapy alone in recurrent cervical cancer is poor.

  4. Uncontrolled vaginal bleeding from cervical cancer occasionally is encountered in the emergency department. In most cases, bleeding can be stabilized with tight vaginal packing after which a transurethral Foley catheter should be placed. Acetone-soaked gauze is the most effective packing for vessel sclerosis and control of hemorrhage from necrotic tumor. Emergent radiotherapy or IR embolization may be necessary.

C. Endometrial carcinoma. Endometrial carcinoma is the most common gynecologic malignancy in the United States. An estimated 43,470 new cases will be diagnosed in 2010, with approximately 90% being adenocarcinomas arising from the lining of the uterus. Risk factors for endometrial cancer include Caucasian race, obesity, early menarche, late menopause, nulliparity, tamoxifen therapy, estrogen replacement therapy, infertility, hereditary nonpolyposis colon cancer (HNPCC), and factors leading to unopposed estrogen exposure. Hysterectomy with bilateral salpingo-oophorectomy effectively reduces endometrial and ovarian cancer risk in women with HNPCC and should be offered after completion of childbearing or at time of colectomy. Complex atypical endometrial hyperplasia, a precursor lesion, progresses to carcinoma in 29% of cases if left untreated. Only 1% to 3% of cases of hyperplasia without atypia progress to carcinoma. Hyperplasia can be treated conservatively with progestins and close observation with follow-up endometrial biopsy. Extrafascial hysterectomy is suggested for persistent hyperplasia in patients who have completed their childbearing. Pregnancy and OCP use appear to be protective.

  1. Presentation and clinical features. The most common symptom is abnormal vaginal bleeding, often in a postmenopausal patient. Approximately three-fourths of patients present with stage I disease. Endometrial sampling should be considered mandatory in all postmenopausal women. Although endometrial carcinoma is rare in women younger than 35 years, patients in this age group who have persistent noncyclic vaginal bleeding, are nonresponsive to medical management, or are morbidly obese should undergo endometrial assessment (ACOG Practice Bulletin 65. *Obstet Gynecol.* 2005;106:413).

  2. Physical examination should include an evaluation for obesity, hirsutism, and other signs of hyperestrogenism. The uterus may be enlarged or of normal size.

  3. Diagnosis is by transcervical aspiration (e.g., Pipelle), which usually is performed as an office procedure, or by hysteroscopy/D&C, which is performed in the operating room. Ultrasonography may assist in diagnosing an intrauterine abnormality.

  4. Treatment generally consists of a laparoscopic or open-staging procedure including pelvic washings, extrafascial total hysterectomy,

TABLE 36-4	Endometrial Cancer Staging	
TNM	FIGO	Definition
T1	I	Tumor confined to the corpus uteri
T1a	IA	Invades one-half or less of the myometrium
T1b	IB	Invades more than one-half of the myometrium
T2	II	Invades cervical stroma but does not extend beyond the uterus
T3	III	Local and/or regional spread as specified
T3a	IIIA	Involves the serosa and/or adnexa
T3b	IIIB	Vaginal and/or parametrial involvement
N1	IIIC IIIC1 IIIC2	Metastasis to the pelvic and/or para-aortic lymph nodes Positive pelvic nodes Positive para-aortic lymph nodes with or without positive pelvic lymph nodes
T4	IVA	Invades the bladder and/or bowel mucosa
M1	IVB	Distant metastasis including intra-abdominal and/or inguinal lymph nodes

FIGO, International Federation of Gynecology and Obstetrics; TNM, tumor, node, metastasis.

bilateral salpingo-oophorectomy, and sometimes omentectomy. Pelvic and para-aortic lymphadenectomy is considered both diagnostic and therapeutic and should be performed in patients who have a tumor of more than 2 cm, deep myometrial invasion, tumor grade of 2 or 3, or suspicious lymph nodes. Intraoperative evaluation of the uterus should be performed by bivalving the uterus and obtaining a frozen section as needed. Adjuvant radiotherapy and/or chemotherapy are used postoperatively in patients with poor prognostic factors who are at high risk for recurrence. Hormonal therapy can also be used.

5. **Prognosis** generally is favorable, with 5-year survival of more than 90% for patients with surgical stage I tumors (Table 36-4). Prognosis depends on the tumor grade, depth of myometrial invasion, adnexal involvement, pelvic cytology, LVSI, and lymph node spread. Rare histologies, such as clear-cell or papillary serous cancers and sarcomas arising from the wall of the uterus, do not share the overall good prognosis

of early-stage adenocarcinomas. African American women have mortality rates nearly twice that of Caucasian women.

D. **Ovarian carcinoma** is the deadliest of all the gynecologic malignancies. There will be approximately 21,880 new cases diagnosed in 2010. More than two-thirds of patients in whom epithelial ovarian cancer is diagnosed eventually die from this disease (13,850 per year in the United States) (*CA Cancer J Clin.* 2010;60:260–267). Besides tumors arising from the ovarian coelomic epithelium, which are the most common, germ cell (often in younger patients) and stromal primary tumors can occur. Two-thirds of epithelial ovarian cancers are diagnosed at advanced stages with extraovarian metastasis. Incidence increases steadily with advancing age to a total lifetime incidence of 1 in 68. Risk factors include nulliparity, late menopause, early menarche, use of infertility drugs, and personal or family history of breast or ovarian cancer. Genetic cancer syndromes including *BRCA1* or *BRCA2* mutations and HNPCC have also been associated with an increased risk of ovarian cancer, and prophylactic removal of ovaries and fallopian tubes decreases the risk of gynecologic cancer in these patients. Use of OCPs, pregnancy, and tubal ligation appear to be protective.

1. **Presentation and clinical features.** Women with early-stage disease are generally asymptomatic. In advanced stages, patients may present with vague abdominal pain or pressure, nausea, early satiety, weight loss, or swelling.

2. **Diagnosis** of ovarian cancer at early stages has proved to be clinically difficult (Table 36-5). No cost-effective screening test has proven to be reliable in detecting stage I disease (confined to the ovaries). Bimanual examination remains the most effective means of screening, followed by surgery for histologic diagnosis. Ultrasonography of the pelvis (preferably transvaginal) and CT scans are effective adjuncts. CA 125 antigen is not effective for mass screening but serves as an effective tumor marker in patients with initial elevations once diagnosis has been established and treatment is initiated.

3. **Treatment** is primarily aggressive surgical debulking for all patients with a good performance status. Complete staging includes pelvic washings on entering the peritoneum, total abdominal hysterectomy, bilateral salpingo-oophorectomy, omentectomy, pelvic and para-aortic lymph node dissection, and peritoneal biopsies. Optimal cytoreduction (residual disease <1 cm) improves response to adjuvant chemotherapy and overall survival. In young women with early-stage disease, fertility-sparing surgery can often be performed with removal of the uterus and contralateral ovary after childbearing age is completed. However, complete staging at initial surgery is still necessary. Patients with disease outside the ovary are treated with 6 cycles of paclitaxel and platinum–based chemotherapy either IV or intraperitoneally. The inclusion of bevacizumab (a humanized monoclonal antibody against vascular endothelial growth factor-A) to primary chemotherapy in ovarian cancer is being evaluated in a phase III trial.

TABLE 36.5	Ovarian Cancer Staging	
TNM	**FIGO**	**Definition**
T1	I	Tumor limited to one or both ovaries
T1a	IA	Limited to one ovary; capsule intact, no tumor on ovarian surface, no malignant cells in ascites or peritoneal washings
T1b	IB	Limited to both ovaries; capsule intact, no tumor on ovarian surface, no malignant cells in ascites or peritoneal washings
T1c	IC	Limited to one or both ovaries with any of the following: capsule ruptured, tumor on ovarian surface, malignant cells in ascites, or peritoneal washings
T2	II	Tumor involves one or both ovaries with pelvic extension
T2a	IIA	Extension and/or implants on uterus and/or tubes; no malignant cells in ascites or peritoneal washings
T2b	IIB	Extension to other pelvic tissues; no malignant cells in ascites or peritoneal washings
T2c	IIC	Pelvic extension with malignant cells in ascites or peritoneal washings
T3	III	Tumor involves one or both ovaries with microscopically confirmed peritoneal metastasis outside the pelvis and/or regional lymph node metastasis
T3a	IIIA	Microscopic peritoneal metastasis beyond the pelvis
T3b	IIIB	Macroscopic peritoneal metastasis beyond the pelvis ≤2 cm
T3c	IIIC	Peritoneal metastasis beyond the pelvis >2 cm and/or regional lymph node involvement
M1	IV	Distant metastasis (excludes peritoneal metastasis)

FIGO, International Federation of Gynecology and Obstetrics; TNM, tumor, node, metastasis.

4. **Prognosis** correlates directly with stage and residual disease after debulking. Median survival depends on optimal cytoreduction at initial laparotomy. Median survival for optimally debulked advanced-stage tumors is nearly 80% at 1 year; the 5-year relative survival rate for all stages is 46% (*CA Cancer J Clin.* 2010;60:260–267).

37 Common Surgical Procedures

Kathryn J. Rowland and Bradley D. Freeman

This chapter reviews concepts, indications, and technical aspects of procedures commonly performed in hospitalized surgical patients, focusing on central venous catheterization, thoracic and peritoneal drainage procedures, airway access, and laparoscopy.

Basic rules govern the successful performance of surgical procedures: (1) Necessary equipment, supplies, lighting, and assistance should be available before starting the procedure; (2) the patient should be positioned to optimize exposure; (3) patient comfort must be ensured, and appropriate analgesia and sedation must be provided so that the patient can cooperate with and tolerate the procedure; and (4) sterile technique should be practiced when appropriate. Adherence to standards regarding consent, time-out, and documentation should be followed, as always.

I. **CENTRAL VENOUS CATHETERIZATION.** Central venous catheterization is commonly used in surgical patients both for diagnosis [central venous pressure (CVP) determination or pulmonary artery catheter for hemodynamic monitoring] and treatment [fluid infusion, administration of vasoactive agents, or mechanical device (e.g., pacemaker or inferior vena cava filter insertion)]. Several approaches to access the central venous system exist, each with advantages and disadvantages. Before placement of a central venous access device (CVAD), the patient should be evaluated for the presence of an indwelling central venous device, such as a transvenous pacemaker, and for signs of central venous obstruction, such as distended collateral veins about the shoulder and neck. **Contraindication:** Venous thrombosis is an absolute contraindication to catheter placement at the affected site. Relative contraindications include coagulopathy [international normalized ratio (INR) >2 or partial prothrombin time (PTT) >2 times control] refractory to correction and thrombocytopenia (platelet count <50,000/μL). For an elective procedure, the INR should be corrected to less than 1.5, PTT to less than 1.5 times control, and platelet count to greater than 50,000/μL.

A. **Types of catheters.** Catheters are classified on the basis of number of lumens, lifespan (short, intermediate, long-term), site of insertion (subclavian, internal jugular, femoral, peripheral), subcutaneous tunneling, anti-infective features (Dacron or silver-impregnated cuff, and/or antibiotic-impregnated catheters), and tip structure (valved, nonvalved). Prior to insertion, one should carefully consider the indications for placement, the expected duration of treatment, and the number of lumens necessary to achieve the treatment goals. Multilumen catheters are associated with slightly higher rates of infection than single-lumen catheters, and the choice of catheters should minimize the number of lumens while allowing for optimal patient care (*Crit Care Med.* 2003;31:2385).

1. **Short-term (nontunneled) CVADs.** The advantages of single-lumen and multilumen nontunneled catheters include low cost, bedside placement and removal, and ease of exchange of damaged catheters. A variety of products are available based upon the clinical need for administration of multiple drugs (**triple-lumen catheter**), the rapid administration of fluids (multiaccess catheter [**MAC**]; Arrow International, Teleflex Medical, Research Triangle Park, NC), hemodialysis or pheresis (**Hemo-Cath;** MedComp, Harleysville, PA; or **Quinton Permcath;** Covidien, Mansfield, MA), or to allow for hemodialysis or pheresis with an additional lumen available for fluid or drug administration (**Mahurkar; Covidien** or **Trialysis;** Bard Access Systems, Murray Hill, NJ).

2. **Intermediate-term, peripherally inserted CVADs.** Peripherally inserted central catheters (**PICCs**) are composed of Silastic or polyurethane and can be kept in place for several days to several months for inpatient or outpatient therapy. These catheters are commonly used for home total parenteral nutrition (TPN) or intravenous antibiotic administration. PICCs can be inserted using local anesthetic at the bedside via cephalic, basilic, or median cubital veins. Proper position should be radiographically documented with a chest radiograph. These catheters have low risk of insertion-related complications, such as pneumothorax, and infection. Disadvantages of PICCs result from their small diameter and length (40 to 60 cm) and include low flow rates, problems with withdrawal occlusion, and risk for thrombophlebitis (*J Vasc Interv Radiol.* 2000;11:1309). Power injectable PICCs allow for more rapid flow rates of fluids and are compatible with the power injectors used for radiocontrast studies. Careful consideration is necessary prior to insertion in renal patients as PICCs can injure the upper-extremity veins, thus limiting suitability for future arteriovenous hemodialysis access.

3. **Intermediate-term, nontunneled CVADS.** These catheters contain a silver-impregnated gelatin cuff (Vitacuff; Vitaphore Corporation, San Carlos, CA), which is designed to be positioned subcutaneously and to serve as a barrier to migration of bacteria from the skin. The gelatin dissolves within a short time, facilitating removal. The **Hohn catheter** (Bard Access Systems, Murray Hill, NJ) is the prototypical CVAD of this type, and it may remain in place for several months.

4. **Long-term, tunneled CVADS.** Tunneled catheters enable indefinite venous access for prolonged nutritional support, chemotherapy, antibiotics, hemodialysis, or blood draws. The subcutaneous portion of the catheter contains a Dacron cuff that functions to induce scar formation, anchoring the catheter in place, and preventing bacterial migration from skin. Most tunneled catheters are manufactured using silicone, which is more flexible and durable than other materials. Examples include the **Hickman** and **Broviac**

catheters (Bard Access Systems, Murray Hill, NJ). The **Groshong catheter** (Bard Access Systems, Murray Hill, NJ) differs by the presence of a slit valve at the tip, which seals it from the bloodstream. Unlike other catheters, which require daily or weekly heparinized saline injections, Groshong catheters are flushed with normal saline with decreased flushing frequency and thus they are well suited for patients with history of heparin allergy or heparin-induced thrombocytopenia.

5. **Implanted venous ports.** Ports are used primarily for chronic therapy (>6 months) for which only intermittent access is needed. Common indications include chemotherapy and frequent hospitalizations (e.g., patients with sickle cell disease or cystic fibrosis). Access is commonly obtained via the internal jugular or subclavian veins, and a reservoir is placed in a subcutaneous pocket created in the infraclavicular fossa. Most models contain a silicone or polyurethane catheter connected to a metal or plastic reservoir with a dense silicone septum for percutaneous needle access. Models vary in height and presence of a dual or single chamber. Advantages of ports over other CVADs include a lower incidence of infection and less maintenance (monthly heparin flushes when not in use). Plastic ports are magnetic resonance scan compatible and are as durable as ports with reservoirs constructed of metal. Power injectable ports compatible with the power injectors used for radiocontrast studies are available. Port access requires skin puncture with a special noncoring (Huber) needle to prevent deterioration of the septum.

B. **Internal jugular approach**

1. **Indications.** The internal jugular vein is easily and rapidly accessible in most patients. Advantages of this site include decreased risk of pneumothorax compared with the subclavian approach and ready compressibility of the vessels in case of bleeding. For the unsedated or ambulatory patient, this may be an uncomfortable site and may hinder his or her neck movement. Maintaining a sterile dressing on the insertion site can be difficult, especially in the presence of a tracheostomy. This is a commonly used site of central venous access for the placement of tunneled catheters and ports where the catheter's exit site is on the chest.

2. **Technique.** Imaging devices (such as ultrasonography) are being increasingly used to delineate the vascular anatomy and enhance the safety of vascular access procedures (*Curr Opin Crit Care.* 2008;14:415; *Crit Care Med.* 2007;35:S186). Ultrasound guidance has been shown to increase both the overall success rate and first attempt success rate at internal jugular central venous cannulation on meta-analysis (*BMJ.* 2003;327:361). If available, such devices should be used, particularly in patients in whom anatomic landmarks are obscure. The pulse of the common carotid artery is palpated at the medial border of the sternocleidomastoid (SCM) muscle at midneck. The internal jugular vein is located lateral to the common carotid artery and courses slightly anterior to the artery as it joins the

subclavian vein (Fig. 37-1). The physician stands at the head of the bed. The patient is placed in the Trendelenburg position at an angle of 10 to 15 degrees, with his or her head flat on the bed and turned away from the side of the procedure. The skin is prepared with a chlorhexidine-based antiseptic solution, which has been shown to be superior to providine–iodine solutions in the prevention of catheter colonization (*Infect Control Hosp Epidemiol.* 2008;29:847). Sterile drapes are applied. One percent lidocaine is infiltrated subcutaneously over the belly and lateral border of the SCM. Two equally effective approaches to the internal jugular vein are described: the central and posterior approaches. For the central approach, a 21-gauge "seeker" needle is introduced approximately 1 cm lateral to the carotid pulse into the belly of the SCM. At a 45-degree angle, the needle is slowly advanced toward the ipsilateral nipple. For the posterior approach, the seeker needle is introduced at the lateral edge of the SCM and directed toward the sternal notch at a 45-degree angle. Constant negative pressure is exerted on the syringe, and entry into the vein is confirmed by the return of venous blood. Pulsatile, bright red blood suggests arterial access and mandates removal of the needle and direct manual pressure to the site for 10 minutes. The vein should be entered within 5 to 7 cm with both approaches. If the vein is not entered, the needle should be withdrawn and redirected for another attempt. Redirection of the needle should be inserted just below the surface of the skin because of the potential of the needle tip to lacerate adjacent vessels if redirected within the subcutaneous tissues. Under ultrasound guidance, the carotid artery (noncompressible, pulsatile) and internal jugular vein (compressible, nonpulsatile) are visualized and the vein is punctured under direct ultrasound guidance. Following venous access with the seeker needle, a 14-gauge needle is then introduced just inferior to the seeker needle and is advanced along the same path until venous blood is aspirated. The **Seldinger technique** is employed, whereby a flexible guidewire is passed into the vein through the 14-gauge needle, and the needle is removed over the wire. It is important to maintain control of the guidewire at all times. In cases of low flow, venous placement can be confirmed at this point by ultrasound visualization of the wire within the internal jugular vein. A nick is then made in the skin at the puncture site with a no. 11 blade to allow passage of the dilator. The dilator is threaded over the wire and creates a tract for the passage of the less rigid central venous catheter. The dilator is removed with the guidewire in place and the catheter is introduced over the wire and advanced to 15 to 20 cm so that its tip is at the junction of the superior vena cava (SVC) and the right atrium. The guidewire is then removed. In patients with difficult anatomy or indwelling devices (vena cava filters, pacemakers), fluoroscopy should be used to guide placement. Aspiration of blood from all ports and subsequent flushing with saline confirm that the catheter is positioned in the vein and that all of its ports are functional. The catheter is then secured to the patient's neck at a minimum of two sites, and a sterile dressing is applied. A chest radiograph is obtained to confirm the location of the catheter tip and to rule out the presence of a pneumothorax.

3. Complications

a. Pneumothorax. All percutaneously placed neck catheters carry a risk of pneumothorax. Every attempt at placement of a central venous catheter, successful or unsuccessful, should be followed by an erect chest radiograph before the catheter is used or catheter placement is attempted at another site. Presence of a small pneumothorax may be observed with serial chest radiographs. Unstable hemodynamics, worsening respiratory status, or expanding pneumothorax mandates tube thoracostomy placement (see Section II.B for procedure details).

b. Carotid artery injury. Carotid artery puncture complicates internal jugular cannulation in as many as 10% of cases, representing 80% to 90% of all insertion-related complications. Inadvertent carotid artery puncture is usually tolerated in the noncoagulopathic patient and treated by direct pressure over the carotid artery. If the carotid artery is punctured, no further attempts at central venous access should be made on either side of the patient's neck and the patient must be observed for the development of a neck hematoma and resultant airway compromise. Although carotid artery puncture is usually benign, it can be life threatening when it results in inadvertent intra-arterial cannulation, stroke, hemothorax, or carotid artery–internal jugular vein fistula. In the hemodynamically unstable or poorly oxygenating patient, it is not always possible to distinguish venous blood from arterial blood by appearance. This can lead to inadvertent cannulation of the carotid artery. If the dilator or catheter is 7 French (F) or smaller, it can usually be removed and direct pressure held over the carotid puncture site without further detrimental sequelae. Catheters larger than 7F should be removed in a setting in which operative repair of the arteriotomy can be performed.

c. Guidewire-related complications. Advancement of the guidewire into the right atrium or ventricle can cause arrhythmia, which usually resolves once the wire is withdrawn. Central venous catheter insertion in patients with indwelling devices (such as vena cava filters or pacemakers) must be performed under fluoroscopic guidance to minimize the possibility of entanglement of the guidewire with these structures.

d. Venous stenosis. Venous stenosis can occur at the site where the catheter enters the vein, which can lead to thrombosis of the vessel. Because the upper extremities and neck have extensive collateralization, stenosis or thrombosis is usually well tolerated.

e. Other. Air embolus, perforation of the right atrium or ventricle with resultant hemopericardium and cardiac tamponade, and injury to the trachea, esophagus, thoracic duct, vagus nerve, phrenic nerve, or brachial plexus can all complicate the placement of central venous catheters.

C. **Subclavian vein approach**

1. **Indications.** The subclavian approach to the central venous system is generally most comfortable for the patient and easiest to maintain. The Centers for Disease Control and Prevention (CDC) published guidelines in 2002 that recommend subclavian access as the preferred site in patients at risk for CVAD infection (*MMWR Recomm Rep.* 2002;51:1). A prospective observational study found that catheter-related bloodstream infection (CRBSI) incidence was lowest in subclavian access, higher in jugular access, and highest in femoral access and recommended that sites for CVAD placement be considered in that order (*Crit Care.* 2005;9:R631). In the presence of an open wound, tracheostomy, and tumors of the head and neck, CVAD should be placed in the subclavian position to minimize infection risk.

2. **Technique.** The subclavian vein courses posterior to the clavicle, where it joins the internal jugular vein and the contralateral veins to form the SVC (Fig. 37-1). The subclavian artery and the apical pleura lie just posterior to the subclavian vein. The patient is placed in the Trendelenburg position with a rolled towel between the scapulas, which allows the shoulders to fall posteriorly. The skin is prepared with a chlorhexidine-based antiseptic solution, draped, and

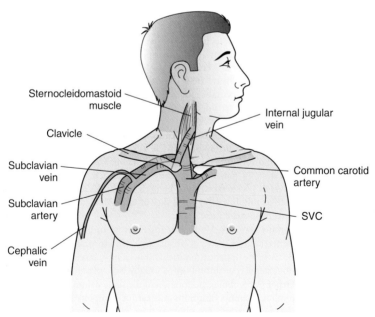

Figure 37-1. Anatomy of the upper chest and neck, including the vasculature and important landmarks. SVC, superior vena cava.

1% lidocaine is infiltrated subcutaneously in the infraclavicular space near the middle and lateral third of the clavicle. The infusion of lidocaine is carried into the deep soft tissue and to the periosteum of the clavicle. A 14-gauge needle is introduced at the middle third of the clavicle in the deltopectoral groove. The needle is kept deep to the clavicle and parallel to the plane of the floor and is slowly advanced toward the sternal notch. Constant negative pressure is applied to the syringe. Once the needle enters the subclavian vein, the guidewire, the dilator, and the catheter are introduced by the **Seldinger technique.** As with the other approaches, all catheter ports are aspirated and flushed to ensure that they are functional. A chest radiograph is obtained to confirm the location of the catheter tip and to evaluate for pneumothorax.

3. **Complications.** The complications of subclavian venous catheterization include those described in the previous section. Puncture of the subclavian artery can be troublesome because the clavicle prevents the application of direct pressure to achieve homeostasis. Therefore, this approach should be avoided in the patient with uncorrectable coagulopathy. If the artery is punctured, the patient should be placed on hemodynamic monitoring for the next 30 to 45 minutes to ensure that bleeding is not ongoing. Inadvertent cannulation of the subclavian artery with the dilator or catheter is a potentially fatal complication. The dilator or catheter should be left in place and angiography performed. Removal of the catheter should be done in the operating room so that open arteriotomy repair may be performed if necessary. Left-sided subclavian catheter placement poses the risk of injury to the thoracic duct, brachiocephalic vein, and SVC with the needle or dilator. Attention must be paid to the final position of the catheter tip when placed on the left side to avoid abutting the SVC wall, which poses the immediate or delayed risk of SVC perforation.

D. **Femoral vein approach**

1. **Indications.** The femoral vein is the easiest site for obtaining central access and is therefore the preferred approach for central venous access during trauma or cardiopulmonary resuscitation. This approach does not interfere with the other procedures of cardiopulmonary resuscitation. It should be remembered that a femoral vein catheter does not actually reach the central circulation and may not be ideal for the administration of vasoactive drugs. The femoral approach is also favored during trauma resuscitation except when there is an injury to the inferior vena cava. The femoral vein catheter inhibits patient mobility, and the groin is a difficult area in which to maintain sterility. Therefore, it should not be used in elective situations, except when upper-extremity and neck sites are not available. This may be the only site available in patients with upper-body burns. Catheters placed at any site during a medical emergency (including cardiopulmonary or trauma resuscitation) when sterile technique cannot be assured should be replaced within 48 hours of insertion to minimize the risk of CRBSI.

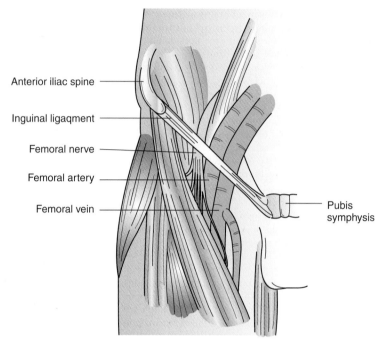

Anterior iliac spine

Inguinal ligaqment

Femoral nerve

Femoral artery

Femoral vein

Pubis
symphysis

Figure 37-2. Anatomy of the femoral vessels.

2. **Technique.** The femoral artery crosses the inguinal ligament approximately midway between the anterosuperior iliac spine and the
pubic tubercle. The femoral vein runs medial to the artery as they
cross the inguinal ligament (Fig. 37-2). The skin is prepared with a
chlorhexadine-based antiseptic solution, draped, and 1% lidocaine is
infiltrated in the subcutaneous tissue medial to the femoral artery and
inferior to the inguinal ligament. The pulse of the femoral artery is
palpated below the inguinal ligament, and a 14-gauge needle is introduced medial to the pulse at a 30-degree angle. It is directed cephalad
with constant negative pressure until the vein is entered. Once the needle enters the femoral vein, the guidewire, the dilator, and ultimately
the catheter are inserted using the **Seldinger technique.** When a femoral pulse cannot be palpated, as in cardiopulmonary arrest, the position
of the femoral artery can be estimated to be at the midpoint between
the anterosuperior iliac spine and the pubic tubercle, with the vein
lying 1 to 2 cm medial to this point. Once the catheter is successfully
placed, all three ports are aspirated and flushed to ensure that they are
functional.

3. **Complications.** Injury to the common femoral artery or its branches
during cannulation of the femoral vein can result in an inguinal or

retroperitoneal hematoma, a pseudoaneurysm, or an arteriovenous fistula. The femoral nerve can also be damaged. Injury to the inguinal lymphatic system can result in a lymphocele. The possibility of injuring peritoneal structures also exists, particularly if an inguinal hernia is present. Errant passages of the guidewire and the rigid dilator run the risk of perforating the pelvic venous complex and causing retroperitoneal hemorrhage. Late complications include infection and femoral vein thrombosis.

E. **Catheter maintenance.** Proper care of access sites and devices is crucial to their long-term function. CVADs require sterile dressing changes at least weekly. Our institution uses sterile, occlusive, transparent dressings; however, this has not been shown superior to the use of sterile, gauze dressings secured with tape (*Cochrane Database Syst Rev.* 2003;(4):CD003827). More frequent dressing changes may be needed for those patients who are immunocompromised. Chlorhexidine gluconate–impregnated sponges (BioPatch; Ethicon Inc, Somerville, NJ) applied to the skin at the site of catheter insertion beneath an occlusive dressing have been shown to reduce CRBSIs (*JAMA.* 2009;301(12):1231–1241). Application of topical antibiotic beneath an occlusive dressing may provide a moist culture medium for bacterial growth and should be avoided. Catheter lumens should be flushed on a regular basis to prevent thrombosis. Heparin has been shown to be superior to saline for decreasing thrombotic occlusions of central venous catheters (*JPEN J Parenter Enteral Nutr.* 2010;34:444) (see Section I.G. for further details).

F. **CRBSIs** occur with a prevalence ranging from 3% to 7% and has a mortality rate of up to 20% (*Infect Control Hosp Epidemiol.* 2000;21:375). CRBSIs prolong intensive care unit stays, increase total hospital days, and have an attributable cost of nearly $12,000 per incidence (*Crit Care Med.* 2006; 34:2084). Catheter colonization—or bacterial growth from the catheter tip—occurs in 20% of central venous catheters.

1. **Epidemiology.** CRBSIs are generally caused by coagulase-negative staphylococci (37%), followed by gram-negative bacilli (14%), enterococci (13.5%), coagulase-positive *Staphylococcus aureus* (12.6%), and *Candida albicans* (5%) (*Am J Infect Control.* 1999;27:520). Treatment of these organisms has become increasingly difficult now that 60% of *S. aureus* isolates and 90% of coagulase-negative *Staphylococcus* isolates are resistant to oxacillin. The percentage of enterococcal isolates resistant to vancomycin has also increased, from 0.5% in 1989 to 28.5% in 2003 (*Am J Infect Control.* 2004;32:470). The majority of catheter infections are monomicrobial.

2. **Pathogenesis.** Infection occurs by two routes. First, endogenous skin flora at the insertion site migrate along the external surface of the catheter and colonize the intravascular tip. Second, pathogens from contamination at the hub colonize the internal surface of the catheter and are washed into the bloodstream when the catheter is infused. Occasionally, catheters may become hematogenously seeded from another focus of infection. Rarely, infusate contamination or break in sterile technique leads to CRBSI.

3. **Definitions and diagnosis.** Catheter colonization is defined as greater than 15 colony-forming units of microorganisms on semiquantitative culture. The definition of CRBSI requires bacteremia or fungemia in a patient with CVAD and meeting of the following criteria: (1) clinical signs of infection (fever, chills, tachycardia, hypotension, leukocytosis), (2) no identifiable source for bloodstream infection other than the CVAD, and (3) isolation of the same organism from semiquantitative culture of the catheter and from the blood (drawn from a peripheral vein taken within 48 hours of each other) (*Clin Infect Dis.* 2009;49:1). Diagnosis of CRBSI with coagulase-negative staphylococci requires two positive blood cultures or a positive catheter culture.

4. **Presentation and treatment.** Catheter infections may manifest with local, regional, or systemic signs. Treatment is based upon consideration of multiple factors, including severity of infection, causative organism, type of catheter, and remaining options for vascular access.

   a. **Local and regional catheter-related infections** (*Clin Infect Dis.* 2009;49:1). Local exit-site infections may present with pain, erythema, induration, or drainage. In general, short-term (non-tunneled) CVADs should be removed if an exit-site infection is present. For long-term (tunneled) CVADs, an uncomplicated exit-site infection (without purulent drainage, in the absence of systemic signs, and with negative blood cultures) can be treated with topical antibiotics, systemic antibiotics for skin flora, and more frequent dressing changes and care. Catheter removal is required if systemic antibiotic therapy fails. Tunnel infection or port abscess, purulent drainage, or systemic manifestations (leukocytosis, positive blood culture) require catheter removal, incision and drainage, and systemic antibiotics.

   b. **Bacteremia** (*Clin Infect Dis.* 2009;49:1). Bacteremia is the most severe manifestation of a catheter-related infection and often presents with fever and leukocytosis. In the setting of bacteremia, indwelling catheters generally should be removed and the patient should be treated with a course of systemic antibiotics. Empiric antibiotic treatment while awaiting culture results should consist of coverage against gram-positive cocci, including methicillin-resistant staphylococci. For lower-extremity CVADs, coverage against gram-negative bacilli and *Candida* should be included as well. In select patients with limited vascular access and other potential sources for infection, salvage of the catheter can be attempted with broad-spectrum antibiotics and antibiotic lock therapy for 10 to 14 days. Persistent bacteremia after 72 hours necessitates catheter removal. The presence of fungemia requires immediate removal of the catheter, with initiation of antifungal treatment. Rewiring of the existing catheter should not be performed in the setting of CRBSI.

5. **Risk factors.** The risk for infection varies with the catheter insertion site, with the femoral vein associated with a much higher infection rate than subclavian vein access (19.8% vs. 4.5%) (*JAMA.* 2001;286:700).

Jugular venous catheterization carries an intermediate risk of infection. The likelihood of infection directly correlates with length of time a catheter has been in position. PICCs in intensive care unit patients have been demonstrated to have similar rates of CRBSI as that of non-tunneled CVADs but have longer time to the development of infection (*Am J Infect Control.* 2010;38:149).

6. **Prevention.** The largest impact in reducing CRBSIs has been achieved via inexpensive interventions and educational initiatives on basic infection control practices. When instituted together, hand hygiene, chlorhexidine-based skin preparation, maximal barrier precautions, avoidance of the femoral vein for insertion, and daily review of the necessity for and removal of all unnecessary central venous catheters have been demonstrated to result in an up to 66% reduction in CRBSI (*N Engl J Med.* 2006;355:2725).

   a. **Antimicrobial-impregnated catheters.** Antimicrobial-coated catheters, ionic silver cuffs, and antibiotic-impregnated hubs have been developed in efforts to reduce CRBSI. In a multicenter, randomized, double-blind, controlled trial, second-generation chlorhexidine-silver sulfadiazine (CHSS)–impregnated CVADs reduced microbial colonization compared to uncoated catheters (*Ann Intern Med.* 2005; 143:570). A subsequent meta-analysis found that rifampin/minocycline–impregnated CVADs reduced the rate of microbial colonization and CRBSI (*J Antimicrob Chemother.* 2007;59:359). Not all studies have supported a decreased rate of CRBSIs with antimicrobial-impregnated catheters over that achieved with educational initiatives and infection prevention bundles of care alone (*Crit Care Med.* 2009;37(2):702). The emergence of resistant organisms resulting from the use of antimicrobial-impregnated catheters remains a potentially important concern. The current data are inconclusive; however, many support the use of antimicrobial-impregnated catheters, especially in high-risk patients.

   b. **Routine (elective) catheter replacement.** Routine catheter replacement (either changing position to a new site or rewiring an existing catheter after an arbitrary length of time) has not been demonstrated to decrease the incidence of catheter-related infections. Thus, CVADs should be left in place until discontinuation is clinically indicated.

G. **Thrombosis** (*J Natl Compr Cancer Netw.* 2006;4:889). Difficulty in aspirating blood or infusing fluid from a previously functional catheter may be indicative of partial or complete catheter blockage. Blockage may be due to kinking of the catheter, occlusion of the catheter tip on a vessel wall, or luminal thrombosis. The spectrum of thrombotic complications ranges from fibrin sleeve formation around the catheter to mural or occlusive thrombus. Although only 3% to 5% of central venous catheters develop clinically significant thromboses, ultrasonography with color Doppler imaging has been found to detect venous thrombosis in 33% to 67% of patients when the indwelling time of the CVAD was greater than 1 week.

A negative Doppler ultrasonography in a symptomatic patient should be followed by venographic assessment because thrombi in the central upper venous system (SVC, brachiocephalic, and subclavian veins) are better detected by venography.

   1. **Intervention** (*Lancet.* 2009;374:159). Inspection of the catheter and repositioning of the patient to exclude mechanical obstruction should first be performed. Empiric thrombolytic intervention with alteplase (2 mL of 2 mg/2 mL alteplase administered into the catheter lumen and allowed to dwell for at least 30 minutes) is generally an effective and safe means of restoring CVAD function and blood flow without resorting to catheter replacement. If this procedure fails or if the patient is symptomatic, imaging with Doppler ultrasonography or venography should be performed. In the presence of a venous thrombosis, the catheter should be removed and systemic anticoagulation should be initiated.

H. **Catheter removal.** Catheters should be removed as soon as they are no longer clinically indicated, given the increased risk of CRBSIs with increased catheter duration (*Surg Infect.* 2010;11(6):529). Proper internal jugular or subclavian catheter removal requires placement of the patient in Trendelenberg positioning (head down). To prevent an air embolus, the patient is instructed to perform the Valsalva maneuver; taking a deep breath in, holding the breath, and bearing down (to create a high intrathoracic pressure) during removal. The catheter tip should always be inspected to verify that it is intact. Manual pressure is applied for 5 minutes while the patient breathes normally (or longer for patients with coagulopathy or for removal of larger-bore catheters). Once hemostasis is obtained, an occlusive dressing is applied. In the absence of clinical suspicion for CRBSI, the catheter tip should not be routinely cultured (*Clin Infect Dis.* 2009;49:1).

II. THORACIC DRAINAGE PROCEDURES

A. **Thoracentesis**
   1. **Indications.** Thoracentesis can provide both diagnostic and therapeutic benefit for patients with pleural effusions. Pleural effusions are categorized as transudative or exudative. Transudative effusions are associated with conditions of increased hydrostatic pressure or decreased colloid osmotic pressure such as volume overload, congestive heart failure, or cirrhosis. Exudative effusions are associated with conditions resulting in inflammation such as infection or cancer. This differentiation is based on gross, microscopic, and biochemical characteristics. Diagnostic thoracentesis is indicated for an effusion of unknown etiology. Pleural fluid lactate dehydrogenase (LDH), protein, pH, glucose, amylase, lipid, Gram stain, culture, and cytology should be performed. A pleural fluid–serum LDH ratio greater than 0.6 and a fluid–serum protein ratio greater than 0.5 indicate an exudative effusion, whereas a fluid–serum LDH ratio less than 0.6 and a fluid–serum protein ratio

less than 0.5 indicate a transudative effusion. Therapeutic thoracentesis is indicated to relieve respiratory compromise resulting from large pleural effusions. For recurrent pleural effusions, when repeated therapeutic thoracentesis is needed, chest tube drainage and pleurosclerosis should be considered.

2. **Technique.** Erect and lateral decubitus chest radiographs or equivalent imaging studies (such as computed tomographic scan) should be obtained to assess the size and location of the effusion as well as whether the effusion is free flowing or loculated. For free-flowing effusions, the patient is seated upright and slightly forward. The thorax should be entered posteriorly, 4 to 6 cm lateral to the spinal column and one to two interspaces below the cessation of tactile fremitus and where percussion is dull. Loculated effusions can be localized by ultrasonography, and the site for thoracentesis is marked on the skin. The site is prepared with chlorhexadine and draped with sterile towels. One percent lidocaine is infiltrated into the subcutaneous tissue covering the rib below the interspace to be entered. The infiltration is carried deep to the periosteum of the rib. Next, with negative pressure placed on the syringe, the needle is advanced slowly over the top of the rib to avoid injury to the neurovascular bundle, which lies just inferior to the rib. The needle is advanced until pleural fluid is returned and is then withdrawn a fraction to allow for injection of lidocaine to anesthetize the pleura. Lidocaine is then infiltrated into the intercostal muscles as the needle is withdrawn. Most thoracentesis kits contain a long, 14-gauge needle inserted into a plastic catheter with an attached syringe and stopcock. The needle–catheter apparatus is introduced at the level of the rib below the interspace to be entered. With negative pressure applied to the syringe, the needle is slowly advanced over the top of the rib and into the pleural cavity until fluid is returned. Aspiration of air bubbles indicates puncture of the lung parenchyma; the needle should be promptly removed under negative pressure. Once the needle is in the pleural space, the catheter is advanced over the needle toward the diaphragm. Special attention is taken not to advance the needle as the catheter is being directed into the pleural space. A drainage bag is attached to the stopcock to remove the pleural fluid. The amount of fluid removed depends on the indication for the thoracentesis. A diagnostic thoracentesis requires 20 to 30 mL of fluid for the appropriate tests; a therapeutic thoracentesis can drain 1 to 2 L of fluid at one time. Care should be taken when draining large volumes of effusions, as fluid shifts can occur and cause hemodynamic instability. A chest radiograph should be obtained after the procedure to evaluate for pneumothorax and resolution of the effusion.

3. **Complications.** Pneumothorax is the most common complication of thoracentesis. Small pneumotharaces (i.e., <10%) are generally well tolerated and can be followed with serial radiographs every 6 hours. Tube thoracotomy (see Section II.B) is indicated for large pneumothoraces. Reexpansion pulmonary edema can occur in situations when a large amount of fluid is removed. Hemothorax, empyema, injury

to the neurovascular bundle, laceration of the lung parenchyma, and subcutaneous hematoma are other potential complications.

B. **Tube thoracostomy**

1. **Indications and contraindications.** Tube thoracostomy is indicated for a pneumothorax, hemothorax, recurrent pleural effusion, chylothorax, and empyema. In an emergent situation such as a tension pneumothorax, a needle thoracostomy using a 14-or 16-gauge needle inserted in the second intercostal space, midclavicular line, can allow for air decompression while awaiting tube thoracostomy.

2. **Tubes.** The size of the thoracostomy tube needed depends on the material to be drained. Generally, a 32F to 36F tube is used for the evacuation of a hemothorax or pleural effusion. In a pneumothorax, a 24F to 28F tube is used. Alternatively, a percutaneous small-bore (18F) chest tube (Thal-Quick; Cook Medical, Bloomington, IN) can be placed by the Seldinger technique.

3. **Anatomy.** Understanding of thoracic anatomy is needed to prevent injuries to the lung parenchyma, diaphragm, intercostal neurovascular bundles, and mediastinum during chest tube placement. Adhesions of the lung to the chest wall may be present and complicate insertion and advancement of the thoracostomy tube. During normal respiration, the diaphragm can rise to the level of the fourth intercostal space; insertion of the chest tube lower than the sixth interspace is discouraged. The tube should be passed over the top of the rib to avoid injury to the intercostal neurovascular bundle, which runs in a groove on the inferior aspect of each rib.

4. **Technique.** The patient is placed in the lateral position with the site of insertion (affected side) up, and the head of the bed inclined 10 to 15 degrees. The patient's arm on the affected side is extended forward or above the head. With the skin prepared and draped, 1% lidocaine is infiltrated over the fifth or sixth rib in the middle or anterior axillary line into the subcutaneous tissue covering the rib below the interspace to be entered, carried deep to the periosteum of the rib. With negative pressure placed on the syringe, the needle is advanced slowly over the top of the rib until a rush of air or fluid is returned. The needle is then withdrawn a fraction to allow for injection of lidocaine to anesthetize the pleura. As the needle is withdrawn, lidocaine is infiltrated into the intercostal muscles. A 2- to 3-cm transverse incision is then made through the skin and subcutaneous tissue. A curved clamp is used bluntly to dissect an oblique tract to the rib (Fig. 37-3A). With careful spreading, the clamp is advanced over the top of the rib. The parietal pleura is punctured with the clamp, and an efflux of air or fluid is usually encountered. A finger is introduced into the tract to ensure passage into the pleural space and to lyse any adhesions at the point of entry (Fig. 37-3B), ensuring that there is no lung adherent to the thoracic wall. With the clamp as a guide, the thoracostomy tube is introduced into the pleural space (Fig. 37-3C); the tube is directed posteriorly or basally for a dependent effusion and apically for a pneumothorax. A

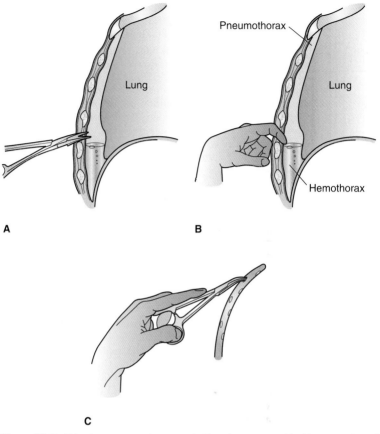

Figure 37-3. Tube thoracostomy placement. **A:** Pleural space entered by blunt spreading of the clamp over the top of the adjacent rib. **B:** A finger is introduced to ensure position within the pleural space and to lyse adhesions. **C:** The thoracostomy tube is placed into the tunnel and directed with the help of a Kelly clamp. The tube is directed posterior and caudal for an effusion or hemothorax and cephalad for a pneumothorax.

clamp placed at the free end of the thoracostomy tube prevents drainage from the chest until the tube can be connected to a closed suction or water-seal system. The thoracostomy tube is advanced until the last hole of the tube is clearly inside the thoracic cavity. When the tube is positioned properly and functioning adequately, it is secured to the skin with two heavy silk sutures and covered with an occlusive dressing to prevent air leaks. A U-stitch around the tube is commonly placed for use as a purse-string suture to close the tract once the tube is removed. A chest radiograph is obtained after the procedure to assess for lung reexpansion and tube position. Under certain circumstances, such as the presence of loculated pleural effusions or prior thoracic surgery, radiographic guidance is required for tube placement.

5. **Complications.** Placement of a thoracostomy tube in the inferior aspect of the chest may result in inadvertent injury to adjacent abdominal organs (such as the spleen, liver). Failure to guide the tube into the pleural space can result in dissection of the extrapleural plane. Extrapleural tube diagnosis can be difficult, but anteroposterior and lateral chest radiographs should reveal a lung that has failed to reexpand and suggest a chest tube placed outside the thorax. The tube should be removed and placed within the thoracic cavity to reexpand the lung. Parenchymal, hilar injuries, or cardiac injuries can occur with overzealous advancement of the tube or dissection of pleural adhesions. Other complications include subcutaneous emphysema, reexpansion pulmonary edema, phrenic nerve injury, esophageal perforation, contralateral pneumothorax, and neurovascular bundle injury. Late infectious complications include empyema, infection along the thoracostomy tube tract, and abscess; following strict sterile technique during tube placement may minimize these complications.

III. PERITONEAL DRAINAGE PROCEDURES

A. **Paracentesis**

1. **Indications.** Paracentesis is a useful diagnostic and therapeutic tool. Diagnostic paracentesis is most commonly indicated in the surgical patient to determine the presence of infection in ascites. Accordingly, ascites should be submitted for cell count, Gram stain, microscopy, and culture. A therapeutic paracentesis is indicated for patients with respiratory compromise or discomfort caused by tense ascites and in patients with ascites refractory to medical management. Relative contraindications include previous abdominal surgery, pregnancy, and coagulopathy.

2. **Technique.** Patients should be in a supine position. The bladder should be empty. Level of the ascites can be determined by locating the transition from dullness to tympany with percussion. Depending on the height of the ascites, a midline or lateral approach can be used. Care must be taken with the midline approach because the air-filled bowel tends to float on top of the ascites. Ultrasound guidance can help in identification of ascites, obtainment of successful ascitic fluid, and avoidance of injury to the bowel (*Am J Emerg Med.* 2005;23:363). The skin at the site of entry should be prepared and draped. One percent lidocaine is infiltrated subcutaneously and is carried to the level of the peritoneum. For the midline approach, a needle is introduced at a point midway between the umbilicus and the pubis symphyses. For the lateral approach, the point of entry can be in the right or left lower quadrant in the area bounded by the lateral border of the rectus abdominis muscle, the line between the umbilicus and the anterior iliac spine, and the line between the anterior iliac spine and the pubis

symphysis. A simple diagnostic tap can be achieved by inserting a 22-gauge needle into the peritoneal cavity and aspirating 20 to 30 mL of fluid. Constant negative pressure should be applied to the syringe, and care should be taken not to advance the needle beyond the point where ascites is encountered. For a therapeutic paracentesis, a 14-gauge needle fitted with a catheter allows for efficient drainage of larger volumes of ascites. With either the midline or the lateral approach, once ascites is returned, the catheter is advanced over the needle and directed toward the pelvis. A drainage bag is attached to the catheter to collect and measure the fluid removed.

3. **Complications.** Injuries to the bowel or bladder can occur with paracentesis. Emptying the bladder prior to the procedure, avoiding the insertion of the needle near surgical scars, and maintaining control of the needle once inside the peritoneum help to minimize these injuries. Intraperitoneal hemorrhage from injury to a mesenteric vessel can occur. Laceration of the inferior epigastric vessels can lead to a hematoma of the rectus sheath or the abdominal wall. In patients with large, recurrent ascites, a persistent leakage of ascites from the site of entry can result. Peritonitis or abdominal wall abscesses can also result. Removal of a large amount of ascites can result in fluid shifts and hemodynamic instability.

IV. EMERGENCY AIRWAY ACCESS

A. Endotracheal (ET) intubation

1. **Indications.** Establishment of a secure airway is the first priority in the management of an acutely ill patient. A thorough description of this topic is beyond the scope of this text. A brief overview of the salient aspects of this technique is provided.

2. **Technique.** Preoxygenation with a bag-valve-mask apparatus and 100% oxygen, suction, adequate sedation, muscle relaxation, an appropriately sized ET tube, and a functional laryngoscope are required. Two types of laryngeal scope blades are available: a straight blade (Miller) and a curved blade (Macintosh). The straight blade may provide better visualization in children, and the curved blade may be better for patients with short, thick necks. The physician should be comfortable using either blade. With the physician at the patient's head, the head is positioned so that the pharyngeal and laryngeal axes are in alignment (Fig. 37-4A). The patient's head and neck are fully extended into the "sniffing" position. With the nondominant hand, the physician opens the patient's mouth with the thumb and the index finger on the patient's lower and upper teeth, respectively. The oropharynx is inspected, and foreign bodies or secretions are removed. The blade of the laryngoscope is introduced and used to sweep the patient's tongue to the side. The blade is then advanced with gentle traction upward and toward the patient's feet. Once the epiglottis is visualized, the tip of the blade is positioned in the vallecula. Great care must be taken not to use the handle as a lever against the patient's teeth and lips,

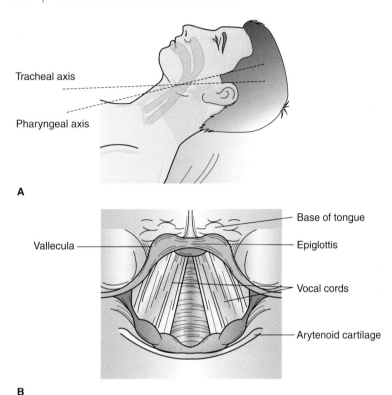

Tracheal axis

Pharyngeal axis

A

Base of tongue

Vallecula

Epiglottis

Vocal cords

Arytenoid cartilage

B

Figure 37-4. Orotracheal intubation. **A:** Fully extending the patient's head into the "sniffing" position aligns the pharyngeal and laryngeal axes. This allows for the best visualization of the airway. **B:** View of the larynx and airway during oral intubation of the trachea.

as this can result in damage and chipping of the teeth. The glottic opening and vocal cords should come into view (Fig. 37-4B). If not, gently increasing the upward and caudal traction or having an assistant place external pressure on the cricoid and thyroid cartilage can be helpful. If the glottic opening still cannot be visualized, the blade should be removed and the patient oxygenated and repositioned prior to additional attempts. Once the glottic opening is adequately visualized, the ET tube is advanced under direct vision until the cuff passes through the vocal cords. The cuff is inserted roughly 2 cm past the vocal cords, and the patient's incisors should rest between the 19- and 23-cm markings on the tube. The stylet and the laryngoscope are carefully removed while maintaining control and position of the ET tube. The cuff is inflated, and proper position is confirmed by auscultating bilateral breath sounds and determining end-tidal carbon dioxide. Once position is confirmed, the ET tube is secured to the patient. An anteroposterior chest radiograph is obtained to confirm position. Ideally, the tip of the ET tube should be 2 to 4 cm above the carina.

3. **Complications.** Chipped teeth, emesis and aspiration, vocal cord injury, laryngospasm, and soft-tissue injury to the oropharynx can all complicate ET intubation.

B. **Cricothyroidotomy**

1. **Indications.** Cricothyroidotomy is indicated when attempts at establishing translaryngeal intubation fail.

2. **Technique.** Most cricothyroidotomies are done in emergent situations. An understanding of the anatomy in the region of the trachea is necessary to minimize complications. The thyroid cartilage is easily identified in the midline of the neck (Fig. 37-5). The cricoid, the only complete cartilaginous ring, is the first ring inferior to the thyroid cartilage. The cricothyroid membrane joins these two cartilages and is an avascular membrane. Inferior to the cricoid and straddling the trachea is the isthmus of the thyroid gland. The thyroid lobes lie lateral to the trachea, and the superior poles can extend to the level of the thyroid cartilage. The area should be prepared, draped, and anesthetized with 1% lidocaine. A vertical skin incision is made. The cricoid cartilage is identified and held firmly and circumferentially in the physician's nondominant hand until the end of the procedure. With a no. 11 or 15 blade, a small, 3- to 5-cm transverse incision is made over the cricothyroid membrane. The incision

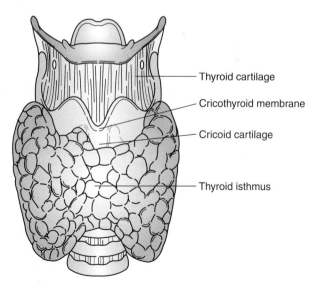

Thyroid cartilage

Cricothyroid membrane

Cricoid cartilage

Thyroid isthmus

Figure 37-5. Anatomy of the larynx.

is carried deep until the airway is entered through the cricothyroid membrane. The index finger of the physician's nondominant hand can be used to identify landmarks as the dissection proceeds should the field become obscured. The tract is widened using a clamp, a tracheal dilator, or the end of the scalpel handle. The tracheostomy tube is inserted along its curve into the trachea and the cuff is inflated. An ET tube can be used if a tracheostomy tube is not immediately available. Proper position should be confirmed with end-tidal capnography.

3. **Complications.** Creation of a false passage when inserting the tracheostomy tube is the most common complication. This should become evident by the absence of breath sounds, lack of end-tidal carbon dioxide, and the development of subcutaneous emphysema. Pneumothorax can also occur. Injury to surrounding structures, such as the thyroid, parathyroids, esophagus, anterior jugular veins, and recurrent laryngeal nerves, can occur in situations of urgency. Subglottic stenosis and granuloma formation are potential long-term complications.

C. **Percutaneous tracheostomy**

1. **Indications.** Percutaneous tracheostomy (PT) has become increasingly popular for the establishment of a nonemergent airway. The advantages of PT over surgical tracheostomy (ST) are primarily related to reduced tissue trauma and the ease of bedside performance, which avoids transportation of critically ill patients to the operating room. Several studies support the cost-effectiveness of this approach (*Crit Care Med.* 2001;29:926). Contraindications include unstable cervical spine, inability to identify anatomic landmarks, refractory coagulopathy, and difficult oropharyngeal anatomy such that reestablishing a translaryngeal airway would be difficult in the event of airway loss. PT should only be performed electively.

2. **Technique.** PT should be performed under bronchoscopic guidance. The patient should be adequately sedated and positioned in a moderate degree of neck extension. An initial 1.5-cm skin incision over the first tracheal ring is made and blunt dissection is performed down to the level of the pretracheal fascia, using a mosquito hemostat. The existing endotracheal tube is withdrawn into the subglottic position, permitting a needle to be introduced between the first and second or second and third tracheal rings midline. A guidewire is inserted through the needle and the needle is then removed, leaving the guidewire in place. Progressive dilation of the tracheal stoma is achieved using beveled plastic dilators over the guidewire (Seldinger technique). Once the stoma has been adequately dilated, the tracheostomy tube is introduced into the trachea over the guidewire, using a dilator as an obturator. The tracheostomy is then secured to the skin, using heavy, nonabsorable, monofilament suture.

3. **Complications.** There are no significant differences in the rate of intraprocedural complications between PT and ST (*Crit Care.* 2006;10:R55). Postoperative complications include accidental decannulation, bleeding, and stoma infection and may be reduced with PT as compared to ST (*Crit Care Resusc.* 2009;11:244). The complications

associated with cricothyroidotomy, including creation of a false passage, pneumothorax, injury to surrounding structures, and long-term subglottic stenosis and granuloma formation, can also occur with PT.

V. LAPAROSCOPY.
An overview of general laparoscopic principles is provided. Readers are referred elsewhere in this manual for information pertaining to specific disease processes.

A. **Advantages.** Laparoscopic procedures may result in less patient discomfort, shorter hospitalizations, and more rapid convalescence than with open techniques.

B. **Contraindications**

1. **Absolute contraindications** include the inability to tolerate general anesthesia and uncorrectable coagulopathy.

2. **Relative contraindications**

   a. **Prior abdominal surgery** may require alternative port locations to avoid intra-abdominal adhesions. Laparoscopic adhesiolysis may be necessary to improve exposure.

   b. **Peritonitis** may limit access secondary to adhesions.

   c. **First- and third-trimester pregnancy.** Laparoscopy is more safely undertaken in the second trimester for conditions that require urgent surgical management (i.e., cannot be safely delayed until after delivery).

   d. **Severe cardiopulmonary disease** may be exacerbated by hypercarbia that occurs secondary to insufflation of carbon dioxide as well as changes in pulmonary and cardiovascular mechanics during periods of increased intra-abdominal pressure. These effects can be minimized using lower intra-abdominal pressures (8 mm Hg) in conjunction with abdominal wall lift devices.

   e. **Massive abdominal distention** may result in an increased risk of iatrogenic bowel injury.

C. **Access and pneumoperitoneum.** A working space is created in the patient's abdomen by insufflating carbon dioxide after access is obtained either by a closed or open technique. While both techniques have been shown to be safe, some studies suggest a lower complication rate with open direct insertion (*Surg Laparosc Endosc Percutan Tech.* 2005;15:80). Optical access trocars have been advocated in the morbidly obese population (*Surg Innov.* 2008;15:126).

1. **Closed technique.** A Veress needle is placed most commonly at the umbilicus through a small skin-stab incision. Two serial clicks are heard as the needle penetrates the fascia and peritoneum, respectively. The surgeon aspirates the needle with a 10-mL syringe partially filled with saline to look for blood or enteric contents. The surgeon injects 3 to 5 mL of saline through the needle. If any resistance is met, the syringe is most likely in the abdominal muscle or omentum and should be repositioned. If no resistance is met, the surgeon aspirates the syringe again and removes the plunger. Observing the saline pass freely into

the abdomen with gravity (drop test) confirms proper intra-abdominal placement. The abdominal cavity is insufflated via an automatic pressure-limited insufflator to 10 to 15 mm Hg. The initial intra-abdominal pressure should be less than 10 mm Hg. As the abdomen expands, pneumoperitoneum is confirmed by percussion. After insufflation, the abdominal wall is stabilized manually, the Veress needle is removed, and the initial trocar and port are inserted blindly in a direction away from critical abdominal structures.

   a. **Elevated pressure** with low flow (1 L/minute) on insufflation usually indicates placement of the Veress needle into a closed space (e.g., pre- or retroperitoneal, within the omentum).

   (1) First, the port's insufflation valve should be confirmed to be open.

   (2) If so, the Veress needle is removed and reinserted with a subsequent drop test.

   (3) If the **needle position is in doubt,** an open insertion technique should be used.

   b. **Return of blood, cloudy or bilious fluid, or enteric contents** after Veress needle placement mandates needle repositioning and inspection of the violated abdominal organ.

2. **Open insertion** of the initial port is by a direct cut down through the abdominal fascia. A Hasson (wedge-shaped) port is placed under direct vision and secured to the abdominal fascia with stay sutures.

3. **Complications**

   a. **Gas embolism is life threatening.** With right ventricular outflow obstruction, expired end-tidal carbon dioxide falls, with concomitant hypotension and a "mill-wheel" heart murmur.

   (1) Insufflation is stopped and the pneumoperitoneum is released.

   (2) The patient should be placed in a steep Trendelenburg position with the right side up to float the gas bubble up toward the right ventricular apex and away from the right ventricular outflow tract.

   (3) Air from the right ventricle is aspirated through a central venous catheter.

   b. **Brisk bleeding** after trocar insertion warrants emergent conversion to open laparotomy. The trocar should not be removed until proximal and distal control of the injured vessel is achieved.

4. **Alternatives to carbon dioxide pneumoperitoneum** have been advocated because of the potentially deleterious effects of hypercapnea. Alternative pneumoperitoneum gases such as nitrous oxide, helium, and argon have been evaluated experimentally. Increased intra-abdominal pressure can occur with any insufflation gas (e.g., compression of the vena cava with decreased venous return to the heart, resultant hypotension, decreased renal blood flow, and diminished urinary output). External abdominal wall lift devices are available to create a working space without pneumoperitoneum.

D. **Port placement.** The location of ports has been standardized for most procedures, and several general rules for port placement have been established. All additional ports should be placed under direct video visualization.

Before inserting the port, the surgeon indents the abdominal wall manually and identifies the location with the video camera. Transilluminating the abdominal wall identifies significant vessels to avoid. The skin and peritoneum are anesthetized locally. The surgeon makes a small stab incision with a no. 11 blade. The trocar is introduced in a direct line with the planned surgical target to minimize torque intraoperatively. The tip of the trocar should be visualized as it passes through the peritoneum.

1. The **camera port** should be behind and between the surgeon's two operative ports to maintain proper orientation.

2. **Working ports** are placed lateral to the viewing port, with the operative field ahead. All ports should be at least 8 cm apart to avoid the interference of instruments with one another. Ports should be approximately 15 cm from the operative field for the site to be reached comfortably by standard 30-cm instruments and to maintain a 1:1 ratio of hand–instrument tip movement.

E. **Exiting the abdomen.** The surgeon should survey the abdomen at the conclusion of the procedure to detect any visceral injury or hemorrhage. The operative site is irrigated, and hemostasis is obtained. Inspection of the peritoneal side of all port sites as the trocars are removed allows verification of hemostasis. Port-site fascial incisions that are larger than 5 mm should be closed with permanent or long-term absorbable suture to avoid the risk of incisional herniation. This can be done through the port-site incision or under video guidance with a fascial closure device (also known as a "suture passer"), which is particularly helpful in obese patients.

F. **Converting to open surgery.** A laparoscopic case may need to be converted to an open case for a number of reasons.

1. **Elective conversion**

   a. **Surgeon experience** is critical. The surgeon's threshold for conversion should be low while gaining experience.

   b. **Failure to progress** is the most common reason to convert. This can be secondary to adhesions, inflammatory changes, poor exposure, or altered or aberrant anatomy. In cases of unclear anatomy, avoiding injuries should take precedence over avoiding laparotomy.

   c. The surgeon may discover **a disease not appropriate for minimally** invasive methods (e.g., gallbladder cancer or colon cancer invading adjacent organs).

   d. **Technical problems or instrument malfunction** may occasionally require conversion. The surgeon must check that all equipment is in working order before starting the operation.

2. **Emergent conversion** should be performed in the event of severe bleeding or complex bowel injuries if repair is beyond the skill level of the surgeon.

G. **Postoperative management** for most laparoscopic procedures is similar to that for open procedures, although laparoscopic surgery is associated with less postoperative pain and shorter hospital length of stay and recuperation time.

Common Postoperative Surgical Emergencies

Elizabeth T. Robertson and Christopher D. Anderson

This chapter explores the common syndromes facing postoperative patients and initial stages of management. Many of these syndromes have different etiologies depending on postoperative day. The topics include altered mental status, oliguria, hypotension, tachycardia, nausea/vomiting, shortness of breath, and chest pain.

I. **ALTERED MENTAL STATUS/COMBATIVE PATIENT.** The physiologic changes from surgical stress can alone affect neurologic function. In addition, after major surgery, patients are placed in unfamiliar surroundings, are woken throughout the night, and are administered novel, powerful medications. All of these must be taken into account and a differential should be generated before the reflexive administration of sedatives or antipsychotics.

A. The patient in **postoperative day 0** is recovering from general anesthesia, whose effects can last up to 48 hours. At the postoperative check, approximately 4 hours after completion of the surgery, mental status should be evaluated.

1. The patient will likely be drowsy but should be arousable to voice or light touch. If he or she is not, narcotics are likely to blame. If his or her respiratory rate is depressed, stimulate the patient and encourage deep breathing. If the patient is obtunded in the early postoperative period, consider naloxone injection and continuous infusion. An arterial blood gas (ABG) can be obtained to determine if the patient needs ventilator assistance to recover from carbon dioxide narcosis. Intensive care monitoring may be required.

2. If the patient responds to stimulation with combativeness, he or she is usually calmed with reorientation. The amnestics administered during general anesthesia can cause a patient to repeatedly lose orientation. In addition, many anesthetic agents agonize the γ-aminobutyric acid receptors, causing disinhibition. If the patient is not easily reoriented by health care workers, a close friend or family member can be more effective.

B. In **postoperative days 2 and 3,** consideration should be given to alcohol withdrawal. Further discussion is available in Chapter 1 Section III.A.4.

C. **Elderly patients** have less neurologic reserve and are the largest population to suffer from mental status changes. Their other organ systems are also delicate, often requiring intensive care unit (ICU) admissions and resultant ICU delirium. The effects of sedative and pain medications can be quite prolonged in this population and additional administration should only be done with careful consideration.

D. Sudden mental status changes in a previously stable patient should be emergently worked up for medical causes. If the patient is completely unresponsive, begin the basic life support (BLS) algorithm. Evaluate for breathing and a pulse and call a code. If the patient is obtunded, but protecting his or her airway, further medical evaluation can commence.

1. Obtain a full set of vital signs. Hypoxia can result in mental status suppression and also agitation. If the patient was complaining of an antecedent headache, hypoxia should be high on the differential. Hypotension and arrhythmias can also cause mental status changes.

2. A fingerstick for blood glucose should be done. With the advent of intensive glucose control, more hypoglycemic events have been noted (*JAMA*. 2008;300:933). Any newly obtunded patient should have a rapid bedside glucose measurement.

3. Consideration should be given to inadvertent or unknown extra administration of narcotic agents. A dose of 0.04 mg of naloxone is a reasonable trial dose.

4. A stat head computed tomographic (CT) scan is reasonable to evaluate for intracranial hemorrhage.

5. A complete blood cell count, basic metabolic profile, ABG, and current type and screen should be obtained to evaluate for hemorrhage, early signs of infection, and electrolyte disturbances as well as preparing for blood resuscitation should that be necessary. An electrocardiogram and serial troponins should be obtained to evaluate for arrhythmias and myocardial infarction (MI).

II. **OLIGURIA.** Low urine output in the postoperative period has several different causes that can be organized by postoperative day. One must consider the operative procedure and the definition of oliguria. Oliguria in a post–renal transplant patient is very different from that in a patient with oliguria after a Whipple procedure. In addition, patient characteristics can change the approach. For example, a patient with chronic kidney disease who is lasix dependent cannot tolerate multiple liters of fluid without close monitoring of his or her pulmonary status.

A. On postoperative day 0, the patient is few hours out from the operating room and has endured a serious trauma. The patient is being actively resuscitated and oliguria is likely due to hypovolemia. Total body fluid is increased, but most of the fluid is being third-spaced from the extensive capillary leak secondary to the systemic inflammatory response. Fluid bolus administration is the usual remedy. A true bolus given in the ICU is 1 L of crystalloid administered on a pressure bag through a large-bore catheter. Transient increases in the central venous pressure and mean arterial pressure can be demonstrated in a hypovolemic patient.

1. Hemorrhage is an important cause of hypovolemia on postoperative day 0. If you have given 1 or 2 L of fluid (or 10 to 20 mL/kg in a

pediatric patient), it is reasonable to check the hemoglobin level. If the hemoglobin level is low, consideration can be given to transfusion and/or return to the operating room for exploration.

2. Mechanical causes of oliguria should also be considered. If the patient has an indwelling Foley catheter, careful examination should be done to evaluate for kinking or inadvertent clamping. The Foley catheter can be flushed to determine if it is clogged. If the patient does not have an indwelling urinary catheter, serious consideration should be given to placing one. This will not only decompress a distended nonfunctional bladder but will also allow for close serial monitoring of urine output to avoid renal compromise.

3. After pelvic surgery ureteral injury can cause oliguria, often along with hematuria. This is most common in a reoperative field. Serum creatinine level can increase due to intraperitoneal urine resorption. Intraperitoneal drain fluid can be evaluated for the creatinine level. CT scan with delayed images can demonstrate ureteral anatomy, but there is often hesitation to administer intravenous dye in patients with an elevated creatinine level. A retrograde ureteropyelogram can provide similar information.

4. An unusual cause of oliguria in the early postoperative period is cardiac insufficiency. Patients who have preexisting congestive heart failure should undergo intensive monitoring with consideration given to a central catheter, CardioQ, or even Swan-Ganz catheter. If a patient with no known cardiac dysfunction is not responding to fluid challenges and has worsening respiratory function, it is reasonable to check troponins, take electrocardiograms (EKGs), and perform cardiac echocardiography to evaluate ventricular volume status.

B. During postoperative days 1 and 2, new-onset oliguria is less likely to be due to fluid sequestration. Fluid mobilization usually occurs by postoperative day 3. Other causes of oliguria should be considered.

1. Ileus and small bowel obstruction can lead to fluid sequestration inside the bowel, as gastrointestinal secretions are not propelled to the colon for usual reabsorption. In addition, distended bowel becomes edematous and pulls fluid from the intravascular space. These patients require nasogastric (NG) tube decompression and volume resuscitation but for slightly different reasons than in the very early postoperative patient.

2. In the first few postoperative days, patients are administered a multitude of agents to manage infection risk, pain, and postoperative nausea. Some of these agents can be nephrotoxic, and a careful evaluation of a patient's medication list can reveal the offending agent.

3. Delayed hemorrhage should be considered, especially if anticoagulation for a patient's preexisting condition has been restarted. Operative site bleeding is less likely than immediately postoperatively, but the risk of gastrointestinal bleeding begins to increase in this stressed population. Hemoccult evaluation of stools and gastroccult evaluation of gastric secretions are reasonable.

C. In postoperative days 3 to 10, one should consider ileus recurrence with fluid sequestration as well as oliguria as an early sign of severe sepsis.

III. **POSTOPERATIVE HYPOTENSION** should immediately raise concerns of postoperative bleeding. There are more mundane causes, but this should always be considered. If hypotension is not quickly resolved, transfer the patient to a higher level of care.

A. First, ensure that the blood pressure reading is accurate. Get a manual blood pressure reading to confirm the noninvasive cuff blood pressure. Be sure to get a full set of vitals as well. If the patient is tachycardic and febrile, you can move quickly along the severe sepsis pathway.

B. Severe hypovolemia can cause hypotension and is usually accompanied by tachycardia. The notable exception to this is the patient on β-blocker, in whom tachycardia is blunted. Oliguria accompanies hypotension in this situation, and the management of hypovolemic shock is covered in Section II.A.

C. Anesthetics and analgesics are also common causes of postoperative hypotension. These drugs vasodilate the patient, and hypotension can be managed with volume administration.

D. After restarting home medications, patients can develop unexpected hypotension. With further investigation, you often discover that the patients do not adhere to their home medication prescriptions and this is the first day they have ever taken all of their antihypertensives together.

IV. **TACHYCARDIA** can be found in most of the other syndrome presentations discussed here. Anyone who is under stress from hypotension, pain, or shortness of breath will likely develop a sinus tachycardia. Tachycardia can be divided into mild (<120) and severe (>130) and management depends on rhythm determination.

A. Mild sinus tachycardia is often due to postoperative pain, atelectasis, and hypovolemia. This patient should have these issues managed and be observed until the tachycardia resolves.

B. Severe sinus tachycardia needs to be proven on an EKG. It can be difficult to identify a supraventricular tachycardia when the heart rate is 150. If it is truly sinus, the patient has potentially suffered a pulmonary embolus (PE) or is in stage 2 shock. These patients need a monitored bed and aggressive work-up with a PE protocol CT scan, blood cultures, chemistry, and hematology laboratory values. Consider invasive monitoring with a central catheter and an arterial catheter.

C. Severe nonsinus tachycardia is managed according to Advanced cardiac life support (ACLS) protocol. These patients should also be managed in a monitored setting. The stress of surgical recovery can induce atrial fibrillation with rapid ventricular response in a patient who has never experienced it before.

V. **NAUSEA AND VOMITING** attributable to anesthesia can affect up to 30% of patients (*Anesthesiology.* 1992;77:162). During postoperative days 0 and 1, aggressive management with antiemetics can be employed. Multimodal therapy with ondansetron, phenergan, compazine, scopolamine, and even decadron can be required. Propofol also has excellent antiemetic effects but should be administered only in a monitored setting by a sedation provider.

A. Patients who have undergone antireflux operations should be aggressively managed with antiemetics before symptoms arise. Any sign of nausea should prompt medication administration. There should be a low threshold to place an NG tube. Even one episode of retching can cause an esophageal wrap to slip.

B. Patients who have undergone extensive intra-abdominal procedures and are more than 24 hours out from anesthesia should be evaluated before administration of antiemetics. Up to 20% of these patients will suffer an ileus requiring nasogastric decompression (*Dis Colon Rectum.* 2000;43:61). Administration of antiemetics will not resolve the symptom long term, and the ileus can progress to a severe state. If the patient is nauseated, distended, burping, and has not passed flatus, you should consider placing an NG tube.

C. A patient with an NG tube in place who complains of nausea should have the NG tube manipulated until functioning properly. This often requires an experienced clinician to coax the tube into doing its job. This may even require replacement of a larger-bore NG tube.

VI. **SHORTNESS OF BREATH** is often thought of as being a primary respiratory problem, but it can be a symptom of systemic illness.

A. **Volume overload** is a common cause of shortness of breath beyond the immediate postoperative period. Patients sequester fluid during and immediately after surgery and mobilization usually begins on postoperative day 2. If the patient is significantly volume expanded and crackles are heard on auscultation, intravenous lasix administration can rapidly relieve symptoms. Chest radiograph will demonstrate volume overload, but even an emergent radiograph in the ICU can take up to 30 minutes.

B. **Reactive airways** are common in postoperative smokers and asthmatic patients. The local trauma of an endotracheal tube can induce bronchospasm (*Anesth Analg.* 1995;80:276). Work of breathing is increased and expiratory wheezes are auscultated. If the patient is able to use an inhaler, this is preferred, but if the patient is tachypneic, nebulized β-agonists and anticholinergics are appropriate.

C. **PE** can cause shortness of breath, but tachycardia or pleuritic chest pain is more common. PE protocol CT scan will definitively diagnose PE, but a patient who is short of breath should not be sent to the scanner alone. If the patient is in extremis, consider intubation before obtaining the radiologic study.

D. **Pneumonia** can cause shortness of breath and is accompanied by fever, elevated white blood cell count, and productive cough. Chest radiograph provides diagnosis, and sputum culture can guide antibiotic therapy.

E. Shortness of breath can also be a result of MI, intra-abdominal complication, systemic sepsis, and fever.

VII. CHEST PAIN. The work-up for chest pain in the postoperative period mirrors the work-up in an emergency department, with the added consideration of incisional pain. Chest pain work-up begins with a close questioning of the patient on the type of pain, which narrows the differential significantly. A substernal heaviness is very different from pain inferior to the xiphoid in a patient with a high midline incision. After a complete history is taken, most chest pain complaints warrant a new set of vital signs, laboratory evaluation, and a chest radiograph.

A. **Myocardial infarction.** Consider serial troponins and EKGs in any patient complaining of chest pain. In our practice, we often "rule out" a high-risk patient with three serial troponins in postoperative day 0. This evaluates a patient for intraoperative ischemia, which is actually rare. Postoperative MIs classically occur on postoperative day 2 and any new development of chest pain should prompt a full work-up for MI.

B. The complete work-up of MI includes serial troponins and EKGs as well as a current set of electrolytes and hemoglobin levels. If your index of suspicion is high, apply oxygen to the patient and administer morphine to manage the pain. Place the patient on telemetry monitoring. Aspirin administration can be lifesaving and nitroglycerin should be considered if the blood pressure could tolerate it. β-Blocker has also been shown to benefit patients with an MI (*Am J Cardiology.* 1999;84:76). If the troponin levels are elevated or the EKG demonstrates new ST depressions, an emergent cardiology consultation should be obtained. Even if the patient is not a candidate for cardiac catheterization, they will assist with follow-up for the post–MI patient.

C. PE is a very common postoperative occurrence, and autopsy studies demonstrate that it is more common than clinicians appreciate (*Chest.* 1995;108:978). Chest pain with a sensation of shortness of breath and low oxygen saturations should raise the possibility of PE. Work-up should begin with a chest radiograph and consideration should be given to a PE protocol CT scan. If a patient has marginal renal function a ventilation-perfusion (VQ) scan is a reasonable option.

D. Other causes of postoperative chest pain include pleural effusion and musculoskeletal pain from intraoperative positioning or referred incisional pain. These can be differentiated with a plain chest radiograph and physical examination.

Index

Note: Page locators followed by f and t indicates figure and table respectively.